Clinical Procedures in Anesthesia and Intensive Care

Clinical Procedures in Anesthesia and Intensive Care

Edited by

Jonathan L. Benumof, MD

Professor of Anesthesia
University of California, San Diego, Medical Center
San Diego, California

with 45 contributors

J. B. Lippincott Company

Philadelphia New York London Hagerstown

Acquisitions Editor: Mary K. Smith
Coordinating Editorial Assistant: Anne Geyer
Project Editor: Anne-Adele Wight
Indexer: Sandi Schroeder
Design Director: Susan Hermansen
Design Coordinator: Kathy Kelley-Luedtke
Interior and Cover Designer: Ellen C. Dawson
Production Manager: Helen Ewan
Production Coordinator: Kathryn Rule
Compositor: Pine Tree Composition, Inc.
Printer/Binder: Arcata Graphics/Halliday

3 5 6 4 2

Library of Congress Cataloging-in-Publicaton Data

Clinical procedures in anesthesia and intensive care / [edited by]
Jonathan L. Benumof.
p. cm.
Includes bibliographical references and index.
ISBN 0-397-50958-2
1. Anesthesia. 2. Critical care medicine. I. Benumof, Jonathan, 1942– .
[DNLM: 1. Anesthesia—methods. 2. Critical Care—methods. WO 375 C641]
RD81.C59 1992
617.9′6—dc20
DNLM/DLC
for Library of Congress 92-4830
CIP

Every effort has been made to ensure drug selections and dosages are in accordance with current recommendations and practice. Because of ongoing research, changes in government regulations, and the constant flow of information on drug therapy, reactions, and interactions, the reader is cautioned to check the package insert for each drug for indications, dosages, warnings, and precautions, particularly if the drug is new or infrequently used.

To those who have a fear
of trying a critical procedure
for the first time

Contributors

Stephen E. Abram, MD
Professor of Anesthesiology
Medical College of Wisconsin
Director, Pain Management Center
Milwaukee County Medical Complex
Milwaukee, Wisconsin

David D. Alfery, MD
Member, Anesthesiology Consultants of Nashville, PC
Chairman, Department of Anesthesia
Parkview Hospital—Centennial Medical Center
Nashville, Tennessee

Isaac Azar, MD
Professor of Clinical Anesthesiology
Mount Sinai School of Medicine
Associate Director
Beth Israel Medical Center
New York, New York

Jonathan L. Benumof, MD
Professor of Anesthesia
University of California, San Diego, Medical Center
San Diego, California

Janna Blanchard, MD
Private Practice
Austin, Texas

Robert A. Boas, MBChB, FFARACS
Clinical Lecturer
School of Medicine
University of Auckland
Auckland, New Zealand

Claire M. Brett, MD
Associate Professor of Anesthesia and Pediatrics
Attending Physician, Pediatric Intensive Care Unit
University of California, San Francisco
San Francisco, California

Jerry M. Calkins, PhD, MD
Clinical Professor
University of Arizona
Chairman
Department of Anesthesiology
Maricopa Medical Center
Phoenix, Arizona

Randall M. Chesnut, MD
University of California, San Diego, Medical Center
San Diego, California

Mary V. Clemency, MD
Assistant Professor of Anesthesiology
Emory University School of Medicine
Grady Memorial Hospital
Atlanda, Georgia

Neal H. Cohen, MD, MPH, FCCM
Professor of Clinical Anesthesia and Medicine
Vice Chairman, Department of Anesthesia
University of California, San Francisco
Director, Critical Care Medicine
University of California, San Francisco
San Francisco, California

John W. Danforth, MD
Assistant Clinical Professor of Medicine
University of California, San Francisco,
School of Medicine
Director, Coronary Care Unit
Director, Clinical Research for the Division
of Cardiology
Pacific Presbyterian Medical Center
San Francisco, California

James W. Davis, MD
Assistant Clinical Professor of Surgery
University of California, San Francisco,
College of Medicine
University of California, San Diego,
Medical Center
San Diego, California

Alan M. Demby, MD
Assistant Professor of Urology
University of California, San Diego,
College of Medicine
University of California, San Diego,
Medical Center
San Diego, California

John C. Drummond, MD, FRCPC
Associate Professor of Anesthesiology
University of California, San Diego
Staff Anesthesiologist
Veterans Affairs Medical Center
San Diego, California

D. Jill Ellis, MD
Assistant Clinical Professor of Anesthesiology
University of California, San Diego
Anesthesiologist
Kaiser Permanente Hospital
San Diego, California

David V. Feliciano, MD
Professor and Vice-Chairman
Department of Surgery
University of Rochester Medical Center
Attending Surgeon and Surgical Intensive Care
Unit Director
Strong Memorial Hospital
Rochester, New York

T. James Gallagher, MD, FCCM
Professor
Departments of Anesthesiology and Surgery
University of Florida, College of Medicine,
Chief, Division of Critical Care Medicine
Medical Director, Hyperbaric Medicine
Shands Hospital, University of Florida
Gainesville, Florida

Nora Goldschlager, MD
Professor of Clinical Medicine
University of California, San Francisco
Director, Coronary Care Unit
San Francisco General Hospital
San Francisco, California

Stephen M. Hahn, MD
Clinical Associate
Medicine and Radiation Oncology Branches
National Cancer Institute
Bethesda, Maryland

Zaharia Hillel, MD, PhD
Associate Professor of Clinical Anesthesiology
Columbia University College of Physicians
and Surgeons
Director, Cardiothoracic Anesthesiology
St. Luke's-Roosevelt Hospital Center
New York, New York

H. Blane Howell, CDR, MC, USNR
Staff Anesthesiologist
Southern Maine Medical Center
Biddeford, Maine

Brigid Doyle Ide, MS, RN
Assistant Clinical Professor
University of Califonia, San Francisco,
School of Nursing
Clinical Nurse Specialist in Cardiology
University of California, San Francisco,
Medical Center
San Francisco, California

Thomas G. Karagianes, MD
Associate Clinical Professor of Anesthesiology
University of California, San Diego,
School of Medicine
Associate Medical Director
Surgical Intensive Care Unit
University of California, San Diego,
Medical Center
San Diego, California

Gershon Levinson, MD
Associate Clinical Professor of Anesthesia
University of California, San Francisco
Staff Anesthesiologist
Children's Hospital of San Francisco
San Francisco, California

Robert C. Mackersie, MD
Assistant Professor of Surgery
University of California, San Diego,
University Hospital
San Diego, California

Lawrence F. Marshall, MD
Professor of Surgery/Neurosurgery
University of California, San Diego,
School of Medicine
Chief, Neurosurgical Services
University of California, San Diego,
Medical Center
San Diego, California

John Paul McGee II, MD
Assistant Professor of Clinical Anesthesia
Northwestern University Medical School
Senior Attending Physician
The Evanston Hospital
Glenview, Illinois

Edward A. Meathe, MS
Principal Engineer
Department of Anesthesiology
University of California, San Diego,
Medical Center
San Diego, California

Frederick G. Mihm, MD
Associate Professor of Anesthesia
Stanford University
Associate Medical Director
Intensive Care Units
Stanford University Medical Center
Stanford, California

Somayaji Ramamurthy, MD
Professor
University of Texas Health Science Center
San Antonio, Texas

Laurence S. Reisner, MD
Professor of Clinical Anesthesiology and
Reproductive Medicine
University of California, San Diego,
Director of Obstetric Anesthesia
University of California, San Diego,
Medical Center

Myer H. Rosenthal, MD
Professor of Anesthesia, Medicine, and Surgery
Medical Director of Intensive Care
Stanford University
Stanford, California

Cairo A. Salvatierra, MD
Tri City Medical Center
Oceanside, California

Theodore J. Sanford, Jr., MD
Clinical Professor of Anesthesiology
University of California, San Diego
Chief Anesthesiology Service
Veterans Administration Medical Center
San Diego, California

Joseph D. Schmidt, MD
Professor and Head, Division of Urology
University of California, San Diego,
Medical Center
San Diego, California

Steven R. Shackford, MD
Professor and Chairman,
Department of Surgery
University of Vermont
College of Medicine
Surgeon-in-Chief
Medical Center Hospital of Vermont
Burlington, Vermont

Persis K. Shroff, MD
Associate Professor of Clinical Anesthesiology
School of Medicine in Shreveport
Louisiana State University Medical Center
Shreveport, Louisiana

George M. Shumaik, MD
Associate Clinical Professor of Medicine
and Surgery
University of California, San Diego,
Department of Emergency Medicine
University of California, San Diego,
Medical Center
San Diego, California

Jonathan H. Skerman, BDSc, DSc
Professor of Clinical Anesthesiology and
Obstetrics and Gynecology
School of Medicine in Shreveport
Louisiana State University Medical Center
Shreveport, Louisiana

Daniel M. Thys, MD
Professor (Pending)
Department of Anesthesiology
College of Physicians and Surgeons
Columbia University
Director
Department of Anesthesiology
St. Luke's/Roosevelt Hospital Center
New York, New York

Jeffrey S. Vender, MD, FCCM
Associate Professor of Clinical Anesthesia
Northwestern University Medical School
Chief, Division of Anesthesiology
Director, Medical/Surgical Intensive Care Unit
The Evanston Hospital
Winnetka, Illinois

C. F. Ward, MD
Anesthesia Service Medical Group
Green Hospital of the Scripps Clinic
San Diego, California

John A. Weigelt, MD
Professor
Department of Surgery
University of Texas Southwestern Medical Center
Medical Director, Surgical Intensive Care Unit
Medical Director, Trauma Department
Parkland Memorial Hospital
Dallas, Texas

Mark H. Zornow, MD
Assistant Clinical Professor of Anesthesiology
University of California, San Diego
San Diego, California

Joanne Zupan, MD
Staff Anesthesiologist
Kaiser Permanente Hospital
San Diego, California

Preface

The purpose of this book is to bring together in one book a description of all the modern clinical procedures that anesthesiologists must be very familiar with (either perform themselves, or be in close practical and/or intellectual contact with) in order to administer high-quality anesthesia and perioperative intensive care. At present, no single text covers all these clinical procedures; the available descriptions are widely dispersed among general and subspecialty anesthesia and surgical textbooks. Some of the procedures presented in this book are performed daily by anesthesiologists (for example, inserting peripheral and central intravenous and arterial catheters, intubating the trachea with a single-lumen tube, delivering epidural and spinal anesthesia). The medical student, intern, or beginning anesthesia resident who has not yet had experience with these common procedures will want to study these chapters in detail before attempting them, and even the experienced anesthesiologist will likely find some new pearls of wisdom and useful alternatives not yet suggested in these chapters. Many procedures (the bulk of the book) are performed less frequently (eg, double-lumen tube intubation, tube thoracostomy, evoked potential monitoring, sympathetic nerve block). For everyone involved with anesthesia and intensive care, these chapters will serve as a good reference for both primary and alternative methods of accomplishing a procedure. Finally, there are some procedures that are very rarely performed by, but must be known to, the members of an anesthesia team (eg, transtracheal jet ventilation, intraosseus infusion, intraaortic balloon counterpulsation) because their life-saving aspects or their comprehension are essential in order for the anesthesia team to care for the patient intelligently.

Although each of the clinical procedures in this book has an important purpose, the purpose can be broadly categorized into either monitoring/diagnosis or the administration of a treatment. The main criterion for inclusion of a procedure in this book was that, for the procedure to be performed successfully, a substantial amount of skill and knowledge was required, and that the procedure had to be at least clearly understood, if not primarily performed, by an anesthesia and/or intensive care team member. For example, measuring systemic arterial blood pressure (monitoring) by applying a noninvasive automatic blood pressure cuff requires a trivial amount of skill and intellectual capacity (therefore is not included in the book), whereas the insertion of an arterial catheter line does (therefore is included in the book). For further example, administration of an antiarrhythmic drug requires no technical skill (is not included in the book), whereas use of an external or transvenous pacemaker does (is included in the book). Thus, although some procedures involve monitoring and still others the administration of a treatment, all involve application of both skill and knowledge.

The 44 chapters are grouped according to the basic system that is being monitored or treated. Section I deals with the preparation of an anesthesia machine and ventilator and all the important monitoring equipment used by anesthesiologists. Section II contains a large number of diagnostic and therapeutic respiratory procedures. Section III contains a wide variety of procedures related to the diagnosis and treatment of diseases of the cardiovascular system. Sections IV and V contain all the important monitoring and therapeutic procedures related to the central and peripheral nervous systems, respectively. Section VI is a potpourri of genital, urinary, gastrointestinal, and miscellaneous procedures.

Within each chapter the procedure is completely described in the text as well as by illustration. The illustrations are extensive (by intention) so that each chapter, and the book as a whole, has a very definite atlas-type quality to it. For the most part, the illustrations and text can be understood independently of one another. In fact, some chapters are so well illustrated that these procedures can be easily referred to at the same time the procedure is actually being performed.

Each chapter is organized in approximately the same way, namely, Introduction, Indications, How to Do the Procedure (along with reasonable alternatives), Discussion of the Procedure, Complications, and References. The various introductions may variously and appropriately involve relevant anatomy, physiology, history, or legal matters, depending on the procedure in question. The How to Do the Procedure section is the core of each chapter. In order to impart to the reader the greatest degree of success in doing the procedure, we have tried to present every little step in the process. The section under Discussion of the Procedure is intended to be scholarly and may focus on the logic behind the procedure, how to interpret the data or results from the monitoring/diagnostic or therapeutic procedure, how the procedure leads to still other procedures, how to do the secondary procedures (eg, endotracheal intubation leads to a discussion of how to set the dials on a mechanical ventilator), and the pitfalls of the procedure. The Indications and Complications sections in each chapter are relatively straightforward. The chapters vary in length according to the complexity of the procedure.

In summary, this volume is intended for everyone in anesthesia and/or intensive care who does not know how to do a particular procedure, or is looking for a new alternative or approach to an old procedure. Therefore, medical students, interns, residents, faculty members, and private practitioners in anesthesia should find this book useful. Many parts of the books should be of strong interest to similar individuals in the disciplines of surgery, intensive care, pediatrics, and internal medicine.

I gratefully acknowledge the scholarly contributions of the authors and the editorial assistance of Mr. Richard Winters.

Jonathan L. Benumof, MD

Contents

Section IV
Central Nervous System Procedures

Section V
Peripheral Nerve Procedures

Section VI
Gastrointestinal, Obstetric, and Renal Procedures

Color Plates

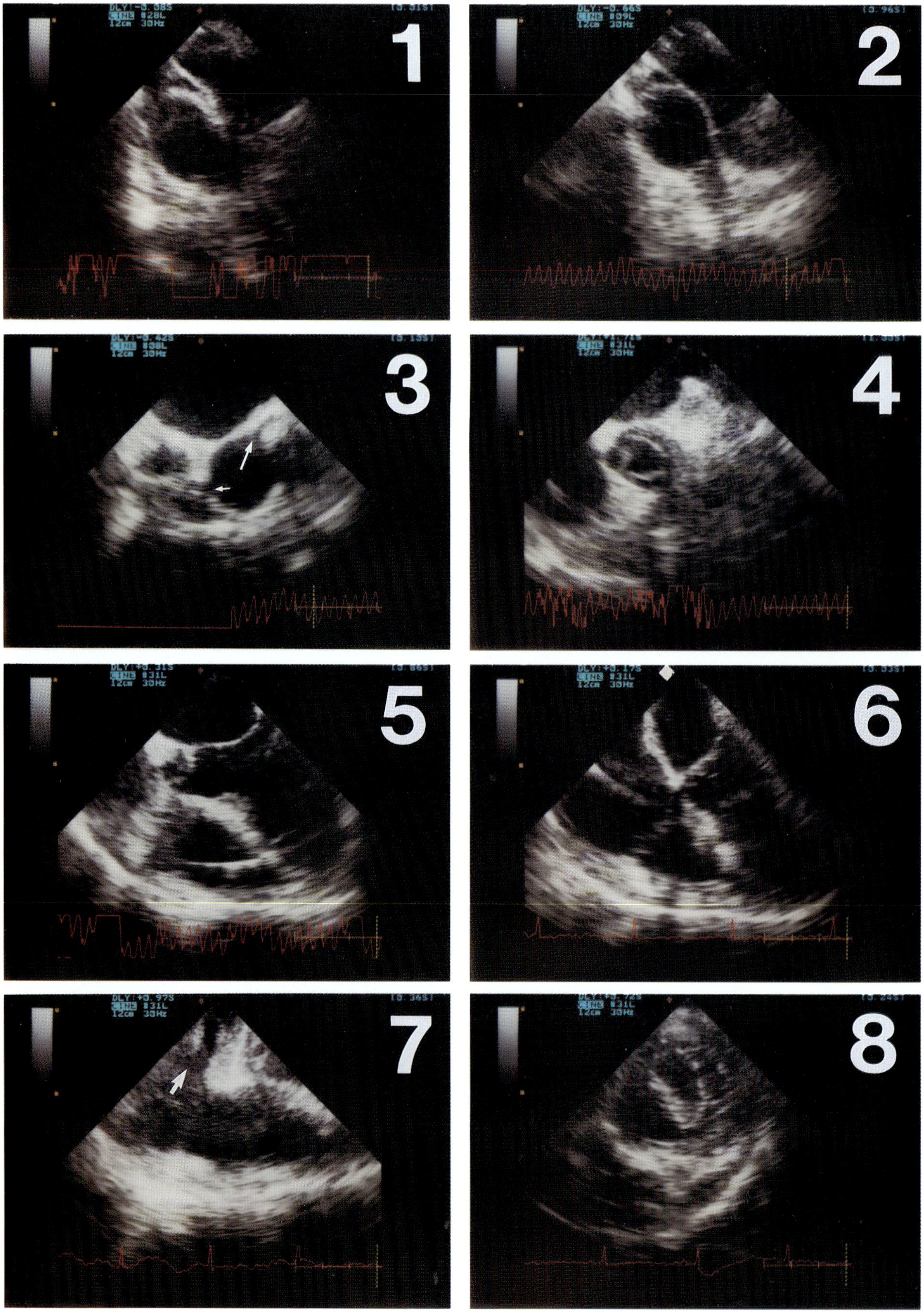
1
2
3
4
5
6
7
8

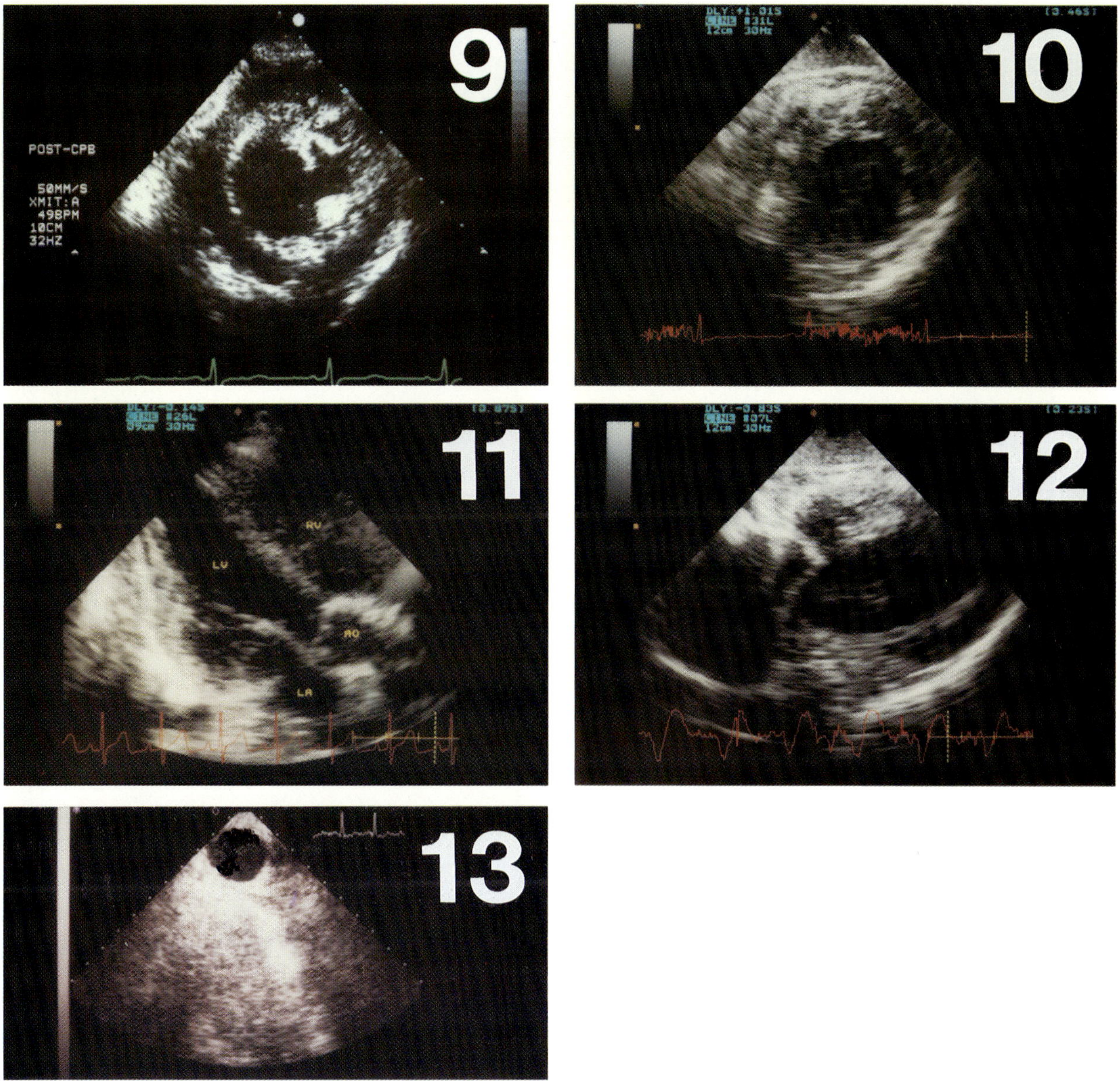

Color Figure 1 • Two-dimensional images of the human heart obtained with a transesophageal transducer. The images in panels 1 through 12 were obtained using scan planes at the depths and orientations in the esophagus indicated by the numbers at the corresponding positions identified in Fig. 23-13. The schematic representation of the video images is also found in the corresponding insets in Fig. 23-13. In panel 3, the long arrow points to the left main coronary artery, and the shorter arrow points to the right coronary artery. The arrow in panel 7 points to the coronary sinus.

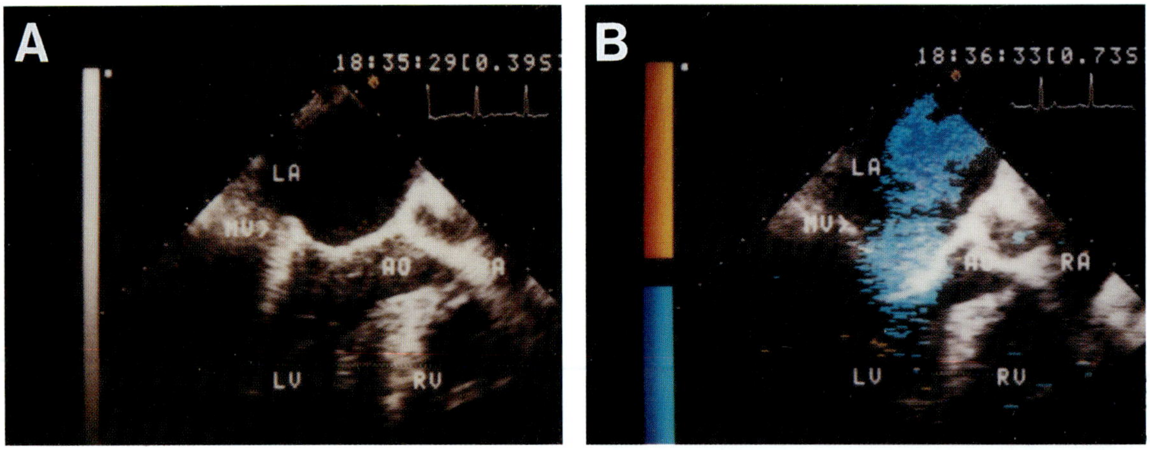

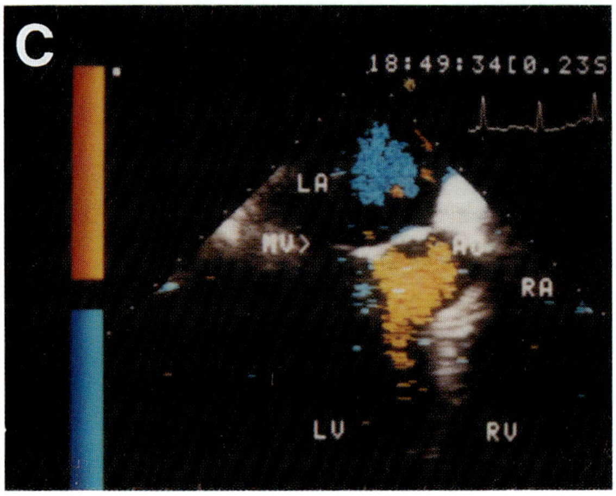

Color Figure 2 • Color-flow Doppler image of a normal heart in a transesophageal four-chamber view. (***A***) Standard 2-D image, (***B***) late diastolic frame showing mitral valve inflow from the left atrium (*LA*) into the left ventricle (*LV*) in blue, and (***C***) midsystolic frame showing blood exiting the LV outflow tract into the aorta (*AO*) in orange-red color and pulmonary venous flow into the LA in blue color. MV = mitral valve; RA = right atrium; RV = right ventricle. The color flow scheme used (see vertical color bars) identifies flow direction as toward (red) and away from (blue) the transducer but does not distinguish between velocity amplitudes. The method maps flow variance with brighter hues.

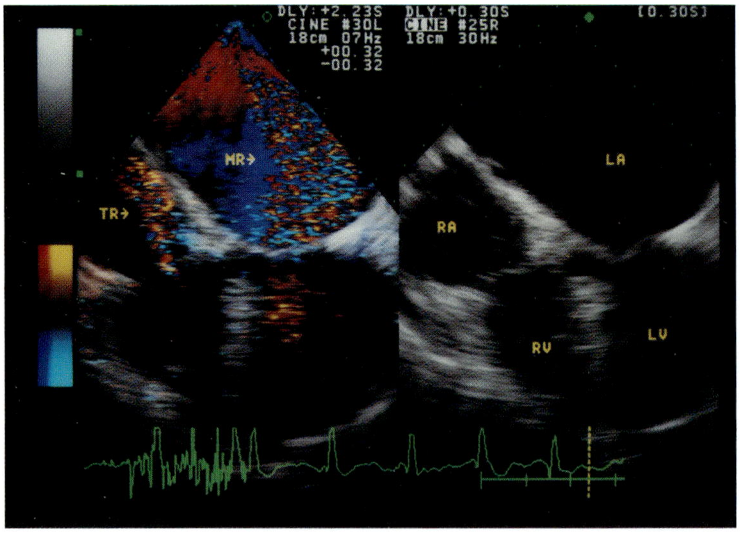

Color Figure 3 • Doppler color-flow imaging of mitral valve regurgitation (MR) and tricuspid regurgitation (TR). On the right panel, the cardiac anatomy in the four-chamber view is identified (LA = left atrium; RA = right atrium; LV = left ventricle; RV = right ventricle). On the left panel, the color map differentiates velocities up to 0.32 mm/sec^{-1}. The MR and TR jets are seen as mosaic mixtures of red, blue, orange, yellow, and cyan pixels consistent with turbulent blood flow. The smooth red and blue colors in the enlarged LA cavity indicate systolic left atrial filling, with swirling.

Left Main Coronary Artery Aneurysm

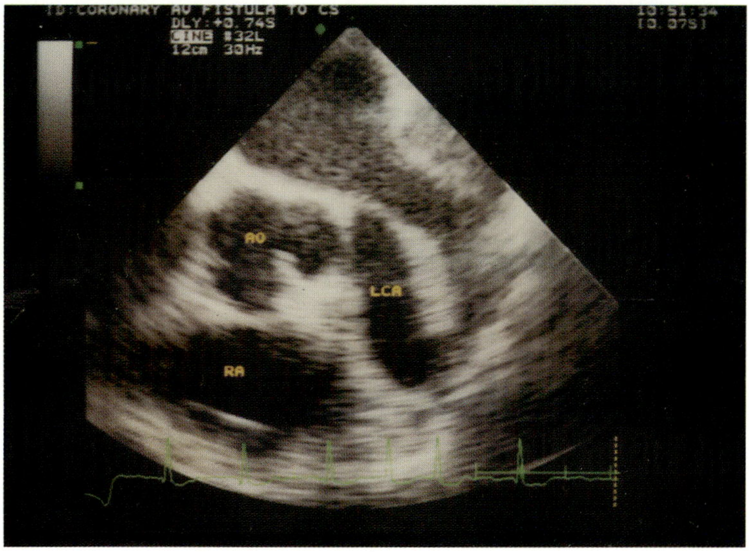

Color Figure 4 • Aneurysmal dilatation of the left main coronary artery (*LCA*) in a patient with a coronary artery–coronary sinus atrioventricular fistula. AO = aorta; RA = right atrium.

Left-to-Right Shunt in ASD

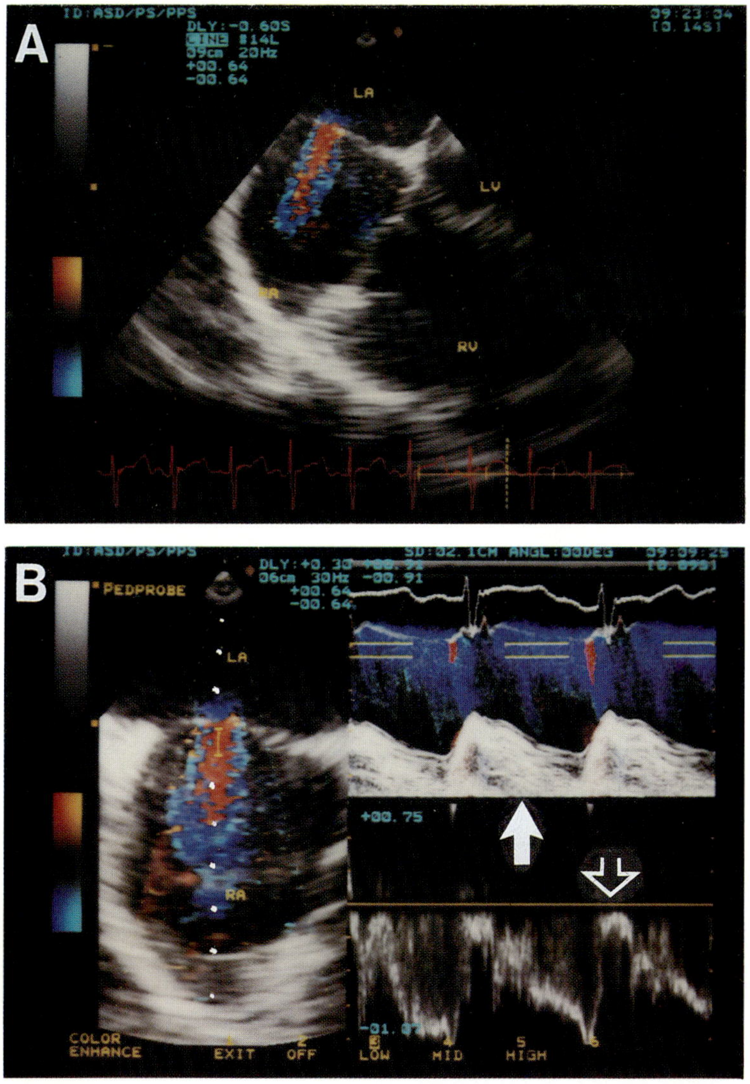

Color Figure 5 • Left-to-right shunt in a pediatric patient with an atrial septal defect. A color-flow map with variance was used. LA = left atrium; RA = right atrium; LV = left ventricle; RV = right ventricle. (***A***) Four-chamber view, note the late diastolic LA to RA flow jet with a clear region of aliasing at its center indicating velocities in excess of 0.64 m/sec^{-1}. (***B***) Combined 2-D, color flow, and M-mode imaging. The solid arrow points to the color M-mode tracing, which demonstrates continuous left-to-right shunt with increased velocity during atrial systole. The open arrow points to the pulsed wave Doppler signal, which indicates shunt flow in excess of 1.0 m/sec^{-1}. These images were obtained with a new 0.6-mm pediatric transesophageal transducer.

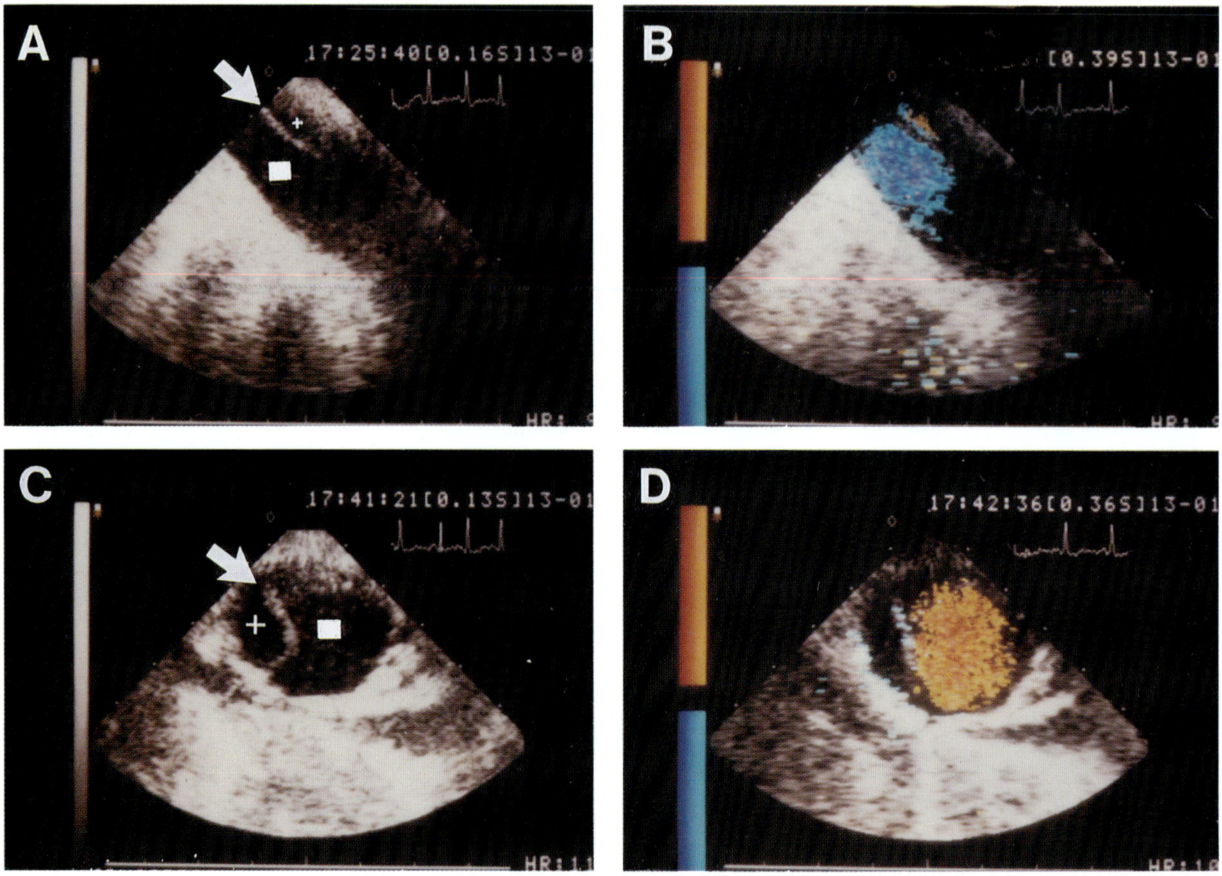

Color Figure 6 • Doppler color-flow study of a patient with a dissection involving the descending thoracic aorta: (***A***) and (***B***) longitudinal view, (***C***) and (***D***) cross-sectional view. The ■ symbol marks the true lumen, and the + symbol marks the false lumen. The arrow points to the dissected wall. Doppler color flow demonstrates blood flow in the true lumen.

Tricuspid Valve Regurgitation

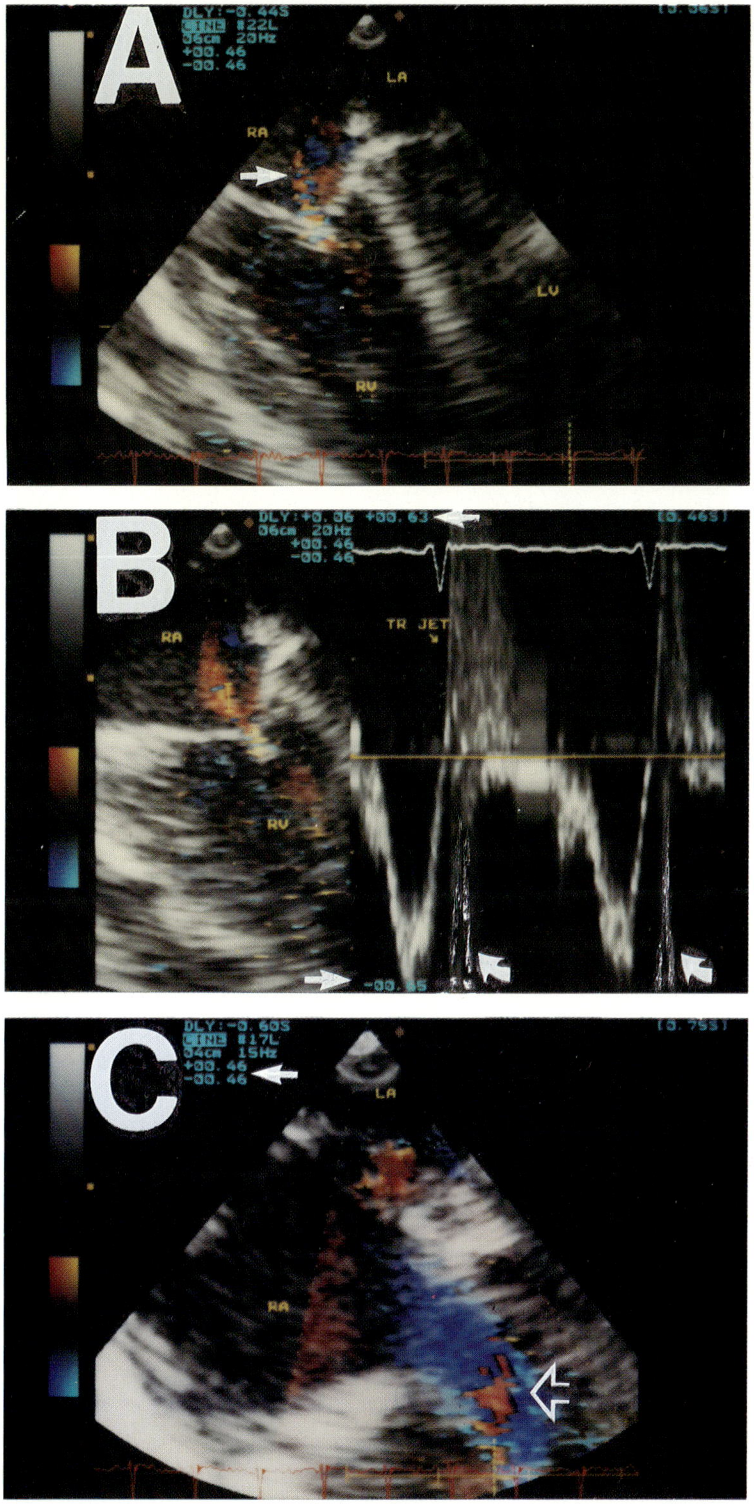

Color Figure 7 • Tricuspid valve regurgitation in a pediatric patient with pulmonic valve stenosis. LA = left atrium; LV = left ventricle; RA = right atrium; RV = right ventricle. (***A***) Four-chamber view with arrow pointing to a small tricuspid valve regurgitation (TR) jet. (***B***) A combined 2-D and pulsed wave Doppler study. With the sample volume just proximal to the tricuspid valve, the maximal velocity that can be measured unambiguously is $\pm$ 0.63 m/sec^{-1} (solid arrows). On the Doppler power spectrum, three peaks can be recognized: (1) a downward peak (Vmax − 0.63 m/sec^{-1}) indicating the normal diastolic ventricular inflow, and (2) a systolic upward peak corresponding to the TR jet. The velocity of this jet exceeds the maximal velocity that can be measured unambiguously. As a result, the highest velocity signals are displayed on the third peak (3), which is synchronous with and in the same direction as the TR jet peak. Its origin, however, is on the lower baseline (*curved arrows*) due to aliasing. (***C***) The 2-D magnification has been increased. The maximum velocity that can now be measured unambiguously is $\pm$ 0.46 m/sec^{-1}. The normal diastolic inflow into the RV is aliased (*open arrow*) because the upper limit of unambiguous velocity detection has been exceeded. (***B***) The inflow Vmax (peak 1) was seen to reach − 0.63 m/sec^{-1}.

Lifescan™ Recording During Carotid Clamping

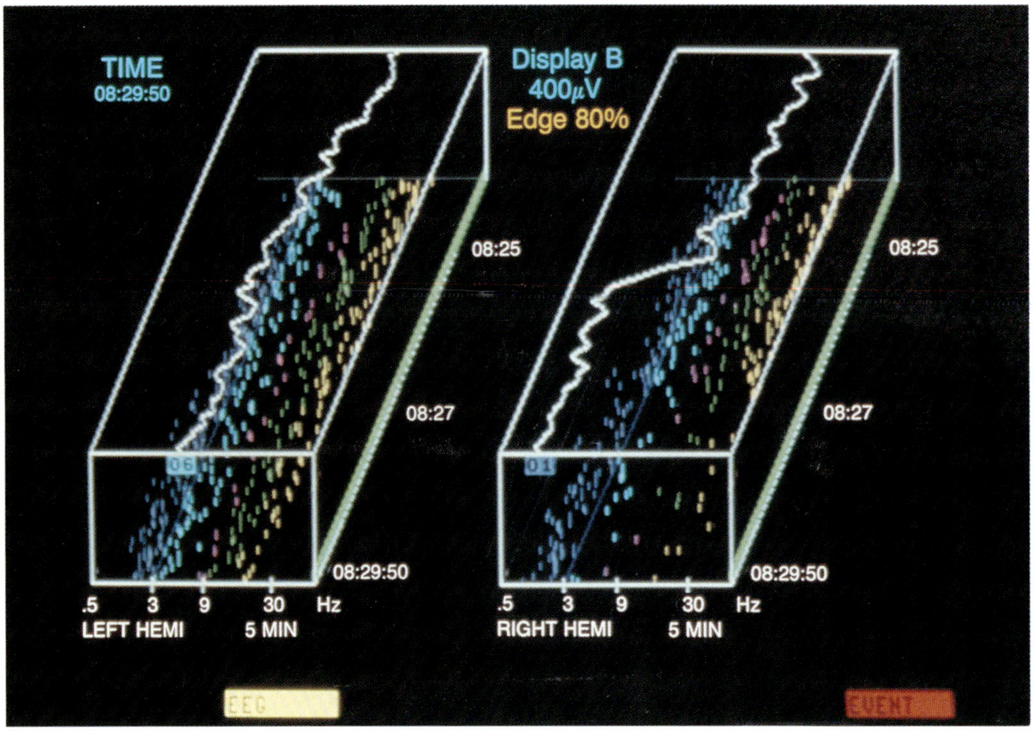

Color Figure 8 • An aperiodic analysis recording obtained from the Lifescan EEG analyzer during cross-clamping of the carotid artery. The white line on the top of each box is the spectral edge (SEF-80). A clamp has been placed on the right carotid artery at 8:25. Note the sudden shift to the left in the right box, while the SEF remains constant in the left. A shunt was placed and the asymmetry resolved. (Courtesy of Diatek Inc, San Diego, California.)

Section I

•

Preparing and Using the Anesthesia Machine and Monitors

Chapter 1

•

Jerry M. Calkins, MD, PhD

Preuse Check of the Anesthetic Delivery System

OUTLINE

I. INTRODUCTION AND INDICATIONS

Anesthesia must be delivered quickly, effectively, and safely, with a minimal amount of stress for patient, surgeon, and anesthesiologist. General anesthesia requires the administration of varying combinations of intravenous pharmacologic agents, together with both respiratory and anesthetic gases in sufficient amounts to produce a state in which the patient is unconscious and pain free, with muscles appropriately relaxed. This anesthetized state must be maintained throughout the operative procedure and must be reversed easily at the termination of surgery.

The association of anesthesia with patient morbidity and mortality during and after surgery has never been doubted. Estimates of the annual anesthesia-related deaths in the United States range from 2000 to 10,000.[1,2] A recent report by Lunn and Mushin suggests at least 55% of these are preventable.[3] In situations where anesthesia was one of several contributing factors, 45% of deaths were preventable. However, in situations where anesthesia alone was the contributing factor, 83% of deaths were considered avoidable.[3]

The results of these and other studies indicate that preventable mishaps can be divided into three categories: human error, the interface of patient and equipment, and equipment failure. All three are a direct result of the complex interactions between anesthesiologist, patient, and equipment.[2–5] Approximately 75% of preventable mishaps have been attributed to human error.[2,4] Avoidable events aggravated by the complex interface between patient and equipment constitute the second largest category and account for 15% of preventable mishaps.[2–4] The third largest group, equipment failure, accounts for the balance of nearly 10%.[2,3]

In addition to categorizing the cause of untoward events, the results of these investigations indicate that nearly 25% of the most frequent and 15% of the associated factors leading to preventable incidents are directly related to either insufficient understanding of equipment design and function or failure to perform normal routine preuse checks, or both. In addition, those events that were related to preexisting equipment failure, equipment faults, and errors in equipment setup were potentially avoidable if equipment operation was adequately assessed prior to use. From these data, it is obvious that a significant number of preventable mishaps might be prevented if each anesthesiologist not only understands how the equipment operates, but also performs a preuse check to insure that it is functioning properly prior to the delivery of each anesthetic.

Manufacturers provide checkout instructions and procedures in their manuals of operation. The Food and Drug Administration (FDA), with the cooperation of the American Society of Anesthesiology (ASA) and the American Association of Nurse Anesthetists (AANA), has also proposed a checkout procedure (see the appendix). Suggested variations to these guidelines exist in various other sources.[5] Even with the widespread availability of this information, evidence exists that some anesthesia providers still fail either to understand fully the functioning of their equipment or to routinely conduct a proper preuse check of their equipment before each case.

The purpose of this chapter is to briefly review the principles of operation of the anesthetic delivery system and to integrate the preuse checkout with these principles. It is the author's intention not only to present the rationale for the preuse checkout (the principles of operation), but to show how, by completing the various steps of the preuse check, appropriate assessment of equipment function and the detection of operational problems can be accomplished prior to the delivery of anesthesia. The discussion of the preuse check includes not only equipment function but also detection of those failures that lead to the most frequent undesired events. Some of the safety instrumentation used to monitor the anesthetic delivery system also is considered.

It is beyond the scope of this chapter to discuss the preuse checkout for all anesthesia equipment (see Chapters 2 and 3 for other anesthesia equipment). However, special consideration is given to the anesthetic delivery system, which consists of an anesthesia machine, ventilator, and patient breathing circuit. It is impossible to include here a discussion of each specific model variation of a piece of equipment from a particular manufacturer. For specific details regarding design and functional variations, the reader is encouraged to use manuals from the manufacturer and other sources of information, such as those given in the references for this chapter.

In this chapter, the FDA proposed procedure, which is reproduced in the appendix, serves as the overall guideline for the preuse check. However, the reader should feel free to modify this procedure according to individual needs and conditions and to develop a reasonable equivalent. Any modification should account for differences in particular equipment design and variations that are applicable to the local clinical practice. However, such modification should receive appropriate peer review. Any modification should not be made without appropriate review of the operator's manual for specific special procedures or precautions. It is also wise to adopt the procedure as an official departmental policy and include it as a written document on each machine and in departmental policy manuals.

A. *Anesthesia Equipment and the Preuse Check*

Functionally, anesthesia equipment can be classified into two major categories (Fig. 1–1).[6] The first category, the anesthetic delivery system, consists of an anesthesia machine, a ventilator, and a patient breathing circuit. The second category, instrumentation, consists of devices for monitoring both the anesthetic delivery system and the status of the patient.

The purpose of the preuse checkout is to assess the operation and function of the anesthetic delivery system just prior to its scheduled use. To understand this preuse check more fully, the operation of the system will be assessed systematically by following the flow of gases through it. This will enable the reader to relate how, by carefully following the preuse check, the most common operational problems can be easily identified. It goes without saying that once identified, the problem must be corrected. This may require removal of equipment from service for a period of time until skilled individuals can repair and correct the problem. The delivery of anesthesia must not proceed until the preuse check has been satisfactorily completed!

As an important part of quality assurance and risk management, it is essential that a note be made on the anesthesia record with the appropriate machine identification number after completing the preuse check. For

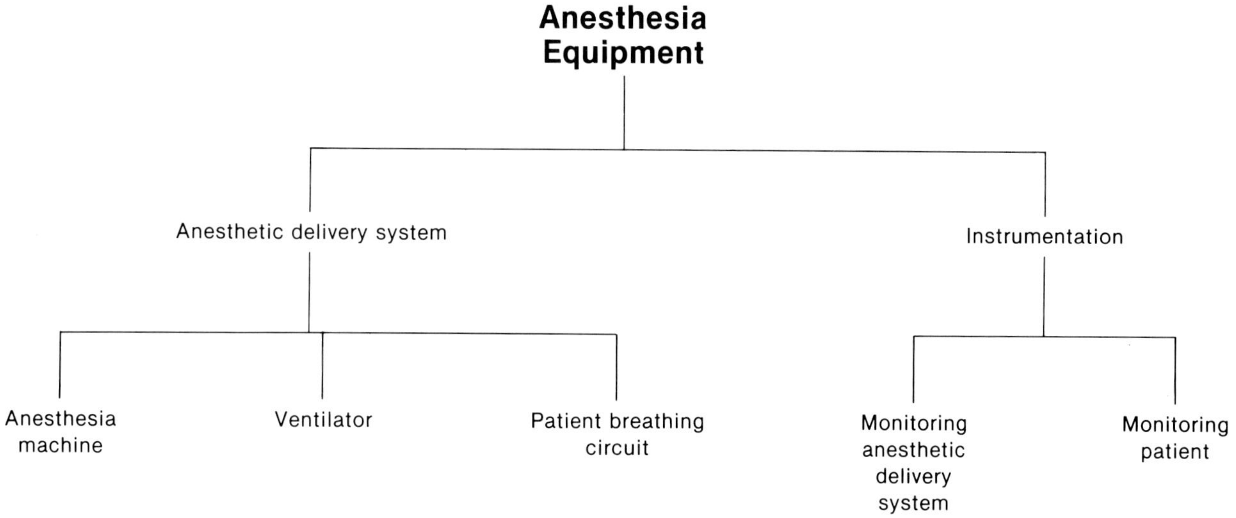

Figure 1–1 • Anesthesia equipment can be classified into particular categories.

example, a control number that is used for maintenance records or the manufacturer's model number can be used. Any problems that are observed must receive appropriate documentation and correction before continuing with the delivery of anesthesia.

If the anesthesiologist uses this same machine in consecutive cases, several steps need not be repeated and/or may be abbreviated after the initial checkout (see the items marked with an asterisk in the Anesthesia Apparatus Checkout Recommendations in the appendix). However, it is highly recommended that the patient breathing circuit and oxygen supply always be verified prior to the induction of any case.

II. How to Check the Anesthetic Delivery System: Current Design, Problems, Checkout

The anesthetic delivery system consists of an anesthesia machine connected to a patient breathing circuit, a ventilator, and airway management equipment (anesthesia mask; endotracheal [ET] tube). The anesthesia machine enables the anesthesiologist to produce a desired oxygen–nitrous oxide mixture (Fig. 1–2), to which is added a variable concentration of an anesthetic vapor. This resultant mixture flows from the machine through the breathing circuit and airway management equipment into the patient by either spontaneous or mechanical ventilation.

A. *Anesthesia Machine: Current Design, Problems, Checkout*

Even the most vocal critics of present-day anesthesia machines will admit that both technology and design have stood the test of time. This has resulted in a gradual evolution of design standardization through the years. Such standardization enables the user, with a minimum of refamiliarization, to encounter a new machine and immediately introduce it into practice.[7]

The importance of this aspect must not be underestimated, since the preuse checkout for one type of machine will follow similar steps for another. However, there may be significant functional design differences between machines. Therefore, a complete understanding of these differences in design and manufacturers' recommendations between designs must be considered.

Ruggedness is an additional asset of current mechanical hardware.[8] The operating room is a hostile environment for equipment. Constant movement of equipment, splashing with water and solvents, impact by heavy objects, and changes in temperature all mean wear and tear. Reliability requires that equipment be free from failure rather than free from inaccuracy (but within certain wide limits). Nevertheless, anesthesia machines generally perform according to design specifications.[7]

Although a machine is rugged, never assume physical breakage cannot occur. The first step in the preuse checkout of the anesthesia machine is visual inspection (step 1, FDA procedure; see the appendix). Pay par-

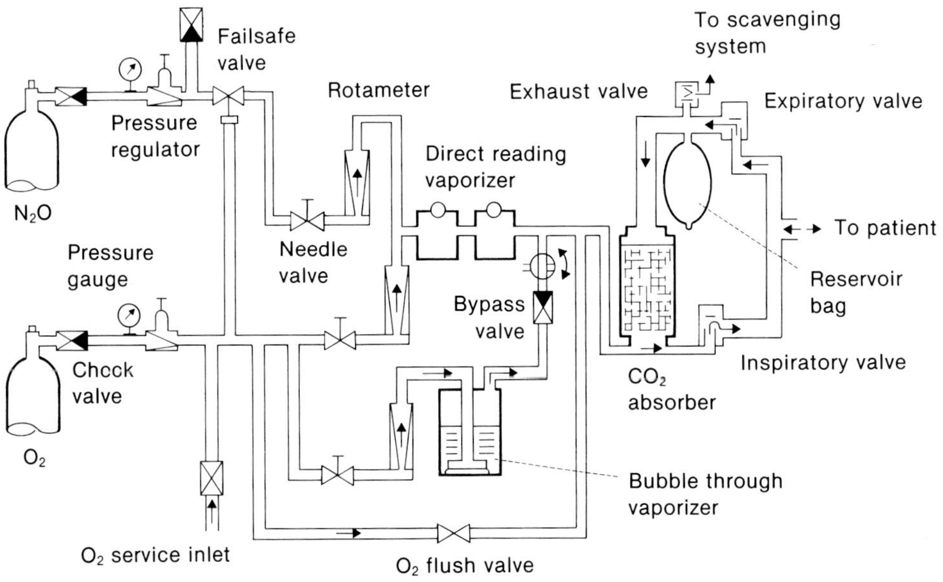

Figure 1–2 • A simplified schematic diagram of an anesthesia machine and patient breathing circuit. The patient breathing circuit is connected to airway management equipment such as an anesthesia mask or endotrachial (ET) tube. (Reprinted with permission of the publisher from C. Waterson. The anesthesia machine: Current design and alternatives. Med Instrum 17(6):379–382, 1983.)

ticular attention to the general appearance and condition of the machine. Are any components (eg, flowmeters, vaporizers, pressure gauges) obviously damaged? Are the gas supply hoses appropriately attached? Visually inspect the patient breathing circuit to determine if there are any damaged components, such as the carbon dioxide absorber and breathing valves. Are the gas cylinders correctly mounted in their respective yokes? Is the cylinder wrench present? Is there a valid inspection sticker present? If not, when was the last documented service performed? Note the last time the machine received appropriate preventive maintenance.

While visually inspecting the machine, the user can also perform a brief electrical inspection. Check the electrical cords to insure that monitors are plugged in appropriately and that the main power cord from the machine has been inserted in an appropriate wall outlet. Also for additional safety, move cords out of the way of the wheels of the machine.

After completion of this visual inspection, any electrical equipment requiring warm-up and the machine master switch, if present, should be turned on (step 2, FDA procedure; see the appendix). Newer-design machines use a single master switch to control all electrical and pneumatic power. If this switch is not turned on, none of the electrical or gas circuits will operate.

Once the general visual inspection is complete and appropriate switches are turned on (step 6, FDA procedure; see the appendix), the user can turn his or her attention to the subsystems of the machine. In its simplest form, the anesthesia machine is composed of two subsystems (see Fig. 1–2). One subsystem, the gas supply and delivery system (see Section III.A.1), consists of tubing and flowmeters interconnected in parallel. The second subsystem, the anesthetic vaporizer (see Section III.A.2), uses various techniques to produce an anesthetic vapor from a volatile liquid. Examples of two of the newer machine designs are shown in Figs. 1–3 and 1–4.

The preuse check of the anesthesia machine is the systematic assessment of these two subsystems. This check is performed to insure patient safety and the proper functioning of the machine. The check is basically a logical sequence of inspection steps that assesses the integrity of the pathway for respiratory gases and anesthetic vapors from the hospital supply through the machine and patient breathing circuit into the patient.

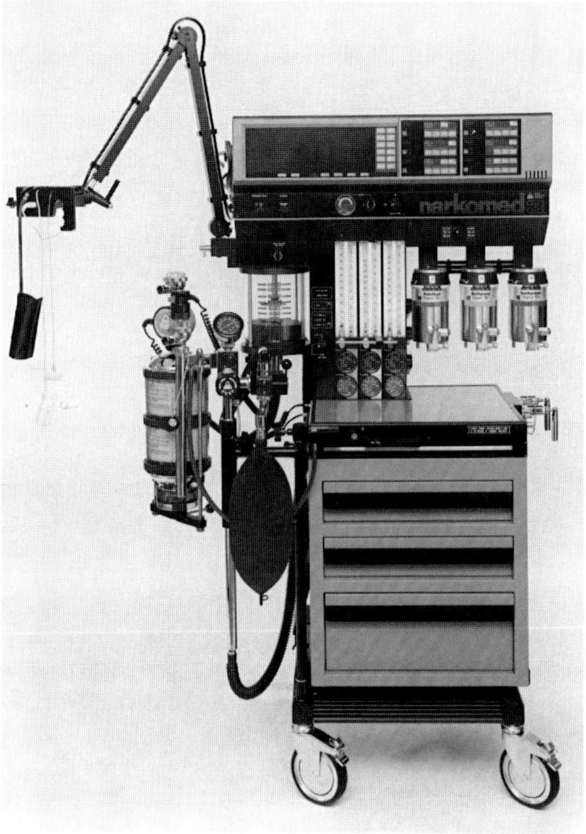

Figure 1–3 • The North American Drager Narkomed 3 anesthesia machine. (Reproduced with permission from North American Drager, Telford, PA.)

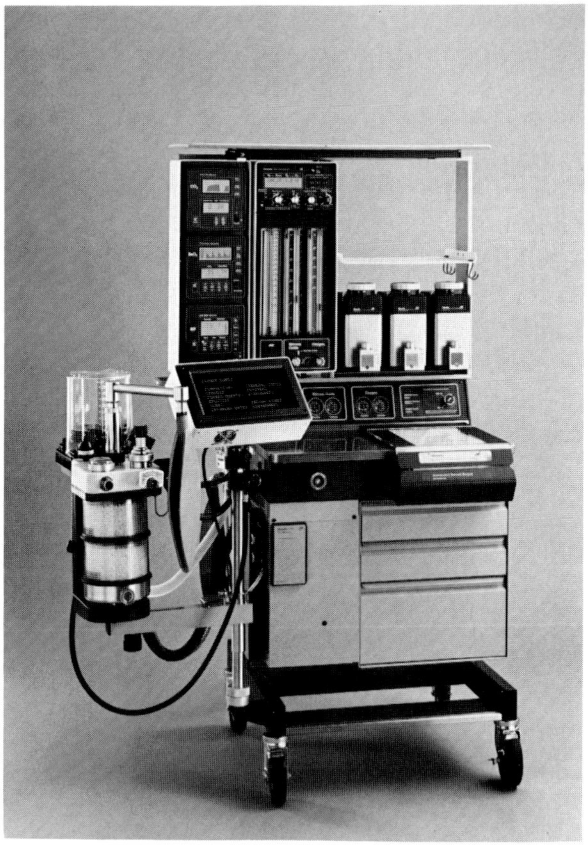

Figure 1–4 • The Ohmeda Modulus II anesthesia machine. (Reproduced with permission from Ohmeda, Madison, WI.)

1. Gas Supply and Delivery: Design, Problems, Checkout

Since catastrophic events occur in anesthesiology when appropriate gas supplies, particularly oxygen, are not being used, one must be extremely careful, consistent, and thorough in assessing the oxygen gas supply to the patient circuit. Machine checkout is to verify not only that the supply is adequate, at the origin, but also that the integrity of the delivery system to the patient is not compromised. The assessment of gas supply is designed to insure that an ample amount exists at the source and that the machine neither leaks nor contains any malfunctioning mechanical components that will compromise an adequate flow of respiratory and anesthetic gases to the patient.

Gases are provided to the anesthesia machine inlet from either a pressurized hospital central supply or small storage cylinders (tanks) attached to the machine (see Fig. 1–2). Although simplistic in concept, both centralized hospital systems and machine cylinders have contributed significantly to problems during anesthesia delivery.

Centralized hospital systems are designed for both main and reserve supply. Each consists of either bulk or cylinder storage, control equipment including valves and pressure regulators, a distribution pipeline, and numerous supply outlets.[9] Design and operation must be such that the necessary supply of gases (oxygen and nitrous oxide) are always available. Gas supplied by the hospital is regulated and maintained at 40–50 psi at the wall outlet. (See Chapter 10 for use of high oxygen wall pressure for transtracheal jet ventilation.)

Numerous accidents involving supply systems have been reported.[10,11] These have included oxygen supply contamination by the inadvertent filling of the oxygen reservoir with nitrogen,[12] faulty oxygen–air mixing valves with loss of oxygen,[13] and loss of oxygen pressure and flow secondary to supply and distribution problems.[10] The most notorious and usually fatal accidents with gas supply have occurred after contamination of oxygen by nitrous oxide.[13-15] The most common cause has been cross-connection of lines after system modifications.[16,17] Other problems have included depletion of the reserve supply before the main supply, improperly adjusted regulators,[18] and leaks. Bulk liquid oxygen systems have been constructed without a means to connect an emergency supply of compressed oxygen to the main pipeline.[19]

To prevent interchanging the gas supply wall outlet with incorrect anesthesia machine inlet (eg, nitrous oxide outlet into the oxygen inlet), noninterchangeable connectors are used at each end of the hose. The two types of noninterchangeable connections most commonly used are the Diameter Index Safety System (DISS) and noninterchangeable quick couplers. Each type of connection incorporates a male and a female end that are designed specifically for each type of gas.

The second source of gas for the anesthesia machine is available from cylinders located in yokes attached to the anesthesia machine. This supply can be used as either the main source, when a central hospital gas supply does not exist, or a reserve source. (See Chapter 10 for use of high oxygen tank pressure for transtracheal jet ventilation.)

Each anesthesia machine has at least one yoke for an oxygen cylinder, and on most there is an additional yoke for nitrous oxide. To prevent incorrect placement of a tank into the wrong yoke, two pins located in the yoke must fit into corresponding holes drilled into the tank. The placement of these pins and holes is unique for each gas. This identification system, which is referred to as the Pin Index Safety System, is standard throughout the United States.[11,14,20] Potential hazards have been reported with cylinders.[21] These include contamination of contents, faulty check valves, improper identification, and improper cylinder testing.[22] Other problems have arisen from perforation of the cylinder thermal relief plug, from errors in color coding, and from placement in the incorrect yoke.[11,20]

To check both the central and cylinder supplies satisfactorily, it is essential that all tanks be turned off initially and that the supply hoses be disconnected from the wall. It is imperative that the central supply line gas supplies be tested (step 11, FDA procedure; see the appendix). This can be accomplished by first looking for obvious problems, inspecting the supply hoses, looking for cracks and any worn places, connecting the supply hoses, and verifying correct color coding and connectors (Figs. 1–5 and 1–6). All low-pressure gas connections to the anesthesia machine should have clearly identifiable color-coded hoses, labels, and noninterchangeable connectors at each end. The user should verify that the supply pressures from the wall are constant and within an acceptable range of 45 and 50 psi. In newer-design machines, pressure gauges labeled *pipeline pressure gauge* and located on the front panel of the anesthesia machine indicate this.

With the gas cylinders that are attached to the machine turned off, verify gas flow by adjusting all gas delivery units to flows within the midrange. The user can verify that oxygen is flowing as indicated with the oxygen analyzer that is located in the circuit. Should the oxygen analyzer immediately go to zero, this indicates that something other than oxygen is in the main oxygen supply line. Other gas monitors (eg, a mass spectrometer) that are used to indicate nitrous oxide can also be used to verify gas concentrations coming from the machine into the circuit. Once this has been accomplished shut off the flow-control valves.

To check the oxygen supply from the attached cylinders (step 5, FDA procedure; see the appendix), dis-

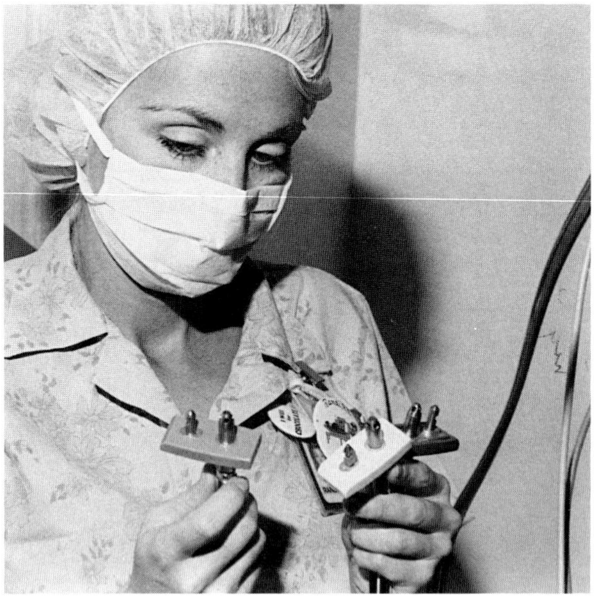

Figure 1–5 • Verify that noninterchangeable connectors are used on the gas supply of color-coded hoses.

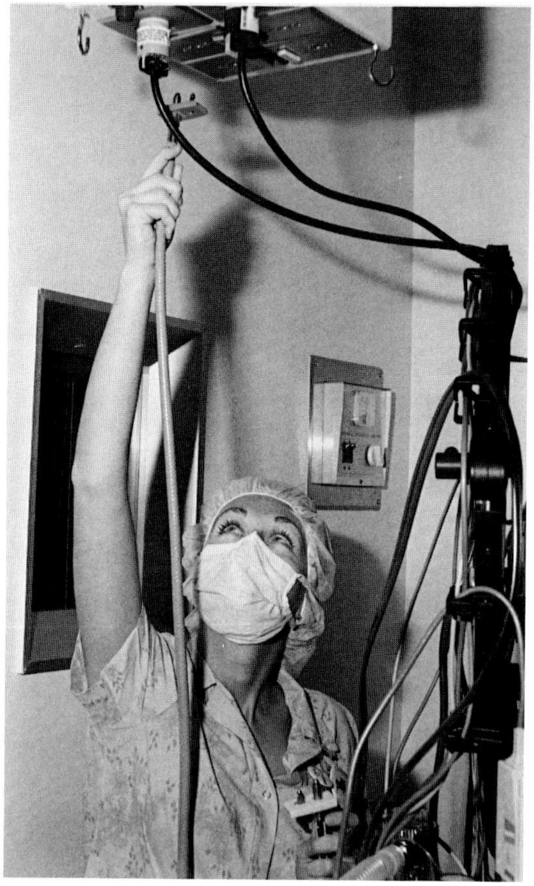

Figure 1–6 • Check connection of noninterchangeable connectors on the gas supply hoses.

connect the pipeline supply, if it is connected (see Fig. 1–6), and turn off cylinders. This must be accomplished to isolate each supply, since both the cylinder and central supply feed into a common manifold (see Fig. 1–2) and would interfere with testing the other system. After completing this operation, note that all supply pressure gauges (central and cylinder) are set to zero. If the pressure gauges have not returned to zero, open either the needle valves for oxygen and nitrous oxide or the oxygen flush valve to empty the system as indicated by a zero pressure on the gauges. These pressure gauges are usually located on the front panel of the machine and are labeled *pipeline pressure* and *cylinder pressure,* respectively.

Once the machine is successfully isolated from the wall supply, verify that the gas cylinders have been inserted appropriately into the corresponding gas yokes. Inspect for any force fits or damage done to the cylinders or the machine yokes. In addition to this visual inspection, verify that a cylinder wrench is attached to the machine and can be quickly used to open and close the valves on the top of the cylinders (Fig. 1–7).

The oxygen cylinder supply check-out is accomplished in several steps. First, visually inspect the yoke and the cylinders to insure that the oxygen cylinder is attached at the oxygen yoke. Next, open the oxygen cylinder valve and check the pressure. Now close the cylinder valve and inspect for a high-pressure leak. If one exists, the needle on the pressure gauge will quickly

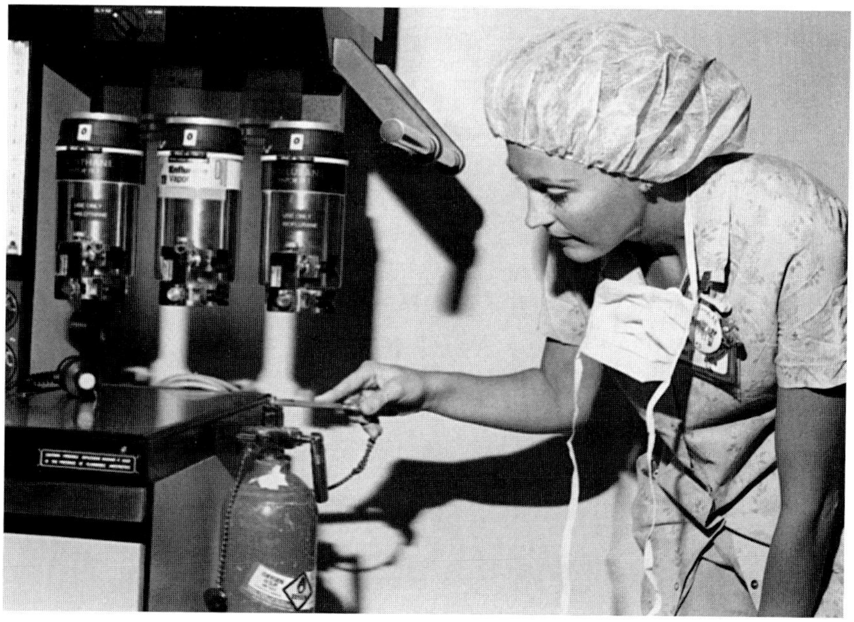

Figure 1–7 • Verify the presence (on the machine) and use of the cylinder wrench.

move toward zero. Empty the system with the flush valve and repeat the procedure using the second oxygen cylinder, if present. Any oxygen cylinder less than 600 psi should be replaced. At least one oxygen cylinder should be nearly full. When using the cylinders, open the less full cylinder (if known) first.

The same procedure is completed for nitrous oxide. However, because of design differences between oxygen and nitrous oxide, to empty the piping system it will be necessary to open and close the flow-control valve for nitrous oxide. Since nitrous oxide is stored as a liquid, a nitrous oxide pressure below 745 psig indicates the cylinder is less than one fourth full. Any additional gas supplies, such as air and helium, should be assessed in a similar manner by repeating these steps.

Machine pressure regulators located near the yoke reduce cylinder pressures to approximately 40 psi before the gas enters the machine (see Fig. 1–2). In some newer designs, a second regulator located just prior to the pressure fail-safe system further reduces both wall and cylinder pressures to 15–20 psi.

Some controversy exists as to whether the oxygen cylinder valve should be left open or closed once the gas supply from the oxygen cylinder has been assessed. Whether this is done or not is a function of both philosophy and the nature of the equipment being used. In some anesthesia machine models, check valves prevent gas flow from a higher positive pressure source to a lower pressure source (eg, from a flowing supply line into an empty cylinder or from a full closed cylinder back into an empty central piping system). Hence, the oxygen cylinder would not be used unknowingly or by accident while the wall supply was being used. However, the safety controversy exists when the cylinder pressure is higher than that at the wall and there are no (or no properly functioning) check valves. In this instance the potential exists for emptying the cylinders first and then using the wall supply. If this occurs and the primary oxygen cylinder is emptied, the user may not know that a change to a second oxygen cylinder is required. Some anesthesiologists feel that if the oxygen cylinder is turned off, then an ample oxygen supply will always be available on the machine. These individuals are relying on anesthesia machine and patient monitors and clinical observation to detect the wall supply is diminishing. If this situation arises, the oxygen cylinder valve can be opened. The procedure used (open or closed oxygen cylinder) is a matter of personal preference and local clinical procedure. However, if the user chooses to leave the oxygen cylinders turned on, he or she should check the operator's manual for the machine and verify the existence of check valves, precautions, and the consequences of leaving the cylinders on.

As a safety feature, anesthesia machine designs employ a pressure safety system (fail-safe system).[8,9] From the supply, the gas flows into the inlet of the anesthesia machine and is directed through the pressure safety system (fail-safe system) toward the flow delivery unit (see Fig. 1–2). The pressure safety system will not allow nitrous oxide to flow unless an oxygen supply pressure exists in the machine.

The fail-safe system begins with the master pressure regulator valve located in the oxygen supply line just distal to the origin of the oxygen (cylinder or wall) (see Fig. 1–2). From the master regulator, a reference pressure is provided to the slave regulator (fail-safe) valve controlling the pressure and flow of the nitrous oxide line. When sufficient oxygen pressure of 40 psi is present in the master regulator, the reference pressure enables the slave regulator valve to open and nitrous oxide to flow. Unfortunately, in some machines pure nitrous oxide can be delivered when only oxygen supply pressure is present. In these systems oxygen flow (which is the important parameter) is not required.

With the exception of the fail-safe system, no other means was available to prevent the delivery of pure nitrous oxide in earlier machines. New ANSI Z-79 standards required a minimum continuous low flow of oxygen varying from 200 to 300 mL/min, as indicated by the low-flow rotameter. Ingenious mechanical linkages, pressure-repeating diaphragm units, and other mechanical devices found in state-of-the-art machines prevent the delivery of gas mixtures with an oxygen concentration below a lower limit.[6] Control of minimum oxygen–nitrous oxide ratios vary from 25:75 to 30:70, depending on the manufacturer.

The appropriate evaluation of the fail-safe system should be accomplished prior to the delivery of anesthesia (step 10, FDA procedure; see the appendix).

To test the pressure safety system, set all gas flows to a midrange on each flowmeter (1 or 2 L/min). Now close the oxygen cylinder and open the oxygen flush valve to release the oxygen pressure. In so doing, verify that all flows fall to zero. Now open the oxygen cylinder and close all other cylinders and bleed the system pressure for these other gases. Close the flow-control valves. In assessing whether the fail-safe system is working or not, keep in mind that oxygen flow is not required for flow from another gas source. Only oxygen pressure is required. This test clearly demonstrates that without oxygen pressure all flows decrease to zero. With oxygen pressure, other gases will flow.

It is obvious that without appropriate gas analysis and alarms on machines, it is possible to provide a 100% nitrous oxide in some of the older-design machines. An assessment of the ratio protection and warning systems, if they are present, can be evaluated in this manner by attempting to create a hypoxic oxygen–nitrous oxide mixture (step 9, FDA procedure; see the appendix). In attempting to create an unsafe mixture, the user can verify a correct change in gas flows as well as produce and silence any alarm.

From the fail-safe system, the gas is directed to the flow delivery unit. Two methods have been used to accomplish delivery and control of the gas mixture: gas proportionating and gas mixing.[8,24] In a gas-proportionating system, the delivered concentration of each gas constituent is a function of a predetermined, precisely controlled ratio of gases that is always independent of the total gas flow. For example, for a final mixture of 70% nitrous oxide and 30% oxygen, the metered ratio of mass delivery will always be 7:3, regardless of the total flow rate. Concentration is only a function of the proportional relationship between constituents. It does not rely on setting individual gas flows. An oxygen–nitrous oxide blender functions like an oxygen–air blender, which is commonly used with mechanical ventilators.

Most current anesthesia machines depend on gas mixing to control the concentration of delivered gases. In this technique, the flow rate of each constituent is independently controlled and measured by a delivery unit consisting of a needle valve and a rotameter. The needle valve functions as a flow controller and a means of turning the gas on and off. The rotameter, which consists of a transparent tube and flow indicator (float, bobbin), acts as a flow-rate monitor.

In a gas-mixing system, each gas has a specific delivery unit. They are connected in parallel and exhaust into a common manifold prior to leaving the machine. The final concentration and total flow, as determined by mixing the component flows, are dependent functions and subject to the accuracy of the control and measurement equipment.

Although simple in design and function, this flow delivery unit has a number of performance-related problems.[9,14,25] Needle valves are prone to leakage and looseness around the stem packing. The closing interface between the tip of the valve stem and its seat leaks as a result of wear. The control knobs may loosen, or they may be accidentally bumped, inappropriately altering flow. Although fine adjustment is possible, it is difficult to reproduce exact flows.

Rotameters also are fraught with mechanical and operational problems.[9,11] In some designs the flow indicators (bobbins, floats) are prone to stick unless the glass tubes are immaculately clean and free of static electricity. Bobbins have been reported to remain hidden after sticking at both the top and the bottom of the tube.[25] Very unusual problems from particulate contamination have been reported.[25] Flowmeters tend to become inaccurate after some use.[26,27] In addition, the design of current gas delivery systems allows inaccuracies of flow because of gas density changes. Backpressure from either obstruction or ventilator cycling is transmitted from the circuit to the flowmeters. This effect is commonly referred to as the "bounding" or "bouncing" bobbin. Other pressure effects, such as altitude, also produce error.[28] The lack of a standard location of the oxygen flowmeter for metabolic gas supply has created difficulties during emergencies.[29] Leaks develop in the manifold as a result of poor assembly or cracked flow tubes.[24,30] Other problems have resulted from mistakes made during routine maintenance. These include improper vertical alignment of flow tubes and the interchange of either flow tubes or indicators, such as high or low flow, or nitrous oxide, for oxygen. When high-flow nitrous oxide and low-flow oxygen have accidentally been used together.[11]

Because of these and other problems with needle valves and rotameters, numerous recommendations and standards have been adopted for the United States.[11,20] ANSI Committee Z-79 standards for reduction of error require that the oxygen flowmeter for metabolic requirements always be located on the extreme right of any group of flowmeters, which is the position nearest to the patient. On machines with both low- and high-flow rotameters in parallel, a distinction between control knobs is necessary. Newer-design machines use low- and high-flow rotameters connected in series rather than in parallel. In this design, only one flow-control knob is used for each gas. Newer flowmeters are designed with improved scales, pin indexing, and unique bore sizes, so that indicators and tubes cannot be interchanged. Floats must be visible at all times, and new static-free, damage-resistant materials are also being used. Fragile components of the flow delivery system are protected by transparent covers. Color coding for gases remains constant throughout the machine.

Needle valve control knobs have been color coded and the design changed so that the tactile senses of the user can be used to distinguish them. On some machines protective guards for control knobs have been added to prevent accidental changing of flows.

Assessment of the flow delivery system includes verification that appropriate gas supply exists and a visual inspection of rotameter and needle valve for any physical damage. During this inspection of the rotameter, insure that the float is at the bottom of the tube when the flow-control valves (needle valves) are closed. In those machines that have a continuous low-oxygen flow, inspect to see that the oxygen is flowing at the manufacturer's recommended minimum amount. This varies between manufactures but usually ranges from 200 to 300 mL/min. Adjust the flow of all the gases through their full range and check for any erratic movements of the floats. Turn the flow-control knobs so there is no longer flow through the rotameter and insure that the floats have returned to the bottom of the flowmeter (Fig. 1–8).

During the administration of anesthesia, it may be necessary to fill the patient breathing circuit with oxygen at a rate higher than what the ordinary gas delivery unit (flowmeters or rotameters) can supply. For example, such a situation exists any time a patient is disconnected and reconnected to the breathing circuit. This higher flow of oxygen is supplied via the oxygen flush valve and line (see Fig. 1–2). The oxygen flush system provides a high flow ranging from 35 to 75 L/min at a high pressure (20–45 psi) directly into the patient breathing system. (See Chapter 10 for use of oxygen flush system for transtracheal jet ventilation.)

High-flow oxygen flush systems have also caused problems. Numerous problems have been reported from valves remaining open or from inadvertent engagement of the valve.[9,11,25] Prior to the mid-1970s, some machines had a three-position rather than a two-position valve. The positions were designated as off or on for either the vaporizer or oxygen flush. Often the anesthesiologist used the flush position and forgot to turn on the vaporizer. The result was that vaporized anesthetic would exhaust to the room. Existing ANSI standards prohibit this design. Other recommendations suggest spring-loaded or self-closing oxygen flush valves. The evaluation of the performance of the flush system is accomplished when the user verifies the integrity of the patient breathing circuit. In general, the flush is evaluated by opening the spring-loaded valve, listening for the rush of oxygen into the circuit, and closing the valve.

2. Anesthetic Vaporizer: Design, Problems, Checkout

Vaporizers are designed to produce an accurate gaseous (vapor) concentration from a volatile liquid anesthetic agent. The accurate concentration of anesthetic vapor can then be safely added to the previously metered oxygen and nitrous oxide as they leave the mixing manifold (see Fig. 1–2).

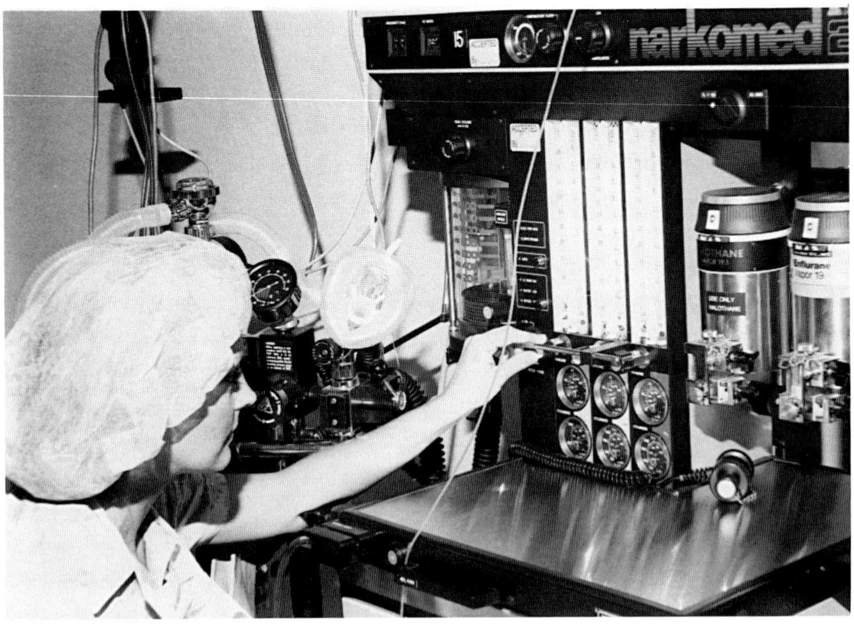

Figure 1–8 • Adjust the flow of all gases through the full range of flows and verify movement of floats from zero to maximum flow and return to zero without erratic movement. A metal bar in front of the flow knobs prevents accidental bumping (and turning) of the flow knobs.

The vaporizer has one of two basic designs: flowmeter controlled or concentration calibrated.[8] In either device, the anesthetic vapor is swept from the vaporizer by a carrier gas consisting either of pure oxygen or of an oxygen–nitrous oxide mixture as it bubbles through or passes over the liquid. The carrier gases are exposed to the volatile liquid in any one of several designs. In all cases, the liquid surface area to gas interface is designed to insure the most efficient vaporization process.

Flowmeter-controlled vaporizers (also called Kettle's, variable bypass wick type, bubble-through) depend on rotameters for their accuracy. This type of vaporizer usually receives an oxygen carrier gas from a separate parallel low-flow oxygen delivery system (see Fig. 1–2). In these vaporizers, the carrier gas becomes saturated with vapor prior to entering the manifold. Within the manifold it is diluted to the desired concentration in proportion to the relative flow rates. Large diluent gas flows are required for accurate delivery of the desired vapor concentration. Ultimately, they can pollute the environment. To use this type of vaporizer, the anesthesiologist must calculate final concentrations delivered to the patient prior to turning on the vaporizer via a separate circuit bypass valve (see Fig. 1–2). This is one disadvantage of these vaporizers.[8,24]

Cooling of the liquid by evaporation leads to a decrease in vapor pressure and hence output concentration. These vaporizers are also sensitive to pressure fluctuations from the circuit.[9] However, later designs placed check valves in the inlet gas circuit to minimize this problem. Since the concentration depends on the accuracy of the rotameters, all previously discussed problems of the gas delivery unit for measuring and controlling flow apply.

To eliminate calculation of final concentrations, the direct reading vaporizers (also called DRV, variable bypass, calibrated, or "TEC-type" vaporizers) were developed. Although the thermodynamic evaporative processes previously described occur, appropriate outlet concentrations are obtained by accurate mechanical inlet flow proportionating.[26] Dilution and temperature compensation are also accomplished within the vaporizer. For operation of the DRV, the anesthesiologist need only dial the desired concentration.

The DRV also has problems.[9] The outlet concentration can vary with flow. This may be negligible in moderate-flow ranges but is of concern in low-flow closed-circuit anesthesia.[8,24] The pressurization of the system by the cycling of the ventilator can also affect output concentration.[9] The rate of heat transfer is not always adequate to overcome cooling caused by evaporation, and a lower than desired vapor pressure results. The performance of the vaporizer deteriorates over time as passages get dirty and components wear. Periodic calibration and cleaning are necessary.[8,31]

Regardless of design, all vaporizers share common difficulties. Vaporizers possess efficiency problems resulting from corrosion, scaling, and fouling.[9] Many earlier designs are not flow, temperature, or pressure compensated, and the delivery characteristics change as these factors change. Inability to prevent wrong anesthetics from being placed in the vaporizers,[32] downstream contamination of in-series vaporizers,[33] and delivery of more than one agent[14,25] are other hazards. All vaporizers suffer from problems with excessive levels that result from overfilling, tipping, or excessive flow. Although not proved to be a hazard, discoloration of agents contained in the vaporizer has caused some concern.

To overcome some of these problems, new designs require that vaporizers be mounted and interlocked to allow easy removal for servicing and to prevent simultaneous delivery of more than one volatile agent. Some manufacturers have also adopted a keyed filler system that prevents filling the vaporizer with the incorrect agent.[6]

The preuse vaporizer check is done in several steps (step 4, FDA procedure; see the appendix). First, visual inspection through the sight glass and manual check of drain valves is necessary to insure that appropriate liquid levels are present in each vaporizer. In the DRV type, the level must be between the minimum and maximum markings. In those machine designs having interlocking vaporizers, the interlock system and the integrity with the vaporizer needs to be verified. This can be accomplished by placing the lock into an appropriate position and verifying that only the specified vaporizer can be turned on and off. Be sure that all other vaporizers are in the off position and cannot be turned on when one is already on.

Verification of correct agent in the vaporizer is more difficult. The DRV-type vaporizer is designed for a specific agent. It has been recommended that the user sniff the inspiratory gas to verify that there is no odor when all vaporizers have been turned off. The sniff test is then repeated when an appropriate vaporizer has been turned on to verify the correct agent. Some anesthesiologists believe that the sniff test of the patient breathing circuit is not necessary and exposes the user to the extra hazards of increased environmental pollution and potential health problems created by increased breathing of an anesthetic agent. Specific gas analyzers are very useful. However, only some mass spectrometers have agent specificity. Most commercial monitors, including infrared techniques, cannot differentiate between specific anesthetic gases. However, they can be useful in verifying vaporizer performance when the identity of the exact agent in use is known.

B. *Patient Breathing Circuit: Design, Problems, Checkout*

The patient breathing circuit is the conduit through which anesthetic and respiratory gases flow to and from the patient. There are numerous variations of both adult and pediatric circuits. Each has presented problems to the user. A complete discussion of the advantages and disadvantages of alternating circuit design is beyond the scope of this chapter. The majority of remarks will be directed to the most common adult circuit, the semiclosed circle absorber system (see Fig. 1–2).

The semiclosed circuit is a closed loop of large-bore, low-pressure tubing divided into an inspiratory and expiratory limb. Contained within this loop are two unit directional valves, a carbon dioxide absorber, circuit gas venting (scavenging), a humidifier, an adjustable-pressure limiting (APL valve, also referred to as the pop-off, relief, or overflow valve), a reservoir bag, and airway management equipment, including masks and ET tubes.

In this circuit, fresh gas is introduced proximal to a unidirectional inspiratory breathing valve and allowed to accumulate in the carbon dioxide absorber as well as either the reservoir bag or ventilator bellows. During inspiration, gas moves through the absorber from either the reservoir bag or ventilator bellows and inspiratory valve into the inspiratory limb of the circuit. The pressure difference between the inspiratory and expiratory limbs keeps the unidirectional exhalation valve closed. During exhalation, the pressure differential reverses. The inspiratory valve closes and the expiratory valve opens, allowing the exhaled gas to travel into the reservoir bag or ventilator bellows and absorber. The APL valve enables the user to control the circuit volume and pressure by regulating gas venting from the circuit. Circuit exhaust is either carried into the room or collected by a gas-scavenging system.

Anesthesia circuits currently contain one or more valves of various designs. These include unidirectional breathing valves and the APL valve. Problems with valves have resulted from missing, dirty, and malfunctioning components; leaking seals; broken, leaking, and dirty valve covers; and improper valve seating.[11,14,25]

There are numerous designs for the unidirectional breathing valves. The disk valve is the most common in current systems. This valve consists of only one movable part, a flat disk. The disk is made of plastic or metal and is held against the valve seat by gravity or a mechanical spring.

The typical APL valve is designed to regulate circuit pressures by manually adjusting the spring tension against a disk. When circuit pressure overcomes the valve resistance, the disk is lifted from its seat and gas is allowed to exhaust from the circuit. The user must continually observe the circuit volume and pressure throughout the delivery of anesthesia so that the APL valve can be adjusted appropriately. Performance of the APL valve is checked when looking for leaks in both the machine and breathing circuit.

The absorber contains a carbon dioxide absorbent that removes carbon dioxide. Because of its simple design, few problems arise. Most problems have resulted from absorbent dust contamination of the breathing circuit, canister leaks, inappropriate bypass valving, and lack of indicator dye for spent material.[11,25] The two major problems with the carbon dioxide absorber are expended soda lime absorbent in the canister and leaks.

Numerous problems have arisen with the tubing and breathing bags. Most incidents with breathing tubes have occurred with the Bain circuit[25] and result from avulsion of the inner tube from the machine end of the circuit. Pinhole leaks have also been reported.

The reservoir or breathing bag is very compliant, with an easily expanded volume. It allows accumulation of gas during exhalation, so that a reservoir is available for the next inspiration; provides a means for visually monitoring the spontaneous breathing pattern of the patient; buffers breathing circuit pressure increases; and provides a means that can be used to ventilate the apneic patient manually.

Few problems have arisen from the tubing and breathing reservoirs used in the semiclosed circuits. Bags containing numerous holes and failed exhaust stopcocks have caused the most frequently repeated mishaps.[25]

There have been numerous investigations to determine the effects of chronic anesthetic gas exposure on congenital birth defects and the carcinogenicity of these agents. Although the data are inconclusive, sufficient information exists from some animal studies to suggest that chronic exposure to these agents may create undesired effects. Current National Institute of Occupational Safety and Health (NIOSH) guidelines for the operating room environment recommend a time average exposure of less than 25 parts per million (ppm) nitrous oxide and 2 ppm volatile anesthetics. Hence, a need for waste-gas scavenging has developed.

Either passive or active scavenging (venting) systems are used in removing circuit exhaust. In passive scavenging, anesthetic waste gases are vented directly into the existing room ventilation system. The scavenging tubing connects the exhaust port of the breathing circuit to the hospital system. In active methods, the anesthetic circuit connects directly to a high-flow vacuum system via an appropriate interface. In active methods, the tubing connects either the ventilator or the APL valve exhaust port of the breathing circuit to the hospital vacuum system. In either situation, common hazards exist. Obstruction of the connecting exhaust tubing is one of the most common. Obstruction results in overpressurization of the circuit.[25] However, a dangerous hazard also results from malfunction of the active system entrainment (vacuum relief) valve, which can produce a vacuum in the breathing circuit.[25]

Humidification of the breathing gas has long been widely accepted. However, not until the introduction of improved humidifier designs and fiber-packed cartridges has serious consideration been given to routine humidification. Mechanical humidifiers employ a number of heat exchanger–evaporator design techniques. Most commonly, these include either heated tubes or plates performing as thin-film evaporators submerged in sterile water and normal saline. In the humidifier, the breathing gas is heated and humidified.

Mechanical and structure failures cause the greatest number of malfunctions in humidifiers.[34] These include connector failures, disconnections, reverse connections, thermal hazards of overheating, electrical problems, and contaminants. Problems with fiber-cartridge designs include gas leaks and the potential for increasing airway resistance.

Although simple in design, breathing circuits are fraught with problems, the greatest being the potential for disconnection at any of the several locations. Numerous investigators have shown that 10% to 15% of preventable mishaps result directly from airway leaks and disconnections.[4,35,36] Causes of leaks and disconnections include poor fit resulting from incorrect size, incorrectly shaped taper, wrong materials, thermal expansion, broken fitting, and absence of a locking device. In addition, lack of standardization and quality control has plagued equipment design and implementation. Appropriate selection of materials is also essential.

The preuse check of the patient breathing circuit is designed to verify both the integrity and function of the circuit. This check is performed in several steps (steps 13, 15, 16, and 17, FDA procedure; see the appendix). First, the various components of the breathing circuit should be inspected visually. This step helps to verify the flow, logic, integrity, and continuity of the breathing circuit. Lack of integrity results in leaks in the circuit ranging from a few hundred milliliters per minute to several liters per minute. One of the most important verifications that the user can make is to assess and test the integrity of the anesthetic delivery system for leaks and particularly the patient breathing circuit. This is accomplished (step 16, FDA procedure; see the appendix) by first closing the APL and sealing the circuit at the patient end, where the mask or ET tube connect (Fig. 1–9). Next, fill the system with oxygen via the oxygen flush valve until the reservoir bag is full, but with a negligible pressure in the system. Now set the oxygen flowmeter to 5 L/min by turning the needle valve and observing the float. Allow the system to pressurize to 20 cm H_2O as indicated by the circuit pressure gauge. Slowly decrease the oxygen flow until pressure no longer rises above approximately 20 cm H_2O. The flow rate necessary to maintain a circuit pressure of 20 cm H_2O approximates the total leak rate. The leak rate should be no greater than a few hundred milliliters per minute for a semiclosed system. Of course, it is much less when using a closed-circuit technique.

One word of caution should be given for those systems having check valves in the inlet gas circuit inside the machine. In such machines check valves make it imperative to measure flow accurately in this step when the pressure just stops rising.

The next step is to squeeze the bag to a pressure of approximately 50 cm of H_2O and verify that the system is tight. If the user is unable to maintain pressure in the system, either find the source of the leak or remove the machine from service until the correction is made. Do not proceed when a significant leak is present!

During the preuse check for leaks, the exhaust valve (APL) and scavenger system performance can also be assessed (step 17, FDA procedure; see the appendix). First, visually inspect the scavenger system and be sure the necessary hoses and bag are attached (Fig. 1–10). It may be necessary to refer to the manufacturer's manual. Next, open the APL valve in a pressurized circuit and observe the release of circuit pressure. This should occur

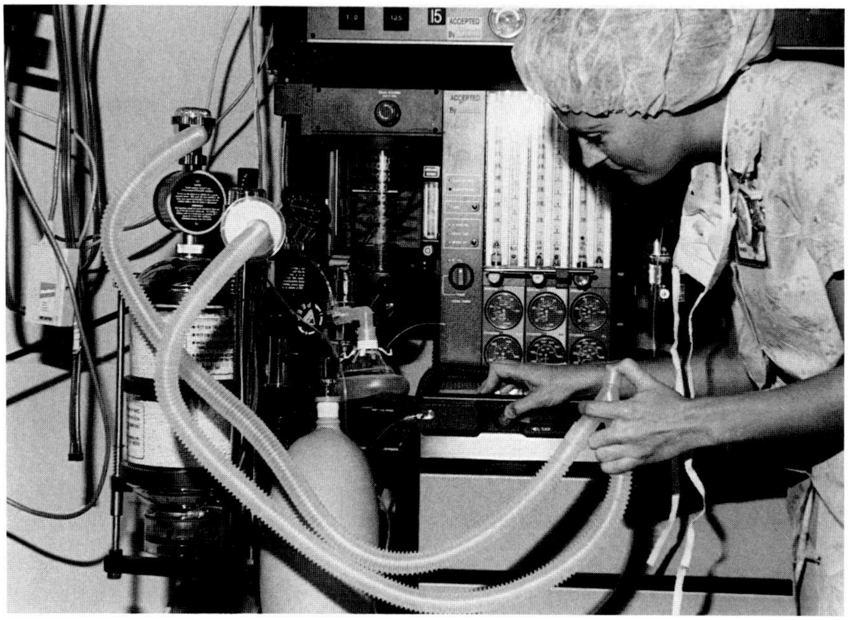

Figure 1–9 • Test the system for leaks by first closing the adjustable-pressure limiting (APL) valve, occlude the circuit at the patient end, and fill the circuit to at least 20 cm H_2O by opening (pressing) the oxygen flush valve.

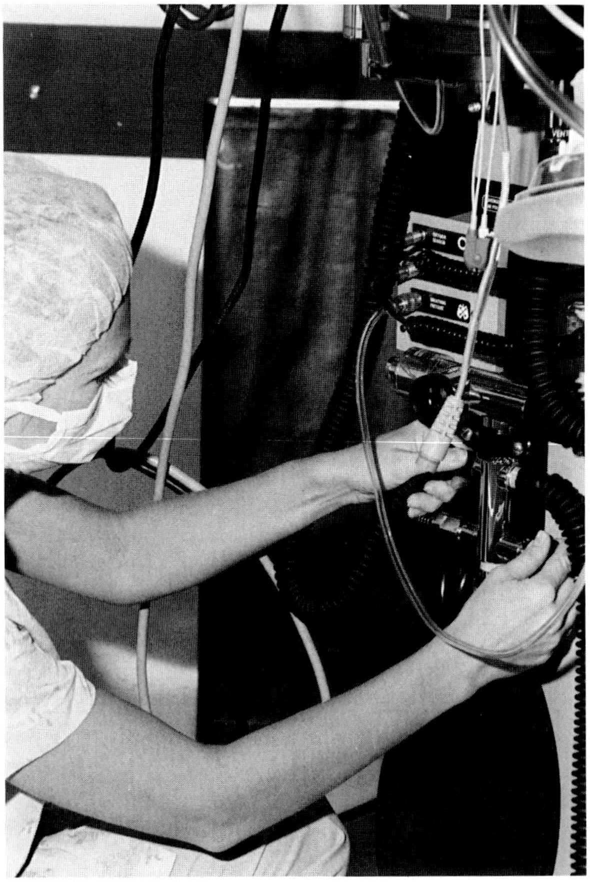

Figure 1–10 • Visual inspection of the scavenger system is essential.

immediately. Any occlusion in the exhaust system will maintain a constant pressure in the circuit. Occlude the breathing system at the patient end and verify that either a negligible positive or negative pressure appears with either a zero or 5-L/min flow and be sure that the exhaust relief valve opens (if present) with flush flow. In the active type of system that uses high vacuum, care must be used to insure that the entrainment reservoir bag operates between half-full to collapsed during each full breathing cycle. This is usually accomplished by adjusting a needle valve at the scavenger manifold located on the machine. This enables the user to assess if the scavenging system is working appropriately.

The function of the unidirectional valves (step 15, FDA procedure; see the appendix) can be carried out by one of two methods. Some individuals recommend inhaling and exhaling through a surgical mask into the breathing system (Fig. 1–11). This enables the user to assess each limb individually for unidirectional flow and to check for any resistance to breathing. Others prefer to pressurize the system by closing the APL valve and sealing the circuit at the patient end at the mask connector to stop all flow exiting the system. By inflating the reservoir bag and squeezing it, the breathing valves will move and the function can be checked (Fig. 1–12). The advantage of breathing into the circuit is that it gives the user an indication of any excessive resistance, which might not be detected by the second method. As a fur-

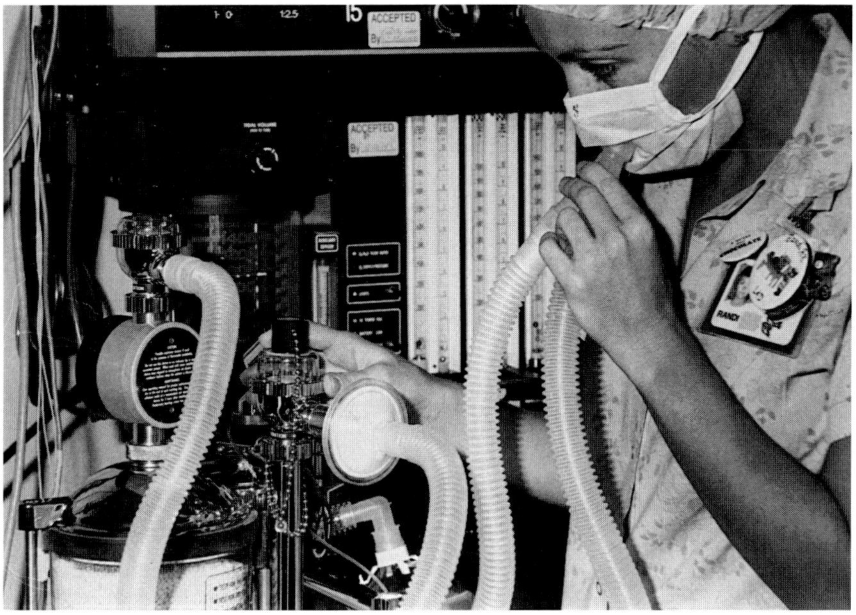

Figure 1–11 • Breathing in the circuit enables the user to assess unidirectional breathing valve function and any breathing circuit resistance that is present.

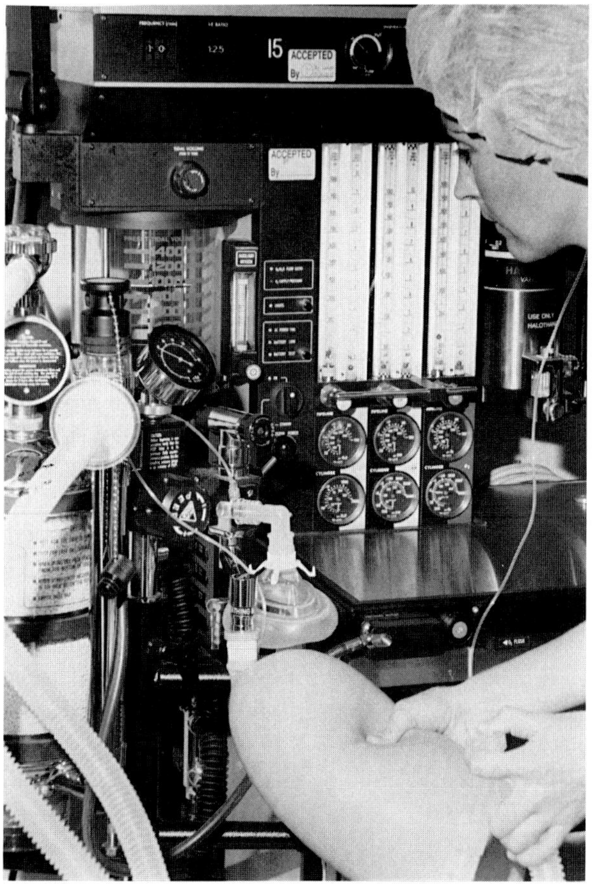

Figure 1–12 • Function of the breathing valves in the patient breathing circuit can be checked by closing the APL valve, occluding the patient connection, pressurizing the circuit, and squeezing the bag.

ther safety consideration, some recommend that a second pressure leak and breathing test be done just prior to the induction of anesthesia to insure no system changes.

Preuse check of the carbon dioxide absorber, humidifier, and airway management equipment begin with visual inspection. For the absorber, be sure that no visible cracks exist in the containers and that the material in the canister has not been used completely (indicated by the amount of colored indicator present). Be certain that the humidifier is attached correctly, has an appropriate amount of water in it, and has the temperature control properly set. Leak testing and function assessment of the breathing circuit must be done with both carbon dioxide absorber and humidifier in the circuit prior to induction of anesthesia. Check the airway equipment for size and function (see Chapters 5–13).

C. *Ventilators: Design, Problems, Checkout*

Ventilators have become an integral part of anesthetic delivery systems. There are two designs for integrating the ventilator into anesthesia delivery.[6,37] In the first design, commonly used in the United States, the ventilator is considered an accessory to the machine. This simplifies the design of the delivery system and enables the easy incorporation of a low-flow closed-circuit technique with rebreathing of gases. In this design, the ventilator either is located within the mainframe of the anesthesia machine or is a free-standing accessory unit awkwardly attached to the machine. In either case, the outlet of the ventilator attaches directly to the patient breathing circuit of the anesthetic delivery system in place of the breathing reservoir bag. In this design a mechanical ventilator functions as a controller for both ventilation and circuit gas volumes by replacing the functions of the reservoir bag and APL valve.

The second design is more popular in Europe.[6,37] The anesthesia system is built around the ventilator. This approach may complicate machine design, with more emphasis on high-flow than on low-flow delivery.

A mechanical ventilator provides a positive force for transporting respiratory and anesthetic gases into a patient. Currently designed ventilators provide positive pressure ventilation at a controlled minute volume (tidal volume times rate). Operational control is accomplished either electronically or mechanically with fluidic–pneumatic systems.

Most ventilators have a bellows contained within another housing. The bellows communicates directly with the breathing circuit and causes a preselected volume of gas (tidal volume) to flow into the patient via the circuit. The flow of gas into the circuit results from collapsing the ventilator bellows bag by pressurizing the surrounding gas volume contained within the bellows housing but outside the bellows.

Some ventilators function with the bellows rising during inspiration and falling with gravity when filling during exhalation. This design poses a significant hazard. During the filling cycle (expiration), the descending bellows will continue to fill even in the event of a circuit leak such as a patient disconnection.[38] Since this ventilator cycles regardless of the magnitude of the leak, the end result may range from mild hypoventilation with dilution of the breathing gas to complete inability to ventilate the patient.[14]

In newer designs, the ventilator bellows functions in reverse. The bellows rises during exhalation and falls during inhalation. For this type of operation, an added safety feature for detecting circuit leaks and particularly complete patient disconnections is inherently present. If there is any sizable leak in the patient breathing circuit, the bellows will not completely fill during exhalation and therefore breathing gas cannot be delivered during inspiration. Hence, the problem is easily detected and corrected.

The ventilator attaches to the patient breathing circuit at the location of the reservoir bag. In machines of earlier design, the process of switching from bag to ventilator requires at least four steps: the bag is removed, the ventilator is turned on, the delivery hose is attached to the circuit in place of the bag, and the APL valve is closed. Failure to perform one or more of these steps often results in a misconnection, leading to a catastrophic event.[38] The most common incident results from underinflation because of failure of the APL valve to close.

Other problems include leaking bellows, resulting in dilution of gas concentrations, and faulty pressure relief valves, resulting in overpressurization. The disconnection of component parts also accounts for numerous mishaps.[27]

Several hazards and deficits of ventilators have been addressed in newer designs. Ventilators are being integrated into the anesthesia machines, reducing the potential for misconnection. The ventilator delivery hose is attached permanently to the patient circuit via a two-way valve. This valve connects either the ventilator or the APL valve and reservoir bag to the patient circuit at any one time. In most of the newer designs, selection of the ventilator automatically isolates the APL valve and reservoir bag from the circuit.

The operator knobs on anesthesia ventilators should clearly indicate the physiologic parameters they influence, such as tidal volume, ventilation rate, and minute ventilation (see Chapters 6 and 14). In many current models, however, more esoteric parameters, such as inspiratory flow, inspiratory time, and expiratory pause, are also controlled by knobs (see Chapters 6 and 14). Although these directly control device function, they must be combined and manipulated to reach the desired integrated output function.

New ventilator designs have incorporated both safety and functional considerations. Control is simpler and easier to accomplish. Safety has been improved with the "rising bellows" during exhalation and the incorporation of alarm systems.

Because of the importance of the ventilator and its attachment to the circuit, appropriate preuse performance must be conducted not only to test the ventilator (step 18, FDA procedure; see the appendix), but also to test the valving arrangement that attaches the ventilator to the circuit. If the switching valve is present, test each function in both bag and ventilator mode. To accomplish this, close the APL valve and, if necessary, occlude the system at the patient end. Test for leaks and pressure relief by appropriate cycling (the exact procedure will vary with the type of ventilator). To initiate this, attach the reservoir bag at the patient end of the breathing circuit and turn the selection valve to the ventilator mode. Now partially fill the breathing circuit and bellows via the oxygen flush valve. Cycle the ventilator and assure appropriate filling and emptying of both the reservoir bag and bellows. Depending on ventilator design, the user may be required to squeeze the reservoir bag in order to fill the bellows; this simulates exhalation.

D. Instrumentation: Checkout

Newer machines have instrumentation, physically integrated into the machine cabinet, that monitors the anesthetic delivery system. These instruments are used to assess system function continually during anesthesia delivery.

Since most new anesthesia delivery systems physically integrate monitors and alarms into the main frames of the anesthesia machine, it is essential that their function be properly assessed (see also Chapter 3). Each machine uses instrumentation that is supplied by the particular manufacturer. Hence, the appropriate manuals that accompany the machines and instruments should be reviewed. However, several principles apply in general.

As previously discussed, by turning on the master switch of the anesthesia machine, the user activates both the flow of gases and the electrical components. Prior to turning on the switch, the user should visually inspect the electrical circuitry for frayed cords to insure that the electrical power is coming from an appropriate outlet. This includes checking that the line isolation monitor light has not switched from green to red once the machine has been turned on. If so, have the machine ground circuits inspected by qualified individuals before proceeding.

Check, connect, and calibrate all electronic monitors, particularly the oxygen sensor and airway pressure and flow monitors. Inspect the final position of all the controls. The oxygen monitor should be calibrated early in the precheck procedure and used to verify the presence of oxygen (Fig. 1–13). To calibrate most oxygen monitors, turn the unit on and be sure the battery is functioning properly. Allow ample time for the monitor to come to a steady state. Place the sensor in room air and read 21%. Replace the oxygen monitor back into the breathing circuit, and fill and empty the system several times with 100% oxygen. Check that the oxygen monitor reading is nearly 100%. If not, adjust the appropriate calibration dial (present in each unit) until it indicates 99%. Place the sensor in room air and read 21%. Once this is accomplished, check both high and low alarms. Airway volume and pressure alarms can be verified during leak–pressure check of the circuit. Performance can be verified by turning the units on and adjusting the range switches.

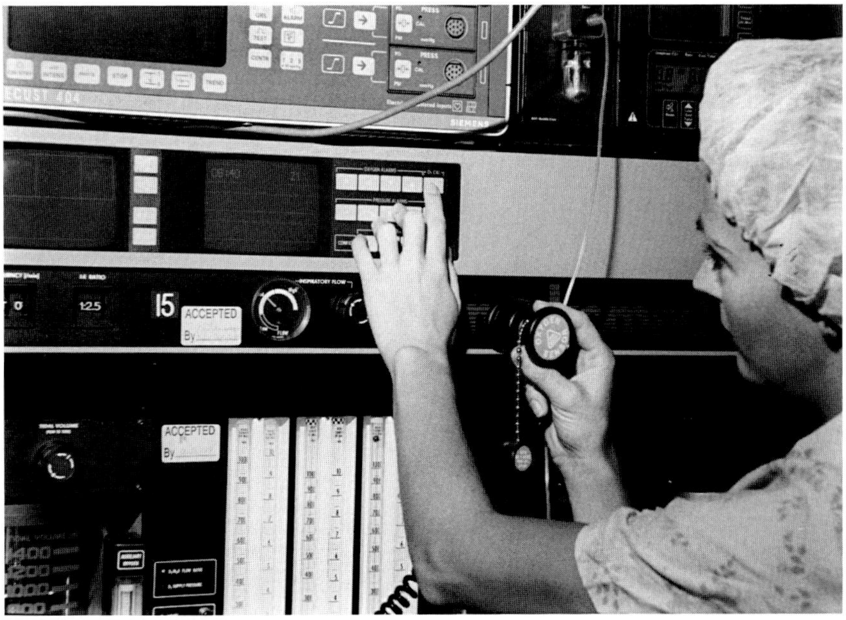

Figure 1–13 • Calibration of the oxygen sensor should occur prior to the preuse check so that it can be used to verify the presence of oxygen in the circuit.

III. Summary

Although quite simple and reliable, the design of today's anesthetic delivery system is still fraught with potential problems that can directly affect performance and patient safety. Thus, newer technologies are continually being sought and implemented to improve safety. Standards for design and function are being written and some have been recently adopted. However, this added safety and sophistication could increase complexity considerably. Therefore, the need to check the function of all equipment prior to induction of any anesthetic is all the greater. The individual must become thoroughly familiar with the design and operation of the anesthesia machine and ventilator being used. This is easily accomplished by reviewing the manuals and material provided by the manufacturer. Take time to learn and know the equipment! Take time to learn how to inspect and conduct a preuse check properly for each day and each case. Know what is required for preventive maintenance. The function and safety of the equipment are the user's responsibility.

IV. Appendix

A. *The FDA Anesthesia Apparatus Checkout Procedure*

In 1984, representatives of the anesthesia medical industry and the FDA met and investigated ways to reduce patient risk during anesthesia.[39] As a result of these meetings, the FDA was asked to take a leading role in the development and issuance of general guidelines for a preuse checkout of the anesthetic delivery system. The objectives of these guidelines were to promote a simple procedure and concept of routine preuse checkout. In addition, these guidelines provide fundamental techniques that could be modified by the user to fit his or her specific situation.

The result of this effort produced the recommended procedure given in this appendix. This procedure was developed as a result of these collaborative efforts. The initial draft was based on a checklist that has been developed over 10 years in the residency program in Massachusetts General Hospital. The resulting revised procedure was evaluated at several hospitals and by the three major manufacturers of anesthesia machines. It was then reviewed again by the FDA Advisory Panel on Anesthesiology and Respiratory Therapy Devices and their consultants. The resulting draft was subsequently published in the *Federal Register* of March 28, 1986.

The version that is given in this appendix is designed to provide a general preuse checkout and inspection procedure to be performed by the user once at the start of each day and in an abbreviated manner before each case. It is designed to insure that the machine, patient breathing circuit, ventilator, and essential safety monitors are correctly interconnected, adjusted, and functioning as expected.

Although this particular checkout has been recommended and issued by the FDA, it is *not* a federal regulation. The user is not legally obligated to follow it. Its sole purpose is for use as a guideline that should be modified as needed to allow for differences in equipment and clinical practice. However, it is suggested that if significant modifications are made, they should be reviewed, approved, and documented by peers as appropriate departmental policies.

Obviously, any modifications to the procedures should be made with close attention to information contained in any operator manuals. The recommendations that are published in this appendix do not relieve the user of the responsibility to be knowledgeable of any special procedures or precautions that are described in the operator manual supplied with the equipment.

B. *The FDA Anesthesia Apparatus Checkout Recommendations**

This checkout, or a reasonable equivalent, should be conducted before administering anesthesia. This is a guideline which users are encouraged to modify to accommodate differences in equipment design and variations in local clinical practice. Such local modifications should have appropriate peer review. Users should refer to the operator's manual for special procedures or precautions.†

*Reprinted from Carstensen P. FDA Issues pre-use checkout. Anesthesia Patient Safety Foundation Newsletter 1(3):13–20, 1986; with permission.

†If an anesthetist uses the same machine in successive cases, the steps marked with an asterisk (*) need not to be repeated or may be abbreviated after the initial checkout.

‡A vaporizer leak can only be detected if the vaporizer is turned on during this test. Even then, a relatively small but clinically significant leak may still be obscured.

1. *Inspect anesthesia machine for*: (*)
   machine identification number
   valid inspection sticker
   undamaged flowmeters, vaporizers, gauges, supply hoses
   complete, undamaged breathing system with adequate CO_2 absorbent
   correct mounting of cylinders in yokes
   presence of cylinder wrench
2. *Inspect and turn on*: (*)
   electrical equipment requiring warm-up.
   (ECG/pressure monitor, oxygen monitor, etc.)
3. *Connect waste gas scavenging system*: (*)
   adjust vacuum as required
4. *Check that*: (*)
   flow-control valves are off
   vaporizers are off
   vaporizers are filled (not overfilled)
   filler caps are sealed tightly
   CO_2 absorber by-pass (if any) is off
5. *Check oxygen (O_2) cylinder supplies*: (*)
   a. Disconnect pipeline supply (if connected) and return cylinder and pipeline pressure gauges to zero with oxygen flush valve.
   b. Open O_2 cylinder; check pressure; close cylinder and observe gauge for evidence of high pressure leak.
   c. With the O_2 flush valve, flush to empty piping.
   d. Repeat as in b. and c. above for second O_2 cylinder, if present.
   e. Replace any cylinder less than about 600 psi. At least one should be nearly full.
   f. Open less full cylinder.
6. *Turn on master switch (if present)*: (*)
7. *Check nitrous oxide (N_2O) and other gas cylinder supplies*: (*)
   Use same procedure as described in 5a. & b. above, but open and CLOSE flow-control valve to empty piping.
   Note: N_2O pressure below 745 psi. indicates that the cylinder is less than 1/4 full.
8. *Test flowmeters*: (*)
   a. Check that float is at bottom of tube with flow-control valves closed (or at min. O_2 flow if so equipped).
   b. Adjust flow of all gases through their full range and check for erratic movements of floats.
9. *Test ratio protection/warning system (if present)*: (*)
   Attempt to create hypoxic O_2/N_2O mixture, and verify correct change in gas flows and/or alarm.
10. *Test O_2pressure failure system*: (*)
   a. Set O_2 and other gas flows to mid-range.
   b. Close O_2 cylinder and flush to release 0_2 pressure.
   c. Verify that all flows fall to zero. Open O_2 cylinder.
   d. Close all other cylinders and bleed piping pressures.
   e. Close O_2 cylinder and bleed piping pressure.
   f. Close control valves.
11. *Test central pipeline gas supplies*: (*)
   a. Inspect supply hoses (should not be cracked or worn).
   b. Connect supply hoses, verifying correct color coding.
   c. Adjust all flows to at least mid-range.
   d. Verify that supply pressures hold (45–55 psi).
   e. Shut off flow-control valves.
12. *Add any accessory equipment to the breathing system*: (*)
   Add PEEP valve, humidifier, etc., if they might be used (if necessary remove after step 18 until needed).
13. *Calibrate O_2 monitor*: (*)
   a. Calibrate O_2 monitor to read 21% in room air.
   b. Test low alarm.
   c. Occlude breathing system at patient end; fill and empty system several times with 100% O_2.
   d. Check that monitor reading is nearly 100%.
14. *Sniff inspiratory gas*:
   There should be no odor.
15. *Check unidirectional valves*: (*)
   a. Inhale and exhale through a surgical mask into the breathing system (each limb individually, if possible).
   b. Verify unidirectional flow in each limb.
   c. Reconnect tubing firmly.
16. *Test for leaks in machine and breathing system*: (*)
   a. Close adjustable pressure limiting (APL) (pop-off) valve and occlude system at patient end.
   b. Fill system via O_2 flush until bag just full, but negligible pressure in system. Set O_2 flow to 5 L/min.
   c. Slowly decrease O_2 flow until pressure *no longer rises* above about 20 cm H_2O. This approximates total leak rate, which should be no greater than a few hundred mL/min. (less for closed-circuit techniques).
   CAUTION: Check valves in some machines make it imperative to measure flow in step c. above when pressure *just stops rising*.
   d. Squeeze bag to pressure of about 50 cm H_2O and verify that system is tight.
17. *Exhaust valve and scavenger system*:
   a. Open APL valve and observe release of pressure.
   b. Occlude breathing system at patient end and verify that negligible positive or negative pressure appears with either zero or 5 L/min. flow and exhaust relief valve (if present) opens with flush flow.
18. *Test ventilator*:
   a. If switching valve is present, test function in both bag and ventilator mode.
   b. Close APL valve if necessary and occlude system at patient end.

c. Test for leaks and pressure relief by appropriate cycling (exact procedure will vary with type of ventilator).
d. Attach reservoir bag at mask fitting, fill system and cycle ventilator. Assure filling/emptying of bag.

19. *Check for appropriate level of patient suction.*
20. *Check, connect, and calibrate other electronic monitors.*
21. *Check final position of all controls.*
22. *Turn on and set other appropriate alarms for equipment to be used.* (Perform next two steps as soon as is practical.)
23. *Set O_2 monitor alarm limits.*
24. *Set airway pressure and/or volume monitor alarm limits* (if adjustable).

V. References

1. Pierce, EC. Historical perspectives. In Pierce EC, Cooper JB (eds). Analysis of Anesthetic Mishaps. International Anesthesiology Clinics 22:2, 1–16. Boston, Little, Brown, 1984.
2. Herr GP. Anesthesia mishaps: Occurrence and prevention. In Katz RL (ed). Semin Anesth 1:1. , Grune & Stratton, 1983, 213–224.
3. Lunn JN, Mushin WW. Mortality Associated with Anaesthesia. London, Nuffield Provincial Hospitals Trust Publishers, 1982.
4. Cooper JB, Newbower RS, Kitz RJ. An analysis of major errors and equipment failures in anesthesia management: Considerations for prevention and detection. Anesthesiology 60:34–42, 1984.
5. Spooner RB, Kirby RR. Equipment-related anesthetic incidents. In Pierce EC, Cooper JB (eds). Analysis of Anesthetic Mishaps. International Anesthesiology Clinics 22:2. Boston, Little, Brown, 1984, 133–147.
6. Calkins JM. Monitoring the anesthetic delivery system. In Blitt CD (ed). Monitoring in Anesthetic and Critical Care Medicine. New York, Churchill-Livingstone, 1984.
7. Saunders RJ, Jewett WR. System integration: The need in future anesthesia delivery systems. Med Instrum 17(6):389–393, 1983.
8. Waterson CK. The anesthesia machine: Current design and alternatives. Med Instrum 17:379–382, 1983.
9. Dorsh JA, Dorsh SE. Understanding Anesthesia Equipment: Construction, Care and Complications. Baltimore, Williams & Wilkins, 1975.
10. Pelton DA. Noninflammable medical gas pipeline systems. In Wyant GM (ed). Mechanical Misadventures in Anesthesia. Toronto, University of Toronto Press, 1978, 8–19.
11. Rendell-Baker L. Problems with anesthetic gas machines and their solutions. In Rendell-Baker L (ed). Problems with Anesthetic and Respiratory Therapy Equipment. Int Anesthesiol Clin 20:3. Boston, Little, Brown, 1982, 1–82.
12. Sprague DH, Archer GW. Intraoperative hypoxia from an erroneously filled liquid oxygen reservoir. Anesthesiology 42:360–362, 1975.
13. Thorp JM, Railton R. Hypoxia due to air in the oxygen pipeline: A case for oxygen monitoring in theatre. Anaesthesia 37:683–687, 1982.
14. Weitzner SW. Equipment hazards: Malfunction and misuse. Semin Anesth 2:205–212, 1983.
15. Feeley TW, Hedley-Whyte J. Bulk oxygen and nitrous oxide delivery systems: Dangers and designs. Anesthesiology 44:301–305, 1976.
16. N_2O asphyxia. Editorial. Lancet 1:845, 1974.
17. Spurring PW, Shenolika BK. Hazards in anaesthetic equipment. Br J Anaesth 50:641, 1978.
18. Finlay J, Pelton DA. Needed: Error protection in hospitals. JAMA 45:64–66, 1971.
19. Feeley TW, McClelland KJ, Malhotra IV. The hazards of bulk oxygen delivery systems. Lancet 1:1416–1418, 1975.
20. Rendell-Baker L. Standards for anesthesia: The issues. In Brown BR (ed). Future Anesthesia Delivery. Contemp Anesth Pract 8:59–86, 1984.
21. Feeley TW, Bancroft ML, Brooks RA, et al. Potential hazards of compressed gas cylinders: A review. Anesthesiology 48:72–74, 1978.
22. Dinnick OP. More problems with piped gases. Anaesthesia 31:79–792, 1976.
23. Davenport HT, Wright BM. Simple oxygen-failure safety device. Br Med J 3:570–571, 1974.
24. Calkins JM, Saunders RJ, Waterson CK. Gas and vapor delivery. In Brown BR (ed). Future Anesthesia Delivery. Contemp Anesth Pract 8:99–107, 1984.
25. Wyant GM. Mechanical Misadventures in Anesthesia. Toronto, University of Toronto Press, 1978.
26. Sadove MS, Thomason RD, Thomason CL, et al. An evaluation of flowmeters. Am Assoc Nurs Anesth J 44:162–165, 1976.
27. Saunders RJ, Calkins JM, Gooden TM. Accuracy in rotameters and linear flowmeters. Anesthesiology 55(suppl):116, 1981.
28. Freidman J, Lightstone PJ. The effect of high altitude on flowmeter performance. Anesthesiology 55(suppl):A117, 1981.
29. Eger EI II, Epstein RM. Hazards of anesthetic equipment. Anesthesiology 25:490–504, 1964.
30. Mulroy M, Ham J, Eger EI. Inflowing gas leak: A potential source of hypoxia. Anesthesiology 45:102–104, 1976.
31. Bjoraker DG. Inability to shut off a halothane vaporizer. Anesthesiology 50:53–54, 1979.
32. Shih A, Wen-Hsien W. Potential hazard in using halothane-specific vaporizers for isoflurane and vice versa. Anesthesiology 55(suppl):A115, 1981.
33. Wickett RE, Jenkins LC, Root LS. Downstream contamination of in-series vaporizers. Can Anaesth Soc J 21:114–116, 1974.
34. Bancroft ML. Problems with humidifiers. In Rendell-Baker L (ed). Problems with Anesthetic and Respiratory Therapy Equipment. Int Anesthesiol Clin 20:3. Boston, Little, Brown, 1982, 83–102.
35. Thomson DM. Simple estimation of leak rates and volumes in gas systems and anaesthetic machines. Lancet 2:1421–1422, 1973.
36. Ruben H, Johansen SH. Factors influencing gas loss through leaks in anaesthetic circuits. Acta Anaesthesiol Scand 11:291–295, 1967.
37. Otto CW. Anesthesia ventilators: Special requirements. In Brown BR (ed). Future Anesth Delivery. Contemp Anesth Pract 8:165–173, 1984.
38. Morse HN. When is an apparatus inherently dangerous? Med Electron Products 15:16–81, 1984.
39. Carstensen P. FDA Issues pre-use checkout. Anesthesia Patient Safety Foundation Newsletter 1(3):13–20, 1986.

Chapter 2

•

Edward A. Meathe, MS

Preparation of the Transducers and Pressure-Monitoring Systems

OUTLINE

I. Introduction

When the clinical situation indicates that the patient's intravascular pressure must be continuously monitored, a cannula is inserted into the appropriate vascular space and the pressure within this space is coupled hydraulically to a mechanical device that converts this pressure into an electrical signal. There are two pivotal elements in such a system, the pressure transducer and the electronic unit, which amplifies, processes, and displays the results. These are the topics of this chapter. Our discussion begins with the hydraulic system and concludes with the electronic processing and display unit. Errors made in the setup, calibration, or interpretation of the results of these systems can alter the perception of the patient's cardiovascular status and may alter patient care.

II. How to Prepare the Transducers and Pressure-Monitoring Systems

A. Transducer Operation

Figure 2–1 shows a schematic diagram of a typical pressure transducer. A flexible diaphragm separates the internal components from the fluid used to couple pressure in the vascular space to the transducer. While the external side of the flexible diaphragm is coupled to the vascular space, the interior of the transducer is maintained at atmospheric pressure by a small vent in the housing. When external pressure on the diaphragm exceeds atmospheric pressure, the diaphragm deforms inward. This motion is coupled via a push rod to a spring on which are mounted four resistive strain gauges. As the spring

Internal Components of a Generic Pressure Transducer

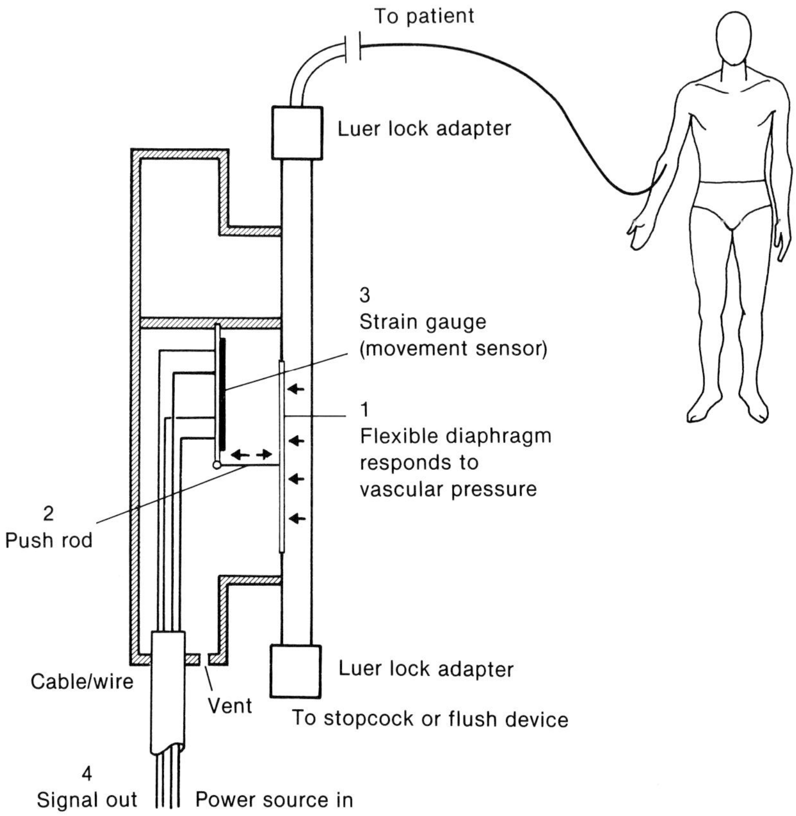

Figure 2–1 • A typical disposable pressure transducer. Vascular pressure is coupled from the patient to the flexible diaphragm of the transducer *(1)* via fluid-filled tubing. The back side of the diaphragm is exposed to atmospheric pressure through a vent in the transducer housing. Vascular pressures exceeding atmospheric pressure cause the diaphragm to deform inward. This motion is coupled via a push rod *(2)* to a set of strain gauges *(3)*. The strain gauges in turn are deformed by this motion, resulting in a change of their electrical resistance. By applying electrical power to the strain gauges the change in resistance can be converted to an electric signal *(4)* suitable for processing by the electronic monitoring system.

bends because of the motion of the push rod, the strain gauges are elongated or contracted; in the process, their resistance to electrical current changes. This change in electrical resistance is directly proportional to the pressure on the external side of the diaphragm.

Two concepts are important to the proper use of pressure transducers and the interpretation of the information obtained from them. First, the signal generated by the transducer is the result of a pressure difference (ie, the pressure on the external surface of the sensing diaphragm [the pressure to be measured] minus the internal pressure within the transducer [atmospheric pressure]). Second, the sensing diaphragm of the transducer is not usually located in the vascular space whose pressure is to be monitored. Instead, a short cannula or longer catheter, along with several feet of tubing and connecting stopcocks, is filled with fluid and used to couple the sensing diaphragm of the transducer to the vascular space. The inherent hydraulic characteristics of this cannula–tubing system often distort the pressure signal as it travels between the vascular space and the transducer, resulting in erroneous values of systolic pressure.

B. *Transducer and Hydraulic System Configuration*

Although it is possible to monitor vascular pressures with catheters in which a pressure transducer is an integral part of the catheter, economic factors generally prohibit their routine use. For the most part, invasive pressure monitoring is accomplished by connecting a discrete pressure transducer to the appropriate vascular space via a length of fluid-filled tubing and cannula or catheter. A typical configuration is shown in Fig. 2–2. The transducer may be designed to be disposable or reusable. Either transducer operates in the fashion described

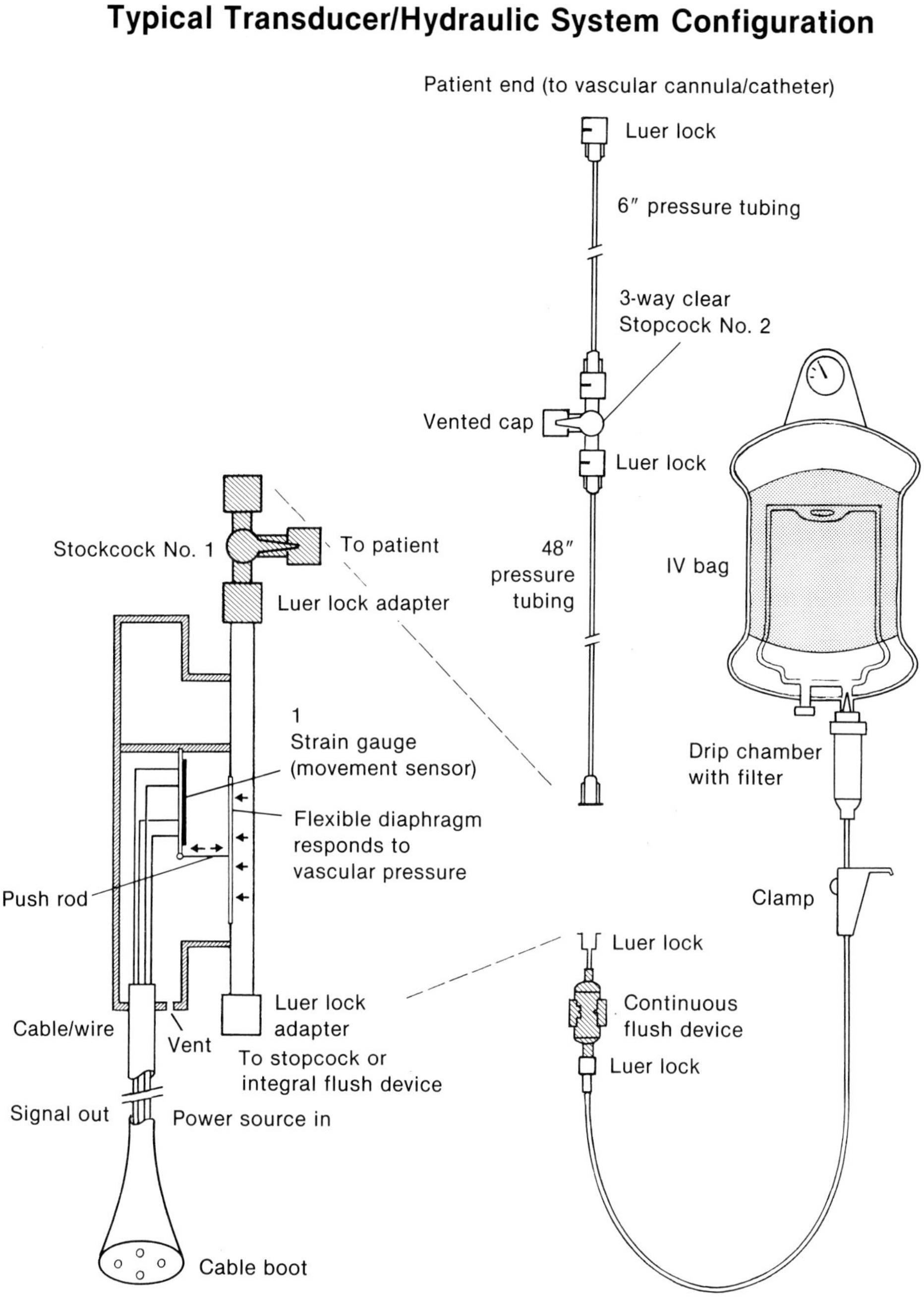

Figure 2–2 • Coupling of the vascular pressure to the transducer is accomplished using fluid-filled pressure tubing—the hydraulic system. The configuration shown here uses a 6-inch length of pressure tubing to connect to the invasive cannula/catheter; it is also used to secure the tubing to the patient. Stopcock No. 2 is used for drawing blood and flushing the hydraulic system. A 48-inch length of pressure tubing connects stopcock No. 2 and the pressure transducer via stopcock No. 1. This permits placing the transducer at a convenient location. Stopcock No. 1 is used to calibrate the system. The other port of the transducer is connected to a pressurized IV bag through a continuous-flush device (CFD). The CFD provides a constant flow of flush solution through the hydraulic system, thus maintaining its patency.

previously. Economy, sterility, and convenience are the factors that usually determine which type of device is selected.

The transducer–hydraulic configuration shown in Fig. 2–2 provides an economical, convenient, and reasonably accurate system for transducing vascular pressures. One port of the transducer is connected to a pressurized bag of heparinized (1–3 units/mL) flush solution via a continuous flush device (CFD). The flush solution is pressurized to a level well in excess of the systolic pressure. The CFD will maintain a continuous flow of flush solution through the transducer, tubing, and cannula of 1–3 mL/min. The CFD can also be activated manually to provide a rapid flush of the system. The other port of the transducer is connected to a Luer lock stopcock (No. 1), a 48-inch length of pressure tubing, another Luer lock stopcock (No. 2), a 6-inch length of pressure tubing, and then to the cannula or catheter. Stopcock No. 1 provides a convenient port for use in calibrating the monitoring system. The 48-inch length of pressure tubing represents a compromise between the ideal situation, from a monitoring accuracy point of view, of no tubing between the transducer and vascular space, and the practical need to locate the transducer such that it can be conveniently mounted and accessed for calibration. Stopcock No. 2 provides access to the vascular space for drawing blood, and in conjunction with stopcock No. 1 is used to flush air bubbles from the system. The 6-inch length of pressure tubing connects the cannula–catheter to the rest of the system and it can be used to secure the tubing in place. The cannula–catheter, tubing, stopcocks, and fluid path of the transducer compose the hydraulic element of the pressure-monitoring system.

Although the hydraulic coupling of the transducer to the vascular space provides an economic and convenient method of monitoring pressure, this very system also provides a mechanism by which the monitored pressure may be distorted significantly. The etiology of this distortion and methods to deal with it are discussed in a later section. However, the following rules should be applied when configuring a pressure-monitoring system to minimize the distortion.

1. The tubing (pressure tubing and catheter–cannula) should have as large an internal diameter as is practical.
2. The total length of all the tubing should be minimized. In practice, a total length of 4–5 feet provides a convenient and reasonably accurate hydraulic system.
3. When filling the hydraulic system with fluid, every effort should be made to remove all bubbles, no matter how small. A good procedure to follow is:
   a. Remove all air from the bag containing the flush solution before connecting it to the continuous flush device.
   b. Follow the transducer manufacturer's instructions for filling the transducer with fluid.
   c. Fill the pressure tubing with fluid. Connect a 12-mL syringe filled with flush solution to the proximal stopcock of the tubing system (stopcock No. 1 in Fig. 2–2). Connect a 3-mL syringe filled with flush solution to the distal stopcock of the system (stopcock No. 2 in Fig. 2–2). Then vigorously flush the solution between the two syringes. This will remove air bubbles from the tubing and stopcocks.

C. *System Calibration*

Regardless of the vascular pressure to be measured, the calibration scenario remains consistent. The first step is to establish a reference point for the pressure measurement. Since the pressure transducer senses the difference between vascular pressure and atmospheric pressure, we normalize the transducer output to atmospheric pressure. This procedure is commonly known as *zeroing* the system. It is accomplished by first configuring the transducer and hydraulic system as shown in Fig. 2–2. The transducer and tubing are then filled with flush solution, taking care to remove all air bubbles from the system. As illustrated in Fig. 2–3, one of the stopcocks in the hydraulic system, usually the one closest to the transducer, is placed at the level of the patient's right atrium. This can be accomplished by securing the transducer in a holder and attaching the holder to an IV pole. Using a carpenter's level, a yardstick with a bubble level attached, or simply careful visual observation, adjust the height of the stopcock to be used in zeroing the system to the level of the patient's right atrium. Open the stopcock such that the transducer's sensing diaphragm is exposed to atmospheric pressure and the path to the patient is occluded. Following the monitor manufacturer's instructions, adjust the zero control of the monitor so that the pressure indicated on the monitor is 0 mmHg (0 torr). The system is now zeroed. Whenever the patient's position is changed, the transducer must be repositioned so that the stopcock used to zero the system remains at the same level as the patient's right atrium.

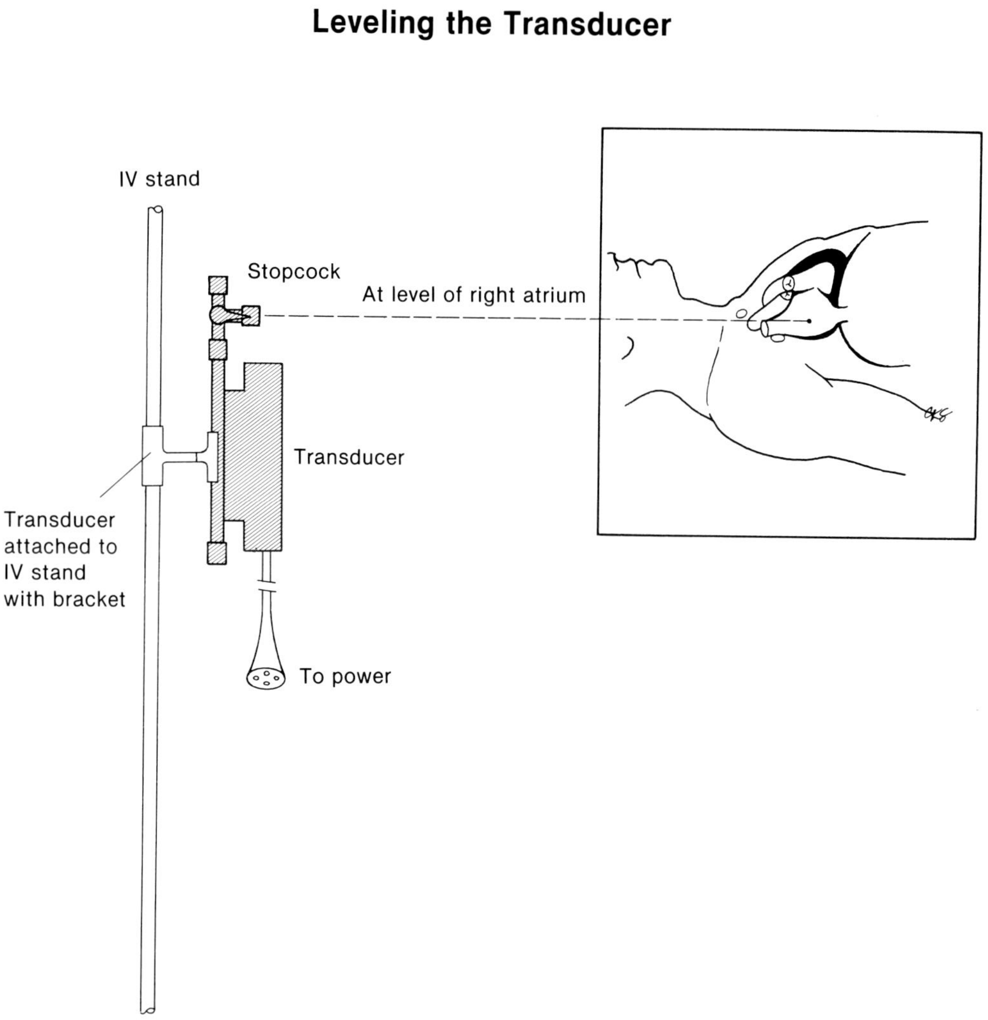

Figure 2–3 • Adjusting the height of the intravascular pressure monitoring transducer such that it is at the level of the patient's right atrium eliminates errors produced by the hydrostatic pressure of the fluid-filled hydraulic system. The stopcock used to "zero" the system should be placed at the level of the patient's right atrium.

The second step of the calibration process is to insure that the system responds accurately to a change in the input (vascular) pressure. This is sometimes referred to as calibrating the *span* or *gain* of the system. It is important to note that the "system" we refer to here begins at the transducer and terminates at the monitor's display of the results. That is, it includes all components of the monitoring system, not just the monitor. The best method for calibrating the gain of the system is to apply a known pressure to the transducer and then to insure that the monitor's display accurately reflects that pressure. This can be done using a standard mercury column manometer. Figure 2–4 shows a manometer adapted for this purpose. A four-way stopcock (stopcock No. 2) is placed on the distal end of the rubber hose connected to the manometer, and it is set so that all three ports are open. To the remaining male port connect a 6-foot length of pressure-monitoring tubing. On the female port, connect a three-way stopcock (stopcock No. 1) attached to a 12-mL syringe. When performing the gain calibration, connect a sterile stopcock (stopcock No. 3) to the distal end of the pressure tubing. Attach this stopcock to the open port of the stopcock used in the zero calibration of the hydraulic system. Again this stopcock should be adjusted such that the transducer will be exposed to the pressure in the mercury manome-

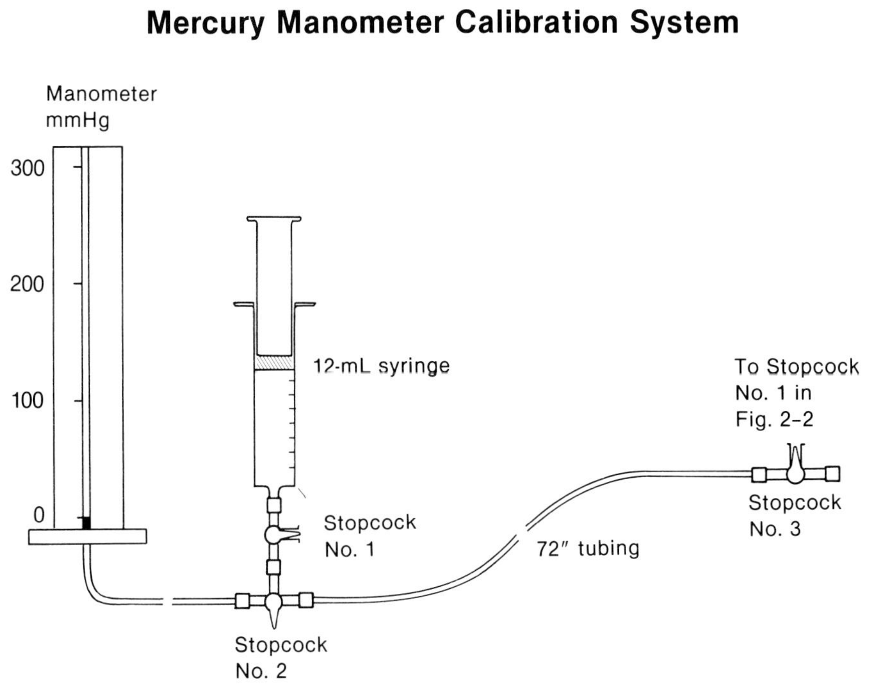

Figure 2–4 • System "gain" calibration can be accomplished using a mercury column manometer. The tubing from the manometer is connected to a four-way stopcock *(No. 2)*. Another port of stopcock No. 2 is connected to a three-way stopcock *(No. 1)*, and then to a 12-mL syringe. A 72-inch length of pressure tubing is connected between the remaining port of stopcock No. 2 and a sterile three-way stopcock *(No. 3)*. This stopcock, which is replaced prior to each calibration sequence, is connected to the stopcock used in calibrating the pressure monitoring system. Stopcock No. 2 is set such that all three ports are in communication with each other. Air is drawn into the syringe, stopcock No. 1 is adjusted such that the syringe is in communication with the manometer and transducer–hydraulic system, and then the syringe is used to pressurize the system. The electronic monitoring system should report the pressure indicated on the manometer.

ter, while the port to the patient is occluded. Occlude the IV tubing that connects the pressurized flush bag to the continuous flush device on the transducer. This will prevent the pressure in the flush bag from interfering with the gain calibration. Adjust stopcock No. 1 in Fig. 2–4 so that the syringe is open to the atmosphere. Fill the syringe with approximately 10 mL of air. Now rotate the lever on stopcock No. 1 so that the syringe is in communication with the mercury manometer and the pressure transducer. Depress the plunger of the syringe until the mercury column indicates an appropriate calibration pressure—200 mmHg when monitoring arterial pressures and 50 mmHg for venous pressures. Adjust stopcock No. 1 so that the syringe and open port are isolated from the transducer. The pressure indicated by the manometer should be stable. If it is decreasing, the system has a leak and should be examined for a loose connection. If it is rising, the cause is most likely that the continuous flush device is open and the pressure in the bag of flush solution is increasing the pressure in the transducer system. Clamp off the flush bag during the gain calibration. Once a stable pressure has been achieved within the transducer system, compare the pressure value displayed on the monitor to that of the mercury manometer. When the difference (error) exceeds 2% of the pressure indicated on the mercury manometer or ±2 mmHg, whichever is greater, then several options are available. If the monitor provides a gain adjustment, set the gain so that the value displayed on the monitor equals the value shown on the mercury manometer. When the monitor provides no gain adjustment, replacing the transducer may resolve the problem. If the transducer is replaced the entire calibration process should be repeated. If the preceding steps do not resolve the discrepancy, then the electronic monitor should be examined by the hospital's clinical engineering service or by the manufacturer.

Current transducers and electronic monitoring systems have gain characteristics that are very stable with regard to time and temperature. Therefore, the

Table 2–1 • Calibration Procedure for Invasive Pressure Transducer and Hydraulic Systems

1. Assemble the transducer, pressure tubing, stopcocks, and flush solution–hydraulic system.
2. Fill the hydraulic system with flush solution, taking care to eliminate all air bubbles.
3. Connect the electric cable of the transducer to the pressure input of the electronic monitor.
4. Place the stopcock to be used to zero the system at the height of the patient's right atrium. Perform the zero calibration following the directions provided by the manufacturer of the electronic monitor.
5. Using a mercury column manometer, perform a gain calibration on the system.

gain calibration is required only once per 8-hour shift in the Intensive Care Unit (ICU) or once for each intraoperative procedure. The calibration of the system's gain on a per-shift basis in the ICU enhances the quality control aspects of the pressure-monitoring process through personnel changes. The zero calibration should be performed during the initial system calibration process as well as about 30 minutes later. This will allow any temperature-induced drift in the transducer or monitor's zero reference point to be corrected. The zero calibration should be checked every few hours, or if the pressure reading on the monitoring system is in question. Whenever the position of the patient is changed, the transducer's height should be adjusted so that the stopcock used to perform the zero calibration is at the level of the patient's right atrium. The calibration procedure is summarized in Table 2–1.

III. DISCUSSION OF THE PROCEDURE

A. *System Components*

All pressure-monitoring systems consist of four components:

1. *Pressure transduction*—conversion of a pressure into an electrical signal.
2. *Pressure signal acquisition*—increasing the amplitude of the electrical signal produced by the transducer to a level suitable for processing.
3. *Pressure signal processing*—calibration of the incoming signal, filtering of the signal, and extraction of pertinent information (eg, systolic, mean, and diastolic pressures).
4. *Information display*—usually in the form of both digital (numeric) and analog (waveform) data.

Regardless of the manufacturer, the system used to monitor vascular pressures will implement components 1, 2, and 4 in a similar manner. However, the advent of the microprocessor has permitted more sophisticated techniques of information extraction to be applied to pressure monitoring. These techniques, or software algorithms, are often specifically designed to process pressure signals from particular vascular locations (eg, in the determination of systolic, mean, and diastolic pressures in the pulmonary artery). The more that the monitoring system automates functions formerly performed by the clinician, the more research and evaluation must go into the initial purchase of the monitoring system. The manufacturer should provide the results of unbiased clinical studies that assess the accuracy of the monitor's signal-processing algorithms. The user should have a clear and well-defined understanding of the clinical needs and standards regarding vascular pressure monitoring.

B. *Overestimation of Systolic Pressure*

Beside errors in system calibration, one of the most common technical problems associated with intravascular pressure monitoring is overestimation of the systolic pressure.[1] This is most often noted when monitoring the arterial pressure; however, it also occurs when monitoring intracardiac ventricular pressures or pressure in the pulmonary artery. An example of this overestimation of systolic pressure, also known as overshoot, is shown in Fig. 2–5. The solid tracing shows radial artery pressure as recorded using a catheter with a pressure transducer mounted at its distal end. This recording is therefore the actual intraarterial pressure. The dashed tracing shows the pressure waveform recorded using a transducer and hydraulic configuration as shown in Fig. 2–2. A 20-μL air bubble was inserted into the fluid path at stopcock No. 1. The significant comparisons to be made in this figure are that the systolic pressure as recorded with the external transducer is 30 mmHg greater than the systolic pressure recorded by the intraarterial transducer; the diastolic pressures recorded by each system are the same; and the mean pressures, although not noted on the recording, are identical.

This artifact in the pressure waveform is produced by the fluid-filled tubing and cannula–catheter. As stated earlier, for the transducer to create an electrical signal, its sensing diaphragm must be moved. The greater the

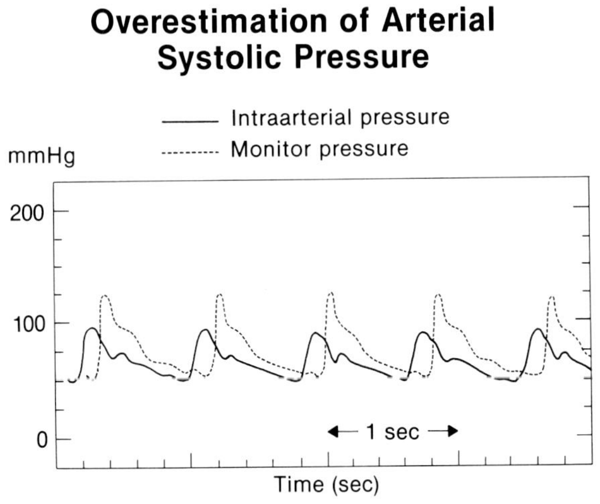

Figure 2–5 • Poor transducer–hydraulic system fidelity can result in the exaggeration of the rapidly changing parts of the vascular pressure waveform—the systolic rise. In the preceding example, the true intraarterial pressure, as measured by a transducer placed directly into the artery, is shown by the solid line (——). The dashed tracing (- - - -) shows the arterial pressure as it appeared on the electronic monitoring system using the transducer–hydraulic configuration shown in Fig. 2-2 with a 20-μL bubble inserted into the fluid path. The diastolic and mean pressures of the two signals are the same; however, the systolic pressure as monitored via the hydraulically coupled transducer is overestimated.

external pressure, the greater the movement, and hence the larger the output signal. For the vascular pressure to produce a deflection in the transducer's sensing diaphragm, the pressure must be coupled from the vascular space via the hydraulic system. Thus, to move the sensing diaphragm, the entire fluid column must also move; in so doing, it must overcome its own inertia, the compliance of the tubing and air bubbles, the resistance of the diaphragm, and the resistance offered by the tubing and stopcocks. For static pressures, the fluid column moves once and then reaches a new point of equilibrium, with the vascular pressure producing a steady-state deflection of the transducer's sensing diaphragm. However, for phasic pressures, pressures whose magnitude is changing rapidly (at the heart rate and faster), the fluid column must respond rapidly and fully to every change in the input pressure. For the moment, let us suppose that we can hold constant the magnitude of the input pressure change and only permit a variation in the rate at which the pressure changes. For slowly changing input pressures, from zero to several pressure cycles per second, a given change of input pressure produces the same deflection of the sensing diaphragm; thus, the monitoring system accurately reproduces the input signal. As the input pressure changes more rapidly, the resistance of the fluid column to movement decreases. Hence, the same input pressure change produces a greater deflection of the sensing diaphragm, and the pressure recorded by the monitor appears to be greater than the input pressure. This discrepancy between transduced and input pressures continues to increase as the rate of change of input pressure increases until it reaches a peak; then it begins to decrease as the rate of change of input pressure continues to increase.

Figure 2–6 illustrates the frequency response of an ideal transducer–hydraulic system, the system shown in Fig. 2–2, and the frequency response of that system with a small bubble in the fluid path. The vertical axis represents the ratio of the magnitude of the pressure pulse as monitored by the transducer–hydraulic system and the magnitude of the pressure pulse within the vascular space. The horizontal axis represents the sinusoidal rate of change (frequency) of the intravascular pressure. An ideal transducer–hydraulic system would exhibit a ratio of 1.0 for all frequencies of input pressure change; that is, the output pressure would always equal the input pressure regardless of the rate of input pressure change. However, our "real-world" systems exhibit a response that, over a range of input frequencies, amplifies the magnitude of the input signal. The optimal frequency response of the transducer–hydraulic system shown in Fig. 2–2 exhibits a peak at a frequency of approximately 20 cycles per second. This is the optimal frequency response because, given the type of transducer, the length of the fluid path (tubing), the diameter of the fluid path, and the absence of air bubbles, it is the best response obtainable for the system. The peak of the curve is called *resonance*, and the rate of change of input pressure at which it occurs is called the *resonant frequency*. The height of the peak, the magnitude of the difference between the input pressure and the transduced pressure, is related to a characteristic called *damping*; the greater the damping, the lower the resonant peak. The accuracy with which a transducer–hydraulic system responds to changing input pressures is called its *fidelity*. All these factors influence the accuracy of the intravascular pressure measurement.[2,3]

When a small air bubble is introduced into the fluid path, the fidelity of the system is reduced. Figure 2–6 shows the frequency response of the transducer–hydraulic system of Fig. 2–2 with a small (20-μL) bubble inserted into the fluid path. The bubble has lowered the resonant frequency and increased the damping of the sys-

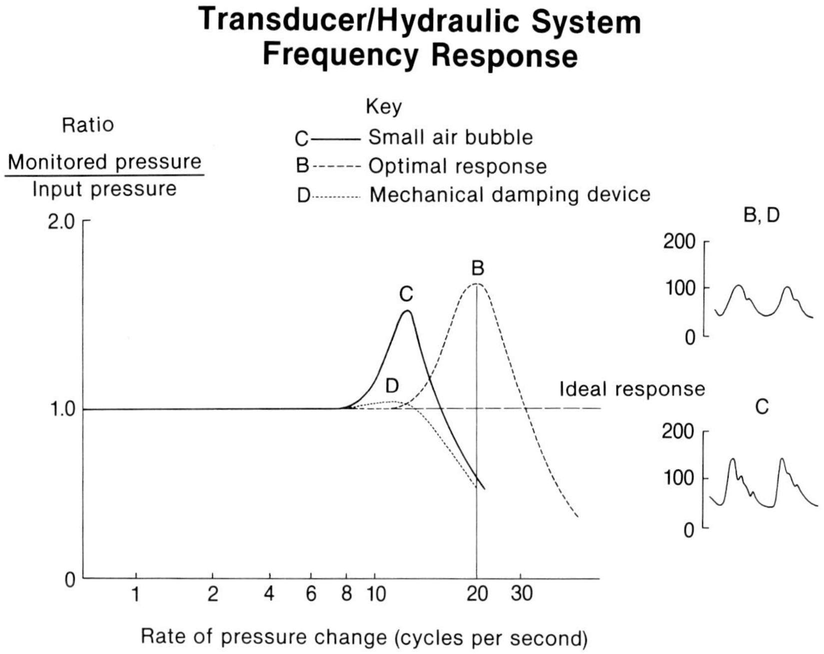

Figure 2–6 • The accuracy of a transducer–hydraulic system's reproduction of input pressure signals can be defined by its frequency response—the ratio of the pulse pressure displayed on the monitor to the input (intravascular) pulse pressure, where the input is sinusoidally varied through a spectrum of frequencies. The ideal response exhibits an output/input ratio of 1.0 for all frequencies. An optimally configured transducer–hydraulic system, such as that shown in Figure 2–2, exhibits a frequency response *(B)* with a resonant frequency of approximately 20 cycles per second. Adding a small bubble to this system produces a frequency response *(C)* with a decreased resonant frequency and increased damping. This system is less able to respond accurately to rapidly changing input pressure signals. The inclusion of a mechanical damping device in this system will selectively increase the damping *(D)*, thus enabling the system to respond more appropriately to the more rapidly changing components of the pressure wave. Significantly, the low-frequency, slow-changing portion of all these frequency responses is the ideal ratio of 1.0.

tem. In effect, it has made the system less able to respond accurately to the more rapidly changing components of the pressure waveform. Since the rapidly changing parts of an arterial pressure wave are located in the systolic rise, the segment between the diastolic pressure and the systolic pressure, this portion of the waveform will be exaggerated, leading to an overestimation of the systolic pressure.

Despite configuring a system that provides optimal fidelity considering the clinical situation, systolic pressures are often overestimated. This can occur because of small, undetected air bubbles within the hydraulic system or simply because the system, even when operating at optimum fidelity, cannot accurately reproduce the rapidly changing portions of a particular vascular pressure waveform. At this point further modification of the system configuration may not be practical. Nonetheless, a device is available that can minimize the waveform distortion. It is a mechanical damping device that, when inserted into the fluid path of the hydraulic system, selectively increases damping. This is accomplished either by placing an adjustable restriction in the fluid path or by inserting an air bubble in parallel with the fluid path.[4] The apparent contradiction between assembling an optimum hydraulic system by eliminating all air bubbles and resolving the problem of "overshoot" by including an air bubble is explained by the location and configuration of the air bubble. Air bubbles in the fluid path cause an increase in system damping and a decrease in the resonant frequency; thus, the system exhibits diminished fidelity. However, if an air bubble is connected to the fluid path via a narrow passage, the effect is to increase the damping without effectively altering the resonant frequency of the system. Such a device is shown in the hydraulic configuration illustrated in Fig. 2–7. Depending on the device selected, the restriction between the fluid path and air bubble may be fixed, thereby providing a fixed amount of compensa-

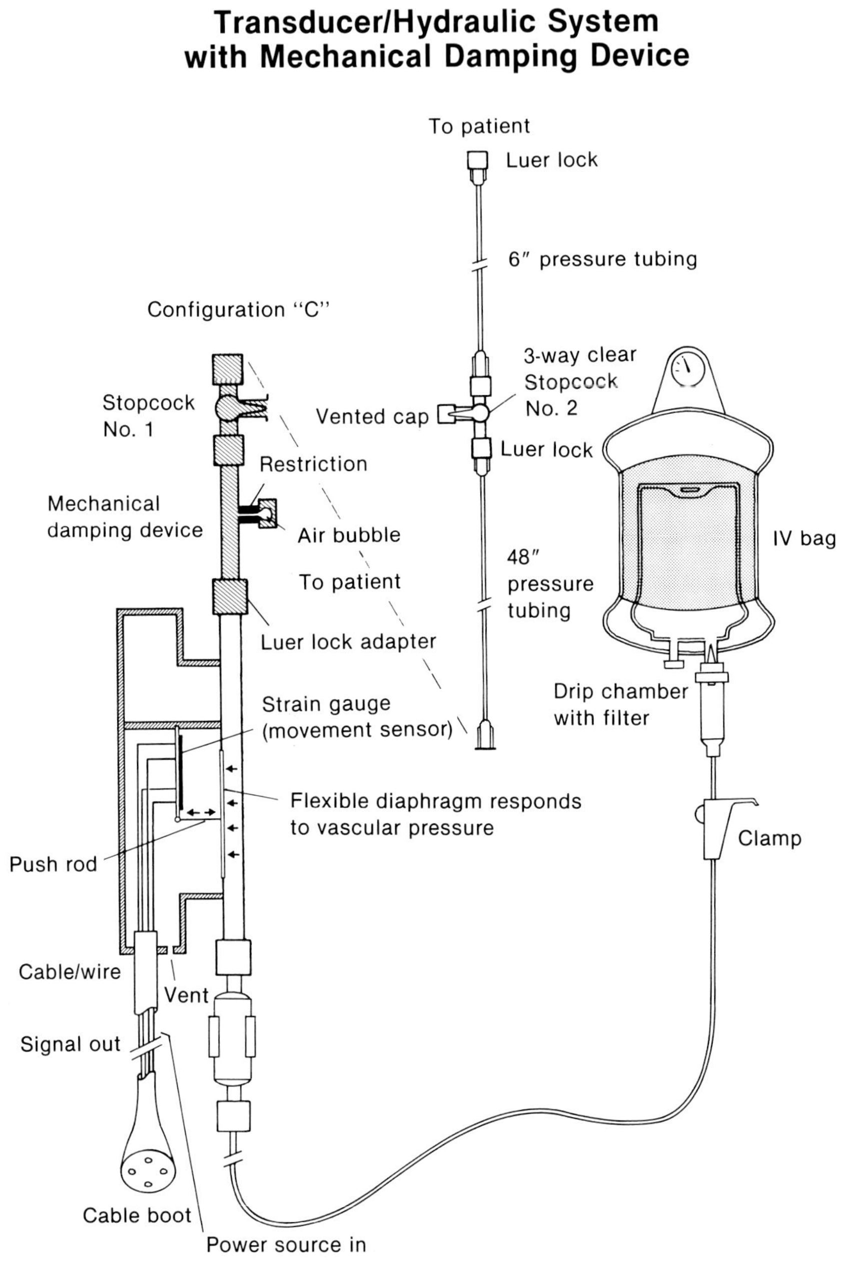

Figure 2–7 • A mechanical damping device can improve the frequency response of a transducer–hydraulic system, and thus the system's accuracy in reproducing the vascular pressure waveform. The device is inserted between the transducer and the monitoring line.

tion, or adjustable, thus allowing the user to alter the compensation. When such a device is inserted into the transducer system shown in Fig. 2–2, the resultant frequency response would be as shown in Fig. 2–6D. It is clear that a mechanical damping device can significantly improve the fidelity of hydraulically coupled pressure-monitoring systems, and hence the accuracy of systolic pressure measurements.

Two significant questions remain in the discussion of overshoot. First, how does the clinician know when overshoot is present? Second, when a mechanical damping device is used, how can the efficacy of the device be assessed? To answer each of these questions would require the direct measurement of vascular pressure (ie, measurement of pressure using a transducer placed directly into the vascular space). In most cases this is not economically or clinically practical. Any other method of measurement, whether indirect (auscultatory, oscillometric, etc) or via a transducer hydraulically coupled to the vascular space, presents its own peculiar sources of error. Bruner et al[5] compared direct (invasive catheter coupled hydraulically to a pressure transducer) and indirect methods of measuring arterial pressure and found little correlation between them. In practice, when assessing the accuracy of a pressure measurement, the clinician must establish his or her own reference measurement or "gold standard." This could be any of the noninvasive methods, either manual or automated, or the occlusion (pulse return) method. In the occlusion method, a pneumatic cuff is placed on the upper arm and inflated until pressure pulses obtained from a distal arterial line are abolished. The pressure in the cuff is slowly released while observing the pressure trace obtained from the arterial line. The pressure present in the cuff when the first pulsation is noticed in the arterial line trace is assumed to represent the systolic arterial pressure. Although any of the clinically practical methods for evaluating the accuracy of the invasive systolic pressure measurement are subject to error, the occlusion method appears to offer the most objectivity. Therefore, overshoot in an invasive arterial systolic pressure measurement can be detected by comparison to the systolic pressure determined by another clinically acceptable method. If significant overestimation of the systolic pressure, greater than 15 mmHg, is present, then insertion of a mechanical damping device into the hydraulic fluid path will reduce or eliminate the overshoot. The efficacy of this device may be evaluated by comparing the compensated intraarterial systolic pressure to the occlusion pressure. If the damping device is adjustable, its effect on systolic pressure may be titrated to the occlusion pressure.

In some cases the fidelity of the transducer–hydraulic system is so compromised that the ratio of monitored pressure to vascular pressure never exceeds 1.0, but it rapidly falls below 1.0 at frequencies above 0.5 cycles per second. An example of the waveform produced by such a system is shown in Fig. 2–8. The solid tracing represents the true intraarterial pressure; the dashed line depicts the arterial pressure as displayed on the monitoring system. Because of poor system fidelity the monitored pressure has had its rapidly changing components attenuated, producing a smooth, damped wave on the monitor. The systolic and diastolic pressures reported by the monitoring system will be lower and higher, respectively, than the actual intraarterial pressures. However, the mean pressure reported by the system will be correct. The cause of this type of compromise in fidelity is often due to clot formation at the tip of the cannula–catheter. It is usually resolved by a gentle flushing of the system. The efficacy of this maneuver can be assessed by observing the return of a "normal" pressure waveform.

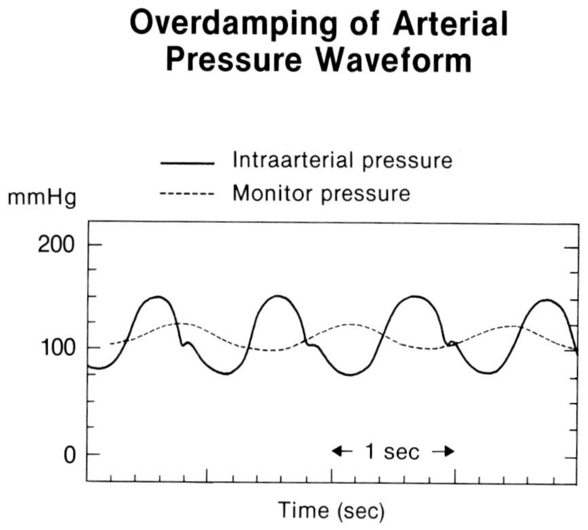

Figure 2–8 • An overdamped pressure waveform results in the underestimation of the systolic pressure and an overestimation of the diastolic pressure; however, the mean pressure is correct. The solid tracing (——) illustrates the true intraarterial pressure; the dashed tracing (- - - -) shows the results of an overdamped transducer–hydraulic system. Overdamping is usually the result of clot formation at the tip of the catheter/cannula.

In both the case of overshoot and overdamping the mean pressure measured by the monitoring system accurately reflects the intravascular mean pressure. Referring to Fig. 2–6, this is because the frequency response of all systems for an unchanging vascular pressure (0.0 cycles per second) is 1.0. This also explains why the normal calibration process will not identify systems prone to overshoot or overdamping. In systems that exhibit overshoot, the systolic pressure is overestimated, but the diastolic and mean pressures are accurate. This is predicted by the system's frequency response, since the ratio of monitored pressure to vascular pressure is 1.0 for unchanging and slowly changing input pressures. Diastolic pressure is the result of the slowly changing portion of the pressure waveform.

C. *Central Vascular Pressure Measurements*

When monitoring central vascular pressures such as central venous pressure (CVP), pulmonary artery pressure (PAP), pulmonary capillary wedge pressure (PCWP), or left atrial pressure (LAP), the measurement of interest is usually the transmural pressure—the pressure difference between the interior of the vascular compartment and the space surrounding the vessel or cardiac chamber. Vascular pressure measurements in the thoracic cavity are confounded by the effects of ventilation and the mechanics of pressure transduction.[6] A typical monitoring scenario is illustrated in Fig. 2–9. A catheter (Swan-Ganz) has been placed in the central circulation such that its distal port lies in a branch of the pulmonary artery. With the catheter's balloon deflated, the distal port couples the pressure in the pulmonary artery to the transducer. When the balloon is inflated, right-sided pressures are occluded and the distal port is coupled, via the pulmonary capillary bed, to the left atrium. The proximal port of the catheter lies in the right atrium and couples the CVP to another transducer.

The heart, its major vessels, and the lungs are enclosed within the thoracic cavity, bounded by the chest wall and diaphragm. The space surrounding these structures is the pleural space, and the pressure within this space the pleural pressure (P_{PL}). Therefore, to determine the transmural central vascular pressure we would have to monitor the difference between the pressure in the vascular compartment and the pleural pressure. For example, in the case of pulmonary artery pressure this would be:

$$PAP_{transmural} = P_{PA} - P_{PL}$$

However, as we concluded in the discussion of transducer operation, the transducer determines the difference between the pressure in the vascular compartment and atmospheric pressure:

$$PAP_{transducer} = P_{PA} - P_{ATM}$$

Monitoring Configuration for Central Vascular Pressure Determination

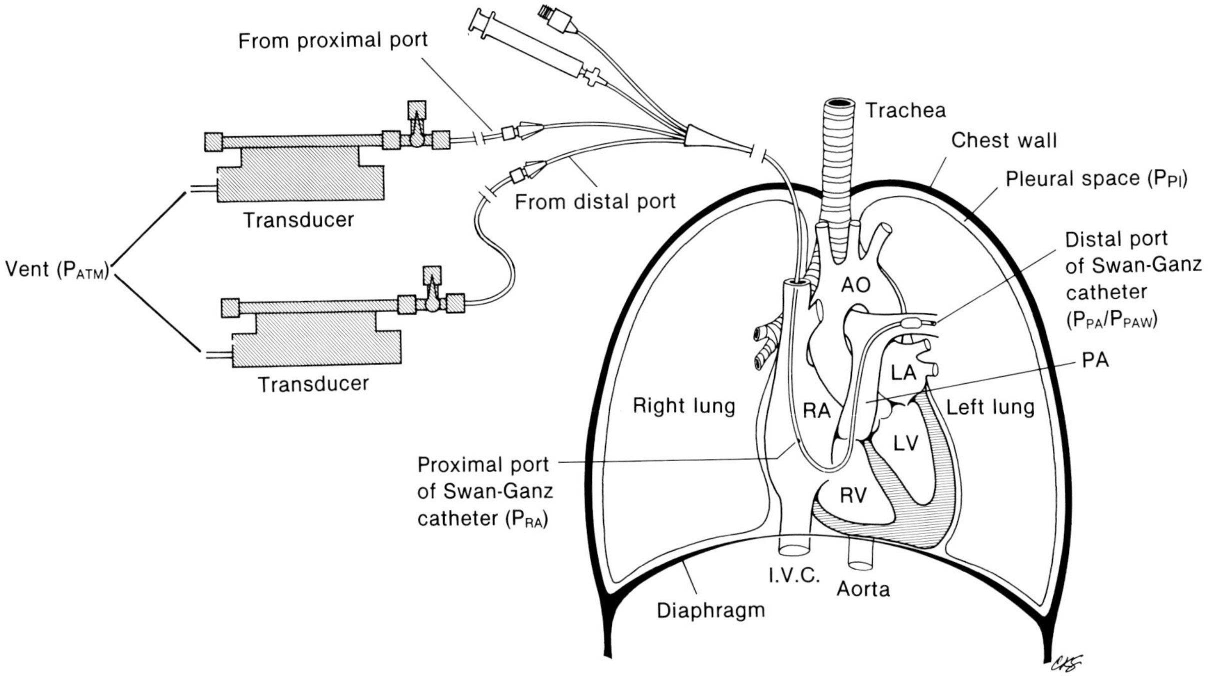

Figure 2–9 • Central vascular pressure determinations are confounded by factors other than the vascular pressures. This figure is a schematic representation of a typical monitoring scenario. A catheter has been placed such that its distal port lies in a branch of the pulmonary artery and its proximal port is within the right atrium. Both ports are connected to pressure transducers via a fluid column (catheter and pressure tubing). The transducers measure the difference between the vascular pressure (P_{PA}, PCWP, or P_{RA}) and atmospheric pressure (P_{ATM}). Pressure within the cardiac chambers and great vessels is also influenced by extramural pressures; that is, the pressure in the pleural space (P_{PL}). The determination of transmural vascular pressures requires that the measurement be made at a point in the ventilatory cycle when the effect of pleural pressure is minimized.

Therefore, for the pressure measured by the transducer to be equivalent to the transmural pressure, the pleural pressure (P_{PL}) must equal atmospheric pressure (P_{ATM}).

Pleural pressure is modulated by ventilation. During spontaneous inspiration the chest wall moves out and the diaphragm descends, creating a decrease in pleural pressure. Exhalation, a normally passive function, results in a return of the pleural pressure to its baseline value. At the end of exhalation, in the absence of continuous positive airway pressure (CPAP) or positive end-expiratory pressure (PEEP), the baseline value of pleural pressure is slightly below atmospheric pressure—approximately 2 cm H_2O less than atmospheric pressure in the supine patient. During a controlled, ventilator-driven inspiration, the lungs are expanded, producing a rise in pleural pressure and an expansion of the thoracic cavity. Exhalation during controlled ventilation follows the same pattern as during spontaneous breathing with the pleural pressure returning to a value slightly less than the atmospheric pressure at the end of exhalation.

The superior and inferior vena cava, right atrium, pulmonary artery, pulmonary veins, and left atrium are relatively thin-walled, compliant vessels and chambers. As such, they transmit external variations in pleural pressure to their interior, thereby modulating the intravascular pressure. An example is shown in Fig. 2–10. The top panel shows the pulmonary artery pressure monitored in a spontaneously breathing patient. With each inspiration the decrease in pleural pressure is coupled to the pulmonary vascular space, producing a transient decrease in mean pulmonary artery pressure. The bottom panel illustrates the response of the monitored pulmonary artery pressure to positive pressure controlled ventilation. With each ventilator-produced inspiration, pleural pressure rises, producing a concomitant rise in the mean pulmonary artery pressure. These variations in vascular pressure synchronous with inspiration are present because the transducer is measuring vascular pressure relative to atmospheric pressure. To assess the transmural vascular pressure, the systolic, mean, and diastolic pressures must be determined at a point in the ventilatory cycle when pleural pressure approximates atmospheric pressure. That is, systolic, mean, and diastolic pressures should be determined at end-exhalation.[7,8]

Systolic, mean, and diastolic pressures are usually determined by the electronic patient-monitoring system. This is accomplished in a number of ways. The most rudimentary is to select the highest and lowest pressure values monitored in a given time interval (eg, 10 seconds) and to average the signal over the same interval. The highest value is reported as the systolic pressure; the lowest value, as the diastolic pressure; and the average value, as the mean pressure. With a spontaneously breathing patient, the systolic pressure reflects transmural systolic pressure, but the diastolic and mean pressures are lower than the transmural pressure. The magnitude of the error depends on the magnitude of the pleural pressure change during inspiration—the greater the change in pleural pressure, the greater the error in the diastolic and mean pressure determinations. For the pa-

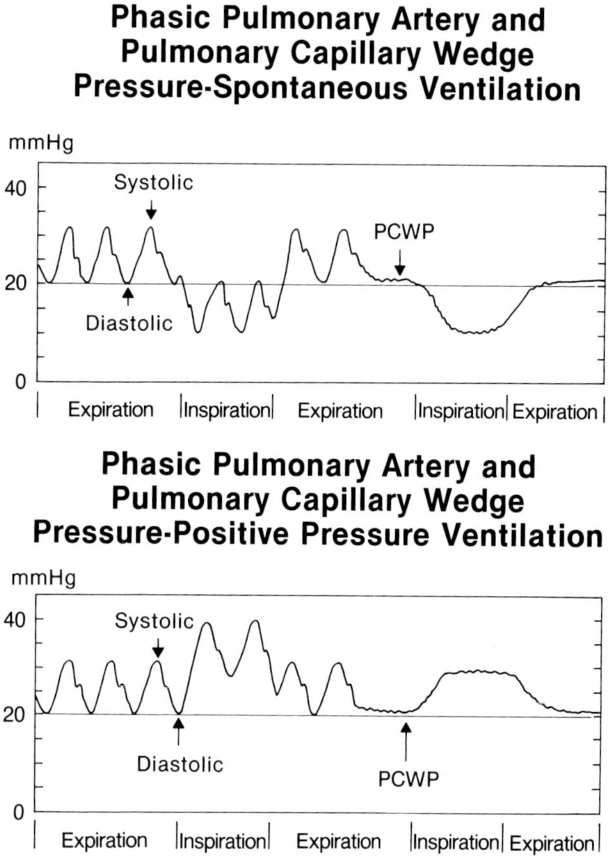

Figure 2–10 • Changes in pleural pressure, synchronous with ventilation, modulate central vascular pressure. The top panel illustrates the effect of pleural pressure changes on pulmonary artery (P_{PA}) and pulmonary capillary wedge (PCWP) pressure during spontaneous ventilation. During each inspiration, the fall in pleural pressure produces a concomitant decrease in the mean P_{PA} and PCWP. The bottom panel illustrates the effect of pleural pressure changes during controlled ventilation. With each ventilator-produced inspiration, pleural pressure rises, producing a rise in the mean P_{PA} and PCWP. In both situations, the determination of transmural pressures requires that the pressure measurements be made at end expiration.

tient whose breathing is controlled by a ventilator, the diastolic pressure determined by the monitor will reflect transmural pressure, and the systolic and mean pressures will be in error. Again, the magnitude of the error depends on the magnitude of the pleural pressure change. Mean pressure, when determined as the average of the vascular pressure over a period of time, will also be in error: greater than the correct value in the case of controlled ventilation, and less than the correct value in the case of spontaneous ventilation.

As patient-monitoring systems become more sophisticated, especially with the advent of the microprocessor, elegant signal-processing algorithms are being used to determine systolic, mean, and diastolic pressures. These signal-processing algorithms are invisible to the clinician and indeed are often promoted by the manufacturer's marketing and sales staff as the solution to accurate vascular pressure monitoring. Regardless of the algorithm used to determine central vascular pressures, systolic, mean, and diastolic pressures must be assessed at the end of exhalation to minimize the effects of pleural pressure. In the absence of a monitoring system sophisticated enough to make this determination, the clinician can determine systolic, mean, and diastolic pressures at the point of end-exhalation by:

1. Observing the pulmonary artery pressure waveform on the monitor's calibrated display screen or calibrated strip-chart recording. Select a pressure pulse occurring just prior to an inspiration (end-exhalation). From this pulse determine the systolic and diastolic pressures. The mean pulmonary artery pressure at end-exhalation can be estimated by the same calculation used to estimate the mean arterial pressure from auscultatory systolic and diastolic measurements (ie, one-third the pulse pressure [systolic–diastolic] added to the diastolic pressure).
2. Observing the CVP, PCWP, or LAP waveform on the monitor's calibrated display screen or calibrated strip-chart recording. Select a portion, approximately the length of one cardiac cycle, of the pressure wave occurring just prior to an inspiration (end-exhalation). Estimate the average pressure occurring during this interval (ie, the mean pressure at end-exhalation).

For the clinician, the ability to monitor vascular pressures accurately now begins with the prepurchase assessment of the patient-monitoring system's signal-processing algorithms and the education of all personnel who use the system in the "anatomy and physiology" of vascular pressure measurement. Not only must these signal-processing algorithms extract the values of interest appropriately, but they must be applied to the correct pressure signals. For central vascular pressures, systolic, mean, and diastolic measurements should be made at the point of end-exhalation. Yet the algorithm that performs this task should not be used in the determination of systolic, mean, or diastolic arterial or intracranial pressures, since the anatomy and physiology of these measurements is different from central pressure measurements.

IV. Complications

A. *Thrombosis and Emboli*

Because of the high incidence of thrombosis with arterial catheters, it is recommended that a continuous flush device always be used to infuse heparinized saline constantly through the catheter. When a thrombus does form, the pressure waveform appears damped. Although a vigorous flush will likely clear the thrombus, it may force it into the aorta, where it may embolize to vital organs. A better procedure is to attempt to aspirate and remove the clot prior to flushing the catheter. Then a gentle flush should complete clearing the system. It is especially important when monitoring the radial artery or umbilical artery pressure in infants or neonates to aspirate clots from the system and never to flush the catheter vigorously, since it is very easy to push a clot to the brain.

Clearing gas bubbles from the hydraulic system not only improves the fidelity of the pressure measurement, but also reduces the risk of inadvertently flushing air into the patient. Avoiding such a scenario in neonatal patients who may have a patent foramen ovale is particularly important. Air bubbles in the hydraulic system should always be aspirated and removed. An air trap can be included in the IV set connecting the flush bag to the transducer in order to stop any air emanating from the pressurized flush bag.

B. *Infection*

Many transducer and hydraulic systems come packaged in sterile containers and are disposable. However, the clinician must still be aware that radial or central catheters are a route of infection.[9,10] Problems with infection are greater when using reusable transducers. When reusable transducers are employed, they should have a sterile disposable dome applied for each patient use. In addition, the transducer should be cleaned and disinfected between uses. This may be done as follows:

1. Using a towel or cloth soaked with a disinfecting solution, wipe the case of the transducer and its electrical cable. Care should be taken not to get fluid on the electrical connections.
2. Remove any blood from the transducer, using hydrogen peroxide.
3. Place several 4 × 4 gauze sponges in a cup or shallow tray. Place the transducer, exposed sensing diaphragm down, on the gauze pads.
4. Fill the container with a high-level disinfecting solution to a depth sufficient to cover the pads and the sensing diaphragm of the transducer, but not deep enough to contact any of the electrical connections. Let the transducer soak in this solution for 30 minutes.
5. Remove the transducer, rinse the sensing diaphragm thoroughly with sterile water, let it dry, place it in a sterile bag, and seal and date the bag. If the transducer is not used within 1 month, repeat the disinfecting procedure.

When the transducer is used again, a new sterile disposable dome should be applied, following the transducer manufacturer's recommendations. Regardless of whether a reusable or disposable transducer is used, the transducer and hydraulic system should be replaced after every 48 hours of patient use.

Stopcocks are an overlooked source of infection in pressure-monitoring systems.[11] When not in use, stopcocks should have a cap placed on each unused port. Following the aspiration of blood through a stopcock, any blood remaining in the stopcock port should be cleared away. Of course, it is especially important to wash your hands before moving on to the next patient.

V. REFERENCES

1. Gardner RM. Direct blood pressure measurement—dynamic response requirements. Anesthesiology 54:227–236, 1981.
2. Kleinman B. Understanding natural frequency and damping and how they relate to the measurement of blood pressure. J Clin Monit 5:137–147, 1989.
3. Boutros A, Albert S. Effect of the dynamic response of transducer-tubing system accuracy of direct blood pressure measurement in patients. Crit Care Med 11:124–127, 1983.
4. Kleinman B, Powell S. Dynamic response of the ROSE damping device. J Clin Monit 5:111–115, 1989.
5. Bruner JMR, Krenis LJ, Kunsman JM, Sherman AP. Comparison of direct and indirect methods of measuring arterial blood pressure, part III. Med Instrum 14:182–188, 1981.
6. Teplick RS. Measuring central vascular pressures: A surprisingly complex problem. Anesthesiology 67:289–291, 1987.
7. Berryhill RE, Benumof JL, Rauscher LA. Pulmonary vascular pressure reading at the end of exhalation. Anesthesiology 49:365–368, 1978.
8. Maran AG. Variables in pulmonary capillary wedge pressure: Variation with intrathoracic pressure, graphic and digital recorders. Crit Care Med 8:102–105, 1980.
9. Buxton AE, Anderson RL, Klimek J, Quintiliani R. Failure of disposable domes to prevent septicemia acquired from contaminated pressure transducers. Chest 74:508–513, 1978.
10. Weinstein RA, Stamm WE, Kramer L, Corey L. Pressure monitoring devices—overlooked source of nosocomial infection. JAMA 236:936–938, 1976.
11. Walrath JM, Abbott NK, Caplan E, Scanlan E. Stopcock: Bacterial contamination in invasive monitoring systems. Heart Lung 8:100–104, 1979.

Chapter 3

•

Edward A. Meathe, MS

Preparing the Monitors

OUTLINE

I. INTRODUCTION

The question of what parameters to monitor and how intensively to monitor them is germane to every area of critical care. Advances in electronic instrumentation and materials technology have provided the clinician with a host of monitoring possibilities. Considerations of patient safety, legal liability, and, increasingly, the cost-to-benefit ratio are important factors in the decision of what, when, and how intensely to monitor.

The American Society of Anesthesiologists (ASA) has established standards for basic intraoperative monitoring (see the appendix). These standards address the monitoring of oxygenation, ventilation, circulation, and temperature. This chapter addresses patient monitoring in these areas. Such monitoring, although specifically designated for intraoperative use, is also applicable for the intensive care unit patient who is supported by mechanical ventilation.

Figure 3–1 illustrates the patient-monitoring connections that would be established during a typical general anesthetic. The electrocardiogram is monitored via lead wires connected to the thorax. Patient oxygenation is monitored in two ways. Inspired oxygen is continuously monitored with a sensor placed in the breathing circuit, usually on the inspiratory limb. Arterial hemoglobin oxygen saturation is monitored with an infrared light source and sensor, which in most cases is applied to the finger. Blood pressure is monitored with a cuff applied to one of the limbs. Inspired and expired gas, usually carbon dioxide but also in some cases the anesthetic gases, are drawn from the airway for analysis. Heart and breath sounds, as well as temperature, may be monitored using an esophageal stethoscope.

Because of advances in sensor technology and electronic instrumentation, especially the microprocessor, what on the surface appears to be an intimidating array of equipment and patient interfaces is in fact easily managed and, for the most part, is considered a standard of care (see the appendix). Operating procedures for these devices have been simplified such that equipment setup and preparation effort are minimal, and calibration for most of these devices is required only periodically. Although straightforward and easy to use, they still have failure modes of which the user should be aware.

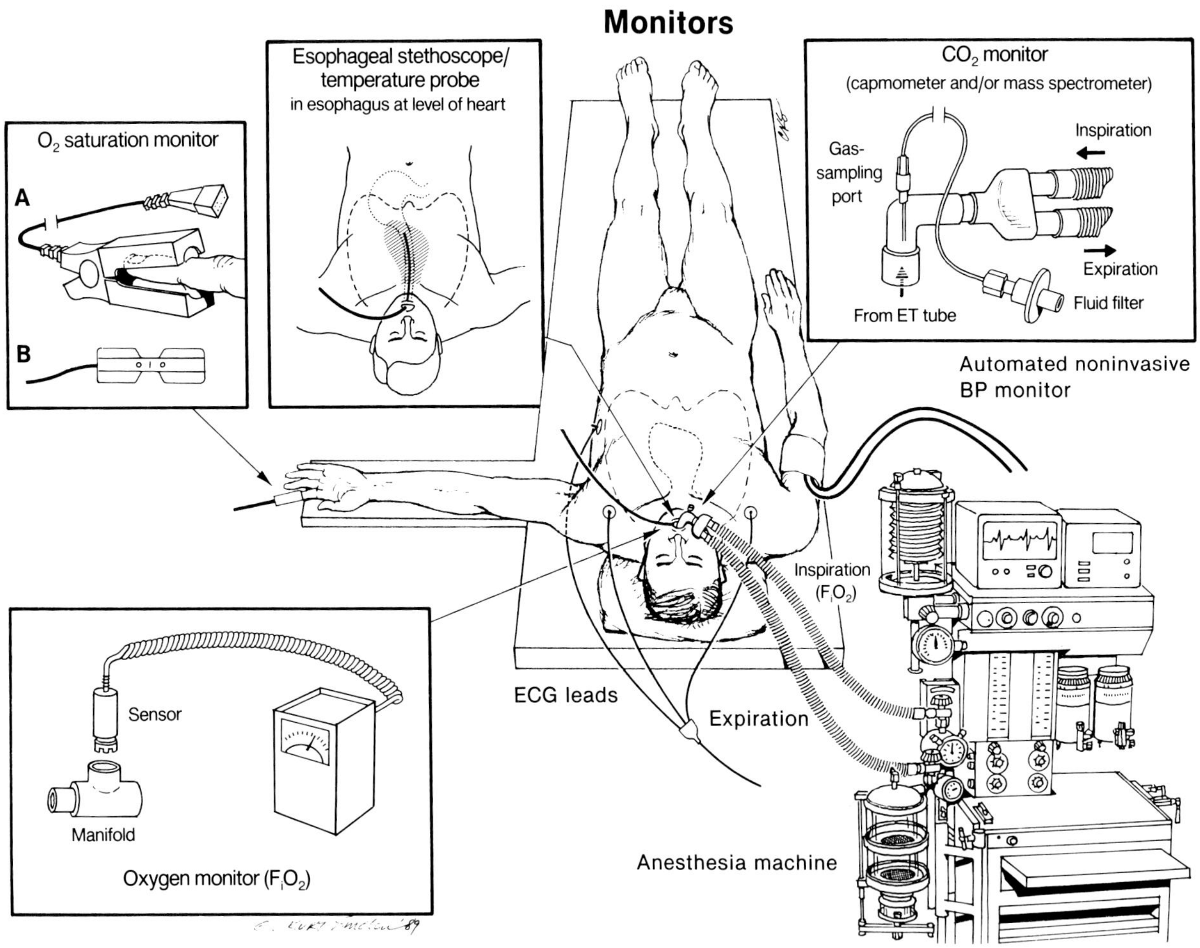

Figure 3–1 • Patient monitoring systems typically used during a general anesthetic procedure. The oxygen concentration of the inspired gas is continuously monitored via an electrode in the breathing circuit; an arterial oxygen saturation sensor is attached to a finger; an esophageal stethoscope permits the monitoring of heart, breath sounds, and temperature; inspired and expired gas are drawn from the airway to determine CO_2 concentration and possibly anesthetic gases, nitrogen, and oxygen; an inflatable cuff is attached to the arm to automatically and noninvasively determine the blood pressure (BP); continuity of the breathing circuit, ventilator, and patient is monitored by a pressure sensor within the anesthesia machine; and three electrodes attached to the patient's thorax provide for monitoring of the electrocardiogram (ECG).

II. How to Prepare the Monitors

A. *Inspired Oxygen Concentration*

The sensor of this monitor is usually placed in the inspiratory limb of the breathing circuit, thus allowing the monitoring of inspired oxygen concentration. This location also permits the sensor to operate in a generally dry gas environment at room temperature. Prior to use, the monitor should be calibrated and its correct operation verified. Although specific details of the calibration process will be spelled out by the manufacturer, a general guideline follows.

1. If the monitor is battery powered, use the battery check feature to verify an adequate power source. If the batteries are low or marginal, they should be replaced.
2. When using a monitor with an analog display (meter) be sure that the needle on the display is pointing to 0% when the device is in "standby" mode. If it is not, use the "zero" adjustment to position the needle at the 0% point.
3. Expose the sensor to 100% oxygen. The monitor should indicate 100% oxygen. If it does not, adjust the calibration control, if available, so that the display indicates 100%.
4. Expose the sensor to room air and allow time for the monitor to stabilize—approximately 30 seconds. The display should read 21% oxygen ±2%. If it does not, recharge or replace the sensor.
5. Verify the operation of the low-oxygen concentration alarm. This can be done quickly by setting the alarm level to a value greater than 25% and then exposing the sensor to room air. If the alarm does not sound, and the monitor correctly indicates an oxygen concentration of 21% ± 2%, then the monitor should be replaced or repaired prior to use.

B. *Arterial Hemoglobin Oxygen Saturation—Pulse Oximetry*

Of all the technology introduced into the critical care environment within the last 5 years, pulse oximetry is perhaps the most widely used. Devices for noninvasively determining the oxygen saturation of hemoglobin have been available for years; however, their bulk, and particularly the size of the sensor, prohibited their acceptance as a routine clinical monitor. The microprocessor and advances in sensor technology have permitted the development of clinically effective and efficient noninvasive hemoglobin saturation monitors—pulse oximeters.

Figure 3–2 illustrates a typical monitoring configuration. A light source (light-emitting diode) and a light sensor (photodiode) are mounted on opposite arms of a clamp-type probe—in this example, a reusable probe. The probe clamps loosely but snugly around a convenient digit, usually a finger. The light source illuminates the underlying tissue bed, while the light sensor receives these signals and sends them back to the monitor. The microprocessor within the monitor isolates the time-varying component and then determines the oxygen saturation percentage and the heart rate. Most systems also provide an indication of the quality of the phasic signal either through a display of the waveform or signal strength. Disposable probes provide a convenient, albeit relatively expensive alternative method for signal acquisition. Their flexibility, however, allows them to be applied at various locations, including the ear, the nose, the tongue, or the foot of a neonate (Fig. 3–3).

Noninvasive pulse oximeters provide for simple and straightforward operation. The instruments are self-calibrating and automatically acquire the arterial signal, adjusting for a wide range of tissue density and perfusion. Monitoring is initiated by connecting the instrument to a properly grounded "Hospital-Grade" electrical outlet, attaching the sensor cable, selecting the sensor probe appropriate for the situation and applying it to the patient, connecting the probe to the sensor cable, and turning on the instrument. The sensor should not be placed on an extremity with an arterial catheter or blood pressure cuff in place, because an occlusion of blood flow would compromise device performance. In patients likely to experience severe vasoconstriction, or in any case where perfusion may be low, using a nasal probe may permit acquisition of an adequate signal long after low perfusion in a digit has made this impossible.

C. *Gas Monitoring—Carbon Dioxide and Anesthetic Gases*

The quantitative monitoring of carbon dioxide at the patient's airway is an excellent method of assessing the adequacy of ventilation. Continual (defined as repeated regularly and frequently in steady and rapid succession) or continuous (defined as prolonged and without interruption) capnography has become a frequent monitoring modality for anesthetized or heavily sedated patients. These are accomplished either through a monitor dedicated to a single patient or via a system designed to monitor several patients sequentially. Although most of

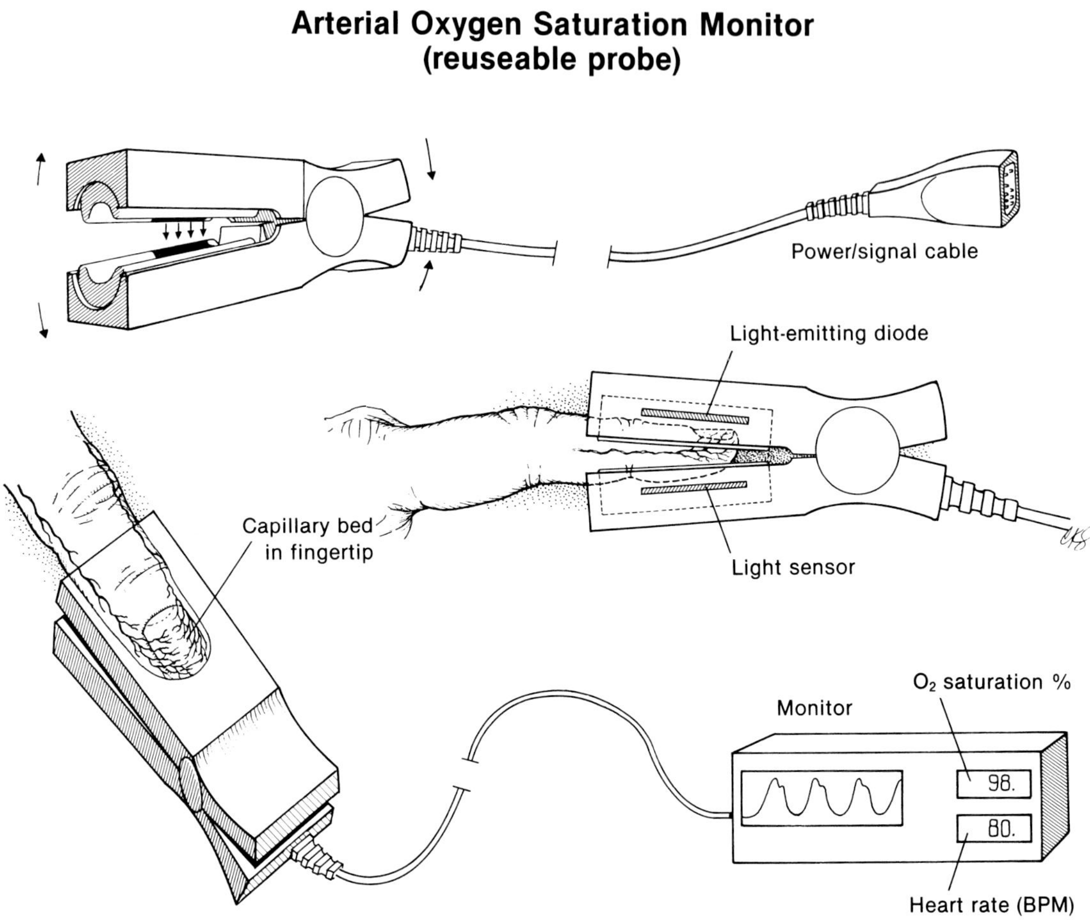

Figure 3–2 • Arterial oxygen saturation is monitored by directing infrared light of two wavelengths through a blood-perfused tissue bed. This is usually accomplished at a finger or other digit. The technique employed depends upon pulsatile blood flow in the digit. Anything that compromises this flow may reduce the accuracy, or even the availability, of the measurement.

these systems monitor only carbon dioxide concentration, several newer devices also monitor anesthetic gases. Since the operating principles are the same for either system, the following discussion focuses on carbon dioxide monitoring, with the understanding that these procedures are also applicable to the monitoring of anesthetic gases.

1. Single-Patient Gas Monitoring

Gas monitoring systems dedicated to use on one patient are of two types: side-stream sampling, where the inspired and expired gas is drawn into the analyzer, and mainstream sensing, where the gas is analyzed while in the breathing circuit. The block diagram of a generic side-stream sampling gas analyzer is shown in Fig. 3–4. Gas is drawn into the system and in many cases passed through a fluid trap to remove liquid water prior to entering the analyzer. The system also provides a mechanism for passing two calibrating gases through the analyzer. These two gases, usually room air (approximately 21% oxygen, 79% nitrogen, 0% carbon dioxide) and a gas containing a known mixture of oxygen, nitrogen, and carbon dioxide (and possibly other gases analyzed by the monitor) are used to adjust the "zero," or reference, point and gain of the monitor, respectively. The precise details of the calibration procedure will be specific to the monitor being used; however, a two-step process is most often involved.

1. While room air is being drawn into the monitor, the system is commanded to perform a "zero" calibration. This procedure is usually automatic and results in the monitor

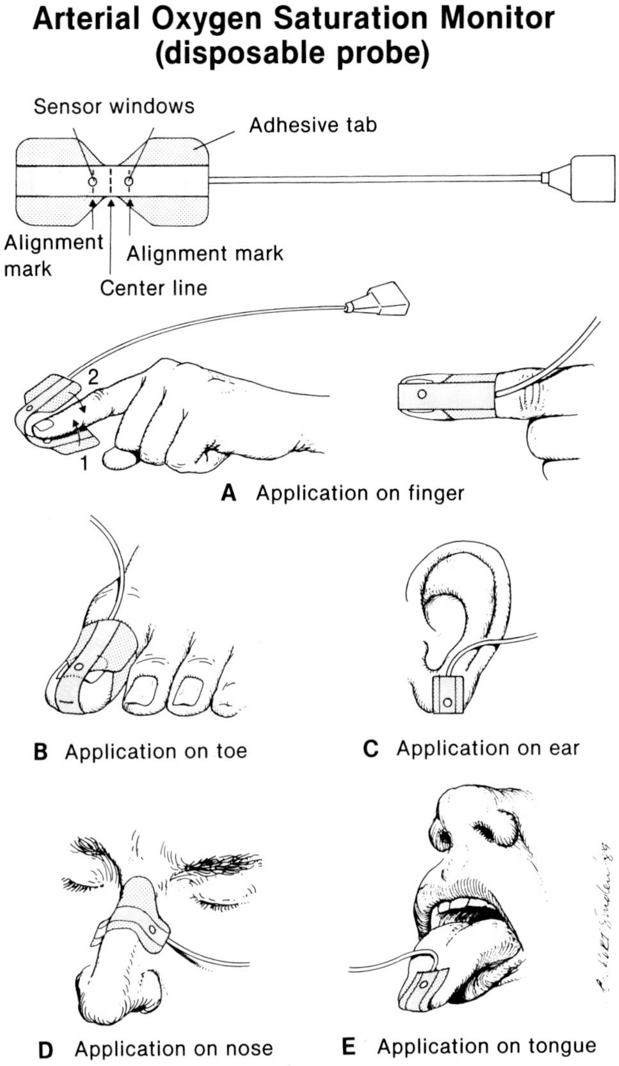

Figure 3-3 • The finger and toe are common sites for the application of the arterial oxygen saturation probe. However, should peripheral vasoconstriction or injury render these sites unusable, the sensor may be applied to other locations as long as they are sufficiently perfused and allow the transmission of the infrared light. Some of these locations are shown in this figure.

internally recording its zero concentration, 0% carbon dioxide or anesthetic gases. If the system requires a manual setting of the zero level then, as room air is flowing through the analyzer, the zero control is adjusted until the display of carbon dioxide or anesthetic gas concentration is zero.

2. A calibration tank containing known amounts of the gases of interest, and a balance gas, is connected to the analyzer. As this gas is passing through the analyzer, the system gain is adjusted for each of the calibration gases.
   a. In many systems the concentration of gases in the calibration tank is entered into the monitoring system. As the calibration gas is flowing through the analyzer, the system is commanded to perform an automatic gain calibration. This results in the system's microprocessor adjusting the gain for each gas so that the output equals the calibration values.
   b. In systems without an automatic gain calibration feature, as the calibration gas is flowing through the analyzer, the user manually adjusts the system gain until the displayed gas concentrations equal those in the calibration tank.

If a mainstream-sensing device is used, then the calibration procedure is again implemented in two steps, although specific details will be peculiar to the device.

1. The zero, or reference, point is established by placing the sensor around a cuvette containing no carbon dioxide. The zero level is then set automatically or manually, depending on the device.
2. The system gain is established by placing the sensor around an optical filter, which simulates a known concentration of carbon dioxide. The system gain is then adjusted so that the display reflects this carbon dioxide concentration.

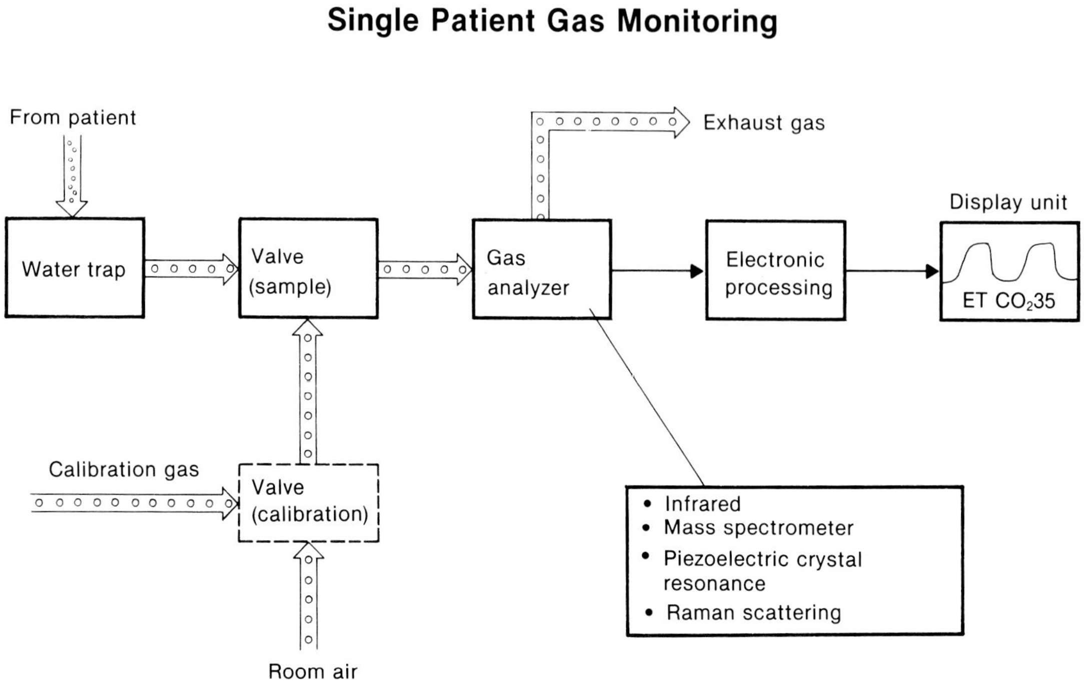

Figure 3–4 • This figure shows typical components found in a single patient gas-monitoring system. Gas is drawn from the patient's airway and passed through a water trap, where liquid is removed. The gas then passes through the analyzer, where the concentration is determined. The output of the analyzer is then processed and displayed as a waveform and digital values. Several different types of analyzers are available. During calibration, gas is drawn from one of two sources: room air for the "zeroing" procedure and a gas cylinder (calibration gas) containing known concentrations of the gas, or gases, detected by the analyzer.

The analyzer itself may use infrared absorption techniques, mass spectrometry, piezoelectric crystal resonance, or Raman scattering.

Following analysis the sample gas is vented from the monitor. This gas may then be returned to the patient's breathing circuit, exhausted to atmosphere, or scavenged in the event anesthetic agents are present in the mixture. The electronic signals generated by the analyzer are processed and the results are displayed. A good display will present both the waveform representing the time-dependent gas concentration and digital values representing the inspired and end-tidal concentrations as well as the respiratory rate.

2. Multiple-Patient Gas Monitoring

Inspiratory–expiratory gas monitoring can also be accomplished using a single analyzer for a number of patients. This is commonly done with a mass spectrometer. The components of such a system are shown in Fig. 3–5. The mass spectrometer, through a system of electronically controlled valves, sequentially samples inspiratory–expiratory gas from each patient connected to the system. The gases within the mixture are identified, their concentration determined, and the results (waveform, inspired, and end-tidal digital values) are sent to the patient's bedside monitor via the electronic processing and control unit. System calibration is performed in a manner similar to that of the single-patient gas monitor, with the exception that the multiple-patient gas monitor performs the entire two-point calibration process automatically.

3. Acquiring the Gas Sample

Acquisition of a sample of the inspired–expired gas for analysis may be accomplished through side-stream sampling or a mainstream sensor. Each of these mechanisms is illustrated in Fig. 3–6. With side-stream sampling, gas is usually withdrawn at the elbow connector located between the proximal end of the endotracheal tube and the ventilator hoses (see Fig. 3–6A). The sampling port extends down the center line of the elbow toward the patient. A length of plastic tubing connects the port of

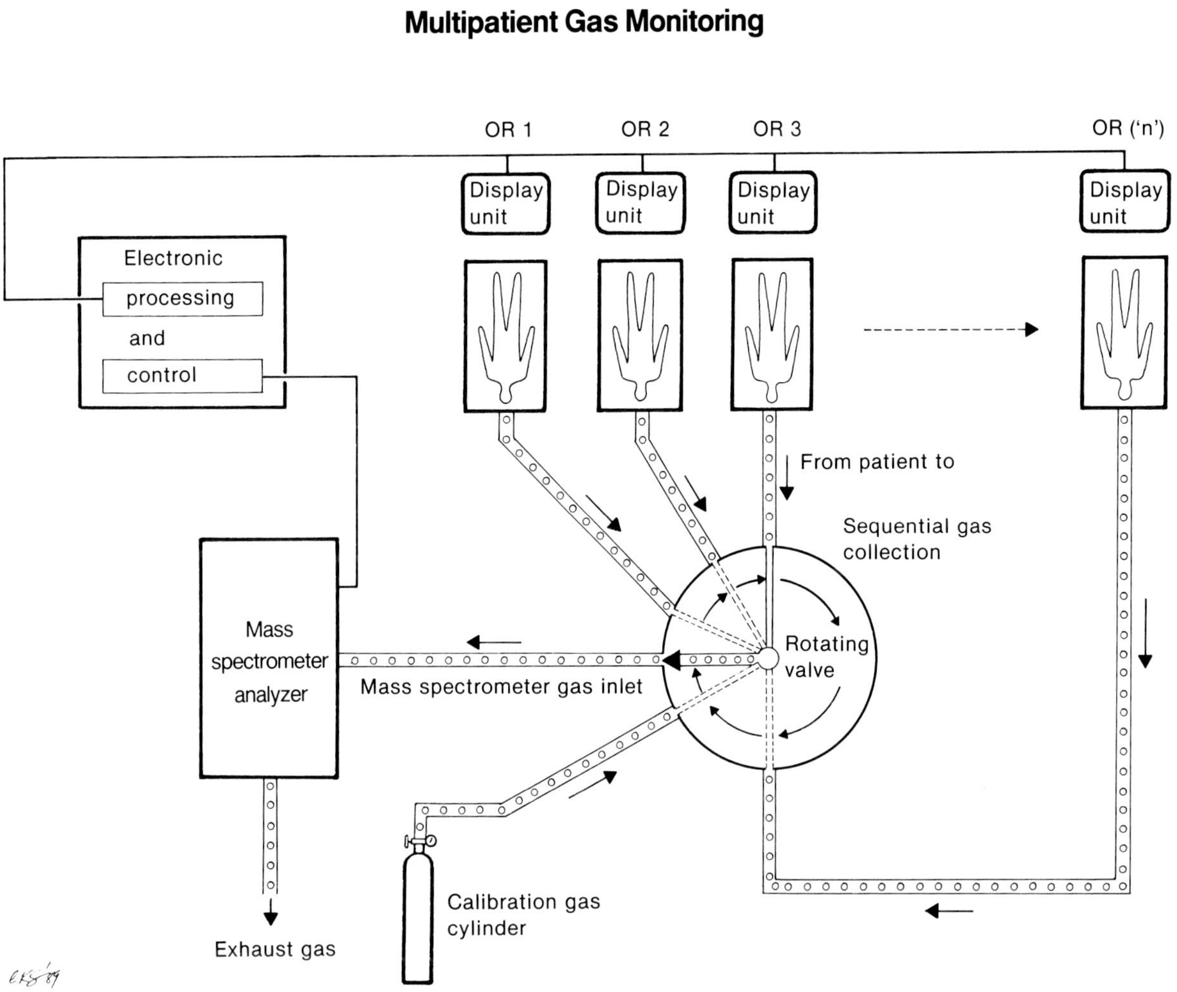

Figure 3–5 • A single mass spectrometer may provide gas monitoring at several locations. Each location has a display unit and sample port. Inspired and expired gas are drawn through the sample port and transported to the mass spectrometer by long sample tubes, often exceeding 100 feet in length. A valve system, either a rotor valve or a series of solenoids, sequentially passes gas from each monitoring location to the mass spectrometer, where the concentration of the gases in the mixture is determined. An electronic processing unit controls the valve sequencing, processes the output of the mass spectrometer, and sends the results back to the appropriate patient location.

the bedside monitor or to a central analyzer. A filter is often placed at the end of the sample tube to stop fluid and particulate matter from entering the analyzer.

When monitoring small infants, particularly neonates, the small tidal volumes can render the end-tidal carbon dioxide, as determined by gas sampling from the elbow, a poor reflection of alveolar end-tidal carbon dioxide. Moving the gas-sampling site closer to the carina will improve this determination. Endotracheal tubes with an integral gas-sampling port are available that facilitate such measurements (see Fig. 3–6B).

Carbon dioxide monitoring can also be performed on awake nonintubated patients by piercing a nasal oxygen prong with an intravenous catheter.[1] Although it does not necessarily reflect the end-tidal carbon dioxide concentration, such a system can function as a respiratory rate (apnea) monitor for use with sedated but nonintubated patients.

Mainstream-sensor gas analysis has been applied to the measurement of carbon dioxide concentrations in inspired–expired gas. This consists of a mainstream sensor placed in the breathing circuit just proximal to the patient's endotracheal tube (see Fig. 3–6). The sensor contains the infrared source and detector necessary to monitor carbon dioxide concentration. Mainstream-sensor gas analysis provides a rapid response to gas concentra-

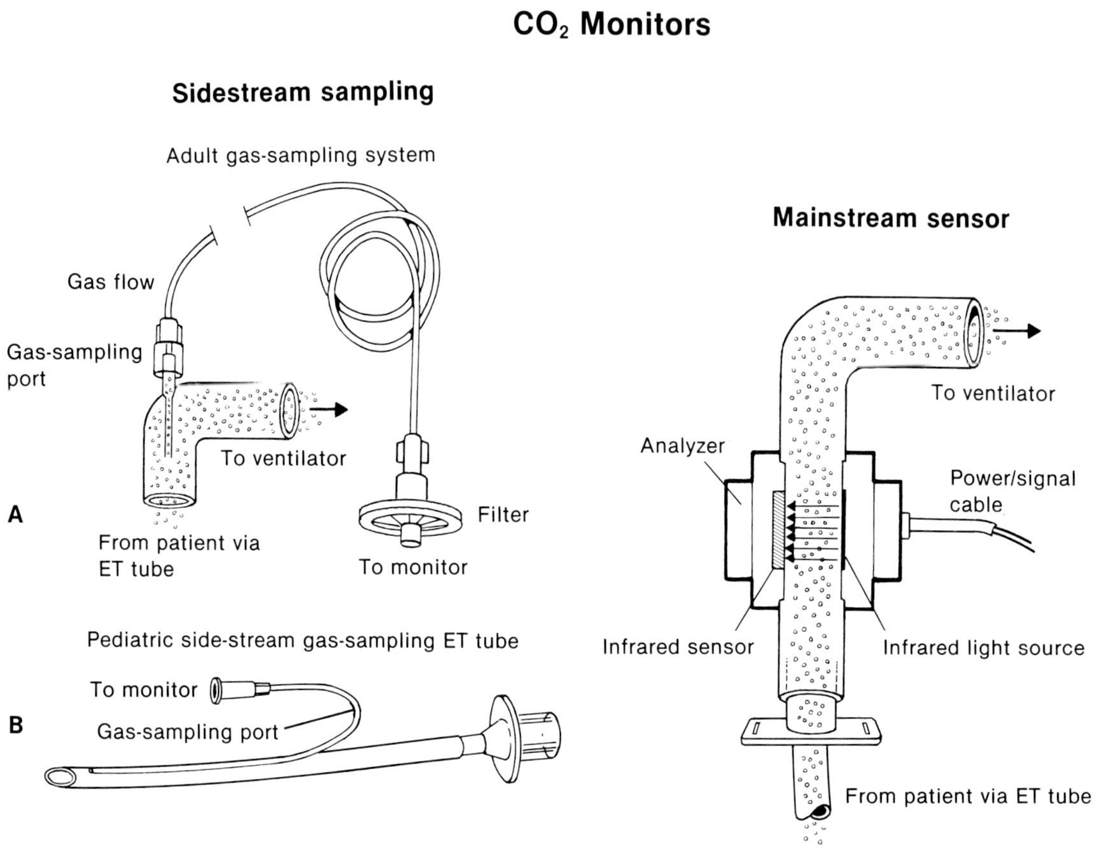

Figure 3–6 • (Left panel) Inspired and expired gas may be sampled from the airway via a sample port. (***A***) The port extends down the midline of the breathing circuit elbow. (***B***) With pediatric patients, from the distal end of an endotracheal (ET) tube. (Right panel) Mainstream gas sensors have the analyzer inserted in the breathing circuit between the ET tube and the elbow.

tion changes and eliminates the requirement of withdrawing gas from the circuit. However, it does add some dead space to the circuit as well as placing additional weight, and possibly torque, on the endotracheal tube. Placing the analyzer near the patient makes it more vulnerable to damage and, hence, costly repairs and equipment unavailability.

D. Monitoring Breath Sounds

Auscultation of breath sounds is accomplished in one of two ways during anesthesia, with either a precordial or an esophageal stethoscope. The most common precordial stethoscope is a heavy metal bell that comes in adult and pediatric sizes. Small circular patches of adhesive material are available to affix the bell to the chest. In anesthetized intubated patients an esophageal stethoscope is often used. This device consists of a catheter (usually 12, 18, or 24 French sizes) with a closed perforated distal end covered by a pliable plastic membrane. The proximal end provides a port for attachment of connecting tubing. Some esophageal stethoscopes also incorporate a temperature probe.

Use of either system is quite straightforward. The precordial stethoscope is affixed to the chest wall and connecting tubing is attached between the stethoscope and the anesthesiologist's earpiece. The esophageal stethoscope is inserted into the esophagus to approximately the level of the heart; connecting tubing is attached between the stethoscope and the anesthesiologist's earpiece. The position of either of the stethoscopes should be adjusted until heart sounds are prominent.

E. Ventilator Disconnect Alarm

When ventilation is controlled by a mechanical ventilator, a device should be incorporated in the system to continuously monitor the integrity of the breathing circuit with the patient and notify the user in the event of a circuit disconnect. This device should be activated automatically when the ventilator is turned on. These devices usually monitor the pressure within the breathing circuit. For the ventilator to inflate the patient's lungs, it must raise the pressure in the breathing circuit. If the patient becomes detached from the circuit or if a partial or whole disconnect occurs within the circuit, the pressure developed within the system will be significantly less during each mechanical breath. When, in a given period of time, the monitor detects no pressure above its alarm threshold, it sounds an alarm. In some systems this alarm threshold can be varied to accommodate differences in patient lung compliance and tidal volume settings.

This alarm system should always be checked prior to connecting the patient to the ventilator. The system may be set up to ventilate an anesthesia breathing bag and then disconnect the bag from the circuit; this should produce an alarm. Alternatively, the ventilator could be operated with an open circuit and no patient connection; the alarm should be activated under this situation.

F. *Automated Noninvasive Blood Pressure*

Manual auscultation of Korotkoff sounds to determine the arterial blood pressure is common practice. This procedure requires the exclusive attention of the clinician during the determination. The absolute values of systolic and diastolic blood pressure determined depend on the observer's hearing acuity and attention, cuff size and placement, and accuracy of the aneroid manometer. During the administration of an anesthetic, the need for a pressure measurement often conflicts with other demands on the anesthetist's time. Today a host of electronic devices is available that automatically determine the arterial blood pressure without the need for intervention by the clinician.

Implementing this monitoring procedure is straightforward. A cuff of the appropriate size is placed on the upper arm, or the leg (ankle or thigh) if the arm is unavailable. If the device monitors Korotkoff sounds, care must be taken to locate the microphone over the artery during application of the cuff. The cuff should not be placed on the same extremity being used for intravenous infusion. The monitor may then be programmed to make a pressure determination when manually requested by the user, or to make pressure determinations at predetermined intervals. These devices do not require calibration before use; however, as with other equipment, regular maintenance accompanied by a system calibration is recommended.

Recent advances in technology have produced two devices that permit the noninvasive acquisition of a continuous blood pressure signal. The first device, the Finapres (manufactured by Ohmeda, Inc.), is based on a method developed by the Czechoslovakian physiologist Penaz. To use this device, a small blood pressure cuff is wrapped around the middle phalanx of a finger and the connecting tubing is attached to the monitor. Since a light source and sensor are incorporated in the cuff to monitor the plethysmogram, care should be taken to follow the manufacturer's recommendations when positioning the cuff. The device does not require a special calibration procedure. Calibration and monitoring are automatically handled by the system, with continuous display of the phasic arterial waveform and numeric values of systolic, mean, and diastolic pressure and heart rate.

The second device, the APM770 (manufactured by Cortronic, Inc.), uses a standard blood pressure cuff attached to the upper arm. The APM770 is self-calibrating and produces a continuous display of the phasic arterial pressure waveform as well as the systolic, mean, and diastolic pressure numeric values. This device has the advantage of also being able to make single-point blood pressure determinations using the oscillometric method.

G. *Monitoring Temperature*

Of all the monitoring procedures employed in anesthesia, temperature monitoring is the easiest to implement. It consists literally of selecting a type of probe applicable to the monitoring site, inserting or attaching the probe, and connecting it to the monitor. Temperature is usually monitored at one of the following sites: esophagus, rectum, nasopharynx, tympanic membrane, or skin.

Esophageal temperature can be monitored with a reusable or disposable temperature probe inserted into the esophagus, or with a temperature probe incorporated into the esophageal stethoscope. The esophageal temperature probe should be placed in the lower one-fourth of the esophagus to obtain the most stable temperature measurement.[2] Measurement of temperature in the upper portions of the esophagus tends to reflect the temperature of the inspired gases, since the probe is located close to the trachea.

Axillary skin temperature can be monitored using the same type of probe that is used in esophageal and rectal temperature monitoring. The arm should be abducted before positioning the probe, then returned to the adducted position. Skin temperature can also be monitored using liquid crystal thermometry. These devices consist of a Mylar strip impregnated with liquid crystals and placed on a black background. At a given temperature some of the crystals reflect or scatter incident light, thus indicating the temperature of the sensing side of the strip. To obtain the best results, the strip should be placed on the skin of the forehead.

Calibration of temperature probes is not required prior to use. However, checking the calibration of a system can be difficult when it is required. The monitor can often be checked by using a device supplied by the manufacturer that simulates the response of the temperature probe at a particular temperature. Plugging this device into the monitor in place of the probe will produce a predictable result. If it becomes necessary to verify operation of the probe itself, it and a reference device, usually a mercury thermometer, must be submerged in a stable temperature water bath. The temperature of the bath should be within the normal body temperature range. The value displayed on the monitor must equal the temperature indicated on the mercury thermometer.

III. Discussion of the Procedures

A. *Inspired Oxygen Concentration*

For the mechanically ventilated patient, or the patient receiving an inhalation anesthetic, insuring an adequate level of inspired oxygen is critical for their safety. The concentration of oxygen being delivered to the patient can be monitored using either the polarographic, paramagnetic, Raman, or mass spectrometer methods. Polarographic monitoring of oxygen concentration is the most common of these methods. Most anesthesia machines are purchased with these self-contained oxygen monitors. The electrode of the analyzer is placed in the circuit between the patient and the ventilator–anesthesia machine (Fig. 3–7). Oxygen molecules diffuse through the membrane located at the tip of the electrode into the electrolyte solution in proportion to their concentration in the gas within the breathing circuit. Once inside the electrolyte solution, the oxygen molecules are reduced, causing a current to flow between the anode and the cathode. The magnitude of current flow is proportional to the oxygen concentration in the electrolyte solution. Thus, current flow is proportional to the partial pressure of oxygen in the ventilator–anesthesia machine circuit. The monitor converts this current into a display that represents the percentage of oxygen in the gas.

Gases other than oxygen, such as nitrous oxide, carbon dioxide, halothane, enflurane, or isoflurane, when present at normal levels, do not influence the performance of the polarographic oxygen monitor significantly. Moreover, noncondensing humidity does not degrade the accuracy of polarographic oxygen sensors. However, the addition of water vapor to a dry gas mixture does lower the true oxygen percentage; yet the monitor does measure the lower oxygen concentration accurately. Condensing humidity conditions, on the other hand, can cause the measured oxygen percentage to be significantly lower than the true oxygen percentage. Variations in the temperature of the gas being monitored may cause slight inaccuracies in the measured oxygen concentration. These are minimal, however, since the monitor compensates for the effects of temperature within its specified operating range. To eliminate potential sources of error, the polarographic oxygen sensor is usually placed in the inspiratory limb of the anesthesia machine or ventilator, such that it is monitoring a generally dry gas mixture at room temperature.

The polarographic oxygen sensor and the galvanic, or fuel cell, type are inherently slow in responding to changes of oxygen concentration. Typically, such a system may take 10 seconds to provide a 90% response to a step change in oxygen concentration. Therefore, these systems can only be used to monitor the average oxygen concentration; they are not able to respond on a breath-to-breath basis.

The monitoring of inspired oxygen concentration has become routine and straightforward. Yet, since it measures the percentage of oxygen in the gas mixture, it cannot guarantee that an adequate supply of oxygen is being delivered to the patient. An input gas mixture of 40 mL/min oxygen and 120 mL/min nitrous oxide produces an F_IO_2 of 25%, whereas input flow rates of 400 mL/min oxygen and 1200 mL/min nitrous oxide produce the same F_IO_2. Yet in the first example, the amount of oxygen supplied to the patient would not provide for the normal oxygen consumption of an adult patient. A monitor to be discussed later, the pulse oximeter, would have detected the inadequacy of this situation.

The F_IO_2 monitor is an indispensable component of any anesthesia machine–ventilator. Insuring that the monitor is in place and functioning properly prior to initiating a procedure significantly increases the likeli-

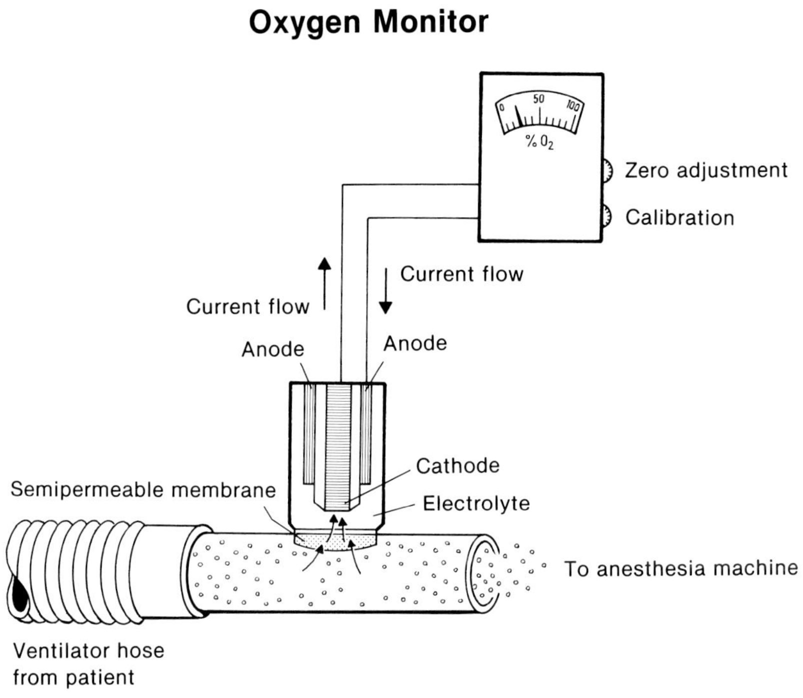

Figure 3–7 • A polarographic sensor is often used to monitor the oxygen within the breathing circuit. It is usually inserted in the inspired limb of the breathing circuit. Oxygen molecules diffuse across the sensor's membrane and enter the electrolyte solution where the oxygen molecules are reduced, producing a current flow between anode and cathode proportional to the oxygen concentration. The monitor measures the magnitude of the current and converts it into an indication of oxygen concentration.

hood of detecting a potentially hypoxic breathing circuit mixture.

B. Arterial Hemoglobin Oxygen Saturation— Pulse Oximetry

The pulse oximeter provides an indication of the patient's blood oxygen content by measuring functional oxygen saturation. Functional oxygen saturation is defined as the percentage of available hemoglobin that is saturated with oxygen. This determination is made by measuring the absorption of two different wavelengths of light (red and infrared) after they have passed through a tissue bed. Absorption of the red wavelength will be significantly different between reduced and oxygenated hemoglobin, whereas absorption of the infrared wavelength will change much less. Since the absorption coefficients of the two types of hemoglobin are known at each wavelength, the percent saturation can be calculated.

The tissue bed in which the monitoring takes place is assumed to be composed of two components: a time-invariant one consisting of various components of the tissue (skin, muscle, bone, fingernail) and venous blood, and another consisting of arterial blood that varies with each arterial pressure wave. Each component attenuates light at the two wavelengths; by subtracting the effects of one component from the other the signal from the arterial blood may be isolated and analyzed.

Although the use of this device is straightforward, several circumstances may interfere with its normal operation. The photodiode light sensors are intended to respond only to incident light from the probe's light-emitting diodes. For this reason the probe attempts to shield the light sensor from ambient light. However, intense light sources—such as bright sunlight, infrared heating lights, operating room lights, or bilirubin lights—may interfere with the measurement. If this becomes, or is likely to become, a problem, the probe should be completely covered with an opaque material, such as a towel, blanket, or drape.

Monitoring of the arterial oxygen saturation and the pulse rate requires the accurate detection of a pulsatile arterial signal. Patient motion can easily interfere with this process. The symptoms of this problem may be an erratic or rapidly changing saturation or pulse rate display, or a pulse rate that does not correlate with other monitors. When this is a problem, insuring good adhesion of the sensor to the monitoring site or changing the monitoring site may resolve the problem. Measurements taken at the nasal bridge are readily affected by motion or ventilation. For the surgical patient, the likelihood of motion artifact is greatly reduced following induction of anesthesia. Selecting a monitoring mode that provides greater filtering (averaging) of the sensor signal, if available, may also reduce the effects of motion artifact.

When these devices are used in the operating room, use of the electrosurgical unit (ESU) can produce significant interference with normal performance. This may be caused by:

1. The ESU cable and the oxygen saturation sensor/probe cable being too close to each other. If possible, separate the cables.
2. The oxygen saturation sensor/probe being too close to the site of electrocautery or the patient return electrode. If possible, move the sensor to a different site.
3. The oxygen saturation sensor/probe not providing sufficient insulation from the ESU signal because of excessive use or moisture. Replace the sensor/probe if possible.
4. The ESU and the oxygen saturation monitor being plugged into the same electrical circuit. Plug them into separate circuits, if possible.
5. The internal electrical design and construction of the oxygen saturation monitor not being sufficient to prevent radiated ESU signals from interfering with normal operation. If aberrant performance during ESU use is the norm, this is most likely the situation. However, the instrument should resume normal operation shortly after ESU use has stopped.

Inadequate perfusion at the monitoring site may result in the absence of a saturation value, a pulse rate, or both. In this case the perfusion is too poor to allow the instrument to detect an acceptable pulse. This may be resolved by moving the sensor/probe to a different site. The bridge of the nose is often a good option in these situations, since the nasal septal anterior ethmoid artery is supplied via the internal carotid artery. In these cases, to verify that the problem does not reside in a defective sensor/probe, test the instrument on yourself. Another source of the problem could be the electrical cable between the monitor and the sensor/probe.

The pulse oximeter measures *functional saturation* (eg, oxygenated hemoglobin expressed as a percentage of hemoglobin available for oxygen transport). Significant levels of dysfunctional hemoglobins, such as carboxyhemoglobin or methemoglobin, may affect the accuracy of the measurement. In addition, cardiogreen and other intravascular dyes may also affect the accuracy of the measurement.

C. Gas Monitoring—Carbon Dioxide and Anesthetic Gases

Infrared absorption is by far the most common method of analysis. This method uses the fact that carbon dioxide absorbs infrared light at specific wavelengths. By comparing the intensity of carbon dioxide–specific infrared light passed through the sample gas with that of light passed through a gas of known carbon dioxide concentration, the concentration of carbon dioxide in the sample gas may be determined. Infrared analysis has been implemented in two ways: (1) transportation of the gas from the airway to a remote analyzer or (2) a mainstream-sensor system with the analyzer mounted in line with the endotracheal tube. With the mainstream analyzer no gas must be withdrawn from the breathing circuit.

Mass spectrometry provides the capability for continuous analysis of multiple gases within a mixture. The mass spectrometer produces a beam of ions from a gas sample, sorts the ions according to their mass-to-charge ratios, and provides output signals that are proportional to the relative amount of each gas in the mixture. Mass spectrometer systems, although very accurate, tend to be bulky and expensive.

A new adaptation of technology to gas monitoring is the piezoelectric analyzer. This device employs a quartz crystal coated with a material that absorbs the gas of interest. The amount of gas absorbed will depend on its concentration in the input mixture. As the crystal's coating absorbs the gas, the crystal's frequency of oscillation changes, with the change in frequency being proportional to the gas concentration. The application of this technology to medical gas analysis is in its infancy.

In a Raman analyzer, the sample gas mixture is illuminated by an intense laser beam. Gas molecules scatter the incident light, causing a shift in the light's frequency (wavelength). The amount of frequency shift depends on the type of molecule producing the scattering. The intensity of the scattered light at that frequency depends on the concentration of the gas in the mixture. This method of analysis is rapid, accurate, and species specific.

All gas monitoring systems are limited in their ability to respond to rapidly changing gas concentrations, such as those generated by high ventilatory rates.[3] This limitation arises from several sources: the type of analyzer, the volume of the analysis chamber, the sample tubing, and the flow rate. In general, mass spectrometers and Raman analyzers provide a more rapid response than infrared analyzers. However, these responses can be diminished significantly by the process of transporting the gas sample from the patient to the analyzer.

Mainstream-sensor gas monitoring systems avoid the problem of gas transport by analyzing the gas in the breathing circuit itself. In theory this technology should provide a better system response than sidestream-sensor systems. However, independent testing has indicated that some sidestream sampling units provide a system response equal to or greater than mainstream-sensor units.[4] The disadvantage of these systems is that they increase the dead space of the breathing circuit, impose an additional mass and possible torque on the endotracheal tube, and place a costly device, the sensor, in a location in which its likelihood of being damaged is increased. At the present time, mainstream-sensor systems provide only the capability of carbon dioxide monitoring.

Sidestream sampling systems, although more convenient, are limited in their ability to respond to rapidly changing gas concentrations by the sample tubing and gas-sampling rate. The side-stream sampling system's ability to respond to rapidly changing gas concentrations is diminished as the length of the sample tubing is increased and as the sampling rate is decreased. The short lengths of tubing (6–8 ft) used with single-patient gas monitoring systems do not significantly limit system accuracy when the ventilatory rate is less than 50 breaths/min.[5] Long sampling lines, such as those associated with central, multipatient mass spectrometer systems, can severely limit the response of gas monitoring systems.[6] Errors of 10% in inspiratory values have been reported at breathing rates of 40 breaths/min when using long sampling catheters under otherwise ideal conditions.[7]

A typical tracing of an inspired/expired carbon dioxide waveform, capnogram, is shown in Fig. 3–8. Inspiration is indicated by a rapid fall in carbon dioxide concentration, eventually reaching the concentration in the inspired gas—usually 0%. Expiration begins sometime before the waveform starts to rise. This is because dead space must be cleared before the expired carbon dioxide reaches the sampling site. After a rapid rise, the waveform reaches a plateau, with the final stable point indicating the carbon dioxide concentration at end-expiration—the alveolar carbon dioxide concentration. When a system is unable to respond to high ventilation rates, the waveform loses the characteristic shape of Fig. 3–8 and begins to assume a more sinusoidal one (Fig. 3–9). The shortened inspiratory time associated with a rapid breathing rate does not allow the system (sample tubing and analyzer) to reach the true inspiratory gas concentration level before exhalation begins and the carbon dioxide concentration starts to rise. Similarly, the shortened expiratory time does not permit the system to respond to the actual end-expiratory gas concentration. The result is an overestimation of the inspired gas concentration and a concomitant underestimation of the end-tidal gas concentration.

The rapid respiratory rate and small tidal volume encountered in monitoring the neonatal patient present special problems for carbon dioxide monitors. Mainstream-sensor units add more dead space to the breathing circuit, as well as placing additional mass, and pos-

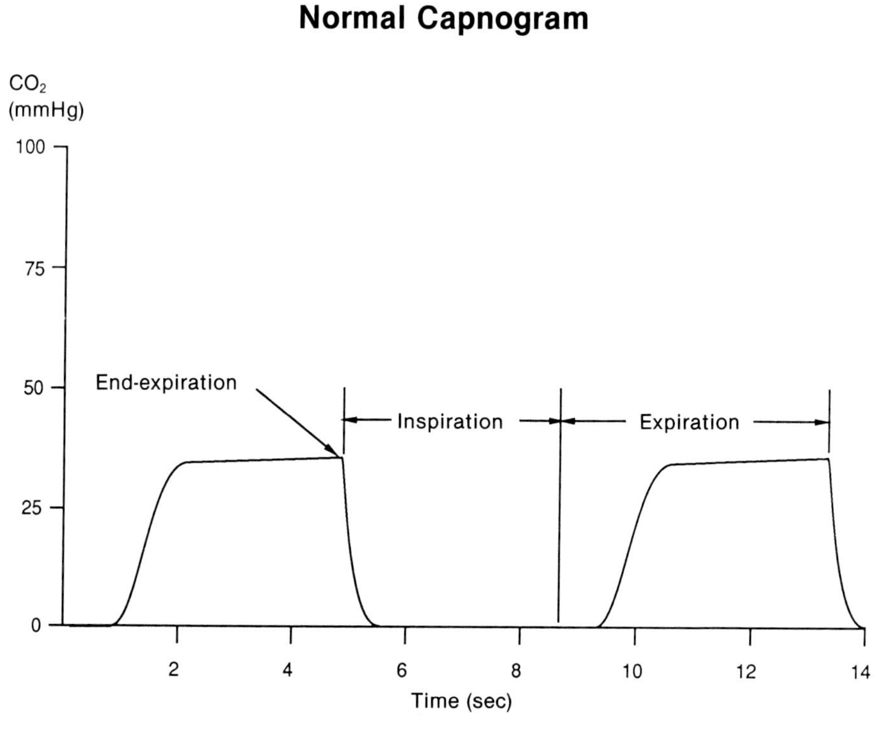

Figure 3–8 • In a normal capnogram, CO_2 concentration falls with each inspiration, approaching a value of 0 mmHg in most situations. With expiration the CO_2 concentration rises until it reaches a plateau at end expiration. The concentration at this point is taken to represent the alveolar concentration.

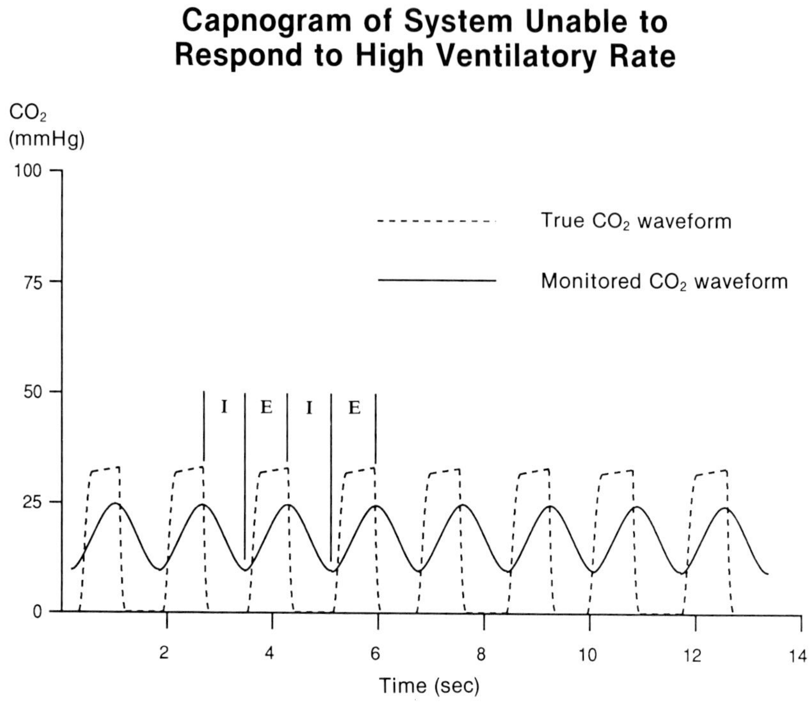

Figure 3–9 • If the patient is being ventilated at a high rate the system may be unable to respond fully to the rapidly changing CO_2 concentration. In these cases, the capnogram may not fall to 0 mmHg during inspiration (*I*), it may not plateau at end exhalation (*E*), and it will have a characteristically sinusoidal shape. Thus, the end-expiratory CO_2 concentration will not reflect the alveolar concentration and it will appear that the patient is rebreathing exhaled gas—inspired CO_2 concentration is greater than zero.

sibly torque, on the endotracheal tube. Sidestream sampling systems suffer from potential problems of inadequate system response necessary to monitor the carbon dioxide waveform accurately. Low-dead-space cuvettes and airway adapters can be purchased for mainstream-sensor units and some side-stream sampling units. This will improve the response of the side-stream sampling unit. Either system may have difficulty in acquiring an end-tidal sample representative of alveolar carbon dioxide concentration. Fresh gas inflow along with low tidal volume may dilute the expired gas when measured at the proximal end of the endotracheal tube. However, an endotracheal tube with a side-stream sampling port located near the tip of the tube is available (see Fig. 3–6B). Sampling the expired gas at this location minimizes the mixing of alveolar and fresh gas.

Capnometers usually report the inspired and end-tidal carbon dioxide concentration as well as the respiratory rate. The inspired concentration is taken as the lowest carbon dioxide concentration in one respiratory cycle, whereas the end-tidal value is represented by the greatest carbon dioxide concentration encountered in that cycle. The respiratory rate (breaths per minute) is calculated by determining the breath-to-breath interval in seconds and dividing it into 60 (sec/min). In patients who are mechanically ventilated, this measurement can be complicated by the patient making spontaneous, yet ineffective, breathing efforts. This results in a transient fall in the carbon dioxide concentration; however, the spontaneous inspiration is too shallow to remove all the carbon dioxide from the area of the sample port. Figure 3–10 illustrates the effect on the capnograph. This situation often causes the monitor to indicate a falsely high inspired carbon dioxide concentration, possibly a lower end-tidal carbon dioxide concentration, and a respiratory rate that is the combination of the rate of mechanical ventilation and the spontaneous rate. It is important, therefore, to monitor the quality and contour of the waveform as well as the numeric values presented by the system.

When nasal cannulae are used to sample inspired and expired gas in the awake nonintubated patient, the results may not necessarily reflect the true end-tidal (alveolar) carbon dioxide concentration.[8-10] End-tidal measurements may be artificially lower because of the oxygen insufflation flow rate through the nasal cannula, the position of the sample tube, the respiratory pattern, or the capnometer gas sample rate. However, despite questions of true end-tidal accuracy, this system does provide an excellent respiratory rate and apnea monitor for the sedated patient.

Condensation of water vapor and coalescence of water aerosols from humidifiers, as well as patient secretions, can cause a significant accumulation of water and secretions in the breathing circuit. This water or the secretions may then be drawn into the sampling line of

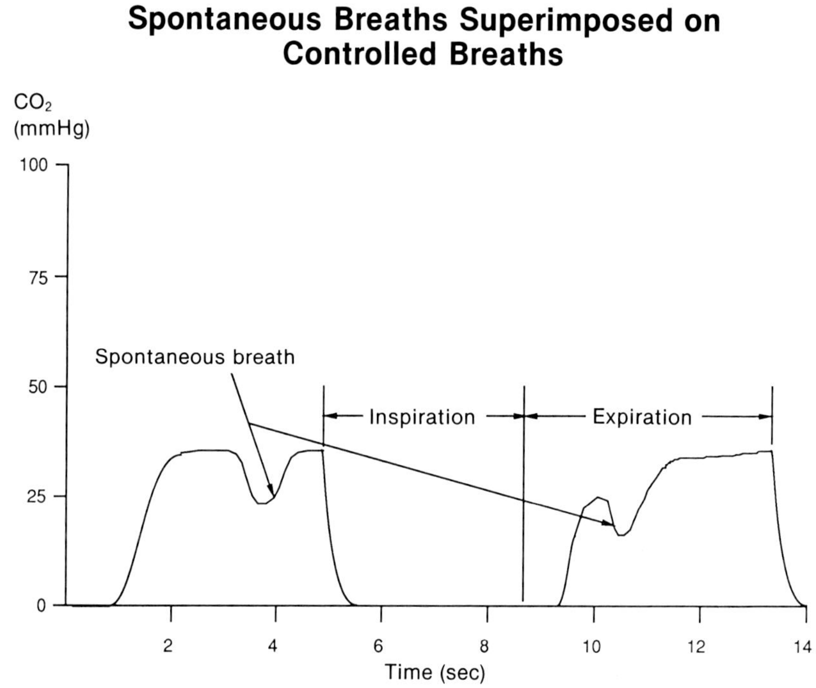

Figure 3–10 • If the patient is making spontaneous breathing efforts while being mechanically ventilated, the capnogram will reflect the effect of both breaths. This may lead to a respiratory rate calculation that is the combination of the mechanical rate and the spontaneous rate—an indication that the patient is rebreathing expired gas (inspired CO_2 concentration greater than zero)—and possibly an artifically low end-expiratory CO_2 concentration.

a side-stream gas monitor, and possibly into the analyzer itself. Liquids can cause corrosion, form residues, and obstruct sample lines that can degrade the performance of the carbon dioxide monitor by interfering with the sample flow or fouling the analyzing chamber. Obstruction of the sample flow will reduce the system's ability to respond accurately to rapidly changing gas concentrations. This is especially true with the long sample line associated with central mass spectrometer systems.[11] Most single-patient gas monitors incorporate either a liquid trap or an in-line filter through which the sample must pass before entering the analyzer. Positioning the sample port upward, away from the patient, along with using center-stream sampling (see Fig. 3–6A), should significantly reduce the frequency with which liquids are drawn into the system. Also, a sample line made from a material permeable to water is available that largely removes water vapor from expired breath.

John Severinghaus reports a problem with the calculation of the partial pressure of carbon dioxide (PCO_2) in some capnometers.[12] This error is related to the manner in which the device calculates PCO_2 relative to the partial pressure of water vapor. Severinghaus indicates that several manufacturers calculate PCO_2 as:

$$PCO_2 = FCO_2 \times P_b$$

where FCO_2 is the fractional concentration of carbon dioxide ($\%CO_2/100$) in dry gas and P_b is atmospheric pressure in millimeters of mercury. This yields the PCO_2 of the dry gas in the analyzer but does not represent the PCO_2 of alveolar gas, which is saturated with water vapor. Alveolar PCO_2 would be determined by the equation

$$PCO_2 = FCO_2 \times (P_b - 47 \text{ mmHg})$$

where the 47 mmHg accounts for water vapor at 37°C. You may ascertain which way your system determines PCO_2 if you know the carbon dioxide concentration in the calibration gas. The procedure is as follows:

1. Perform a system calibration using the calibration gas of known carbon dioxide concentration.
2. With the system in the monitoring mode, reread the calibration gas.
   a. If the carbon dioxide value indicated by the system equals $FCO_2(P_b - 47 \text{ mmHg})$, the system corrects for the missing water vapor.
   b. If the carbon dioxide value indicated by the system equals $FCO_2(P_b)$, the system does not correct for the missing water vapor.

If the results of this step correlate with step 2b, then Severinghaus recommends the following correction procedure. This procedure can be used if the system in question permits the user to enter the carbon dioxide concentration of the calibration gas.

1. Determine the PCO_2 reading when dry calibration gas is passed through the monitoring system—PCO_{2dry}. Sample this gas for a long enough period of time for the sample line and analyzer to dry out completely. Note PCO_{2dry} when the system is dry and the reading is stable.
2. Sample expired gas from a patient for several minutes, thus allowing the sample system to become wet.
3. Quickly switch the sample line from the patient to the calibration cylinder. Note the PCO_2 value indicated on the monitor after several seconds—PCO_{2wet}. After approximately 15 seconds the value will slowly rise to equal PCO_{2dry}.
4. Determine the dry/wet ratio:

$$\text{(dry/wet) ratio} = PCO_{2dry}/PCO_{2wet}$$

5. Determine the "compensated" calibration value for the cylinder as:

$$\text{Comp } CO_2 = \text{Actual \% } CO_2 \times [(P_b - 47)/P_b] \times \text{(dry/wet) ratio}$$

6. Enter this Comp CO_2 value as the new (compensated) value of the calibration gas.

D. *Monitoring Breath Sounds*

A major cause of inadequate sound intensity and fidelity is a poorly fitting earpiece. The use of a cast acrylic earpiece, either ready-made or custom-fitted, or a rubber molded earplug can improve sound quality significantly. To maintain the highest fidelity, the length of the connecting tubing and its softness should be kept to a minimum. Finally, the hearing acuity of the clinician may also impose a limitation in detecting heart and breath sounds.

Electronic devices that amplify and differentiate heart and breath sounds are now available as an adjunct to the completely acoustic stethoscopes. These devices place a microphone on the chest wall or in the esophageal stethoscope, amplify and filter the detected sound, and often transmit the sound to the anesthetist via infrared or radio waves. This transmission modality does not require the anesthetist to be tethered to the patient to monitor heart and breath sounds. It also permits more than one person to monitor at the same time. Some of these devices permit the balancing of heart and breath sound intensity, thus allowing users to adjust the sounds to accommodate their hearing acuity and patient-to-patient variability.

E. *Ventilator Disconnect Alarm*

When under general anesthesia, the patient's head, airway, and the breathing circuit connection are often obscured from view by surgical drapes and the ether screen. Therefore, the presence of a functional ventilator disconnect alarm is imperative. To accommodate differences in patient lung compliance and tidal-volume settings, the disconnect alarm threshold can often be varied. Prior to initiating mechanical ventilation, the proper functioning of this system should be verified by a simulation of a patient disconnection from the ventilator.

F. *Automated Noninvasive Blood Pressure*

Three major techniques are used in automated noninvasive blood pressure monitors: oscillometry, auscultation of Korotkoff sounds, or the ultrasonic detection of arterial wall movement under the cuff. Oscillometry requires only a standard blood pressure cuff, whereas the other techniques require the proper placement of a microphone or Doppler probe. By far the most common technique is oscillometry. In this method, the device monitors the small intracuff pressure oscillations as cuff pressure is reduced from a suprasystolic value to zero. Figure 3–11 illustrates this technique. The intracuff pressure is increased until it exceeds the systolic pressure. The intracuff pressure is then slowly released, while the system monitors the small pressure oscillations (pulses) that occur with each heartbeat. When the intracuff pressure reaches the systolic pressure, the amplitude of the intracuff pulse noticeably increases. The pulse amplitude continues to increase until the intracuff pressure equals the mean arterial pressure, at which time the pulse amplitude is at its maximum. As the intracuff pressure continues to decrease, the pulse amplitude decreases. At the point where the intracuff pressure approximates the arterial diastolic pressure, the amplitude of the intracuff pulse decreases significantly. With this technique, the determination of the mean arterial pressure is relatively straightforward. The accuracy of the systolic and diastolic determinations depends on the signal quality and the robustness of the computer algorithm used by the monitoring system.

The accuracy of these determinations can be significantly affected by the size and application of the cuff,

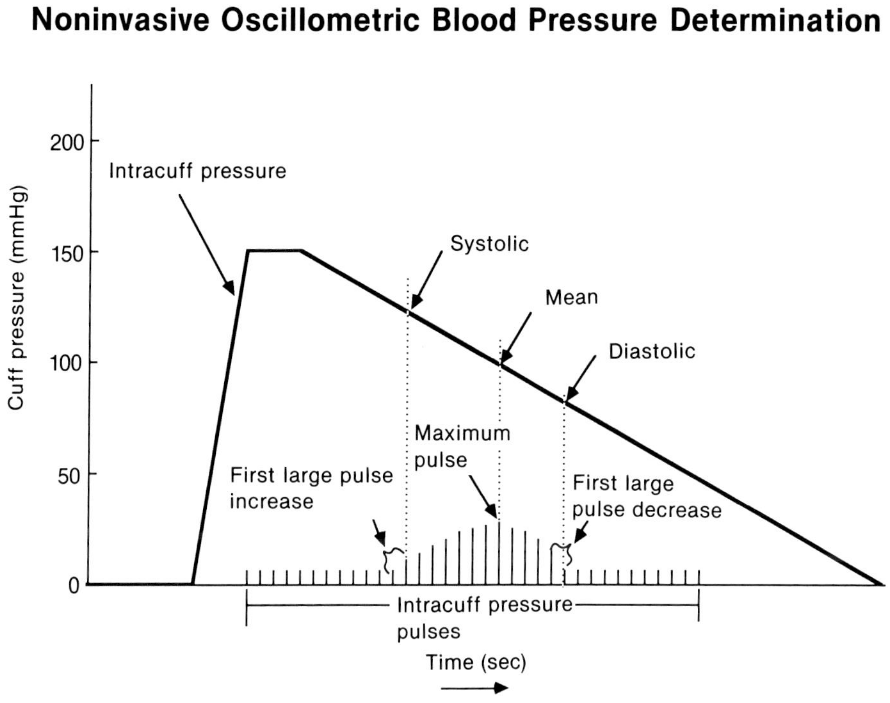

Figure 3–11 • The noninvasive determination of blood pressure by the oscillometric method depends upon the detection of small intracuff pressure pulses as the pressure within the cuff is decreased. The first large increase in intracuff pulse amplitude indicates the intraarterial systolic pressure. Intracuff pressure at the time of maximum pulse amplitude is the mean intraarterial pressure. The intraarterial diastolic pressure is indicated by the first large decrease in pulse amplitude.

spurious intracuff pressure pulses, and the computer algorithm used by the monitor. Using a proper size and snugly applied cuff, the tissue pressure around the deep arteries beneath the cuff equals cuff pressure. A cuff that is too narrow requires an internal pressure greatly in excess of systolic pressure to occlude the artery. A general rule is that the minimum width of the cuff should be one-third the circumference of the limb on which it is placed. If the cuff is applied too loosely, an intracuff pressure greatly in excess of the systolic pressure is required to occlude the artery. Although the cuff should be applied snugly, excessive tightness can cause venous congestion and discoloration of the limb. The patient's extremity should be observed for signs of impeded blood flow, especially when pressure determinations are made frequently.

Because the pressure determination requires the monitoring of small intracuff pressure pulses, anything that produces spurious intracuff pulses may jeopardize the accuracy of the determination. In some cases, it may prevent the monitor from making any determination. The most likely cause of spurious pulses is patient motion. The monitor may not operate effectively on patients who are experiencing convulsions or tremors. When used in the operating room, inadvertent bumping of the cuff or limb by the surgeon can also produce these spurious pulses.

The computer algorithm (program) used by the system determines how the device responds to artifacts such as patient motion. Many systems stop the cuff deflation process momentarily, or even increase intracuff pressure, when spurious intracuff pressure pulses are detected. The deflation is resumed after a few seconds, with the assumption that the artifact has stopped. If the artifact continues for too long, the algorithm will stop the determination and deflate the cuff. In the presence of a motion artifact, even if the device completes its determination, the results may be erroneous. If this is suspected, a manual determination should be made, or if the artifact has stopped, the device can be commanded to make another determination. Should the patient be experiencing arrhythmias, this may increase the determination time or even prohibit one from being made.

If the cuff is not at heart level, the difference in the reading due to hydrostatic pressure should be noted. For every inch the cuff is above heart level, a value of 1.8 mmHg should be added to the displayed readings. If the cuff is below heart level, 1.8 mmHg should be subtracted from the displayed readings.

The Finapres monitor is based on the arterial wall unloading technique described by Penaz.[13] With this method, the volume of the finger's artery is kept constant throughout the cardiac cycle by applying an external pressure equal to the intraarterial pressure. Finapres senses finger volume using a light source and sensor incorporated within the finger cuff to monitor the plethysmogram and holds it constant by adjusting the pressure within the cuff. Thus, the pressure within the cuff reflects the intraarterial pressure. Proper functioning of this unit requires sufficient arterial volume in the peripheral arteries. Factors that may influence digital blood flow are hypothermia, hypovolemia, low cardiac output, pain, high or low blood pressure, vasoconstrictor drugs, and arterial spasm. Any of these factors may compromise the performance of this unit. Several papers have been published concerning the performance of this device.[14–17]

The APM770 operates on the principle that arterial pressures (stresses) and the resulting displacements (strains) of an artery segment conform to a nonlinear elasticity stress–strain relationship. A calibration process performed at the beginning of monitoring determines this relationship for the patient in question. The systolic, mean, and diastolic pressures of an occlusive cuff measurement cycle, as well as a short sequence of displacement waveforms measured at a low cuff pressure, are used to compute a specific elasticity relationship for the relevant range of pulsatile displacements and corresponding pressures of the artery at the monitoring site. The system uses this relationship to convert ongoing displacements into a pressure waveform, while a low reference cuff pressure is held constant.[18] During the period of use the cuff is maintained at a constant pressure of between 15 and 20 mmHg. No papers have been published yet concerning the clinical use of this device. However, its ability to operate continuously and display results at low intracuff pressure, to use a standard blood pressure cuff, and to perform single-point oscillometric blood pressure determinations makes the device clinically attractive.

G. *Monitoring Temperature*

The thermistor, the thermocouple, and the liquid crystal are types of temperature probes in common use. The thermistor probe consists of a semiconductor element that changes its electrical resistance nonlinearly as a function of its temperature. The device is linearized over a range of temperatures by placing a resistor in parallel with the thermistor. Simple electronic circuitry is then all that is needed to transform the resistance change of the thermistor into an indication of temperature. Two major types of thermistors are in widespread medical use. It is imperative that the clinician insure that the thermistor probe is compatible with the monitoring system, despite the fact that the probe connector and monitor receptacle are a match. Using a probe unfamiliar to the monitor will result in erroneous results.

The thermocouple probe consists of two dissimilar metals joined together. This junction produces a potential that changes with its temperature. Measuring this potential in reference to another junction held at a different temperature allows the system to monitor temperature. The thermocouple probes are often less expensive than thermistor probes.

Liquid crystal temperature strips operate by reflecting or scattering light when they are at a particular temperature. By placing liquid crystals having different temperature sensitivities on a single strip, skin temperature can be indicated. Although this system does not require electrical or electronic components to operate, it does require light and therefore is difficult to use in dark rooms. In addition, the temperature range and resolution are limited compared to thermistor and thermocouple systems.

Although we often seek an indication of core temperature, what we get is an indication of the temperature at the location of the sensor. Rectal temperature seldom reflects core temperature in the anesthetized patient, particularly when core temperature is changing rapidly.[19] Esophageal temperature, on the other hand, tends to reflect core temperature changes.[20] A well-placed tympanic probe will produce a temperature that correlates well with cerebral temperature. Although the absolute skin temperature is lower than core temperature, it tends to reflect changes in core temperature, especially in patients undergoing anesthesia.

IV. COMPLICATIONS

A. *Arterial Hemoglobin Oxygen Saturation—Pulse Oximetry*

The noninvasive determination of arterial oxygen saturation by pulse oximetry poses little direct hazard to the patient. All sensor/probe sites, especially on infants, should be checked frequently for skin abrasion or circulatory impairment. When using an electrosurgical unit with any electronic monitoring system that provides a potential pathway for stray ESU current to return to the ESU, the user should exercise caution in insuring that the ESU is configured properly and being used correctly and that the ESU patient return pad is completely and securely attached to the patient.

B. *Gas Monitoring—Carbon Dioxide and Anesthetic Gases*

Mainstream sensors are heated to prevent water vapor from condensing on the windows of the cuvette. These sensors should not become hot enough to burn patients during any monitoring procedure. However, users should minimize or aviod, if possible, prolonged contact of the sensor unit with the patient to prevent heat or pressure injuries.

Several infection control issues are associated with breathing circuit gas monitoring.[21] If the airway adapter, whether mainstream or side stream, is to be reused, it should be cleaned and subjected to high-level disinfection between uses. The sample tubing and any associated filter should be disposed of as infectious waste after use. Some gas monitoring systems have a reverse-flow feature to force liquids and secretions drawn into the sample tube back into the breathing circuit. This is in an effort to maintain an unobstructed sample line. Reverse flow is an undesirable feature because of possible cross-infection. Even when the sample tubing is changed between patients, the possibility exists of forcing contaminants from within the analyzer back into the breathing circuit.

When using sidestream sampling systems that incorporate a fluid trap to prevent liquid from entering the analyzer, the liquids in the trap should be considered infectious and should be treated as such. The trap should be emptied and cleaned or changed after each use. When the trap is changed, the surfaces surrounding it should be disinfected. Personnel who clean the system should wear protective gloves whenever changing or replacing airway adapters, mainstream sensors, sample tubing, fluid traps, and filters.

When used in the presence of anesthetic gases, the exhaust gas from sidestream sampling monitors should be scavenged. Although the exhaust gas could be returned to the circuit, it would then present a possible cross-infection hazard. Exhaust gas, when vented to the atmosphere, presents the possibility of contaminated aerosols placing attending personnel at risk of infection. Although this has not been proven, it is desirable to place a bacterial filter between the patient and the monitoring system.

C. *Automated Noninvasive Blood Pressure*

Placing the cuff on an extremity being used for intravenous infusion will interrupt the infusion during each determination. If the cuff is applied too tightly, this may cause venous congestion and a reduction in intravenous flow.

When the blood pressure is being monitored at frequent intervals, the extremity should be observed for signs of impeded blood flow. This is especially true for those devices that continuously monitor the pressure by maintaining a constant pressure in the cuff. The Finapres maintains the finger under a pressure equal to the mean arterial pressure; yet even though the finger tends to turn a dusky color because of impeded venous return, the device appears to be well tolerated.[22] The monitor has been used on a patient for up to 7 hours without harm. It has also been used during cardiopulmonary bypass.[23] Although there are no published reports concerning clinical efficacy of the APM770 continuous noninvasive blood pressure monitor, the low intracuff pressure (15–20 mmHg) would reduce the likelihood of venous congestion.

D. *Monitoring Temperature*

The use of the nasopharyngeal route for monitoring temperature is not recommended because of the dangers of epistaxis and trauma to the posterior nasopharyngeal mucosa. Thermistor and thermocouple probes, by their very nature, are electrical conductors and therefore potential sources of electrical burns in conjunction with electrosurgical unit use. Burns have been reported when using these devices.[24,25] Cleaning of reusable probes, especially those with seams in their outer covering, may cause a deterioration of the seam and subsequently increase the likelihood of electrical burns. Single-use, electrically insulated disposable probes significantly reduce the likelihood of such occurrences.

V. APPENDIX

A. *Standards for Basic Intraoperative Monitoring (Approved by ASA House of Delegates October 21, 1986)*

These standards apply to all anesthesia care although, in emergency circumstances, appropriate life support measures take precedence. These standards may be exceeded at any time based on the judgment of the responsible anesthesiologist. They are intended to encourage high quality patient care, but observing them cannot guarantee any specific patient outcome. They are subject to revision from time to time, as warranted by the evolution of technology and practice. This set of standards addresses only the issue of basic intra-operative monitoring, which is one component of anesthesia care. In certain rare or unusual circumstances, (1) some of these methods of monitoring may be clinically impractical, and (2) appropriate use of the described monitoring methods may fail to detect untoward clinical developments. Brief interruptions of continual† monitoring may be unavoidable. *Under extenuating circumstances, the responsible anesthesiologist may waive the requirements marked with an asterisk (*); it is recommended that when this is done, it should be so stated (including the reasons) in a note in the patient's medical record.* These standards are not intended for application to the care of the obstetrical patient in labor or in the conduct of pain management.

STANDARD I

Qualified anesthesia personnel shall be present in the room throughout the conduct of all general anesthetics, regional anesthetics, and monitored anesthesia care.

Objective

Because of the rapid changes in patient status during anesthesia, qualified anesthesia personnel shall be continuously present to monitor the patient and provide anesthesia care. In the event there is a direct known hazard (eg, radiation), to the anesthesia personnel that might require intermittent remote observation of the patient, some provision for monitoring the patient must be made. In the event that an emergency requires the temporary absence of the person primarily responsible for the anesthetic, the best judgment of the anesthesiologist will be exercised in comparing the emergency with the anesthetized patient's condition and in the selection of the person left responsible for the anesthetic during the temporary absence.

†Note that "continual" is defined as "repeated regularly and frequently in steady rapid succession" whereas "continuous" means "prolonged without any interruption at any time."

STANDARD II

During all anesthetics, the patient's oxygenation, ventilation, circulation and temperature shall be continually evaluated.

OXYGENATION

Objective

To insure adequate oxygen concentration in the inspired gas and the blood during all anesthetics.

Methods

1. Inspired gas: During every administration of general anesthesia using an anesthesia machine, the concentration of oxygen in the patient breathing system shall be measured by an oxygen analyzer with a low oxygen concentration limit alarm in use.(*)
2. Blood oxygenation: During all anesthetics, adequate illumination and exposure of the patient is necessary to assess color. Although this and other qualitative clinical signs may be adequate, there are quantitative methods, such as pulse oximetry, that are encouraged.

Ventilation

OBJECTIVE

To insure adequate ventilation of the patient during all anesthetics.

Methods

1. Every patient receiving general anesthesia shall have the adequacy of ventilation continually evaluated. While qualitative clinical signs such as chest excursion, observation of

the reservoir breathing bag and auscultation of breath sounds may be adequate, quantitative monitoring of the carbon dioxide content and/or volume of expired gas is encouraged.

2. When an endotracheal tube is inserted, its correct positioning in the trachea must be verified. Clinical assessment is essential and end-tidal carbon dioxide analysis, in use from the time of endotracheal tube placement, is encouraged.
3. When ventilation is controlled by a mechanical ventilator, there shall be in continuous use a device that is capable of detecting disconnection of components of the breathing system. The device must give an audible signal when its alarm threshold is exceeded.
4. During regional anesthesia and monitored anesthesia care, the adequacy of ventilation shall be evaluated, at least, by continual observation of qualitative clinical signs.

CIRCULATION

Objective

To insure the adequacy of the patient's circulatory function during all anesthetics.

Methods

1. Every patient receiving anesthesia shall have the electrocardiogram continuously displayed from the beginning of anesthesia until preparing to leave the anesthetizing location. (*)
2. Every patient receiving anesthesia shall have arterial blood pressure and heart rate determined and evaluated at least every five minutes. (*)
3. Every patient receiving general anesthesia shall have, in addition to the above, circulatory function continually evaluated by at least one of the following: palpation of a pulse, auscultation of heart sounds, monitoring of a tracing of intraarterial pressure, ultrasound peripheral pulse monitoring, or pulse plethysmography or oximetry.

BODY TEMPERATURE

Objective

To aid in the maintenance of appropriate body temperature during all anesthetics.

Methods

There shall be readily available a means to continuously measure the patient's temperature. When changes in body temperature are intended, anticipated or suspected, the temperature shall be measured.

VI. REFERENCES

1. Goldman JM. A simple, easy, and inexpensive method for monitoring ETCO2 through nasal cannulae. Anesthesiology 67:606, 1987.
2. Whitby JD, Dunkin LJ. Temperature differences in the oesophagus. Preliminary study. Br J Anaesth 40:991–995, 1968.
3. Scamman FL. Accuracy of a central mass spectrometer system at high respiratory frequencies. Anesthesiology 65:A136, 1986.
4. Carbon Dioxide Monitors. Health Devices, Plymouth Meeting, Emergency Care Res Inst (ECRI), 15:255–285, 1986.
5. From RP, Scamman FL. Ventilatory frequency influences accuracy of end-tidal CO_2 measurements. Anesth Analg 67:884–886, 1988.
6. Lerou JGC, Egmond J, Kolmer HHB. Evaluation of long sampling tubes for remote monitoring by mass spectrometry. J Clin Monit 6:39–52, 1990.
7. Scamman FL, Fishbaugh JK. Frequency response of long mass spectrometer sampling catheters. Anesthesiology 65:422–425, 1986.
8. Urmey WF. Accuracy of expired carbon dioxide partial pressure sampled from a nasal cannula. I. Anesthesiology 68:959–960, 1988.
9. Dunphy JA. Accuracy of expired carbon dioxide partial pressure sampled from a nasal cannula. II. Anesthesiology 68:960–961, 1988.
10. Goldman JM. Reply. Anesthesiology 68:961–962, 1988.
11. Carlon GC, Kopec IC, Miodownik S, et al. Frequency response of the peripheral sampling sites of a clinical mass spectrometer. Anesthesiology 72:187–190, 1990.
12. Severinghaus JW. Water vapor calibration errors in some capnometers: Respiratory conventions misunderstood by manufacturers? Anesthesiology 70:996–998, 1989.
13. Penaz J. Photoelectric measurement of blood pressure, volume and flow in the finger. Digest 10th Int Con Med Biol Engr, Dresden, 104, 1973.
14. Wesseling KH, de Wit B, Settels JJ, Klawer WH. On the indirect registration of finger blood pressure after Penaz. Funkt Biol Med 1:245–250, 1982.
15. Molhoek PG, Wesseling KH, Settels JJM, et al. Evaluation of the Penaz servo-plethysmo-manometer for the continuous, noninvasive measurement of finger blood pressure. Basic Res Cardiol 79:598–609, 1984.
16. Wesseling KH, Settels JJ, van der Hoeven GMA, et al. Effects of peripheral vasoconstriction on the measurement of blood pressure in the finger. Cardiovasc Res 19:139–145, 1985.
17. Kurki T, Smith NT, Head N, et al. Noninvasive continuous blood pressure measurement from the finger: Optimal measurement conditions and factors affecting reliability. J Clin Monit 3:6–13, 1987.
18. Principles of Operation of the APM770 Blood Pressure Monitor. Cortronic Corporation. 1989.
19. Morris RH. Operating room temperature and the anesthetized, paralyzed patient. Arch Surg 102:95–97, 1971.
20. Severinghaus JW. Temperature gradients during hypothermia. Ann NY Acad Sci 80:515–521, 1959.
21. CO_2 Monitoring and Infection Control. Health Devices, Plym-

outh Meeting, ECRI, 15:272–273, 1986.
22. Gravenstein JS, Paulus DA, Feldman J, et al. Tissue hypoxia distal to a Penaz finger blood pressure cuff. J Clin Monit 1:120–125, 1985.
23. Smith NT, Wesseling KH, de Wit B. Evaluation of two prototype devices producing noninvasive, pulsatile, calibrated blood pressure measurement from a finger. J Clin Monit 1:17–29, 1985.
24. Schneider AJL, Apple HP, Braun RT. Electrosurgical burns at skin temperature probes. Anesthesiology 47:72, 1977.
25. Parker EO. Electrosurgical burn at the site of an esophageal temperature probe. Anesthesiology 61:93–95, 1984.

Section II

•

Respiratory Procedures

Chapter 4

•

Jeffery S. Vender, MD, FCCM
Mary V. Clemency, MD

Oxygen Delivery Systems, Inhalation Therapy, Respiratory Therapy

OUTLINE

I. INTRODUCTION

Many patients suffer from acute and chronic dysfunction of the cardiopulmonary system. Appropriate management of the surgical and critical care patient necessitates an understanding of both prophylactic and therapeutic techniques to support gas exchange and pulmonary function. Oxygen therapy is one of the most commonly employed medical interventions. An understanding of the oxygen delivery systems and devices is essential for optimal care. Bronchial hygiene is now a cornerstone in prophylactic care of the perioperative surgical patient. The bronchial hygiene techniques employed are supportive of the natural cough mechanism. Finally, many medications that are specifically intended to treat pulmonary pathophysiology can be delivered by inhalation therapy with both greater efficiency and less toxicity than oral or parenteral methods. This chapter is an overview of the various procedures and techniques employed in the respiratory care of our patients.

II. OXYGEN DELIVERY SYSTEMS

A. *Indications*

Oxygen is perhaps the most common drug used in anesthesia and critical care. The primary indication for oxygen therapy is to prevent or treat hypoxemia. Ultimately, the therapeutic goal is to prevent or correct tissue hypoxia. Hypoxia is oxygen deficiency at the tissue level. The most common cause of decreased oxygen tension (PO_2) in the peripheral tissues is decreased oxygen delivery (DO_2). Oxygen delivery depends on cardiac output (CO), hemoglobin concentration (Hgb), and arterial oxyhemoglobin saturation (SaO_2) according to the equation DO_2 (mL/min) = CO (mL/min) × Hgb (g/dL) × SaO_2 × 1.34 (mL/O_2/gHb). Hypoxia is possible if DO_2 is decreased because of depressed myocardial function, anemia, or hypoxemia or if cellular utilization is altered (eg, increased metabolic rate, cyanide poisoning). A balance must be maintained between tissue oxygen supply and demand. Supplemental oxygen may increase SaO_2, improving DO_2 until anemia is corrected or cardiac function improves.

Oxygen therapy plays its major and most effective role, however, in correcting hypoxemia. Hypoxemia is a relative deficiency of dissolved oxygen in the arterial blood. The most common causes of hypoxemia are decreased alveolar oxygen tension (P_AO_2), increased true shunt, and decreased mixed venous oxygen content. Hypoxemia due to a decreased P_AO_2 is significantly responsive to oxygen therapy.

Common causes of a decreased P_AO_2 include hypoventilation, low $\dot{V}/\dot{Q}$ mismatch, and breathing a diminished inspired oxygen fraction. Clinical conditions commonly associated with a decreased P_AO_2 include COPD, retained secretions, and mild pulmonary edema. Oxygen administration increases P_AO_2, which in turn increases arterial oxygen tension (P_aO_2) and SaO_2. Decreases in P_AO_2 are responsive to oxygen therapy. Even small increases in the F_IO_2 will improve hypoxemia due to a decreased P_AO_2.

With true intrapulmonary shunting, oxygen therapy is of limited benefit. The larger the shunt, the less responsive the hypoxemia is to an increase in F_IO_2. This problem is referred to as "refractory" to oxygen therapy. Therapy for this problem is usually aimed at methods of decreasing the shunt (eg, CPAP and removal of mucous plug).

Decreased mixed venous oxygen context ($C\bar{v}O_2$) can cause hypoxemia. This hypoxemia is due primarily to exaggerating the effects of a preexisting shunt by shunting more desaturated blood. Decreased $C\bar{v}O_2$ is due to a decreased arterial oxygen content, cardiac output, or increased oxygen consumption.

In addition to treating hypoxemia, oxygen therapy can be beneficial for decreasing myocardial work and the work of breathing. Hypoxemia is commonly associated with tachycardia and hyperventilation. Normalization of these compensatory mechanisms without any deterioration in oxygenation is often associated with oxygen therapy.

B. *Types of Oxygen Delivery Systems*

Almost all oxygen delivery systems are nonrebreathing gas systems that deliver the entire inspiratory atmosphere to the patient exclusive of any contribution from exhaled gases. Nonrebreathing systems eliminate exhaled carbon dioxide from the inspiratory gas system. To accomplish this, one-way valves to vent exhaled gases and inspiratory gas flow sufficient to meet peak flow rate and minute volume must be present. Various methods to meet ventilatory gas demands are available. The use of an inspiratory reservoir and one-way valves that allow for inspiratory entrainment of room air are typical of nonrebreathing systems.[2,13,25]

Nonrebreathing systems are divided into two types, low-flow–variable-performance systems and high-flow–fixed-performance systems, according to the manner in which each system meets the patient's inspiratory demands.

1. LOW-FLOW OXYGEN SYSTEMS

A low-flow–variable-performance system depends on room air (RA) entrainment to meet the patient's peak inspiratory and minute ventilatory demands that are not met by the inspiratory gas flow or oxygen reservoir alone. Low-flow devices include nasal cannulae, simple face masks, and tracheostomy collars. Low-flow systems are characterized by the ability to deliver high and low F_IO_2s and the ability to humidify inspired gases. These systems do not insure accuracy of the F_IO_2. The fraction of inspired oxygen (F_IO_2) becomes unpredictable and inconsistent when these devices are used for patients with abnormal or changing ventilatory patterns. Low-flow systems produce F_IO_2 ranging from 21% to 80%. The F_IO_2 may vary with the size of the oxygen reservoir, oxygen flow, and the patient's ventilatory pattern (eg, tidal volume, peak inspiratory flow, respiratory rate, and minute ventilation). With a normal ventilation pattern, these devices can deliver a predictable and consistent F_IO_2.

It is imperative to understand and appreciate the fact that low-flow systems do not mean low F_IO_2s. As stated, with changes in tidal volume, respiratory rate, oxygen reservoir size, and so on, the F_IO_2 can vary dramatically at comparable oxygen flow rates. The following is a theoretical mathematical estimate of an F_IO_2 produced by a low-flow system (eg, nasal cannula) in two different clinical conditions.

Example 1 is based on the textbook "normal" patient and ventilatory pattern. The following assumptions are used for the F_IO_2 calculation: the anatomic reservoir for a nasal cannula consists of nose, nasopharynx, and oropharynx and is approximately one-third of the entire normal anatomic dead space (includes trachea)—for example, 1/3 × 150 mL = 50 mL; a nasal cannula oxygen flow rate of 6 L/min (100 mL/sec); a tidal volume (V_T) of 500 mL; a respiratory rate of 20/min; inspiratory time of 1 sec; and expiratory time of 2 sec. If the terminal 0.5 sec of the 2-sec expiratory time has negligible gas flow, then the anatomic reservoir (50 mL) will completely fill with 100% oxygen, assuming an oxygen flow rate of (100 mL/sec).

Using the preceding "normal" variables, the F_IO_2 can be calculated for a 500-mL V_T, 1-sec inspiratory time as follows:

- 50 mL oxygen—anatomic reservoir (50 mL)
- 100 mL oxygen—oxygen flow rate 6 L/min (100 mL/sec)
- 70 mL oxygen—350 mL entrained room air (0.2 F_IO_2) = 0.2 × 350 mL = 70 mL oxygen

The total oxygen inspired contains 220 mL of 100% oxygen. Therefore, the F_IO_2 is 0.44 (220 mL O_2/500 mL V_T).

To show the marked variability in F_IO_2 with low-flow systems at similar oxygen flow rates, all the same assumptions will be used but the V_T will be decreased by 50% (250 mL). The final F_IO_2 is calculated as follows:

- 50 mL O_2—anatomic reservoir
- 100 mL O_2—oxygen flow rate 6 L/min (100 mL/sec)
- 20 mL O_2—100 mL entrained room air (0.2 F_IO_2) = 0.2 × 100 mL = 20 mL O_2

This total oxygen inspired (1 second) contains 170 mL of 100% oxygen. But with the reduction in tidal volume, the F_IO_2 is 0.68 (170 mL O_2/250 V_T).

This 50% variability in F_IO_2 at 6 L/min oxygen flow clearly demonstrates the effects of a variable ventilatory pattern. In general, the larger the V_T or faster the respiratory rate, the lower the F_IO_2. The smaller the V_T or lower the respiratory rate, the higher the F_IO_2. With a stable, unchanging ventilatory pattern, oxygen reservoir size and oxygen flow rate, low-flow systems can deliver relatively consistent F_IO_2s.

Low-flow oxygen devices are the most commonly employed oxygen delivery systems because of simplicity, ease of use, familiarity, economics, availability, and patient acceptance. In most clinical situations, unless contraindicated (see High Flow Systems and Devices), these systems should be used first.

2. HIGH-FLOW OXYGEN SYSTEMS

High-flow–fixed-performance systems are nonrebreathing systems that provide the entire inspiratory atmosphere needed to meet the peak inspiratory flow and minute ventilatory demands of the patient. To meet the patient's peak inspiratory flow, the flow rate and reservoir are very important. Flows in excess of 30–40 L/min (or four times the measured minute volume) are often necessary. In critically ill patients with strong ventilatory drives, peak flows far in excess of normal might be necessary to insure a constant F_IO_2. The system determines the inspired F_IO_2. These systems employ air entrainment devices or air–oxygen blenders to provide the desired F_IO_2 and required flow. High-flow devices include aerosol masks and T-pieces that are powered by air-entrainment nebulizers or air–oxygen blenders and Venturi masks (see Oxygen Delivery Devices). The advantage of high-flow systems is the ability to deliver predictable consistent and measurable high and low F_IO_2s, despite the patient's ventilatory pattern, and to control the humidity and temperature of the delivered gases. The primary limitations of these systems are economics, bulkiness, and patient tolerance.

There are three primary indications for high-flow oxygen devices:

1. Patients who require a consistent, predictable, minimal F_IO_2 to reverse hypoxemia yet prevent hypoventilation due to a dependence on hypoxic ventilatory drive benefit from high-flow oxygen devices.
2. The patient with increased minute ventilation and abnormal respiratory pattern needs a predictably and consistently high F_IO_2.
3. The critically ill patient requiring management in the intensive care setting often benefits in multiple ways (see Section II.A, "Indications").

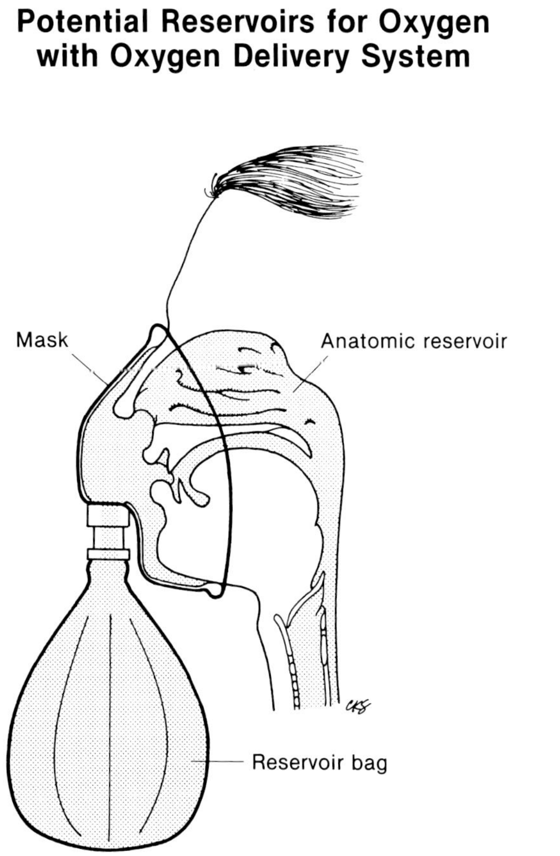

Figure 4–1 • The three reservoirs of low-flow oxygen therapy.

C. *Oxygen Delivery Devices*

1. Low-Flow Devices

a. Nasal Cannulae

Because of their simplicity and the ease with which patients tolerate them, nasal cannulae are the most frequently used oxygen delivery devices. This device consists of two prongs, one inserted into each naris, which deliver 100% oxygen. To be effective, the nasal passages must be patent, but the patient need not breathe through the nose. The flow rate settings range from 0.25 to 6 L/min. The nasooropharynx serves as the oxygen reservoir (Fig. 4–1). Gases should be humidified to prevent mucosal drying if the oxygen flow exceeds 4 L/min. For each 1-L/min increase in flow, the F_IO_2 is assumed to increase 0.04 (Table 4–1).

Thus, F_IO_2s of 0.24–0.44 can be delivered predictably if the patient breathes at a normal minute ventilation with a normal respiratory pattern. Increasing flows to >6 L/min will not significantly increase the F_IO_2 above 0.44 and is often poorly tolerated by the patient.

The components needed for nasal cannula assembly include nasal cannula prongs, delivery tubing, adjustable restraining headband, oxygen flowmeter to provide a controlled gas delivery from a wall outlet, and a humidifier, especially if flow rates are 4 L/min or more.

Procedurally, the initiation of any oxygen therapy should be preceded by a review of the chart, documentation of the oxygen concentration and device ordered, and an explanation to the patient of the oxygen delivery device. If a humidifier is used, it should be filled to the appropriate level with sterile water and connected to the flowmeter.

The nasal prong should be secured in the patient's naris and the cannula secured around the patient's head by a restraining strap.

Avoidance of undue cutaneous pressure is essential. Gauze may be needed to pad pressure points around the cheeks and ears during prolonged use. The flowmeter should be adjusted to the prescribed liter flow to attain the desired F_IO_2 (see Table 4–1).

Table 4-1 • Approximate F_IO_2 Delivered by Nasal Cannula*

Flow Rate (L/min)	Approximate F_IO_2
1	0.24
2	0.28
3	0.32
4	0.36
5	0.40
6	0.44

*Based on normal ventilatory patterns.

Although nasal cannulae are simple and safe, several potential hazards and complications do exist. All oxygen therapy is a fire hazard. Oxygen is not explosive, but it does support combustion. Nasal trauma from prolonged use or pressure from the nasal prongs can cause tissue damage. With poorly humidified high gas flows, dehydration of the airway mucosal surface can occur. This mucosal dehydration can result in mucosal irritation, nosebleeds, laryngitis, earache, substernal chest pain, and bronchospasms.[2,11,13] Finally, because this is a low-flow system, it is imperative to remember the F_IO_2 can be inaccurate and inconsistent, leading to the potential for under- and overoxygenation. This problem is of special concern with overoxygenation in COPD patients with increased hypoxic drive to breathe. Underoxygenation will potentiate any problems associated with hypoxemia.

b. Simple Face Mask

To provide a higher F_IO_2 than nasal cannula with low-flow systems, the size of the oxygen reservoir must increase (see Fig. 4–1). A simple face mask consists of a mask with two side-ports. The mask serves as an additional 100–200-mL oxygen reservoir. The side-ports allow RA entrainment and exit for exhaled gases. The mask has no valves. An F_IO_2 of 0.40–0.60 can be achieved predictably when patients exhibit normal respiratory patterns. Gas flows >8 L/min do not significantly increase the F_IO_2 above 0.60, because the oxygen reservoir is filled. A minimum flow of 5 L/min is necessary to prevent CO_2 accumulation and rebreathing. The actual delivered oxygen is dependent on altered ventilatory patterns similar to those of nasal cannulae.

The equipment needed is identical to that used for nasal cannula oxygen administration. The only difference is the use of a face mask. The predicted F_IO_2 can be estimated from the oxygen flow rate (Table 4–2). Appropriate mask application is needed with all masks to maximize the F_IO_2 and patient comfort. The mask should be positioned over the nasal bridge and on the forehead, restricting oxygen escape into the patient's eye, which can cause ocular drying and irritation. The use of face masks has the added risk of aspiration because of concealed vomitus. Appropriate positioning on a side or in the Fowler's position minimizes the risk, but close observation is essential to prevent this problem. If F_IO_2s above 0.60 are required, a partial rebreathing mask, nonrebreathing mask, or high-flow system should be employed. All oxygen devices that deliver higher F_IO_2s increase the potential of oxygen toxicity (see Complications).

c. Partial Rebreathing Mask

To deliver an F_IO_2 above 60% with a low-flow system, the oxygen reservoir system must be increased (see Fig. 4–1).[2] A partial rebreathing mask adds a reservoir bag with a 600–1000-mL capacity. Side-ports allow entrainment of RA and the exit of exhaled gases. The distinctive feature of this mask is that the first 33% of the patient's exhaled volume fills the reservoir bag. This volume is from the anatomic dead space and contains little carbon dioxide. During inspiration the bag should not completely collapse. A deflated reservoir bag will result in a decreased F_IO_2 because of entrained RA. With the next breath, the first exhaled gas (which is in the reservoir bag) plus fresh gas are inhaled—thus the name *partial rebreather.* Fresh gas flows should equal or exceed 8 L/min and the reservoir bag must remain inflated during the entire ventilatory cycle to insure the highest F_IO_2 and adequate carbon dioxide evacuation. F_IO_2 will vary, depending on the flow rate (Table 4–3). A F_IO_2 of 0.60–0.80+ can be delivered with this device if the mask is applied appropriately and the ventilatory

Table 4-2 • Approximate F_IO_2 Delivered by Simple Face Mask*

Flow Rate (L/min)	F_IO_2
5–6	0.4
6–7	0.5
7–8	0.6

*Based on normal ventilatory patterns.

Table 4–3 • Approximate F_IO_2 Delivered by Mask with Reservoir Bag*

Flow Rate (L/min)	F_IO_2
6	0.6
7	0.7
8	0.8
9	0.8+
10	0.8+

*Based on normal ventilatory patterns.

pattern is normal. This mask's rebreathing capacity allows oxygen conservation and thus may be useful during transportation, when oxygen supply may be limited. Complications with partial rebreathing oxygen delivery systems are similar to those with other low-flow systems mask devices.

d. Nonrebreathing Mask

A nonrebreathing mask (Fig. 4–2) is similar to a partial rebreathing mask but adds three unidirectional valves. One valve is located on each side of the mask to permit the venting of exhaled gases and prevent RA entrainment. The third unidirectional valve is situated between the mask and the reservoir bag and prevents exhaled gases from entering the bag.

The bag must be inflated throughout the ventilatory cycle to insure the highest F_IO_2 and adequate carbon dioxide evacuation. Typically, the F_IO_2 is 0.80–0.90+. Fresh gas flow is usually 15 L/min (range 10–15 L/min). If room air is not entrained, a F_IO_2 approaching 1.0 can be achieved. If fresh gas flows do not meet ventilatory needs, many masks have a spring-loaded tension valve that permits RA entrainment if the reservoir evacuates. This is often needed to meet the increased inspiratory drive of critically ill patients. This spring valve is often called a safety valve. The spring valve tension should be periodically checked. If such a valve is not present, one of the unidirectional valves on the mask should be removed to allow RA entrainment if needed to meet ventilatory demands. If the total ventilatory needs are met without RA entrainment, the rebreathing mask performs like a high-flow system.

The operational application of a nonrebreathing mask is similar to that of other mask devices. To optimize the system, the mask should fit snugly (without excessive pressure) to avoid air entrainment around the mask, which would dilute the delivered gas and lower the F_IO_2. If the mask fit is appropriate, the reservoir bag

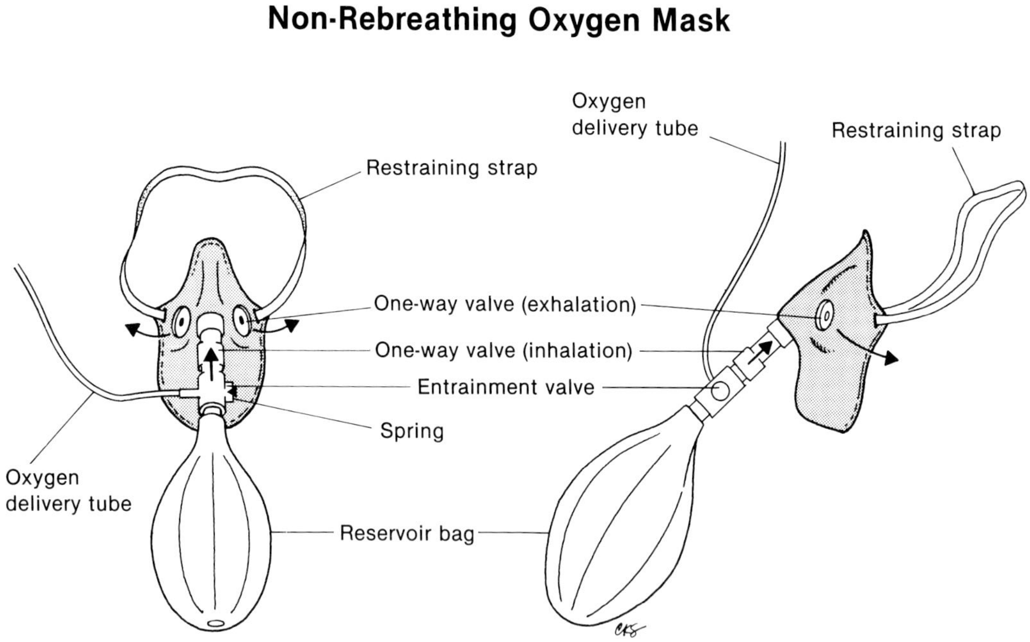

Figure 4–2 • A nonrebreathing oxygen mask. In addition to the exhalation valve, the mask has a one-way inhalation valve.

will respond to the patient's inspiratory efforts. The high flows often employed increase the potential for several problems. Gastric distention, cutaneous irritation, and distention of the venting valves in the open position allowing RA entrainment can all occur with excessive gas flows.

e. *Tracheostomy Collars*

Tracheostomy collars are used primarily to deliver humidity to patients with artificial airways. Oxygen may be delivered with these devices, but like the nasal cannula, the F_IO_2 is unpredictable, inconsistent, and dependent on ventilatory pattern.

2. HIGH-FLOW DEVICES

a. *Venturi Masks*

As discussed earlier, high-flow systems have flow rate and reservoirs large enough to provide the total inspired gases reliably. Most high-flow systems use gas entrainment to provide the flow and F_IO_2 needs. Venturi masks entrain air via the Bernoulli principle and constant pressure-jet mixing.[3] This physical phenomenon is based on a rapid velocity of gas (eg, oxygen) moving through a restricted orifice. This produces viscous shearing forces, which create a decreased pressure gradient (subatmospheric) downstream relative to the surrounding gases. This pressure gradient causes room air to be entrained until the pressures are equalized. Figure 4–3 illustrates the Venturi principle.

By altering the gas orifice or entrainment port size, the F_IO_2 will vary. The oxygen flow rate determines the total volume of gas provided by the device. It provides predictable and reliable F_IO_2s of 0.24–0.50 that are independent of the patient's respiratory pattern. These masks come in two varieties:

1. A fixed F_IO_2 model that requires specific inspiratory attachments that are color-coded and have labeled jets that produce a known F_IO_2 with a given flow.
2. A variable F_IO_2 model (Fig. 4–4) that has a graded adjustment of the air entrainment port that can be set to allow variation in delivered F_IO_2.

To use any air entrainment device properly to control the F_IO_2, the standard air–oxygen entrainment ratios and minimum recommended flows for a given F_IO_2 must be used (Table 4–4). The minimum total flow requirement should result from entrained RA added to the fresh oxygen flow and equal three to four times the minute ventilation. This minimal flow is required to meet the patient's peak inspiratory flow demands. As the desired F_IO_2 increases, the air–oxygen entrainment ratio decreases with a net reduction in total gas flow. Therefore, the higher the desired F_IO_2, the greater the probability of the patient's needs exceeding the total flow capabilities of the device.

Venturi masks are often useful when treating COPD patients who depend on hypoxic ventilatory drive and accurate F_IO_2s.[10] The Venturi mask's ability to deliver a high flow with no particulate H_2O makes it beneficial in treating asthmatics in whom bronchospasm may be precipitated or exacerbated by aerosolized H_2O administration.

Several specific concerns regarding the application of a Venturi mask must be recognized to provide appropriate function. Obstructions distal to the jet orifice can produce back-pressure and an effect referred to as ''Venturi-stall.'' When this occurs RA entrainment is compromised, causing a decreased total gas flow and an increased F_IO_2. Occlusion or alteration of the exhalation ports could produce this situation. Aerosol devices should not be used with these devices. Water droplets

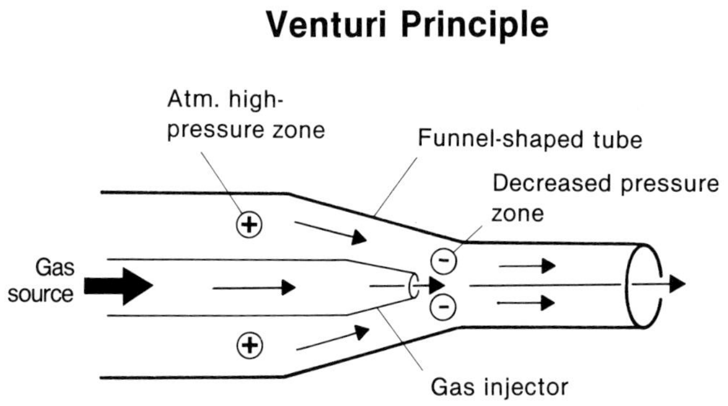

Figure 4–3 • Illustration of the Venturi effect.

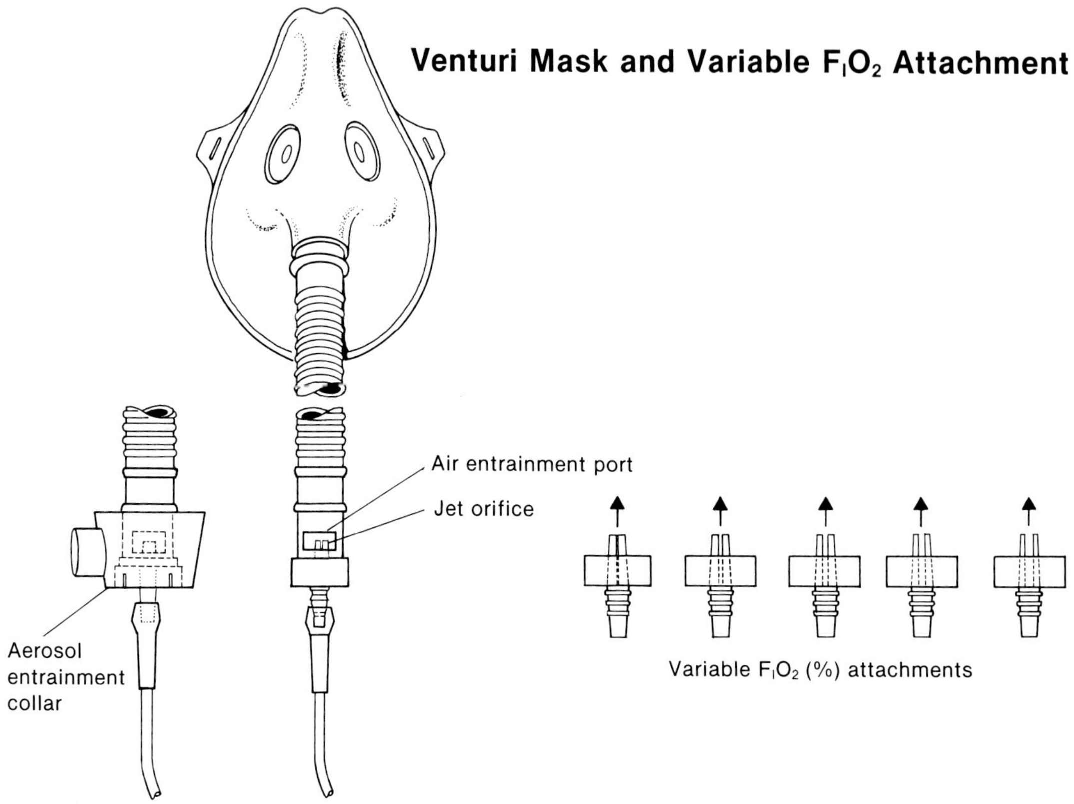

Figure 4–4 • Air entrainment Ventimask. Specific F_IO_2 levels are provided by the various jet orifices.

can occlude the oxygen injector. If humidity is needed, a vapor-type humidity adapter collar should be used.

b. Aerosol Masks/T-Pieces with Nebulizers or Air–Oxygen Blenders

F_IO_2s greater than 0.40 with a high-flow system are best provided by large-volume nebulizers and wide-bore tubing. Aerosol masks, in conjunction with air entrainment nebulizers or air–oxygen blenders, deliver consistent and predictable F_IO_2s regardless of the patient's ventilatory pattern. A T-piece is used in place of an aerosol mask for patients with an artificial airway.

Air entrainment nebulizers can deliver F_IO_2s of 0.35–1.00 and produce an aerosol. The maximum gas flow through the nebulizer is 14–16 L/min. Similar to the Venturi masks, less room air is entrained with higher F_IO_2s. As a result, total flow at high F_IO_2s is decreased. To meet ventilatory demands, two nebulizers may feed a single mask to increase the total flow, and a short length of corrugated tubing may be added to the aerosol mask side-ports to increase the reservoir capacity (Fig. 4–5). If the aerosol mist exiting the mask side-ports disappears during inspiration, room air is probably being entrained and flow should be increased.

Circuit resistance can increase from water accumulation or kinking of the aerosol tubing. The increased pressure at the Venturi device will decrease RA entrainment, increase F_IO_2, and decrease total gas flow. Thus, if a predictable F_IO_2 above 0.40 is desired, an air–oxygen blender should be used. Air–oxygen blenders can deliver consistent and accurate F_IO_2s from 0.21 to 1.0 and flows

Table 4–4 • Approximate Air Entrainment Ratio and Gas Flow (F_IO_2)*

F_IO_2 (%)	Ratio	Recommended O_2 Flow (L/min)	Total Gas Flow (to port) (L/min)
24	25.3:1	3	79
26	14.8:1	3	47
28	10.3:1	6	68
30	7.8:1	6	53
35	4.6:1	9	50
40	3.2:1	12	50
50	1.7:1	15	41

*Varies with manufacturer.

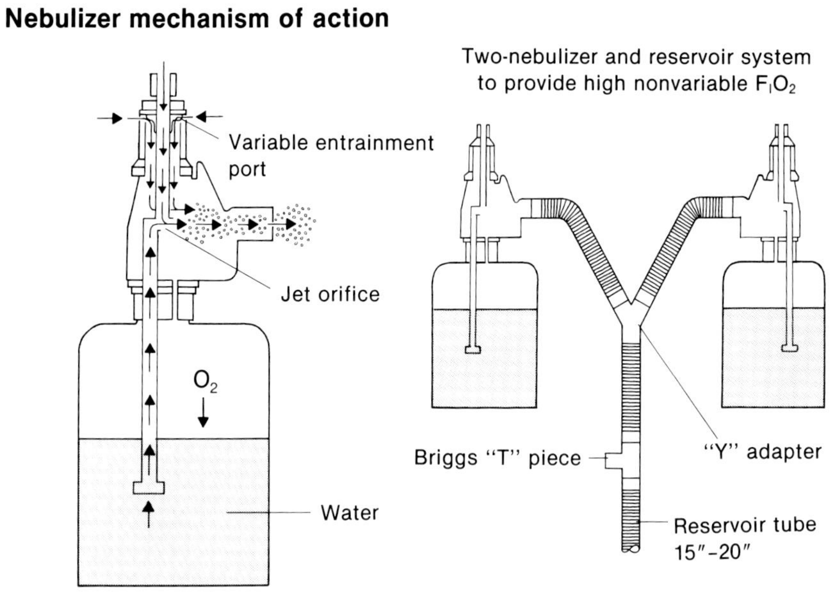

Figure 4–5 • Single- and double-(tandem) unit mechanical aerosol systems.

up to 100 L/min. The higher flows tend to produce excessive noise through the long-bore tubing. They usually are used in conjunction with humidifiers. Air–oxygen blenders are recommended for patients with increased minute ventilation who require a high F_IO_2 and for whom bronchospasm may be precipitated or worsened by a nebulized H_2O aerosol.

With artificial airway, a 15–20-in reservoir tube should be added to the Brigg T-piece to prevent the potential of entraining air into the system.

D. Humidifiers

Humidity is the water vapor in a gas. When it is 100% saturated at 37°C, air contains 43.8 mg H_2O/L. The amount of water vapor a volume of gas contains depends on the temperature. The vapor pressure exerted by the water vapor is equal to 47 mmHg. Alveolar gases are 100% saturated at 37°C. When the inspired atmosphere contains less than 43.8 mg H_2O/L or has a vapor pressure below 47 mmHg, a gradient exists between the respiratory mucosa and the inhaled gas. This gradient causes water to leave the mucosa and to humidify the inhaled gas.

Room air that has relative humidity of 50% at 21°C has a relative humidity of 21% at 37°C. Under normal conditions, the lungs contribute approximately 250 mL/H_2O/day to saturate inspired air 100%.

The administration of dry oxygen lowers the water content of the inspired air. The use of an artificial airway bypasses the nasopharynx and oropharynx, where a significant amount of warming and humidification of inspired gases is accomplished. As a result, oxygen administration and the use of artificial airways increase the demand on the lungs to humidify the inspired gases.

This increased demand ultimately leads to mucosal drying, inspissated secretions and decreased mucociliary clearance. To prevent these complications, a humidifier or nebulizer should be used to increase the water content of the inspired gases.

A humidifier increases the water vapor in a gas. This can be accomplished by passing gas over heated water (heated passover humidifier); by fractionating gas into tiny bubbles as gas passes through water (bubble humidifiers); by allowing gas to pass through a chamber that contains a heated, water-saturated wick (heated wick humidifier); and by vaporizing water and selectively allowing the vapor to mix with the inspired gases (vapor phase humidifier).

Bubble humidifiers can be used with nasal cannulae, simple face masks, partial and nonrebreathing masks, and air–oxygen blenders. They increase the relative humidity of gas from 0 to 70% at 25°C, which is approximately equal to 34% at 37°C.[4,5]

A heated humidifier should be used when delivering dry gases to patients with endotracheal tubes, as it allows delivery of gases with an increased water content and relative humidity exceeding 65% at 37°C. When heated humidifiers are used, proximal airway temperature should be monitored to insure a gas temperature that will allow maximum moisture-carrying capacity yet prevent mucosal burns.

A nebulizer increases the water content of the inspired gas by generating aerosols (small droplets of particulate water) of uniform size that become incorporated into the delivered gas stream and then evaporate into the inspired gas as it is warmed in the respiratory tract. There are two basic kinds of nebulizers, pneumatic and electric. Pneumatic nebulizers operate from a pressurized gas source and are either jet or hydro. Electric nebulizers are powered by an electrical source and are referred to as "ultrasonic." There are several varieties of both types of nebulizers, and they depend more on design differences than on the power source. A more in-depth discussion of nebulizers is available elsewhere.[2,11] The resultant humidity ranges from 50% to 100% at 37°C, depending on the device used. If heated, the relative humidity of the gas can exceed 100% at 37°C. Air entrainment nebulizers are used in conjunction with aerosol masks and T-pieces.

There are three general purposes for aerosol therapy. Like humidifiers, aerosol therapy increases the water content of the inspired gases. The aerosol increases the water content of desiccated and retained secretions enhancing bronchial hygiene. As used under inhalation therapy, aerosols can be used to deliver medications to the tracheobronchial tree. The success of aerosol therapy depends on proper technique of administration and an appropriate indication for use.

The aerosol generated by the nebulizer can precipitate bronchospasm of hyperactive airways.[2,13] Prophylactic bronchodilator therapy should be entertained prior to or during the aerosol treatment. Fluid accumulation and overload have been reported. This is more common in pediatrics and with continuous rather than intermittent therapy. Dry secretions are hydrophilic and can swell because of the absorbed water content. If secretions swell, they can obstruct airways. Mobilization of secretions will limit this problem. Therapeutic aerosols have been implicated in nosocomial infections.[12] Cross-contamination between patients must be avoided.

E. Manual Resuscitation Bags

Manual resuscitation bags are used primarily for resuscitation and manual ventilation of ventilator-dependent patients. These bags can deliver F_IO_2s above 0.90 and tidal volumes up to 800 mL when oxygen flows to the bag are 10–15 mL/min. Factors that promote the highest F_IO_2s include the use of an oxygen reservoir, connection to an oxygen source, and slow rates of ventilation that allow the bag to refill completely. Positive end-expiratory pressure valves (PEEP valves) should be used for patients who require more than 5 cm H_2O PEEP. Be aware of differing capabilities among various resuscitation bags in delivery of maximum F_IO_2.[6–8]

F. Complications

Complications related to oxygen delivery can be divided into two groups: complications related to the oxygen delivery systems (see sections that discuss the specific devices) and pathophysiologic complications related to oxygen therapy.

More common problems due to oxygen delivery devices include pressure sores on the cheek and the ears when using nasal cannulae, and on the nose when using a face mask; mucosal drying from high flows of dry gas; aspiration after vomiting into a face mask; and carbon dioxide rebreathing when masks are supplied with inadequate inspiratory flows. Careful surveillance and appropriate use of each device should prevent these complications. All oxygen therapy can support combustion and is a fire hazard.

Pathophysiologic complications related to oxygen therapy can lead to serious consequences. The three major complications encountered in adults are hypoventilation, absorption atelectasis, and oxygen toxicity.[2,11,14]

Hypoventilation that is related to oxygen therapy is peculiar to COPD patients who rely on hypoxic ventilatory drive. They typically have a chronically elevated arterial carbon dioxide tension (P_aCO_2), a normal pH, and a P_aO_2 usually below 60 mmHg. Because the increased P_aCO_2 is compensated by an increased bicarbonate ion concentration in the arterial blood and the cerebral spinal fluid, the patient may become desensitized to ventilatory stimulation from changes in the P_aCO_2. Instead, the chemoreceptors in the aortic and carotid bodies control ventilation. They are sensitive to P_aO_2 below 60 mmHg. When worsening hypoxemia is treated with supplemental oxygen, the goal is to raise the P_aO_2 just to the patient's chronic level. Thus, the minimum F_IO_2 needed to accomplish this goal should be delivered. If oxygen administration raises P_aO_2 to a level above the patient's chronic state (P_aO_2 55–60 mmHg), the patient's hypoxic drive will be blunted and hypoventilation will result. If hypoventilation is not reversed rapidly, respiratory failure necessitating mechanical ventilation will ensue.

Absorption atelectasis occurs when high alveolar oxygen concentrations cause alveolar collapse. Nitrogen, already at equilibrium, remains within the alveoli and "splints" alveoli open. When high F_IO_2s are administered, nitrogen is washed out of the alveoli, which then are filled primarily with oxygen. In areas of the lung with reduced ventilation–perfusion ratios, oxygen will be absorbed into the blood faster than ventilation can replace it. The affected alveoli become smaller and smaller until surface tension becomes so great as to cause their collapse. Progressively higher fractions of inspired oxygen above 0.50 cause absorption atelectasis in normal individuals. Fractions of inspired oxygen of 0.50 or more may precipitate this phenomenon in patients with decreased ventilation–perfusion ratios.

The third pathophysiologic complication of oxygen therapy, oxygen toxicity, becomes clinically important after 8–12 hours of exposure to high F_IO_2. Oxygen toxicity probably results from direct exposure of the alveoli to a high F_IO_2. Normal lungs appear to tolerate F_IO_2s of less than 0.6. In damaged lungs F_IO_2s greater than 0.50 can result in toxic alveolar oxygen concentration. As most oxygen therapy is delivered a 1 atm barometric pressure, the F_IO_2 and the duration of exposure become the determining factors in the development of most clinically significant oxygen toxicity.

The mechanism of oxygen toxicity is related to the significantly higher production of oxygen free radicals including superoxide anions (O_2^-), hydroxyl radicals (OH^-), hydrogen peroxide (H_2O_2), and single oxygen. These radicals affect cell function by inactivating sulfhydryl enzymes, disrupting DNA synthesis and disrupting cell membranes' integrity. Vitamin E, superoxide dismutase, and sulfhydryl compounds promote normal, protective free radical scavenging within the lung. During periods of lung tissue hyperoxia, these protective mechanisms are overwhelmed and toxicity results.[9]

The classical clinical manifestations of oxygen toxicity include cough, substernal chest pain, dyspnea, rales, pulmonary edema, progressive arterial hypoxemia, bilateral pulmonary infiltrates, decreasing lung compliance, and atelectasis. These signs and symptoms are nonspecific, and thus oxygen toxicity is frequently difficult to distinguish from severe underlying pulmonary disease. Often, only subtle progression of arterial hypoxemia heralds the onset of pulmonary oxygen toxicity.

Pathologically, there are two distinct phases of classical oxygen toxicity. The early, or exudative, phase, observed during the first 24–48 hours, is characterized by the destruction of type I pneumocytes and the development of interstitial and intraalveolar hemorrhage and edema. The late or proliferative phase, which begins after 72 hours, is characterized by resorption of early infiltrates, hyperplasia, and proliferation of type II pneumocytes and increased collagen synthesis. Once oxygen toxicity progresses to the proliferative stage, permanent lung damage may result from scarring and fibrosis.

The treatment for oxygen toxicity is prevention. Oxygen therapy should be directed at improving oxygenation with the minimum F_IO_2 needed to obtain an SaO_2 of greater than 90%. Inhalation treatments and raised expiratory airway pressure may be useful adjuncts in improving pulmonary toilet, decreasing $\dot{V}/\dot{Q}$ mismatch, and improving arterial oxygenation and may be used to maintain adequate oxygenation at a F_IO_2 of 0.50 or less.

III. TECHNIQUES OF RESPIRATORY CARE

The provision of adequate pulmonary gas exchange is implicit in our teaching and management of respiratory care. For optimal gas exchange to occur, the airways must be maintained clear of foreign material (secretions). The various therapeutic techniques available are aimed at the mobilization and removal of pulmonary secretions. In addition, various therapies are intended to optimize breathing efficiency.

Critically ill patients have multiple factors contributing to the presence of increased secretion. Alterations in the mucociliary escalator system due to smoking, stress, high F_IO_2s, anesthesia, foreign bodies in the trachea (eg, endotracheal tube), various tracheobronchial diseases, and abnormalities in mucus production are all recognized contributors to retention of airway secretions. To help compensate for these deficiencies, the patient must be able to promote an adequate cough. Unfortunately, in the critically ill patient or the individual with an artificial airway, an adequate cough is often absent. If any of these problems are present, there will be an increased tendency to retain secretions.

Retained secretions will promote several potential complications. Occlusion of the airway will promote ventilation–perfusion inequalities and eventually absorption atelectasis. This produces a progressively worse hypoxemia that is less responsive to oxygen therapy (see Section II.A). Retained secretions and distal airway occlusion will promote an increased incidence of stasis pneumonia. In addition, retained secretions will increase the patient's work of breathing due to an increased airway resistance associated with the airway inflammation and partial airway occlusion; and a reduced pulmonary compliance due to the atelectasis and reduced lung volumes.

Many of the fundamental practices of respiratory care are aimed at the provision of optimal airway care, tracheobronchial toilet, and the prevention and management of retained secretions. Because dehydration is a common cause of retained secretions, adequate hydration and humidification of gas delivery are essential. Humidity and aerosol therapy were discussed in the oxygen (gas) delivery section of this chapter. The remainder of this section will address other techniques commonly employed in respiratory care. These include airway suctioning, chest physical therapy, and incentive spirometry. Intermittent positive pressure breathing (IPPB) will be discussed separately, since it is used for both the promotion of tracheobronchial toilet and the delivery of medication (see Inhalation Therapy).

A. Suctioning

Airway suctioning is very commonly employed in respiratory care to promote optimal tracheobronchial toilet and airway patency in critically ill patients. Because of the "perceived" simplicity and limited complications, airway suctioning is frequently employed. Unfortunately, if proper indications and technique are not appreciated, the potential for significant complications does exist!

1. Indications

Suctioning of the airway should not be done without appropriate clinical indications. The audible (auscultatory) or visible presence of airway secretions is the most common indication. Increasing peak inspiratory pressures in mechanically ventilated patients are often indicative of retained secretions. "Routine" prophylactic suctioning is unwarranted except in neonates, where the small airway diameters can be acutely obstructed by a small accumulation of secretions.

In addition to removal of secretions, suction catheters are employed as aids in evaluating airway patency. If an artificial airway appears to be occluded, an attempt to pass a lubricated suction catheter can help assess airway patency. Several causes of artificial airway occlusion include mucus plugging, foreign body obstructions, kinking, and cuff herniations. If the suction catheter cannot be passed and ventilation is obstructed, several successive maneuvers are advisable. The cuff should be deflated and the airway repositioned; if improvement is inadequate, then the airway should be removed, adequate ventilation–oxygenation should be provided by air-mask-bag unit (AMBU), and the artificial airway should be replaced.

The actual provision of airway suctioning depends on an appreciation of the available equipment, the appropriate techniques, and the potential complications.

2. Equipment

Numerous commercial suction catheters exist.[2,13,16] The ideal catheter is one that optimizes secretion removal and minimizes tissue trauma. Several specific features of the catheters include the material of construction, frictional resistance, size (length and diameter), shape, and position of the aspirating holes. An opening at the proximal end of the catheter to allow the entrance of room air, neutralizing the vacuum without disconnecting the vacuum apparatus, is ideal. The proximal hole should be larger than the catheter lumen. Tracheal suctioning can occur only with occlusion of this proximal opening.

The conventional suction catheter has both side- and end holes (Fig. 4–6).

The Argyle Aero-Flo catheter provides a distal orifice, multiple side-holes, and a flared end. Report-

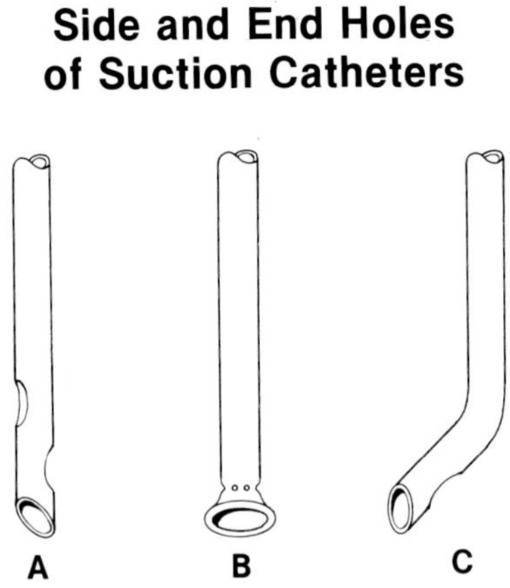

Figure 4–6 • Three suction catheters: (***A***) conventional catheter. (***B***) Argyle Aero-Flo catheter (distal orifice, multiple side-holes; flared end decreases tissue trauma but increases insertion difficulty). (***C***) Condé angle-tipped catheter (increases cannulation of left mainstem bronchus).

edly, this catheter is not as efficacious as the conventional one for removing secretions. The flared tip is to minimize tissue trauma, but it increases the overall catheter diameter, potentially making insertion more difficult and traumatic. Other catheters are designed with special anatomic or physiologic needs in mind. The Cordé angle-tipped catheter is shaped to increase the selective cannulation of the left mainstem bronchus. This is facilitated by turning the head to the right during suctioning. Newer systems have been developed to provide a "closed system" for suctioning. These self-contained catheters allow suctioning of the patient without discontinuation of mechanical ventilation. This can limit some of the complications associated with suctioning and ventilator disconnection.

The length of the typical catheter should pass beyond the distal tip of the artificial airway. The diameter of the suction catheter is very important. The optimal catheter diameter is approximately one-half the internal diameter of the artificial airway. Too large a catheter can produce an excessive vacuum and evacuation of gases distal to the tip of the airway, promoting atelectasis due to inadequate space for entrainment of air around the suction catheter. If too small a catheter is employed, removal of secretions can be compromised. To aid in determining the appropriate size of catheter (French sizes), one must convert the internal airway diameter (millimeters). The conversion can be approximated from:

3. TECHNIQUE

The technique of suctioning is very important for the optimal removal of secretions and limitation of complications. This is a "sterile" procedure necessitating appropriate care in handling the catheter. Gloves and hand washing are necessary, unless a closed system is employed. Other necessary equipment includes a vacuum source, sterile rinsing solution, AMBU-oxygen system, and lavage solution. The optimal vacuum pressure should be adjusted for age.

Prior to suctioning, the patient should be preoxygenated by increasing the F_IO_2 or manual resuscitator ventilatory assistance. This will minimize the hypoxemia induced by F_IO_2 disconnection and application of the suction vacuum. After preoxygenation, the sterile catheter is advanced past the distal tip of the artificial airway without the vacuum. When the catheter can no longer easily advance, it should be slightly withdrawn and intermittent vacuum pressure applied while the catheter is removed in a rotating fashion. This technique reportedly reduces mucosal trauma and enhances secretion clearance. The vacuum time should be limited to 10–15 seconds and discontinuation of ventilation and oxygenation should not exceed 20 seconds. After removal of the catheter, reoxygenation and ventilation are essential. Throughout the procedure, patient stability and tolerance should be monitored. If signs of patient distress or arrhythmia develops, immediately discontinue the procedure and reestablish oxygenation and ventilation. Suctioning is repeated until secretions have been adequately removed. After airway suctioning, oropharyngeal secretions should be suctioned and the catheter should be disposed.

Optimization of secretion removal necessitates adequate hydration and humidification of delivered gases. Occasionally, secretions can become quite viscous. Instillation of 5–10 mL of sterile normal saline can aid removal.

In critically ill patients, using a "closed-system" or swivel adapter to allow simultaneous suctioning and ventilation will limit the consequences of airway disconnection and enhance sterility. These disposable systems are usually more costly but are used for 24 hours.

When an artificial airway is absent, nasotracheal suctioning techniques are employed. This is technically less effective, is more difficult, and has the potential for additional complications. After appropriate lubrication, the catheter is inserted into a patient's nasal passage (often through a previously placed nasopharyngeal airway). The catheter is advanced into the larynx. Breath sounds from the proximal end of the catheter are often used as an audible guide. Upon entry into the larynx, the patient often coughs. The vacuum is connected and suctioning of the trachea is accomplished as previously described.

4. COMPLICATIONS

Complications of suctioning can be significant,[2,17] and to limit them proper technique must be followed. Although it is used to remove secretions, the suction vacuum will also remove oxygen-enriched gases from the airway. If inappropriately applied and monitored, suctioning can produce significant hypoxemia. The use of arterial oxygen monitors (eg, pulse oximetry) can often help detect alterations in arterial oxygenation (SaO_2) and heart rate and the presence of arrhythmias.

Cardiovascular alterations are common. Dysrhythmias and hypotension are the most frequent cardiac complications. Arterial hypoxemia (and eventually myocardial hypoxia) and vagal stimulation secondary to tracheal suctioning are two recognized precipatory etiologies for cardiovascular complications. In addition, coughing induced by stimulation of the airway can reduce venous return and ventricular preload. Avoidance of hypoxemia, prolonged suctioning (greater than 10 seconds), and appropriate monitoring will help reduce the incidence and significance of these complications.

As discussed earlier, inappropriate suction catheter size can produce an excessive evacuation of gas distal to the artificial airway because of inadequate space for proximal air entrainment. This will lead to hypoxemia and atelectasis. This is best avoided by reducing the catheter size to one-half the internal diameter of the airway. Pre- and postsuctioning auscultation of the lungs will help detect significant atelectasis. After suctioning, several hyperinflations of the lungs can help reinflate atelectatic lung segments.

Mucosal irritations and trauma are common with frequent suctioning. The incidence and severity of trauma depend on the frequency of suctioning; technique; catheter design; absence of secretions, allowing more direct mucosal contact; and amount of vacuum pressure applied. Blood in the secretions is usually the first sign of tissue trauma. Meticulous technique is essential to limit this very common complication.

Airway reflexes can be irritated by direct mechanical stimulation. Wheezing due to bronchoconstriction can necessitate bronchodilator therapy.

Nasotracheal suctioning can induce several additional complications. Nasal irritation, epistaxis, and laryngospasm are all noted complications. Laryngospasm can be life threatening if it is not recognized and appropriately managed.

B. *Chest Physical Therapy*

Chest physical therapy (CPT) techniques are an integral part of respiratory care. Chest physical therapy plays an important role in the provision of bronchial hygiene and optimization of ventilation. The mucociliary escalator systems and cough can be aided by adjunctive techniques. This section will discuss postural drainage techniques, percussion and vibration therapy, and incentive spirometry. Other breathing exercises and coughing techniques are covered in more extensive reviews of respiratory care.

1. Postural Drainage

The fundamental goal behind postural drainage is to move loosened secretions toward the proximal airway for eventual removal. Pulmonary drainage takes advantage of the fact that liquids flow in the direction of gravity. Flow of secretions is optimized by liquefaction (see Humidifiers).

The primary indications for pulmonary drainage are malfunctioning of normal bronchial hygiene mechanisms and excessive or retained secretions.[2,11,18,20] In patients with ineffective lung volumes and cough, pulmonary drainage can be used prophylactically to prevent accumulation of secretions. Several clinical conditions typically benefiting from pulmonary drainage are bronchiectasis, cystic fibrosis, COPD, asthma, lung abscess, spinal cord injuries, atelectasis, pneumonia, and healing after thoracic and abdominal surgery.

To administer postural drainage appropriately, the practitioner must be able to visualize the location of the involved lung segments and the proper position to optimize drainage into the proximal airway. The lungs are divided into lobes, segments, and subsegments (Table 4-5).

Precise anatomic descriptions of the various pulmonary subsegments and positions are beyond the scope of this section. The large posterior and superior basal segments of the lower lobe are commonly involved in hospital patients with atelectasis and pneumonia. In the typical hospital patient, these segments are most gravity dependent, causing stasis of secretions. (Fig. 4-7).

Table 4-5 • Lung Segments

Left	Right
Upper lobe	***Upper lobe***
Apical	Apical-posterior
Posterior	Anterior
Anterior	
Middle lobe	***Lingula***
Lateral	Superior
Medial	Inferior
Lower lobe	***Lower lobe***
Superior	Superior
Medial basal	Anterior basal
Anterior basal	Lateral basal
Lateral basal	Posterior basal
Posterior basal	

Dependent Lung Segments

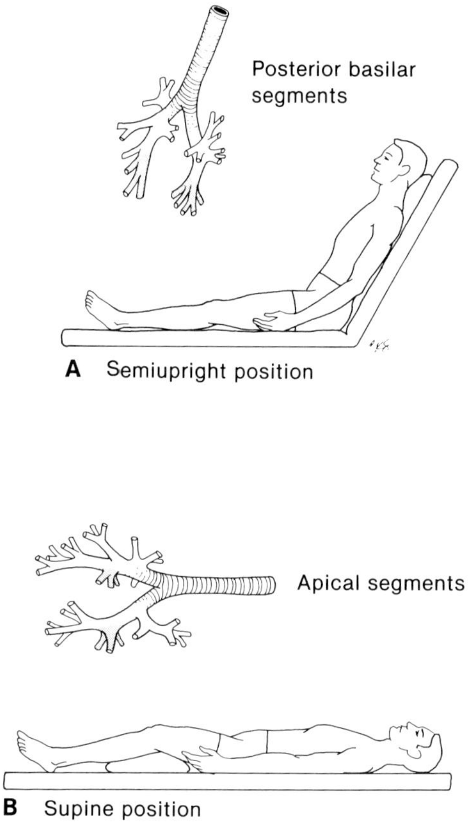

Figure 4–7 • Lung segments typically at risk for retained secretions, atelectasis, and pneumonia due to body position during convalescence. (***A***) Posterior basilar segment of the lower lobe. (***B***) Apical segment of the lower lobe.

Appropriate patient positioning can enhance gravitational flow. Commonly employed positions for postural drainage are demonstrated in Fig. 4–8.

Postural drainage should be done several times per day. For optimal results, postural drainage should follow humidity treatments and other bronchial hygiene therapies. Postural drainage should precede meals by 30–60 minutes, and the treatment should not exceed 30 minutes.

Postural drainage can produce physiologic and anatomic stresses that are potentially detrimental to specific patients.[19] Alterations in the cardiovascular system from abrupt changes in position are well recognized. Hypotension or congestive heart failure due to changes in preload can be induced by positional change. Ventilation–perfusion relationships are altered by changes in position. Ideally, if the diseased pulmonary segment is positioned to optimize pulmonary drainage (uppermost position), blood will preferentially flow to the gravity-dependent, nondiseased segments, improving the ventilation–perfusion relationships. The head-down position, which is commonly used, is best avoided in patients with the intracranial disease. The decreased venous return from the head could increase intracranial pressure.

Continual assessment of patient tolerance during the procedure is necessary. Vital signs, oxygenation monitoring, general appearance, level of consciousness, and subjective comments by the patient are all part of the appraisal process.

Postural Drainage: Use of Various Positions to Drain Different Segments

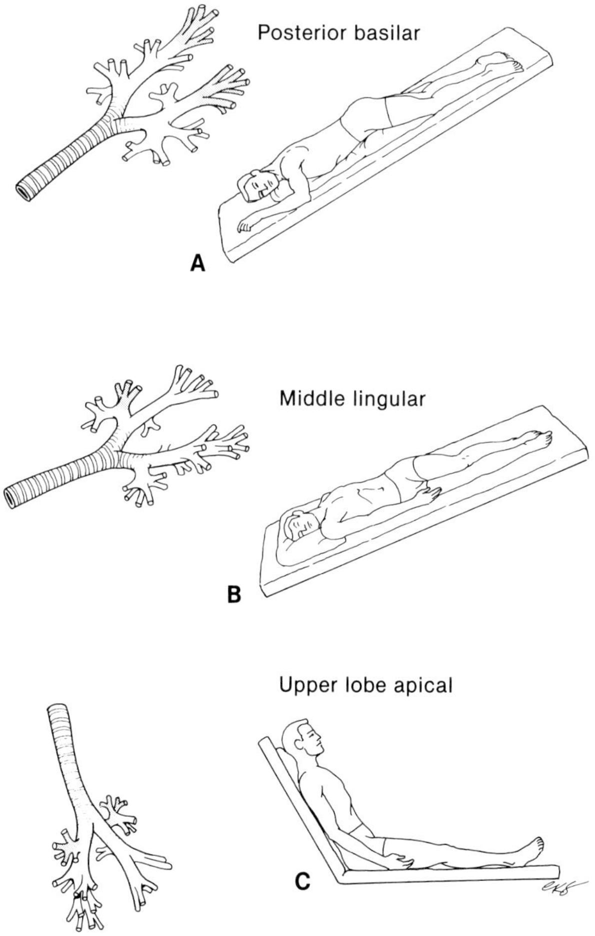

Figure 4–8 • Common position for optimizing postural drainage of the posterior basilar (***A***), middle lingular (***B***), and upper lobe apical (***C***) segments.

2. Percussion and Vibration Therapy

Percussion and vibration therapy are used in conjunction with postural drainage to loosen and mobilize secretions that are adherent to the bronchial walls.[2,21] Percussion involves a manually produced, rhythmic vibration of varying intensity and frequency. In a "clapping" (cupped hands) motion, a blow is delivered during inspiration and expiration over the affected area while in the appropriate position for postural drainage (Fig. 4–9).

Mechanical energy is produced by compression of the air between the cupped hand and the chest wall. Proper percussion should produce a popping sound (similar to striking the bottom of a ketchup bottle). Proper force and rhythm can be accomplished by placing the hands no further than 5 inches from the chest and then alternating a flexing and extending of the wrists (similar to a waving motion). The procedure should last 5–7 minutes per affected area.

Like all respiratory care, percussion therapy should not be performed without a medical order. Therapy should not be performed over bare skin, surgical incisions, bony prominences, kidneys, and female breasts or with hard objects. If a stinging sensation or reddening of the skin develops, the technique should be reevaluated.

Chest Percussion with Cupped Hand-Clapping Motion

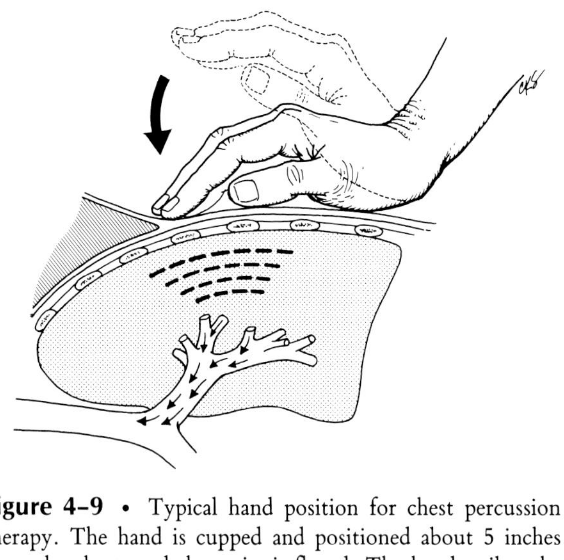

Figure 4–9 • Typical hand position for chest percussion therapy. The hand is cupped and positioned about 5 inches from the chest, and the wrist is flexed. The hand strikes the chest in a waving motion.

Special care must be given to the "fragile" patient. Fractured ribs, localized pain, coagulation abnormalities, bony metastases, hemoptysis, and empyemas are relative contraindications for percussion therapy.

Vibration therapy is used to promote bronchial hygiene in a fashion similar to chest percussion. Manually or mechanically gentle vibrations are transmitted via the chest wall to the affected area during exhalation. Vibrating frequencies in excess of 200/min can be achieved if the procedure is done correctly. In patients receiving IPPB, all chest physical therapy procedures should be performed during the IPPB.

3. Incentive Spirometry

In the 1970s, alternative methods for prophylactic bronchial hygiene were developed to replace the more costly and controversial use of IPPB. Incentive spirometry (IS) was developed after several techniques utilizing expiratory maneuvers (eg, blow and glove bottles) and carbon dioxide–induced hyperventilation were found either to be clinically ineffective or to cause other risks.[2,11,13]

Incentive spirometry was developed with an emphasis on sustained maximal inspiration (SMI). Normal spontaneous breathing patterns have periodic hyperinflations that prevent the alveolar collapse associated with shallow tidal ventilation breathing patterns. Narcotics, sedative drugs, general anesthesia, cerebral trauma, and abdominal or thoracic surgery can all promote shallow tidal ventilation breathing patterns. Complications from this breathing pattern include atelectasis, retained secretions, and pneumonia.

The physiologic principle of SMI is to produce a maximal transpulmonary pressure gradient by generating a more negative intrapleural pressure. This pressure gradient produces alveolar hyperinflation with maximal air flow during the inspiratory phase.[23]

The indications for IS and SMI are primarily related to bronchial hygiene. These techniques should be employed perioperatively in surgical patients at an increased risk of pulmonary complications. Incentive spirometry involves the patient in their care and recovery, which can be psychologically beneficial while also being cost advantageous relative to the equipment and personal costs associated with other forms of respiratory care (eg, IPPB).

The goals of IS and SMI therapy are to optimize lung inflation to prevent atelectasis; optimize the cough mechanism by providing larger lung volumes; and provide a baseline standard to assess the effectiveness of therapy or detect the onset of acute pulmonary disease (as noted by a deteriorating performance). To optimally achieve these goals necessitates patient instruction and supervision. It is now well recognized that preoperative education enhances the effectiveness of postoperative bronchial hygiene therapy (eg, IS and SMI). The purpose of IS and SMI is not to replace an adequate cough and deep-breathing regimen, but to provide the tool to support the patient who for various reasons is ineffective in spontaneous ability to provide bronchial hygiene. Appropriate instruction for proper breathing techniques can help produce an effective cough mechanism.

Various models of incentive spirometers are clinically available.[11] The devices vary in how they function, guide the therapy, or recognize the achievements. Each manufacturer provides instructions for use that should be followed. The devices are aimed at generating the largest inspiratory volumes over 5–15 seconds. The actual device used or rate of flow is not as important as the frequency of use and the attainment of maximal inspiratory volumes and sustained inspiration. Certain devices can give feedback that could be confusing to the patient. Maximal benefit with most devices can only be achieved with user education. This education is the shared responsibility of all those who are caring for patients at risk of compromised bronchial hygiene.

The administration of IS and SMI therapy necessitates a physiologically and emotionally stable patient. Patient cooperation and motivation are very important. To be optimally effective, the patient should be free of acute pulmonary disease and have a forced vital capacity of more than 15 mL/kg and a spontaneous respiratory rate of less than 25/min. The actual therapy follows an explanation of the device, why the therapy is needed, and the techniques to attain optimal benefit. Therapy should be done every waking hour. Typically, the patient should do four to five SMIs at a 30–60-second interval. The patient should be coached to inspire slowly while attaining maximal inspiratory volumes.

Periodic assessment of performance is necessary. Although the effectiveness of IS and SMI for therapeutic bronchial hygiene is undetermined, it appears to be a very cost-effective technique for prophylactic bronchial hygiene.

There are no significant complications associated with IS and SMI therapy. The only contraindications are patients who are uncooperative, physically disabled with acute pulmonary disease, or unable to generate minimum volumes for lung inflation (eg, 12–15 mL/kg).

C. *Intermittent Positive Pressure Breathing*

In the past four decades, very few respiratory care therapies have been as controversial as intermittent positive pressure breathing (IPPB).[2,11,13,25] Objective data assessing therapeutic benefit relative to cost and alternative therapies have been less than confirmatory.[23,24] Numerous conferences have been sponsored by medical organizations to evaluate literature supporting and opposing IPPB. The inconclusive result of these efforts has significantly reduced (and in some situations, eliminated) the use of IPPB. Alternative techniques (previously discussed) have been substituted. The present use of IPPB appears to be restricted to practitioners, who prescribe it with specific indications and goals in mind. This section is intended to define IPPB, recognize its indications, and describe the technique of administration and potential side-effects and complications. An extensive historical and in-depth analysis of IPPB controversies is beyond the scope of this section.

1. INDICATIONS

Intermittent positive pressure breathing is the therapeutic application of inspiratory positive pressure to the airway and is distinctly different from intermittent positive pressure ventilation (IPPV) or other means of prolonged and continuous ventilation.

The clinical indications of IPPB are subjective and unproven. It is easier to assess IPPB if the indications are described as clinical goals. The fundamental basis and singular goal of IPPB is to provide larger tidal volume (V_T) than the spontaneously breathing patient, in a physiologically tolerable manner. If this goal is achieved, IPPB could be employed to (1) improve and promote the cough mechanism; (2) improve distribution of ventilation; and (3) enhance delivery of inhaled medications.

Bronchial hygiene can be compromised in patients with a reduced or inadequate cough mechanism. An adequate vital capacity (15 mL/kg) is necessary to generate the volume and expiratory flow needed to produce an effective cough. Although IPPB can increase V_T significantly, effectiveness will still depend on the pressure and flow patterns generated, as well as on an understanding of cough technique. Therefore, if cough is improved, one can indirectly see the benefit of IPPB for removal of secretions and limiting complications associated with this problem.

The increased V_T produced by IPPB can be used to improve the distribution of ventilation. If areas of hypoventilation exist, the increase in V_T could improve ventilation to perfusion mismatch. As in most respiratory care therapies, the efficacy depends on the underlying patient's condition, patient selection, optimal technique, and frequency of application. Continual assessment of the therapy is mandatory. Theoretically, if ventilation increases, atelectasis could be prevented or treated.

Pulmonary care often uses inhalation therapy for therapeutic administration of medications. The beneficial effects of these pharmacologic agents often necessitate a reasonable distribution of ventilation. In patients unable to provide an adequate inspiratory volume, IPPB can enhance drug delivery and distribution. Where the patient is capable of an adequate cough and spontaneous deep breath, a hand nebulizer is as efficacious as IPPB. IPPB is rarely used solely for delivery of medication. If spontaneous V_T is inadequate for drug delivery, the cough mechanism and distribution of ventilation are also compromised.

2. Administration

Similar to all respiratory care therapies, IPPB necessitates a medical order. The effectiveness of IPPB depends upon the individual administering the therapy.[11] It is incumbent for that individual to (1) understand the appropriate operation maintenance and clinical application of the mechanical device employed; (2) select the appropriate patient; (3) provide the necessary patient education to optimize the effort; (4) assess the effectiveness relative to goals and indications; and (5) identify complications or side-effects associated with the therapy.

The basic concepts and components of IPPB machines are well described in the literature. The generic device uses a gas pressure source, a main control valve, a breathing circuit, and an automatic cycling control. Typically, IPPB is delivered via a pressure-cycled ventilator. Positive pressure (eg, 30–50 cm H_2O) is used to expand the lungs. To be effective, the increase in V_T from the IPPB treatment must exceed the patient's limited spontaneous vital capacity by 100%. A prolonged inspiratory effort to the preset pressure limit should be emphasized. Therapy is typically 6–8 breaths/min, lasting a total of 10 minutes.

Keys to successful therapy include: (1) machine sensitivity to the patient's inspiratory effort; (2) a tight seal between the machine and patient, since these are pressure-limited devices; (3) a progressive increase in the inspiratory pressure as tolerated by the patient in an effort to achieve a desired exhaled volume; and (4) a cooperative, relaxed, and well-educated patient. The patient should be monitored for efficacy, intolerance, and complications of therapy.

The physiologic side-effects and complications associated with IPPB are well described in the literature.[11] The incidence and significance of these problems depend on the individual patient and administrator. If understood and recognized, many of the reported problems can be prevented or readily reversed.

Both hyperventilation and variable oxygenation can result from IPPB therapy. Hypocarbia due to an increased V_T and respiratory frequency can produce altered electrolytes (K^+), dizziness, muscle tremors, and tingling and numbness of the extremities. Proper patient instruction and a 5–10-minute rest period after therapy can minimize this problem. Hypoxemia and hyperoxia due to inaccurate F_IO_2s can be a concern in patients dependent on "hypoxic respiratory drive" (carbon dioxide retainers).

The use of IPPB can increase mean intrathoracic pressure, resulting in a decreased venous return. Like other forms of positive pressure ventilation, a decreased venous return (preload) can produce a decreased cardiac output and subsequent vital sign changes (hypotension, tachycardia). In addition to cardiovascular changes, IPPB can impede venous drainage from the head. This is a potential but limited concern in patients with intracranial pressure, if IPPB is appropriately administered in the sitting position.

Barotrauma is a concern with all forms of positive pressure ventilation (PPV). The exact etiologic mechanism of PPV in the development of pneumothorax and ruptured lobes is unclear. Clearly, PPV results in increased intrapulmonary volume and pressure, but these same conditions tend to promote a better cough mechanism that causes sudden marked changes in pressure and lobe rupture. Any chest pain complaints must be evaluated to rule out barotrauma prior to proceeding with an IPPB treatment.

Other reported complications include, but are not limited to, gastric insufflation and secondary nausea and vomiting, psychological dependency, nosocomial infections, altered airway resistance, and adverse reactions to administered medications. The incidence and significance of these adverse effects are often the result of inappropriate administration, patient noncompliance, and simple lack of attention to detail. Some of the complications are due to patient selection. Asthmatics reportedly tolerate IPPB poorly and have an increased airway resistance and higher incidence of barotrauma. Often effective goal achievement (improved cough) results in complications. As noted, barotrauma and even hemoptysis have been attributed to the production of an improved cough mechanism.

There are few definite contraindications to IPPB. Relative contraindications of IPPB are focused on its lack of documented efficacy. Untreated pneumothorax is a definite contraindication to IPPB. Good clinical contraindications are lack of a definite indication for IPPB or an available, less expensive alternative therapy.

IV. INHALATION THERAPY

Inhalation therapy is often used synonymously with the term *respiratory care.* In a general context, inhalation therapy can be thought of as the delivery of gases for ventilation and oxygenation, as aerosol therapy, or as a means of delivering therapeutic medications.

Therapeutic aerosols have been used for centuries. Simple vaporization of water has long been a remedy for the common cold. Therapeutic aerosols have been employed in the treatment of pulmonary patients with bronchospastic airway disease, chronic obstructive pulmonary disease, and pulmonary infection. The basic goals of aerosol therapy are to improve bronchial hygiene, humidify gases delivered through artificial airways, and deliver medications. The first two goals were discussed earlier in this chapter.

The advantages to delivering drugs by inhalation are multiple. Easier access, rapid onset of action, reduced extrapulmonary side-effects, reduced dosage, coincidental application with aerosol therapy for humidification, and psychological benefits have all been cited.[2,11,13] In the nonintubated patient, aerosol therapy necessitates patient cooperation. Often, skilled help and complex special equipment are necessary. The equipment is a potential source of nosocomial infections.[12] Aerosol therapy has many of the same disadvantages noted with humidification. Although drug usage is often reduced, precise titration and dosages are difficult because of variable degrees of drug deposition in the airway.

This section will provide an overview of inhalation pharmacology. The basic principles, devices for medication delivery, and specific pharmacologic agents employed will be discussed. For a more comprehensive topic review and specific drug information, one should refer to available reference texts.

A. *Basic Pharmacologic Principles*

The basic pharmacology of inhalation therapy necessitates a brief pharmacologic review. A medication is a drug that is given to elicit a physiologic response and is used for therapeutic purposes. Unfortunately, undesired responses (side-effects) are also produced. The medication can interact with receptors by direct application (topical effect) or absorption into the bloodstream.

Various routes of pharmacologic administration are used for respiratory care. Subcutaneous, parenteral, gastrointestinal, and inhalation administrations are all commonly employed in the management of pulmonary diseases. Inhalation therapy employs the increased surface area of the lung parenchyma as a route of medication administration. This necessitates the drug reaching the alveolar and tracheobronchial mucosal surfaces for systemic capillary absorption.

Although inhaled medications can have topical effects, the primary reasons for the inhalation of medications is convenience, a safe method for self-administration, and maximal pulmonary benefit with reduced side-effects. If the drug depends on systemic absorption, the drug's distribution and blood concentration are important. Blood concentration is altered by several mechanisms, such as dosage, route of administration, absorption, metabolism, and excretion. Alteration in liver and kidney function can produce unexpected drug levels and side-effects.

If multiple drugs are employed for respiratory care, various drug interactions can occur. *Potentiation* is the result of one drug with limited activity changing the response of another drug; *synergism* is two drugs with similar action resulting in a greater response than the sum of the individual drugs. If the response of the two drugs is the sum of the individual medications, they are *additive. Tolerance* necessitates increasing drug levels to elicit a response, and *tachyphylaxis* results in the inability of larger doses to produce the expected response. Finally, the nomenclature for drug dosages should be understood. Two common methods expressing drug dosage are *ratio strength* (drug dilutions) and *percentage strength* (percent solutions). The following facts are necessary to understand this often confusing topic. A *solution* is a homogeneous mixture of two substances. A *solute* is the dissolved drug, and a *solvent* is the fluid in which the drug is dissolved. A gram of water equals 1 mL of water and 1 g equals 1000 mg. *Ratio strength* is expressed in terms of parts of solute to the total parts of solvent (or grams of solute/grams of solvent). A 1:1000 solution is 1 g of a drug in 1000 g of solvent (or 1000 mg/1000 mL = 1 mg/1 mL). *Percent strength* is expressed as the number of parts of solute in 100 parts of solvent (or grams of solute/100 g of solvent). A 1% solution is 1 g of drug in 100 g of solvent.

B. Aerosolized Drug Delivery Systems

Therapeutic aerosols are commonly employed in respiratory care. As stated earlier, inhalation delivery of drugs can often produce therapeutic drug effects with reduced toxicity. The effectiveness of aerosols is related to the amount of drug delivered to the lungs. Actual pulmonary deposition of aerosolized drugs is a result of drug sedimentation due to gravity, inertial impact due to airway size, and directional change of air flow and kinetic energy.[2] Aerosol delivery also depends on particle size, pattern of inhalation, and degree of airway obstruction. Particle size should be smaller than 5 μm; otherwise, the upper airway is not penetrated. The route of administration is preferably through the mouth, since the nose acts as a barrier. The ideal pattern of inhalation should be large volume, slow inspiration (5–6 seconds), and accentuated by an inspiratory hold (10 seconds). If airway obstruction is significant, adequate deposition of drugs can be limited. If the obstruction is not relieved, larger dosages or increased frequency of administration could be necessary. The most common methods for aerosolized drug delivery are metered-dose inhalers (MDI), gas-powered nebulizers, and IPPB (discussed earlier).

The MDI is a convenient and commonly employed method of aerosolized drug delivery (Fig. 4–10).[11,13] These prefilled drug canisters are activated by manual compression and deliver a predetermined unit (metered) of medication. Appropriate instruction is necessary for optimal utilization.[27] With the canister in the upside-down position, the device should be compressed only once per inhalation. The patterns of inhalation should be as described earlier. It is imperative that the tongue not obstruct flow, but it is controversial whether the device should be placed in the mouth or held several centimeters from the lips with the mouth wide open. If multiple doses are prescribed, an interval of several minutes between puffs is advisable.

Several problems with MDI drug delivery have been previously recognized. Manual coordination is necessary to activate the canister. Arthritis can cause difficulty, as can misaiming the aerosol. Pharyngeal deposition can lead to local abnormalities (eg, oral candidiasis secondary to aerosolized steroids). Systemic effects due to swallowing the drug can be reduced if the pharynx is rinsed after inhalation to reduce pharyngeal deposition.[13] The newer MDI devices have been designed to reduce some of these problems.

The gas-powered nebulizers can be hand-held or placed in line with the ventilatory circuit (Fig. 4–11).[11,13] The hand-held devices are typically employed on more acutely ill individuals and as an alternative to an MDI. The full hand-held system uses a nebulizer, a

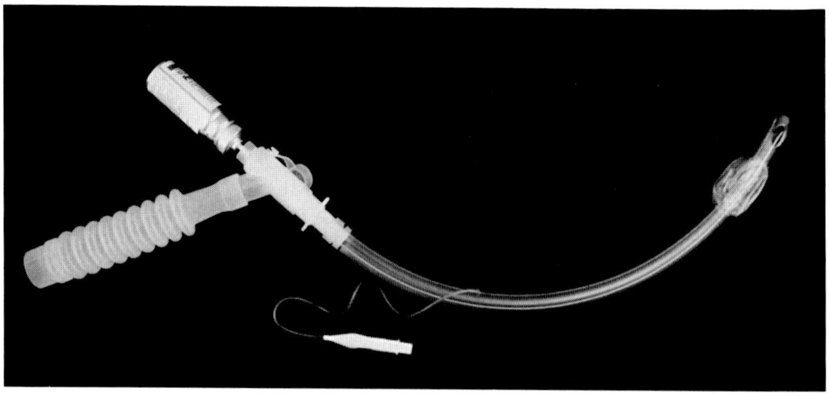

Figure 4–10 • Metered dose inhaler.

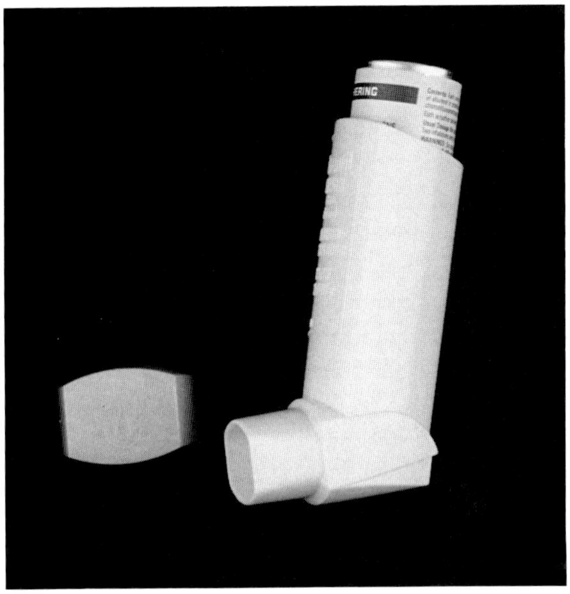

Figure 4–11 • Hand-held nebulizer.

pressurized gas source, and a mouthpiece or face mask. The mouthpiece is preferable, since some drugs could be deposited in the lung.

These systems are more expensive, cumbersome, and often less efficient than MDIs. Supervision is usually necessary for appropriate drug preparation and administration. Typically, the drug is diluted in saline. The drug is usually more concentrated, since a majority of the drug is never aerosolized or is lost during exhalation. Only the drug that is inspired could reach the lung.

The total volume to be nebulized is usually 4–6 mL (see Pharmacologic Agents) at gas flows of 6–8 L/min (device dependent). The treatment time is usually 5–10 minutes. During the course of treatment, the patient's vital signs and subjective tolerance must be monitored. Aerosolization of medication for drug delivery is different from aerosol therapy for humidification (see Humidifiers).

Both the MDI and the gas-powered nebulizers can be used in-line with an artificial airway and/or ventilator circuit (Fig. 4–12). The drug delivery system is positioned in the inspiratory limb, as proximal to the artificial airway as possible. In-line drug delivery is usually less efficient in ventilated patients than in spontaneously breathing, nonintubated patients because of the breathing pattern, drug deposition on the endotracheal tube, and airway disease.

C. *Pharmacologic Agents*

Numerous drugs are used in the management of pulmonary diseases. Nebulized (aerosolized) drug delivery is commonly employed to improve mucociliary clearance (mucokinetics) and relieve bronchospastic airway disease. The major drugs employed for inhalation therapy can be categorized by their ability to affect these two issues. In addition, certain antiinflammatory, antiasthmatic drugs are given by aerosol. The following reviews some of the commonly employed *aerosolized* drugs and is not meant to be a comprehensive review of respiratory

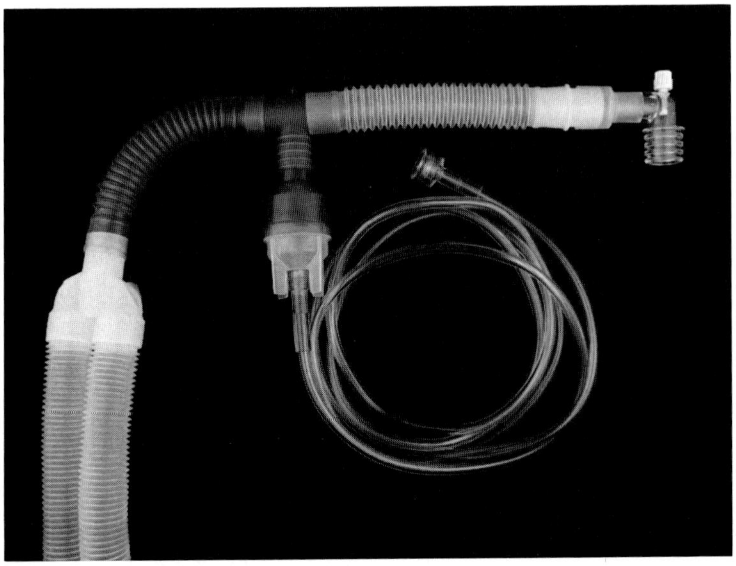

Figure 4–12 • In-line metered dose inhaler.

pharmacology. All listed dosages are meant to be representative for adult patients (if needed, specific product literature should be referred to, prior to use).

1. Mucokinetic Drugs

Mucokinetic drugs are employed to enhance mucociliary clearance. These agents can be classified according to their mechanism of action. Hypoviscosity agents are the most commonly employed mucokinetic agents. Saline, sodium bicarbonate, and alcohol are the specific agents most commonly used. The mechanism of action for each drug varies but tends to effect mucus viscosity by disrupting the mucopolysaccharide chains that are the primary composition of mucus. The other category of mucokinetic aerosol agents is made up of the mucolytics. The following is a brief synopsis of the various drugs in these two groups.[26]

a. Hypoviscosity Agents

Saline is the most commonly employed mucokinetic agent. It can be used as a primary drug or solvent. The mechanism of action is reduced viscosity by dilution of the mucopolysaccharide strands. The indication for use is thick, tenacious mucus secretions. The typical concentration is 0.45% to 0.9% NaCl. The two major side-effects associated with aerosolized saline are overhydration and the promotion of bronchospasm in patients with hyperactive airway disease (especially in newborns).

Alcohol (ethyl alcohol, ethanol) decreases the surface tension of pulmonary fluid. The typical concentration is 30% and the dosage is 4–10 mL. The primary indication is pulmonary edema. This agent should be administered by side arm nebulization or IPPB, but not as a heated aerosol. The contraindication is a hypersensitivity to alcohol or its derivative. Side-effects include airway irritation, bronchospasm, and local dehydration.

b. Mucolytic Agents

Acetylcysteine 10% (Mucomyst) is an effective mucolytic. The mechanism of action is the lysis of the disulfide bonds in mucopolysaccharide chains reducing the viscosity of the mucus. The indication is the management of viscous, inspissated, mucopurulent secretions. The actual effectiveness in the treatment of mucostasis is inconclusive, and each individual must be monitored to determine the benefit of therapy. The usual dosage is 2–5 mL every 6 hours. Hypersensitivity is a contraindication. In general, acetylcysteine is relatively nontoxic. Side-effects include unpleasant taste and odor, local irritation, inhibition of ciliary activity, and bronchospasm. For these reasons, pretreatment with a bronchodilator is recommended. Other reported side-effects include nausea, vomiting, stomatitis, rhinorrhea, and generalized urticaria. Acetylcysteine is incompatible with several antibiotics. The drug should be avoided or used with extreme caution in patients with bronchospastic airway disease. Other special concerns are a need for refrigeration, reactivity with rubber, and limited use after opening (96 hours).[25]

2. Bronchodilators and Antiasthmatic Drugs

Acute and chronic bronchospastic airway diseases afflict many individuals. Many drugs, varying primarily by their mechanism of action and route of delivery, are available to manage this problem. This section will deal only with aerosolized drugs that are commonly employed in the therapy of bronchospastic airway disease[32] (Table 4–6).[28,29] The drug groups will be divided by their mechanism of action: sympathomimetics, anticholinergics, steroids, and cromolyn. A comprehensive review of these drugs, the various mechanisms for bronchodilation, and the management of specific pathophysiologic problems is beyond the scope of this chapter.

a. Sympathomimetics

Sympathomimetics include the beta-adrenergic agonists and methylxanthines (not available in aerosol). The primary mechanism of action of the beta-adrenergic agonists is to stimulate the enzyme adenyl cyclase to increase the conversion of adenosine triphosphate (ATP) to cyclic adenosine monophosphate (cAMP). The cAMP causes bronchial smooth muscle relaxation and inhibits antigen-induced release of medicators that induce some of the pathophysiologic responses seen in allergic asthma. In general, the response of sympathomimetic drugs is classified according to whether the effects are alpha, beta-1, or beta-2. Beta-2 receptors are responsible for bronchial smooth muscle relaxation. The common side-effects associated with beta-adrenergic agonists are due to their additional beta-1 and alpha effects. Beta-1 effects cause an increase in heart rate, arrhythmias, and cardiac contractility; alpha effects increase vascular tone. Potent beta-2 stimulants can produce unwanted symp-

Table 4–6 • Aerosolized Bronchodilators and Antiasthmatic Drugs

Sympathomimetics (Trade)	Method	Dosages*	Mechanism
Isoetharine hydrochloride 1%	Nebulized	0.25–0.5 mL in 4.0 mL	Beta-2 agonist increase in cyclic AMP
(Bronkosol)	MDI	2 puffs (340 μg/puff) q.i.d.	
Metaproterenol sulfate 5%	Nebulized	3.0 mL in 2.5 mL	
(Alupent)	MDI	2 puffs (0.65 mg/puff) q.i.d	
Albuterol	MDI	2 puffs (90 μg/puff) q.i.d.	
(Ventolin, Proventil)	Nebulized	2.5–5 mg in 4 mL q.i.d.	
Racemic epinephrine 2.25% (Vaponepherine)	Nebulized	0.5 mL in 3.5 mL	Weak beta-2 and mild alpha mucosal vasoconstrictor
Isoproterenol (0.5%)	Nebulized	0.25–0.5 in 3.5 mL	Prototype beta-agonist
Isuprel	MDI		Significant beta-1 side effects
Anticholinergic			
Ipratropium bromide	MDI	2 puffs (18 μg/puff) q.i.d.	Cholinergic blocker increasing beta stimulation
Antiallergy Agents			
Cromolyn sodium 1%	Nebulized	20 mg q.i.d. in 2–4 mL	Suppression of mast cell response to Ag–Ab reactions
(Intal)	MDI	2 puffs (800 μg/puff) q.i.d.	Used prophylactically
Beclomethasone acetonide (Vanceril, Beclovent)	MDI	2 puffs (42 μg/puff) q.i.d.	Antiinflammatory Inhibit leukocyte migration Potentiate effects of beta-agonists
Dexamethasone sodium phosphate (Decadron)	Nebulized	0.25 mL (1 mg) in 2.5 mL	

*Dosages may vary – references to specific drug inserts are recommended.

toms: anxiety, headache, nausea, tremors, and sleeplessness. Prolonged utilization can lead to receptor down-regulation and reduced drug response. Ideally, the more pure the beta-2 response, the better the therapeutic benefit relative to side-effects. The following sympathomimetics are commonly employed in clinical practice.[2,13,23,25]

Isoetharine hydrochloride 1% (Bronkosol) is available in a 1% solution. Its primary action is beta-2 with weak beta-1 (therapeutic doses) and no alpha effects. The nebulized dosage is usually 0.25 to 0.5 mL in 4.0 mL normal saline. The bronchodilatory effects are weaker than isoproterenol and last 1–3 hours. The drug is available in an MDI. Typical dosage of the MDI is two puffs (340 μg/puff) four times a day.

Metaproterenol sulfate 5% (Alupent) is very similar to isoetharine, but the duration of action is approximately 5 hours. The dosage is 0.3 mL (5%) in 2.5 cc normal saline. Metaproterenol is available in an MDI.

Albuterol (Ventolin, Proventil) is a newer sympathomimetic agent available in an MDI. It is a strong beta-2 with limited beta-1 properties. Its beta-2 duration of action is approximately 6 hours.

Racemic epinephrine 2.25% (Vaponephrine) is a mixture of levo and dextro isomers of epinephrine. It is a weak beta and mild alpha drug. The alpha effects provide mucosal constriction. In the aerosol form, this drug acts as a good mucosal decongestant. The drug does have minimal bronchodilatory action. Cardiovascular side-effects are limited. Typical dosage is 0.5 mL (2.25%) in 3.5 mL saline, given as frequently as every hour in adult patients. Racemic epinephrine is commonly mixed with 0.25 mL (1 mg) dexamethasone for the management of postextubation swelling and croup.

Isoproterenol (Isuprel) is the prototype pure beta-adrenergic bronchodilator. Bronchodilation depends on adequate blood levels. In addition, isoproterenol is a pulmonary and mucosal vascular dilator. This causes an increased rate of absorption, higher blood levels, and increased beta-1 side-effects. These side-effects can be quite significant and often reduce the utilization of this agent in patients with cardiac disease; arrhythmias, myocardial ischemia, and palpitations can all occur. If the pulmonary vasculature vasodilates to areas of low ventilation, then the potential to augment ventilation–perfusion mismatch and increase intrapulmonary shunt exists. Typical dosage is 0.25 to 0.5 mL (0.5%) in 3.5 mL saline. The effect lasts 1–2 hours. Isoproterenol is also available as an MDI.

b. *Anticholinergic Agents*

Anticholinergic drugs play an increasing role in the management of bronchospastic pulmonary disease. These drugs inhibit acetylcholine at the cholinergic receptor site, reducing vagal nerve activity. This produces bronchodilation (preferentially in large airways) and a reduction in mucus secretion. Major side-effects include dry mouth, blurred vision, headache, tremor, nervousness, and palpitations.

Ipratropium bromide (Atrovent) is a newer commercially available anticholinergic. Its effects are primarily beta-2. It is available as an MDI. The standard dosage is 36 μg, q.i.d (18 μg/puff). Hypersensitivity to the drug is a contraindication. Caution should be exercised in patients with narrow angle glaucoma.

c. *Antiallergy and Asthmatic Agents*

The two main groups of aerosolized agents in this category are cromolyn and steroids. These drugs are often used in concert with other medications.

Cromolyn sodium 1% (Intal) is primarily used prophylactically to prevent bronchospasm in exercise-induced asthma.[13] The drug is not effective in the management of acute bronchospasm. The mechanism of action is suppression of mast cell response to antigen–antibody reactions. Cromolyn sodium is available in a powder (spinhaler), liquid, and MDI for inhalation therapy. The typical dosages are 20 mg q.i.d. via nebulizer or 2 puffs q.i.d. (800 μg/puff) with the MDI. The MDI appears to be tolerated best. Hypersensitivity is a contraindication. Side-effects include local irritation, allergic symptoms—rash, urticaria—and airway hyperactivity (most common with the powder).

Steroids are commonly used for maintenance therapy in patients with chronic asthma.[30,31] The mechanism of action is attributed to their antiinflammatory properties, reducing leakage of fluids, inhibiting migration of macrophages and leukocytes, and possibly blocking the response to various mediators of inflammation. Recently, steroids have been reported to potentiate the effects of the sympathomimetic drugs.[13]

Dexamethasone sodium phosphate (Decadron) is the prototypic steroid for respiratory care. It is used most often for its antiinflammatory action and for postextubation with racemic epinephrine. The typical dosage is 0.25 mL (1 mg) in 2.5 mL saline. The side-effects of steroids are related to their chronicity of use and degree of systemic absorption. Because of its systemic effects, dexamethasone is used on a limited basis as an aerosol.

Beclomethasone acetonide (Vanceril, Baclovent) is an aerosolized steroid that is highly active topically and that has limited systemic absorption or activity. The typical dosage is 2 puffs (42 μg/puff) t.i.d. or q.i.d. Hoarseness, sore throat, and oral candidiasis are reported side-effects. The candidiasis can be managed with topical antifungal drugs. Mild adrenal suppression is reported with high doses and caution is advised when switching from oral to inhaled steroids.

The preceding pharmacologic agents are representative of those commonly employed by aerosol in respiratory care. Other drugs (eg, antiviral and antibiotic drugs) are beyond the scope of this chapter. Appropriate pharmacologic management necessitates assessing response to therapy. Objective and subjective relief of symptoms and improvement in pulmonary function while minimizing side-effects of these drugs are the endpoints of good inhalation therapy.

V. References

1. American College of Chest Physicians—Heart, Lung and Blood Institute. National Conference on Oxygen Therapy. Chest 85:234–247, 1984.
2. Shapiro BA, Harrison RA, Kacmarek RM, Canc RD. Clinical Application of Respiratory Care. Chicago, Year Book Medical Publishers, Inc., 1985.
3. Scacci R. Air entrainment masks: Jet mixing is how they work; The Bernoulli and Venturi Principles are how they don't. Respir Care 24:928–931, 1979.
4. Klein EF, Shah DA, Shah NJ, Modell JH, Desautels D. Performance characteristics of conventional and prototype humidifiers and nebulizers. Chest 64:690–696, 1973.
5. Hall TO. Aerosol generators and humidifiers. In Barnes TA (ed). Respiratory Care Practice. Chicago, Year Book Medical Publishers, Inc., 1988, 356–404.
6. Carden E, Friedman D. Further studies of manually operated self-inflating resuscitation bag. Anesth Analg 56:202–206, 1977.
7. Barnes TA, Watson ME. Oxygen delivery performance of four adult resuscitation bags. Respir Care 27:139–146, 1982.
8. Barnes TA, Watson ME. Oxygen delivery performance of old and new designs of the Laerdal, Vitalograph and AMBU adult manual resuscitators. Respir Care 28:1121–1128, 1983.

9. Deneke SM, Fanburg BL. Normobaric oxygen toxicity of the lung. N Engl J Med 303:76–86, 1980.
10. Gibson RL, Comer PB, Beckham RW, et al. Actual tracheal oxygen concentrations with commonly used oxygen equipment. Anesthesiology 44:71, 1976.
11. Burton GL, Hodgkin JE (eds). Respiratory Care, 2nd ed. Philadelphia, JB Lippincott, 1984.
12. Craven DE, Goulartet A, Maki BJ. Contaminated condensate in mechanical ventilator circuits. A risk factor for nosocomial pneumonia? Am Rev Respir Dis 129:625–628, 1984.
13. Kacmarek RM, Stoller JK (ed). Current Respiratory Care. Toronto: BC Decker, 1988.
14. Fisher AB. Oxygen therapy: Side effects and toxicity. Am Rev Respir Dis 122:61, 1980.
15. Marini JJ. Postoperative atelectasis: Pathophysiology, clinical importance, and principles of management. Respir Care 29: 516–522, 1984.
16. Chapman GA, Kim CS, et al. Evaluation of the safety and efficiency of new suction catheter design. Respir Care 31:889–895, 1986.
17. Demers RR. Complications of endotracheal suctioning procedures. Respir Care 27:453–457, 1982.
18. Harris JA, Jerry BA. Indications and procedures for segmental bronchial drainage. Respir Care 20:1164, 1975.
19. Tyler ML. Complications of positioning and chest physiotherapy. Respir Care 27:458, 1982.
20. Zadai CL. Physical therapy for the acutely ill medical patient. Phys Ther 61:1746–1754, 1981.
21. Radford R. Rational basis for percussion—augmented mucociliary clearance. Respir Care 27:556, 1982.
22. Martin RJ, Roger RM, Grant BA. The physiologic basis for the use of mechanical aids to lung expansion. Am Rev Respir Dis 122:105–107, 1980.
23. Ziment I. Why are they saying bad things about IPPB? Respir Care 18:677, 1973.
24. Murray JF. Review of the state of the art of intermittent positive pressure breathing therapy. Am Rev Respir Dis 110:193, 1974.
25. Eubanks DH, Bone, RC. Comprehensive Respiratory Care. St Louis, CV Mosby, 1985.
26. Barton AD. Aerosolized detergents and mucolytic agents in the treatment of stable chronic obstructive pulmonary disease. Am Rev Respir Dis 110:104–110, 1974.
27. Self TH, Brooks JB. Necessity of teaching patients correct bronchodilator inhalation technique. Immunol All Pract 4:40–44, 1982.
28. Weinberger M, Hendeles L, Ahrens R. Pharmacologic management of reversible obstructive airway disease. Med Clin North Am 65:529, 1981.
29. McFadden RR. Aerosolized bronchodilators and steroids in the treatment of airway obstruction in adults. Am Rev Respir Dis 122:89, 1980.
30. Morse HG. Mechanisms of action and therapeutic role of corticosteroids and asthma. J Allergy Clin Immunol 75:1–14, 1985.
31. Newhouse MT, Dolovich MB. Control of asthma by aerosols. N Engl J Med 315:870–874, 1986.

Chapter 5

•

John P. McGee II, MD
Jeffery S. Vender, MD, FCCM

Nonintubation Management of the Airway

OUTLINE

I. Introduction

A patent airway is the first principle of resuscitation and life support, and airway management is an essential skill for those caring for critically ill patients. Respiratory care, nursing, intensive care, and emergency room physicians should all be competent in the essentials of airway care.

Too frequently, inexperienced personnel believe airway care necessitates intubation of the trachea. The focus of this chapter is on the nonintubation skills and tools of airway care. Airway care can be divided into the establishment and maintenance of the airway and of breathing (respiratory support). Airway establishment and maintenance are achieved by anatomic manipulation of the head and neck or the use of artificial airway devices. Respiratory support techniques control the atmosphere the patient breathes and allow for manual ventilatory assistance.

A. *Airway Anatomy*

Nonintubation airway management is dependent on the patency of the oropharynx, nasopharynx, and larynx. A thorough understanding of airway anatomy is necessary to appreciate the therapeutic maneuvers and devices employed in airway care (Fig. 5–1). Very detailed reviews of airway anatomy can be found in various atlases and texts.[1–3]

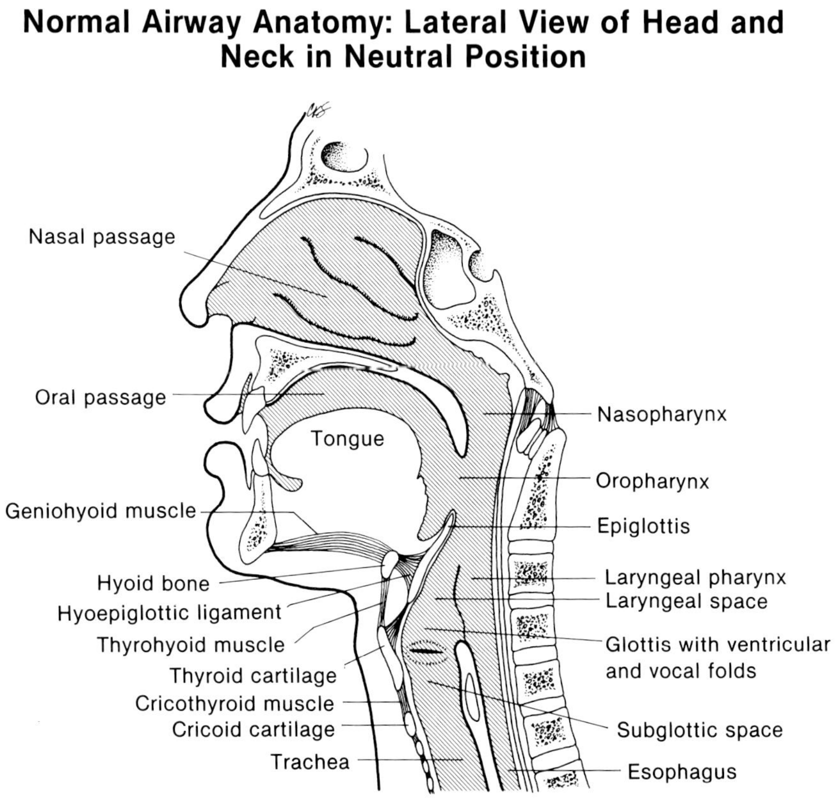

Figure 5–1 • Normal airway anatomy: lateral view of head and neck in neutral position. The various sections of the airway are labeled. Note that (1) the tongue could easily obliterate the airway at the oropharynx by falling backward; (2) the muscular line from mentum to hyoid bone (geniohyoid muscle) to thyroid cartilage (thyrohyoid muscle and membrane) to cricoid (cricothyroid muscle) has a folded and right-angled character. This line can be straightened by extending the head and pulling the jaw forward (anteriorly), thus pulling the epiglottis and tongue away from the posterior pharyngeal wall.

Gas passes to the larynx by two routes. One is through the nares, warmed and humidified by the turbinates, into the nasopharynx via the choanae, to the oropharynx, laryngopharynx, and larynx. The nasal passages can be obstructed by choanal atresia, septal deviation, mucosal swelling, or foreign material (eg, mucus, blood). The other route is through the mouth, between the palate and tongue to the oropharynx, laryngopharynx, and larynx. The common pathway, the oropharynx and laryngopharynx, can be occluded by a relaxed tongue and epiglottis protruding posteriorly and caudad against the inferior pharyngeal constrictor and the laryngeal introitus. Airway manipulations and devices can treat this cause of obstruction fairly efficiently in most cases. Laryngeal obstruction due to spasm must be treated by positive airway pressure, deeper anesthesia, muscle relaxants, or endotracheal intubation.

Laryngeal closure can occur from intrinsic or extrinsic muscles of the larynx. Tight airway closure (laryngospasm, effort closure) is accomplished by the external laryngeal muscles forcing the mucosal folds of the quadrangular membrane into apposition by contracting the cylindrical section of airway from the hyoid bone to the cricoid cartilage (Fig. 5–2). Muscle groups also extend from the thyroid cartilage to the hyoid and cricoid. During their contraction the interior mucosae and soft tissue are forced into the center of the airway (ventricular and vocal folds), and the thyroid shield is deformed (compressed inward), providing a spring to rapidly open the airway once these muscles relax.[1] The larynx closes at the level of the true cords by action of the intrinsic muscles of the larynx (especially interarytenoid and cricothyroid) during phonation, but this closure is not so tight as the laryngeal spasm referred to earlier.

Opening the larynx is achieved by elongating and unfolding the airway section from hyoid to cricoid cartilage.[1,3] Muscles tether the hyoid bone and the tongue to the chin (geniohyoid, digastric, hyoglossus, and genioglossus). Other muscles tether the cricoid and thyroid to the sternum and first ribs (sternothyroid). The "strap muscles" tether the hyoid bone to the sternum and rib (sterno- and omohyoid). When the head is tilted to extend the chin and the mandible is displaced forward on the temporomandibular sliding joint (a jaw-thrust maneuver), maximum stretch occurs at the hyoid–thyroid–cricoid area. The hyoid bone is pulled anteriorly along with the epiglottis and root of the tongue, opening up the oropharynx. The ventricular and vocal folds flatten against the sides of the thyroid, opening the laryngeal airway.

The inferior and middle constrictors close the superior part of the esophagus (cervical sphincter), thus preventing regurgitation. Muscle relaxants often will open the airway by relaxing the intrinsic and extrinsic laryngeal muscles closing the airway, but they will also relax the pharyngeal constrictors, permitting regurgitation (and aspiration) if gas has been forced into the stomach during attempts at ventilation or if the patient has an incompetent lower esophageal sphincter mechanism (hiatus hernia, achalasia, esophageal dysmotility). These two problems, airway patency versus airway protection, represent the major dilemma of airway management without an endotracheal tube.

B. *Upper Airway Obstruction*

Upper airway obstruction is a common airway emergency necessitating nonintubation airway manipulation and airway devices. Soft tissue obstruction of the pharynx and larynx are the usual causes of upper airway obstruction. Lower airway obstruction is not dealt with in this chapter.

The causes of soft tissue upper airway obstruction at the pharynx include hypopharyngeal obstruction due to loss of muscle tone from a central nervous system abnormality (anesthesia, trauma, coma), expanding space-occupying lesions (tumor, mucosal edema, hematoma), and foreign substances (teeth, vomitus, foreign body). Laryngeal obstruction is most often related to increased muscle activity from attempted vocalization or a reaction from foreign substances (secretions, foreign bodies, tumors). Recognition of upper airway obstruction is essential and is dependent on observation, suspicion, and clinical data.

The presentation of airway obstruction can be partial or complete. Partial airway obstruction is recognized by noisy inspiratory sounds. Depending on the magnitude, cause, and location of the obstruction, the tone of the sounds can vary. Snoring is the typical sound of partial airway obstruction in the hypopharynx. Stridor or crowing suggest glottic (laryngeal) obstruction or laryngospasm. In addition, signs and symptoms of hypoxemia and/or hypercarbia should make one suspicious of an airway obstruction.

Complete airway obstruction is a medical emergency. Signs of complete obstruction in the spontaneously breathing individual are inaudible breath sounds or the inability to feel air movement; use of accessory neck muscles; sternal, intercostal, and epigastric retrac-

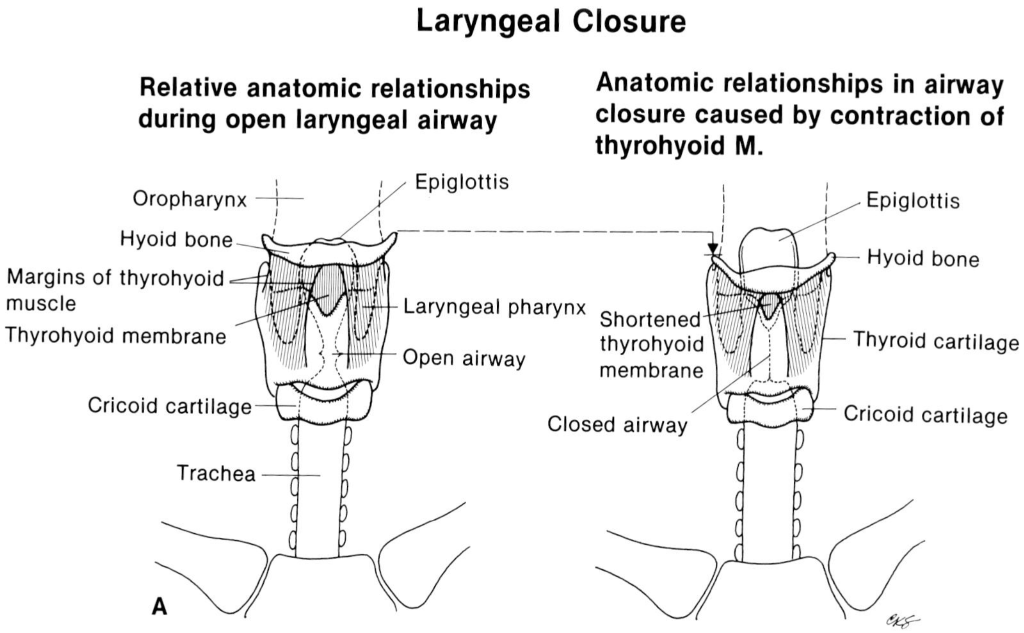

Figure 5–2 • Laryngeal closure (***A***) The left panel is a schematic frontal view of the airway at the larynx. The right panel shows contraction of the thyrohyoid muscle, which approximates the hyoid bone to the thyroid cartilage, forcing the ventricular and vocal folds into apposition.

(continued)

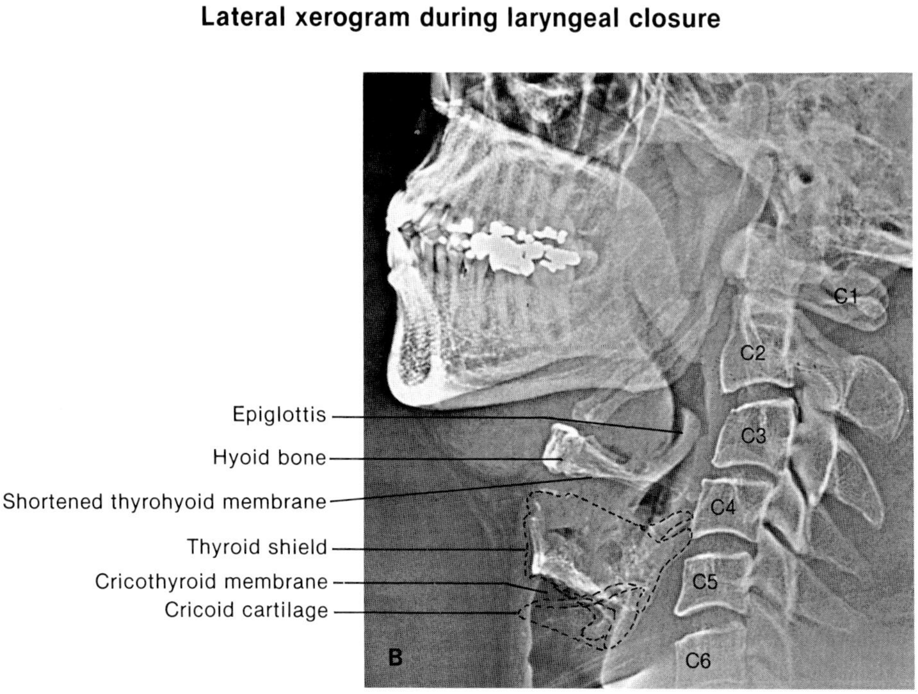

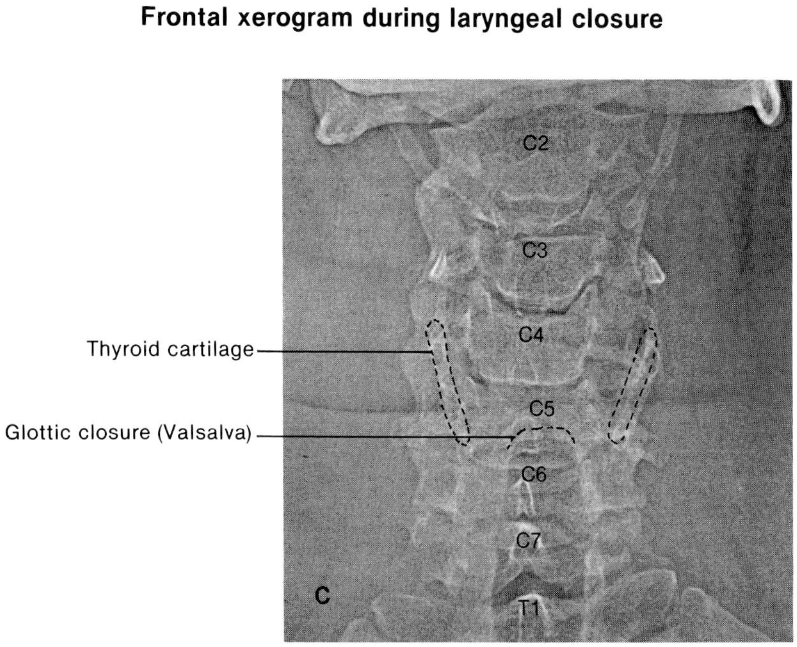

Figure 5–2 *(continued)*
(***B*** and **C**) Lateral and frontal xerograms during Valsalva laryngeal closure. Note thyrohyoid approximation in lateral view and abrupt airway cutoff in frontal view.

tion; absence of chest expansion on inspiration; and agitation.

Relief of airway obstruction is the focus of this chapter. Rapid, simple maneuvers should take precedence in the management of this problem.

II. How to Manage the Airway Without Intubation

A. *Simple (Noninstrumental) Airway Maneuvers: Head Tilt, Chin Lift, Jaw Thrust*

The sections on airway anatomy and airway obstruction constitute essential background to the understanding of airway maneuvers. When muscles of the floor of the mouth and the tongue relax, the tongue and epiglottis lie close to or on the back wall of the oropharynx, causing soft tissue obstruction.[4–6] It is also possible for the epiglottis to overlie the glottic opening and to obstruct it.[7] This is exaggerated by flexing the head and neck and/or opening the mouth (Fig. 5–3).[7,8] The distance between the mentum (chin) and the thyroid notch is relatively short in the flexed position. Any maneuver that increases this distance will straighten out the mentum–geniohyoid–hyoid–thyroid line, thus elevating the hyoid bone further from the pharynx.[4] The hyoid elevates the epiglottis via the hyoepiglottic ligament.[9] There are two maneuvers to lengthen this anterior neck distance. The first maneuver (head tilt) is to tilt the head back on the atlantooccipital joint while keeping the mouth closed (teeth approximated). This distance may be further augmented by elevating the occiput 1–4 inches above the level of the shoulders (sniffing posi-

Head and Neck in Neutral (and Flexed) Positions

Lateral xerogram of head and neck in neutral position

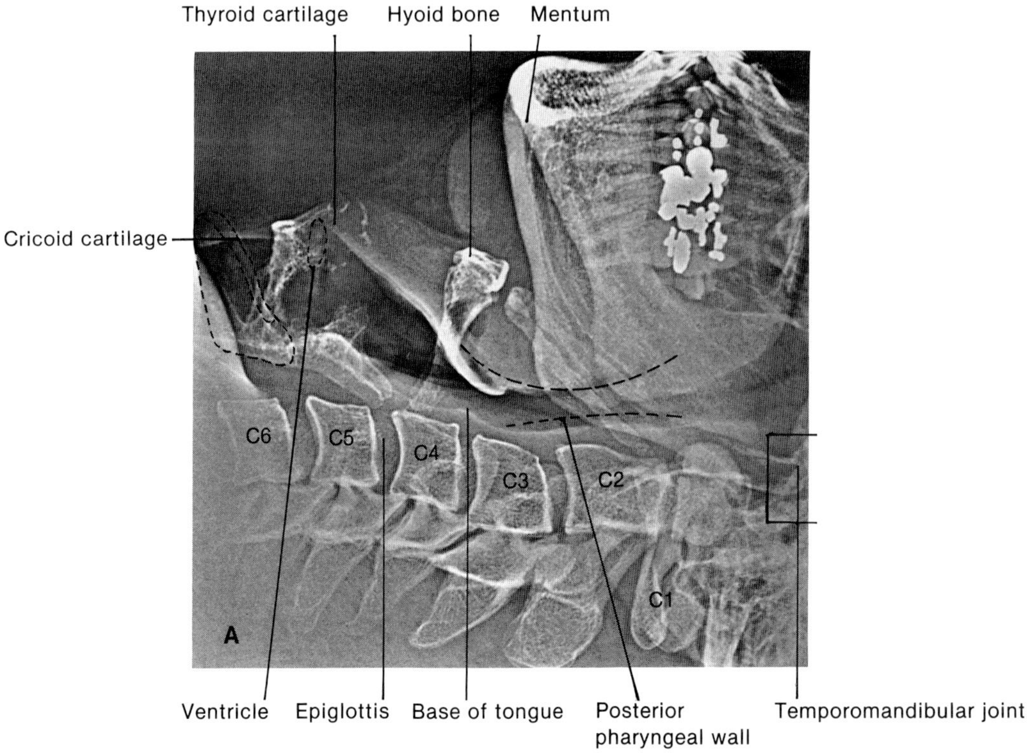

Figure 5–3 • Head and neck in neutral position. Patient awake and supine. (*A*) Lateral xerogram of head and neck in extended position: lateral view. Note mentum, temporomandibular joint, base of tongue, pharyngeal wall, hyoid bone, epiglottis, thyroid, cricoid cartilage. Note proximity of epiglottis to posterior pharyngeal wall.

(continued)

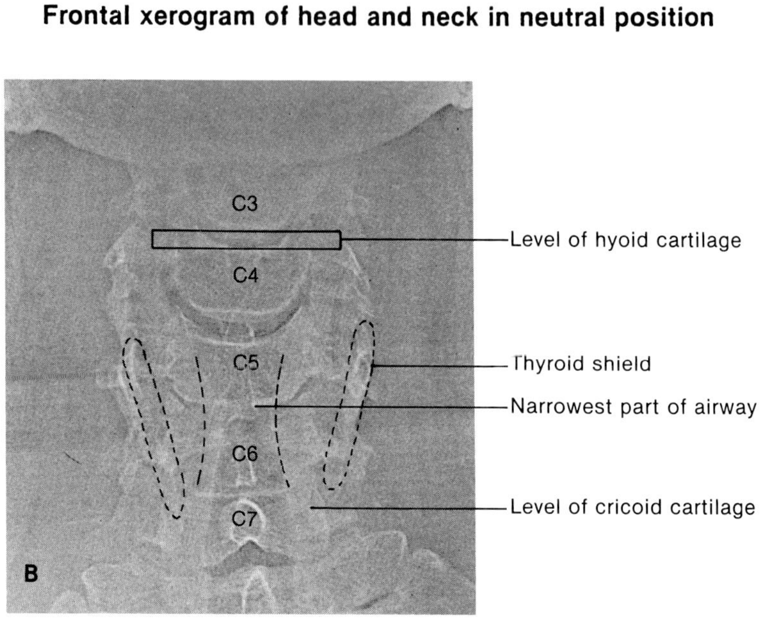

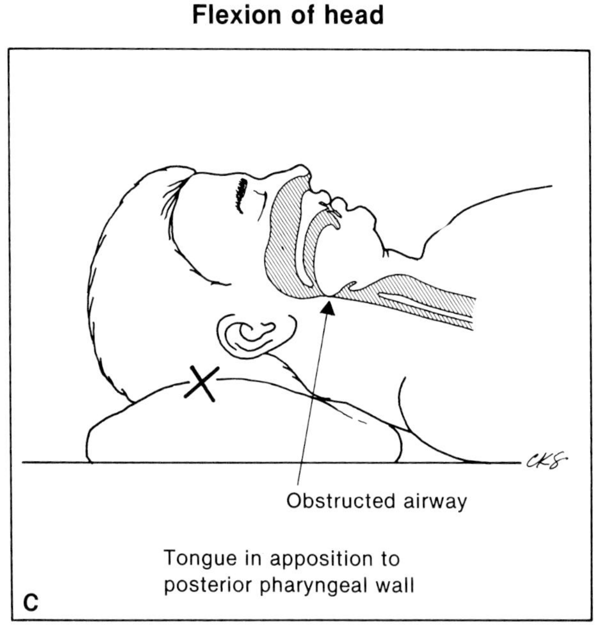

Figure 5–3 *(continued)*
(***B***) Frontal view. Note airway narrowest at the level of the vocal cords (C5). (***C***) The flexed head with tongue falling back into the pharynx.

tion), so long as the larynx and posterior pharynx stay in their original position. In some patients the cervical spine is stiff enough that elevating the head also elevates the C4–5 laryngeal area, leaving the airway unchanged. In children under 5 years of age the upper cervical spine is more flexible and can bow upward, forcing the posterior pharyngeal wall upward against the tongue and epiglottis, thereby exacerbating the obstruction. Therefore, a child's airway is usually best maintained by leaving the head in a more neutral position than that described for an adult. The head tilt is the simplest first airway maneuver in resuscitation[5,6,8] (Fig. 5–4). Head tilt may be accomplished by a chin or neck lift. Extreme caution should be exercised in suspected neck injuries or cerebrovascular disease. The head tilt by chin lift is reportedly more effective than the head tilt by neck lift.[5] In the

Head and Neck in Extended Position

Lateral xerogram of head and neck in extended position

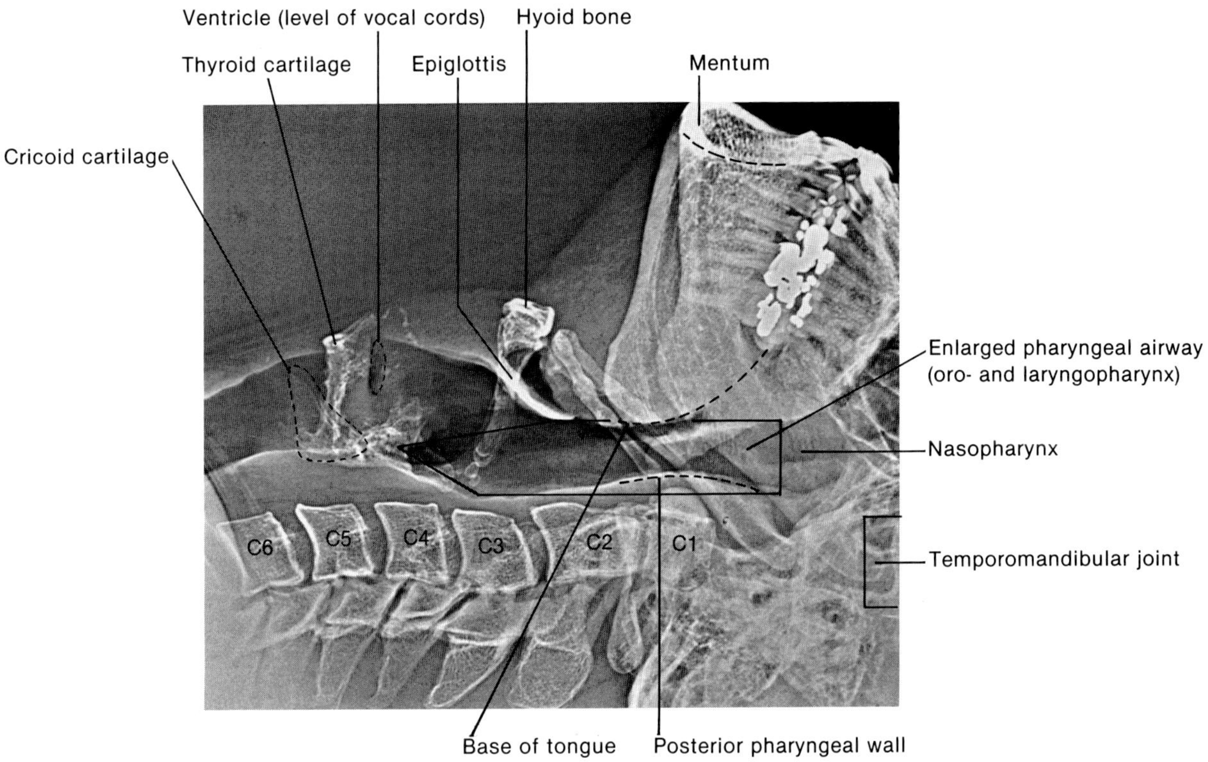

Head tilt and chin lift to obtain extended position

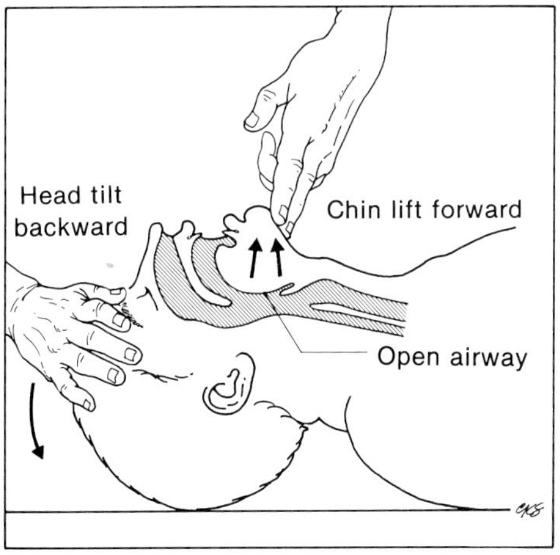

Figure 5–4 • Lateral xerogram of head and neck, extended position. Labeling as in Fig. 5–3. Note enlarged pharyngeal airway and hyoid bone moved anteriorly and elevated (opposite C2–3). Note thyroid shield and level of vocal cords now elevated to C4–5. The drawing shows the head being tilted backward and the chin being lifted forward, both of which greatly open the airway.

latter, the mouth opens and the slack geniohyoid allows the hyoid bone (and epiglottis) to remain close to the pharyngeal wall.

The second maneuver (jaw thrust) more directly lifts the hyoid bone and tongue away from the posterior pharyngeal wall by subluxating the mandible forward onto the sliding part of the temporomandibular joint.[5] The occluded teeth prevent the movement of the mandible, so the thumbs depress the mentum while the fingers grip the rami of the mandible and lift it upward to protrude the mandibular teeth in front of the maxillary teeth after the mouth opens slightly. This is called the *jaw thrust maneuver* and reliably opens the airway (Fig. 5–5). In most people the mandible is readily drawn back into the joint by elasticity of the joint capsule and masseter muscle; consequently, this position is difficult to maintain with one hand.

Some 20% of patients occlude the nasopharynx with the soft palate during exhalation, when the muscles are relaxed.[5] If the mouth and lips are closed, exhalation is impeded. In these cases an airway device is required to allow free exhalation. Without an airway device, the mouth must be opened slightly to assure that the lips are parted. These three maneuvers done together are known as the *triple airway maneuver* (head tilt, jaw thrust, open mouth)[5] (Table 5–1; see Fig. 5–5). The triple airway maneuver is the most reliable manual method to achieve upper airway patency.

B. *Heimlich Maneuver*

As previously noted, the various airway maneuvers can help obtain airway patency but do not relieve airway obstruction due to foreign material lodged in the upper airway. A foreign body obstruction should be suspected with a witnessed aspiration, and when the patient cannot talk, when ventilation is absent, or when positive pressure ventilation meets resistance after routine airway maneuvers have been done. Prior to the insertion of artificial airway devices, a manual effort (finger sweep) should be made to evacuate any foreign material present in the oropharynx. A Heimlich maneuver is indicated when coughing or traditional means are unable to relieve *complete* airway obstruction due to foreign material.[5,9] The Heimlich maneuver (subdiaphragmatic ab-

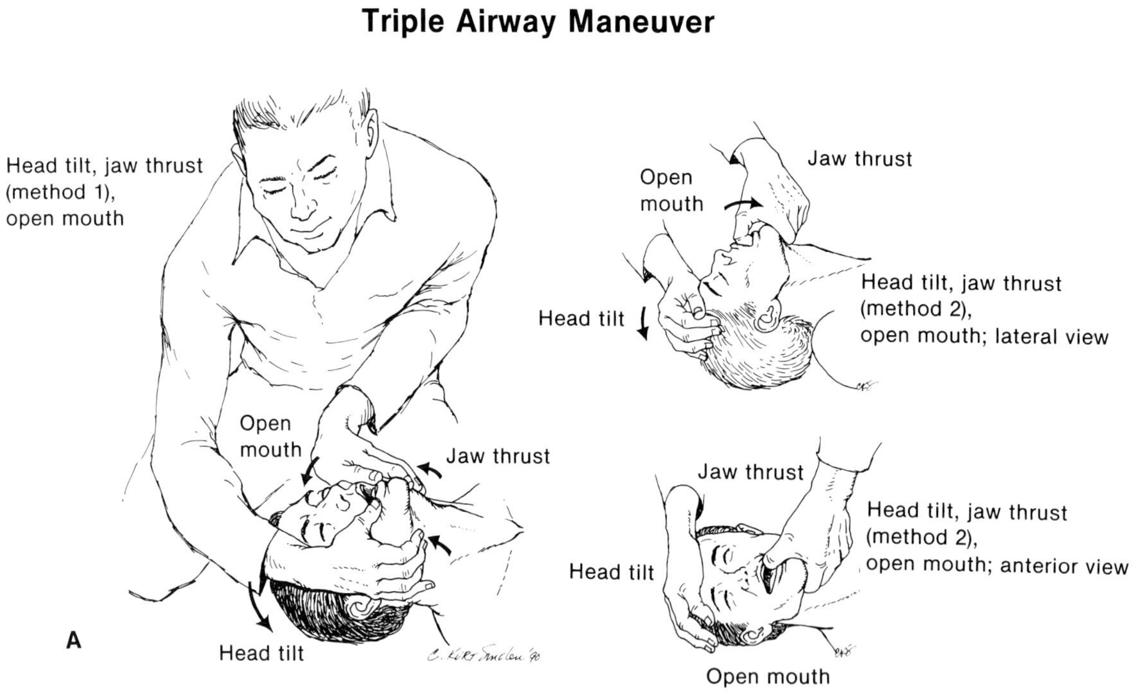

Figure 5–5 • (***A***) Triple airway maneuver. Note that (1) the head is extended on the atlantooccipital joint; (2) the mouth is opened to get the teeth out of occlusion as well as to open the oral fissure; and (3) the mandible is forced upward, forcing the condyles to slide anteriorly at the temporomandibular joint.

(continued)

Lateral xerogram of jaw protrusion

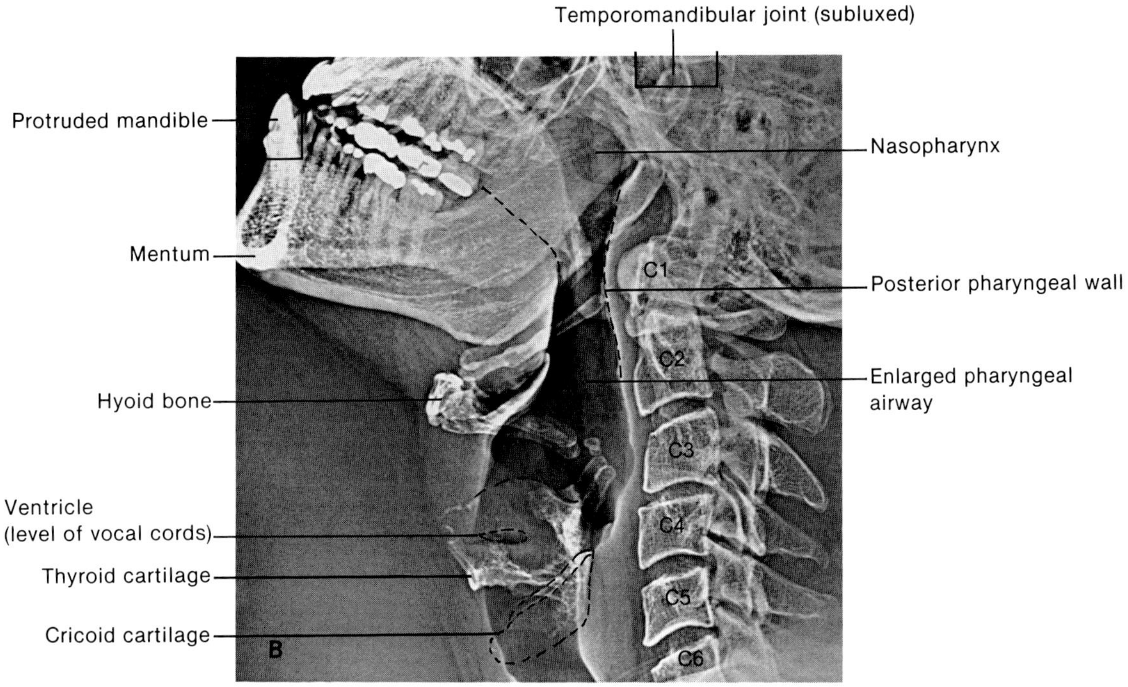

Frontal xerogram of jaw protrusion

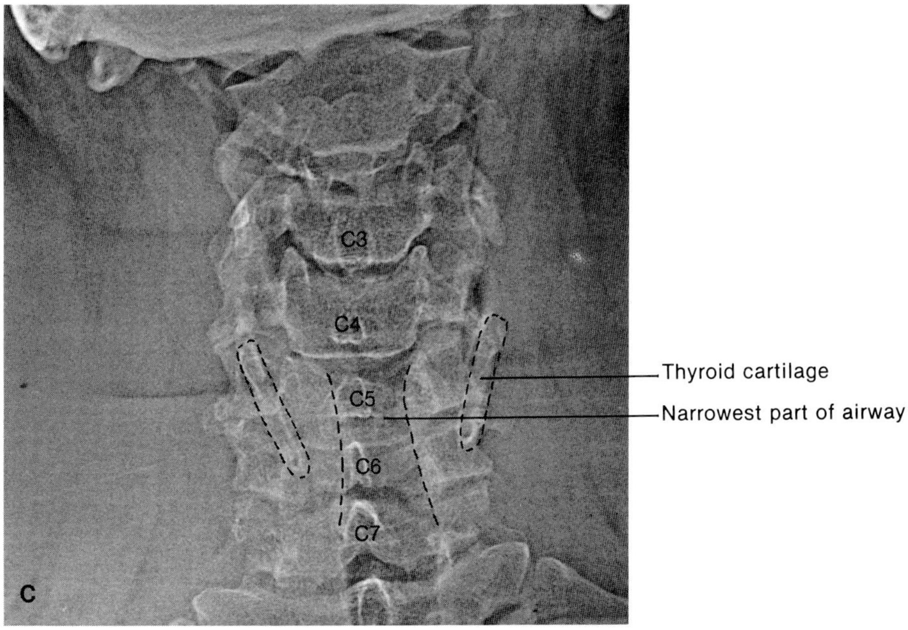

Figure 5–5 *(continued)*
(***B***) Lateral xerogram of jaw protrusion. Note temporomandibular joint with condyle on sliding portion of joint and lower incisors protruding. Note enlarged pharyngeal airway and elevated hyoid, thyroid (opposite C4), and cricoid (opposite C5). (***C***) Frontal xerogram of jaw protrusion. Note that the airway shadow is widened. Although the narrowest part of the airway remains at about the C5–6 border, the thyroid cartilage has moved cephalad.

dominal thrusts) is a recently recommended alternative to back blows (Fig. 5-6 and Table 5-2). In emergency situations one technique should not exclude the other alternatives. The Heimlich maneuver is not advocated by all authorities.[10]

Table 5-1 • Simple (Noninstrumental) Airway Maneuvers

Head Tilt	
Procedure:	
1. With the patient supine and operator at the patient's side; place one hand under the neck and the heel of the other hand on the forehead.	
2. Extend the head by displacing the forehead back and lifting the occiput up (neck lift).	
Indication:	Soft tissue upper airway obstruction
Contraindications:	Fractured neck Basilar artery syndrome Infants (relative)
Complications:	Sore neck Pinched nerve
Chin Lift	
Procedure	
1. With the patient supine and operator at the head of the patient; place one hand on the forehead, with the first two fingers of the other hand over the underside of the chin.	
2. Simultaneously tilt the forehead and exert upward traction on the chin.	
Indication:	Alternative to neck lift for head tilt
Contraindications:	Same as head tilt
Complications:	Same as head tilt
Jaw Thrust	
Procedure:	
1. From above the patient's head, place thumbs on the maxilla and fingers behind the angle of the mandible (bilaterally), opening, lifting, and displacing the jaw forward.	
2. Retract the lower lip with thumbs.	
3. Tilt the head backward (unless contraindicated).	
Indication:	Head tilt contraindicated (eg, fractured neck) or ineffective
Contraindications:	Fractured jaw Dislocated jaw Awake patient
Complications:	Dislocated jaw Damaged teeth
Open Mouth	
Procedure:	Open lips with thumbs after subluxating jaw as part of triple airway maneuver.
Indication:	Expiratory obstruction after head tilt
Contraindications:	Worsening of inspiratory airway
Complications:	None

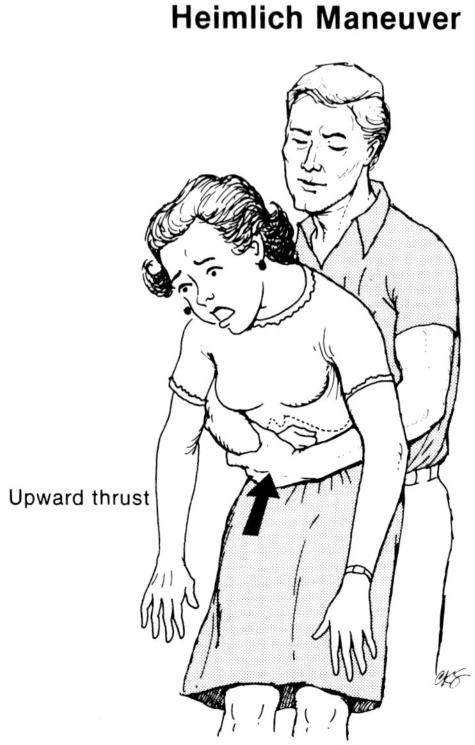

Figure 5-6 • Heimlich maneuver. Opening an airway obstructed by a laryngeal foreign body by compressing the lungs through external pressure on the abdominal viscera (forcing the diaphragm cephalad).

C. *Artificial Airway Devices*

When airway maneuvers are inadequate to establish airway patency, it is often necessary to employ artificial airway devices. The following addresses the various available devices and discusses techniques of insertion, maintenance, indications, contraindications, and complications.

1. Oropharyngeal Airways

An oral airway can be used as a bite block to prevent occlusion of the teeth, but more often it is used to provide a patent airway. The airways range in size from 0 for neonates to 4 for adults. The airways are usually made of plastic, metal, rubber, or elastomeric.[11] They should be wide enough to contact two or three teeth on the mandible and maxillae and be slightly compressible, so that the pressure of a clenched jaw is distributed over all the contacted teeth while the lumen remains patent. The airway is designed with a straight bite section to

Table 5-2 • The Heimlich Maneuver

Procedure:
In the upright patient, wrap both arms around the chest with the right hand in a closed fist in the low sternal–xiphoid area and the left hand on top of the fist. With a rapid forceful thrust, compress upward, increasing subdiaphragmatic pressure and creating an artificial cough.
Indication:
Complete upper airway obstruction by a foreign body threatening asphyxia
Contraindications:
Fractured ribs (relative)
Cardiac contusion (relative)
Partial airway obstruction
Complications:
Fractured ribs, sternum
Liver or spleen trauma

contact the teeth, a flange at the buccal (proximal) end to prevent swallowing or overinsertion of the airway, and a distal semicircular section to follow the curvature of the mouth, tongue, and posterior pharynx so that the tongue is displaced anteriorly (concave side against the tongue) (Fig. 5–7). In addition, an air channel is often provided to facilitate oropharyngeal suctioning.

There are several types of oral airways; the flange, straight section, and pharyngeal curve are the same in all types described herein (see Fig. 5–7).[11]

1. The Guedel airway has a plastic elliptical tube with a central lumen reinforced by a harder inner plastic tube at the level of the teeth and by plastic ridges along the pharyngeal section.
2. The Berman airway consists of two horizontal plates joined by a median ridge.
3. The Ovassapian airway has a large anterior flange to control the tongue and a large opening at the level of the teeth, open posteriorly, to allow a fiberscope and endotracheal tube to be passed through it and later disengaged from the airway.
4. The Berman-type airway has a hinged lower section meant to lift the base of the tongue (see Fig. 5–7).

The use of an oral airway is straightforward, but it is essential to do it correctly. The patient should be comatose or adequately anesthetized to allow depression of the pharyngeal and laryngeal reflexes. The mouth is opened and a tongue blade is placed at the base of the tongue and drawn upward, lifting the tongue off the posterior pharynx (Fig. 5–8A). The airway is placed so that the oropharyngeal tube is just off the posterior wall of the oropharynx with 1–2 cm protruding above the incisors (Fig. 5–8B). (If the flange is at the teeth when the tip is just at the base of the tongue, the airway is too small.) A jaw-thrust maneuver is done with the fingers of both hands to lift the tongue off the pharyngeal wall; the thumbs then tap the airway down the last 2 cm so that the curve of the pharyngeal airway lies behind the base of the tongue (Fig. 5–8C). The condyles of the jaw are then allowed to reduce back into the temporomandibular joint. The mouth should be inspected so that neither tongue nor lips are caught between teeth and airway. An alternative method of insertion is to insert the airway backward (convex side toward the tongue) until the tip is close to the posterior wall of the oropharynx (past the uvula) and then to rotate it 180° (Fig. 5–8D). Rather than pushing the tongue straight downward, the tip rotates and sweeps under it from the side. This method is not as reliable as the tongue–blade-assisted method mentioned earlier and has the added risk that the twisting motion can catch gapped teeth and loosen them in patients with poor dentition. If the airway is too short, the tongue may still obstruct the airway at the level of the oropharynx. If it is too long, it may reach to the level of the laryngopharynx, where it contacts the epiglottis. In the lightly anesthetized or awake patient, this stimulation will cause coughing or laryngeal spasm. The best treatment for this problem is to withdraw the airway 1–2 cm. A topical anesthetic spray of the pharynx (Cetacaine, tetracaine 0.5%, lidocaine 4%) and/or a water-soluble local anesthetic lubricant on the airway will reduce the chance of laryngeal activity but should be avoided in the patient with gastric contents.

Indications for use of an oropharyngeal airway consist of an obstructed upper airway (complete or partial) in the unconscious patient and a need for a bite block in the unconscious patient; it can also be used as an adjunct for oropharyngeal suctioning. There are two important contraindications to its use. First, awake or lightly anesthetized patients may have reactive airways, and an oral airway can cause retching or vomiting. Second, patients with caps on any of the front four teeth risks fracturing the caps if they bite down hard on the airway (this is only a relative contraindication). Although the use of a nasopharyngeal airway avoids this risk, it exposes the patient to the risk of epistaxis (see later).

There are three major complications to the use of oral airways: trauma, airway hypersensitivity, and air-

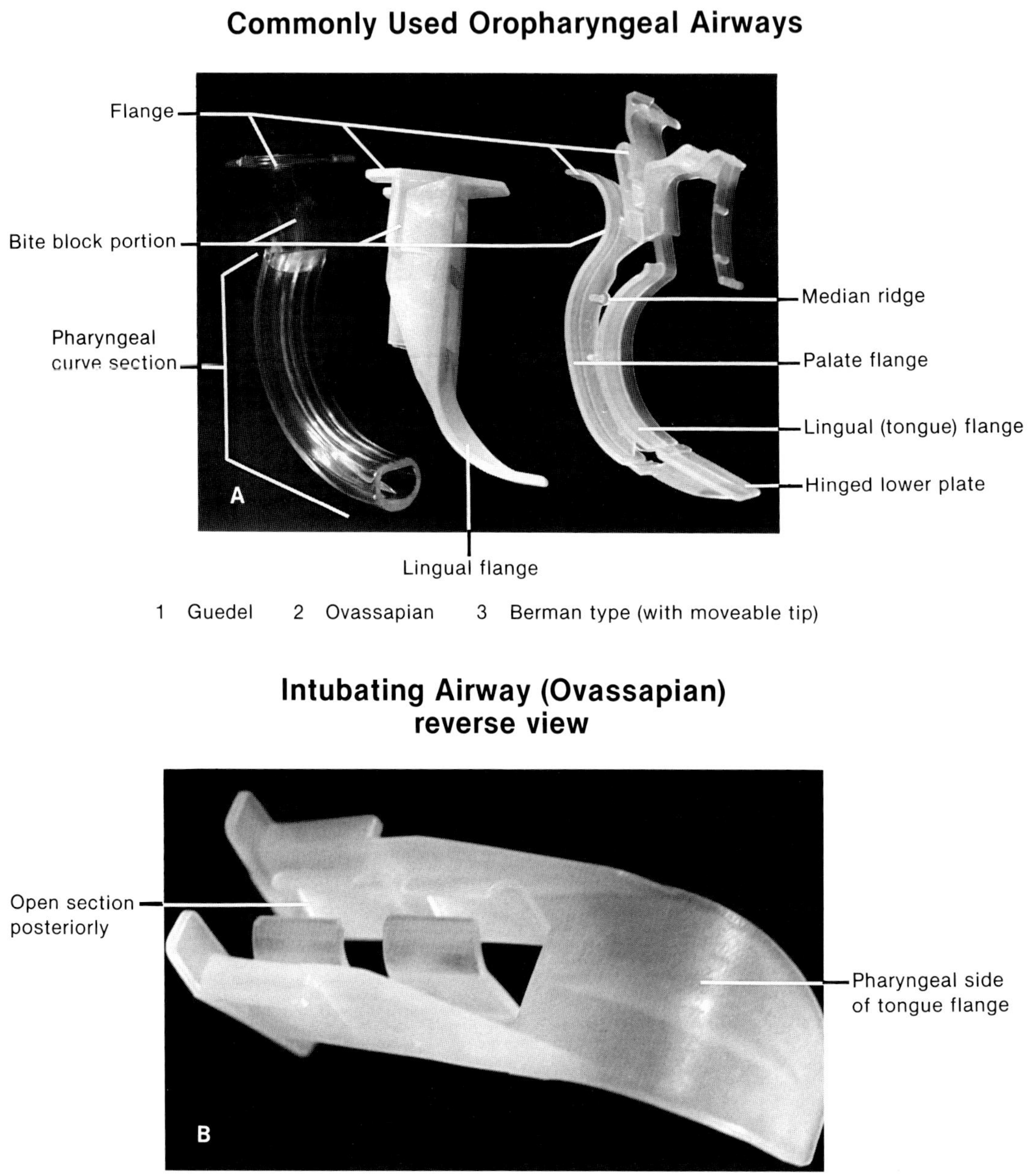

Figure 5–7 • Commonly used oropharyngeal airways. All oral airways have a flange to prevent overinsertion, a straight bite block portion, and a pharyngeal curve section. *(1)* The Guedel airway is totally (circularly) enclosed so that soft tissue cannot restrict the central airway. A small suction catheter (less than 14 gauge) can usually be inserted through the Guedel airway into the lower oropharynx, but the oral cavity must still be suctioned around it to remove oral secretions. *(2)* The Ovassapian airway has a large anterior flange to control the tongue. The airway is open posteriorly so that an endotracheal (ET) tube can be inserted through the airway with the fiberoptic technique and the assembly later separated. *(3)* Berman-type airway has anterior and posterior flanges and central ridge. This model has a hinge so that the lower plate can be pulled up to elevate the tongue. *(4)* Posterior view of Ovassapian airway showing open posterior section allowing airway to be disengaged from the ET tube after successful intubation.

Oropharyngeal Airway Insertion Technique

Retract tongue with tongue blade

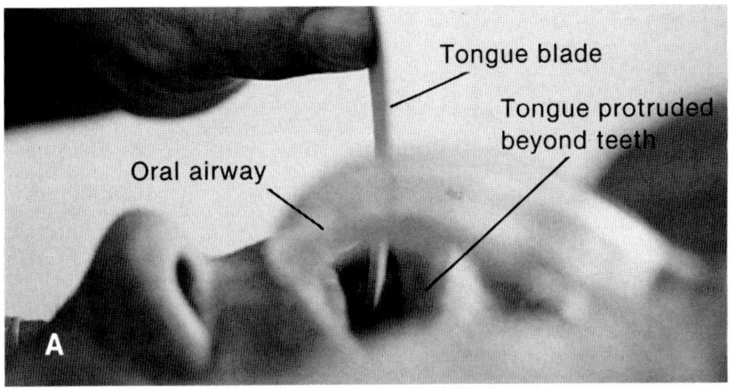

Insert oropharyngeal airway

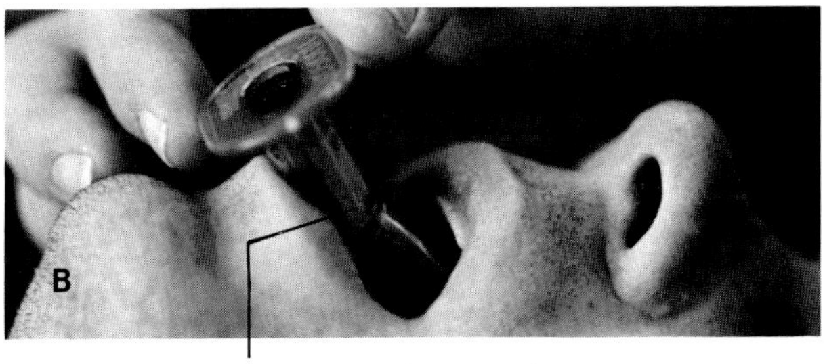

Tap Oropharyngeal Airway into Place

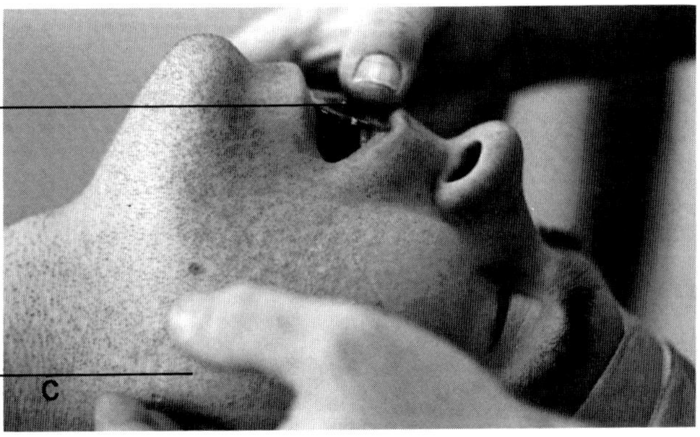

Alternative method of oropharyngeal airway insertion

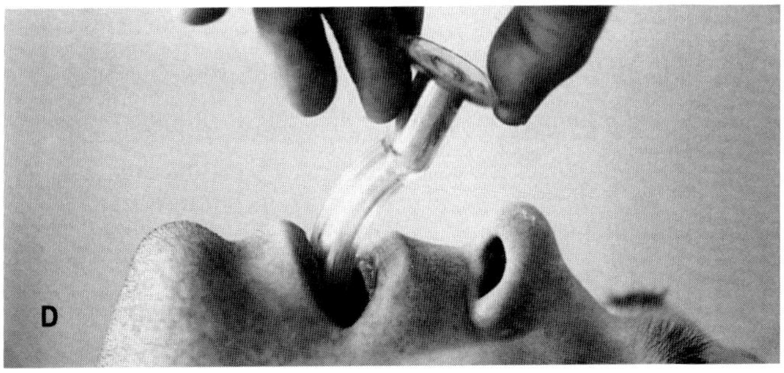

Airway is placed with concavity initially facing the palate and is then rotated 180°

Figure 5–8 • Oropharyngeal airway insertion technique. Parts ***A*–C** illustrate standard technique; ***D*** is an alternative when no tongue blade is available. (***A***) The tongue blade is placed deep in the mouth with the left hand and the tongue is pulled forward and depressed. The airway is inserted with the concave side toward the tongue. (***B***) The oral airway has been placed by the right hand so that the junction of the bite block section and pharyngeal curve is at the lower incisors. (***C***) A jaw thrust maneuver is done with fingers at the angle of the jaws while the thumb taps the airway into place. When the jaw is allowed to relax, inspect the lips so that they are not caught between the teeth and airway. (***D***) As an alternate technique, the airway is placed in reverse manner (concave toward palate) and then spun into place. The junction of the bite block section and the pharyngeal curve should be near the incisors before the spin move is done.

way obstruction. Minor trauma, including pinching of the lips and tongue, is common. Potential ulceration and necrosis of oropharyngeal structures from pressure and long-term (days) contact has been reported.[12] This problem necessitates constant surveillance during the length of use. Dental injury can occur from twisting of the airway, involuntary clenching of the jaw, or direct axial pressure. Dental damage is most common in patients with periodontal disease, dental caries, pronounced degrees of dental proclination, and isolated teeth.[11,13]

Airway hyperactivity is potentially lethal. Oro pharyngeal and laryngeal reflexes can be stimulated by the placement of an artificial airway. Coughing, retching, emesis, and laryngospasm are common reflex responses. Any airway that contacts the epiglottis or vocal cords can stimulate this response, but the problem is more common with larger oral airways. These problems should be first managed by partial withdrawal of the airway. In cases of laryngospasm it might be necessary to apply mild positive airway pressure and, in trained hands, to cautiously administer small doses of succinylcholine for prompt cessation. Finally, airway obstruction is also a potentially lethal complication. An oral airway that is too short might be ineffective; too long an airway could force the epiglottis against the posterior pharyngeal wall. If it is incorrectly inserted, the airway can displace the tongue into the posterior pharynx, obstructing the airway.

2. *Nasopharyngeal Airway*

The nasopharyngeal airway provides an alternative airway device for treating soft tissue upper airway obstruction. A nasal airway is less stimulating than an oropharyngeal airway and therefore better tolerated in the awake, semicomatose, or lightly anesthetized patient. In conditions of poor dentition, limited mouth opening, or oropharyngeal trauma, the nasal airway is often preferable. Nasopharyngeal airways are pliable bent cylinders made of plastic or soft rubber in variable widths or lengths (Fig. 5–9). A flange or movable disk prevents the outside end from passing beyond the nares. The concavity is meant to follow the hard palate and posterior wall of the nasooropharynx. The airway is beveled on the left side to aid in following the airway and minimizing mucosal trauma as it advances. A narrow nasopharyngeal tube is often desired to minimize nasal trauma but may be too short to reach behind the tongue. An endotracheal tube of the same diameter may be cut to a longer length and softened in hot water to provide a longer airway. A safety pin or 15-mm adapter should be inserted in the cut endotracheal tube to prevent its migration into the nasopharynx (see Fig. 5–9).

The nose should be inspected to determine its size, its patency, and the presence of nasal polyps or marked septal deviation. Vasoconstriction of the mucous membranes can be accomplished with cocaine or Neo-Sy-

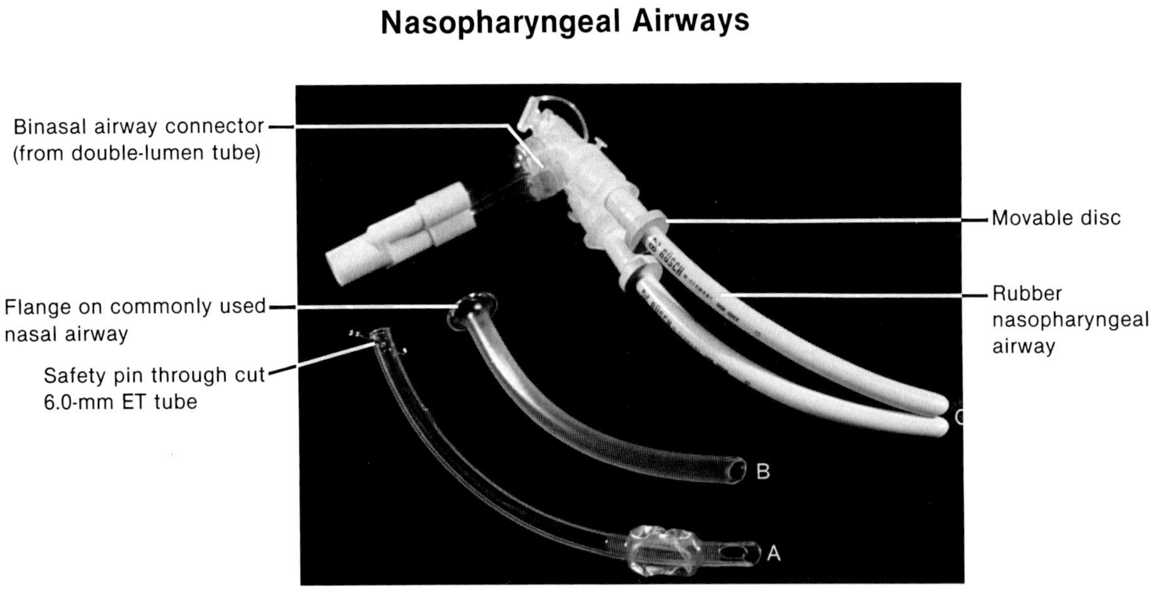

Figure 5–9 • Nasopharyngeal airways. (*A*) Endotracheal (ET) tube 6 mm in length cut with safety pin to prevent overinsertion (note added length). (*B*) Clear nasal airway with flange at proximal end. (*C*) Binasal airway. Two standard airways (these have movable disks to prevent overinsertion) connected to double-lumen tube adapter.

Insertion of Nasopharyngeal Airway

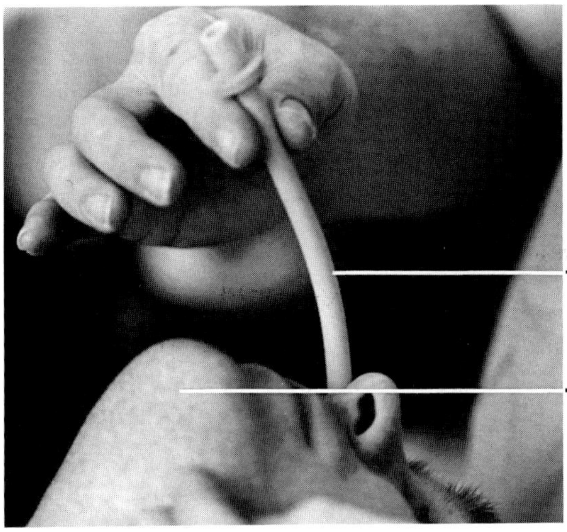

Figure 5–10 • Insertion of nasopharyngeal airway. The airway is oriented concave to hard palate and inserted straight back.

nephrine drops or spray. Cotton swabs can be saturated in the solution and gently passed parallel to the palate into the nasopharynx (occasionally this must be done in stages over 3–5 minutes). If three cotton swabs can be accommodated in the nasal passage to the nasopharynx, a 7.5 airway will usually pass. The airway is generously lubricated with a water-soluble anesthetic ointment. The ointment may also be squirted into the nose. The swabs are removed and the airway is gently passed with the concave side against the hard palate (Fig. 5–10), through the nose parallel to the palate, passing under the inferior turbinate, until resistance is met in the posterior nasopharynx (anterior wall of the retropharyngeal space). The tube must bend 60° to 90° here to proceed down the pharynx. Usually this can be done with continuing pressure on the airway. However, sometimes it is helpful to rotate the airway 90° counterclockwise, bringing the bevel against the posterior nasopharyngeal mucosae, and to resume gentle pressure. As the tube makes the bend, it can be rotated back to the original position. If the patient coughs or reacts as the nasal tube is inserted to its full extent, it should be withdrawn 1–2 cm. If the patient's airway is still obstructed after insertion, a longer airway should be tried (unless laryngeal spasm is suspected).[11]

The indications for a nasopharyngeal airway consist of upper airway obstruction in awake, semicomatose, or lightly anesthetized patients; in patients who are not adequately treated with oropharyngeal airways; in patients with dental indications or oropharyngeal trauma; and in patients in whom there is a need to facilitate oro- and laryngopharyngeal suctioning. The contraindications consist of nasal airway occlusion, nasal fractures, marked deviated septum, coagulopathy, prior transphenoidal hypophysectomy or Caldwell-Luc procedures (nose packed), CSF rhinorrhea, and adenoid hypertrophy (relative, usually in pediatrics).

The complications of nasopharyngeal airways consist of failure of passage of the airway, epistaxis, submucosal tunneling, and pressure sores.[13,14]

If the tube will not pass through the nose with moderate pressure, then a narrower airway should be tried; the nose should be redilated with cotton swabs; or the other naris should be tried. If the tube will not pass the bend at the nasopharynx, then turn the tube 90° and gently push; then turn it 180° and try again. Alternatively, withdraw the tube 1–2 cm and pass a suction catheter through the nasal airway as a guide into the oropharynx, then push the airway forward over the suction tube. Finally, one can try the other naris. In a few patients, the longest available nasal tube will not reach to behind the tongue and the airway remains obstructed. Cutting a 6.0 endotracheal tube at 18 cm will provide a long enough airway for this problem. A safety pin through the proximal end provides a flange to prevent migration of the tube into the naris. Epistaxis is usually self-limiting and resolves spontaneously. If the anterior plexus is bleeding, apply pressure to the nostrils. If the posterior plexus is bleeding, leave the airway in, suction the pharynx, ventilate the patient, and consider intubation of the trachea if bleeding does not stop rapidly. Position the patient on his or her side to avoid aspiration of blood. A formal nasal pack or otolaryngology consultation may be necessary. The solution to submucosal tunneling in the retropharyngeal space is simply to withdraw the airway. The other nostril may be used for the nasopharyngeal tube, or an oropharyngeal airway may be used. The patient should be frequently observed for pressure sores of the ala nasi or for evidence of sinusitis, and upon extubation some mucosal ulceration may be observed.

3. Binasal Airway

The use of two nasopharyngeal airways joined together by an adapter (see Fig. 5-9) has been previously described.[15,16] This technique allows for spontaneous and potentially low positive pressure ventilation if the mouth is occluded. To allow for assisted ventilation, the tubes must be positioned near the larynx, and the surrounding soft tissues must help seal the hypopharynx. The use of two tubes provides enough bulk to seal within the hypopharynx as well as enough cross-sectional area to minimize airway resistance. (Two 6.0-mm airways will have a cross-sectional area exceeding that of an 8.0-mm airway.) Although gastric inflation is possible, excessive gas flow can exit the mouth.[15]

D. *Nonintubation Ventilation*

Despite a patent airway, ventilation can be inadequate. Ventilatory assistance can be achieved through several alternatives other than intubation. Standard cardiopulmonary resuscitation courses have long taught the effectiveness of mouth-to-mouth and mouth-to-nose ventilation. Mouth-to-artificial-airway using an S-tube (double [flange opposed to flange] Guedel airway) overcomes many of the esthetic objections to the previous techniques. More sophisticated approaches to ventilatory assistance (as in anesthesia) typically include the use of mask and bag systems.

1. Masks

Face masks differ in material, shape, type of seal, and transparency. The mask is composed of three parts: the body, seal (or cushion), and connector (or collar). The body is the main structure of the mask. Since the body rises above the face, all face masks increase dead space. A more malleable body allows for a better fit to the face and a reduced dead space. The added dead space is usually not significant when ventilation is spontaneous, and it is never significant if ventilation is controlled. Respiratory gas analysis (capnography) can verify adequate ventilation. The seal is the actual rim of the mask that comes in contact with the face. The two types of seals are a cushion rim that is often inflatable and a rubber or plastic edge that is a noninflatable flexible extension of the body. The connector is at the top of the body and provides a 22-mm female adapter for a breathing circuit or ambu-bag elbow. A collar with hooks allows for a mask retaining strap to be attached to help hold the mask to the face. The precise application of the straps (eg, crossed [ipsilateral strap to contralateral hook] versus uncrossed) is a matter of individual preference and is usually the result of the best seal and ventilation arrangement following multiple trials.

The Ohio anatomic mask has a body contoured to a Caucasian face, with a sharp notch for the nose, a double curve to fit the malar eminence of the cheek, and a curved chin section (Fig. 5-11) It is made of conductive rubber, is slightly malleable, and has a high-pressure, low-volume cushion. Its disadvantages include poor fit on a face with a broad, flat bridge of the nose and poor malleability to different-sized faces. The correct size is important, and several sizes should be readily available. It is opaque, so that vomitus cannot be detected readily, and it requires extensive aeration with the seal cushion collapsed after ethylene oxide sterilization because the ethylene oxide absorbed in the rubber can cause a chemical burn on the skin. Disposable transparent plastic masks have been made with high-volume low-pressure cushions that apply a seal to the face much more easily.

The base of the body is flat; the large, flexible cushion fits a wide variety of faces. The cushion may be factory sealed or have a nipple for the injection of air. A progression of this style is the "easy-seal" mask having a reinforced flexible disk for a body and a large floppy cushion comprising the entire undersurface of the disk except for the 22-mm adapter air passage. This mask is used in arrest situations but has not commonly been used to administer anesthesia.

The proper method of use of a face mask depends on obtaining a good sealed fit between the mask and the patient's face, and success in doing this is fundamental to administering adequate ventilation and inhalation anesthesia. The mask should comfortably fit both the hand of the user and the face of the patient. An anatomic

Face Masks

Front view

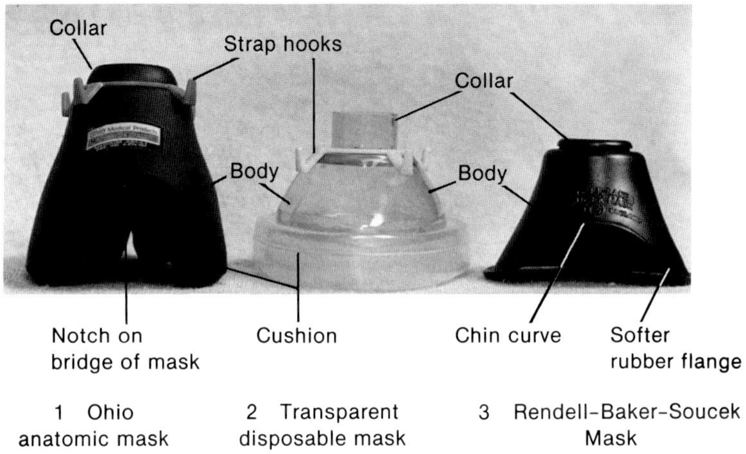

Side view

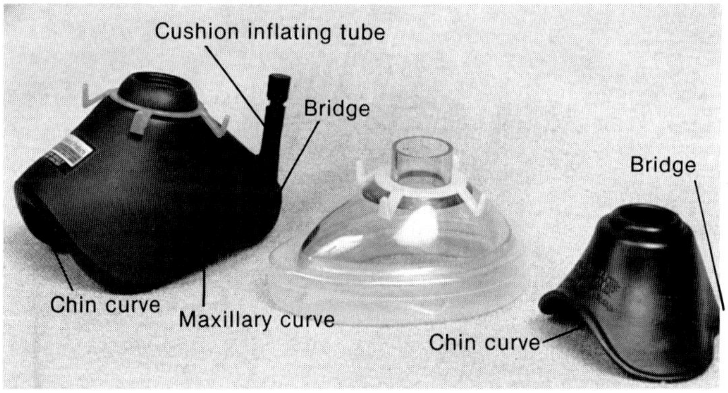

Figure 5–11 • Face masks. Front view, side view. *(1)* Ohio anatomic mask. *(2)* Transparent disposable mask. *(3)* Rendell–Baker–Soucek mask. Top panel shows front view and bottom panel shows side view. Note the various parts of the masks and different cushions and contours; strap hooks can also be put on the Rendall–Baker–Soucek mask if desired.

mask (Ohio) is meant to fit at the bridge of the nose, the alveolar ridge of the mandible, and along the malar eminences. Although the body of the mask is formed so that a cushion is not essential for a seal much of the time, the cushion should be inflated to equalize pressure all along the contact points of the face. If the mask is too long, the face can be elongated 1–2 cm by placing an oral airway. If the mask is too short with the oral airway in place, the oral airway can be removed and a nasal airway placed. The mask can also be moved 1–2 cm along the bridge of the nose to make a small mask fit at the chin.

Several methods are described for holding the mask. Regardless of the precise method, multiple trials with close monitoring for leaks are necessary. Our preferred method follows. The left hand grips the mask with the thumb and index finger around the collar (Figs. 5–12 and 5–13). The left side of the mask fits into the palm. The middle finger can be on the mask or chin, depending on the span of the user's hand, the size of the mask and face, and the ease of fit. The proximal interphalangeal joints of the fingers and the distal interphalangeal joint of the thumb should be at the midline of the mask, allowing the pads of the fingers to put pressure on the right side of the mask. The mask must be sealed at all four sides. The seal at the bridge of the

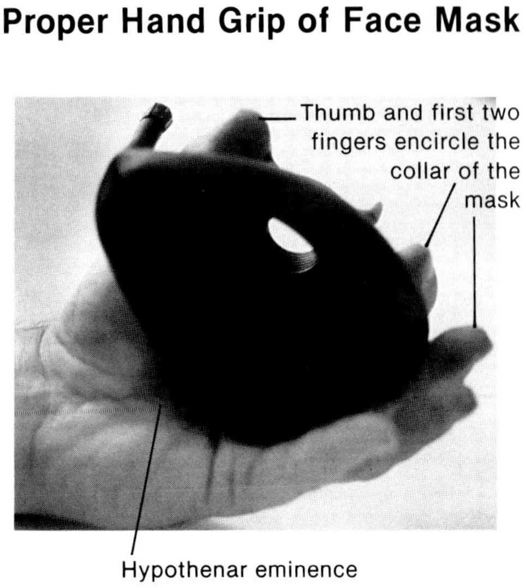

Figure 5–12 • Proper hand grip of face mask. Note hypothenar eminence extends down from mask while thumb and two fingers encircle collar.

nose is accomplished first by spreading the sides of the mask at its bridge and placing it on the bridge of the nose so that the mask does not put pressure on the eyes. The nose will subsequently be sealed by downward pressure of the thumb. The mask is lowered on to the face and the fit of the chin section is noted. If the chin section is at the level of the teeth, either a larger mask is used or the current one is slid down the face. If the chin section hits the mentum instead of the alveolar ridge, the sides of the mask may not seal (on the Ohio anatomic mask especially). An oral airway is used to lengthen the face 1–2 cm to let the chin section of the mask fall into the alveolar ridge of the mandible. Alternatively, a smaller mask can be used. The chin section is sealed by pulling the mandible up into the mask with the fingers and by rotating the wrist to push the bridge down as the mandible is pulled up. The left side of the mask is sealed by gathering skin of the cheek against the side of the mask with the hypothenar eminence. The right side of the mask is sealed by finger pressure on the right side of the mask by the thumb and the distal phalanges of the first two fingers and by pronating the left forearm to rotate the mask onto its right side. The sides of the mask are somewhat malleable to adjust to narrow or wide faces. In edentulous patients the cheeks are too hollow to allow a perfect fit. Buccal gauze sponges can be placed between the alveolar ridges and cheeks to fill out the face, but there is a small risk of a sponge being dislodged into the oropharynx, with consequent obstruction. In addition, edentulous patients have a loss of vertical dimension to the face that can be restored in part by an oral airway. In rare situations it might be beneficial to leave the dentures in place (although the dentures could dislodge and obstruct the airway, break, or be lost). Another alternative is to use a mask sufficiently large to fit over the chin so that the seal is along the caudal part of the chin, the cheeks are entirely within the mask, and the mask seals laterally along the mandible. (These maneuvers to make a difficult mask fit possible are often best side-stepped by endotracheal intubation, but clinical judgment must determine when this is the case.) Mask-retaining straps can be placed at the occiput and connected to the mask collar to put pressure at various angles to assist the seal. The tension on the straps should be no more than necessary to achieve a seal, and the tension should be released and the mask moved slightly every 15–30 minutes to allow perfusion of the underlying skin. External gauze sponges may be used to protect the skin from excessive pressure by a strap. When straps or gauze sponges are employed, extreme care must be given to avoid ocular trauma.[5,16] An additional maneuver to compensate for mask leaks is to increase fresh gas flow.

The preceding detailed procedures are important if black Ohio anatomic masks are used. The transparent masks with high-volume, low-pressure cuffs deform to seal more easily and contact a larger amount of facial skin, minimizing the chance of pressure ischemia in a long case. The chin and cheek areas seal more easily, but the size of the cushion occasionally results in pressure on the eye globe if the mask is high on the bridge of the nose. The thumb can pull the mask caudad to roll the cushion away from the eye. The cushions may be factory sealed or inflatable. The latter should be filled sufficiently so that the edge of the body of the mask does not contact the face. Some masks do not have cushions (Rendell-Baker–Soucek masks), but the rubber or plastic is usually tapered and flexible, so that it deforms along the face to give a larger area of contact than just the edge.

A face mask is indicated to seal a patient's airway to a mixture of gases to either ventilate, oxygenate, or anesthetize him in a number of situations without endotracheal intubation. These situations include preoxygenation with spontaneous ventilation, ventilation prior to intubation (including resuscitation situations), ventilation or oxygenation when placement of an endotracheal tube cannot be confirmed (visually or by capnography) and the patient's vital signs deteriorate, and delivery of anesthetic gases. The contraindications consist of situa-

Sealing and Holding the Mask to the Face

Application of mask to face

A

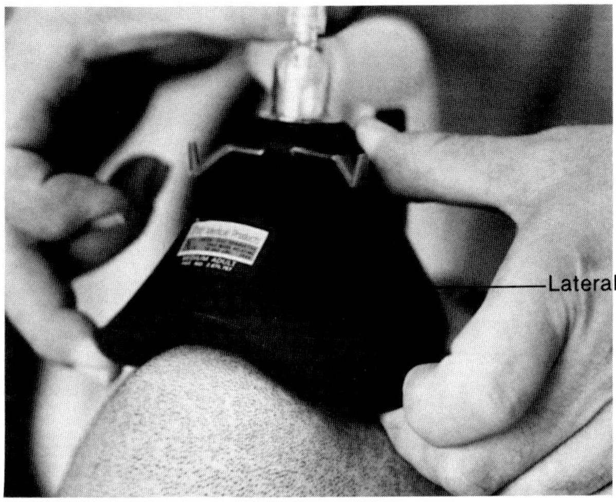

Application of mask to face

Standard one-handed grip of mask to face: side view

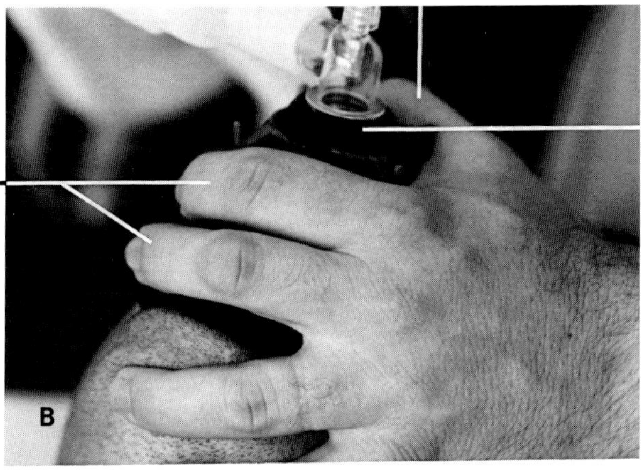

One-handed mask grip—maintaining jaw thrust

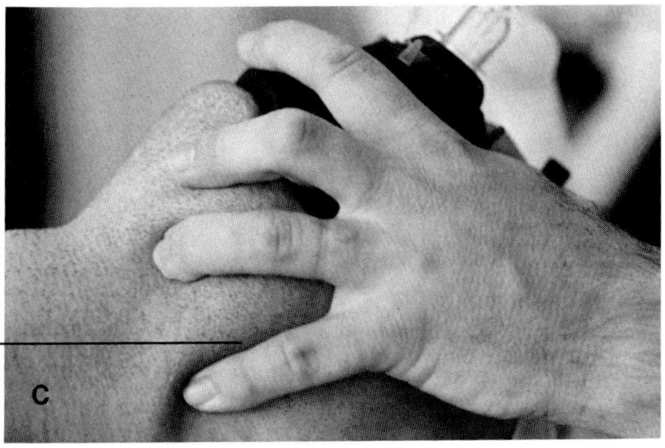

Caudad-side view

Figure 5-13 • Sealing and holding the mask to the face. (***A***) Application of mask to face. Fingers spread the bridge and lateral sides of the mask as it is lowered onto face. (***B***) Side view of standard one-handed grip of mask to face. The thumb and first two fingers encircle the collar of the mask while the last two fingers pull mandible up into mask and extend the head. (***C***) One-handed mask grip: maintaining jaw thrust. Caudad–sideview of handgrip shows little finger at the angle of the jaw maintaining backward and upward pull to maintain jaw thrust. Note that because of the increased span required of the hand, only the first finger is now on the mask, while the second and third fingers pull the mandible into the face and extend the head. (The exact position of the four fingers depends slightly on the size of the left hand.) To avoid teeth grating on one another, this technique usually requires the prior insertion of an oral airway.

tions when there is a large likelihood of gastric contents soiling the trachea, such as a full stomach, hiatus hernia, esophageal motility disorders, and pharyngeal diverticula (eg, Zenkers), and there is also a need for general anesthesia. In addition, whenever there is a likelihood of gas inflating the stomach (such as with a weakened cricopharyngeal sphincter [eg, with prolonged neuromuscular paralysis or bulbar neurologic disease]), a need for high airway pressures (eg, decreased compliance of lungs or chest wall, obesity [twice ideal body weight], marked kyphoscoliosis, marked bronchospasm), or an adverse position (eg, marked head down, fracture table, lithotripsy, CT scan, prone), then use of a mask for positive pressure ventilation is inadvisable. Mask ventilation is also contraindicated whenever there is a need to avoid the head and neck manipulation (head tilt) that may be necessary to maintain the airway, or whenever there is a need to avoid touching the neck (surgery of the head and neck) or an inability to seal the mask (eg, facial trauma and edentulous mouths with alveolar recession). Lack of integrity of the dermis, resulting in marked bullae from friction (eg, epidermolysis bullosa) is a contraindication to the use of a face mask. Finally, inability to sustain adequate assisted or spontaneous ventilation is a relative contraindication to further use of a face mask.

There are several complications from using a face mask. First, a poor mask fit can result in gas leaks that can lead to a waste of gases, a loss of the reservoir bag filling as a means of monitoring ventilation, the inability to maintain positive pressure, and potentially compromised ventilation and oxygenation. Various techniques to manage this problem were described earlier under methods of managing a face mask. Second, pressure from a malpositioned mask or too tight a seal, especially with the use of straps, can cause skin, nerve, and ophthalmic injury. Appropriate mask selection, application, and vigilance constitute the best means of avoiding this problem. Gastric distention and aspiration constitute a potentially lethal problem with positive pressure ventilation by mask. Transparent masks allow for earlier recognition of regurgitation. Finally, reactions to the residue from the sterilization process can cause a contact dermatitis. Allergies to the mask material have been reported.

2. Respiratory (Resuscitator) Bags

The air-mask-bag unit (AMBU) was developed in 1955 by Rubin.[17] The AMBU has provided an alternative means of artificial ventilation to the standard anesthesia bag and circuit. The bag can be used with a mask or endotracheal tube. Its advantage is in being self-inflating, thus avoiding the need for compressed gas. The disadvantage is that the "feel" of the airway (compliance and resistance) is poor and the delivery of high concentrations of oxygen more complex. Various types of hand resuscitator units exist. They use various valve systems to insure nonrebreathing and the units vary to a minor or moderate extent in size, weight, percentage of oxygen delivery, volume, reinflation time, cycling rate, number of parts, and so on.[18]

Criteria for selection of an AMBU should include easy, foolproof assembly; a nonsticking valve system to prevent rebreathing while allowing exhalation; various sizes; a closable pressure pop-off valve; standard 15/22-mm connection; capability to deliver 95% oxygen and 0–12 cm H_2O positive end-expiratory pressure (PEEP); airway pressure monitor; sterilizability; and performance under varying common environmental conditions.[19] Limited complications have been associated with the use of AMBU bags. Inaccurate inspired oxygen due to inadequate oxygen inflow rate and valve locking due to mechanical malfunction or excessive oxygen flow rates are some of the reported problems.

3. Determining the Effectiveness of Nonintubation Ventilation and Use of Supplemental Airway Maintenance Techniques

The mask seal should be sufficient to permit a 20-cm H_2O positive pressure with a minimal leak. It is important to limit positive airway pressure to 25 cm H_2O to avoid inflating the stomach, which will in turn restrict diaphragmatic movement and increase the chance of regurgitation through the esophageal sphincters.[5,16,20] The effectiveness of ventilation should be judged by exhaled tidal volume, movement of the chest, good bilateral breath sounds, vital signs, and available monitors of oxygenation and ventilation. If the patient cannot be ventilated with 25 cm H_2O positive pressure, either the airway is obstructed at the pharynx by the tongue, the airway is obstructed at the larynx by cord spasm, the patient has sufficient muscle tone to prevent chest expansion, or there is a decrease in pulmonary compliance or increased airway resistance. The oral airway will correct the first; a small dose of succinylcholine will decrease laryngeal spasm and muscle tone, and definitive treatment of the compliance and resistance issue depends on the etiology. Tracheal tug (caudad movement of the larynx or paradoxical movement of the chest) suggests airway obstruction. A naso- or oropharyngeal airway may open the pharyngeal airway at the cost of laryngeal spasm, which is again treated with a small dose of succinylcholine. Paralysis should be a temporary expedient in treating laryngeal spasm, with deeper anesthesia being the more definitive treatment. The known presence of anatomic airway obstruction (tumor or polyp) precludes the use of muscle relaxants, since loss of muscle tone may cause nearly untreatable airway obstruction.

Occasionally, the airway is sufficiently difficult to require the triple airway maneuver to be maintained during ventilation or anesthesia. Since the jaw tends to slide back into the temporomandibular joint, the force required to maintain the position is difficult to maintain constantly, but this must be done. Placement of an oral airway as previously described can be very helpful in this regard. After the oral airway is set in place with the thumbs, the last three fingers of the left hand pull the mandible tightly against the oral airway so that the friction of the incisors on the airway is sufficient to prevent the mandible from slipping back into joint. The right hand places the mask at the bridge of the nose while the thumb and first finger of the left hand receive the mask and adjust it to the face; the left hand now squeezes the mandible–airway–face mask together as a unit. If pressure is relaxed, the jaw can be felt to slide back into joint (if it does so, the triple airway maneuver is repeated). The tension on the jaw can be adjusted by grip strength, by backward weight of the anesthetist, or by the left little finger placed below the angle of the jaw to keep the mandible protruded. (This last maneuver usually requires a rather large hand; see Fig. 5–13C.) This position may not only clear the tongue from the pharynx but may partly treat a laryngeal spasm by exerting force on the hyoid bone, elevating the epiglottis and unfolding the vestibular and vocal folds. It is tiresome to maintain this position, and the pressure required creates a risk of local skin or nerve injury. If after 5–10 minutes the patient will not maintain his airway without a jaw-thrust, his trachea should be intubated. Positive airway pressure can be maintained throughout the respiratory cycle (PEEP or CPAP [continuous positive airway pressure]) to lessen soft tissue obstruction. The pop-off valve is closed to maintain about a 15-cm positive pressure during expiration (no greater than 20 cm). Inspiration can still be assisted to 25 cm H_2O.

The difficulty in maintaining a mask fit and a patent airway with one hand is occasionally so great that the patient's safety is best served if the mask fit and airway are controlled by two hands while a second person ventilates the patient's lungs by squeezing the bag.[16] The two-handed airway technique uses the fingers to perform a jaw-thrust maneuver while the thumbs hold the mask in place by pressure on the lateral sides of the mask (Fig. 5–14).

The confirmation of adequate ventilation is of primary importance to patient safety. Clinical observation

Holding the Mask to the Face with Two Hands

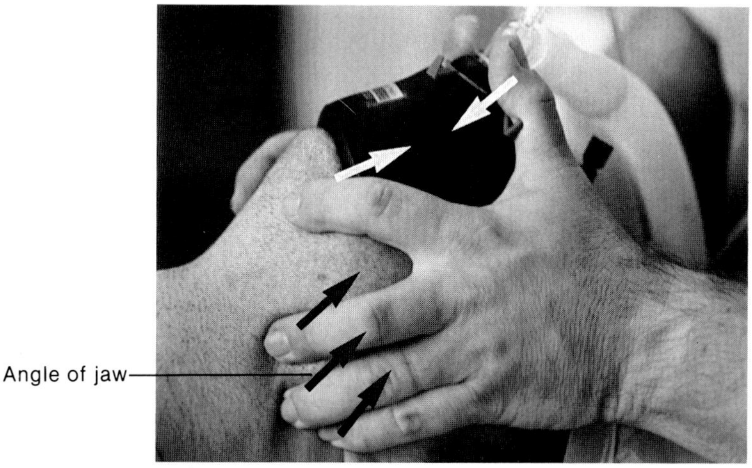

Figure 5–14 • Holding the mask to the face with two hands. Note thumbs hooked over collar of the mask, with lower fingers maintaining jaw thrust (if needed) and upper fingers pulling mandible into the mask and extending the head. *(Arrows indicate direction of force.)*

is key in the assessment of the airway. There are several additional techniques to monitor the adequacy of the airway and of the ventilation. First, the fingers of the left hand supporting the mandible are used to sense the vibration of airflow in the mouth and pharynx. The distal interphalangeal joint should be at the rim of the mandible so that the pads of the fingers contact the soft tissue of the floor of the mouth. They also sense anesthetic depth (muscle tone, swallowing prior to vomiting). Second, the right hand on the anesthesia reservoir bag senses emptying and filling of the bag during the respiratory cycle. The lower the fresh gas flow, the more sensitive is this monitor. With experience, this technique helps assess airway resistance and compliance. Third, pretracheal (or precordial) stethoscopes are basic monitors that should not be neglected. The stethoscope can be attached to the skin over the sternal notch by double-sided adhesive disks, usually permitting both tracheal sounds and heart tones to be heard. Fourth, capnography offers positive evidence of ventilation when a normal capnogram can be seen. Occasionally, a poor mask fit and a gas leak (with high compensatory flows) prevent a good capnogram even with adequate ventilation. Placing an aspirating catheter into a nasal prong and connecting it to a capnometer can give a trend index of ventilation even in a sedated patient. Finally, the pulse oximeter offers reassurance that the oxygenation is adequate when the SaO_2 is above 95%. When below 90%, it strongly suggests that the ventilation may be inadequate (airway obstruction, esophageal ventilation, laryngeal spasm, retained secretions).

III. Discussion: Specific Clinical Situations

Airway maintenance without endotracheal intubation is a necessity of the practice of anesthesia, respiratory care, emergency medicine, and critical care. Occasionally, nonintubation techniques are desirable, since they avoid the sympathetic responses to tracheal intubation (tachycardia, hypertension, coughing). Some of the risks of nonintubation of the airway are laryngeal spasm, aspiration of gastric contents, and sudden unexpected airway obstruction. It is not well suited to prolonged positive pressure ventilation. It requires constant monitoring by precordial/pretracheal stethoscope, watching and feeling a reservoir bag, respiratory gas analysis, pulse oximetry, vital signs, and an educated hand. Airway maintenance during a prolonged steady state (30 minutes to 3 hours) presents a different set of problems and vigilance requirements from that of airway maintenance in a transitional period between a natural airway and the placement or removal of an endotracheal tube. Three situations requiring airway maintenance without endotracheal intubation that deserve special mention are during sedation, during transitional periods surrounding endotracheal intubation, and during induction and maintenance of a general anesthetic.

A. *During Sedation*

Sedation is used to allay patient anxiety or minimize discomfort from position or duration of the procedure, when the stimuli of surgery have been largely ablated by a regional anesthetic block or local anesthetic infiltration. Mild sedation during which the patient can converse easily requires no special airway management, although supplemental oxygen per nasal cannula or clear plastic oxygen insufflation mask should always be used. Sedation to the point of somnolence and stertor requires some intervention to assure adequacy of ventilation and oxygenation, and moderate patient discomfort often requires sedation to this level. Chin lift or jaw thrust usually results in increased patient awareness and clearing of the stertor, reassuring the anesthetist that the patient is not overly sedated. If stertor returns, turning the head 45° to one side or the other may help. (The epiglottis may be the cause of this stertor,[21] and mild twisting of the neck may open a sufficient airway.) Monitoring with pretracheal stethoscope or pulse oximetry may provide enough reassurance to continue with present conditions. The patient may allow an anesthesia mask (attached to a circle system) to lie over his nose and mouth (secured loosely with a head strap). This arrangement permits monitoring of respiration via the reservoir bag, and perhaps capnography, and continued sedation with 25% to 50% nitrous oxide. In patients whom a mask will not fit closely at all (edentulous being the most common), sedation can be temporarily deepened, the nares anesthetized, and a small nasal airway inserted into which a 15-mm adapter (which goes to an oxygen source) has been inserted. A more complete seal and wider airway can be used by using two nasal airways (see Binasal Airway). The anesthesia circle system can then be connected, respiration monitored, and sedation continued with nitrous oxide. Since a mask or nasal airway used in this way may not have a tight fit to the face, scavenging of nitrous oxide is probably incomplete and controlled ventilation impossible. These techniques have less hemodynamic disturbances than do endotracheal intubation, but they require monitoring and the ability to revise techniques as determined by the level of sedation. Because of field avoidance, mask techniques are usually not feasible during monitored anesthesia care for cataract surgery. An oral airway is usually not successful, since it is more stimulating than the nasal airway and may induce retching with this level of sedation.

Complications of mild sedation are usually minimal. Any nasal airway technique may cause epistaxis, usually treatable with nasal pressure. Airway obstruction can go undetected if monitoring is not adequate. Any patient sedated to the point of dozing requires constant airway monitoring. The availability of pulse oximeters has simplified this task, although they monitor oxygenation rather than carbon dioxide levels. Capnography done by aspirating gas from one prong of a nasal prong set or from a catheter inserted through a plastic mask so that the end of it sits close to the nose will give at best a count of respiratory rate. The entrainment of room air along with expired gas by the capnometer pump makes the end-expired carbon dioxide of little value other than a trend monitor of rate, since decreased ventilation is accompanied by a increased entrainment of room air, resulting in a decreased end-tidal carbon dioxide level.

B. *Transitional Airway Techniques*

Prior to intubation of the trachea, the patient usually has received a neuromuscular blocker or, in the case of cardiopulmonary arrest, has no muscle tone. The larynx is open and laryngeal spasm is not a consideration. The techniques of airway maintenance, triple airway maneuver, obtainment of mask seal, limitation of ventilatory pressures to 25 cm H_2O, and early use of oropharyngeal airways are usually sufficient to permit ventilating the patient. Airway maintenance from extubation to smooth spontaneous ventilation is complicated by the presence of a reactive larynx capable of spasm. Therefore, the timing of extubation is an important consideration. Extubation can be either at a deep stage of anesthesia with minimal airway reactivity or during very light anesthesia (nearly awake) so that there is full control of reflex activity (and usually some coughing and straining). The middle ground of moderate anesthetic depth is at an increased risk of laryngospasm. The correct timing is confirmed as follows: the patient should be breathing spontaneously and be considered to have an empty stomach. The oropharynx is suctioned to remove pooled secretions. If smooth, spontaneous ventilation continues, the tube is moved slightly and the cuff is deflated. If the patient continues to breathe smoothly, the trachea is extubated. If, on the other hand, coughing and straining ensue, extubation must wait until the patient again breathes smoothly for two or three cycles. In either event, an inspiratory breath is augmented maximally and the endotracheal tube is withdrawn at end inspiration, allowing rapid expiratory airflow or a cough to clear retained secretions from around the vocal cords. A triple airway maneuver is done immediately (within 5 seconds),[21] spontaneous ventilation is confirmed, and a mask with 100% oxygen is applied to the face. If secretions are copious or intraoral blood is expected, the patient should be put into a position to optimize drainage (head down or lateral).

Laryngeal spasm can be treated with positive pressure if it seems to improve breath by breath.[22,23] A small dose of succinylcholine (10 mg) will remedy the situation more completely at the risk of some muscle ache postoperatively. If obstruction continues, laryngoscopy should be done to investigate the cause, and reintubation should be considered. Special attention must be given to patients with full stomachs, since they are at increased risk of aspiration.

During emergence, the patient usually passes through a stage of generalized increased muscle tone, especially masseter spasm. The force of contraction can put extreme pressure on the central incisors of the mandible with damage to caps or teeth with periodontal disease. An airway should never be removed by force, since lateral stresses may dislodge teeth. Either wait for jaw relaxation or open the jaw with firm pressure on the mandibular ramus between the clenched teeth and the buccal mucosae. Two techniques can be used to minimize the danger to teeth. The first is to have an acrylic tooth guard made by the dental service prior to operation to distribute the forces over more teeth. The other is to place a nasopharyngeal tube prior to extubation of both the endotracheal tube and oral airway so that the teeth are in occlusion when the masseter tightening occurs. The disadvantage of this method is the possibility of epistaxis and the risk that the nasopharyngeal airway will be too short to provide an adequate airway.

C. *Induction and Maintenance of Anesthesia Without Muscle Relaxation*

The major difference between airway management during an inhalation anesthetic without muscle relaxation and with muscle relaxation is that the larynx is responsive to irritation and can obstruct. Spasm can occur in response to irritation of the epiglottis and laryngeal introitus from oro- or nasopharyngeal airways, pungent anesthetics, secretions, and surgical stimulation if the anesthesia level is inadequate.[23] If the airway must be maintained over 30 minutes, anesthesiologist fatigue can be a problem, and vigilance for a sudden change in airway patency is always imperative.

Aspiration prophylaxis directed toward increasing the pH of gastric contents (0.3 *M* sodium citrate, H-2 blockers), decreasing secretion volume (ranitidine or cimetidine), or speeding gastric emptying (metoclopromide) is a prudent but not required precaution before undertaking an inhalation anesthetic by mask. Control of secretions with an antisialagogue (glycopyrrolate, scopolamine, atropine) should be done, since secretions can stimulate the larynx. Mild sedation with a narcotic will suppress some cough reflexes, although heavy sedation will make spontaneous ventilation more difficult. Since regurgitation is always a fear with this technique, people with a risk of full stomach or those in whom the esophageal sphincters (cardiac or cricopharyngeal) are weakened (eg, recent food ingestion, hiatus hernia, pregnancy from 3 months gestation to 2 weeks postpartum) are not good candidates for mask ventilation. Prolonged muscle paralysis is also a relative contraindication, since the cricopharyngeal sphincter (being striated muscle) is weakened. Patients with an esophageal pouch or Zenkers diverticulum also should not receive an anesthetic by mask, since the contents of the pouch might be regurgitated into the pharynx. Ventilation with more than 20 cm H_2O airway pressure is associated with air passing the cricopharyngeal sphincter and entering the esophagus and stomach.[5] Patients who cannot be ventilated satisfactorily with 20 cm inspiratory pressures when paralyzed or breathing spontaneously with augmented ventilation (obese, head down position, bronchospasm, tense abdominal distention) should have the trachea intubated.

Before beginning, the room and equipment should be arranged to provide all needed material within reaching distance. Because the left hand will be on the patient's face or chin nearly continuously, charting, machine changes, reaching for drugs will be done with the right hand. The anesthesia machine should be just off the corner of the OR table, the anesthetic chart should be taped to the writing surface, and the anesthetic cart should be immediately behind the anesthetist. All controls and surfaces should be reachable with the right hand while the left hand remains on the headboard of the operating table at the level of the patient's head. Several towels should be available to elevate the patient's head, and a head strap (mask retaining strap) should be on top of the towels.

Equipment for intubation should be checked and ready as for any anesthetic. A Yankaur or ''tonsil'' suction should be attached to a suction line for induction and maintenance to allow one-handed manipulation. It is changed to a soft 18-gauge suction catheter for emergence, when muscle tone and light or no anesthesia precludes the pharyngeal placement of a rigid suction catheter. A selection of masks of at least two sizes and two bridge configurations should be available. Clear plastic masks are preferable, since the airway can be observed, although the black rubber anatomic models may fit better and be easier to use. Masks must fit both the anesthetist's hand and the patient's face without use of marked pressure, so that a variety of masks for trial is more important here than when less than 5 minutes of mask ventilation is anticipated prior to endotracheal intubation. An assortment of oral airways (nos. 3, 4, 5 for most adults) and nasal airways (6.5–8.0 mm) should be available. Since commercial nasal airways are occasionally too short, a 6.0- or 6.5-mm endotracheal tube can be cut at 18 cm, a safety pin put through it at the 17-cm mark, and the tube softened in hot irrigating solution prior to use.

All drugs expected to be used should be drawn up in labeled syringes. Those in which repeated small doses may be given throughout the induction period should be fitted with small needles (22–25 gauge) to minimize backup into the syringe if it is left in the IV line (Pentothal or succinylcholine are the most common drugs used in this way).

Preoxygenation should be done unless the patient has strong objections to it. For intravenous induction, Pentothal is the most commonly used drug; it can be used in two ways. First, a large bolus dose (after a 50-mg test dose) of 4–5 mg/kg can be given; an oral airway can be placed early; and the patient can be ventilated with increasing concentrations of inhalation anesthetic to 2–3 minimal anesthesia concentration (MAC) within 2–3 minutes and delivered in high gas flows to allow rapid changes in inspired concentration. Ventilation is best controlled until incision, when the increased stimulus is usually sufficient to promote spontaneous ventilation. Attempts to achieve spontaneous ventilation before the onset of surgical stimulation usually require that the level of anesthesia be too low for the patient to lie quietly with the incision. The initial high induction dose of drug allows the oral airway to be placed early without stimulating a laryngeal response.

Second, a small dose of Pentothal (3 mg/kg) or other induction agent can be titrated in 50-mg increments to allow spontaneous or assisted ventilation while the inhalation anesthetic is gradually increased in 0.25–0.50-MAC increments until the patient breathes smoothly and the blood pressure has decreased by 20%. This procedure takes time, during which the room should be quiet and the patient should be undisturbed. Hastening the process by rapid escalation of inspired anesthetic concentrations or early instrumentation of the airway usually produces coughing and laryngeal irritation and spasm. Passage through the second stage of delirium or breath holding may be hastened by increasing the nitrous oxide concentration to 70% to use the second gas effect, or by using small doses of Pentothal. Head position and neck flexion maneuvers (to test muscle tone) should be tried before inserting artificial airways, as should gentle positive airway pressure (assisted ventilation at no more than 25 cm H_2O and/or constant airway positive pressure of 10–15 cm H_2O augmented during inspiration to 20–25 cm H_2O). In general, nasal airways are better tolerated than oral, but at the risk of epistaxis. Reactivity to oropharyngeal airways can be lessened by topical anesthesia of the pharynx and epiglottis by preinduction gargling with viscous lidocaine. A postinduction spray with 4% lidocaine (200 mg maximum) or Cetacaine can be helpful. The mask must not be off the face for more than 20 seconds to avoid rapid decreases in anesthetic level. The fingers of the left hand holding the mandible and mask will perceive muscle tightening as an early sign of lightness or overstimulation, and swallowing as a prelude to vomiting. In general, smaller airways are tried first in nonparalyzed patients to avoid laryngeal irritation. Despite the best plans, laryngeal irritation frequently presents with "crowing," stertor, or obstruction. Crowing can usually be remedied by deepening the anesthetic (Pentothal 50–100 mg and/or increasing the inhalation agent); stertor or obstruction may be from the tongue, necessitating airway maneuvers or devices, but may also be from laryngeal spasm, where muscle relaxation (10–20 mg succinylcholine) will temporarily cure the problem. A succinylcholine infusion is usually more titratable than the bolus injections.

Despite the stated drawbacks, no agent is more effective than succinylcholine in restoring a patent airway if the patient's airway was previously normal. Large airway tumors, especially if pedunculated, can act as a ball-valve with relaxation of the airway musculature; muscle relaxants should not be used in these patients. Occasionally, a patient does not breathe smoothly, regardless of depth of anesthesia, or coughs repeatedly unless paralyzed. It is better to intubate the trachea than to continue to administer an anesthetic to a completely paralyzed patient with a mask.

An inhalation induction is most commonly done on children to avoid the discomfort of an awake placement of an IV. In an adult, an inhalation induction is occasionally necessary. There are two approaches to this situation. One is to preoxygenate the patient and rapidly turn the vaporizer to 4–5 MAC for the minute required to induce anesthesia. This approach is more likely to cause bradycardia and coughing, but frequently works well in children (the vagal reflex should be blocked with adequate doses of atropine). The other approach is to preoxygenate the patient and to begin a rhythmic monologue while introducing the inhalation agent slowly and in small concentrations, encouraging the patient to breathe smoothly, and predicting the sensations (dizziness, tingling at the lips, etc) just as he or she is about to experience them. The anesthetist gradually increases the concentration of inhalation anesthetic from 0.5 MAC to 2 MAC in 10 L O_2. As the patient nears the second stage of anesthesia, heralded by uneven respiration and increased muscle tone, the nitrous oxide is rapidly increased to 70% to hasten passage through the second stage. The inhalation anesthetic is usually raised to 3–4 MAC temporarily. As the patient resumes a smooth respiratory pattern, the blood pressure will have decreased by 20% and the fresh gas flows will be reduced to 2–4 L/min of N_2O in O_2 (50% each) with volatile inhalation agent at a concentration of 1–2 MAC. After the incision, the level is titrated against respiration and blood pressure.

The most important feature of unintubated airway management during the maintenance of anesthesia is monitoring the progress of the operation and the state of the airway. Increasing levels of stimuli must be anticipated and the anesthetic deepened prior to its occurrence, usually by increased concentration of inhaled volatile anesthetic. The use of intravenous narcotics as the major component of obtaining increased depth of anesthesia is usually self-defeating, since ventilation decreases and the uptake of inhalation anesthetic decreases. If the increased stimulus is unheeded and laryngeal spasm occurs, succinylcholine is the fastest way to regain control of the airway. Positive pressure on the airway may suffice but often requires high airway pressures leading to gastric inflation. The smooth conduct of an inhalation anesthetic by mask requires more vigilance, anticipation, and knowledge of the individual surgeon than does one by endotracheal tube, but the practitioner of the art of anesthesia and the patient can be greatly rewarded.

Fatigue is a common problem if the operation lasts more than 1 hour and the airway is difficult to manage. There are many ways to minimize fatigue. The patient's head should be at a level between the anesthesiologist's waist and shoulders. The anesthetist should sit on a variable-height chair or stand so as to accomplish this. The elbow of the anesthetist's left arm should be kept into his or her left side to minimize shoulder strain, and weight can substitute for muscle power if the left arm is allowed to extend and the anesthetist leans backward. Resting the elbow on the table next to the patient's head will also relax the shoulder. The right hand may hold the mask temporarily to give the left hand a rest if the patient is breathing spontaneously. A head strap can assist the anesthetist's forearm muscles. Strapping the mask does not free the left hand for other than the briefest of times (15–30 seconds) because the pads of the fingers are irreplaceable monitors. The left hand still provides extension of the head, sometimes required to maintain a patent airway even with artificial airways in place. Vaseline gauze can be placed between the mask and skin to improve the seal or minimize friction on the dermis, especially important in cases of epidermolysis bullosa. The length of time the inhalation anesthetic can be safely administered depends in great part on the ease in holding the airway.

There are no outcome studies concerning the relative safety of giving anesthetics by mask versus endotracheal tube in situations where either is applicable. Airway problems such as aspiration, inadequate ventilation, and esophageal intubation constitute the major part of anesthetic catastrophes. The patient, the anesthetist's airway skills, and the ability to confirm endotracheal intubation (capnography) interact in any given situation to determine the best approach. Airway skills remain a primary skill of the anesthesiologist. An understanding of the anatomy, airway maneuvers, and devices and the appropriate use of the bag and mask are essential to the safe administration of anesthesia and care of critically ill patients.

IV. References

1. Fink BR, Demerest RJ. Laryngeal Biomechanics. Cambridge, MA, Harvard University Press, 1978.
2. Applebaum EL, Bruce DL. Tracheal Intubation. Philadelphia, WB Saunders, 1976.
3. Ferner H. Pernkopf Atlas of Topographical and Applied Human Anatomy: Head and Neck. Philadelphia, WB Saunders, 1980.
4. Standards and guidelines for cardiopulmonary resuscitation and emergency cardiac care. JAMA 244:453, 1980.
5. Safar P, Bircher NG. Cardiopulmonary Cerebral Resuscitation. Philadelphia, WB Saunders, 1988, 13–94.
6. Safar P, Ajuto-Escarraja L, Chang F. A study of upper airway obstruction on the unconscious patient. J Appl Physiol 14:760, 1959.
7. Boidin, MP. Airway patency in the unconscious patient. Br J Anaesth 57:306–310, 1985.
8. Morikawa S, Safar P, DeCarlo J. Influence of head position upon upper airway patency. Anesthesiology 22:265, 1961.
9. Heimlich HJ. A life-saving maneuver to prevent choking. JAMA 234:398, 1975.
10. Redding JS. The choking controversy: Critique of evidence on the Heimlich maneuver. Crit Care Med 7:745, 1979.
11. Dorsch JA, Dorsch SE. Understanding Anesthesia Equipment. 2nd ed. Baltimore, Williams & Wilkins, 1984.
12. Moore W, Rauscher L. A complication of oropharyngeal airway placement. Anesthesiology 16:643, 1955.
13. Stauffer JL, Silvestri RL. Complications of endotracheal intubation, tracheostomy, and artificial airways. Respir Care 27:417, 1982.
14. Zwillich C, Pierson DJ. Nasal necrosis: A complication of nasotracheal intubation. Chest 64:376, 1973.
15. Weisman H, Bauer RO, Huddy RA, Elam JO. An improved binasopharyngeal airway system for anesthesia. Anesth Analg 51:11, 1972.
16. Finucane BT, Santori AH. Principles of Airway Management. Philadelphia, FA Davis, 1988.
17. Rubin H. A new non-rebreathing valve. Anesthesiology 16:643, 1955.
18. Stephenson HE. Cardiopulmonary resuscitation. In Burton GC, Hodgkin JE (eds). Respiratory Care. Philadelphia, JB Lippincott, 1984, 897.
19. LaBouef LL. Assessment of eight resuscitators. Respir Care 80:1136, 1980.
20. Pontoppidan J, Gefin B, Lowenstein E. Acute respiratory failure in the adult. N Engl J Med 287:690, 1972.
21. Hanning, CD. Obstructive sleep apnea. Br J Anaesth 63:477–488, 1989.
22. Fink BR. The Human Larynx. New York, Raven Press, 1975.
23. Fink BR. Etiology and treatment of laryngeal spasm. Anesthesiology 17:569, 1956.

Chapter 6

•

Jonathan L. Benumof, MD

Conventional (Laryngoscopic) Orotracheal and Nasotracheal Intubation (Single-Lumen Type)

OUTLINE

I. Introduction and Indications
- A. Indications for Tracheal Intubation of the Awake Patient in Respiratory Failure
  1. Objective Quantitative Criteria
  2. Subjective Qualitative Criteria
  3. Other Criteria
  4. Integration of the Objective and Subjective Criteria
- B. Indications for Tracheal Intubation of the Generally Anesthetized Patient
  1. Primary Need for a Guaranteed Airway
  2. Secondary Need for a Guaranteed Airway
     - a. Inadequate Mask Ventilation
     - b. The Surgical Procedure Is Changed After the Induction of Anesthesia
     - c. A Major Complication Occurs

II. How to Do Conventional (Laryngoscopic) Orotracheal and Nasotracheal Intubation (Single-Lumen Tube)
- A. Conventional (Laryngoscopic) Orotracheal Intubation
  1. Prelaryngoscopy Maneuvers
  2. Laryngoscopy
  3. Tracheal Intubation
  4. Securement of the Tube
- B. Conventional (Laryngoscopic) Nasotracheal Intubation
  1. Prelaryngoscopy Maneuvers
  2. Laryngoscopy
  3. Tracheal Intubation
  4. Securement of the Tube

III. Discussion of the Procedure: Conventional Mechanical Ventilation, Weaning, and Extubation of the Trachea
- A. Initial Ventilator Settings: Intermittent Mandatory Ventilation
- B. Goal 1: $F_IO_2 < 0.5$ and P_aO_2 Acceptable
  1. Why This Goal Is No. 1: Oxygen Toxicity
  2. How to Achieve Goal 1
- C. Goal 2: $F_IO_2 < 0.5$, PEEP < 10 cm H_2O, and P_aO_2 Acceptable
  1. Why This Goal Is No. 2: Match Ventilation to Perfusion
  2. How to Achieve Goal 2
- D. Goal 3: $F_IO_2 < 0.5$, PEEP < 10 cm H_2O, IMV < 1 Breath/Min, and P_aO_2 Acceptable
  1. Why This Goal Is No. 3: Conversion from Intermittent Mandatory to Spontaneous ventilation
  2. How to Achieve Goal 3
- E. Summary of Mechanical Ventilation and Weaning Procedure
- F. Other New Mechanical Ventilation and Weaning Modes
- G. Extubation of the Trachea

IV. Complications

V. References

I. Introduction and Indications

Tracheal intubation achieves four main goals (Table 6–1): it guarantees patency of the upper airway (provided the tracheal tube itself is kept clear of secretions), protects the airway from gastric contents, allows mechanical positive pressure ventilation to be administered, and permits suctioning of the tracheobronchial tree for removal of secretions. Tracheal intubation may be required to achieve one, or any combination, of these four goals.

Two major categories of patients require tracheal intubation; the two categories usually emphasize different tracheal intubation goals. First, awake patients who have impending respiratory failure, or are in respiratory failure, require tracheal intubation (see Section A, immediately following). In this group of patients, the usual purposes of tracheal intubation, in descending order of importance, are to provide mechanical ventilation, tracheobronchial tree suctioning capability, airway patency, and airway protection. Since the degree of respiratory failure in awake patients is amenable to quantification, the most important indications for tracheal intubation in most of these patients are the objective tests of respiratory function. However, in some patients, the gross appearance of the patient alone is sufficient indication.

Second, generally anesthetized patients who have a primary need for a guaranteed airway (eg, patients who undergo neurosurgical, cardiothoracic, ear, nose, mouth, and throat procedures, and major intraabdominal procedures) or patients who develop a secondary need for a guaranteed airway (for example, if ventilation via mask is inadequate, the procedure is changed after induction of anesthesia, or a major complication occurs [eg, malignant hyperthermia]) require tracheal intubation (see Section B). In this group of patients, the usual purposes of tracheal intubation, in descending order of importance, are to provide airway patency, mechanical ventilation, airway protection, and ability to remove secretions. Airway protection is more important in patients who are thought to have gastric contents (ie, full stomachs) and in patients undergoing intraabdominal procedures. A severely poisoned patient (eg, drug overdose; see Chapter 43) is equivalent to a generally anesthetized patient with a full stomach and requires tracheal intubation for airway protection, patency, and mechanical ventilation. Since generally anesthetized patients are usually intubated to provide a guaranteed airway, the most important indication for tracheal intubation in these patients is preoperative knowledge of the surgical procedure and intraoperative recognition of the signs of airway obstruction.

Table 6–1 • Goals of Tracheal Intubation

Guarantees patency of the upper airway
Protects the airway from gastric contents
Allows mechanical positive pressure ventilation
Permits suctioning of the tracheobronchial tree

A. *Indications for Tracheal Intubation of the Awake Patient in Respiratory Failure*

In the absence of frank cardiopulmonary arrest, the diagnosis of impending or actual respiratory failure in awake patients is based on objective quantitative criteria, or subjective qualitative criteria, or both. There are many causes of respiratory failure, and detailing them is beyond the scope of this book. For our purposes, it is sufficient to classify the cause of respiratory failure as acute vs. chronic lung disease (Fig 6–1). The treatment of respiratory failure is mechanical ventilation. The following discussion of indications for tracheal intubation of the awake patient in respiratory failure emphasizes this primary goal of tracheal intubation.

1. Objective Quantitative Criteria

The three right-hand columns in Table 6–2 describe a deterioration in the results of respiratory function testing from an acceptable range to an unstable, possible intubation status requiring close monitoring and intensive nontracheal intubation support (see Chapter 4), to probable intubation and mechanical ventilation necessary status.[1] The respiratory function testing is divided into mechanical, oxygenation, and ventilation categories. In practice, P_aO_2 and P_aCO_2 are used most often as indicators of tracheal intubation (see Fig. 6–1), and vital capacity, peak inspiratory force, and respiratory rate are used most often as indicators of tracheal extubation.

The trend of the data in Table 6–2 is as important as the data themselves. For example, progressively increasing P_aCO_2 from a normal P_aCO_2 in a patient without previous lung disease is more important than an already high P_aCO_2 in a patient with emphysema. Thus, a P_aO_2 of 50 mmHg and a P_aCO_2 of 65 mmHg might

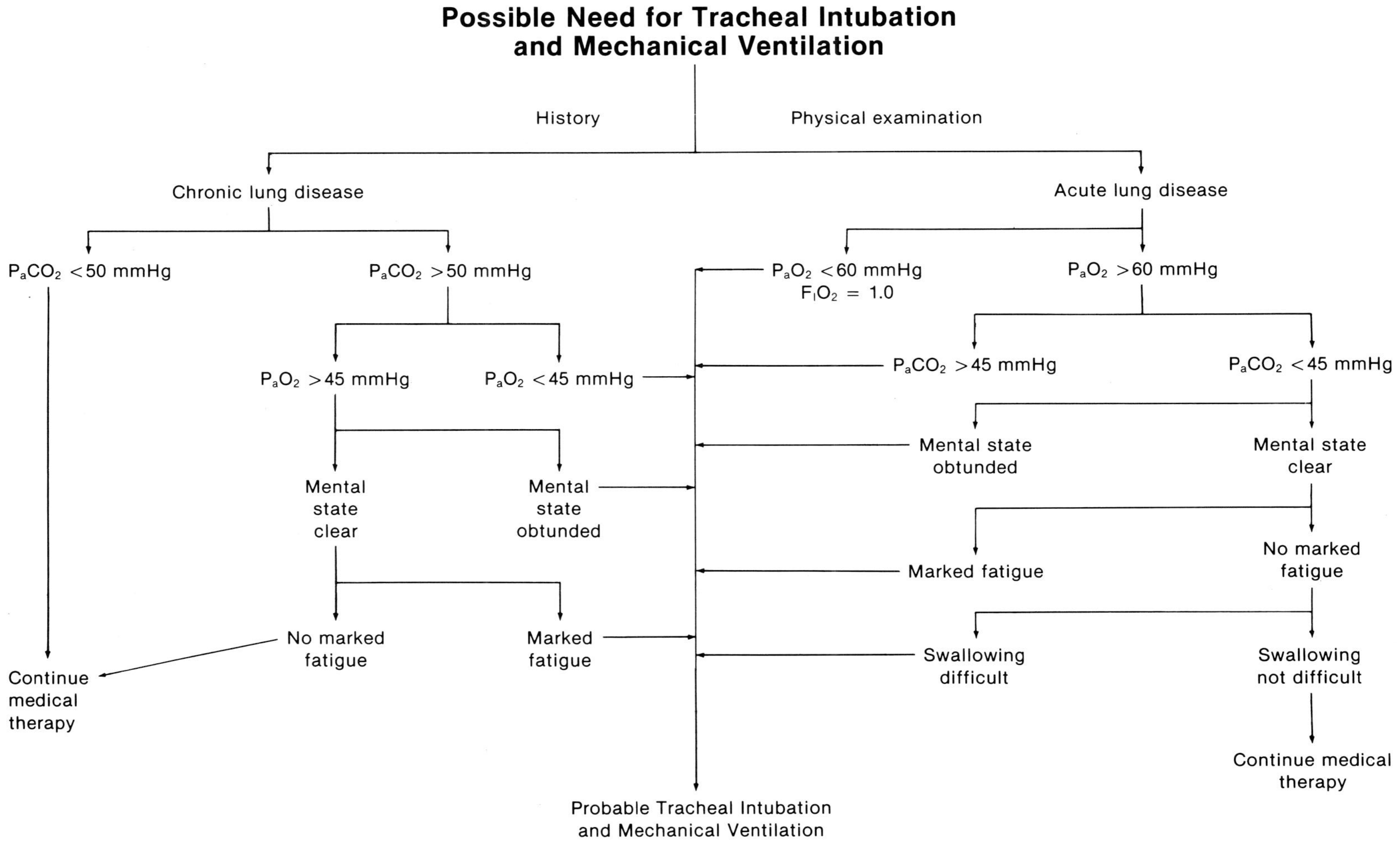

Figure 6–1 • Algorithm for institution of tracheal intubation and mechanical ventilation in patients with acute (right-hand side) and chronic (left-hand side) lung disease. Note that hypoxemia (P_aO_2 <60 mmHg on F_IO_2 of 1.0), hypercapnia (P_aCO_2 >50 mmHg), and subjective qualitative signs (obtunded mental state, marked respiratory fatigue, difficulty in swallowing) can each be independent indications for tracheal intubation and mechanical ventilation. (See text for explanation of medical therapy.)

Table 6-2 • Objective Quantitative Criteria for Tracheal Intubation.

Respiratory Function: *Category*	*Variable*	Acceptable Range	Possible Intubation Chest PT, Oxygen, Drugs, Close Monitoring	Probable Intubation and Ventilation
Mechanics	Vital capacity (mL/kg)	65–75	65–15	<15
	Inspiratory force, (mL H_2O)	100–50	50–25	<25
Oxygenation	A-aDO_2 (mmHg) room air	<38	38–55	>55
	F_IO_2 = 1.0	<100	100–450	>450
	P_aO_2 (mmHg)			
	room air	>72	72–55	<55
	F_IO_2 = 1.0	>400	400–200	<200
Ventilation	Respiratory rate, (breaths/min)	10–25	25–40 or <8	>40 or <6
	P_aCO_2 (mmHg)	35–45	45-60	<60

PT = physical therapy; A-aDO_2 = alveolar-arterial partial pressure of oxygen difference; P_aO_2 and P_aCO_2 = arterial partial pressure of oxygen and carbon dioxide, respectively; F_IO_2 = inspired concentration of oxygen.
(Adapted from Pontpoppidan H, Geffin B, Lowenstein E. Acute respiratory failure in the adult [second of three parts]. N Engl J Med 287:743–752, 1972.)

be normal for a chronic obstructive pulmonary disease (COPD) patient, but these same values would indicate a marked degree of respiratory embarrassment for a previously normal patient. Thus, knowledge of the patient's usual state of health is very helpful in making the decision to intubate the trachea.

2. Subjective Qualitative Criteria

On occasion, one simply needs to look at the patient to determine whether tracheal intubation is necessary. The grossly observable indications for tracheal intubation consist of a depressed level of consciousness and signs of respiratory fatigue. Deterioration in the patient's level of consciousness is an ominous sign for four reasons: a decrease in sensorium (1) decreases the patient's ability to cooperate with needed treatments, (2) may indicate cerebral hypoxia, (3) diminishes or abolishes reflexes preventing aspiration of gastric contents, and (4) may cause upper airway obstruction. Changes in sensorium generally occur very slowly, but in selected patients, expected changes may be a factor in the decision to intubate. Signs of increased work of breathing and impending fatigue are listed in Table 6–3.[2-6] With acute neuromuscular disease, inability to swallow is an indicator for tracheal intubation. The grossly observable signs closely interact with the objective quantitative criteria (see Section I.A.4 and Fig. 6–1) to determine the need for tracheal intubation.

3. Other Criteria

The chest radiograph may reveal readily reversible pathology (eg, a pneumothorax) that can be quickly treated and obviate the need for intubation. As with all other data, the trend in changes in the chest radiograph is important. Consideration should also be given to the contribution of the cardiac output and fluid balance to impaired gas exchange. For example, pulmonary edema

Table 6–3 • Signs of Respiratory Distress and Impending Fatigue[2-6]

Look of anxiety → Frowning
Signs of sympathetic overactivity → Dilated pupils, forehead sweat
Dyspnea → Decreased talking
Use of accessory muscles → Holds head off pillow
Mouth opens during inspiration → Licking of dry lips
Self PEEP → Pursed lips, expiratory grunting, groaning
Cyanosed lips
Restlessness and fidgeting → Apathy and coma

may be very responsive to pharmacologic manipulation of the cardiac output, intravascular volume, and urinary output, and such treatment may quickly obviate the need for tracheal intubation.

4. INTEGRATION OF THE OBJECTIVE AND SUBJECTIVE CRITERIA

Figure 6–1 shows a tracheal intubation logic tree for acute and chronic lung disease. In acute lung disease, hypoxemia is the most important, hypercapnia is the next most important, and the subjective qualitative criteria are the least important indicators of tracheal intubation. Nevertheless, the algorithm shows that each of the three indicators can independently be a primary reason for tracheal intubation. In chronic lung disease, hypercapnia is the most important indicator of tracheal intubation; the other indicators, in order of importance, are hypoxemia and the subjective qualitative criteria. Nevertheless, this algorithm also shows that all three indicators can be independently a primary indication for tracheal intubation. Thus, in both of the algorithms presented in Fig. 6–1, tracheal intubation is still indicated in patients with a P_aO_2 greater than 50–60 mmHg and a P_aCO_2 less than 45–50 mmHg, provided one of the subjective qualitative criteria is present in sufficient magnitude.

The postoperative patient emerging from anesthesia often has a significant element of several of these objective and subjective indications for continued tracheal intubation and mechanical ventilation. These elements include residual anesthesia and/or paralysis (mental state obtunded, weak breathing muscles, no swallowing), objective deterioration in lung function, and need for a smooth transition into a postoperative period that will include many other intensive therapies for other major organs.

In Fig. 6–1, medical therapy may include incentive spirometry, coughing routines, frequent tracheal suctioning (even fiberoptic bronchoscopy), chest physical therapy (chest percussion and vibration in various postures), humidification of the inspired gases, ambulation, increased nutrition, administration of antibiotics, bronchodilators, steroids, diuretics, inotropic drugs, and cessation of smoking. These vigorous attempts to improve regional ventilation, together with the controlled administration of oxygen to relieve tissue hypoxia, may be successful in avoiding tracheal intubation in patients who have only marginal indications for tracheal intubation. Indeed, Campbell[7] has reported that only eight of 70 acutely hospitalized patients with chronic lung disease treated in this manner required tracheal intubation. Similarly, Zwillich et al[8] have reported that only 26 of 304 patients with chronic airway obstruction and acute respiratory failure treated in this manner required tracheal intubation.

B. *Indications for Tracheal Intubation of the Generally Anesthetized Patient*

1. PRIMARY NEED FOR A GUARANTEED AIRWAY

Many surgical procedures require that the patient be tracheally intubated (Table 6–4). All surgical procedures that are performed under general anesthesia and that prevent the anesthesiologist from having access to and/or control over the patient's natural airway require tracheal intubation. These procedures consist of all neurosurgical, ear, nose, mouth, and tracheal procedures; all procedures performed in the prone position; most procedures performed in the lateral decubitus position; and any procedure that involves turning the patient so that the anesthesiologist is not at the patient's head. Intrathoracic and intraabdominal procedures require tracheal intubation because of both mechanical and physiologic impediments to adequate gas exchange. Surgical procedures of a very long duration usually require tracheal intubation because the ability of one individual to maintain an adequate airway decreases with time. Finally, procedures that require a great deal of the anesthesiologist's attention and time for nonrespiratory matters (eg, those involving massive blood loss or extensive monitoring) re-

Table 6–4 • Primary Need for a Guaranteed Airway in the Generally Anesthetized Patient

- I. Prevention of loss of control over airway in patients under general anesthesia
    1. Surgical procedures: neurosurgical, ear, nose, mouth, tracheal
    2. Patient position: prone or lateral decubitus position and procedures that require turning the patient so that the anesthesiologist is not at the head of the patient
- II. Gas exchange is expected to be impaired
    1. Intrathoracic procedures
    2. Intraabdominal procedures
- III. Prolonged general anesthesia
- IV. Complicated anesthetics requiring a great deal of nonairway attention

quire tracheal intubation so that the anesthesiologist's hands and attention are not tied to maintaining a nonguaranteed airway. As noted earlier, the patient emerging from anesthesia for a very major surgical procedure often requires continued tracheal intubation and mechanical ventilation for multiple reasons.

2. Secondary Need for a Guaranteed Airway

When a secondary need for a guaranteed airway arises, it is usually unexpected and may not be planned for. For example, ventilation by mask may become inadequate, the surgical procedure may be changed, or a major surgical or anesthesia complication may occur (Table 6–5). Consequently, the difficulty of tracheal intubation under these circumstances may be increased.

a. Inadequate Mask Ventilation

Airway obstruction is the most common serious cause of inadequate ventilation via a mask, and major airway obstruction unrelieved by such maneuvers as anterior jaw dislocation and insertion of a naso- and/or oropharyngeal airway is an absolute indication for tracheal intubation. The obstruction can be at any level of the airway and may cause preferential ventilation of the esophagus (pathway of least resistance), resulting in distention of the stomach. Stomach distention, in turn, will impair ventilation of the lungs further. Patients under general anesthesia who are breathing via an anesthesia mask make up the largest group with this indication for tracheal intubation. However, respiratory failure patients who are narcotized by carbon dioxide retention, patients who are excessively intravenously sedated or narcotized while under regional anesthesia, patients who are poisoned or have taken a drug overdose, and head-injured patients are also in this category.

Table 6–5 • Secondary Need for a Guaranteed Airway

1. Inadequate mask ventilation
2. Surgical procedure is changed after anesthesia is induced
3. A major anesthetic or surgical complication occurs

Total airway obstruction is characterized by lack of breath sounds, which may be coupled with continuing, sometimes strenuous but ineffectual efforts at breathing. Excessive diaphragmatic activity causes abdominal movements and chest retraction, but they do not represent movement of air. The diagnosis is made by absence of breath sounds, failure to observe movement of the breathing bag or failure to feel the movement and warmth of air at the airway outlet, and absence of a carbon dioxide excretion waveform (if an end-tidal CO_2 monitor is being used).

Partial upper airway obstruction is characterized by restriction of air movement with inspiration, which prolongs the inspiratory phase; diminished tidal exchange and breath sounds; excessive diaphragmatic activity; retraction of the upper chest; discrepancy between the movements of the breathing bag and the chest wall; and various characteristic sounds. Partial obstruction caused by the tongue causes a rough, irregular, stuttery noise frequently associated with "stertorous" respiration. The relative size of the tongue to the oropharynx can be determined by having the patient open his or her mouth widely and say "ah." If the uvula and tonsilar pillars are obscured by the tongue, then the tongue is very large in relation to the oropharynx.[9,10] Partial laryngospasm usually causes a high-pitched whistle or squeak. Partial obstruction by the lips is most noticeable during expiration and is accompanied by a low-pitched, rough, fluttery sound. Pharyngeal secretions cause a gurgling, bubbling noise. Partial obstruction at the trachea due to foreign materials and secretions produces a rattly or sloshy noise.

Lower-airway obstruction is characterized by diminished tidal exchange, excessive intercostal and diaphragmatic activity, active inspiration and expiration during spontaneous respiration, and most important, adventitious breath sounds consisting of rales, rhonchi, or wheezing. Bronchiolar secretions cause rhonchi, and bronchiolar constriction causes wheezing. Alveolar obstruction may be associated with all types of adventitious sounds, but rales are most common. With lower-airway obstruction, the breathing bag classically empties and refills slowly, and moderate changes in compliance can be felt by squeezing the reservoir bag.

Very obese patients may be predictably difficult to ventilate by mask because of the difficulty in raising the heavy chest wall and displacing the massive abdominal wall. Dentureless patients may be difficult to ventilate by mask because of large air leaks between the sunken cheeks and the mask. Although such maneuvers as changing the size of the mask, pressing the mask closer to the face, and changing the contour of the patient's face (eg, placing saline-soaked gauze rolls in the buccal pouches to round out the cheeks) may sometimes diminish or eliminate the air leak, tracheal intubation is often necessary.

b. *The Surgical Procedure Is Changed After the Induction of Anesthesia*

Change in the planned surgical procedure most frequently follows diagnostic procedures such as conversion of a breast biopsy into a mastectomy, conversion of a dilatation and curettage of the uterus to a hysterectomy, and conversion of a bronchoscopy or mediastinoscopy to a lung resection.

c. *A Major Complication Occurs*

The occurrence of a major anesthetic or surgical complication—such as a high or total spinal anesthetic, massive blood loss, malignant hyperthermia, or wearing off of a regional anesthetic (patient experiences undue pain)—often requires tracheal intubation (along with other important treatments).

In summary, both awake and anesthetized patients may require tracheal intubation. In awake patients, this decision will be based on objective quantitative and subjective qualitative criteria, and trends in all of these data. In anesthetized patients, the need for tracheal intubation is usually identified preoperatively but may occasionally arise unexpectedly after the induction of anesthesia. Thus, tracheal intubation may be either an expected, elective, planned procedure or an unexpected, nonelective, emergency procedure. The exact set of circumstances under which the need for tracheal intubation arises often determines the technique by which tracheal intubation is accomplished. Orotracheal intubation is especially indicated when speed of intubation is the primary consideration. Nasotracheal intubation is especially indicated for many surgical procedures involving the face and mouth; it may also be indicated to increase the comfort of intubations of very long duration (days). Decision-making logic algorithms have been developed to determine the best method of tracheal intubation under all circumstances,[11-13] especially regarding whether a difficult tracheal intubation is suspected[12] or unsuspected.[13] Chapters 7–13 describe all the techniques one may use to accomplish the difficult tracheal intubation.

II. How to Do Conventional (Laryngoscopic) Orotracheal and Nasotracheal Intubation (Single-Lumen Tube)

A. *Conventional (Laryngoscopic) Orotracheal Intubation*

The oral route is the easiest and most frequently used approach for tracheal intubation and should be the first technique learned. It is very commonly used for the administration of anesthesia, resuscitative efforts, and other short-term situations requiring airway intubation. Visualization of the glottis is obtained by the introduction of a laryngoscope through the mouth. A tracheal tube is then inserted through the glottis into the trachea under direct vision. The laryngoscope is removed, and the tube is secured to the face or teeth.

1. Prelaryngoscopy Maneuvers

Table 6–6 lists the materials that are to be present and immediately available for conventional oro- and nasotracheal intubation. The materials are grouped according to the temporal sequence of intubation events. Whenever there is a choice in size, the size that is thought to be the right one (medium in Table 6–6), one size larger (large in Table 6–6), and one size smaller (small in Table 6–6) should be available. The equipment listed in Table 6–6 is the minimum equipment essential for performing tracheal intubation, preventing a major complication, or both.

Table 6–7 lists the proper temporal sequence of essential prelaryngoscopy maneuvers. If the intubation is being performed in an intensive care location, adequate access to the patient's head must be arranged and may include removal of the headboard of the bed. The height of the surface upon which the patient rests (bed, operating room table, gurney, etc) should be adjustable (to the level of the intubationist's intercostal margin), and the surface should be nonmovable (rolling parts locked). An experienced aide should be in constant attendance to hand items, such as suction lines, airways, tubes, drugs, and so on, to the intubationist.

Table 6–6 • Minimal Essential Equipment for Tracheal Intubation

I. Preoxygenation and ventilation
   1. Oxygen source should be turned on and attached to a self-inflating ventilation bag
   2. Small, medium, and large anesthesia masks must be present
   3. Small, medium, and large oropharyngeal and nasopharyngeal airways
   4. Tongue depressor

II. Preparation of the endotracheal tube
   4. Small, medium, and large orotracheal tubes
   5. Small, medium, and large nasotracheal tubes
   6. Malleable stylet
   7. Three-way stopcock connected to 10-mL syringe
   8. 4% xylocaine jelly and ointment

III. Anesthesia
   9. Intravenous anesthetics and muscle relaxants
   10. Syringes and needles
   11. 4% xylocaine multidose and two ampules of neosynephrine
   12. Atomizer and local anesthetic

IV. Laryngoscopy
   13. Suction apparatus should be turned on and hard plastic suction catheter attached
   14. Magill forceps
   15. No. 3 and No. 4 Miller blades with functioning light source
   16. No. 3 and No. 4 Mackintosh blades with functioning light source
   17. Towels or pillows to put patient's head in "sniff" position

V. Fixation of the endotracheal tube
   18. Tincture of benzoin
   19. Adhesive and umbilical tape

VI. Determination of endotracheal tube location (see next section)
   20. Stethoscope
   21. End-tidal CO_2 monitor
   22. Pulse oximeter

Suctioning the pharynx may be necessary at any time in any patient, but it is most likely to be necessary in patients who have eaten recently (stomach contents), who have suffered airway trauma (blood), who have had a cardiac and/or pulmonary arrest (stomach contents and secretions), and who have had a failure in an immediate previous intubation attempt (secretions). A curved, clear, hard plastic suction catheter should be used.

The correct head position for laryngoscopy is extremely important. Successful direct laryngoscopy requires aligning the oral, pharyngeal, and laryngeal axes (Fig. 6–2A) such that the passageway from the incisor teeth to the glottis is almost a straight line. To bring the laryngeal axis in line with the pharyngeal axis, the neck first must be flexed on the chest by elevating the head about 10 cm with pads under the occiput (shoulders remaining on the table) (see Fig. 6–2B). To bring the oral axis in line with both the pharyngeal axis and laryngeal axis, the head must also be extended on the neck (extension of the junction of the spine and skull [atlanto-occipital joint]) (see Fig. 6–2C). This position of the head is commonly called the sniff position. The upper airway is maximally patent in the sniff position and is the reason that long-distance runners instinctively assume this head position. Thus, the same positioning movements that make the airway largest also make the airway straightest. Full extension of the head, without elevation of the occiput (Fig. 6–2D), is contraindicated because this position increases the lips-to-glottis distance; rotates the larynx anteriorly, unaligning the oral axis from the pharyngeal and laryngeal axes; and may necessitate subsequent leverage on the maxillary teeth or gums with the laryngoscope blade to expose the larynx.

From the moment a resuscitator begins laryngoscopy to the initiation of positive pressure ventilation via the tracheal tube, a period of time must pass. The duration of this period is directly proportional to the degree of difficulty of exposure of the larynx and inversely proportional to the skill of the intubationist. Since even skilled intubationists may require 30 seconds to 1 minute for this period, preoxygenation with 100% O_2 ventilation via face mask is almost always indicated (see below). Preoxygenation may be either with positive or negative pressure breathing. If the tidal volume is large and the rate is rapid (ie, minute ventilation is high), then the duration of preoxygenation need only be for 1 minute,[14] whereas if the tidal volume is small and/or the rate is slow (ie, minute ventilation is low), then the duration of preoxygenation should be for 3–4 minutes.[15] A note

Table 6–7 • Prelaryngoscopy Maneuvers

1. Equipment and suction available (Table 6–6)
2. Clear access to patient's head
3. Place patient's head in sniff position
4. Preoxygenate
5. Have adequate help available

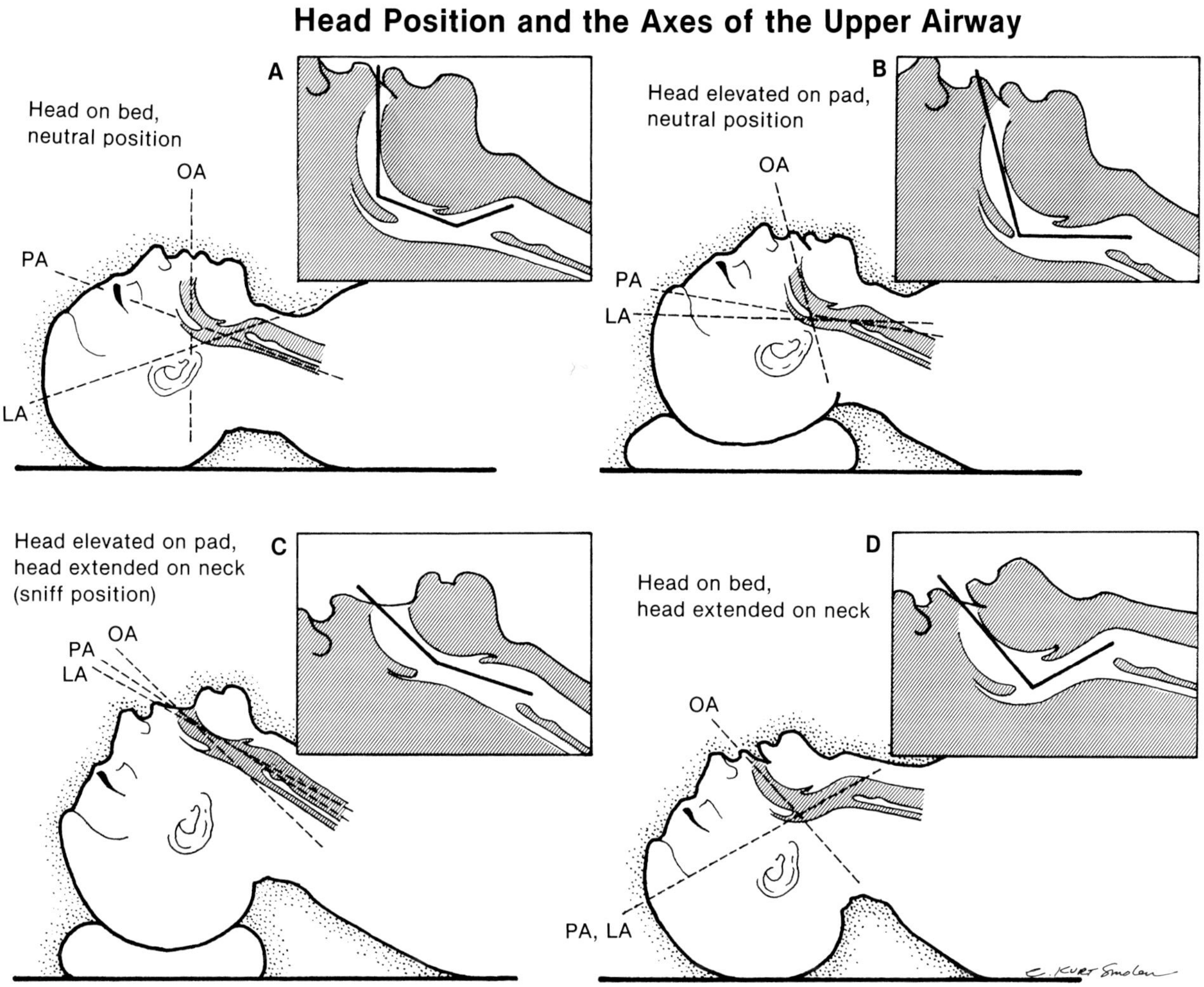

Figure 6–2 • This schematic diagram shows the alignment of the oral axis (*OA*), pharyngeal axis (*PA*), and laryngeal axis (*LA*) in four different head positions. Each head position is accompanied by an inset that magnifies the upper airway (the oral cavity, pharynx, and larynx) and superimposes, as a variously bent bold line, the continuity of these three axes within the upper airway. The upper left panel (***A***) shows the head in a neutral position with a marked degree of nonalignment of the LA, PA, and OA. The upper right panel (***B***) shows the head resting on a large pad that flexes the neck on the chest and aligns the LA with the PA. The lower left panel (***C***) shows the head resting on a pad (which flexes the neck on the chest), as well as concomitant extension of the head on the neck, which brings all three axes into alignment (sniff position). The lower right panel (***D***) shows extension of the head on the neck without concomitant elevation of the head on a pad and results in nonalignment of the PA and LA with the OA.

of caution about preoxygenation is necessary: in instances of poor ventilation via mask the P_aO_2 actually may decrease during attempts to preoxygenate. Ventilation via mask may be inadequate because of the presence of a large mask leak or airway obstruction or some combination of both (see Chapter 5). The immediate assessment of the adequacy of ventilation in the urgent clinical situation is a matter of experience and medical judgment. With regard to the ability to ventilate a patient mechanically, anesthesiologists have found the esophageal obturator airway to be inferior to the black rubber mask–oropharyngeal airway system.[16]

2. Laryngoscopy

The laryngoscope handle is held in the left hand. There are two ways to open the mouth wide. First, extension of the head on the neck (by the right hand) causes the

Opening the Mouth for Laryngoscopy: Extraoral Technique

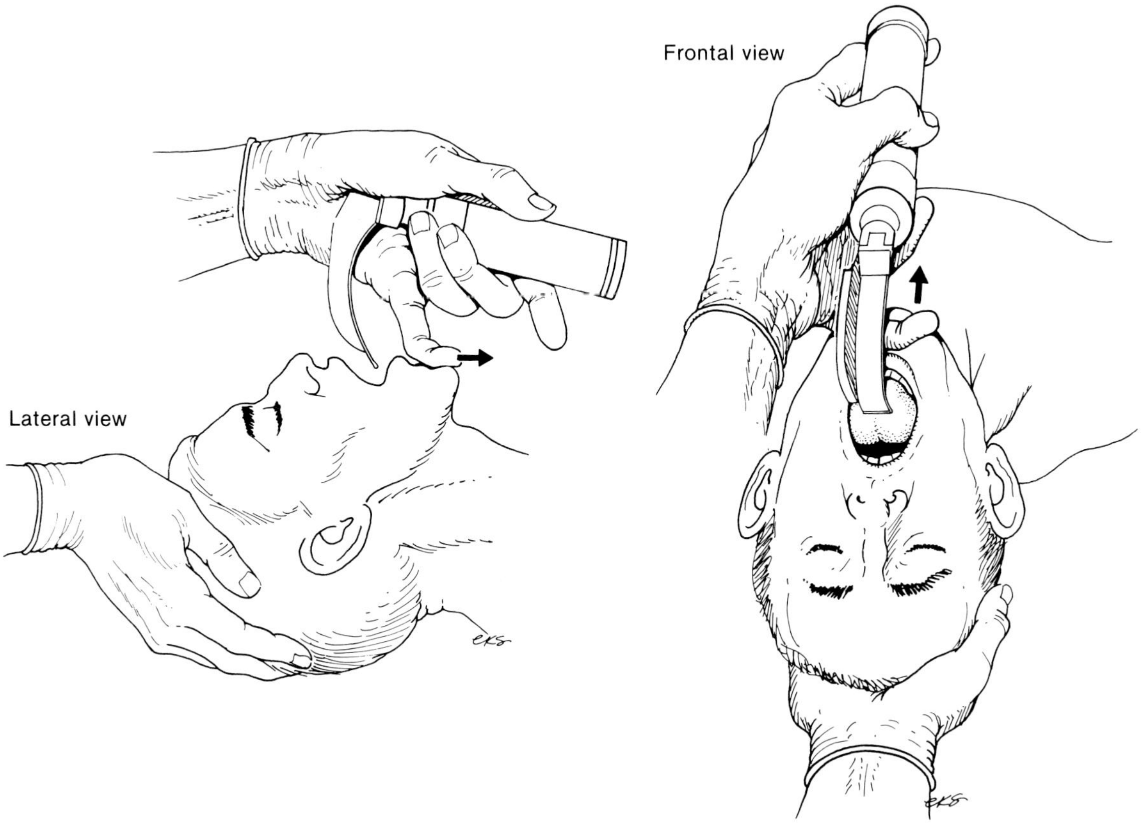

Figure 6–3 • The mouth can be opened wide by concomitantly extending the head on the neck with the right hand while the small finger and medial border of the left hand pushes the anterior aspect of the mandible in a caudad direction (extraoral technique). As the blade approaches the mouth, it should be directed toward the right side of the mouth. Gloves should be worn during laryngoscopy because the hands may come into contact with patient secretions.

lips to part and the mouth to open (Fig. 6–3). If the small finger and medial border of the left hand (which also holds the laryngoscope handle) simultaneously push in a caudad direction on the anterior aspect of the mandible, the mouth will open further. Second, the thumb of the right hand can press down (caudad direction) on the right lower posterior molar teeth, and the index finger of the right hand can simultaneously press up (cephalad direction) on the right upper posterior molar teeth (Fig. 6–4). The two forces in opposite directions on the upper and lower molar teeth will cause the mouth to open widely.

There are three basic types of laryngoscope blades: the curved blade (Macintosh), the straight blade (Jackson or Wisconsin), and the straight blade with curved tip (Miller). Each of these blades has a flange on the left side of the blade for keeping the tongue out of the line of sight (see remaining Chapter 6 figures). The flange of the blade also houses the light source. Each blade has an open right side for visualization of the larynx and for insertion of the endotracheal tube (see remaining Chapter 6 figures).

Following opening the mouth, and with the laryngoscope held in the left hand, the laryngoscope blade is inserted into the right side of the mouth (Fig. 6–5A). During the insertion of the laryngoscope, the patient's right lower lip should be pulled away from the lower incisors (with the right hand or by an assistant) to prevent injury to the lower lip by catching the lower lip between the laryngoscope blade and the incisor teeth (this complication is avoided in Figs. 6–5A and 6–9A). The blade is then simultaneously advanced forward

Opening the Mouth for Laryngoscopy: Intraoral Technique

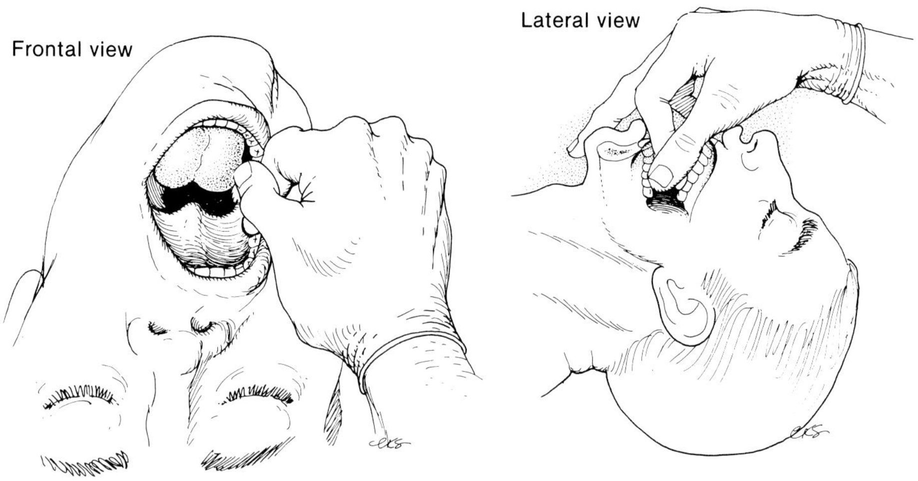

Figure 6-4 • The mouth can be opened wide by pressing the thumb of the right hand on the right lower posterior molar teeth in a caudad direction while the index finger of the right hand simultaneously presses on the right upper posterior molar teeth in a cephalad direction (intraoral technique). Gloves should be worn during laryngoscopy because the hands may come into contact with patient secretions.

Conventional Laryngoscopy with a Curved Blade

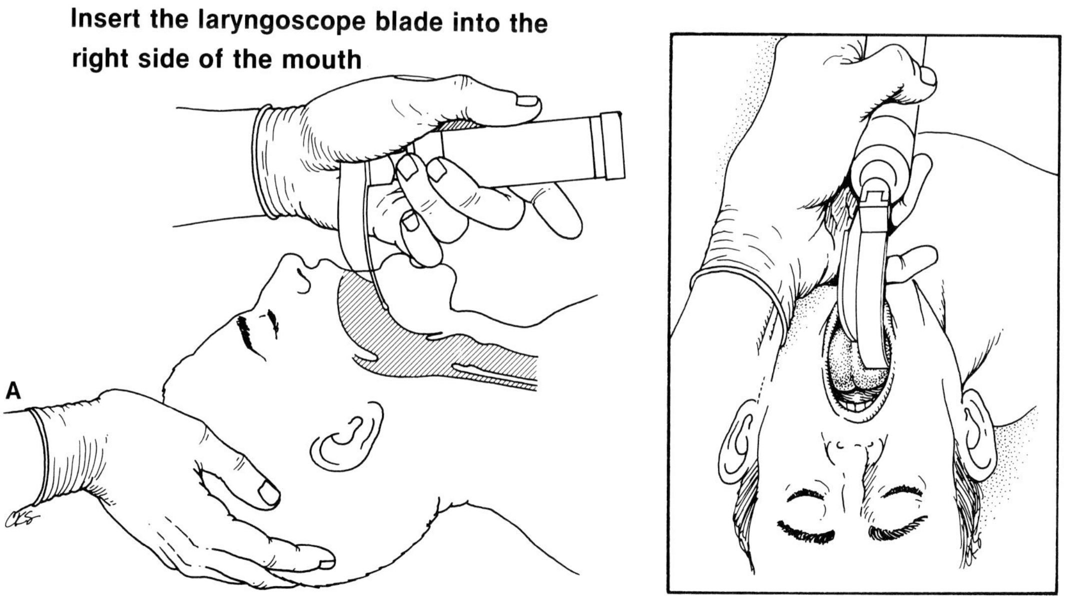

Figure 6-5 • This four-part schematic diagram shows how to perform laryngoscopy with a Macintosh blade; parts ***A*** and ***D*** have both lateral and frontal views, whereas parts ***B*** and ***C*** are just lateral views. (***A***) The laryngoscope blade is inserted into the right side of the mouth so that the tongue is to the left of the flange.

(continued)

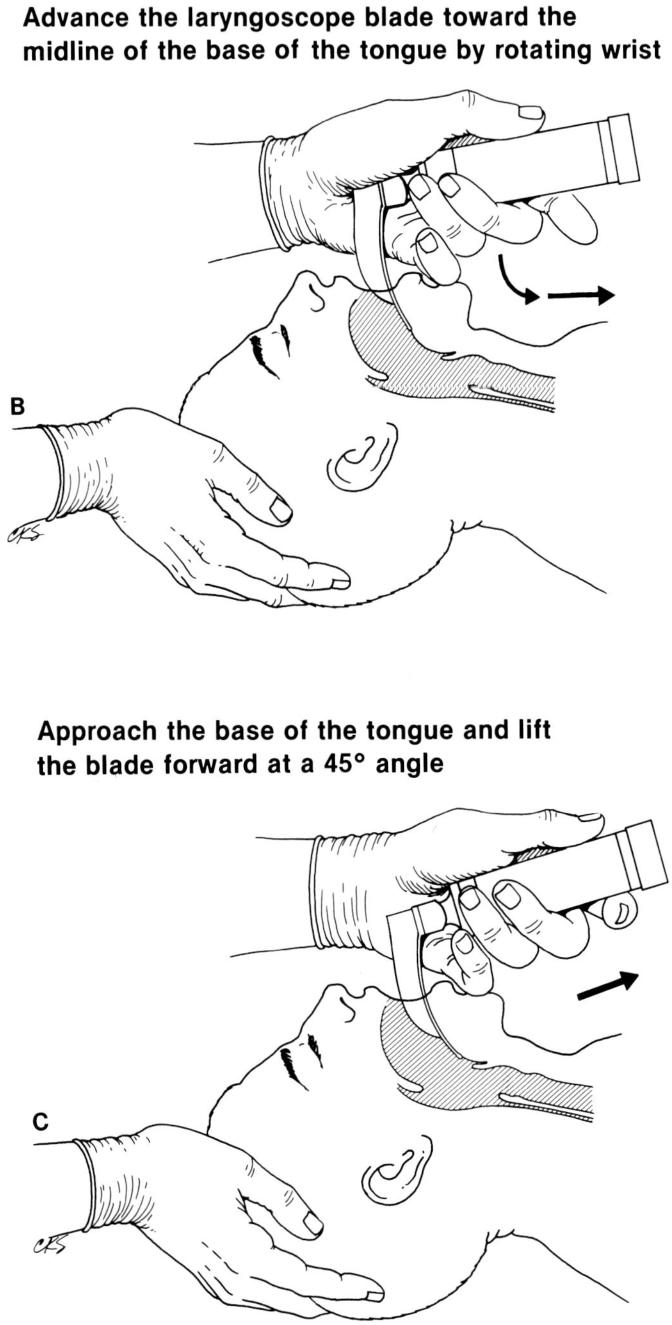

Figure 6–5 *(continued)*
(***B***) The blade is advanced around the base of the tongue, in part by rotating the wrist so that the handle of the blade becomes more vertical (see arrows and part **C**). (***C***) The handle of the laryngoscope is lifted at a 45° angle as the tip of the blade approaches the base of the tongue, thereby exposing the epiglottis.

(continued)

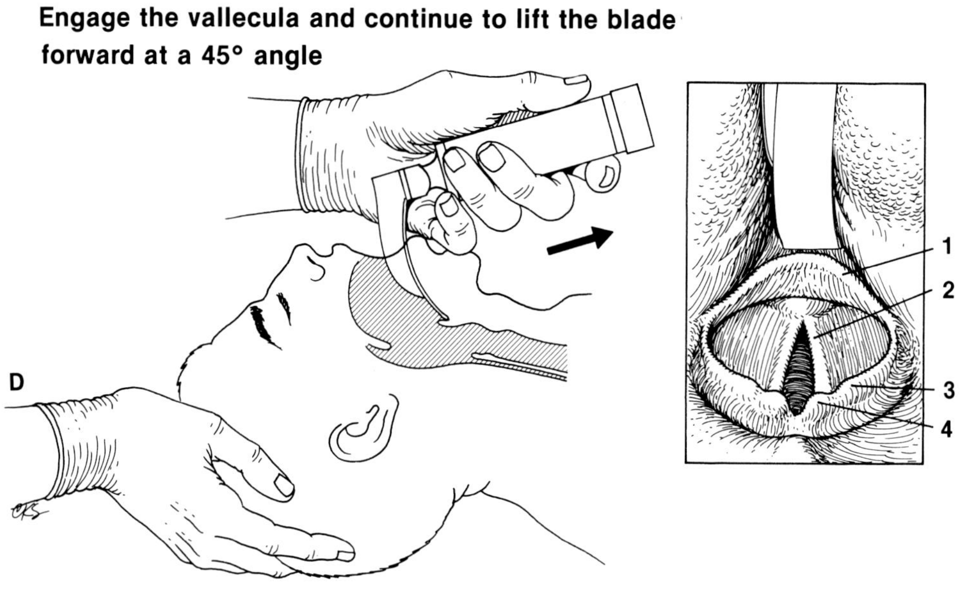

Figure 6–5 *(continued)*
(***D***) The laryngoscope blade is placed in the vallecula with continued lifting of the laryngoscope handle at a 45° angle, resulting in exposure of the laryngeal aperture. 1 = epiglottis, 2 = vocal cords, 3 = cuneiform part of arytenoid cartilage, and 4 = corniculate part of arytenoid cartilage.

toward the base of the tongue (partly by rotating the left wrist; *arrows* in Fig. 6–5B) and swept centrally toward the midline so that the tongue is completely pushed over to the left side of the mouth by the flange of the laryngoscope blade. After the blade has been applied to the base of the tongue, the laryngoscope is lifted to expose the epiglottis (Fig. 6–5C). Hereafter, the left wrist of the operator should remain straight, all lifting being done by the left shoulder and arm. If the laryngoscopist follows a natural inclination to rotate and flex the wrist further, thereby raising the laryngoscope like a lever whose fulcrum is the upper incisor or gum, broken teeth or gum bleeding is likely to result. With the patient in a sniff position, the direction of force necessary to lift the mandible and tongue, and thereby expose the glottis, is along an approximately 45° straight line above an imaginary line from the patient's ear to feet. Careful study of Figs. 6–2C and 6–5 will make this consideration obvious.

Once the epiglottis is visualized, the next step depends on the type of laryngoscope blade being used. If the blade is curved (Mackintosh), the tip should be placed in the vallecula (space between the base of the tongue and the pharyngeal surface of the epiglottis) (Fig. 6–5D). Subsequent forward and upward movement of the blade (exerted along the axis of the handle, not by pulling back on the handle) stretches the hyoepiglottic ligament, causing the epiglottis to move upward, exposing first the arytenoid cartilages and then, with favorable anatomy, allowing more and more of the glottic opening and vocal cords to come into view (see Fig. 6–5D). Insertion of a blade too far into the vallecula, as well as continued rotation of the handle to the vertical, may push the epiglottis down over the glottic opening, resulting in limited exposure of the larynx (Fig. 6–6). If the blade is straight (Jackson, Wisconsin, or Miller), the tip should extend just behind (posterior to) or beneath the laryngeal surface of the epiglottis (Fig. 6–7). As with a curved laryngoscope blade, subsequent forward and upward movement of the straight blade (exerted along the axis of the handle, not by pulling back on the handle) will expose the glottic opening (see Fig. 6–7). With either laryngoscope blade, depression or lateral movement of the thyroid cartilage externally on the neck with the right hand may facilitate exposure of the glottic opening.

Curved blades are thought to be less traumatic to the epiglottis for two reasons. First, the tip of a curved blade does not have to touch the epiglottis. Second, the pharyngeal surface of the epiglottis is innervated by the

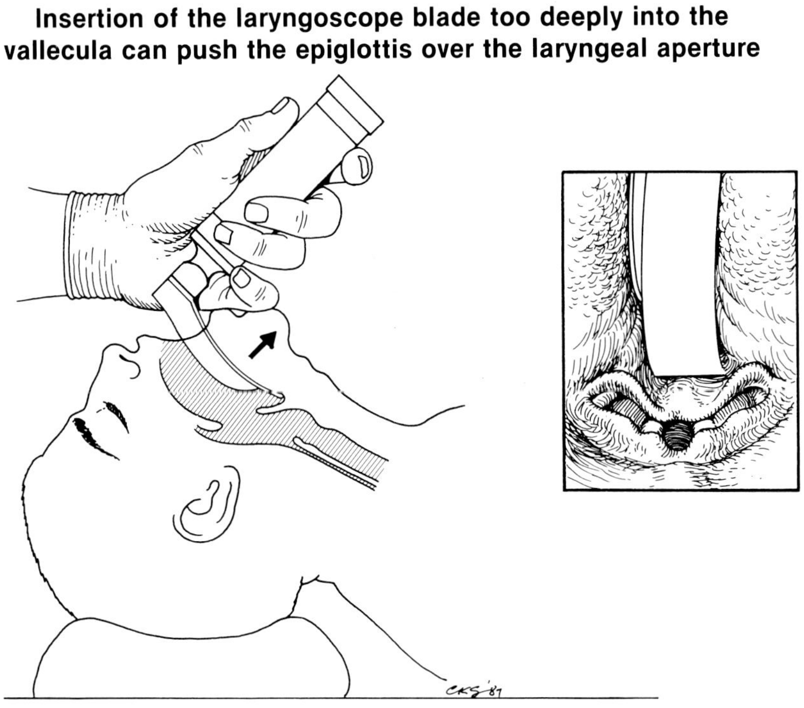

Figure 6–6 • Insertion of the laryngoscope blade too deeply into the vallecula may push the epiglottis down over the laryngeal aperture, diminishing exposure of the vocal cords.

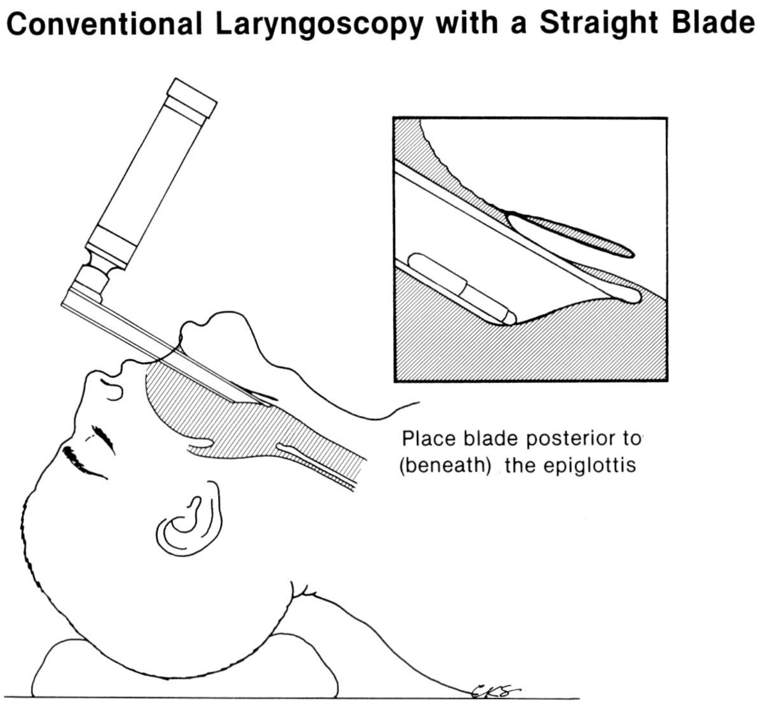

Figure 6–7 • A straight laryngoscope blade (Miller) should be passed underneath the laryngeal surface of the epiglottis; then the handle of the laryngoscope should be elevated at a 45° angle, similar to the lifting that takes place in the use of a curved laryngoscope blade.

glossopharyngeal nerve, whereas the laryngeal surface of the epiglottis is innervated by the superior laryngeal nerve. Stimulation of the laryngeal surface of the epiglottis is thought to predispose to laryngospasm and bronchospasm more than stimulation of the pharyngeal surface of the epiglottis. Curved blades are also thought to be less traumatic to the teeth and to provide more room for passage of the tracheal tube through the oropharynx. On the other hand, straight blades definitely provide a better view of the glottis in patients with a long, floppy epiglottis or an anterior larynx. Therefore, straight blades are the blade of choice in infants, pediatric patients, and patients with an anterior larynx.

Four major common problems are encountered in performing laryngoscopy. First, with either laryngoscope blade, inserting the blade too deeply into the pharynx may elevate the entire larynx, so that the opening of the esophagus will be visualized rather than the glottic aperture (Fig. 6–8). The tracheal and esophageal openings are differentiated as follows: the esophagus is located just to the right of the midline and posteriorly, and the esophageal opening is round and puckered, with no structures around it (see Fig. 6–8). The glottis is located in the midline, has a triangular shape, and contains the prominent knobs of the arytenoids posteriorly and the pale white vocal cords laterally. The dark cavity of the trachea can be seen beyond the glottis (see Figs. 6–5D and 6–9A).

Second, it is very important to keep the tongue completely to the left side of the mouth with the flange of the laryngoscope blade. Many unsuccessful or difficult intubations result from the tongue flopping over the flange of the blade toward the right side of the mouth, thus establishing a narrow "tunnel" through which the vocal cords must be visualized and the endotracheal tube passed (see Fig. 6–9B). Vision is obscured further when part of the narrow tunnel is subsequently occupied by the endotracheal tube. Thus, with a tunnel view, the endoscopist can partially visualize, but not instrument, the larynx. Therefore, all of the tongue must be to the left of the blade (see Fig. 6–9A).

A third common error in performing laryngoscopy is getting too close to the objects being viewed. In the properly positioned patient with the vocal cords exposed, the mouth is only 6–8 in from the cords. This is barely the distance that most people require to focus their eyes on a close object. Yet the beginner at intubation is often seen with one eye virtually in the patient's mouth, as if taking aim with a shotgun. This close distance compromises vision, which is better at a slightly greater distance, and denies the advantage of depth perception, which depends greatly on the use of both eyes.

Insertion of the Laryngoscope Blade Too Deeply into the Pharynx Elevates the Larynx and Exposes the Esophagus

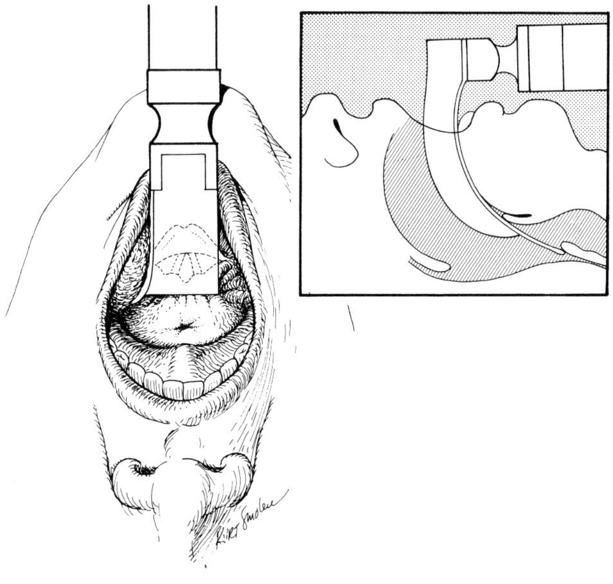

Figure 6–8 • Too deep insertion of the laryngoscope blade into the pharynx may result in elevation of the entire larynx so that the opening of the esophagus rather than the glottic aperture will be visualized. The esophagus is located just to the right of the midline and posteriorly, and the esophageal opening is round and puckered with no structures around it.

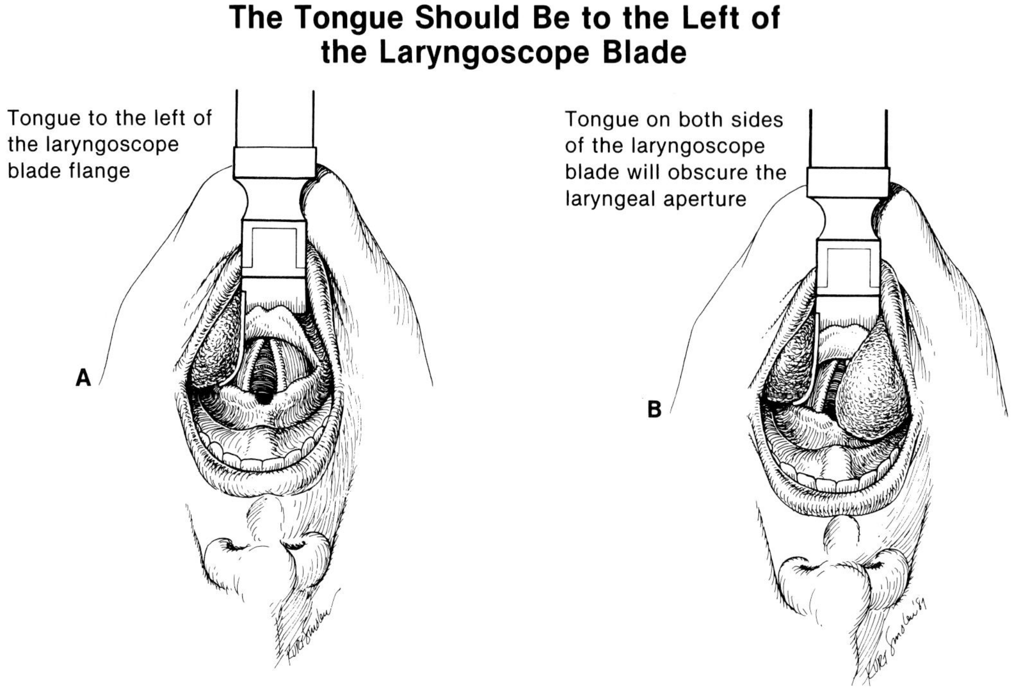

Figure 6–9 • (***A***) The flange on the laryngoscope blade should keep the tongue completely to the left side of the mouth. If this is accomplished, then the tongue will not obstruct the view of the vocal cords. (***B***) If the tongue slips over the laryngoscope blade and occupies part of the right side of the mouth, then the view of the vocal cords will be obscured by the part of the tongue that is on the right side of the mouth.

In barrel-chested and obese patients and large-breasted women, it may be difficult to insert the blade of a laryngoscope correctly into the mouth and avoid interruption of this procedure by anterior chest wall obstruction to movement of the handle of the laryngoscope. In these patients further initial skull–spine extension (atlanto-occipital joint) or 90° rotation of the laryngoscope to the right will permit easier introduction of the blade of the laryngoscope into the mouth and avoid anterior chest wall obstruction to the movement of the handle of the laryngoscope. Finally, one can insert an unattached blade into the right side of the mouth until it is possible to reattach the handle without experiencing chest wall obstruction.

3. Tracheal Intubation

The actual insertion of the tracheal tube is usually easy once the vocal cords are exposed (and the tongue is out of the way) (see Fig. 6–9A). The endotracheal tube used should be a clear plastic one that is tissue implantable (has the marking Z79) and has a large-volume low-pressure cuff on it. Adult female and male tracheas readily accept tracheal tubes with internal diameters of 7–8 and 8–9 mm, respectively (see Chapter 8 for pediatric sizes). If it is thought that fiberoptic bronchoscopy will be necessary subsequently for either diagnosis and/or therapy, the larger size should be used. If it is thought that the space between the upper and lower teeth will be small and that the cuff of the tube may come in contact with the teeth, then the distal tube and cuff should be lubricated to facilitate the cuff sliding by the teeth. The tip of the endotracheal tube should be introduced into the right corner of the mouth and passed along an axis that intersects the line of the laryngoscope blade at the glottis. In that way, the tube does not interrupt the view of the vocal cords. The common error of trying to use the laryngoscope blade as a midline guide, under which the tube is passed, violates this principle, obscures vision, and is a significant source of difficulty for the inexperienced operator. The tube tip is passed through the cords, stopping 2 cm after the tube cuff disappears from sight or when the external markings are at the 21- and 23-cm marks at the incisors in adult women and adult men, respectively; when these external markings are at the lower incisors, the tip of the tube is at the midtrachea.[17] It is of paramount importance that the endoscopist not take his or her eye off the laryngeal aperture until the cuff disappears beyond the vocal cords.

A precurved stylette should be placed in the endotracheal tube whenever a curved laryngoscope blade is used, because the glottic opening can be unexpectedly anterior and therefore unvisualized. To intubate an unvisualized glottis and trachea, the tube must pass along, but to the right of, the curved route made by the blade (as described earlier), and when the styletted tube reaches the end of the blade, it must dip around the epiglottis (by gentle probing) until it "falls into" the glottic opening (as indicated by a loss of resistance). I always use a stylette because if the larynx is anterior (expectedly or unexpectedly), no time will be lost in locating and then placing a stylette in an endotracheal tube. This is an avoidable delay that can only harm the patient. In general, when intubation speed is important (as in a patient with a full stomach), an endotracheal tube should always be styletted. A stylette should be malleable and lubricated and never extend beyond the end of the lumen of the tube. Occasionally, a curved styletted endotracheal tube will impinge on the anterior tracheal wall as it is being inserted. Under these circumstances, while the endotracheal tube is through the vocal cords, the stylette should be withdrawn, which will give the tip of the endotracheal tube its inherent flexibility and permit further passage caudad.

The laryngoscope is removed from the mouth with the left hand. The cuff of the tube is blown up until a moderate tension is felt in the pilot balloon to the cuff. The tube should then be connected to a source of ventilation with 100% O_2 and held in place by one hand. The thumb and index finger should hold the tube or the corrugated tubing while the other three fingers are in contact with the cheek. In this way, if the patient's head were to be turned to one side suddenly, the hand and the tube would follow (rather than remain stationary, which would pull the tube outward).

The next, and most important, task is to ascertain that the tube has indeed been inserted into the tracheobronchial tree rather than the esophagus (Table 6–8). Simple, but not fail-safe, signs of tracheal intubation consist of breath sounds over the chest, lack of breath sounds over the stomach, lack of gastric distention, the rise and fall of the chest, the filling out during inspiration of the intercostal spaces, large spontaneous exhaled tidal volumes, respiratory gas moisture in the endotracheal tube that disappears on inhalation and reappears on exhalation, the sound of air exiting from the endotracheal tube when the chest is compressed, manual squeezing of a reservoir bag that has an appropriate compliance, and pulsing pressure on the suprasternal notch and feeling the pulse transmitted to the pilot balloon of the cuff, or conversely, palpation of a transmitted pulse from the endotracheal tube pilot tube to the cuff to the supersternal notch. The only fail-safe, but invasive, methods of definitively determining tracheal intubation are direct observation of the endotracheal tube going through the vocal cords and the use of a fiberoptic bronchoscope. Direct visualization of the tube lying in the glottic opening may be enhanced by pressing the concavity of the tube posteriorly, which may pull the glottic opening posteriorly and into better view. The fiberoptic bronchoscope allows visualization of the cartilaginous rings of the trachea and the tracheal carina. However, the fiberoptic bronchoscope cannot be regarded as a practical method of determining tracheal intubation. The only noninvasive fail-safe method of determining tracheal location of an endotracheal tube is to observe a CO_2 excretion waveform with each breath (except in cardiac

Table 6–8 • Signs of Tracheal Intubation

A. Nonfailsafe signs
   1. Breath sounds over chest
   2. No breath sounds over stomach
   3. No gastric distension
   4. Chest rise and fall
   5. Intercostal spaces filling out during inspiration
   6. Large spontaneous exhaled tidal volumes
   7. Respiratory gas moisture disappearing on inhalation and reappearing on exhalation
   8. Hearing air exit from the endotracheal tube when the chest is compressed
   9. Reservoir bag having the appropriate compliance
   10. Reciprocating pulsed pressures to and from supersternal notch and to and from balloon on the pilot tube of the endotracheal tube

B. Failsafe Signs
   1. Endotracheal tube visualized between vocal cords*
   2. Fiberoptic visualization of cartilaginous rings of trachea and tracheal carina
   3. CO_2 excretion waveform*
   4. Progressive arterial desaturation by pulse oximetry

*Best practical signs.

arrest, where no carbon dioxide is excreted).[18] Consequently, it is hoped that end-tidal carbon dioxide monitoring will be used wherever and whenever tracheal intubation is being performed. Finally, an esophageal intubation will result in progressive and inexorable arterial desaturation. Therefore, pulse oximetry is very useful as a late monitor of esophageal intubation.

If there is no CO_2 excretion waveform, breath sounds cannot be heard, and/or no chest movement occurs, pull the endotracheal tube out, ventilate the patient with a mask and bag system several times with 100% O_2, and reattempt tracheal intubation again after inspecting the tube for plugs. Changes in the curvature of the endotracheal tube and in the position of the head and neck, and the need for anterior tracheal pressure, should be considered and coordinated during the period of mask ventilation.

The next task is to ascertain that the tip of the endotracheal tube is above the carina and that ventilation is symmetrical. This is done by observing equal expansion of both hemothoraces and by stethoscopic examination for breath sounds throughout both peripheral lung fields. However, hearing uniform breath sounds throughout all lung fields does not guarantee that the tube does not lie in a mainstem bronchus (if it does, it almost always will be in the right mainstem bronchus). If there is any question about a mainstem bronchus intubation, one should retract the tube about 1 cm at a time and reexamine the breath sounds. In one study an insertion depth of 21 cm in adult women and 23 cm in adult men resulted in no incidence of mainstem bronchial intubation.[17] Simultaneous palpation of pulsed pressures both in the cuff in the suprasternal notch and the pilot balloon of the cuff (as described earlier) is another simple way of determining the location of the tube in the trachea. Fiberoptic bronchoscopy is another, but complex, way of determining the location of the tube in the trachea. Outside of the operating room, it is always advisable to confirm endotracheal tube position by chest x-ray. Ideally, the tip of the tube should be at the clavicular (midtracheal) level.

When the tracheal tube is placed, and during taping of the endotracheal tube, the marking of the endotracheal tube at the level of the lower teeth must be noted. This is important for four reasons. First, as discussed earlier, if the tube is inserted to the 21-cm mark in adult women and to the 23-cm mark in adult men, then there will be virtually no incidence of mainstem bronchial intubation.[17] Second, during taping of the tube to the face, anxious beginners have a tendency unwittingly to advance the tube further into the trachea. Third, the patient may cough or make bucking or vomitinglike movements after intubation and, unless the tube has been continuously secured, the patient may self-extubate the tracheal tube. Movement of the initial marking outward facilitates this diagnosis. Fourth, following intubation of the trachea and the initiation of positive pressure ventilation, if the left chest suddenly stops moving or no left chest breath sounds can be heard, there are two likely causes, which the mark of the tube at the teeth can help to determine: (1) the tube has advanced into the right mainstem bronchus, causing left lung atelectasis, or (2) a left pneumothorax, possibly under tension, has developed. If the tube was marked when ventilation was normal bilaterally and this mark subsequently advanced into the patient's mouth, bronchial intubation would be much more likely than pneumothorax, whereas the converse would be true if the mark were stationary. Similar considerations apply to apparent absent ventilation of the right lung.

4. Securement of the Tube

After the mark of the tube at the lower teeth level has been noted, the tube should be tightly secured in place. This is important not only to prevent accidental extubation, but also to minimize tube movement within the airway. Taping the tube to the skin with adhesive tape is the most common method of securing the tube. Figure 6–10 suggests two different ways to tape the tube in place. The securement of the tube in place can be increased by having the lateral ends of the tape shown in Fig. 6–10 completely encircle the jaw and neck. (Place the tape all the way around the posterior neck over to the contralateral neck and jaw.) Application of tincture of benzoin to the skin before the tape is applied will help provide a stronger bond between the tape and skin. In cases of prolonged intubation, changing the tape and reapplying it to a new area on the face every 2 days will help prevent maceration of the skin. In patients with beards or in whom the adhesive tape fails to stick to the skin, the tube can be tied into place with a length of umbilical tape that encircles the tube with a nonslipping knot and then encircles the neck with another nonslipping knot. Adhesive tape may be used over the umbilical tape for added security. Another very reliable method of securing an orotracheal tube is to wire the tube to a tooth. One or two layers of adhesive tape is wrapped around the tube at the level of the lower incisor teeth. Stainless steel wire (25–28 gauge) is passed around a

Securing the Endotracheal Tube with Tape

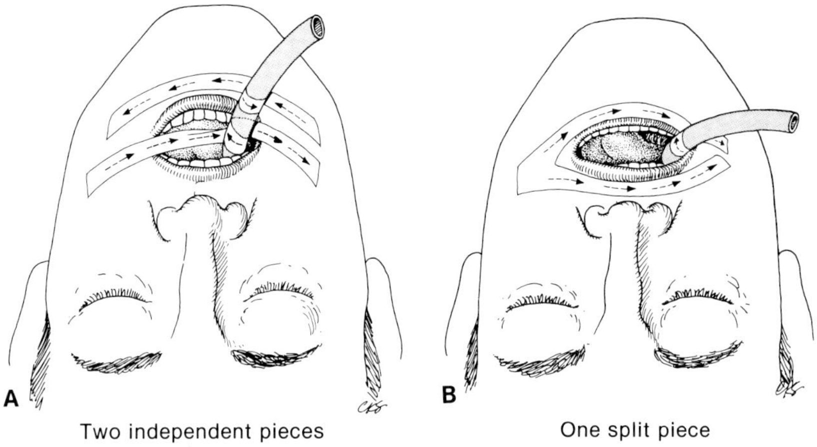

Figure 6–10 • This schematic diagram depicts two ways of taping an oral endotracheal tube in place. (***A***) Thin (½-in) tape can be brought from one lateral jaw around the tube over to the other lateral jaw, both above the upper lip and below the lower lip. Securement of the tube is increased by placing tincture of benzoin over the skin prior to taping, and taping all the way around the back of the neck over to the contralateral jaw. (***B***) Thick (1 in) tape can be brought from a lateral jaw to the angle of the mouth, the tape split in half, with the upper half crossing above the upper lip as an anchor to the skin and with the lower half wrapped around the tube and then over to the contralateral jaw, holding the tube in place. The same, but oppositely directed, taping procedure may be done starting from the contralateral jaw with the thick unsplit tape.

lower incisor tooth and twisted around the tape on the tube. Finally, in anesthetized patients a suture may be passed through the gum and then either around a ring of adhesive tape on the endotracheal tube (as with wire) or through the wall of the endotracheal tube and then tied to the tube. A bite block, rolled gauze, or oral airway (used in the vast majority of tracheal intubations for anesthesia) should be placed between the teeth to prevent the patient from biting down and occluding the lumen of an oral tube. Finally, the mouth and pharynx should be suctioned. The tube cuff then should be deflated so that a gas leak occurs during a positive pressure inspiration and reinflated to a just-seal volume during the next few peak positive pressure inspirations.

B. Conventional (Laryngoscopic) Nasotracheal Intubation

Intubation by the nasal route is a more difficult procedure than oral intubation. On the other hand, nasal tubes are thought to be better tolerated than oral tubes. Therefore, nasal tubes are considered the tube of choice for long-term mechanical ventilation. The tracheal tube is inserted into a nostril and then passed through the nasal cavity and nasopharynx to the oropharynx. Once the tube has been passed into the oropharynx, it can be guided into the glottis with conventional direct laryngoscopic vision and without any special grasping aid, or it can be grasped additionally by a forceps (Magill) and manually directed into the glottis.

1. Prelaryngoscopy Maneuvers

Prior to insertion of the nasotracheal tube into the nose, the nasal mucosa should be sprayed with a vasoconstrictor drug. Vasoconstriction of blood vessels in the nasal mucosa minimizes bleeding due to the trauma of passing a nasotracheal tube through the nose, and it increases the diameter of the nasal passages by constricting (shrinking) the nasal mucosa. In addition, softening the tip of the nasotracheal tube by soaking it in warm saline may decrease the incidence of mucosal damage and bleeding. The nares selected should be the one that the patient thinks offers the least resistance to breathing while the other nares is occluded. However, if both nares offer equal resistance, then the right nares should be chosen if the bevel of the nasotracheal tube, when introduced through the right nares, will face the flat nasal septum, reducing damage to the turbinates. If it is thought that the bevel will not damage the turbinates, then the left nares should be chosen, because entry of the tube into the oropharynx from the left side will permit more room for the laryngoscopic blade and Magill forceps on the right side of the oropharynx. In the vast majority of adults, tubes with an internal diameter of 7.0–7.5 mm will pass through the nares. The other pre-laryngoscopy maneuvers described under direct-vision orotracheal intubation (positioning of the head, suctioning, preoxygenation) should be performed for direct-vision nasal intubation. The nasotracheal tube should be lubricated and passed through the nose in one smooth posterior, caudad, medially directed movement until resistance to forward movement significantly decreases as the tube enters the oropharynx (usually at the 15–16-cm mark).

The pathway that the nasotracheal tube takes should be visualized as a U lying on its side. The curve of the tracheal tube should be aligned to facilitate passage along this curved course. As the tube passes through the nose into the nasopharynx, it must turn downward to pass through the pharynx. In making this turn, it may impact against the posterior nasopharyngeal wall and resist any attempt to push it further. The tube should be pulled back a short distance, and the patient's head should be extended further to facilitate attempts to pass this point smoothly and atraumatically. If this is not done, and the tube is forced, the mucosal covering of the posterior nasopharyngeal wall may be torn open and the tube may be passed into the submucosal tissues.

2. Laryngoscopy

The laryngoscopy for nasal intubation is identical to that described for oral intubation.

3. Tracheal Intubation

Once the tube is in the oropharynx, the tip of the tube must be aligned with the glottic opening. If the tip of the tube is excessively anterior, posterior, or lateral to the glottic opening, it will not enter this orifice. If necessary, the tube must be withdrawn slightly, before any of the corrective measures, described next, are taken. Lateral tip location, as indicated by either direct vision or by observing bulging soft tissue in the lateral neck, can be corrected in either direction by twirling or rotating the adapter of the tube at the nose. If the bulge is on the right, the proximal end of the tube is rotated in a counterclockwise direction and is advanced again. If the bulge is on the left, the proximal end of the tube is rotated in a clockwise direction. Alternatively, this problem can be identified by noting the rotation of a curved adapter, whose curve lies in the same vertical plane as the concave curve of the tube, away from the midline. Anterior tip location, as indicated by either direct vision or bulging soft tissue under the mandible, can be corrected by flexion of the head or by picking up the larynx and trachea externally (anterior displacement). Both of these maneuvers cause the tip of the tube to become more posterior in relation to the glottis. Posterior tip location almost always means esophageal intubation and is indicated either by direct vision or by loss of breath sounds heard or felt from the tube. Posterior tip location can be corrected by extending the patient's head, which will cause the tip of the tube to become more anterior in relation to the larynx. Posterior direction can also be corrected by using a ring tube (Endotrol™). A ring tube has a cord that runs from the anterior surface of the tip of the tube up the length of the tube to a ring on the proximal end of the tube. Pulling on the ring causes anterior bending of the tip of the tube. Finally, posterior tip location can be corrected by pushing the larynx down (posterior displacement), which will cause the larynx to become more posterior in relation to the tip of the tube. The procedures described earlier for correction of the anterior, posterior, and lateral malpositions of the tube tip can be performed more precisely under direct vision compared to blind attempts (see Chapter 7) and result in success more easily.

Since one hand must hold the laryngoscope and another hand may be necessary for manipulation of the head or larynx, an assistant may be necessary to push the tube into the larynx when the appropriate elements are lined up correctly. In addition, if the tube is in the midline but too posterior and this is not corrected by extension of the head, force on the anterior trachea, or use of the ring on an Endotrol tube, the tube must be grasped in the pharynx with a Magill forceps (avoiding the cuff on the tube) and directed anteriorly through the vocal cords (Fig. 6–11). The advantage of the design of

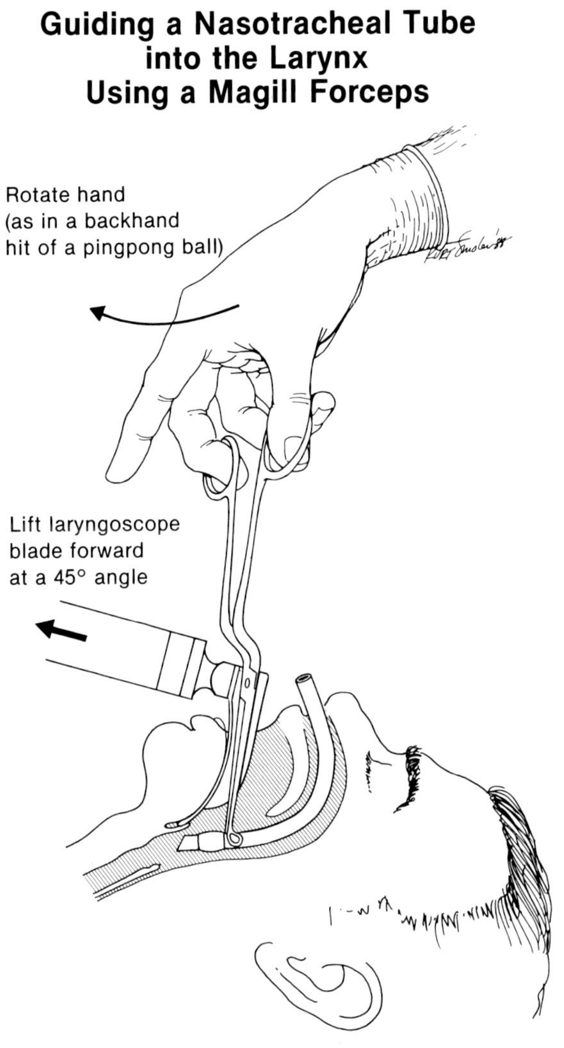

Figure 6–11 • A nasotracheal tube can be guided under direct vision (laryngoscopic control) through the laryngeal aperture by a Magill forceps by simply rotating the hand as one would do using a backhand motion in hitting a pingpong ball. The Magill forceps should grab the nasotracheal tube proximal to the cuff of the endotracheal tube.

these forceps is that when the grasping ends are parallel to the long axis of the tracheal tube, the handle is outside of the right side of the mouth and at a right angle to the long axis of the tube. Since the handle is outside the right side of the mouth, it is away from the line of sight. Since the forceps are grasped parallel to the long axis of the tube, a backhand motion of the right hand will pass the tube toward the glottic opening (see Fig. 6–11). Thus, the intubationist can have the larynx exposed by the laryngoscope held in the left hand, the tube in full view, and a means (the forceps) of manipulating the alignment of the tube and a means of advancing the tube. However, it is often desirable to have an assistant advance the proximal end of the tube so that the intubationist is free to simply guide the tube into the larynx without having to pull it along with the Magill forceps.

In some patients, as the tube enters the trachea, the tube's anterior curvature may direct it against the anterior tracheal wall and interfere with passage past this point. To resolve this difficulty, the head must be lifted (flexed) slowly as the tube is advanced. A nasotracheal tube should be advanced until the cuff is 2 cm below the vocal cords or until the external markings are 24 cm for women and 26 cm for men (3 cm more than for oral tubes) at the nares. The tube's correct placement must be verified as in any intubation (see orotracheal intubation), but this is particularly critical with nasal intubations because the relationship to external tube markings and the location of the tube tip is not as firmly established as it is for orotracheal tubes. If nasal bleeding occurs, it is probably wise to leave the tube in place to act as a tamponade. If the bleeding is severe, the tube can be retracted and the cuff inflated to act as a better tamponade.

4. SECUREMENT OF THE TUBE

The nasotracheal tube can be secured with adhesive tape as described for orotracheal tubes. In addition, a nasotracheal tube can be secured by a suture through the nasal septum and then tied, after being tightly wound around an adhesive band on the tube or passed through the wall of the tube by a needle and then tied.

III. DISCUSSION OF THE PROCEDURE: CONVENTIONAL MECHANICAL VENTILATION, WEANING, AND EXTUBATION OF THE TRACHEA

The most important reason for tracheal intubation of an awake patient in respiratory failure and for continued tracheal intubation in an immediate postoperative patient is to provide mechanical ventilation. Since the administration of mechanical ventilation is often the main reason for the implementation of tracheal intubation, this discussion of the tracheal intubation procedure will focus on how to do conventional mechanical ventilation, how to terminate mechanical ventilation (wean the patient from mechanical ventilation), and finally how to extubate the trachea.

The use of positive end-expiratory pressure (PEEP), constant positive airway pressure (CPAP), and intermittent mandatory ventilation (IMV) of either a spontaneously breathing or apneic patient, and an increased understanding of the toxicity of unnecessarily high inspired concentrations of oxygen (F_IO_2) constitute the cornerstones of modern clinical mechanical ventilation management. This section describes step by step the current practice of mechanical ventilation, weaning, and extubation.[19-22] The recommendations for initial ventilator settings (see Section III.A) are based on the assumption that the patient's lungs are very disordered and therefore require a considerable amount of support. In addition, it is assumed that a volume-limited ventilator is being used, the patient is adequately sedated, and the endotracheal tube and chest tubes are functioning properly.

A. *Initial Ventilator Settings: Intermittent Mandatory Ventilation*

Intermittent mandatory ventilation (IMV) means that the ventilator delivers a positive pressure breath a mandatory number of times per minute while the patient does as much spontaneous breathing as desired between these mechanical breaths. The IMV mode of ventilation is presently the most commonly used and preferable ventilation mode for multiple reasons. First, because the patients are allowed to, and usually are doing some spontaneous ventilation, they can generate a more negative pleural pressure that better maintains venous return and cardiac output (compared to simple intermittent positive pressure ventilation [IPPV]). Second, and consequently, less intravenous fluid is usually required to maintain systemic pressure and perfusion. Third, since it is not necessary to eliminate these spontaneous breaths, sedation requirements are minimized and paralysis requirements are eliminated. Fourth, the patients benefit psychologically because they know they are breathing on their own. Fifth, the respiratory muscles remain coordinated because they are exercised. Finally, when the weaning stage is reached, IMV allows a gradual transition from ventilator dependence to independence. A number of other mechanical ventilation modes also facilitate mechanical ventilation and/or the transition from mechanical ventilation to weaning (pressure support [PS], mandatory minute ventilation [MMV], inverse ratio ventilation [IRV], and airway-pressure-release ventilation [APRV]) that have been introduced recently. These are briefly mentioned in Section III.F and much more extensively in Chapter 14.

With conventional IMV, it is possible for the ventilator to begin to deliver a mechanical breath just as the patient is completing a spontaneous inhalation. This results in the stacking of a machine breath on top of a spontaneous breath and can lead to overdistention of the lungs and high peak inspiratory pressures. This problem can be overcome by use of synchronized IMV (SIMV). With SIMV, the ventilator intermittently senses the onset of a spontaneous breath a mandatory number of times per minute and immediately causes a machine (positive pressure) breath to occur. Consequently, the machine breath overrides the spontaneous breath and stacking of breaths cannot take place.

Mechanical ventilation is initiated with a tidal volume of 12 mL / kg of lean body weight, an IMV respiratory rate so that the arterial carbon dioxide tension (P_aCO_2) is 40 mmHg (usually requires an initial rate of 8–12 breaths/min) and an inspired oxygen fraction (F_IO_2) of 1.0 (Table 6–9). Although patients may breathe spontaneously during IMV (which is especially helpful with regard to lowering pleural pressure and maintaining cardiac output), IMV used in this way should be regarded as providing total and full ventilatory support (ie, the IMV breaths determine the minute ventilation, not the spontaneous breaths).[23,24] One hundred percent oxygen should be used initially to update and document the level of right-to-left shunting and alveolar to arterial oxygen tension difference while minimizing the risk of unexpected hypoxemia. One hundred percent oxygen for a short period of time is not toxic (see Section III.B).

A tidal volume of 12 mL / kg is considered to be large tidal volume ventilation. Large tidal volume ventilation is desirable because it prevents the development of miliary or microatelectasis that is associated with con-

Table 6–9 • Initial Ventilator Settings

1. IMV or SIMV mode
2. Tidal volume 12 mL/kg
3. Respiratory rate so that P_aCO_2 = 40 mmHg (usually 8–12 breaths/min)
4. F_IO_2 = 1.0
5. I:E = 1:2–3
6. Inspiratory flow rate 30 L/min

stant small tidal volume ventilation (eg, 6 mL/kg).[25] The miliary or microatelectasis associated with small tidal volume ventilation results in a progressive increase in the alveolar to arterial oxygen tension difference and a progressive decrease in compliance. These deleterious changes associated with small tidal volume ventilation can be reversed by intermittent sighs. Large tidal volume ventilation therefore functions as very frequent intermittent sighs and thereby minimizes the development of atelectasis. A smaller tidal volume of 8–10 mL/kg should be used in patients with bullous or cystic disease of the lung in an effort to minimize peak inspiratory pressures and risk of tension pneumothorax.

The respiratory rate should be set so that the patient has a normal arterial carbon dioxide tension (usually 8–12 breaths/min). Certainly, hypercapnia should be avoided in the vast majority of patients, since the accompanying acidosis is dangerous and the hypoventilation necessary to produce hypercapnia may also cause atelectasis and hypoxemia. Mild degrees of hypercapnia (P_aCO_2 of 40–50 mmHg) are indicated for patients who are chronic carbon dioxide retainers; mild hypercapnia helps to avoid changing the arterial and cerebrospinal fluid pH and bicarbonate levels from the values that the patient normally lives with. Hypocapnia should be avoided for multiple reasons. First, hypocapnia may cause a decrease in cardiac output via several mechanisms. To produce hypocapnia, an increased amount of positive pressure ventilation, which will decrease venous return, will have to be used. Hypocapnia also causes a withdrawal of sympathetic tone that will decrease the inotropic state of the heart. Hypocapnia and alkalosis may decrease the level of ionized calcium, which will also decrease the inotropic state of the heart. Second, hypocapnia will shift the oxygen–hemoglobin dissociation curve left, which increases the hemoglobin affinity for oxygen. At the tissue level the increased hemoglobin–oxygen binding impedes the delivery of oxygen to the tissues. Third, hypocapnia and alkalosis will increase oxygen consumption. The increase in oxygen consumption is due to a pH-mediated uncoupling of oxidation from phosphorylation; the uncoupling requires more oxygen to be passed along the respiratory chain to generate the same amount of adenosine triphosphate.[26,27] Quantitatively, at a P_aCO_2 of 40 mmHg, oxygen consumption is 250 mL/min, whereas at a P_aCO_2 of 20 mmHg, oxygen consumption is 350 mL/min. Thus, hypocapnia may increase tissue oxygen demand (increased oxygen consumption) when it is impossible to increase tissue oxygen supply (left-shifted oxygen–hemoglobin dissociation curve and decreased cardiac output). Fourth, hypocapnia may cause ventilation-perfusion abnormalities by inhibiting hypoxic pulmonary vasoconstriction and/or causing bronchoconstriction and decreased lung compliance. Fifth, hyperventilation with alkalosis may cause ventricular irritability (perhaps due in part to a concomitant hypokalemia). However, using hyperventilation with hypocapnia to decrease an elevated intracranial pressure in head-injured patients may be a benefit that supersedes the previously cited physiologic disadvantages.

Large tidal volume ventilation usually makes it possible to achieve normocapnia with relatively slow respiratory rates (8–12 breaths/min). This is highly desirable in two ways. First, slow rates allow a decrease in the inspiration-to-expiration ratio (I:E ratio). A long expiratory time increases venous return and augments cardiac output; it facilitates full expiration and avoids air-trapping and obstructive lung disease. The I:E ratio should be approximately 1:2 or 1:3 (except when airway resistance is very high and an even longer exhalation period and lower I:E ratio are required). Second, slow respiratory rates also allow slower inspiratory flow while maintaining an appropriately low I:E ratio. The slower the inspiratory flow, the more laminar and less turbulent is the air stream. This decreases airway resistance, reduces airway trauma, and allows for a more even distribution of inspired gas to regions of lung with different time constants. The inspiratory flow should be approximately 30 L/min.

B. Goal 1: $F_IO_2 < 0.5$ and P_aO_2 Acceptable

1. WHY THIS GOAL IS NO. 1: OXYGEN TOXICITY

An inspired oxygen fraction (F_IO_2) greater than 0.5 is toxic to the lungs,[28,29] and the first and compelling goal is to get the inspired oxygen fraction below 0.5 with the patient having an acceptable P_aO_2 (Table 6–10). The mechanism of oxygen-induced lung damage is the local accumulation of toxic, tissue-reactive free radicals such as superoxide and hydrogen peroxide, which damage the pulmonary tissues. For the purposes of this discussion an acceptable P_aO_2 is defined as one that will be above the steep part of the oxygen–hemoglobin dissociation curve, and for all patients this will be a value greater

Table 6–10 • Mechanical Ventilation and Weaning Plan

Goal # (temporal sequence to be followed)	Goal		Achieved primarily by
1.	$\downarrow F_IO_2 < 0.5$	$P_aO_2 > 60$ mmHg	PEEP titration
2.	$\downarrow F_IO_2 < 0.5$, $\downarrow$PEEP < 10 cm H_2O,	$P_aO_2 > 60$ mmHg	Respiratory care regime
3.	$\downarrow F_IO_2 < 0.5$, $\downarrow$PEEP < 10 cm H_2O, $\downarrow$IMV < 1 b/min,	$P_aO_2 > 60$ mmHg	Patient having adequate breathing power

than 60 mmHg. A P_aO_2 value that is above the steep part of the oxygen–hemoglobin dissociation curve provides some margin of arterial oxygenation reserve and protects against decreases in $P_{\bar{v}}O_2$. In addition, a P_aO_2 greater than 60 mmHg will not cause or promote ventricular arrhythmias.

The rate of onset of oxygen-induced pulmonary damage is proportional to both the inspired tension of oxygen and the duration of the exposure. In normal human volunteers, the first symptom after 6 hours of exposure to 100% oxygen is substernal distress, which begins as a mild irritation in the area of the carina and may be accompanied by occasional coughing. As exposure continues, pain becomes more intense and the urges to cough and breathe deeply also become more intense. When the inspired oxygen tension has been 1.0 for greater than 12 hours, the pain, dyspnea, and paroxysmal coughing are severe. As toxicity progresses, these symptoms are accompanied by objective signs of lung compromise, such as a decreased vital capacity, reduced lung compliance, and deterioration in blood gases. Finally, in animals, after days to weeks, acute respiratory failure occurs, and unless gas exchange is supported by mechanical ventilation, death ensues.

Pathologically, in animals, the lesion progresses from a tracheobronchitis (exposure for 12 hours to a day), to pulmonary interstitial edema (exposure for a few days to a week), to pulmonary fibrosis (exposure greater than a week).[30] Often these pathologic changes are indistinguishable from the pathology of the adult respiratory distress syndrome. Dose–time toxicity curves for humans indicate that oxygen toxicity does not occur when the inspired oxygen fraction is less than 0.5 (even for long periods of time).

2. How to Achieve Goal 1

Positive end-expiratory pressure (PEEP) is the treatment of choice of arterial hypoxemia due to right-to-left shunting through low ventilation-to-perfusion and atelectatic lung regions. PEEP increases end expiratory lung volume (FRC), thereby preventing closure of airways at end exhalation, and recruits alveoli and airways during inspiration. The prevention of airway closure and recruitment of alveoli increases ventilation-to-perfusion relationships and reverses atelectasis.[19] The beneficial effect of the application of PEEP and the deleterious effect of removal of PEEP on arterial oxygenation can be observed within minutes.[31,32] The endpoint for PEEP application is the lowest level of PEEP that provides an adequate P_aO_2 on an F_IO_2 less than 0.5.[33] Increasing PEEP beyond this level to obtain optimal values for various other endpoints, such as the production of maximum oxygen transport,[34] maximum static pulmonary compliance,[34] shunt less than 15%,[35,36] minimal arterial-to-end-tidal carbon dioxide gradient,[37] decreased mixed venous oxygen tension,[38] and minimal F_IO_2,[39] will not be clinically helpful and may cause harm (see later), and may decrease the cardiac output period.[33] In addition, most of these other endpoints require invasive monitoring, vary independently of the PEEP level (ie, they have multiple determinants and therefore have a fair amount of background variation), and/or respond sluggishly to changes in lung pathology.

The decrease in inspired oxygen concentration below 50% is achieved by performing a dose (PEEP)–response (P_aO_2) titration. PEEP is progressively added (range 0–20 mmHg) until the P_aO_2 is relatively normal for that patient (or at least above 60 mmHg) with an F_IO_2 of less than 0.5. PEEP should be raised in 2.5–5.0-cm H_2O increments and the patient allowed to stabilize with regard to respiratory mechanics (peak inspiratory pressure, compliance), hemodynamics (pulse rate and rhythm, systemic and central filling pressures, and cardiac and urine output), and gas exchange (arterial blood gases). Usually, each PEEP increment requires 0.5–1.0 hour to complete. Consequently, the performance of a PEEP–F_IO_2/P_aO_2 titration usually takes only several hours.

In many patients there appears to be a certain critical level of PEEP, above which there is a sudden and dramatic improvement in P_aO_2. In the vast majority of patients, levels of 5–12 cm H_2O are sufficient for substantial reversal of intrapulmonary shunting; it is seldom necessary to go as high as 15 cm H_2O. Of course, as the PEEP titration is being performed, other respiratory care modalities (see later) such as suctioning, turning, administration of antibiotics, and so on (see next section and Chapter 4) are instituted. The advent of fiberoptic bronchoscopy has eliminated the need for super-PEEP (PEEP more than 20–25 cm H_2O) because regions of collapsed lung that are resistant to opening by PEEP are usually obvious on chest radiograph and can be suctioned and lavaged open under direct vision.

As the PEEP requirement increases, cardiovascular support and therefore monitoring requirements (central venous and pulmonary capillary wedge pressure, cardiac and urine output) generally increase.[40] It may be expected that hypovolemic patients will have a decrease in cardiac output as soon as PEEP is applied. Normovolemic patients will maintain cardiac output within normal limits up to a PEEP of 10 cm H_2O because compensatory peripheral venoconstriction maintains venous return. However, normovolemic patients will have a progressive decrease in cardiac output with a progressive increase in PEEP greater than 10 cm H_2O. Postpneumonectomy patients with an increased pulmonary vascular resistance may be expected to have a greater decrease in cardiac output at any given level of PEEP compared to patients with normal lungs.[41] Again, in all patients, using IMV mode with some spontaneous ventilation protects the cardiac output.

The first cardiovascular support response to PEEP-induced impaired hemodynamics should be a moderate augmentation of intravascular volume.[42] If fluid infusion does not restore satisfactory hemodynamics, then inotropes should be used to provide cardiovascular support. In patients with acute hypoxemic respiratory failure, dobutamine causes an increase in cardiac output with a decrease in pulmonary capillary wedge pressure and end-diastolic and end-systolic ventricular volumes (resulting from decreased afterload), whereas dopamine increases cardiac output, pulmonary capillary wedge pressure, and end-diastolic and end-systolic volumes (resulting from increased afterload).[43] Since even small increases in pulmonary capillary wedge pressure may increase the accumulation of pulmonary water in permeability pulmonary edema,[44–46] dobutamine appears to be the inotrope drug of choice.[43]

C. *Goal 2: F_IO_2 <0.5, PEEP <10 cm H_20, and P_aO_2 Acceptable*

1. WHY THIS GOAL IS NO. 2: MATCH VENTILATION TO PERFUSION

If a patient requires more than 10 cm H_2O of PEEP to have a P_aO_2 greater than 60 mmHg on an F_IO_2 of less than 0.5, then the ventilation-perfusion mismatch is so great that it is illogical to make the patient spontaneously ventilate with such disordered lungs. In other words, lungs that have F_IO_2 and PEEP requirements greater than 10 cm H_2O and 0.5, respectively, are inefficient to the point that the work of breathing is likely to be excessive, and the patient will fatigue and fail. When the PEEP requirement is less than 10 cm H_2O, the F_IO_2 is less than 0.5, and the P_aO_2 is adequate, the lungs are fulfilling their basic gas exchange function in a reasonably efficient manner and it now makes sense to ask the patient to do some of the work of breathing on his or her own.

2. HOW TO ACHIEVE GOAL 2

The second goal is to get the PEEP requirement to be less than 10 cm H_2O; of course, it is assumed that what was achieved before (F_IO_2 less than 0.5, acceptable P_aO_2) is retained. This second goal is achieved primarily by instituting an intensive and aggressive respiratory care regimen (see Table 6–10) using coughing routines, frequent tracheal suctioning, fiberoptic bronchoscopy, chest physical therapy (chest percussion and vibration in various postures), humidification of the inspired gases, half-hourly to hourly turnings of the patient, care of the diseased lung in a nondependent position as much of the time as possible, incentive spirometry, administration of antibiotics chosen according to culture and sensitivity studies, and in selected patients, administration of bronchodilators ($beta_2$- agonists, aminophylline, steroids), diuretics, and inotropic drugs. Although there is no hard data to prove that any one of these respiratory care treatments is beneficial when used alone, there is a widespread consensus that when used together, and in the context of the other care necessary in the postoperative management of respiratory failure, they produce a clearing of atelectasis, eradication of infection, and a decrease in the PEEP requirements.[47,48]

The only way patients can remove secretions from the tracheobronchial tree by themselves is by coughing, and effective voluntary coughing is the most efficient method of mobilizing and removing secretions.[49] However, many patients cannot or will not cough (because of depression by drugs, pain, or disease) and the secretions must be mechanically removed. Consequently, tracheal suctioning is often necessary and certainly mandatory whenever secretions are heard in the tracheobronchial tree by auscultation. The patients should be preoxygenated, and the maximum duration of suctioning should be 10 seconds. Various angle-tipped catheters can improve the accuracy of cannulation of the mainstem bronchi,[50] and flexible fiberoptic bronchoscopy can be used for visually directed endobronchial suctioning (see Chapter 13).[51] Certainly, flexible fiberoptic bronchoscopy should be used whenever roentgenologically observable lobar obstruction is resistant to other standard medical therapy.[52] A balloon-tipped fiberoptic bronchoscope permits application of positive pressure to specific regions of the lung, in addition to enabling suction and lavage.[53]

Physically trying to shake the secretions loose from their alveolar and bronchial attachments by vibration and percussion, in conjunction with postural gravity drainage of the lungs, may increase the removal of

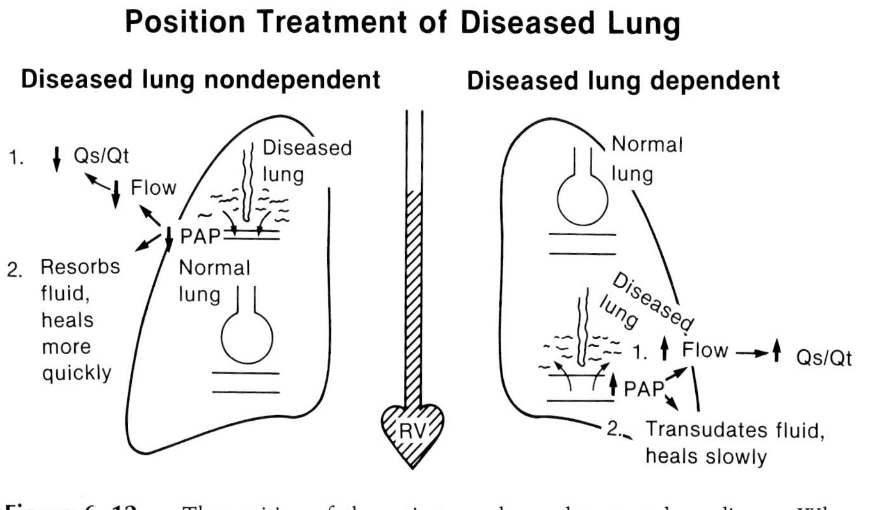

Figure 6–12 • The position of the patient can be used to treat lung disease. When diseased lung is placed in a nondependent position (left panel), it experiences a low pulmonary artery pressure. The low pulmonary artery pressure means that blood flow to the region will be decreased passively, which will cause a decrease in shunt (Q_s/Q_t) through the diseased lung. In addition, the low pulmonary artery pressure causes the nondependent lung to have a propensity to resorb fluid and therefore to heal more quickly. Conversely, when diseased lung is placed in a dependent position (right panel), it experiences a high pulmonary artery pressure. The high pulmonary artery pressure means that blood flow to the region will be increased passively, which will cause an increase in Q_s/Q_t through the diseased lung. In addition, the high pulmonary artery pressure causes a propensity to transudate fluid, resulting in more slowly healing lung or even a progressive deterioration in the lung. (Reproduced with permission from Benumof JL. Anesthesia for Thoracic Surgery. Philadelphia, WB Saunders, 1987, Fig. 19–11, p. 459.)

secretions. External pressure may be applied to specific chest regions during exhalation to increase the expiratory flow of gas and may increase the removal of secretions. Chest physical therapy appears to be especially beneficial for patients who are acutely ill, have large volumes of secretions, and cough ineffectively.[54] Chest physical therapy is also beneficial in patients with lobar atelectasis.[55] It is not beneficial in patients who do not have airway secretions. Chest physical therapy in acutely ill patients may be associated infrequently with bronchoconstriction and hypoxemia.[54]

Dependent lung experiences higher pulmonary vascular pressures, and nondependent lung experiences lower pulmonary vascular pressures. The level of pulmonary vascular pressure has two important consequences for diseased lungs (Fig. 6–12). First, dependent lung has a propensity to transudate fluid, whereas nondependent lung has a propensity to absorb fluid. Consequently, if diseased lung is placed in a dependent position, it may heal more slowly or actually become more diseased. Conversely, if diseased lung is placed in a nondependent position, it may heal more quickly. Second, dependent lung has a higher blood flow and nondependent lung has a lower flow. Consequently, if diseased lung is placed in a dependent position, it will have a higher shunt, because it is mechanically forced to have a higher blood flow. Conversely, if diseased lung is placed in a nondependent position, it will have a lower shunt, because it is mechanically forced to have a lower blood flow. Thus, diseased lung should be in a nondependent position for as much time as possible.[56-59] Frequent turning of the patient allows all parts of the lung to be placed in a nondependent position for their proportional share of the time.

Using the previously described respiratory care regimen usually allows the physician, within a few days, to decrease PEEP to less than 10 cm H_2O with continued maintenance of an adequate P_aO_2 with a low F_IO_2. Once the PEEP requirement is less than 10 cm H_2O, no special attempt is made to reduce it further. Maintenance of some PEEP is desirable in terms of maintaining normal-functional residual capacity and lung compliance and providing a subjective sensation of good lung expansion. The achievement of a F_IO_2 less than 0.5 and PEEP less than 10 cm H_2O with an acceptable P_aO_2 means that the blood and gas within the lungs is matched well enough so that the lungs perform their basic gas exchange function in a reasonably efficient manner. The patient is now a candidate for weaning from mechanical ventilation.

D. Goal 3: F_IO_2 < 0.5, PEEP < 10 cm H_2O, IMV < 1 Breath/Min, P_aO_2 Acceptable

1. WHY THIS GOAL IS NO. 3: CONVERSION FROM INTERMITTENT MANDATORY TO SPONTANEOUS VENTILATION

Goals 1 and 2 were concerned with avoiding oxygen toxicity and matching ventilation to perfusion. Once ventilation-perfusion matching is achieved, it is reasonable to begin converting a patient who, in theory, required full ventilatory support (100% dependent on the ventilator) to one who requires no ventilatory support (no dependence on the ventilator). The use of IMV weaning allows a gradual transition from 100% to 0% ventilator dependence. During the transition, IMV is providing a progressively decreasing amount of partial ventilatory support.[23]

2. HOW TO ACHIEVE GOAL 3

The third goal is to retain what was achieved before (F_IO_2 less than 0.5, PEEP less than 10 cm H_2O, and P_aO_2 acceptable) and now get the IMV rate to be less than 1 breath/min (see Table 6–10). This weaning process is accomplished by a progressive decrease in the IMV rate. The rapidity by which the IMV rate can be reduced is dictated by and is directly proportional to the vital capacity (VC) and peak inspiratory force (PIF). Both of these breathing power indices can be rapidly and easily measured at the bedside with a spirometer (VC) and a dry gas manometer (PIF). The vital capacity is the volume exhaled forcefully after a maximal inspiration. The vital capacity maneuver requires cooperation, adequate lung compliance, and muscle strength. Since the vital capacity requires patient cooperation, it can give some indication of how much cooperation with breathing treatments will occur after extubation. The peak inspiratory force is the negative pressure generated at the airway when inspiration is artificially obstructed. This is a good indication of thoracic muscle strength. It may be more reliable than the vital capacity because it does not depend on patient motivation and may even be performed in the presence of coma. However, it provides little indication of subsequent voluntary activity. A poor vital capacity (dependent on cooperation, lung compliance, and muscle strength) coupled with a good peak inspiratory force (dependent on muscle strength) means that the patient is cooperating poorly, has poor lung compliance, or both.

The minimally adequate VC is 15 mL/kg (normal range: 50–70 mL/kg) and the minimally adequate PIF is −20 to −25 cm H_2O (normal range: −80 to −100 cm H_2O). The IMV rate may be decreased in increments of 1 breath/min in patients who just achieve these minimal values (see next paragraph for stabilization and monitoring process). Values much greater than these minimal ones (more positive VC and more negative PIF) mean that the IMV rate can be decreased more rapidly, and values much below these minimal ones (less positive VC and less negative PIF) mean that the IMV rate must be decreased much more slowly. When the decrease in IMV rate is begun, the head of the bed should be elevated as much as possible to reduce the pressure of the abdominal contents on the diaphragm and to allow the patient to reestablish contact with his or her environment.

As the IMV rate is decreased, the patient is monitored by the spontaneous respiratory rate, VC, PIF, and P_aCO_2. When the rate of IMV withdrawal is appropriate and is being tolerated, the patient's spontaneous respiratory rate remains constant or increases only slightly, the VC and the PIF remain constant or improve, and the arterial blood gases do not deteriorate. Conversely, when the IMV withdrawal rate is too rapid and is not being tolerated, the spontaneous respiratory rate increases greatly (and is usually the first indication of intolerance), the VC and PIF decrease, the arterial blood gas values deteriorate, and the patient may become hypertensive and tachycardic (stress response) and may have arrhythmias. In patients who have a fresh incision and multiple indwelling catheters (nasogastric, urinary, and endotracheal tubes, intravenous and arterial lines), the pain input is high, and spontaneous respiratory rates are often between 20 and 30 breaths/min at the beginning of, and during, weaning.

The inability of a patient who has met the first two goals to tolerate the IMV withdrawal (which is unusual) is usually because either the total clinical status requires full ventilatory support (eg, the patient's lung function is ordinarily marginal or the patient is malnourished or has a neuromuscular problem) and/or the weaning system that is being used results in an intolerable increase in the work of breathing. Increased work in breathing is best indicated by negative fluctuations in inspiratory pressure greater than 2 cm H_2O during spontaneous breathing and usually indicates inadequate inspiratory flow. Patients who fail to wean or take a very long time to wean should be started on an intensive nutritional regimen.[60]

When P_aO_2 is adequate (with the F_IO_2 less than 0.5 [Goal 1], the PEEP less than 10 cm H_2O [Goal 2], VC greater than 15 mL/kg, PIF greater than −20 cm H_2O, IMV less than or equal to 1 breath/min, spontaneous respiratory rate less than 20–30 breaths/min, and P_aCO_2 approximately 40 mmHg [Goal 3]), when no other major organ systems are in acute major failure or are unstable, and when the chest radiograph is reasonably equivalent to the premorbid findings or is rapidly improving and no new changes have appeared (such as infiltrates or pneumothorax), the patient is ready for extubation. Throughout this entire mechanical ventilation and weaning process analgesics and sedatives must be administered and titrated so that the patient is comfortable, is not bucking on the endotracheal tube, and is without active expiratory efforts.

E. Summary of Mechanical Ventilation and Weaning Procedure

The logic of the preceding approach is that the patient's lungs are first required to have the ventilation and perfusion matched well enough—as indicated by an adequate or reasonable P_aO_2, with an F_IO_2 less than 0.5, and a PEEP level of less than 10 cm H_2O—so that the lungs function as an efficient gas exchange organ. Next, the patient's lungs are required to sustain this efficient gas exchange without respirator aid, as indicated by an adequate or reasonable VC, PIF, spontaneous respiratory rate, and P_aCO_2 on a low IMV. Finally, the process requires that no new complicating factor has occurred, as indicated by lack of new chest radiographic findings, by resolution of old chest radiographic findings, and by the absence of any significant disorder or complication in any of the other major organ systems.

F. Other New Mechanical Ventilation and Weaning Modes

In the past few years a number of new mechanical ventilation modes have been introduced. The new modes are an outcome of microprocessor technology that enable the ventilator to monitor breath-by-breath flow, pressure, volume, and respiratory mechanics. The ability to sense and transduce these variables accurately, and online, allows the interaction between patient and ventilator to be much more sophisticated than ever before (see Chapter 13).

Pressure support (PS) ventilation is a ventilatory mode that provides additional inspiratory gas flow through a demand valve in response to a spontaneous breath. This additional gas flow keeps a positive inspiratory airway pressure (which usually has a maximum of up to 20 cm H_2O above PEEP level) during inspiration and is discontinued when the patient's own inspiratory flow rate diminishes considerably, the exact point being determined differently in different ventilators. Thus, "supported" tidal volumes may vary according to the patients inspiratory flow pattern. Pressure support usually reduces the work of breathing,[61,62] since the patient has only to trigger the demand valve, while part or all the "spontaneous" breath itself is being supplied by the ventilator. When high levels of PS are used, it resembles the assist-control pressure-limited mode,[63] although the inspiration is not terminated once the preset pressure is achieved, as in true pressure-limited devices. Some patients find PS to be a more comfortable ventilatory mode, since it reduces the work of breathing and allows the patient to have more control over peak inspiratory flow rate, flow waveform, inspiratory time, and tidal volume.[64] Pressure support may also be used as a weaning mode by gradually decreasing its level as the patient's own tidal volume improves. However, although perfectly practical in most cases, it does not seem to offer any improvement over existing weaning techniques and does require a reliable endogenous respiratory drive for ventilation. In addition, PS may lead to a potentially harmful increase in airway pressure[63] as each and every breath is augmented by positive pressure.

Mandatory minute volume (MMV) and minimal ventilation (MiMv) are both methods that ensure the delivery of a preset minute volume, either by spontaneous breathing or by assistance from the ventilator itself. The difference between the two is that inadequate spontaneous ventilation on a MMV ventilator is supported by independent positive-pressure breaths, whereas during MiMv the mechanical assistance is only in the form of pressure support (ie, the patient has to generate a spontaneous breath to be assisted). Current microprocessor ventilators supply MMV by continuously comparing the accumulating minute volume with the preset value and supplementing any deficit by mandatory mechanical breaths. The potential benefit of the MMV is clear: the patient is guaranteed a minimal minute ventilation regardless of her or his own spontaneous effort or drive and the weaning process becomes "automatic" (ie, the patient passes "from artificial to spontaneous breathing without any attention to the controls being required"[65]). There are, however, no data describing such "automatic weaning" in groups of patients, probably because MMV has two main disadvantages that stem from the characteristics of its main parameter, namely, the minute volume. The first one is that it is difficult to estimate the right value of minute volume, as it would vary greatly according to the patient's deadspace ventilation and carbon dioxide level. If the preselected minute volume value is too high, the patient will remain assisted by the ventilator, although he or she may be ready for extubation. A high preset minute volume value may also render the patient apneic because of a too low P_aCO_2 level. If the preselected minute volume value is too low, then the patient might be hypoventilated, distressed, and hypercarbic. The second problem associated with having minute volume as the preselected parameter is that minute volume is composed of both rate and tidal volume. Indeed, the patient may achieve the preselected minute volume value by shallow hyperventilation, which is not clinically acceptable and might signify impending respiratory catastrophe. Thus, it is difficult to see the practicality of MMV at this stage.

Two other new ventilatory modes that are specifically aimed at patients in the adult respiratory distress syndrome are inverse ratio ventilation (IRV)[66] and airway pressure release ventilation (APRV).[67] Inverse I:E ratio of up to 4:1 is claimed to achieve better oxygenation either by a straightforward increase in mean airway pressure or by a progressive alveolar recruitment and stabilization. Airway pressure release ventilation is the intermittent release of CPAP to ambient pressure for 1 second. Consequently, the pressure waveform of IRV closely resembles that of APRV. The major difference between the two methods, besides the dominant airway pressure being "inspiratory" with IRV and "expiratory" with APRV, is that with IRV the patients do not breathe spontaneously, whereas, with APRV the patient is allowed to breathe spontaneously. Thus, mean airway pressure is lower with APRV than with IRV. The technical details, indications, and clinical efficacy of these modes need to be further evaluated.

G. *Extubation of the Trachea*

Additional criteria for extubation are that the patient should be alert, cooperative, and eager to be extubated. Prior to extubation of the trachea, the pharynx, nose, nasogastric tube (if present), and endotracheal tube should be suctioned. Suctioning is followed by several positive pressure sighs with 100% oxygen. Extubation of the trachea should be accomplished by inflating the patient's lungs with 30 cm H_2O pressure, holding the pressure constant while the endotracheal tube cuff is rapidly deflated, and then immediately pulling the endotracheal tube out of the trachea (Fig. 6–13). This maneuver insures that the first event following extubation is a forceful exhalation from total lung capacity (because of the elastic recoil of the chest wall); the forceful exhalation will blow out any material that has lodged on top of the endotracheal tube cuff and/or vocal cords that could not be reached by any of the other suction avenues (see Fig. 6–13).

The patient is then asked to breathe deeply and is observed for any laryngospasm or stridor. Humidified oxygen with an F_IO_2 0.1 greater than that used while the patient was intubated is administered by green face mask. Nasal prongs are most comfortable and do not interfere with eating, but they also do not provide an F_IO_2 greater than 0.3. When a higher F_IO_2 is required (which is usually the case), a face mask should be used, which, with flow rates of 5–10 L/min, can yield an F_IO_2 of 0.3–0.5. F_IO_2 between 0.5 and 1.0 can be obtained by using a tight-fitting face mask, a face mask with a rebreathing bag, or both (see Chapter 5). Of course, the expected F_IO_2 of all devices depends on appropriate positioning of the device on the patient's face. Arterial blood gases should be measured 0.5–1.0 and 4–6 hours postextubation, and a chest radiograph should be obtained 4–6 hours postextubation. Respiratory care measures instituted during the mechanical ventilation and weaning process are continued. In addition, incentive spirometry, which emphasizes a long increase in inspiratory transpulmonary pressure and lung volume, is the most cost-effective respiratory care measure and should be begun every hour. However, if a patient is experiencing significant postoperative pain, then it is unreasonable to expect good cooperation in performing this deep-

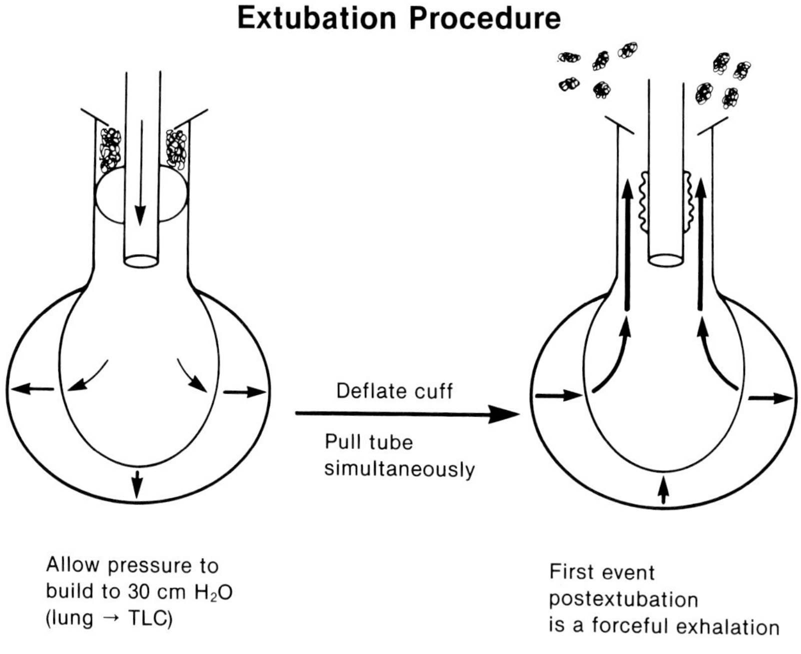

Figure 6–13 • The proper extubation procedure consists of allowing airway pressure to build up to 30 cm of water so that the lung approaches total lung capacity (TLC) (left panel). Then, simultaneously, the endotracheal tube cuff is deflated and the endotracheal tube is pulled out (right panel). This procedure forces the first postextubation event to be a forceful exhalation (cough) due to the forceful elastic recoil of the lung from total lung capacity. The forceful exhalation can blow out of the airway any secretions and/or material lodged between the endotracheal tube cuff and the vocal cords, or on the vocal cords per se. In the author's experience this greatly diminishes the incidence of postextubation laryngospasm, breath holding, and choking-type respiration. (Reproduced with permission from Benumof JL. Anesthesia for Thoracic Surgery. Philadelphia, WB Saunders, 1987, Fig. 19–12, p. 463.)

breathing maneuver; consequently, pain management must be effective. The patient should be postured upright, should be encouraged to cough, and should be encouraged to ambulate as soon and as much as possible. The nasogastric, urinary, extraperipheral intravenous and arterial catheters and pleural tubes should be removed after 6–8 hours of trouble-free extubation.

IV. COMPLICATIONS

The complications of mechanical respiratory support can be divided into those due to tracheal intubation (Table 6–11) and those due to mechanical ventilation (Table 6–12).[8,68] Although the list in Tables 6–11 and 6–12 of possible complications of mechanical respiratory support

Table 6–11 • Complications of Tracheal Intubation

During Intubation

1. Trauma to the cervical spinal column, eye, nose, teeth, lips, tongue, larynx, and trachea
2. Aspiration (blood, tooth, laryngoscope bulb, gastric bulb, gastric contents, and partial dentures)
3. Esophageal intubation
4. Endobronchial intubation
5. Reflexes
   a. Sympathetic (hypertension, tachycardia, myocardial ischemia)
   b. Vagal (hypotension, bradycardia, cardiac arrest, laryngospasm, bronchospasm)

With Endotracheal Tube in Place

1. Bronchospasm
2. Tracheomalacia
3. Tracheal perforation (by cuff, by tip of the tube)
4. Inadequate secretion removal (possible obstruction of the tube)
5. Obstruction of the tube (secretions, kinking, biting)
6. Trauma to all areas of contact (exacerbated by patient movement)
7. Excessive inflation of cuff causing tube lumen narrowing
8. Ruptured cuff

Complications Peculiar to Nasotracheal Intubation

1. Epistaxis
2. Turbinate fracture
3. Intracranial placement through a basilar skull fracture
4. Dislodgment of pharyngeal tonsils (adenoids)
5. Pressure necrosis
6. Auditory tube obstruction
7. Maxillary sinusitis
8. Bacteremia

During Extubation

1. Trauma to glottis by persistent inflated cuff
2. Aspiration of supraendotracheal tube cuff secretions
3. Laryngospasm
4. Respiratory obstruction by immediate edema of any part of the airway previously in contact with the endotracheal tube

After Extubation

1. Sore throat (common), dysphagia
2. Aphonia
3. Paralysis of the hypoglossal and/or lingual nerves
4. Vocal cord paralysis; if bilateral, causes respiratory obstruction
5. Ulceration, inflammation, infection, edema of any part of the airway previously in contact with the endotracheal tube
6. Laryngeal granulomas and polyps
7. Laryngotracheal membranes and webs
8. Tracheal stenosis
9. Sinusitis
10. Muscular aches (due to depolarizing muscle relaxant)

(Blanc VF, Tremblay NAG. The complications of tracheal intubation: A new classification with a review of the literature. Anesth Analg 53:202–213, 1974.)

Table 6–12 • Complications of Mechanical Ventilation

Complications Attributable to Operation of the Ventilator

1. Machine failure or disconnection
2. Alarm failure
3. Alarms not turned on
4. Inadequate humidification
5. Excessive inspired oxygen concentration

Medical Complications of Positive Pressure Breathing

1. Inadequate positive pressure breathing—alveolar hypoventilation
2. Excessive positive pressure breathing—alveolar hyperventilation
3. Massive gastric distention
4. Pneumothorax, pneumomediastinum
5. Atelectasis
6. Pneumonia
7. Hypotension and decreased cardiac output
8. Increased ventilatory dead space
9. ADH secretion and water retention

ADH = antidiuretic hormone.

(Zwillich CW, Pierson DJ, Creagh CE, et al. Complications of assisted ventilation: A prospective study of 354 consecutive episodes. Am J Med 57:161–170, 1974.)

appears formidable, most of the serious complications are individually infrequent to rare events; more important, most are avoidable. Proper technique and adequate anesthesia should make the actual insertion of the endotracheal tube uncomplicated. Adequate sedation to minimize movement of the patient's head, using a just-seal volume of air in the endotracheal tube cuff, and frequent suctioning and turning of the patient will make the presence of an endotracheal tube more benign. The volume of air in the endotracheal tube cuff should be checked for a minimum-volume ("just-") seal 1 hour after each inspired oxygen concentration change and only after the mouth has been suctioned. The endotracheal tube should be suctioned whenever breath sounds indicate the presence of tracheal or bronchial secretions. However, it is impossible to know about or eliminate pressure on the tissues in all areas of contact. Indeed, minor sequelae such as throat discomfort, edema of the glottis (not resulting in respiratory obstruction), and slight mucosal damage at the cuff site occurs in virtually all patients intubated for 48 hours or more.[69,70] In addition, the patient is predisposed to a much higher incidence of both minor and major complications if the duration of intubation is lengthened, if severe systemic illness is present, or if intubation is performed under emergency conditions.

With regard to nasal tubes, epistaxis may follow avulsion of the nasal mucosa covering the turbinates. Proper shrinkage of the nasal mucosa with cocaine or phenylephrine; use of small, generously lubricated nasotracheal tubes; and softening of the tip of the nasotracheal tube by dipping it in warm saline should minimize this complication. If bleeding occurs, the nasotracheal tube should be left in place to provide a tamponade effect. In some instances, the tube may be withdrawn so that only the cuff remains in the naris and subsequent cuff inflation tamponades the bleeding site. Perforation and dissection of the posterior pharyngeal wall creating a false passage may occur especially if force is used to advance the tracheal tube through the nasopharynx. Pharyngeal tonsils (adenoids) may be prominent, especially in children, producing resistance to passage through the nasopharynx or bleeding if they are traumatized. Again, gentle advancement and avoidance of excessive force should minimize this hazard. Necrosis of the external nares reflects excessive pressure from the nasotracheal tube and may be minimized by proper fixation of the tube.[71] Ulceration of the inferior turbinate may be more likely when a large tracheal tube is placed.[72] Auditory tube obstruction by the nasotracheal tube may impair hearing. Maxillary sinusitis resulting from impaired drainage due to obstruction by the nasotracheal tube may be manifested by facial pain, nasal stuffiness, purulent secretions, or fever.[73]

Bacteremia may occur following nasotracheal intubation, reflecting the entrance of normal upper-airway flora into the circulation via traumatized nasal mucosa or the transport of flora from the nose into the trachea by the tube and the subsequent entrance into the circulation via the vascular tracheal mucosa.[74] When nasotracheal intubation is necessary in patients with heart disease, prophylactic antibiotics may be indicated.

Life-threatening airway obstruction due to airway edema may occur following extubation. Edema is most prone to develop above the vocal cords (supraglottic), at the level of the vocal cords (glottic), and below the vocal cords (subglottic). Supraglottic swelling can occur on the lingual surface of the epiglottis and in the aryepiglottic folds. These structures are then displaced medially into the laryngeal inlet, producing obstruction. Glottic swelling can occur in Reinke's space, just beneath the mucous membrane of the vocal cords. Marked edema of both true vocal cords will obstruct the glottis. The subglottic region is an especially dangerous location for the development of edema. The mucous membrane in this location has a loose submucosal tissue that allows the development of edema, and the region is entirely surrounded by the cricoid cartilage, which does not allow swelling except at the expense of the airway lumen. The danger is greater in infants and children because of the small area in this location and the relatively greater loss of airway from even small amounts of edema. Intravenous dexamethasone may be of value in the prevention and treatment of traumatic laryngeal edema.[75]

V. REFERENCES

1. Pontpoppidan H, Geffin B, Lowenstein E. Acute respiratory failure in the adult (second of three parts). N Engl J Med 287:743–752, 1972.
2. Campbell EJM, Agostini E, Davis EN. The Respiratory Muscles: Mechanics and Neural Control. 2nd ed. London, Lloyd Luke, 1970.
3. Knelson JH, Howatt WF, Demuth GR. The physiologic significance of grunting respiration. Pediatrics 44:393, 1969.
4. Cohen BM. The interrelationship of the respiratory functions of the nasal and lower airways. Bull Physiopathol Respir 7:895, 1971.
5. Mueller RE, Petty TL, Filley GF. Ventilation and arterial blood-gas changes induced by pursed-lips breathing. J Appl Physiol 28:784, 1970.
6. Schmidt RW, Wasserman K, Lillington GA. The effect of air flow and oral pressure on the mechanics of breathing in patients with asthma and emphysema. Am Rev Respir Dis 90:564, 1964.
7. Campbell EJM. The J. Burns Amberson Lecture. The management of acute respiratory failure in chronic bronchitis and emphysema. Am Rev Resp Dis 96:626, 1967.
8. Zwillich CW, Pierson DJ, Creagh CE, et al. Complications of assisted ventilation. A prospective study of 354 consecutive episodes. Am J Med 57:161–170, 1974.
9. Mallampati RS, Gatt SP, Gugino LD, et al. A clinical sign to predict difficult tracheal intubation: A prospective study. Can Anaesth Soc J 32:429–434, 1985.
10. Samsoon GLT, Young JRB. Difficult tracheal intubation: A retrospective study. Anaesthesia 42:487–490, 1987.
11. Smith RB. Tracheal intubation. In Bready LL, Smith RB (eds). Decision Making in Anesthesiology. Philadelphia, BC Decker, 1987, 14–15.
12. Holmgreen WC. Difficult intubation: Suspected. In Bready LL, Smith RB (eds). Decision Making in Anesthesiology. Philadelphia, BC Decker, 1987, 16–17.
13. Holmgreen WC, Nishioka GJ. Difficult intubation: Unsuspected. In Bready LL, Smith RB (eds). Decision Making in Anesthesiology. Philadelphia, BC Decker, 1987, 18–19.
14. Gold MI, Duarte I, Muravchick S. Arterial oxygenation in conscious patients after 5 minutes and after 30 seconds of oxygen breathing. Anesth Analg 60:313–315, 1981.
15. Gambee AM, Hertzka RE, Fisher DM. Preoxygenation techniques: Comparison of three minutes and four breaths. Anesth Analg 66:468–470, 1987.
16. Bryson TK, Benumof JL, Ward CF. The esophageal obturator airway: A clinical comparison to mask-oral airway ventilation. Chest 74:537–539, 1978.
17. Owen RL, Cheney FW. Endobronchial intubation: A preventable complication. Anesthesiology 67:255, 1987.
18. Garnett AR, Ornato JF, Gonzalez ER, Johnson EB. End-tidal carbon dioxide monitoring during cardiopulmonary resuscitation. JAMA 257:512–515, 1987.
19. Shapiro BA, Cane RD, Harrison RA. Positive end-expiratory pressure therapy in adults with special reference to acute lung injury: A review of the literature and suggested clinical correlations. Crit Care Med 12:127–141, 1984.
20. Benumof JL. Update on mechanical ventilation. An epitome. Western J Med 128:147, 1978.
21. Weisman IM, Rinaldo JE, Rogers RM, et al. State of the art: Intermittent mandatory ventilation. Am Rev Resp Dis 127:641, 1983.
22. Downs JB, Klein EF Jr, Desautels D, et al. Intermittent mandatory ventilation: A new approach to weaning patients from mechanical ventilators. Chest 64:331–335, 1973.
23. Shapiro BA, Cane RD. The IMV-AMV controversy: A plea for clarification and redirection. Editorial. Crit Care Med 12:472–473, 1984.
24. Cane RD, Shapiro B. Mechanical ventilatory support. JAMA 254:87–92, 1985.
25. Pontoppidan H, Geffin B, Lowenstein E. Acute respiratory failure in the adult (3 parts). N Engl J Med 287:690, 143, 799, 1972.
26. Patterson RW. Effect of P_aCO_2 on O_2 consumption during cardiopulmonary bypass in man. Anesth Analg 5:269–273, 1976.
27. Cohen PJ, Alexander SC, Smith TC, et al. Effects of hypoxia and normocarbia on cerebral blood flow and metabolism in conscious man. J Appl Physiol 23:183, 1967.
28. Winter PM, Smith G. The toxicity of oxygen. Anesthesiology 37:210, 1972.
29. Lambertsen CJ. Effects of oxygen at high partial pressure. In Fenn WO, Rahn H(eds). Handbook of Physiology. Section 3, Respiration. Vol. 2. Baltimore, Williams & Wilkins, 1965, 1027–1046.
30. Nash G, Blennerhasset JB, Pontoppidan H. Pulmonary lesions associated with oxygen therapy and artificial ventilation. N Engl J Med 276:368, 1967.
31. De Campo T, Civetta JM. The effect of short-term discontinuation of high-level PEEP in patients with acute respiratory failure. Crit Care Med 7:47–49, 1979.
32. Rose DM, Downs JB, Heenan TJ. Temporal responses of functional residual capacity and oxygen tension to changes in positive end-expiratory pressure. Crit Care Med 9:79–82, 1981.
33. Albert RK. Least PEEP: Primum non nocere. Chest 87:2–3, 1985.
34. Suter PM, Fairley HB, Isenberg MD. Optimum end-expiratory pressure in patients with acute pulmonary failure. N Engl J Med 292:284–289, 1975.
35. Gallagher TJ, Civetta JM, Kirby RR. Terminology update: Optimal PEEP. Crit Care Med 6:323–326, 1978.
36. Kirby RR, Downs JB, Civetta JM, et al. High-level positive end-expiratory pressure (PEEP) in acute respiratory insufficiency. Chest 67:156–163, 1975.
37. Murray IP, Modell JH, Gallagher TJ, et al. Titration of PEEP by the arterial minus end-tidal carbon dioxide gradient. Chest 85:100–104, 1984.
38. Hurewitz A, Bergofsky EH. Adult respiratory distress syndrome. Med Clin N Am 65:33–51, 1981.
39. Weisman IM, Rinaldo JE, Rogers RM. Positive end-expiratory

pressure in adult respiratory failure. N Engl J Med 307:1381–1384, 1982.
40. Powers SR Jr, Mannal R, Neclerio M, et al. Physiologic consequences of positive end-expiratory pressure (PEEP) ventilation. Ann Surg 178:265–272, 1973.
41. Lores ME, Keagy BA, Vassiliades T, et al. Cardiovascular effects of positive end-expiratory pressure (PEEP) after pneumonectomy in dogs. Ann Thorac Surg 40:464–468, 1985.
42. Jardin F, Farcot J, Boisaute L, et al. Influence of positive end-expiratory pressure on left ventricular performance. N Engl J Med 304:387, 1981.
43. Molloy DW, Ducas J, Dobson K, et al. Hemodynamic management in clinical acute hypoxemic respiratory failure. Dopamine vs. dobutamine. Chest 39:636–640, 1986.
44. Prewitt RM, McCarthy J, Wood LDH. Treatment of acute low pressure pulmonary edema in dogs. J Clin Invest 67:409–418, 1981.
45. Cooligan T, Light RB, Wood LDH. Plasma volume expansion in canine pneumococcal pneumonia. Am Rev Respir Dis 126:86–90, 1982.
46. Molloy W, Ghignone M, Girling L, et al. Dobutamine and lasix in the treatment of oleic acid pulmonary edema in dogs. Fed Proc 42:733, 1983.
47. Petty TL. Critical care for chronic air-flow limitation: Emphysema, chronic bronchitis, and cystic fibrosis. Sem Resp Med 3:263–274, 1982.
48. O'Donohue WJ. National survey of the usage of lung expansion modalities for the prevention and treatment of postoperative atelectasis following abdominal and thoracic surgery. Chest 87:76–80, 1985.
49. Oldenberg FA, Dolovich MB, Montgomery JM, et al. Effects of postural drainage, exercise and cough on mucus clearance in chronic bronchitis. Am Rev Resp Dis 120:739–745, 1979.
50. Wang KP, Wise RA, Terry PB, et al. A new controllable suction catheter for blind cannulation of the main stem bronchi. Crit Care Med 6:347–348, 1978.
51. Fulkerson WJ. Current concepts: Fiberoptic bronchoscopy. N Engl J Med 311:511–515, 1984.
52. Wanner A, Landa JF, Neiman RE Jr, et al. Bedside bronchofiberoscopy for atelectasis and lung abscess. JAMA 244:1281–1283, 1973.
53. Millen JE, Vandree J, Glauser FL. Fiberoptic bronchoscopic balloon occlusion and reexpansion of refractory unilateral atelectasis. Crit Care Med 6:50–55, 1978.
54. Kirilloff LH, Owens GR, Rogers RM, et al. Does chest physical therapy work? Chest 88:436–444, 1985.
55. Marini J, Pierson D, Hudson L. Acute lobar atelectasis: A prospective comparison of fiberoptic bronchoscopy and respiratory therapy. Am Rev Resp Dis 119:971–978, 1979.
56. Remolina C, Khan AU, Santiago TV, et al. Positional hypoxemia in unilateral lung disease. N Engl J Med 304:523–525, 1981.
57. Fishman AP. Down with the good lung. N Engl J Med 304:537–538, 1981.
58. Seaton D, Lapp NL, Morgan WKC. Effect of body position on gas exchange after thoracotomy. Thorax 34:518–522, 1979.
59. Douglas WW, Rehder K, Beynen FM, et al. Improved oxygenation in patients with acute respiratory failure: The prone position. Am Rev Resp Dis 115:559–566, 1977.
60. Larca L, Greenbaum DM. Effectiveness of intensive nutritional regimes in patients who fail to wean from mechanical ventilation. Crit Care Med 10:297–300, 1982.
61. Kanak R, Fahey RJ, Vanderwarf C. Oxygen cost of breathing. Changes dependent upon mode of mechanical ventilation. Chest 87:126, 1985.
62. MacIntyre NR. Respiratory function during pressure support ventilation. Chest 89:677, 1986.
63. Banner MJ, Kirby RR. Similarities between pressure support ventilation and intermittent positive-pressure ventilation (letter). Crit Care Med 997–998, 1985.
64. Banner MJ, Kirby RR. Pressure support ventilation (letter). Crit Care Med 14:665–666, 1986.
65. Hewlett AM, Platt AS, Terry VG. Mandatory minute volume. A new concept in weaning from mechanical ventilation. Anaesthesia 32:163, 1977.
66. Gurevitch MJ, Van Dyke J, Young ES, et al. Improved oxygenation and lower peak airway pressure in severe adult respiratory distress syndrome. Treatment with inverse ratio ventilation. Chest 89:211, 1986.
67. Stock MC, Downs JB, Frolicher DA. Airway pressure release ventilation (APRV): A new ventilatory mode during acute lung injury (ALI). Crit Care Med 14:366, 1986.
68. Blanc VF, Tremblay NAG. The complications of tracheal intubation: A new classification with a review of the literature. Anesth Analog 53:202–213, 1974.
69. Campbell D. Trauma to larynx and trachea following intubation and tracheostomy. J Laryngol 82:981–986, 1968.
70. Baron SH, Kohlmoos HW. Laryngeal sequelae of endotracheal anesthesia. Ann Otol 60:767–791, 1961.
71. Zwillich C, Pierson DJ. Nasal necrosis: A complication of nasotracheal intubation. Chest 64:376, 1973.
72. Sherry KM. Ulceration of the inferior turbinate: A complication of prolonged nasotracheal intubation. Anesthesiology 59:148, 1983.
73. Arens JF, LeJeune FE, Webre DR. Maxillary sinusitis, a complication of nasotracheal intubation. Anesthesiology 40:415, 1974.
74. Berry FA, Blenkenbaker WL, Ball CG. A comparison of bacteremia occurring with nasotracheal and orotracheal intubation. Anesth Analg 52:873, 1973.
75. Biller HF, Harvey JE, Bone RC, et al. Laryngeal edema—an experimental study. Ann Otol 79:1084–1087, 1970.

Chapter 7

•

C. F. Ward, MD
Cairo A. Salvatierra, MD

Special Intubation Techniques for the Adult Patient

OUTLINE

I. INTRODUCTION

If a physician does not think that the trachea can be intubated with a conventional laryngoscopic approach (see Chapter 6), or actually fails to intubate the trachea conventionally, then there are four special (nonlaryngoscopic) ways to intubate the trachea. This chapter describes three of those special techniques: blind nasotracheal intubation, retrograde technique, and high-intensity illumination technique. Chapter 12 describes the fourth special technique, namely, use of a fiberoptic instrument. All three of the techniques described in this chapter can be used with either bloody or nonbloody airways, and all have had a high success rate.

II. Blind Nasotracheal Intubation

A. *History*

In 1920, I. W. Magill intubated a 27-year-old woman with a single large-bore catheter for nasal surgery. The term *large-bore* described what was different about this intubation, for Elsberg, and Meltzer and Auer, had previously reported that endotracheal intubation and insufflation were practicable using a small-bore tube. Magill and Rowbotham reported this single-tube technique in 1921, and 7 years later, Magill commented that "strangely enough" such a large-bore tube, passed through the nose, would easily enter the trachea. He referred to this as *blind intubation,* thus coining a phrase that has obviously stood the test of time and remains in use six decades later.

Oral endotracheal intubation for the administration of anesthesia predated blind nasotracheal intubation, however, having been accomplished by Macewen in 1878. In 1912, Elsberg adopted Chevalier Jackson's laryngoscope to precisely intubate the trachea under direct vision, thus giving this technique almost a 10-year head start over the blind nasal single-tube technique. By 1928, cuffed oral tubes, based on Dorrance's design, were described by Waters and Guedel, and these tubes became far more popular in the United States. Thiopental, a rapid-acting central nervous system and respiratory depressant, was introduced in 1934 by Lundy. Macintosh created the less-stimulating curved laryngoscope blade in 1943, and blind nasal intubation suffered a final major blow (as an intubating method of choice) when the ultra-short–acting barbiturate thiopental was combined with succinylcholine in a light-anesthesia–apneaor-otracheal induction sequence in 1952. The historical decline of blind nasotracheal intubation as a primary intubation mode has therefore occurred primarily because of operating room intubation considerations. For those with greater interest in this remarkable history of endotracheal intubation, an excellent reference, from which the preceding was derived, is Volume 2 of *Essays on the First Hundred Years of Anaesthesia* by W. S. Sykes.[1]

As time passed, endotracheal intubation escaped the operating room, and even the hospital, as basic and advanced cardiopulmonary resuscitation (CPR) became the template for care of the critically ill and intubation outside the surgical theater became common. Those charged with such areas of care quickly discovered that oral intubation of a badly injured, intoxicated patient in a cervical collar with a full stomach, firmly clenched teeth, and an empty intravascular compartment was a far cry from the operating room situation. Blind nasal intubation was one answer to this and indeed became so even for operating room intubation of the same sort of patient. However, for the majority of elective operating room nasal intubations, the intravenous induction sequence is so ingrained that most are probably still done under direct vision with tube passage assisted by forceps or a tube hook (see Chapter 6). Fiberoptics notwithstanding, there are still indications for blind nasal intubation, the most certain being the perceived anatomic inability to open the mouth and an absolute absence of either a fiberoptic scope or experienced fiberoptic endoscopist. Certainly, blind nasal intubation is a skill that should never be allowed to atrophy just because more elegant options have become available. For the majority of anesthesia locations throughout the world, fiberoptic endoscopy is not, and never will be, a viable option.

Learning a technique that has been reborn is usually best accomplished by returning to the original descriptions. In this case, the date is 1928, making the review difficult for those without access to a major library. However, in 1944, Elder published a more obtainable discussion,[2] and from it a number of interesting points can be gleaned. The procedure, as presented by Elder, is described later. If we compare this report to Magill's, published 16 years earlier, very little seems to have changed.

Obviously, the tracheal catheters being discussed are not easily comparable to current plastic tubes. The author mentions adequate rigidity, length, and curvature, with the expectation that each parameter is adjustable to some degree. Not mentioned in the body of the paper, but obvious from the drawings, the catheters are not equipped with a cuff and attendant pilot balloon, and the operator must therefore insert a connector preintubation to avoid catheter disappearance in the nostril. This may also explain the author's suggestion that a "12-mm" (probably outside diameter) catheter is tolerated, even desirable, for the average man.

The patient was positioned as Magill described for "sniffing the morning air," and the most patent nasal passage was anesthetized with 20% cocaine. This is truly an industrial concentration and only 0.25 mL was used, delivered by atomizer, with the patient encouraged to breathe deeply and inhale the cocaine into the lower airway. Once either the right or left nostril was chosen, a bevel was cut in the catheter tip to position the bevel toward the septum and avoid the inferior turbinate.

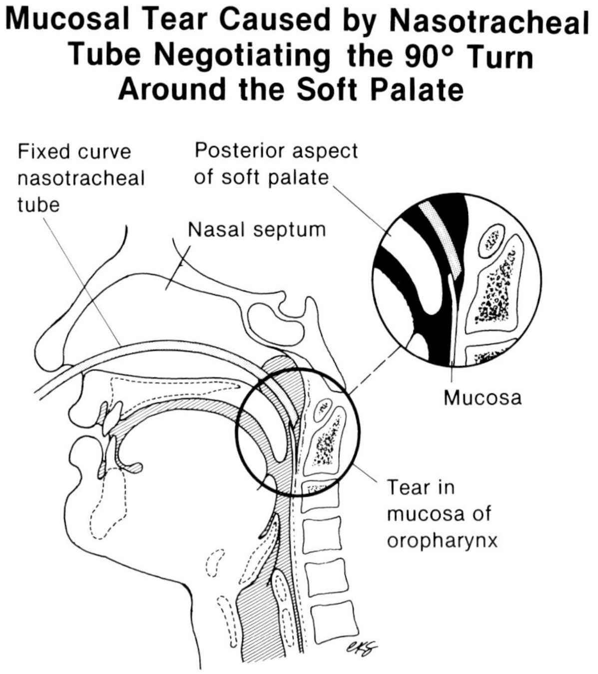

Figure 7–3 • The 90° radius of curvature around the posterior edge of the soft palate may occasionally cause the tip of the nasotracheal tube to tear the mucosa of the oral pharynx. The tear in the mucosa may create a new plane of advance into the retropharyngeal and mediastinal space.

5. Negotiating the Nasopharyngeal Curve

Often, a tube, particularly if warmed in hot water, will negotiate the turn at the posterior choana with ease. On occasion, however, progress ceases here and the next step is a function of touch and experience. If the obstruction seems shallow, it may actually be a cuff-destroying septal spur. This may resist all attempts to coax the tube by, no matter how many different angles are tried. If this is the case, it is better to admit defeat before the bleeding starts and try the other nostril. Further on, a problem area for passage of a tube with a fixed radius of curvature is encountered whenever a much different radius must be traversed. This first occurs at the posterior edge of the soft palate, where an abrupt 90° small radius curve must be negotiated as the oropharynx is entered (Fig. 7–3). It would seem that this might represent an absolute obstacle beyond which the tube simply might not go without some assistance, but another, fortunately rare, undesirable option is for the tube almost to make the turn and create a new plane of advance in the retropharyngeal space through a mucosal tear (see Fig. 7–3). It can be surprisingly easy to pass the tube down to the mediastinum in this space, although obviously never into the airway, and it is important to be aware of this should the tube pass this first turn but respiration be impossible to hear by listening to or by observing the tube.

If the issue is the small radius curve, then technology has something to offer, in the form of a tube with the capability to decrease the manufactured curve. This tube, an Endotrol™, has a pull ring that enters the tube side-wall near the proximal end; traction on this ring reduces the radius of curvature of the tube and markedly facilitates this turn (Fig. 7–4). To some degree, this process is made easier by the fact that these tubes seem to have an inherently decreased radius of curvature and are more supple. As soon as the tip negotiates the turn (Fig. 7–5), traction must be released; otherwise the distal tip may unexpectedly appear in the mouth, having made a very small radius and embarrassing 180° turn.

6. Redirecting the Tube When It Does Not Enter the Trachea

After entering the oropharynx, the tube is advanced easily, with breath sounds monitored all the while, on occasion simply sliding into the trachea without further manipulation (Fig. 7–5 inset and Fig. 7–6). For those other occasions when it does not, the tip can go to one of the four sites mentioned by Elder. Entry into the esophagus is usually marked by complete cessation of breathing sounds and a visible oscillation of the larynx as the tube slides behind it (Fig. 7–7). Either pyriform sinus being entered results in a marked diminution in breath sounds and a palpable external bulge near the hyoid laterally as the tube leaves the midline (Fig. 7–8). The tube resists further advance, as it does when it enters the vallecula. However, impacting the vallecula causes more visible rocking laryngeal movement and is generally more uncomfortable for the patient (Fig. 7–9). The most common and often most troublesome site of obstruction is supraglottic, where breath sounds are well heard, but any attempt to advance the tube meets resistance and the patient may seem to be in respiratory distress transiently.

The solution to esophageal intubation is further neck extension and traction on the pull ring if an Endotrol tube is used. The tube can then be advanced a few centimeters, after which extension and traction should be released to prevent subsequent supraglottic obstruc-

(Text continued on p. 156)

Flexible-Tipped Nasotracheal Tube

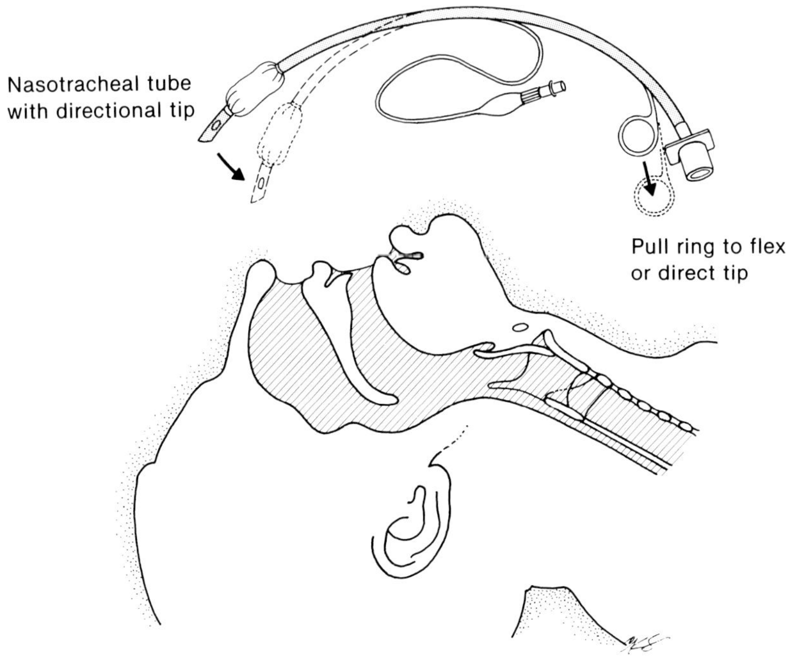

Figure 7–4 • A flexible-tipped NT tube can greatly help the tip of the NT tube negotiate the tight radius of curvature around the soft palate. Pulling on the ring (which connects a pull line to the tip of the endotracheal tube) causes the radius of curvature of the tube to diminish, helping the tube to make the turn around the soft palate.

Manipulation of Tip in Nasopharynx

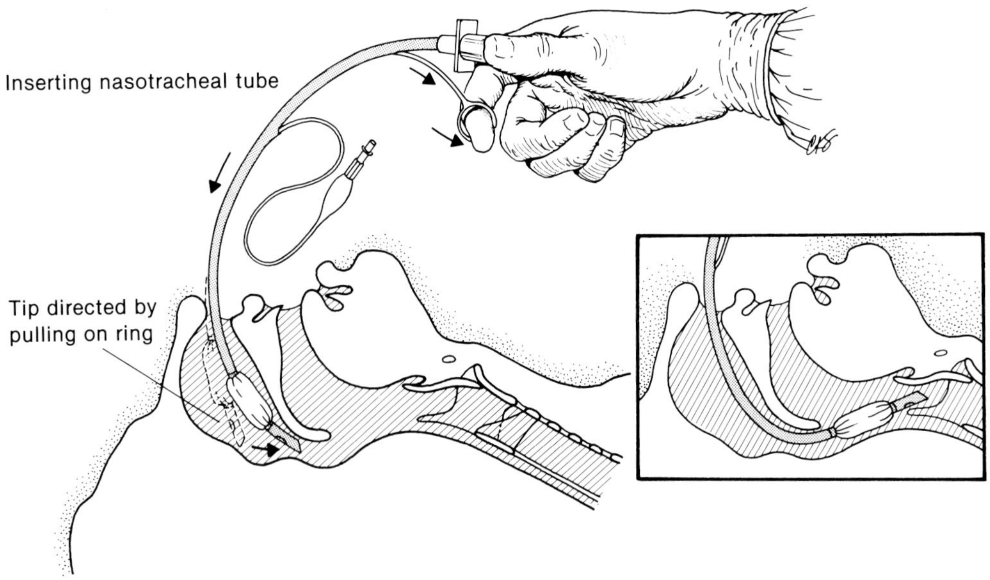

Figure 7–5 • As the tip of the tube approaches the oro pharynx, pulling on the ring will direct the tip of the tube around the soft palate and into the trachea (see inset).

Nasotracheal Tube in Trachea

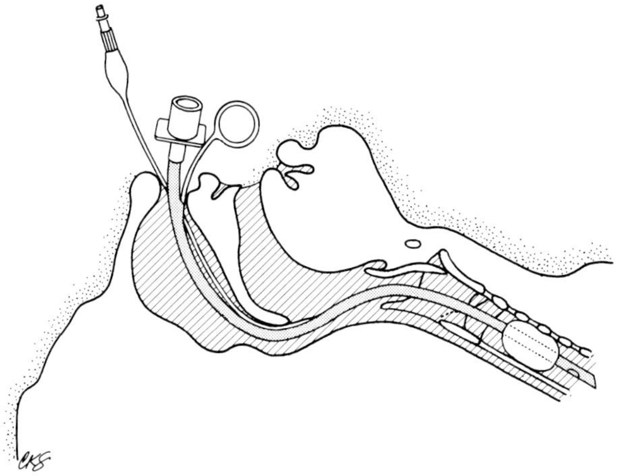

Figure 7–6 • Nasotracheal tube in proper position in the trachea. (Note: The traction ring should be cut free if it enters the nose. Failure to do this may place the tube on continuous tension anteriorly.)

Endotracheal Tube in Esophagus

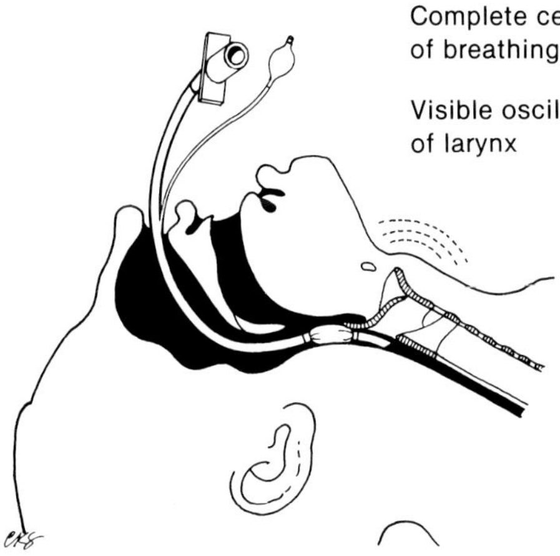

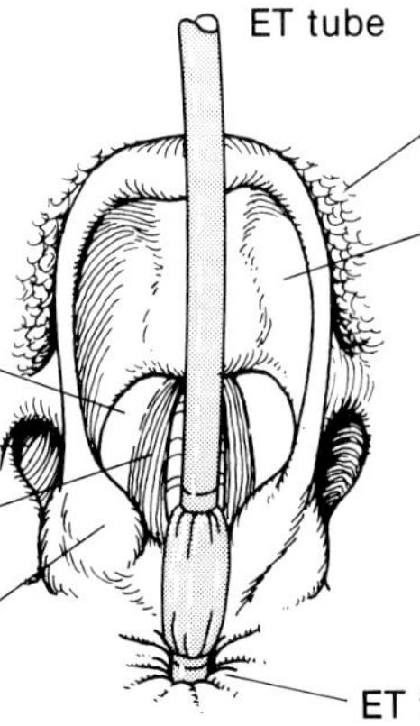

Figure 7–7 • Schematic diagram of an endotracheal tube located in the esophagus. (***A***) Sagittal view. (***B***) Internal view.

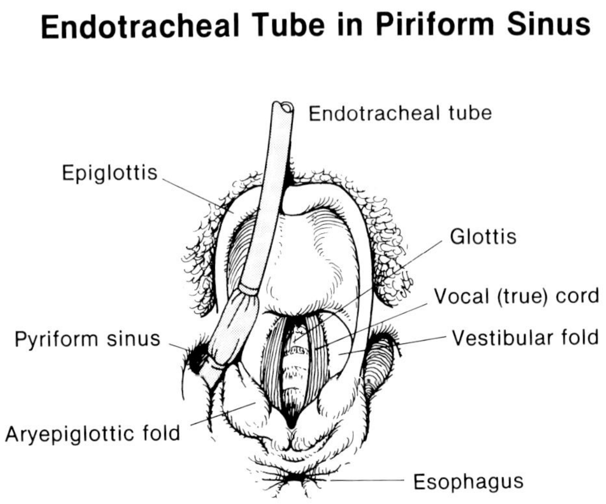

Figure 7–8 • Internal view of an endotracheal tube tip located in the piriform sinus.

tion. Entry into either pyriform sinus is remedied by tube withdrawal and a small rotation toward the midline, followed by readvancing the tube. It is at this point that observation of the "tee" connector proves useful. Escape from the vallecula involves tube withdrawal and neck flexion followed by reintroduction. This same maneuver works equally well for a supraglottic snag (Fig. 7–10), often facilitated by a 90° to 180° counterclockwise rotation to direct the tube tip away from the anterior commissure and tracheal rings. No matter which technique is chosen, true tracheal placement is confirmed by auscultation, chest movement, patient oxygenation, and respiratory gas analysis. If an Endotrol tube was used, the pull ring should be cut free from the tube following tracheal entry, as it enters the side wall in a typical 7.0-mm ID tube at 27 cm, and insertion of the tube to, or beyond, this depth applies traction to the ring with the nostril and flexes the tip into the tracheal wall.

On occasion, after trying all the preceding maneuvers, one is still left with an elongated nasopharyngeal airway and a virgin larynx. A useful technique[4] here may be to insert a suction catheter, typically 14 French, through the tube and possibly directly into the larynx, after which the tube itself may follow (Fig. 7–11). From patients in respiratory distress who demand to remain sitting upright while breathing, one discovers that this technique often seems nearly effortless in this position, in particular if the patient sits just slightly forward (see Fig. 7–11).

7. The Inspired Gas Mixture

Noteworthy in most descriptions of blind nasal intubation is the assumption that the patient will breathe room air spontaneously, thus allowing the operator to listen directly or indirectly to gas movement, occasionally aug-

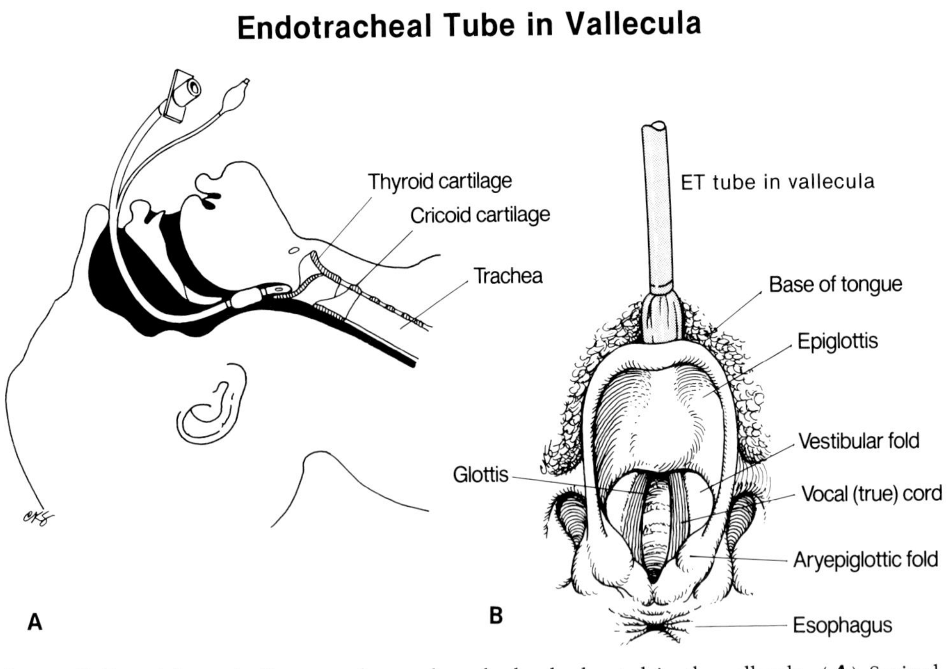

Figure 7–9 • Schematic diagram of an endotracheal tube located in the vallecula. (***A***) Sagittal view. (***B***) Internal view.

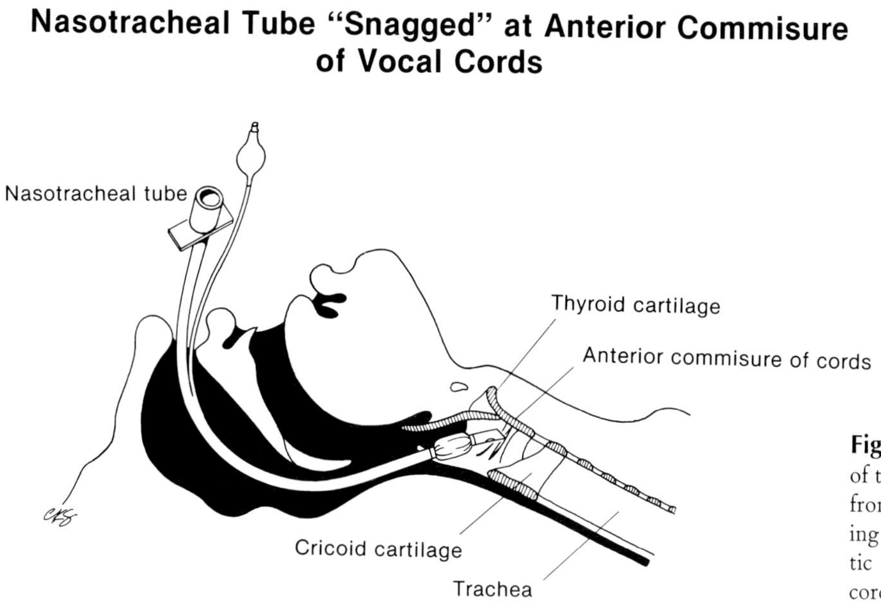

Figure 7–10 • Schematic diagram of the prevention of a nasotracheal tube from passing into the trachea by hanging up ("snagging") on the supraglottic anterior commissure of the vocal cords.

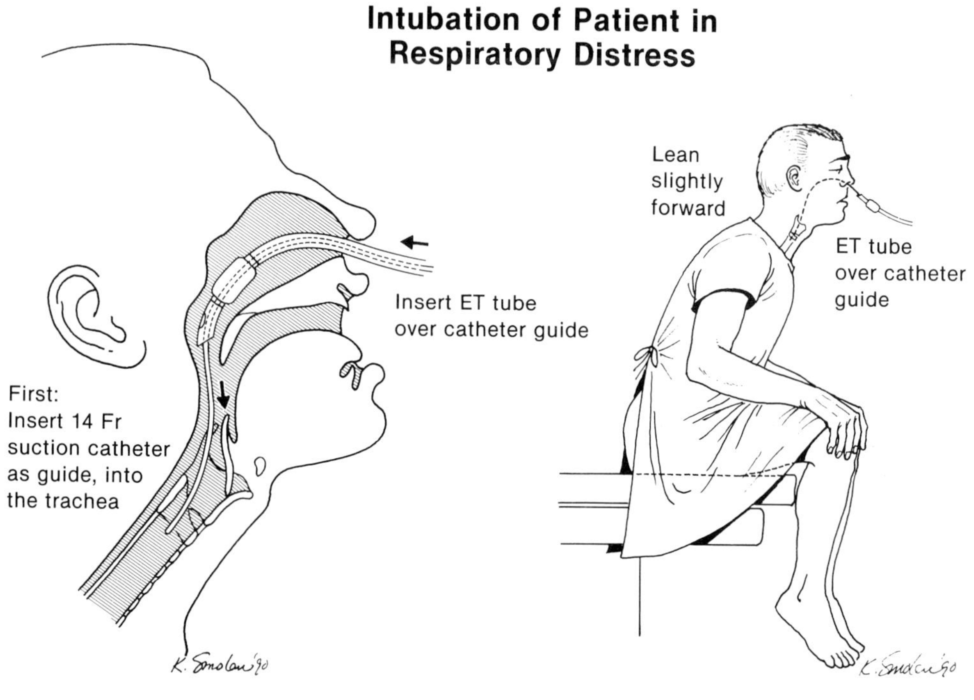

Figure 7–11 • Intubation of the patient in respiratory distress may be facilitated by passage of an endotracheal tube over a catheter guide (such as a nasogastric tube) (left panel) and/or by having the patient lean forward in the sitting position (right panel).

mented by a noise-producing device on the proximal end of the tube.[5] In most circumstances, this assumption holds true, but not invariably. For those patients who require supplemental oxygen, this tradition of listening to respiration must be replaced with noisy oxygen insufflation or some form of circuit attached to the tube. Elder's 1944 review mentioned adding carbon dioxide to inspired gases to increase ventilation; in general, that is not possible for most anesthesia machines today. However, a Mapelson circuit (B–F), with fresh gas flow less than twice minute ventilation will allow for carbon dioxide rebreathing while providing more than 95% oxygen. For patients not already at the end of their respiratory reserve or suspected of increased intracranial pressure, this can be used to assist intubation. The eye then replaces the ear, assisted by a hand placed gently on the anterior neck, and the added advantage of a "sealed" airway is obtained, such that the operator is never rewarded by tracheal entry with a forceful expectoration nearly directly into his or her ear. One can obviously administer anesthetics via the tube in the same manner, but issues of respiratory depression and an adequate, but not too deep, or light, plane of anesthesia make this much more involved. Blind intubation of an apneic patient can be accomplished, but once respiration ceases, the oxygen clock is running (although more slowly than imagined for preoxygenated patients). For most inexperienced practitioners, this will prove to be a stressful exercise, with a lower probability of success. Absent some strong, unusual indication for paralysis, spontaneous respiration should be preserved during this technique. Whenever available, respiratory gas analysis for carbon dioxide should accompany intubation to insure tracheal placement. In fact, if available, this should be included in an ongoing fashion during intubation whenever a breathing circuit is employed.

An interesting variant of blind nasotracheal intubation involves the use of the lighted stylet, which is available in a 33-cm model with increased malleability. (The interested reader should consult the section concerning this technique.) The stylet can, if desired, be passed through a self-sealing flexible bronchoscope port in a circuit elbow so that oxygen can be administered and carbon dioxide sampled during the intubation.

C. *Complications*

Given the anatomy, bacteremia from nasal intubation seems inevitable. Most patients tolerate this without problems, but those lacking an adequate immune system or those with blood flow turbulence-inducing cardiac abnormalities may not. Such patients should receive prophylactic antibiotics suitable for upper airway flora prior to intubation. Two anatomic abnormalities of the heart do not require such coverage: (1) an atrial septal defect closed without a patch and (2) a ligated patent ductus arteriosus. The issue of mitral valve prolapse is currently unclear, but most patients should probably receive coverage.

Once in place, the tube itself obstructs drainage from the ipsilateral maxillary sinus and middle ear. Prolonged nasal intubation and fever of unknown origin require an index of suspicion, such that sinusitis and otitis are both part of the differential diagnosis. In fact, a preexisting problem of this sort may pose a relative contraindication to nasal intubation. One tell-tale indication of sinus problems may be a history of a Caldwell-Luc or nasoantral window procedure in the past. A recent upper respiratory infection, especially with loss of vocal resonance, may pose a theoretical problem, but the issue has not been studied.

Blood supply to cartilage is always tenuous. Pressure from a nasal tube can cause necrosis of the nares, and since cartilage does not regrow, this can be truly disfiguring. Every attempt should be made to avoid conforming the nose to the tube, rather than vice versa, and the nose should be inspected daily during prolonged intubation. If skin breakdown is noted, the tube should be moved.

Bleeding from the nose can vary from annoying to life threatening. Nasal intubation probably should be treated with the same care as epidural catheterization. If the clotting mechanism is suspect for the back, it is equally so for the nose.

Although it is a disease of children, adults now do present for surgery with cystic fibrosis. This disease commonly has associated nasal polyps; if polyps are present, nasal intubation is contraindicated. This also applies to the triad of aspirin allergy, polyps, and asthma and to any history of isolated nasal polyps. In fact, the possibility of nasal pathology, known or otherwise, suggests that examining the nose with a light and speculum would be generally prudent before undertaking a plastic assault. In the current era of illicit drug use, the preintubation discovery of a nasal septal defect might save a great deal of postintubation explanation.

Blind nasal intubation is traditionally avoided in midface LaFort II and III fractures, and one only needs to see one radiograph of a nasogastric tube in the skull to guess why. In fact, one suspects that a gentle blind nasal intubation can be done in this situation, especially if the tube can be flexed, but the admonition remains. As always, this is a matter of priorities. A unstable cervical spine and decaying respiratory status may force the issue, regardless of the usual warnings.

Most patients who require emergent intubation are evaluated in the supine position, thereby making the detection of cerebrospinal fluid rhinorrhea fairly difficult. If, however, this is noted, or the patient is otherwise suspected of having a cribriform plate or anterior cranial fracture, nasal intubation is generally contraindicated. As just mentioned, there may be situations when the airway will take priority, but options should be briefly explored prior to pursuing this route.

Common sense and liability would suggest that prior nasal surgery, especially reconstructive surgery, or nasal trauma would probably contraindicate elective blind nasal intubation, as would a history of epistaxis.

III. RETROGRADE INTUBATION

A. *History*

The title *retrograde intubation* is a misnomer. Intubation certainly does not occur from below to above. Rather, following percutaneous insertion, a guide is passed retrograde from the larynx into, and then out of, the naso- or oropharynx. Inevitably, the question is, "If intubation is not retrograde, how did the term come about?" The answer is simply that the first case report in 1960,[6] which described passing the guide via a tracheostomy stoma, was so labeled. The concept of percutaneous guide insertion actually was presented in 1963 by Waters,[7] who used the far more precise phrase *guided blind endotracheal intubation* to describe passage of an epidural catheter via the cricothyroid membrane to assist tracheal intubation. As is true for many original reports, this is worth reading, for the author's clinical observations are excellent, the technique is well described, and the two patient photographs included, with chief complaint of trismus, are paradigms of understatement.

As originally described, a Tuohy needle was passed through the cricothyroid membrane, bevel cephalad, through which was passed an epidural catheter. The needle was then removed, the catheter was retrieved from the oropharynx with a transnasopharyngeal plastic tube with distal dressmaker's hook, and both catheter and tube were withdrawn from the nose. Subsequent nasal intubation was done using the epidural catheter as a continuous guide to the larynx. Waters pointed out that the tube should not be excessively large, that the catheter should be stiff yet flexible, and that laryngeal spasm was possible during the procedure. This report also required that the catheter pass directly through the endotracheal tube lumen, because Waters used Magill tubes. Four years later, two American authors suggested using a catheter-through-the-needle, central venous pressure catheter in the same fashion, but included the modification of passing the guide through a Murphy side-hole *only* with the guide then outside the tube lumen.[8] Obviously, these authors were solving the problem posed by the minimal distance between the true cords and the cricothyroid membrane, which allowed only about 1.5 cm of tube to enter the trachea before further progress was arrested by the guide passing through the tracheal entry site. By threading the guide through the side-hole, an extra 1 cm of intubation was gained. However, this improvement was submerged in this four-page article and did not resurface until 1974, when Bourke and Levesque[9] made special mention of this anatomic limitation and again suggested threading the guide through the side-hole, only this time from the outside in and then up the tube lumen. This advance was then partially combined with a Seldinger technique of lumen access in 1981 for intubation in a 12-kg child using a 20 gauge needle and 0.021-in guide wire.[10] The word *partially* applies because the Seldinger technique actually involves a needle, guide wire, and catheter specifically chosen to fit together.

When used in the airway, the catheter or tube clearly has no systematic relationship to the much smaller guide. Furthermore, ideally the guide and appropriate tube would be radially centered in the airway. Obviously, this is not the situation here. The guide originates from the anterior wall of the larynx and is usually held in a bow-string fashion by manual tension against the anterior aspect of the anatomy it traverses. It is usually held in tension because it is too supple to direct the tube otherwise. However, the most common problem with this technique is that a tube may "hang up" at or near the glottis. One obvious way to minimize this is to employ a tube that is slightly smaller than usual. Beyond this an impressive variety of tube and guide manipulations have been suggested to deal with this snag (see Section III.B.5) usually along commonsense lines, such as realization of guide tension and slight withdrawal and readvancement of the tube. Akinyemi,[11] from the same hospital as Waters, further suggested that posterior manual displacement of the larynx could be useful.

Two indirect solutions to the guide-tube mismatch have been proposed by several authors.[12,13] One of these solutions represents almost a two-stage approach, wherein the retrograde guide provides a path into the larynx for a second antegrade guide that enters the actual trachea (see Section III.B.5). Another solution consists of passing a stiff, antegrade guide through the tube but not down the wire, so that it can be passed beyond the retrograde guide insertion point. The tube is then passed over both the retrograde and antegrade guide (see Section III.B.5).

B. *How to Do Retrograde Intubation*

1. Head Position, Skin Preparation, Anesthesia

The patient should be placed in the traditional sniffing position with support not only beneath the skull but beneath the neck as well. If necessary, this can be modified with a slight cervical extension to gain access to the anterior neck. An overaggressive approach to this should be avoided, as the patient in question may have less than an optimum airway under the best of circumstances and attempts to intubate cannot be allowed to take precedence over breathing. The operator should stand to the patient's side (generally the right for right-hand-dominant individuals). The neck should be prepared as for a surgical procedure. The skin over the cricothyroid or cricotracheal membrane is then anesthetized with subcutaneous 1% lidocaine. Further local anesthesia is delivered intratracheally with a short 20-gauge needle and syringe after air aspiration has insured tracheal entry. It can be expected that injection of any liquid into the unanesthetized trachea will cause significant cough and moderate laryngeal movement. Therefore, the needle should be held firmly and the injection should be rapid. As needed, the superior laryngeal nerves (between the greater cornu of the hyoid bone and the superior cornu of the thyroid cartilage), glossopharyngeal nerves (fold of tissue between the base of the tongue and the anterior pillar), and pharynx (spray) can be anesthetized as well.

2. Choice of the Entry Site/Needle/Retrograde Guide

The needle entry site is traditionally the cricothyroid membrane (Fig. 7–12), but as noted later, the cricotracheal membrane may eventually prove superior. If the cricothyroid membrane is chosen, the entry site should be closest to the cricoid cartilage itself to avoid the nearby arteries. The needle used to puncture the membrane is dictated by the guide to be used. Options include epidural catheters in various sizes, vascular access

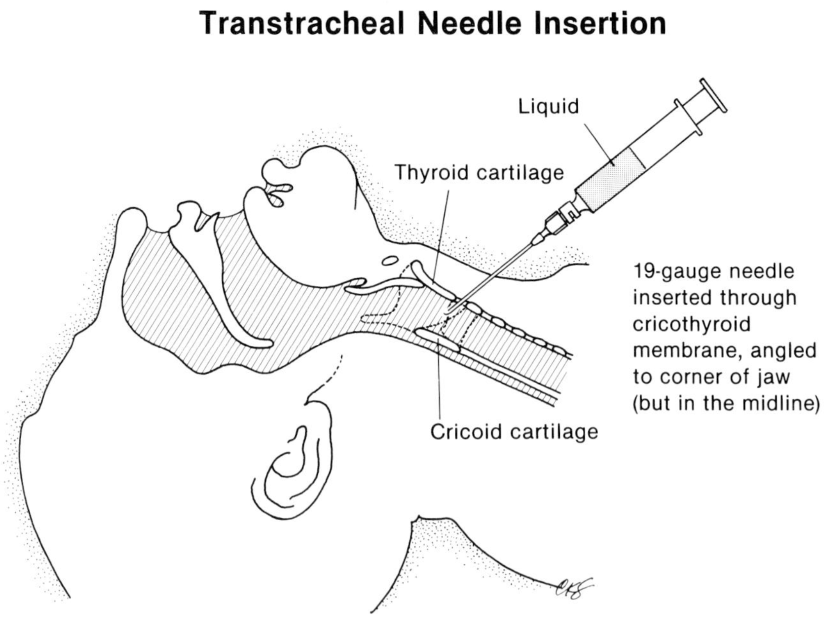

Figure 7–12 • Passage of a transtracheal needle through the cricothyroid membrane. The needle is angled slightly cephalad (30°).

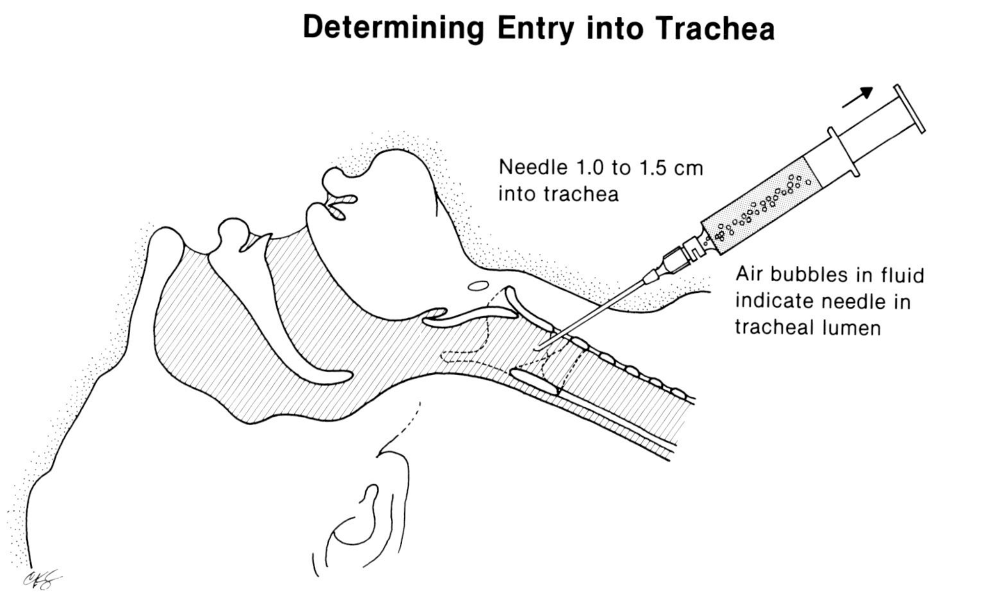

Figure 7–13 • Entry into the trachea is documented by aspiration of air into an attached fluid-filled syringe.

guide wires (a J-tip might be beneficial), and a length of 125 cm or more if either is to fit up the entire length of the suction port of a fiberoptic bronchoscope, or large-sized synthetic suture, probably chosen for a monofilament construction and distinctive color. If a large-bore Tuohy needle is chosen, a small transverse incision over the puncture site will ease introduction. For smaller, sharply beveled thin-wall needles, this is unnecessary.

3. INSERTION OF THE NEEDLE/RETROGRADE GUIDE

The needle is directed in the midline in a slightly cephalad direction (30°) (see Fig. 7–12) and entry is documented by aspiration of air into an attached fluid-filled syringe (Fig. 7–13). The guide is then inserted via the needle until it exits the mouth or nose or until the patient spits it out (Fig. 7–14). On occasion it will be

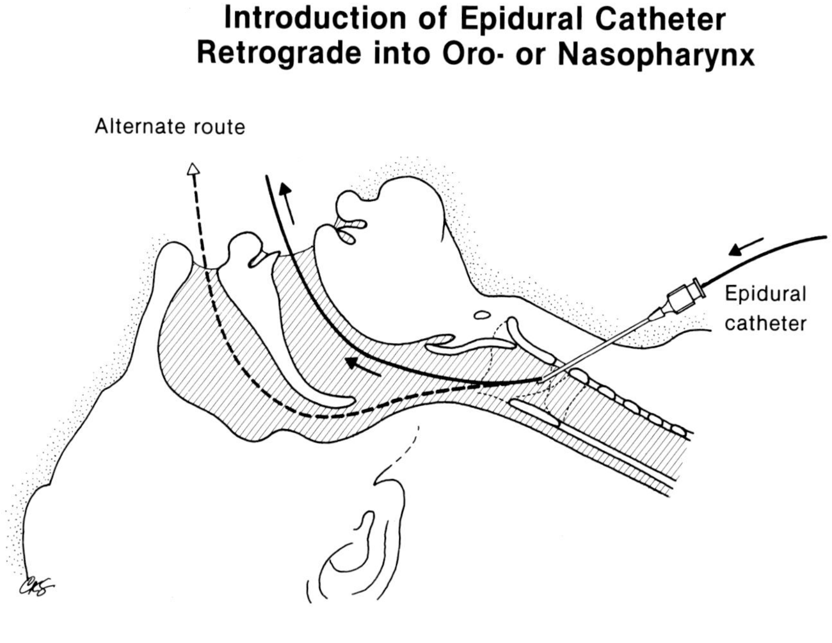

Figure 7–14 • The retrograde guide (in this case an epidural catheter) is passed into the transtracheal needle into the oropharynx or the nasopharynx.

necessary to search the posterior oropharynx for the guide with tongue blade and long, blunt forceps when the guide does not appear and *if* the mouth can be opened. Once the guide has been delivered, the needle is removed from the neck and a clamp is applied to the guide near the puncture site to stabilize it (Fig. 7–15).

4. Passing the Tube Over the Naked Retrograde Guide

Next, the endotracheal tube can be passed over the retrograde guide while both ends of the retrograde guide are pulled tight. Pulling both ends of the retrograde guide tight provides a nonbuckling sling for the endotracheal tube into the trachea. However, the technique as just described does involve significant tension on the retrograde guide. Thus, the possibility certainly exists that the tube will snag at the glottis, especially if the tube is simply passed over the naked retrograde guide. Whereas conventional intubation under direct vision is based on raising the epiglottis from view and placement of the tube in the center of the trachea, the guided blind technique essentially demands that the tube be off center and approach the laryngeal aperture just under the posterior epiglottic surface and perhaps off to one side. Experience suggests that brute force is rarely the answer, especially for smaller tubes, as downward pressure on the tube simply flexes it like a plastic spring until it buckles.

The best first step when the snag occurs may well be to simply relax tension on the guide so that the tube aligns more posteriorly in relation to the larynx. Second, one can reassess the tube and perhaps reduce its size. Another suggested maneuver[14,15] is to withdraw the tube initially and then try 90° counterclockwise rotation (see the next paragraph) while maintaining gentle downward pressure, or to displace the larynx posteriorly with manual pressure. Finally, the head can be gently lifted and the neck flexed in an attempt to align the airway with the natural arc of the tube. Frequently the eventual solution combines all three techniques, just as for nasal intubation (see Chapter 6 and the previous section).

The problem of a tube that reaches the general area of the cords but that does not pass through the cords can be influenced by minor variations in technique and deserves further comment. When the retrograde concept was conceived, the path for the guide was always through the tube lumen. The tube then traveled with its manufactured curved, beveled tip to the pa-

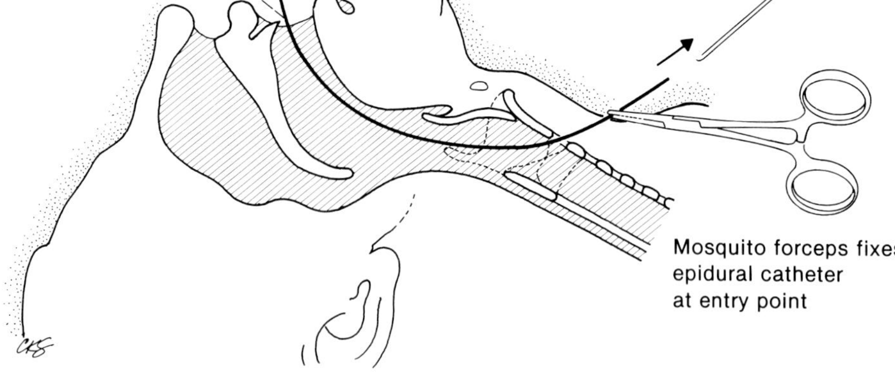

Figure 7–15 • Once the guide has been delivered out of the mouth, the needle is removed from the neck and a clamp is applied to the guide near the puncture site in the neck in order to stabilize it.

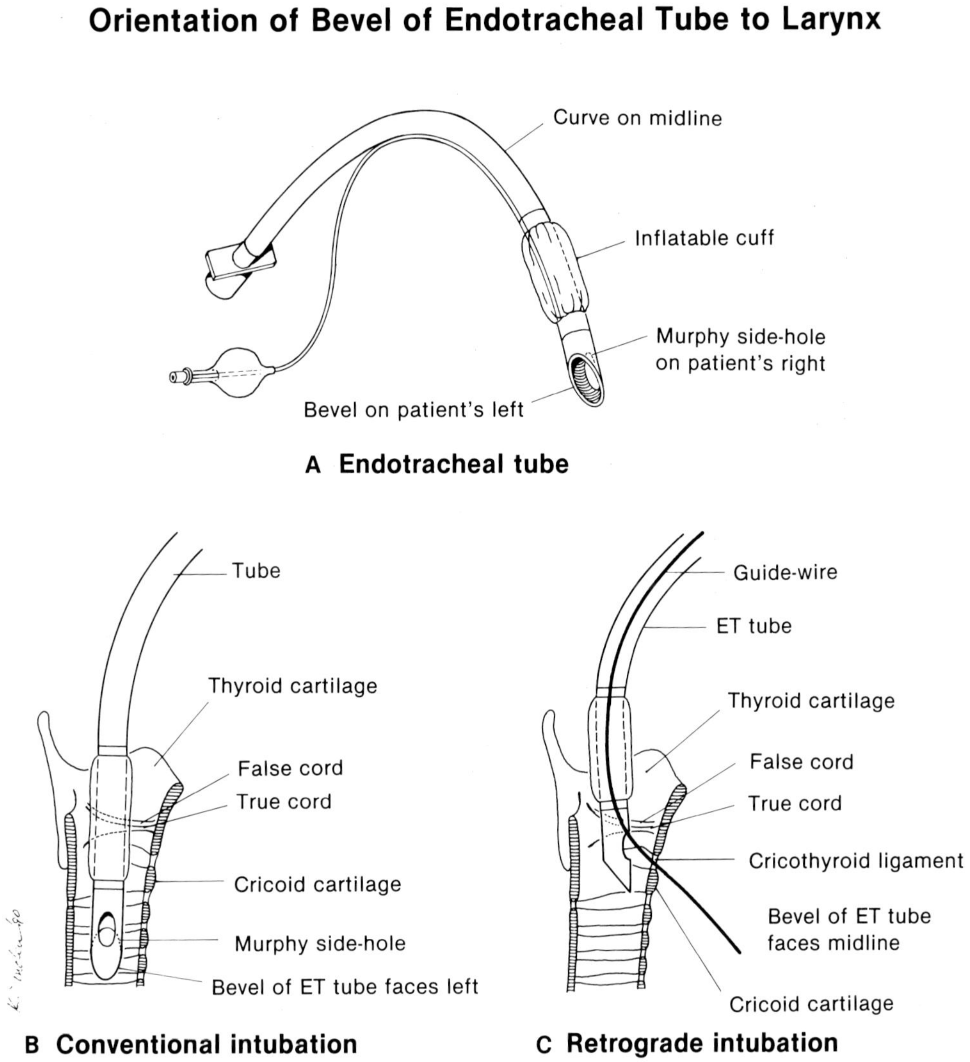

Figure 7–16 • This schematic diagram depicts the orientation of the bevel of an endotracheal tube (***A***) during a conventional intubation (***B***) and during a retrograde intubation (***C***) when the retrograde guide is passed through the Murphy side-hole of the endotracheal tube. In a conventional intubation the face of the bevel of an endotracheal tube faces left and the very tip of the tube (end of the bevel) is at the 3 o'clock position and may impact upon the right vocal cord (which is also at the 3 o'clock position). In a retrograde intubation in which the retrograde guide is passed through the Murphy eye, the face of the bevel of an endotracheal tube faces midline posteriorly; in other words, the very tip of the bevel is at the 12 o'clock position.

tient's right (Fig. 7–16A–B). In distinction, passing the guide through the Murphy side-hole (Figs. 7–16C and 7–17) should reorient the tube 90° counterclockwise from this, so that the tube enters the airway with the bevel tip *in the midline* (see Fig. 7–16C), theoretically directing this tip away from the right vocal cord and arytenoids. Passing the retrograde guide through the Murphy side-hole also gains an extra 1 cm of intratracheal (sublaryngeal) endotracheal tube that is below the point of entry of the retrograde guide (see Fig. 7–16C). If bevel orientation can indeed be an impediment to retrograde intubation, then tubes without the side-hole and tip bevel may result in a higher success rate and cause much less mucosal trauma.

5. ANTEGRADE GUIDE OVER RETROGRADE GUIDE

If the tube fails to pass, the most frequently suggested next step (or this could be the first step) is to pass ante-

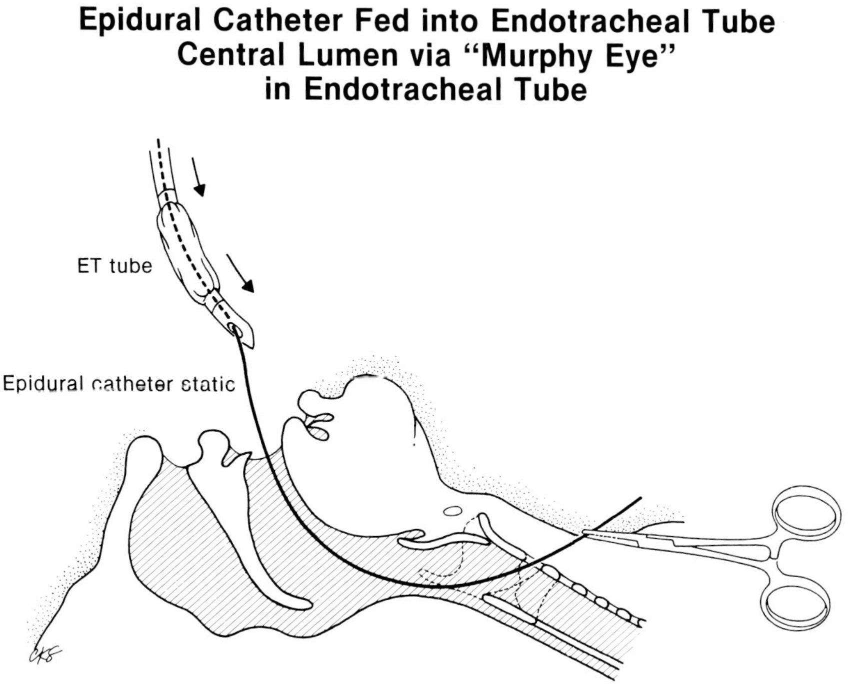

Figure 7-17 • Threading the retrograde guide into the endotracheal (ET) tube via the Murphy side-hole of an ET tube.

grade another piece of equipment slightly larger than the retrograde guide over the retrograde guide until it abuts the entry site of the retrograde guide. This equipment, whether it is a suction catheter, the sheath from the guide wire, a modified Eschmann stylet,[16] or even a fiberoptic endoscope (using the suction channel),[17] when passed over the retrograde wire itself stiffens the tube path and allows for much less tension to be placed on the retrograde guide. Following the passage of the stiffer antegrade guide, the retrograde guide can be withdrawn from above or cut flush with the skin and the antegrade large-bore guide can be further advanced endotracheally, followed in turn by the endotracheal tube. An important caveat for this bidirectional guide technique is that the antegrade guide will be shorter than its predecessor; otherwise the retrograde guide will simply be lost to view as the second guide slides over it. Withdrawal of the first guide through the mouth would then become impossible.

If tube size permits, a better technique might be to pass the antegrade guide down, not the retrograde guide, but in parallel through the tube and then out into the trachea proper (Fig. 7-18). Ideally, this second guide should have an open central lumen, as suggested by Juneja and Trop* through which oxygen can be insufflated and carbon dioxide sampled to provide better oxygenation and to insure that the antegrade guide truly enters the trachea prior to removal of the retrograde wire or catheter. If this is impossible, the same two advantages of an open lumen antegrade guide can be almost achieved by connecting the tube itself to a right-angle swivel of the sort used for fiberoptic bronchoscopy. The guides can then extend through the self-sealing bronchoscope orifice while the patient is connected to a breathing circuit and associated carbon dioxide sampling device.

6. Use of Retrograde Thread to Pull the Tube Tip into the Trachea

Recently, two reports have appeared suggesting still more modification of the technique, so that the retrograde guide no longer plays a simply passive role in the entrance of the endotracheal tube into the trachea but rather pulls the endotracheal tube into the trachea (Fig. 7-19). Harrison and Wise[18] actually sew a retrograde nylon thread guide through the side-wall of an armored tube and place a knot in midthread so that traction can be applied to the tube (Fig. 7-20). The tube is then pulled gently into the oropharynx and into the esophagus (see Fig. 7-19D). The tube is then withdrawn while listening for breath sounds; once they are heard, the thread is put on tension and the airway is entered from behind the epiglottis (see Fig. 7-19E). The tube is

*Juneja and Trop. Personal communication.

Nasogastric Tube as Guide to Distal Airway

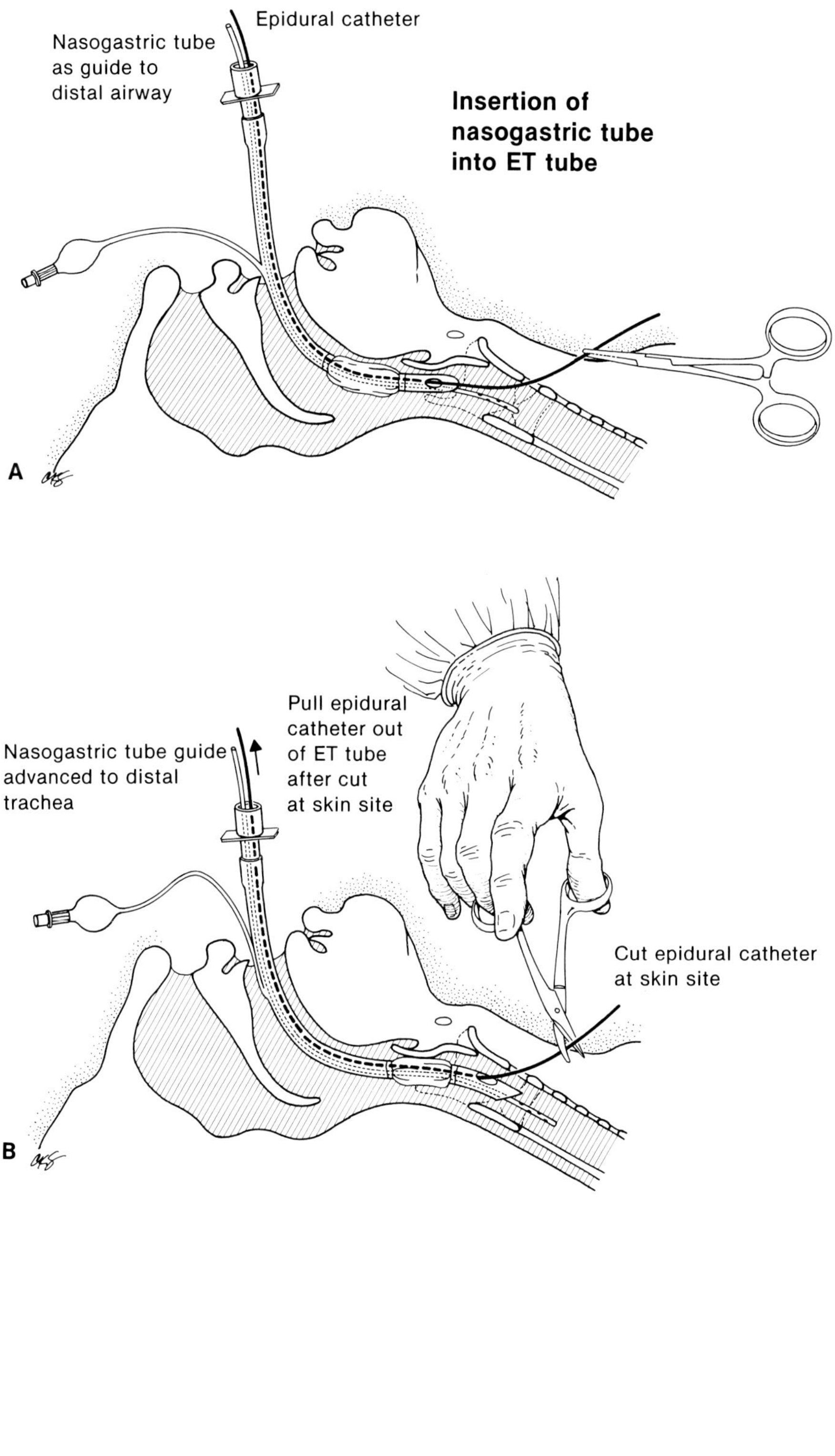

Figure 7–18 • Use of a nasogastric tube as a guide to the distal airway. (***A***) The nasogastric tube is passed down the ET tube distal to the point of the entry of the retrograde guide. (***B***) The retrograde guide is pulled out of the ET tube after it is cut at the neck skin level.

(continued)

Nasogastric Tube Removed from Endotracheal Tube

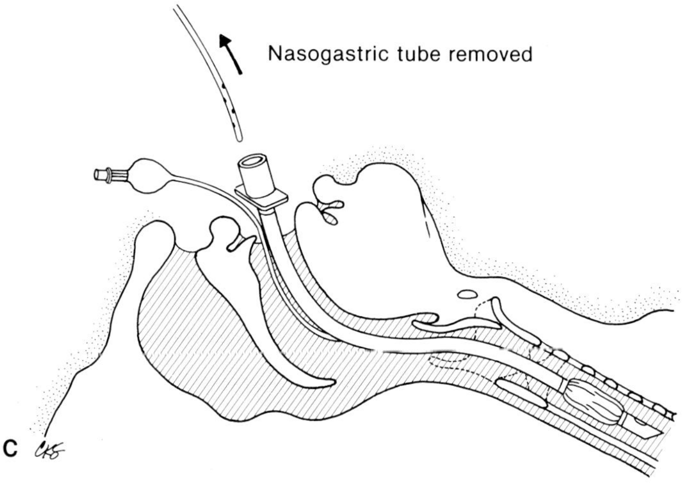

Connection to Ventilation System

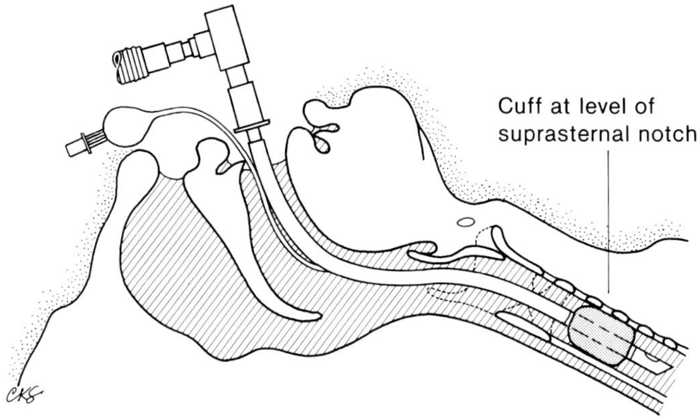

Figure 7–18 *(continued)*
(***C***) The ET tube is pushed further into the trachea over the nasogastric tube and then the nasogastric tube is removed. (***D***) The ET tube is then connected to the ventilation system.

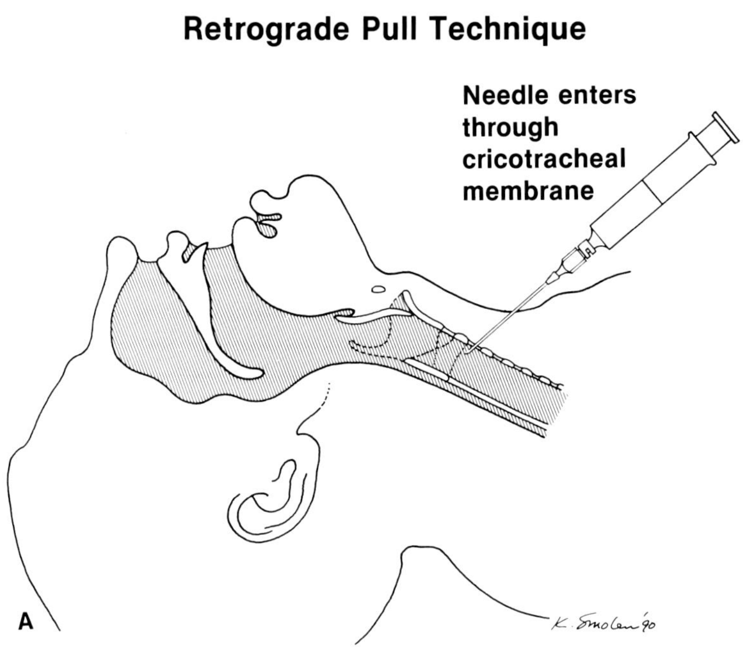

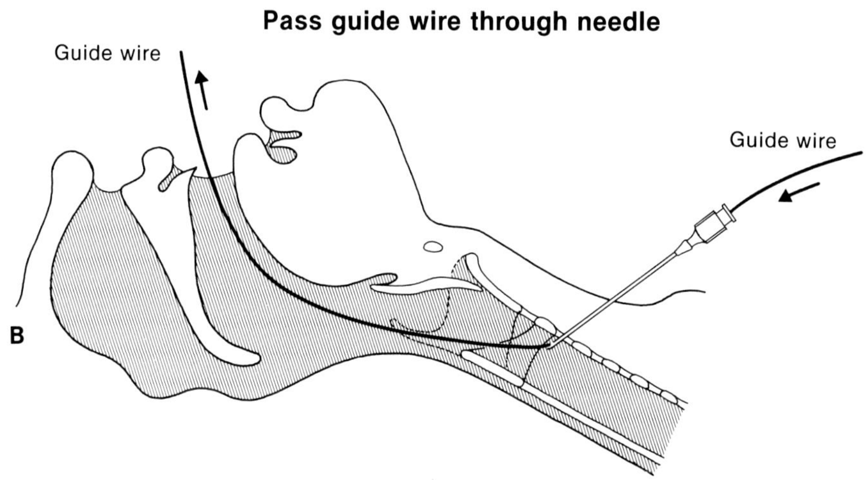

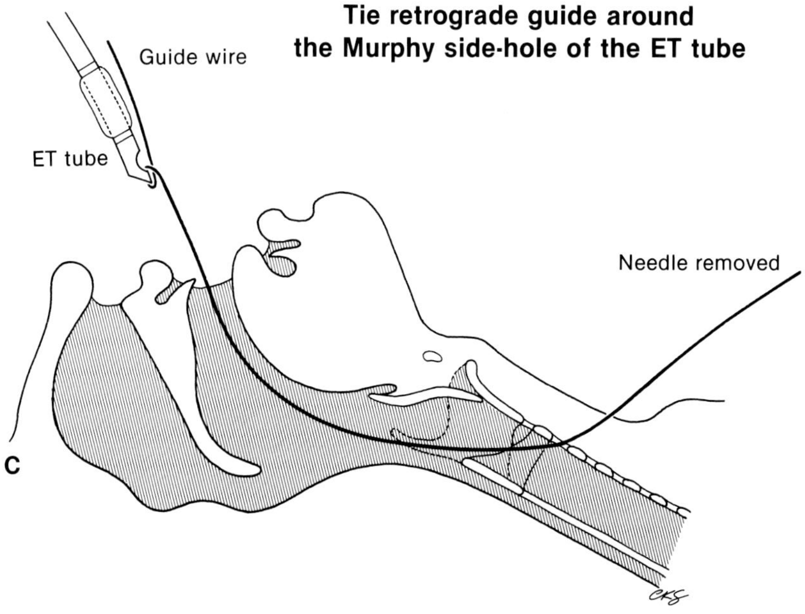

Figure 7–19 • This schematic diagram depicts the sequence of events in a retrograde pull technique. (***A***) The trachea is identified through the cricothyroid membrane puncture. (***B***) The retrograde guide is passed through the needle into the oral airway. (***C***) The retrograde guide is tied around the Murphy side-hole of the endotracheal (ET) tube.

(continued)

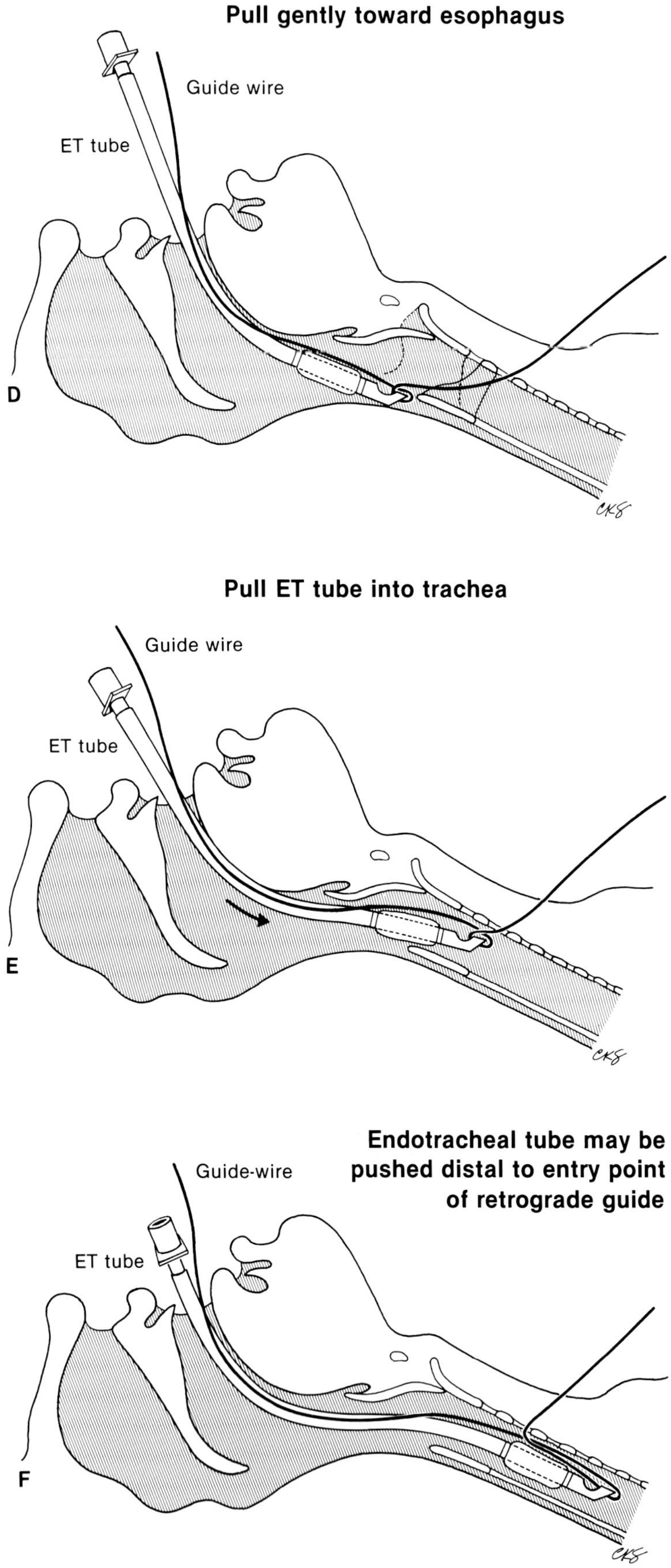

Figure 7–19 *(continued)*
(***D***) The ET tube is then gently pulled toward the esophagus. (***E***) When the ET tube reaches the area of the esophagus, the ET tube is pulled into the trachea by the retrograde guide. (***F***) The ET tube may be pushed distal to the entry point of the retrograde guide.

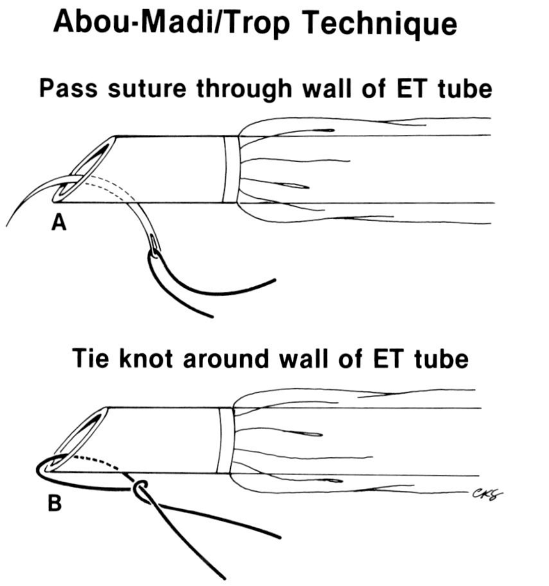

Figure 7–20 • This schematic diagram depicts the Abou-Madi Trop technique of passing a suture through the wall of an endotracheal (ET) tube (***A***) and then tying a knot around the wall of the ET tube (***B***).

passed into midtrachea with the thread left attached (see Fig. 7–19F). When the patient is extubated, this very long thread attached to the tube exits from the mouth and can remain in the airway, thus allowing for reintubation if required. Abou-Madi and Trop[19] proposed a further variant wherein the guide, after it is retrieved from the pharynx, is passed through the Murphy side-hole from the inside out and then over the tip longitudinally, back inside, and then up the tube (Fig. 7–21). This forms a slipknot at the tip of the tube, so that it can be pulled tramlike, as with Harrison and Wise, into the airway. More interestingly, these authors enter the airway via the *cricotracheal* membrane (see Fig. 7–19), which avoids any of the laryngeal anatomy, including the cricothyroid arteries, and allows for a bit more tube insertion before the retrograde guide entry site is reached. A long-standing ''rule'' of most authors has been that the guide, whatever it may be, should pass in only one direction, from the prepared neck to the contaminated pharynx, but never the reverse. Traction techniques violate this concept, although it is not clear that this means infection will actually result.

7. USE OF RETROGRADE GUIDE TO AID CONVENTIONAL LARYNGOSCOPY

If one harkens back to the Waters paper, trismus was the original indication for this technique. Should the indication be instead a difficult intubation where the patient's mouth can be opened, a retrograde guide can serve usefully as an aid to intubation under not quite direct vision by demonstrating the correct path, as well as assisting an antegrade guide or tube to travel down that path. This may seem a cluttered combination of maneuvers, but unusual upper airway anatomy (eg, a tumor) might allow the combination to work where either component alone would fail.

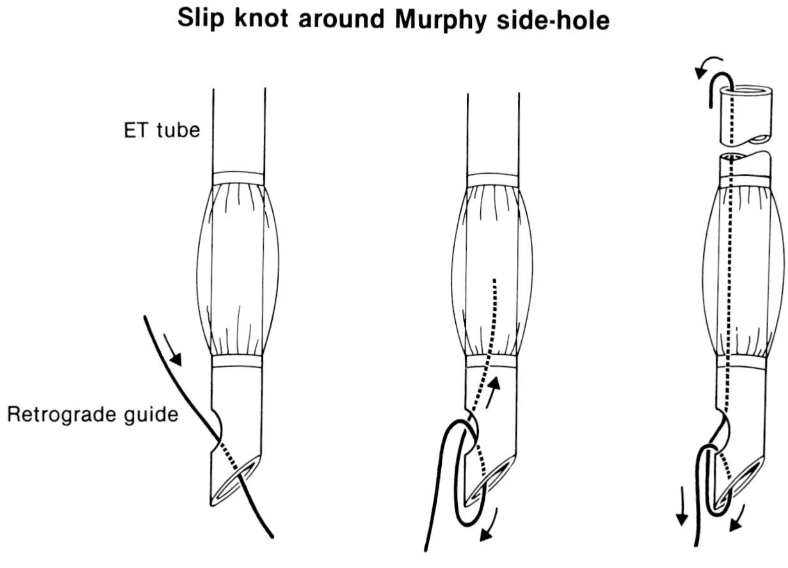

Figure 7–21 • This schematic diagram depicts tying a slip knot around the Murphy side-hole and exiting the retrograde guide through the lumen ET tube.

C. Complications

The most general concern about this technique involves bleeding in and around the airway. Unfortunately, most reports about guided intubation do not document complications in detail. However, the most aggressive circumstance imaginable would use this technique just prior to systemic heparinization. As it happens, a report of that very situation, using 14-gauge needles for puncture, presented 25 patients, only one of whom developed a small peritracheal hematoma, and even this situation did not require therapy.[20] At that, this one patient developed the hematoma only following the development of postbypass disseminated intravascular coagulopathy. Assuming the worst case, where peritracheal bleeding is arterial, manual compression should be maintained for at least 5 minutes or until bleeding stops. In fact, the most recent publication concerning this technique does suggest that bleeding is the most frequent complication and that the technique should be avoided in patients with a preexisting history of hemorrhaging diathesis[19]. Subcutaneous emphysema is probably also of concern, but the literature does not document this as a problem.

IV. Illumination Intubation

A. History

All too frequently, what is "new" in the world is only the old information one does not know. This may be the case with tracheal transillumination as an aid to intubation. Given his other remarkable contributions to the specialty, it is not surprising that Sir Robert Macintosh first reported this concept in early 1957 as an aid to intubation.[21] The primary message of this first report was to describe the construction of the prototype equipment and to very briefly describe its use. A similar report appeared in *Anesthesiology* two years later,[22] again presenting a prototype, this time from Japan, only to be followed within a month by yet a third presentation.[23] This "American" version added the use of a readily available commercial malleable stylet, which, interestingly, looks basically the same as its 1990 kindred, minus smooth plastic insulation. In 1978, Ducrow,[24] expanding on a Macintosh suggestion of intubation without endoscopy, reported orotracheal intubation in anesthetized paralyzed patients, utilizing the illuminated stylet, with no attempt to visualize the glottis whatsoever. In fact, this description seems related to the much older technique of tactile intubation. Reading Ducrow's paper, one is struck by the inclusion of several seemingly unnecessary steps involving an additional guide. Examining the photograph in the paper subtly teaches another point about advances in technology. The tubes Dr. Ducrow used were red rubber; enthusiasm for this technique rose fairly abruptly when clear plastic tubes became widely used, although no particular author pointed out how dramatically such tubes increased the transillumination effect.

An unusual variation on the illuminated stylet was described in 1985,[25] when Heller and Cotton described early experience with a plastic endotracheal tube containing an integral fiberoptic strand to allow for confirmation (not initial placement) of tube position in the infant midtrachea, versus either the esophagus or a mainstem bronchus. From this sequence, one can see that what has evolved over the years is the use of the stylet, with clear tubes, without laryngoscope, not only to place the tube in the trachea, but to demonstrate that nontracheal placement can be identified this way. For extremes of physical habitus, such as the very thin or morbidly obese, obvious questions arise concerning the latter point. An edifying study,[26] using preplaced tubes in adult cadavers, demonstrated 96% accuracy in determination of tube position (trachea, esophagus, upper airway) by physicians and paramedics in an average time of less than 5 seconds. Confusion was occasioned only by thin body habitus, an observation also borne out by Heller and Cotton, who noted that their illuminated tube could not differentiate esophageal from tracheal placement in infants. Clearly, then, the message is that transillumination can identify tube location in two planes almost without exception, whereas the third plane, that of anterior–posterior depth, may be problematic for smaller and thinner patients. The issue of the obese patient has not been specifically addressed in the literature, but one can anticipate a patient with such redundant tissue overlying the anterior neck as to preclude light transmission. Unfortunately, even after manual displacement of such tissue from the neck, actually attempting the technique may be the only way to sort out the possible from the impossible.

Technique development has been assisted by subtle design changes, currently manifest as a device with uniform polymer armor from bulb to battery case (Tube-

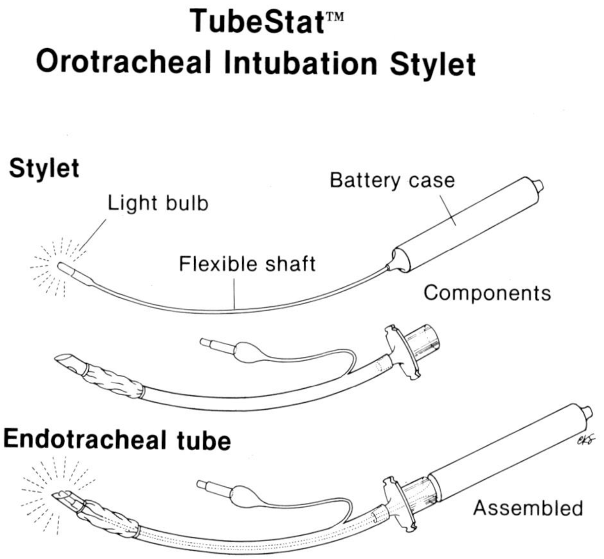

Figure 7–22 • A schematic diagram of the TubeStat® Orotracheal Intubation Stylet, which consists of the stylet (upper panel), the ET tube (middle panel), and the components assembled together (bottom panel) with the ET tube over the stylet.

Stat®, Concept, Inc., Clearwater, FL) (Fig. 7–22). The encasement is not only to ease extraction of the device postintubation, but to insure that that process is complete. The inevitable report of a retained part,[27] which could actually have been published as a title and a single picture, about the earlier naked, noncovered version appeared in 1984. One is struck by how distinctly a light bulb can be seen on the chest radiograph included in this paper, and the points made by the authors are still valid 6 years later—no excessive bends should be made in the malleable stylet, and the device is not meant to withstand great force.

When this concept is first discussed, those with experience tinkering about home or car will draw to mind the simple workshop version of this light, which is commercially available for less than $5. This familiarity is not necessarily an advantage, because it makes all the more painful the $27-plus price tag for the medical version. The batteries in the dedicated airway device are sealed and nonreplaceable but should last for a reasonable time with occasional use. In fact, the manufacturer's recommendation for "limited reuse" are such that per-use costs would be in the vicinity of $1 or so. In this era of HIV infection there may be concern about reuse of an airway device, but consider that fiberoptic bronchoscopes are not throw-away items. If one can be cleaned satisfactorily, so can the other.

For those interested in having their "own" lightwand, nondisposable versions, made of aircraft-quality metal surrounding a fiberoptic bundle, have been available for several years from Anesthesia Medical Specialties, Inc. of Santa Fe Springs, CA, although for some reason this version has not appeared in the literature concerning this technique. This company supplies several different sizes of the device, at about three times the price of the disposable version, including one that is much smaller than the limited-reuse version and would therefore allow for use in a smaller tube than 5 mm ID.

B. *How to Do Illumination Intubation*

1. LEARNING THE CONCEPT

One of the first three reports dealing with illumination intubation stated that the indication for a lighted stylet was to compensate for a laryngoscope bulb failure during endoscopy. Obviously, this inferred a typical direct visualization of the airway by endoscopy. Although this is not the thrust of most recent work, this approach is an excellent place to begin to learn the technique. However, the trainee should not intubate the trachea; rather, he or she should observe the light transmission as the tube is placed. The stylet bulb should be beyond the distal end of the tube cuff, or if the tube is uncuffed, just within the lumen. As the endoscopist inserts the tube, the transillumination will appear abruptly as the bulb passes the bulk of the tongue and epiglottis, just superior to the thyroid cartilage. The larynx itself, once entered, produces a jack-o-lantern effect, which is prominent if room lights are at all dimmed.[28] If the tube enters the esophagus, this internal illumination is much decreased; if deviation occurs laterally, the light appears well off the midline. Given that the light source is within the tube lumen, transillumination of the larynx suggests that the tube has passed the glottis. It can then be slipped off the stylet and advanced into the trachea proper.

Following this observational period, the novice will have some feeling for the sight picture during this procedure. Obviously, the illuminated stylet can then be used as just that and further experience can be gained by noting the appearance of the larynx during intubation.

Alternatively, one can move forward to intubation without laryngoscopy.

2. Anesthesia

It is a given that anesthesia is required to intubate the trachea under most elective circumstances. It is not a given that this requires anesthesia for the entire organism, but it certainly is required for at least the upper segment of the airway, from the posterior third of the tongue to the midtrachea. Further, as this technique generally involves inserting the tube and stylet, and frequently a gloved hand, into the mouth, patient cooperation is obligatory. Cooperaton can be assured with general anesthesia, but this need not be necessary for the technique per se.

3. Preparing the Lighted Stylet and Tube

For orotracheal intubation without laryngoscopy, the "intubationist" should stand at the side facing the patient, who is placed in a neutral to minimally head-elevated position.[29] For those who are right-hand dominant, this should be the patient's right side. The stylet should be lightly lubricated and inserted into the endotracheal tube, size 5.0 mm or larger (bulb diameter 3.76 mm) until the bulb is just within the tube lumen. The stylet should then be flexed through roughly a 90° small radius arc, just proximal to the top of the tube cuff (Figs. 7–23 to 7–25). The limited-reuse stylet is available in two lengths, 25 and 33 cm. The longer, and much more flexible, model is for nasotracheal intubation and comes with a sliding endotracheal tube adapter that allows for adjustment to various tube lengths, which is obviously more necessary for nasal than for oral intubation. The malleability of the longer device allows the tube to negotiate the very-small-radius turn at the posterior border of the palate without impediment. Obviously, the increased flexibility implies a different purpose, changing from *direction* to *confirmation* of tube position. Very few practitioners, authors included, have extensive experience with styleted tubes for nasal intubation, but reasoning from experience with fiberbronchoscopes, it seems essential that the stylet be very well lubricated before insertion and that, furthermore, the minimum acceptable tube size be somewhat larger than 5.0 mm in this setting. In any case, be certain that the

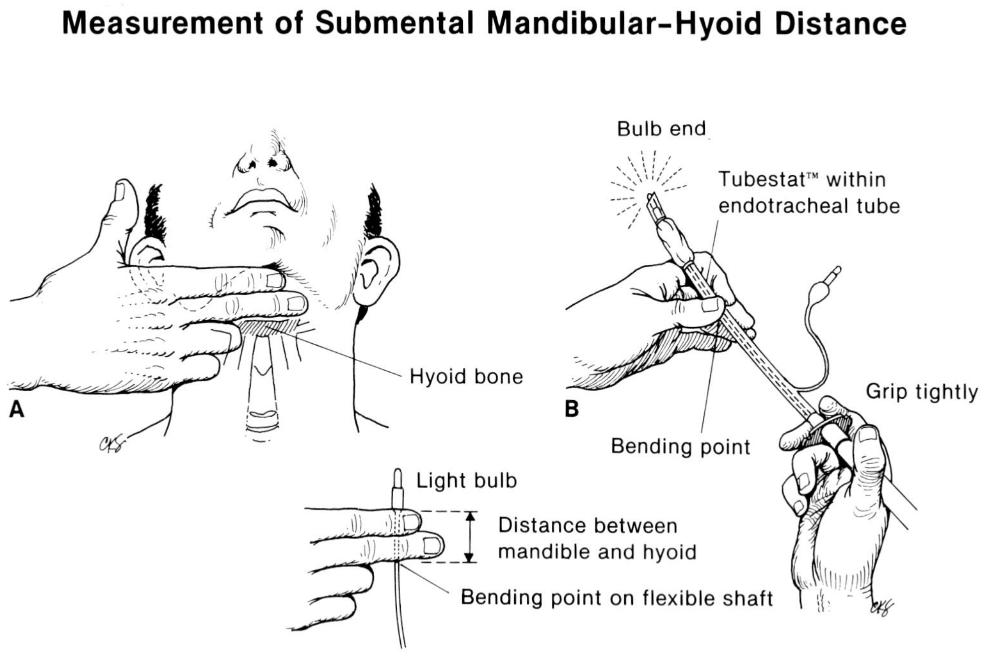

Figure 7–23 • The distance from the tip of the lighted stylet at which a bend is put in is equal to the submental mandibular–hyoid distance. (***A***) Measurement of the submental mandibular–hyoid distance. (***B***) Bending of the flexible shaft of the lighted stylet at a distance from the tip of the stylet that corresponds to the submental mandibular–hyoid distance.

Bend in Light Wand and Mouth Entry

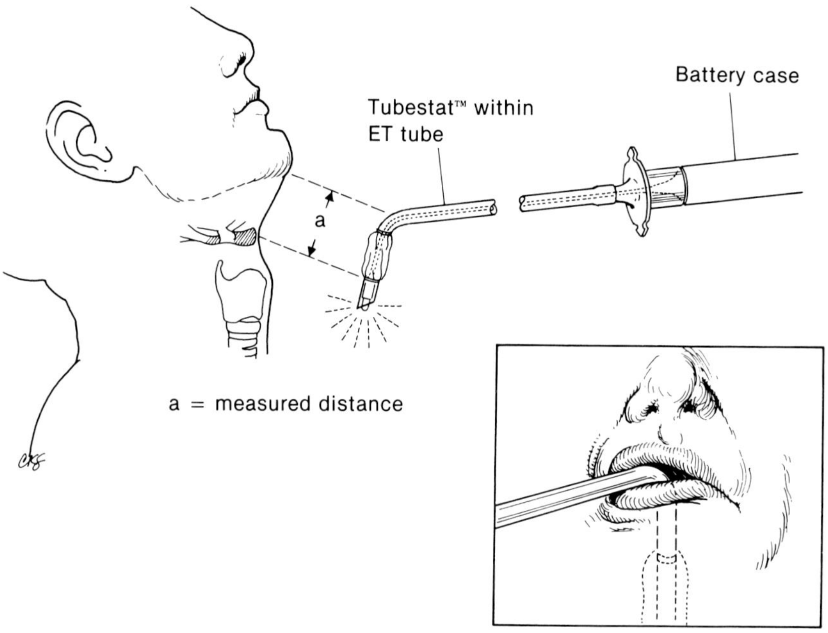

Figure 7–24 • Schematic diagram showing the bend in the light wand in relation to entry of the light wand into the mouth.

Head Position and Bend in Light Wand

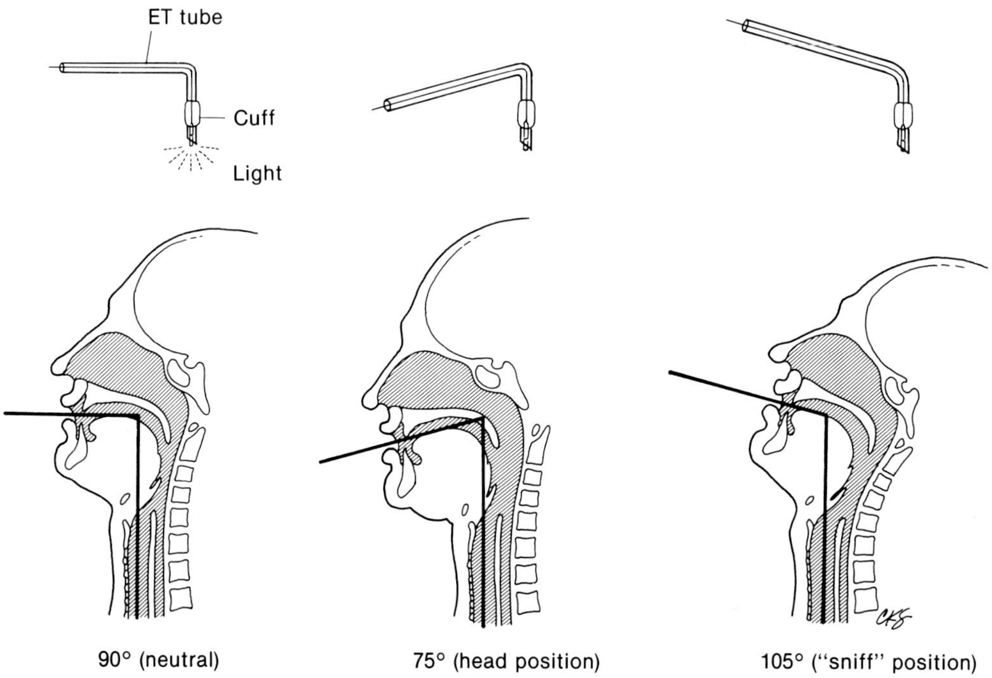

Figure 7–25 • Schematic diagram of head position and the appropriate bend in the lighted stylet.

stylet can be withdrawn from the selected tube while it is shaped roughly, as it will be in the nose. Intubating the trachea with this equipment only to find out that immediate extubation is the sole way to remove the stylet might serve as a low-water mark for a month's worth of clinical achievement.

4. Inserting the Lighted Stylet and Tube

A patient who is voluntarily cooperative should be asked to stick out his or her tongue. If the patient is involuntarily cooperative, it is helpful to grasp, with a gloved left hand and gauze, either the mandible or the tongue and to exert gentle traction until the airway opens (Fig. 7–26). If this procedure is employed following previous direct attempts to intubate the patient, do not be surprised at copious secretions that make grasping the tongue the hardest part of the task. For occasions when this sequence can be anticipated, prior administration of an antisialagogue is recommended.

The tube and stylet are then inserted, looking for the sight picture described earlier (Fig. 7–27). The roughly 30-cm length of the straight segment of the lightwand can make insertion into the mouth awkward in the sagittal plane, so that insertion from the side of the mouth is much easier. If the light then first appears in the esophagus, a combination of anterior lift and gradual withdrawal may allow for a sensation of an abrupt "give" as the tube moves into the glottic orifice with resultant laryngeal transillumination.

A variation of this process has been suggested by Williams,[30] who developed the Airway Intubator™ to assist in fiberoptic intubation but has since pointed out that this same device can be useful with the lightwand as well.

5. Threading the Tube Off the Stylet

Next, the tube can be slipped off the stylet with the left hand (Fig. 7–28). Some consideration of the bend in the

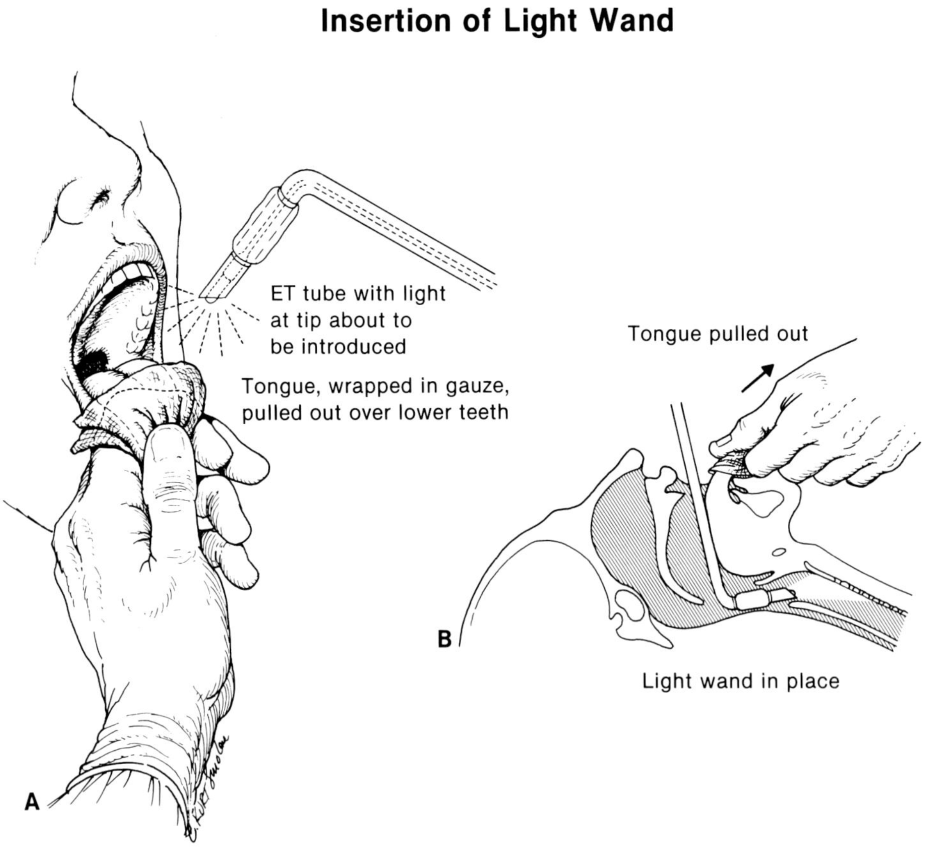

Figure 7–26 • The introduction of the bent light wand into the mouth may be facilitated by pulling the tongue forward (***A***). Lighted stylet in place with the tongue pulled forward (***B***).

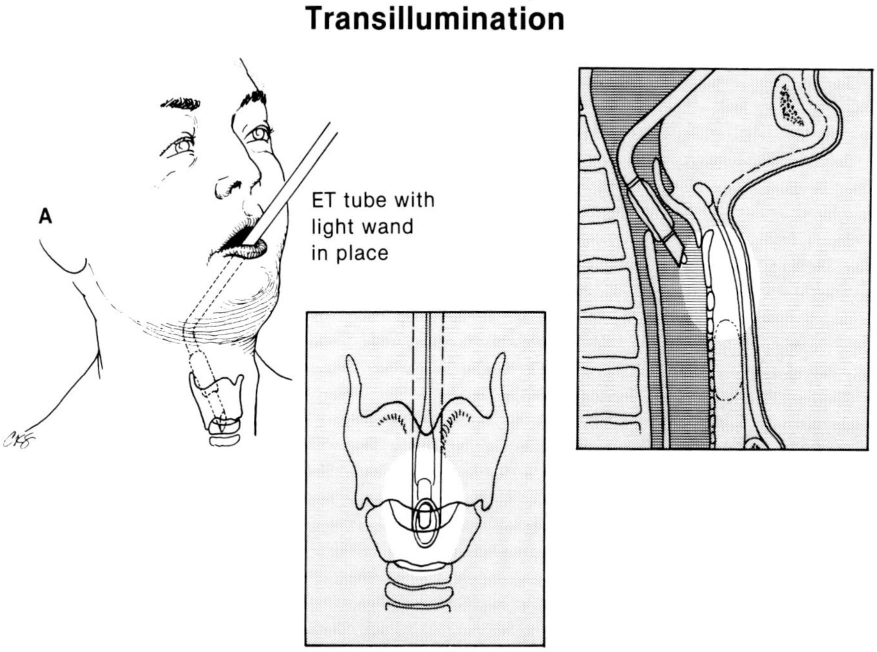

Figure 7–27 • Schematic diagram of transillumination of the neck (left panel) from both anterior view (middle panel) and side view (right panel).

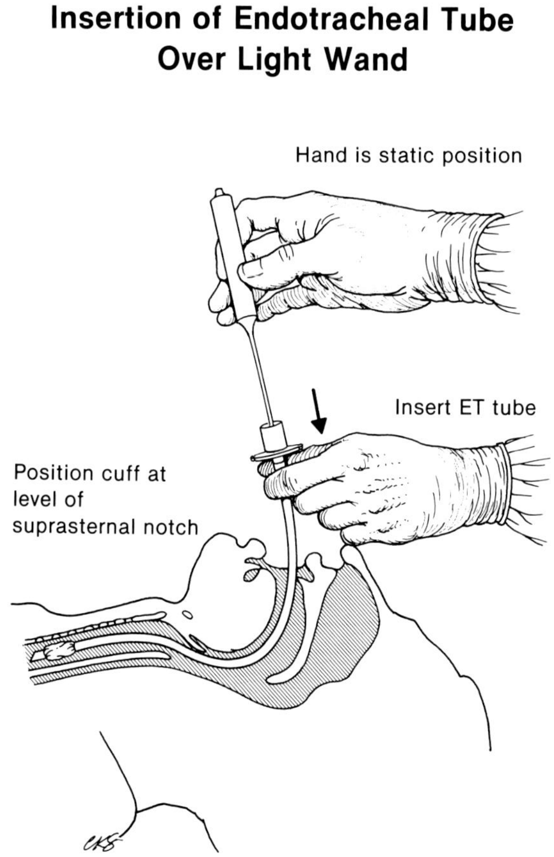

Figure 7–28 • Once the lighted stylet enters the trachea, the ET tube is advanced over the lighted stylet further into the trachea.

stylet, now sitting in the larynx, endorses the idea that the light is essentially pointed at the anterior wall of the thyroid cartilage. This, in turn, makes the final step tube advancement off the immobile stylet, much as in starting an IV. This configuration further means that the more familiar maneuver of advancing both tube and stylet as a unit will be not only unsuccessful but traumatic to the anterior larynx. When the tube is advanced into the trachea, the light in the neck may seem to separate and form an expanding illuminated dumbbell as the tube enters the chest. The usual steps to confirm bilateral gas exchange then ensue. Chest wall movement, auscultation, oxygenation, and end-tidal gas analysis are the final arbiters of correct placement.

The previously mentioned sequence has an attractive simplicity to it, but a caveat is in order. The potential for misadventure during airway transgression in a dark room is very real. Even with some dim background lighting, such as from a radiograph view box, cyanosis can go undetected. This is hardly a controversial view, since it can easily go undetected even in well-illuminated environments. Highly pigmented patients will progress to frank hypoxia with absolute certainty when this new device is initially employed unless oximetry is employed throughout. The good news is that each attempt at intubation takes little time. The bad news is that it is all too easy to persist in multiple attempts and to allow the oxygen reserve to evaporate.

C. Complications

To the degree studied by reports in the literature thus far, except for bulb loss, the spectrum of complications for this technique is indistinguishable from that for conventional direct laryngoscopy techniques. It can be surmised that the lack of required cervical spine movement might actually lessen problems in some patients,[31,32] but data are lacking at the moment.

Obviously, one complication is failure of the technique. As with any other motor skill, the ability to use the technique improves with practice. The author has experienced one complete failure that required subsequent bronchoscopy. In this situation, the epiglottis of this anesthetized and paralyzed patient was noted to actually touch the posterior oropharyngeal wall, so that the bronchoscope tip itself had to be used to gently elevate the tissue until the glottis could be seen. Clearly, the combination of anatomy, drugs, and patient position was at its absolute worst in this case, but it was interesting to note that despite several unsuccessful attempts to reach the larynx with the stylet, the actual tube position was really never in doubt and the attempts took very little time.

The critical aspect of this technique that differs from nearly all other intubation methods is light transmission from inside a human to the outside world. Therefore, anything that interferes with this process decreases the effectiveness of the technique. Severe anterior neck scarring, including flexion contractures, qualifies under this heading, as does excess cervical adipose tissue, although the latter can sometimes be displaced enough to get the job done when room lights are well dimmed. Copious bleeding within the airway might also fit into this category if blood covered the bulb inside the endotracheal tube.

V. References

1. Sykes WS. Essays on the First Hundred Years of Anaesthesia. Huntington, NY, Robert E. Krieger Publishing Company, 1972.
2. Elder CK. Naso-tracheal intubation: advantages and technic of "blind intubation." Anesthesiology 5:392–399, 1944.
3. Katz RI, Hovagim AR, Finkelstein H. A comparison of cocaine, lidocaine with epinephrine and oxymetazoline for prevention of epistaxis on nasal intubation. Anesth Analg 67:S110, 1988.
4. Meyer RM. Suction catheter to facilitate blind nasal intubation. Anesth Analg 68:701, 1989.
5. Jantzen JAH. Tracheal intubation-blind but not mute. Anesth Analg 64:651, 1985.
6. Butler FS, Cirillo AA. Retrograde tracheal intubation. Anesth Analg 39:333–338, 1960.
7. Waters DJ. Guided blind endotracheal intubation. Anaesthesia 18:158–162, 1963.
8. Powell WF, Ozdil T. A translaryngeal guide for tracheal intubation. Anesth Analg 46:231–234, 1967.
9. Bourke D, Levesque PR. Modification of retrograde guide for endotracheal intubation. Anesth Analg 53:1013–1014, 1974.
10. Borland LM, Swan DM, Leff S. Modification of retrograde guide for endotracheal intubation. Anesthesiology 55:577–578, 1981.
11. Akinyemi OO. Complications of guided blind endotracheal intubation. Anaesthesia 34:590–592, 1979.
12. Dhara SS. Guided blind endotracheal intubation. Anaesthesia 35:80, 1980.
13. King HK. Translaryngeal guided intubation using a sheath stylet. Anesthesiology 63:576, 1985.
14. Cossham PS. Difficult intubation. Brit J Anaesth 57:239, 1985.
15. Cooper CMS, Murray-Wilson A. Retrograde intubation. Anaesthesia 42:1197–1200, 1987.
16. Freund PR, Rooke A, Schwid H. Retrograde intubation with a modified Eschmann stylet. Anesth Analg 67:605–606, 1988.
17. Lechman MJ, Donahoo JS, Macvaugh H. Endotracheal intubation using percutaneous retrograde guidewire insertion followed by antegrade fiberoptic bronchoscopy. Crit Care Med 14:589–590, 1986.
18. Harrison CA, Wise CC. Retrograde intubation. Anaesthesia 43:609, 1988.
19. Abou-Madi MN, Trop D. Pulling versus guiding: A modification of retrograde guided intubation. Can J Anaesth 36:336–339, 1989.
20. Casthely PA, *et al.* Retrograde intubation in patients undergoing open heart surgery. Can J Anaesth 32:661–664, 1985.
21. Macintosh R, Richards H. Illuminated introducer for endotracheal tubes. Anaesthesia 12:223–225, 1957.
22. Yamamura H, Yamamoto T, Kamiyana. Device for blind nasal intubation. Anesthesiology 20:221, 1959.
23. Berman RA. Lighted stylet. Anesthesiology 20:382–383, 1959.
24. Ducrow M. Throwing light on blind intubation. Anaesthesia 33:827–829, 1978.
25. Heller RM, Cotton RB. Early experience with illuminated endotracheal tubes in premature and term infants. Pediatrics 75:664–666, 1985.
26. Stewart RD, et al. Use of a lighted stylet to confirm correct endotracheal tube placement. Chest 92:900–903, 1987.
27. Stone DJ, et al. A complication of lightwand-guided nasotracheal intubation. Anesthesiology 61:780–781, 1984.
28. Rayburn RL. Light wand intubation. Anaesthesia 34:677–678, 1979.
29. Williams RT, Stewart RD. Transillumination of the trachea with a lighted stylet. Anesth Analg 65:542–543, 1986.
30. Williams R. Lighted stylet and endotracheal intubation. Anesthesiology 66:851–852, 1987.
31. Ellis DG, et al. Guided orotracheal intubation in the operating room using a lighted stylet: A comparison with direct laryngoscopic technique. Anesthesiology 64:823–826, 1986.
32. Fox DJ, Castro T, Rastrelli AJ. Comparison of intubation techniques in the awake patient: The flexi-lum surgical light versus blind nasal approach. Anesthesiology 66:69–71, 1987.

Chapter 8

•

David D. Alfery, MD

Changing an Endotracheal Tube

OUTLINE

I. Introduction

This chapter discusses what to do when it becomes necessary to change an in-dwelling endotracheal tube (ET). The first section addresses the indications for changing a tube, both the immediate and absolute and those that are less urgent and relative. Next, the three general techniques available for changing an ET are described step-by-step. These consist of direct laryngoscopy, use of a tube changer, and use of a fiberoptic bronchoscope (FOB). The FOB technique is further divided into passage of the instrument alongside the existing ET or passage through the ET. The last section discusses the general principles one should use no matter which method is chosen. Finally, each technique is examined in terms of its advantages and disadvantages, along with its potential complications.

II. Indications

A. Immediate/Absolute

There are several situations where the indication for changing an ET is immediate and urgent (Table 8–1). In general, these are situations where adequate ventilation, oxygenation, or both are not being provided to the patient. Occlusion may occur due to secretions or blood clots that cannot be removed from a kink within the oropharynx. A leaking ET may result from

Table 8-1 • Indications for Changing an Endotracheal Tube

- I. Immediate/Absolute
  - A. Occlusion—unable to ventilate
    1. Kinking
    2. Secretions
  - B. Leak—unable to temporize
    1. Ruptured cuff
    2. Split tube
  - C. Tube bitten off
- II. Not Immediate/Relative
  - A. Occlusion—able to temporize and ventilate
    1. Kinking
    2. Secretions
  - B. Leak—able to temporize and ventilate
    1. Ruptured cuff
    2. Split tube
    3. Tube too short
  - C. Methods for improving patient's condition or comfort
    1. Replace small tube with normal-sized tube
    2. Increase size to allow bronchoscopy
    3. Remove nasotracheal tube causing maxillary sinusitis
    4. Replace orotracheal with nasotracheal tube for patient comfort

a ruptured cuff or a split along the length of the tube. Rarely, an ET may be bitten off by the patient.

B. *Not Immediate/Relative*

Most often the indications for changing an ET are relative and do not require immediate action. There are many situations that allow adequate ventilation and/or oxygenation to be maintained by using some temporizing maneuver but that can be expected to deteriorate over time if the ET is not changed (see Table 8–1). For example, most situations causing obstruction to ventilation occur gradually. Similarly, when a leak occurs adequate ventilation can usually be maintained by increasing the ventilation rate and tidal volume while attempting to minimize the leak by adding air to the cuff. An ET that has been cut too short and is leaking at the glottis can be advanced distally a few centimeters by flexing the neck.[1]

There are other situations in which changing an ET is done to allow improvement in the patient's condition. A small tube placed emergently may need to be replaced with a normal-sized tube. At times, a large ET is required to permit therapeutic or diagnostic bronchoscopy during mechanical ventilation. Maxillary sinusitis is frequently seen following prolonged nasotracheal intubation, and its treatment requires removal of the tube to allow drainage of the sinus. Finally, some tubes are changed to provide patient comfort. For example, patients may be more comfortable with a nasotracheal than an orotracheal tube.

III. TECHNIQUES

A. *Direct Laryngoscopy*

The method for changing an ET that anesthesiologists are most familiar with is probably direct laryngoscopy. It can be used for changing orotracheal tubes, changing nasotracheal tubes, or substituting one for the other. When time permits, it is advisable to give an antisialagogue prior to doing this procedure to minimize secretions and aid visualization. In addition, consideration should be given to the possible frequent need for sedation or paralysis.

After suctioning the patient and a period of ventilation with 100% oxygen, a laryngoscope blade is placed into the mouth and positioned in the hypopharynx valleculae, as one would for any intubation. The existing tube is visualized entering the glottis and any remaining secretions are suctioned (Fig. 8–1A). The replacement ET is positioned as near to the glottis as possible (Fig. 8–1B) and the existing ET is pulled out by an assistant. If a nasotracheal tube is being placed, it may be helpful to use a pair of Magill's forceps (see Chapter 6). Immediately after the existing tube is withdrawn (Fig. 8–1C), the replacement tube is inserted through the glottis and secured in place (Fig. 8–1D).

B. *Tube Changers*

Changing an ET using a tube changer (also called *tube exchanger*) involves applying the Seldinger technique[2] to the airway. Regardless of the type of tube changer chosen, the technique is as follows: an external physical landmark, such as the teeth or nares, is chosen, and the depth of insertion of the existing ET is noted (Fig. 8–2A). Following a period of ventilation with 100% oxygen, a lubricated tube changer—often manufactured as small (for 4.0–6.0 mm inner diameter [ID] tubes),

(Text continued on p. 181)

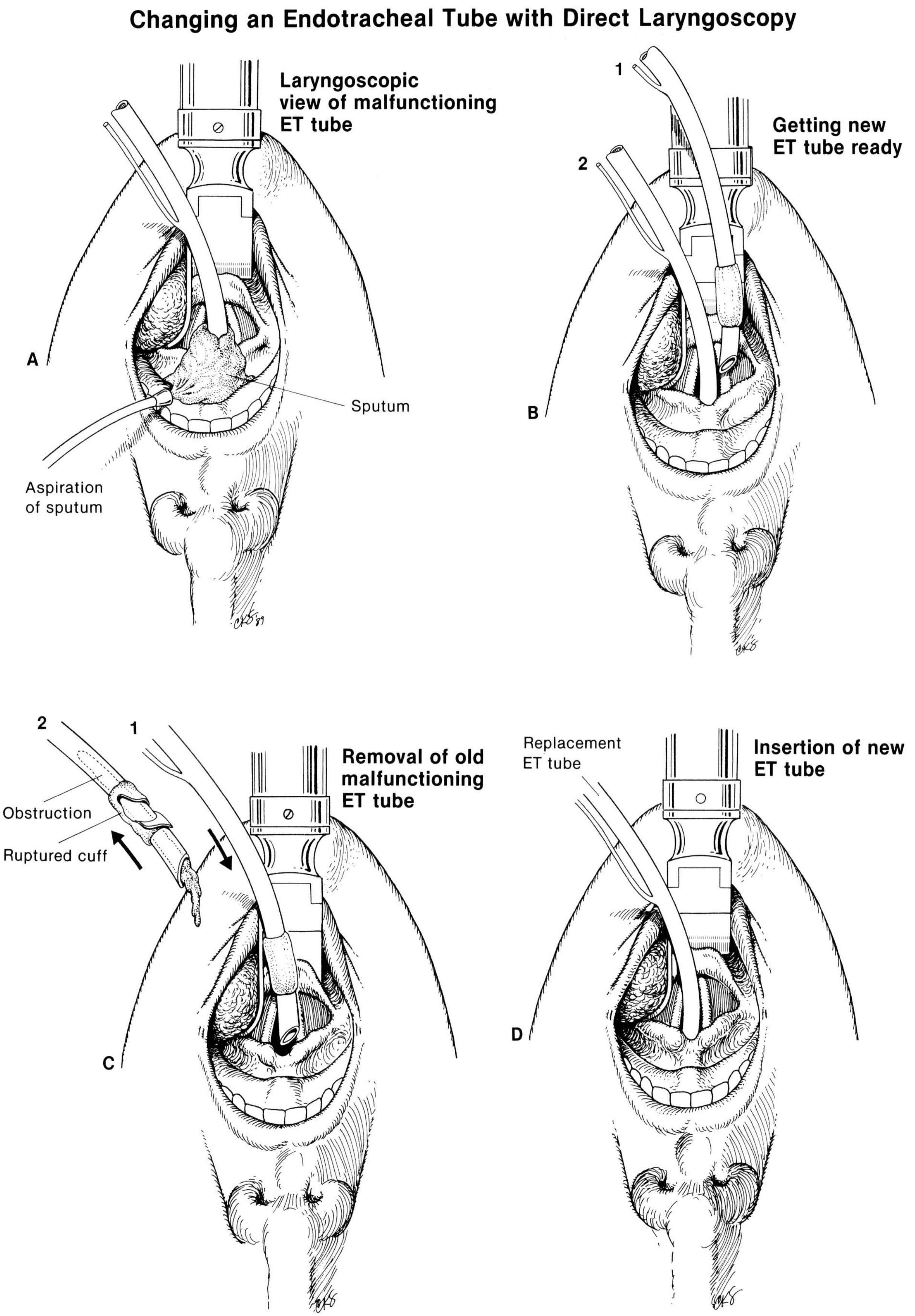

Figure 8–1 • Changing an endotracheal tube (ET) with direct laryngoscopy. See text for details. 1 refers to new ET and 2 refers to malfunctioning ET.

Changing an Endotracheal Tube with a Tube Changer

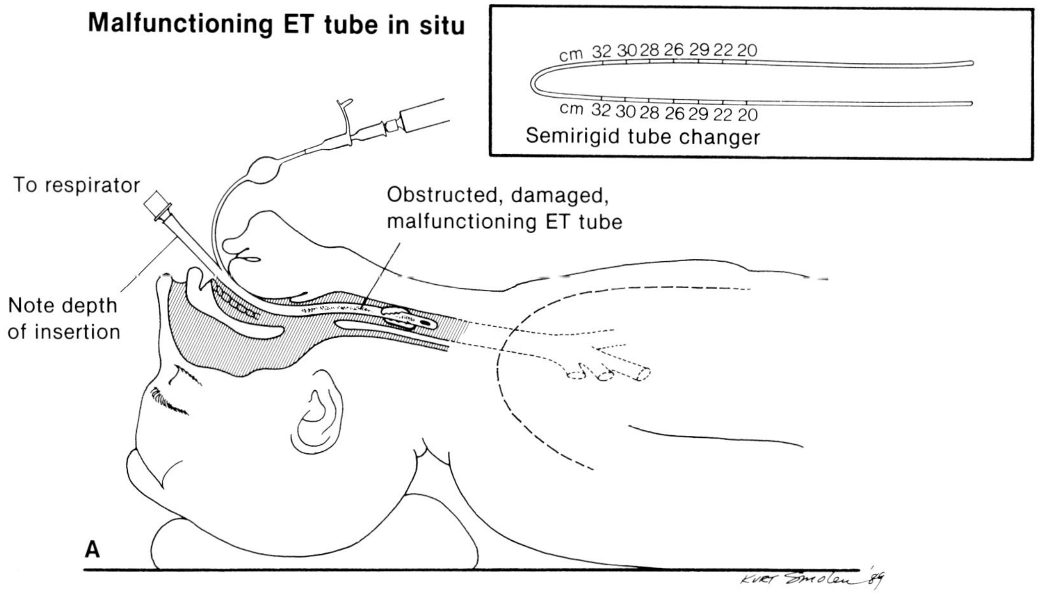

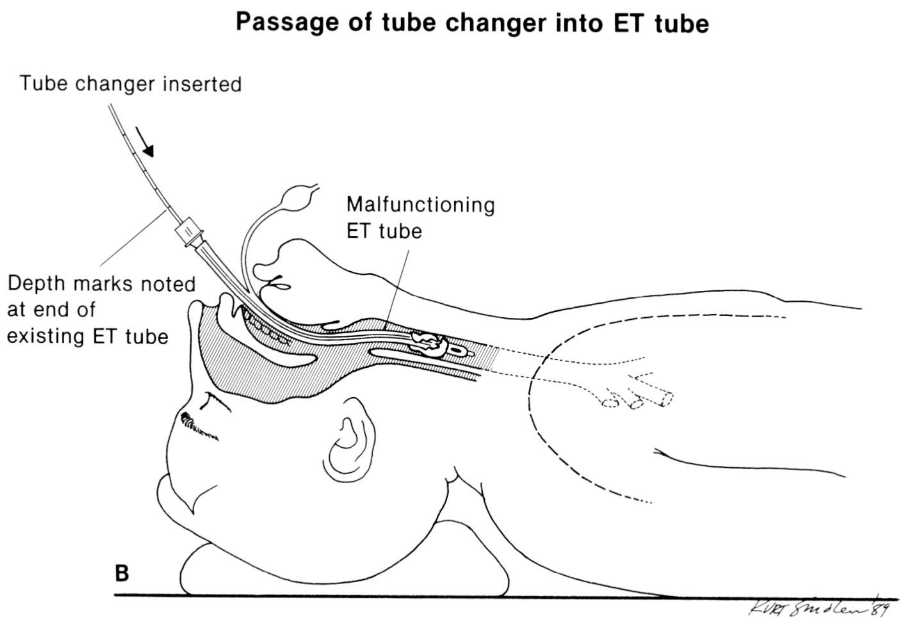

Figure 8–2 • Changing an ET with a tube changer. See text for details.

(continued)

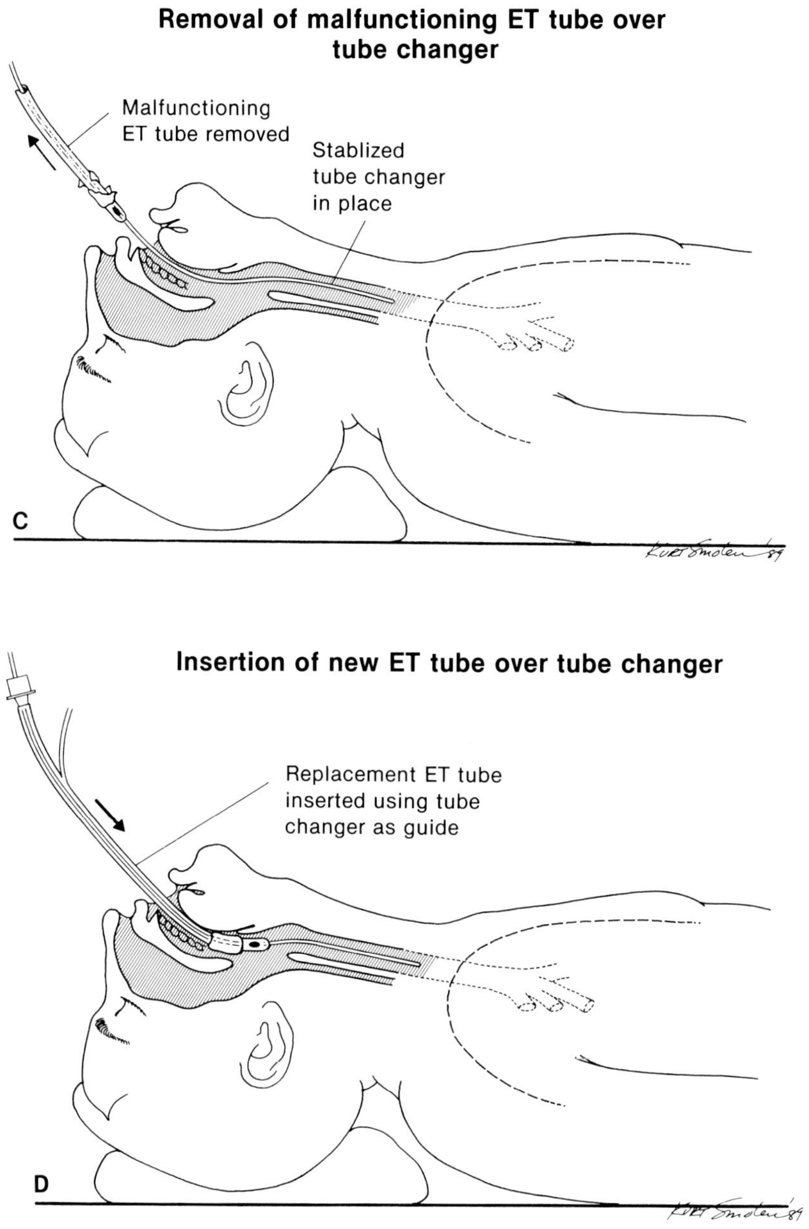

Figure 8–2 *(continued)*

medium (for 6.0–8.5 mm ID tubes), and large (for 7.5 10.0 mm ID tubes)—is inserted into the tracheal tube and advanced until it reaches the end of the existing tube (Fig. 8–2B). It may be necessary to remove the adapter from the end of the existing ET to allow passage of the tube changer. If an ET that is too short is being replaced, then the end of the tube changer must be gently passed distal to the tip of the ET. It is imperative to use a tube changer with a soft or rounded tip when it is advanced past the distal end of the ET. Most tube changers commercially available (eg, Sheridan T.T.X.™) have depth marks printed on their sides to aid in precise placement (see Fig. 8–2A inset). The tube changer is held firmly in place, the cuff of the existing ET is deflated, and the tube is withdrawn (Fig. 8–2C). Care is taken to not alter the tube changer position, and the depth marks are used to verify that its position has been stationary. A new ET is placed over the tube changer (Fig. 8–2D) and advanced until the ET depth marks coincide with the changer depth marks, and both are properly positioned in relation to the original reference landmark chosen (Fig. 8–2E). The tube changer is then removed (Fig. 8–2F) and proper tube position is confirmed by auscultation.

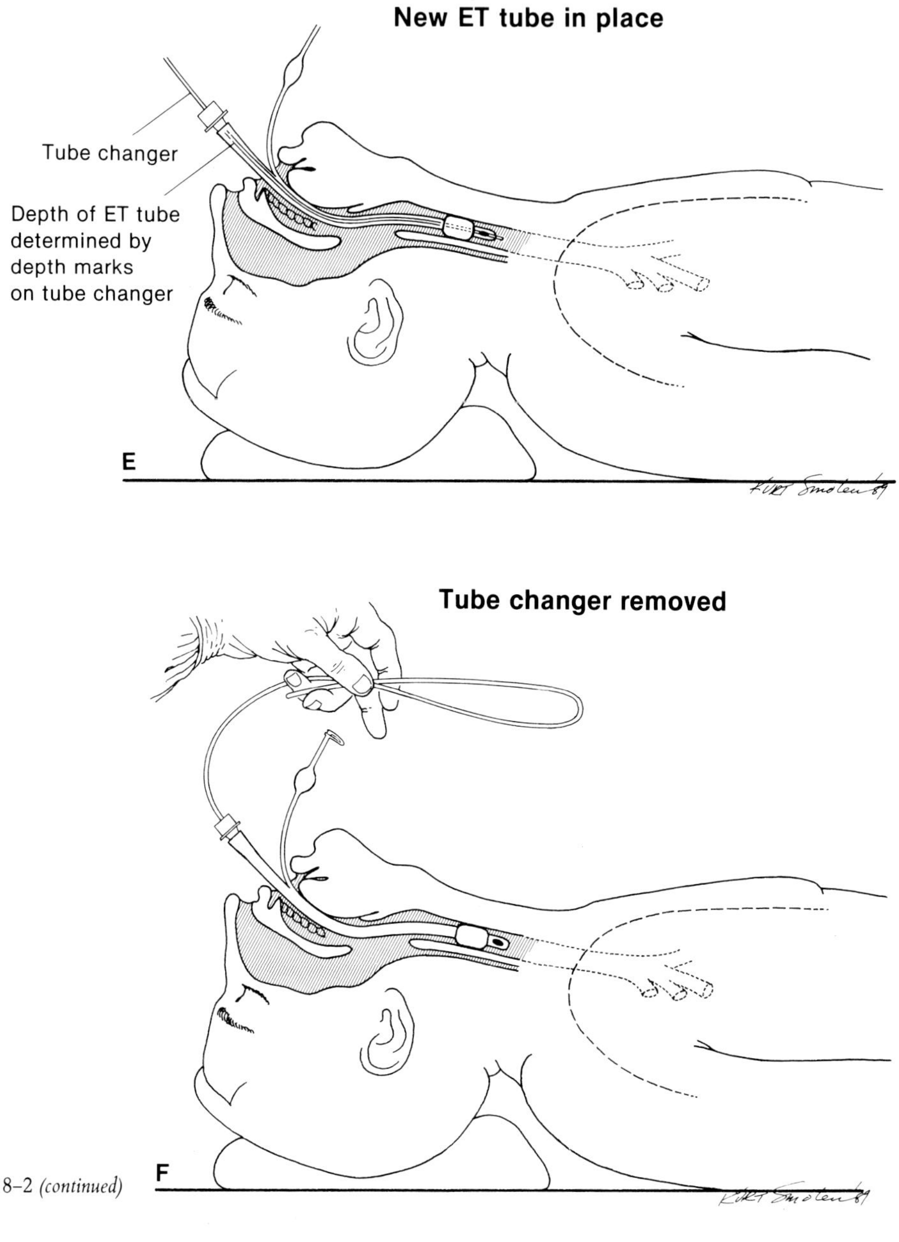

Figure 8-2 *(continued)*

C. *Fiberoptic Bronchoscope*

1. Passage Alongside an Existing Endotracheal Tube

The FOB can be used to change an ET by passing it alongside an existing ET and then using the FOB as the guide for a Seldinger technique.[3-8] As with direct laryngoscopy, it is advisable to give an antisialagogue prior to performing the technique in order to minimize secretions and aid visualization. In addition, sedation may be required. Either the oral or the nasal route may be chosen for this technique. If the replacement tube is to be passed through the nose, it is necessary to topicalize (with local anesthetic spray/ointment) and vasoconstrict (with alpha-agonist spray/ointment) the nasal mucosa prior to passage.

With the patient being ventilated with 100% oxygen, the technique is as follows: the replacement ET is passed over a lubricated FOB to the proximal end of the FOB and secured with tape. The FOB is then passed

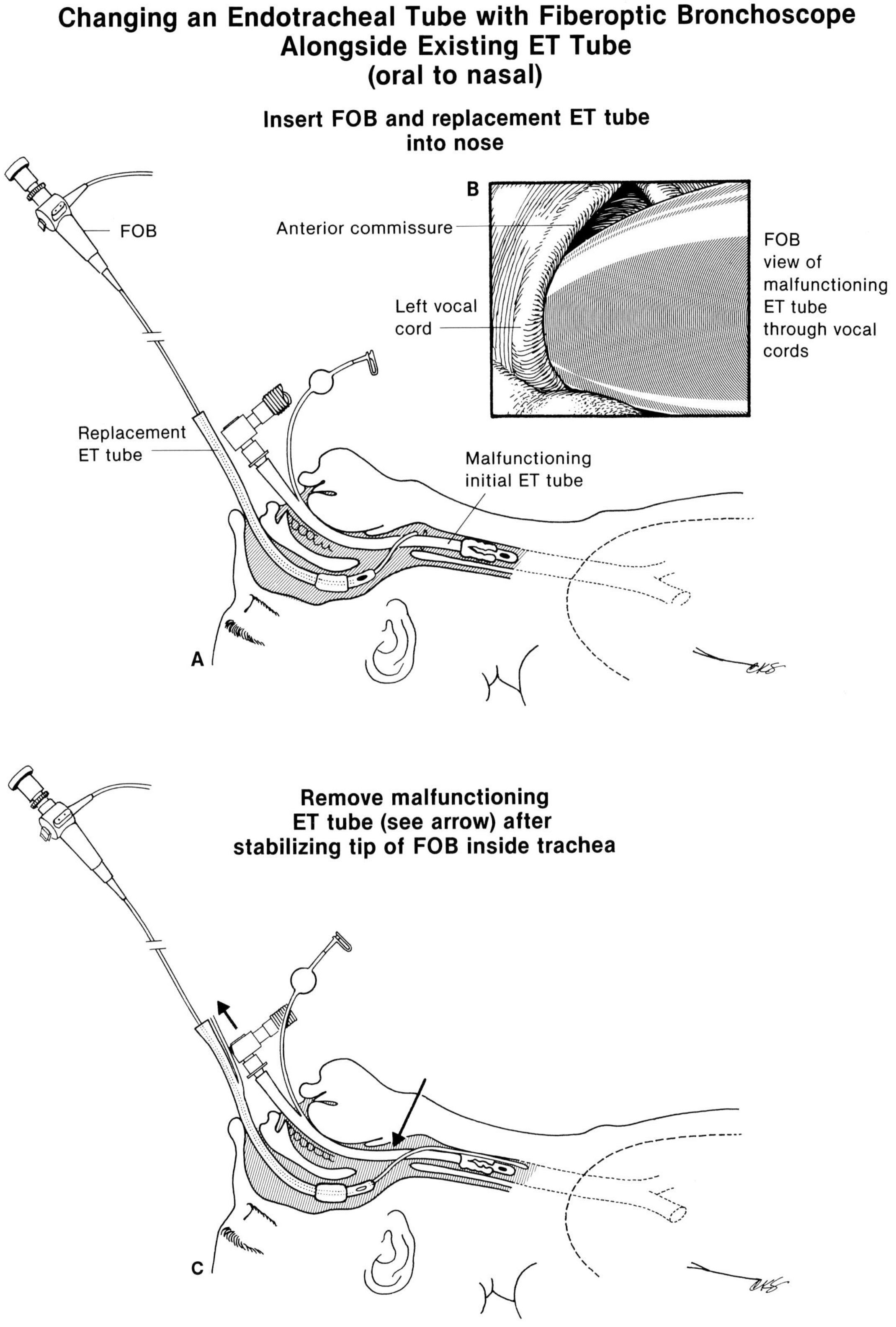

Figure 8-3 • Changing an ET with a fiberoptic bronchoscope passed alongside an existing tube. See text for details.

(continued)

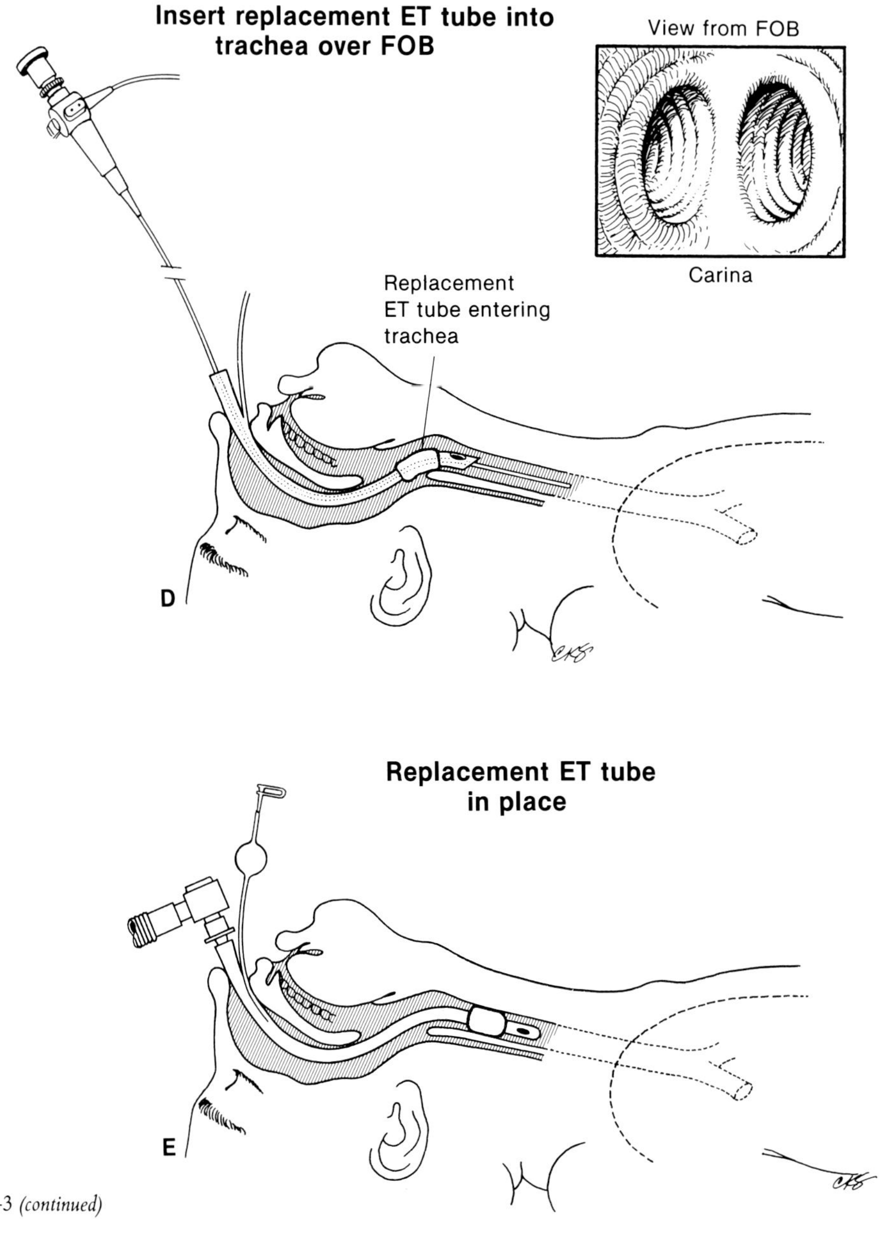

Figure 8–3 *(continued)*

orally or nasally into the hypopharynx. If the nasal route is chosen, to minimize bleeding I prefer to advance only the FOB through the naris until I have successfully entered the trachea. However, if edema or soft tissue structures preclude adequate visualization of the supraglottic area (as is often the case), it may be necessary to blindly insert the replacement ET into the oro- or hypopharynx in order to help clear the way for visualization of the malfunctioning ET tube in the vocal cords (Fig. 8–3A). Identification of supraglottic structures and their relation to the existing ET can be greatly facilitated by having an assistant pull the tongue and/or jaw of the patient forward. After the glottis has been identified (Fig. 8–3B), topical anesthesia is applied to the vocal cords via the suction port of the FOB. The tip of the FOB is then passed alongside the existing ET through the glottis. Since most existing tubes are forced posteriorly against the arytenoid cartilage and posterior commissure because of their natural bend from passage through the pharynx, it may be easiest to enter the glottis *anteriorly* (Fig. 8–3C). In addition, using a narrow-diameter FOB will facilitate passage. After entering the glottis, the cuff of the existing ET is deflated and the tip of the FOB is advanced beyond the distal end of the existing ET but still above the carina. Passage to this distal position may minimize the chance of dragging out the end of the FOB when the existing ET is removed (see Fig. 8–3C). Immediately following removal of the original ET, the replacement tube is passed over the FOB into the trachea (Fig. 8–3D). The position of the replacement ET is confirmed above the carina with the FOB prior to its removal (see Fig. 8–3D inset) and the ET secured in place (Fig. 8–3E).

2. PASSAGE THROUGH AN EXISTING ENDOTRACHEAL TUBE

A second technique using an FOB and the Seldinger technique (with the FOB as the guide) involves passage of the FOB through an existing ET.[9] This technique may be chosen when one is unsuccessful in passing the FOB alongside the existing ET or when the only route available for changing an ET is via the current path (eg, replacing a nasal tube in a patient with a deviated nasal septum and wired jaws). The following items are required for this technique: an FOB, a replacement ET, a small surgical forceps, a No. 11 surgical blade, and a Kocher (or similar large) surgical clamp.

The No. 11 scalpel is placed in the jaws of the small forceps so that its cutting edge is directed outward and its tip is within the grasp of the jaws (Fig. 8–4A). Covering the point of the scalpel with the end of the jaws of the clamp will prevent damage to the FOB. The ET is then changed as follows: The replacement ET is passed over a lubricated FOB and secured at the proximal end of the FOB by tape. Moistened gauze sponges are placed over the lips to help protect them from laceration should the blade slip during the procedure. The ET that is to be replaced should be cut as short as possible in order to allow adequate distal passage of the FOB and to minimize the time it will take to cut along the length of the tube. Following a period of ventilation with 100% oxygen, the airway connector of the ET is removed and the proximal end of the tube is grasped with a sturdy (eg, Kocher) clamp. The FOB is then quickly passed into the existing ET as far distally as possible

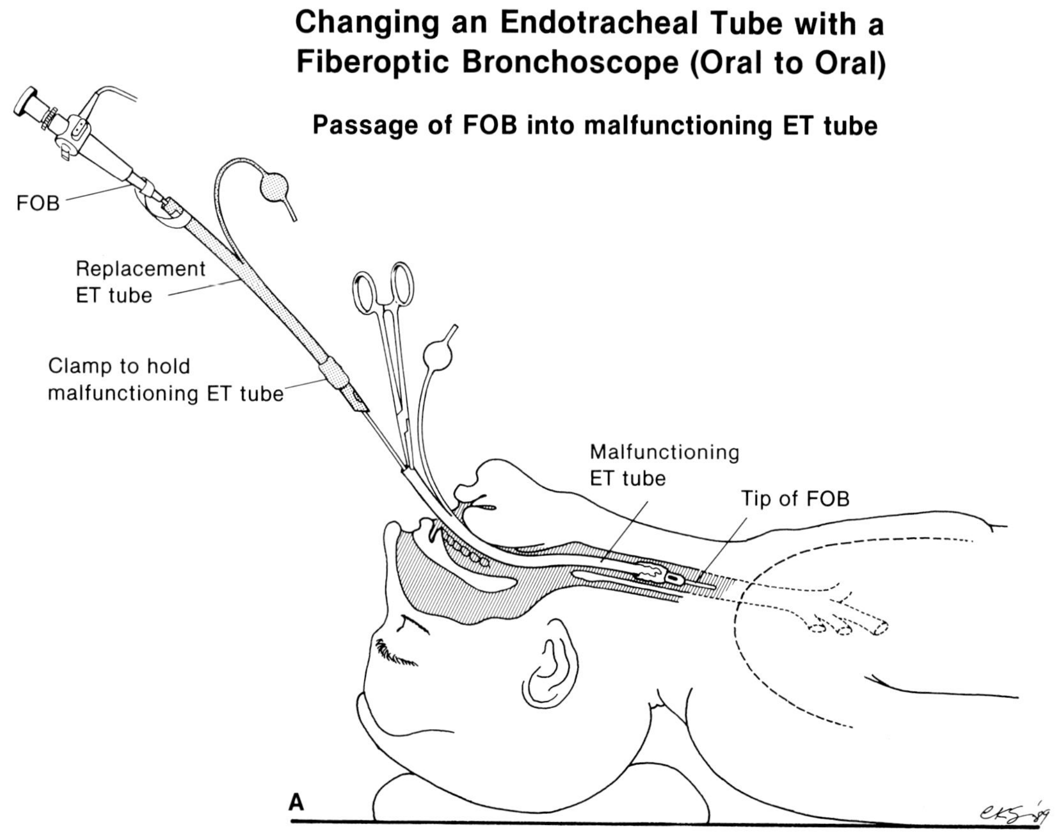

Figure 8–4 • Changing an ET with a fiberoptic bronchoscope passed through an existing tube. See text for details.

(continued)

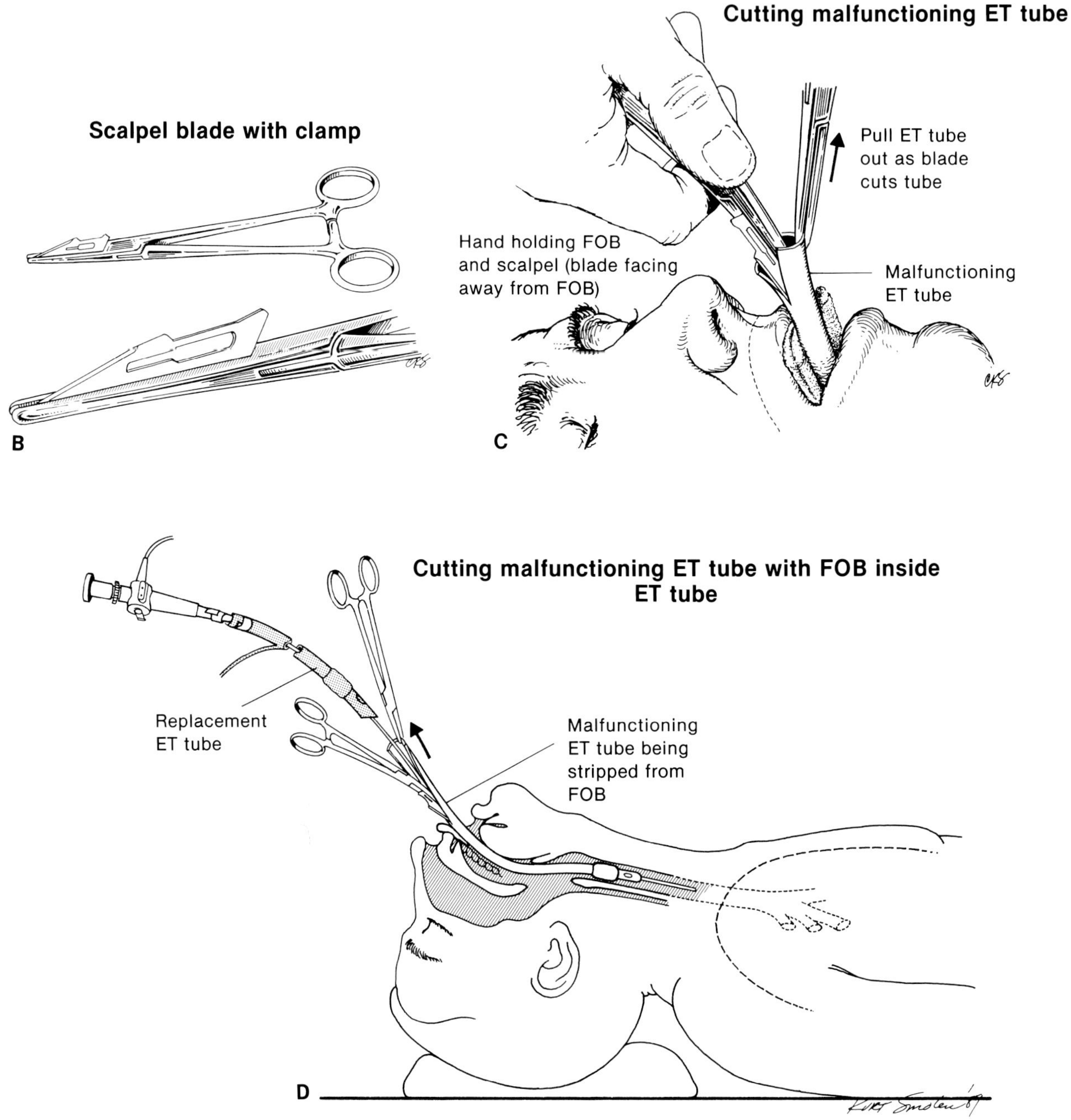

Figure 8–4 *(continued)*

(Fig. 8–4B). An assistant is used to hold the proximal end of the FOB and can frequently confirm the continued position of the FOB within the trachea. The small forceps with the scalpel blade is placed beside the FOB just above the end of the existing ET. The sharp edge of the scalpel should be directed opposite (180°) away from the FOB. The forceps and the FOB are grasped together and held firmly in the same hand so their relative positions remain constant (Fig. 8–4C). The cuff of the existing (malfunctioning) ET is deflated and it is slowly withdrawn by pulling up on the large surgical clamp that holds the proximal end of the existing ET (Fig. 8–4D). Countertraction on the small forceps with scalpel and FOB prevents outward slippage of the FOB. As the malfunctioning ET is removed, the scalpel slices it open along its entire length (Fig. 8–4E). After the original ET is removed, the position of the FOB within the trachea is confirmed and the replacement ET is

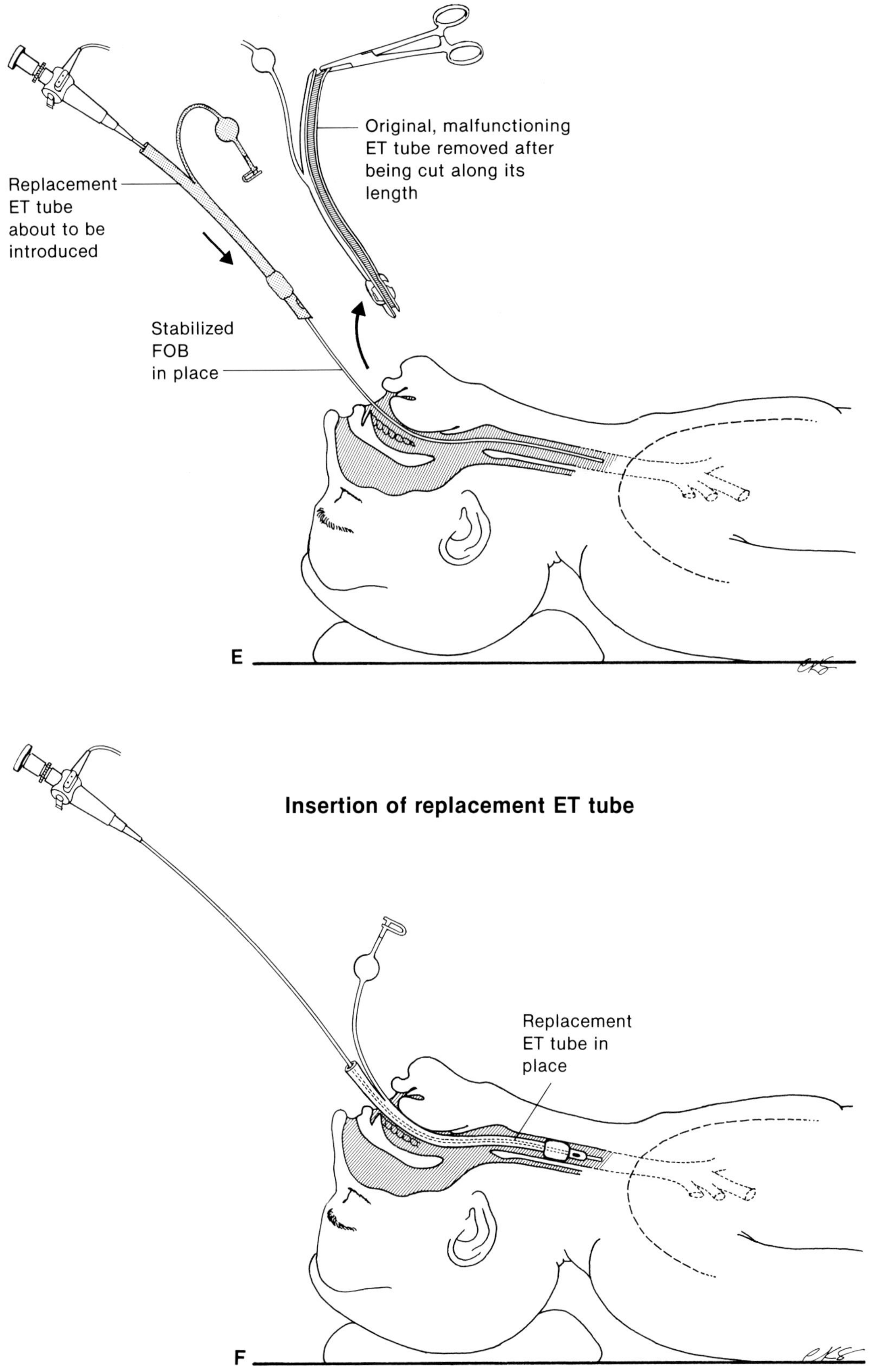

Figure 8–4 *(continued)*

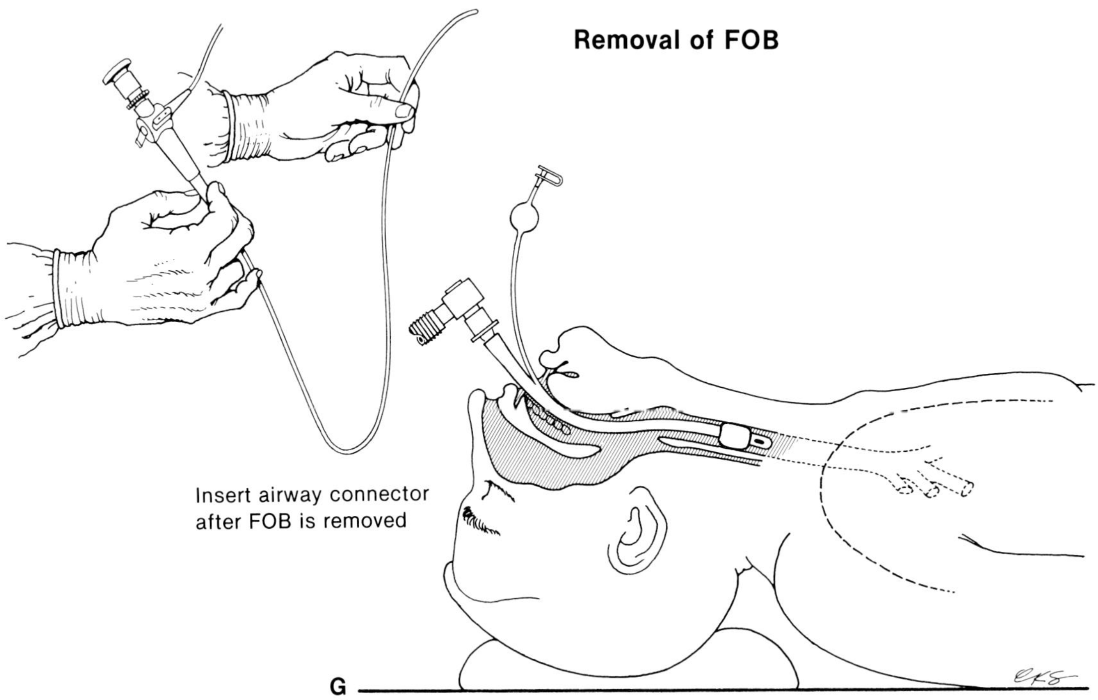

Figure 8–4 *(continued)*

passed distally into the trachea over the FOB (Fig. 8–4F). The proper position of the new ET is confirmed by FOB visualization, the FOB is removed, and the replacement ET is secured in place (Fig. 8–4G).

IV. Discussion and Complications

A. *General Considerations*

1. Initial Assessment and Maneuvers

When one is called on to change an ET an evaluation must be done to determine first, whether the ET really needs to be changed, and second, the urgency of the situation. This assumes, of course, that the patient requires further intubation (see Chapter 6). To determine urgency several questions must be quickly answered. Most important is whether the patient can be adequately oxygenated and ventilated at least for the short term. This usually depends on whether the problem with the ET has developed acutely (eg, complete obstruction) or slowly (eg, slight but steady cuff leak) and whether temporizing maneuvers can improve the situation. In general, one should hand-ventilate the patient with 100% oxygen using an increased minute ventilation as the problem is being sorted out. Measurement of arterial oxygen saturation by pulse oximetry, evaluation of capnograph waveform, and, if possible, sign communication with an awake patient can all help determine the urgency of the situation. Other measures that may temporize or correct the problem include:

1. Deflating an overinflated, herniated cuff.
2. Irrigating the ET to suction inspissated secretions.
3. Manually unkinking a tube that is kinked in the oropharynx.
4. Ventilating by hand using higher airway pressures to overcome partial obstruction.
5. Increasing the minute ventilation in a patient with a leaking ET.
6. Advancing a tube that is leaking because its tip is at the glottis and the cuff is in the pharynx, making an airtight seal impossible (this diagnosis can be made by gentle laryngoscopy [visualizing the cuff in the pharynx or above the vocal cords]; it is necessary to first deflate the cuff before advancing the ET).
7. Flexing the head and neck in order to advance a tube that is too short and just at the glottis.
8. Taping a split tube to occlude the leak.
9. Cutting a split tube shorter.

Number 6 is a common problem for which nurses call physicians to the bedside. Occasionally, a "leaking cuff" is actually a problem caused by a leaking pilot balloon. Measures that can correct this problem include:

1. Placing a closed stopcock on the pilot balloon after the cuff is inflated.
2. Clamping the pilot tube after the cuff is inflated.
3. Cutting off the defective pilot balloon, inserting a blunt needle into the pilot tube, and using a closed stopcock to prevent the escape of air from the cuff.

Many times the maneuvers used to "temporize" a situation will essentially correct the problem and eliminate the need to change the ET (Table 8–2).

2. SECONDARY CONSIDERATIONS

If it is determined that the ET does in fact need to be changed and that the need for changing it is not immediate, several items should be addressed. First, the circumstances and details of the initial intubation should be noted. In particular, if it was done in the operating room, the anesthetic record should be reviewed to determine the difficulty of the intubation. Other questions to be answered are

1. Was the intubation traumatic?
2. Were the vocal cords visualized?
3. Which laryngoscope blade was used if direct laryngoscopy was used?
4. Was one technique attempted and then abandoned in favor of another?
5. Was the patient paralyzed?
6. Was mask and bag ventilation possible?

Table 8–2 • Measures to Temporize or Correct the Problem

1. Increase inspired oxygen concentration
2. Deflate overinflated, herniated cuff
3. Irrigate and suction endotracheal tube
4. Manually unkink endotracheal tube
5. Hand-ventilate with higher airway pressures
6. Increase minute ventilation
7. Advance tube into proper position (may need to deflate cuff first)
8. Flex neck
9. Tape a split tube
10. Shorten a split tube
11. Place stopcock on pilot balloon
12. Clamp pilot tube
13. Insert blunt needle and stopcock into pilot tube

Second, one should determine what has changed since the initial intubation. In particular, what is the status and condition of the upper airway? For example, progression of a superior vena cava syndrome may prevent direct laryngoscopy from being done safely. Similarly, surgery on the oral and pharyngeal cavities may preclude direct laryngoscopy. Knowledge of the current respiratory status allows one to estimate the time frame for a safe period of interrupted ventilation during the changing of the ET. Patients requiring high levels of positive end-expiratory pressure with elevated inspired oxygen concentrations may be at increased risk for this procedure.

Finally, the overall medical condition of the patient is addressed. What is the cardiovascular status in terms of the ability to tolerate sedation or the stress of the technique to be chosen? Is the patient paralyzed? Are tube feedings being given or is the stomach full due to ileus? What is the level of consciousness? What are the current medications? For example, a patient requiring a high dose of lidocaine for arrhythmia control may not be an appropriate candidate for a technique that requires topicalization of the airway.

After these questions have been answered, one should establish that adequate help and equipment are present. At a minimum there should be a nurse or respiratory therapist to help monitor the patient and provide a second pair of hands. Other personnel may be required, depending on the anticipated difficulty or problems of the tube change. For all ET changes the same equipment required for an elective intubation is required (see Chapter 6), including adequate suction and patient monitoring. If a full stomach is suspected and the need to change the tube is urgent, suction should be applied to the nasogastric tube if one is in place and cricoid pressure should be applied until the new ET is secured. All the equipment expected to be used should be checked; in addition, those items that would be required if the chosen technique failed and an alternative were required should be present. For example, the ability to provide jet ventilation should be available when a tube changer is used (see later). Ideally, a pulse oximeter should be used to continually assess arterial oxygen saturation. Finally, 100% oxygen should be given prior to and during (when possible) the period of changing an ET in order to increase the margin of safety.

B. *Choice of Technique and Management of Complications*

When choosing a technique for changing an ET, it is helpful to use an algorithm that addresses several key questions (Fig. 8–5). In addition, knowing the advantages and disadvantages of each technique influences the choice. Finally, the individual skill and experience of the anesthesiologist, as well as the equipment available (or not available) for use, will determine which route is chosen.

When called on to evaluate a patient for an ET change, after determining that an urgent situation is not present, one should ask if the patient really requires intubation. If the answer is yes, one should attempt to remedy the problem by using one or more of the maneuvers listed in Table 8–2. If one determines that the ET does require changing, the major question is whether direct laryngoscopy is safe. If it is, then any of the techniques previously described may be chosen. If direct laryngoscopy can be used, it can, of course, be used alone or be performed in conjunction with a tube changer or an FOB. Using laryngoscopy in conjunction with one of these other techniques just increases its safety. If direct laryngoscopy is deemed unsafe, then one is left with the choice of using either a tube changer or an FOB alone. If an FOB is chosen, one must decide whether to use it by passing alongside or through the existing ET.

1. Direct Laryngoscopy

The majority of anesthesiologists are most familiar with direct laryngoscopy, since it is done so frequently in the operating room. The greatest advantage of this technique is the speed with which it can be done in an urgent situation, since so little equipment is required.

However, the technique has some serious potential disadvantages. First, and most important, this is the only technique that involves at least temporary loss of access to the lower airway in every patient. If an incorrect judgment is made about the ability to visualize the glottis and successfully pass the replacement ET after the original one has been removed, the condition that caused the laryngoscopy failure (eg, supraglottic edema) may also prevent successful bag and mask ventilation. Second, this technique may require head manipulation in some situations (eg, unstable cervical spine fracture) where such movement is hazardous. Third, direct laryn-

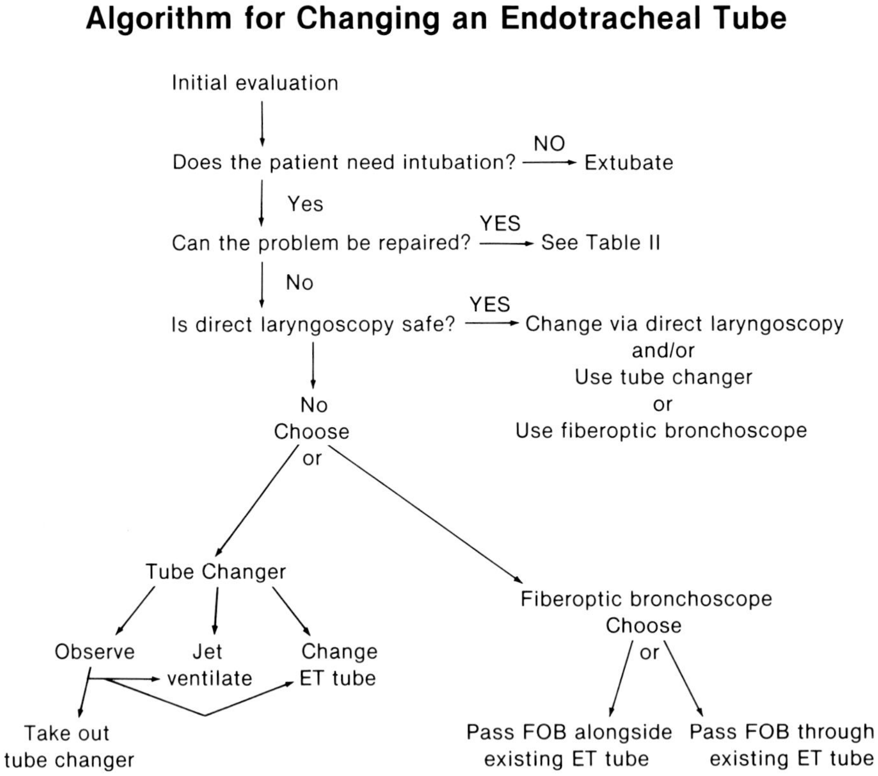

Figure 8–5 • Algorithm for changing an ET.

goscopy involves a significant stress on the cardiovascular system.[10] Either this stress or the sedation that may be given to blunt it may be deleterious in a marginal patient. Finally, there is evidence that there is an increase in the overall complication rate when this method is used. Watson et al reported a series of 15 adult patients in whom ET change was attempted using an FOB.[4] In three of the 15 patients, direct laryngoscopy was required. One of the three patients aspirated stomach contents and a second became hypotensive. In contrast, there was only one minor complication in the 12 FOB tube change patients.

One must be prepared to deal with the situation where the original ET has been removed and the replacement ET has not been passed successfully. Should this occur, several options should be considered, their potential need having been addressed and prepared for prior to the attempt at changing the ET. Ventilation with bag and mask should always be used to oxygenate the patient. Following this, a second attempt at intubation, either nasally or orally and either with attempted visualization or blind, should be tried. If attempts to intubate or ventilate the patient fail, there are three alternatives:

1. Emergency cricothyrotomy can be done (see Chapter 10).
2. Emergency tracheostomy can be performed (see Chapter 10).
3. Transtracheal ventilation can be done via a 14 gauge catheter placed through the cricothyroid membrane (see Chapter 9).[11]

Obviously, both techniques 1 and 2 take considerable skill and time to perform and carry with them serious potential morbidity. Technique 3 is preferable to the other two and can be accomplished reasonably quickly. After passage of the catheter a jet ventilator can be attached directly to the catheter (most preferred system); alternatively, the catheter can be attached to the anesthesia circle system for ventilation via the oxygen flush valve on the anesthesia machine (see Chapter 9).[12] If the latter method is chosen, a 3-mL syringe is attached to the 14 gauge catheter and the proximal airway connector from a 7- or 8-mm ET is inserted into its barrel. Alternatively, a larger syringe can be used and the distal end of an ET can be placed in its barrel and the cuff inflated. The anesthesia circuit is then attached and the patient is ventilated by intermittently pushing the oxygen flush button on the anesthesia machine. This temporizing maneuver allows a more controlled approach to subsequent securing of the airway.

2. TUBE CHANGERS

Use of tube changers has become popular because of their relative simplicity, their widespread availability, and their potential for providing ventilation. Various items have been used as tube changers, including suction tubing, oxygen tubing, pressure monitoring tubing, intravenous tubing, ureteral catheters, esophageal bougies, Fogarty catheters, nasogastric tubes, gum-elastic bougie endotracheal tube introducers, and the plastic conduit that envelopes long-line CVP catheters.[13-17] Recently, a number of manufacturers have introduced disposable tube changers in a variety of sizes and configurations, and some include a center channel along the length of the device. These all function essentially as stylets and are acceptable for changing either nasal or oral tubes.

The primary advantage of a tube changer is the ease with which it is used. Using a calibrated tube changer takes the guesswork out of determining proper depth of insertion. They can be especially useful in situations where direct laryngoscopy is not safe and where the use of an FOB passed alongside the tube may be especially difficult (eg, following surgery to the oral or pharyngeal cavity). Of special importance is the ability to provide jet ventilation by modifying some of the commercially available tube changers (see later)[15,17]

Tube changers have several disadvantages. These devices cannot be used when changing from an orotracheal to a nasotracheal tube and vice versa. A catheter that is too stiff can damage the mucosa of the trachea and can even perforate it. Conversely, a device that is too flexible may not offer sufficient guidance to the replacement ET or may be pulled out when the original ET is removed. Finally, when dealing with almost total ET occlusion, one may not be able to pass a tube changer through the ET.

Several complications are associated with the use of tube changers. If the tube changer is pulled out by the ET that is being replaced, correct placement of a new ET will be unsuccessful. Should this occur, direct laryngoscopy must be performed, as discussed earlier. Using a tube changer leaves the advancing edge of the replacement ET exposed. Occasionally, this edge gets hung up on the glottis or epiglottis and prevents the ET from entering the larynx. In this case, the ET should be rotated while gently trying to insert it. Grasping the thyroid cartilage externally and pushing it from one side to the other or anteriorly–posteriorly (as one would when doing a blind nasal intubation) may aid in allowing the ET to slip past the area of obstruction (see Chapter 6). Adding direct laryngoscopy (in this case combined with a tube changer in place) may also allow successful intubation. If one is still unable to pass the ET, jet ventilation can be carried out if the tube changer has been previously modified to allow this.[15,17] For example, the Sheridan T.T.X.™ tube changers come in several sizes, each with a hollow center channel. Depending on size, the end of this channel will allow the placement of a 14 gauge intravenous catheter (Fig. 8–6) or the proximal airway adapter of a small (2.5 or 3.0 mm) ET (Fig. 8–7). Similarly, a nasogastric tube can be modified in these ways (Figs. 8–8 and 8–9). Placement of the catheter or ET adaptor is accomplished by inserting it into the main lumen of the nasogastric tube after the proximal 6 cm of the nasogastric tube has been cut off; This maneuver forces the sump lumen closed while the main lumen remains patent. These systems can then be hooked up to a jet ventilator (see Fig. 8–9) or attached to an anesthetic circle system (see Figs. 8–7 and 8–8) with oxygen flush for ventilation as described earlier. After a period of ventilation and stabilization, an attempt to pass the ET by direct laryngoscopy (with the tube changer still in place) should again be made.

The ability to provide jet ventilation with a modified tube changer (called a jet style)[15] provides it with a unique advantage over other techniques—namely, the ability to temporize in the midst of an unsuccessful ET change. Furthermore, this system can be helpful in situations where the ability to tolerate extubation is in question but a trial of extubation is deemed warranted.[15] For example, a postoperative patient recovering from head and neck surgery where some degree of airway swelling is expected may require ET removal because of intolerance of the tube after full emergence from anesthesia. Following insertion of the jet stylet and ET extubation, the patient may be observed for a trial period prior to removing the tube changer. If reintubation is required it can be quickly accomplished (with or without concomitant jet ventilation), since the tube changer is still in place.

Finally, tube changers can cause perforation of a major airway. This might result in subcutaneous and/ or mediastinal emphysema as well as pneumothorax. Surgical consultation is warranted if this complication is suspected.

3. FIBEROPTIC BRONCHOSCOPE

Use of the FOB to change an ET offers several distinct advantages.[3,4,7,8] Whether the FOB is passed alongside or through the existing ET, the *in situ* FOB allows immediate confirmation of successful placement of the new ET within the trachea as well as precise positioning of the new ET. With the FOB technique there is a minimal need for sedatives and little hemodynamic insult, especially when combined with topicalization of the airway. Some authors believe that the period of apnea is minimized when using an FOB, but this contention has not been studied. An important advantage of passing the FOB alongside the existing ET is eliminating the need for cutting open the ET along its length. However, some situations may prevent successful passage of the

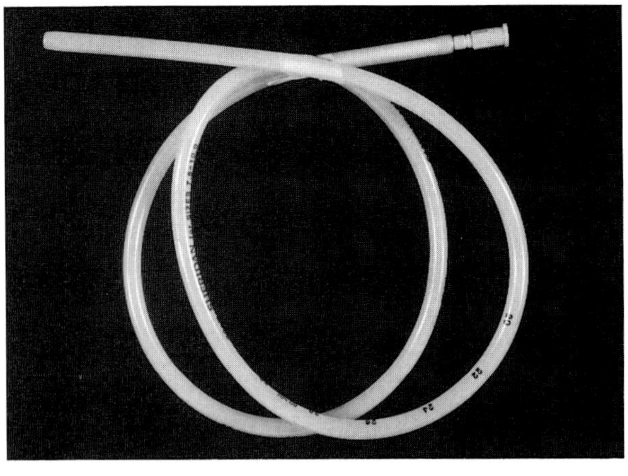

Figure 8–6 • A Sheridan TTX™ tube changer has been modified to allow jet ventilation by placing a 14 gauge catheter in the end.

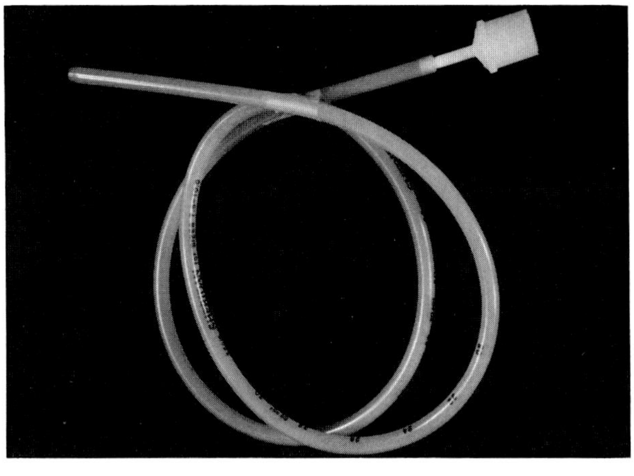

Figure 8–7 • A Sheridan TTX™ tube changer has been modified to allow jet ventilation by placing the proximal airway adapter of a small ET (4.0–6.0 mm ID) in its end.

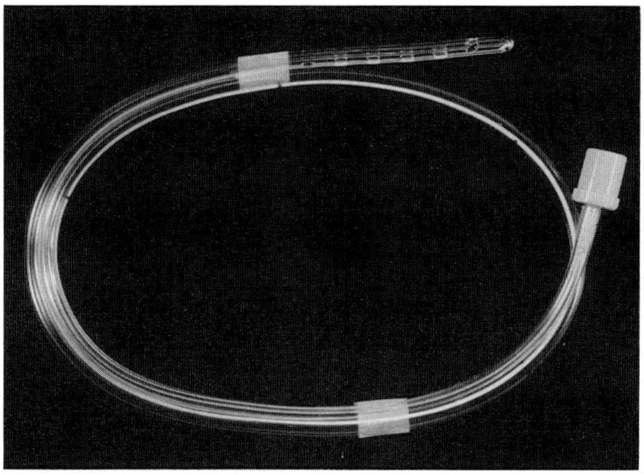

Figure 8–8 • A nasogastric tube has been modified to allow jet ventilation by placing the proximal airway adapter of a small ET (4.0–6.0 mm ID) in the end of the main lumen. The main and sump lumina have had the proximal 6 cm cut off and the insertion of the endotracheal tube adaptor has pressed closed the sump lumen.

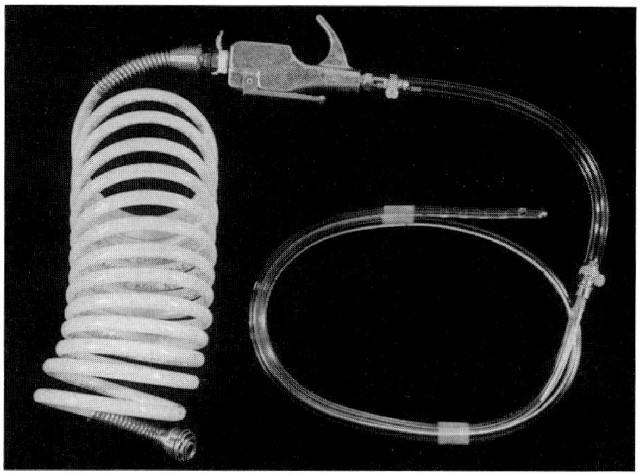

Figure 8–9 • A nasogastric tube, which has been previously modified (as in Fig. 8–8) but using a 14 gauge catheter, is attached to a jet ventilator. See text for details.

FOB into the trachea alongside of the existing ET. These include soft tissue swelling or other alterations in anatomy that prevent adequate visualization, the lack of room in the larynx to accommodate both the FOB and the existing ET, and an inexperienced endoscopist. Indeed, this procedure is considerably more difficult to master than standard intubation using an FOB. In one series, fully one-fifth of attempted tube changes using this technique were unsuccessful.[4] Ovassapian et al recommend placing the tip of the FOB just above the vocal cords when one is unable to pass it alongside the ET.[8] They then recommend that the FOB be quickly inserted into the trachea as soon as the existing ET is withdrawn. I disagree with this approach, given the potential loss of airway control that it entails and the fact that there are alternatives (such as the tube changer with jet ventilation capability) that are safer.

The primary disadvantage of the FOB passed through the ET approach is the potential difficulty in cutting off the existing ET. One should practice this technique on a mannequin prior to attempting it on a patient, since it takes considerable manual dexterity as well as strength to perform. It is possible, however, that there is less chance of the FOB being pulled out of the trachea when using this approach, since the ET cuff will not drag along the side of the FOB. Furthermore, there are situations where the FOB through the ET is the only route available for its use, such as a patient with a wired jaw, nasotracheal tube in place, and deviated nasal septum. Both techniques require considerable expertise with the bronchoscope as well as additional personnel to aid in the procedure.

As with using the tube changer, the primary hazard when using the FOB is that the tip will come out of the trachea when the existing malfunctioning ET is removed. Obviously, in this circumstance the replacement ET cannot be properly positioned. This complication should be immediately apparent during the procedure, since it is advisable to have an assistant maintain visual confirmation of the FOB tip within the trachea as the tube change takes place. If, however, one does not successfully intubate the trachea with the replacement ET, ventilation by bag and mask must be done. Then either a second attempt at FOB placement should be done (preferably via an anesthesia mask with endoscopy port) or placement should be attempted via direct laryngoscopy.

V. REFERENCES

1. Conrardy PA, Goodman LR, Lainge F, et al. Alternation of endotracheal tube position. Crit Care Med 4:8–12, 1976.
2. Seldinger SI. Catheter replacement of the needle in percutaneous angiography: A new technique. Acta Radiol 39:368–376, 1953.

3. Rosenbaum SH, Rosenbaum LM, Cole RP, et al. Use of the flexible fiberoptic bronchoscope to change endotracheal tubes in critically ill patients. Anesthesiology 54:169–170, 1981.
4. Watson CB. Use of fiberoptic bronchoscope to change endotracheal tube endorsed. Anesthesiology 55:476–477, 1981.
5. Watson CB, Prough DS, Balestrier FJ. Bronchoscopic tube change in critically ill patients. Crit Care Med 8:246, 1980.
6. Lee KC, Weedman D, Peters WJ. Use of the fiberoptic bronchoscope to change endotracheal tubes in patients with burned airways. Case report. J Burn Care Rehabil 7:348–350, 1986.
7. Watson CB. Fiberoptic bronchoscopy in anesthesia. Anesth Rev 9:17–26, 1982.
8. Ovassapian A, Dykes MHM. The role of fiberoptic endoscopy in airway management. Sem Anesth 6:93–104, 1987.
9. Hudes ET, Fisher JA, Guslitz B. Difficult endotracheal reintubations: A simple technique. Anesthesiology 64:515–517, 1986.
10. Derbyshire DR, Chmielewski A, Fell D, et al. Plasma catecholamine responses to tracheal intubation. Br J Anaesth 55:855–860, 1983.
11. DeLisser EA, Muravchick S. Emergency transtracheal ventilation. Anesthesiology 55:606–607, 1981.
12. Stinson TW. A simple connector for transtracheal ventilation. Anesthesiology 47:232, 1977.
13. Finucane BT, Kupshik HL. A flexible stilette (sic) for replacing damaged tracheal tubes. Can Anaesth Soc J 25:153–154, 1978.
14. Desai SP, Fencl V. A safe technique for changing endotracheal tubes. Anesthesiology 53:267, 1980.
15. Badger RC, Chang J. A jet-stylet endotracheal catheter for difficult airway management. Anesthesiology 66:221–223, 1987.
16. McCarroll SM, Lamont BJ, Buckland MR, et al. The gum-elastic bougie: Old but still useful. Anesthesiology 68:643–644, 1988.
17. Arndt GA, Ghani GA. A modification of an Eschmann endotracheal tube changer for insufflation. Anesthesiology 69:282–283, 1988.

Chapter 9

•

Persis K. Shroff, MD
Jonathan H. Skerman, BDSc, MScD, DSc
Jonathan L. Benumof, MD

Transtracheal Ventilation

OUTLINE

I. Introduction

When a patient cannot be ventilated via a mask, or intubated, and there is no immediately available alternative plan, then death is inevitable.[1] For the purpose of this chapter, *cannot ventilate by mask* means that a reasonably experienced practitioner of medicine cannot cause a life-sustaining amount of gas exchange despite the use of anterior jaw thrust, oropharyngeal or nasopharyngeal airways, or all three. *Cannot intubate* means that the same medical practitioner cannot pass an endotracheal tube through the vocal cords within a life-sustaining period of time. The incidence of the cannot-ventilate, cannot-intubate situation has ranged from 0.01 to 2.0/10,000 anesthetics.[1-6] There is widespread agreement in the literature that percutaneous transtracheal jet ventilation (TTJV) using a large intravenous catheter placed through the cricothyroid membrane is a very simple, relatively safe, extremely effective treatment of choice for the desperate cannot-ventilate-by-mask, cannot-intubate situation.[7-11] Compared to stab cricothyroidotomy and tracheostomy, establishment of percutaneous TTJV is much quicker, simpler, and therefore more efficacious.

Provision of a quick, relatively atraumatic means of oxygenation transtracheally is not a recent concept. As early as 1667, the procedure of oxygen insufflation was demonstrated in dogs,[12] and again in 1909 the life of paralyzed dogs was maintained by insufflating air

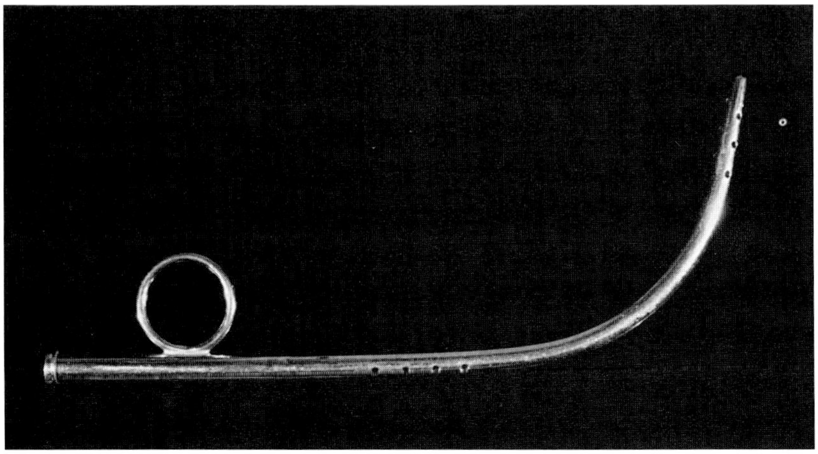

Figure 9–1 • A pre-World War I hollow metal insufflator with perforations in the midportion surface of the device as well as at the tip to permit insufflation of air. Note that both a skin and a cricothyroid membrane incision were required before it could be inserted.

through the trachea[13] (Fig. 9–1). With the beginning of World War I, various surgical devices were designed to allow direct but sometimes ineffective placement of a transtracheal insufflation device through a skin and cricothyroid membrane incision; of course, these devices were only used whenever there was a source of oxygen or air available. During this era, subsequent expansion and development of the concept was continued by surgeons whereby a bougie device allowed double concentric tubes to be inserted directly into the trachea, with the outer tube providing a means of attachment or fixation to the neck—not dissimilar to that provided in tracheostomy kits currently used today (Fig. 9–2).

Another quarter of a century was to pass before a series of experiences with diffusion respiration was described.[14] With diffusion respiration (apneic insufflation) it became clear that although no ventilation occurred (carbon dioxide removal), adequate oxygenation could be maintained for many minutes, provided the airway was patent, nitrogen in the airway was replaced by oxygen, the alveolar space was continuously filled with oxygen (which had to be supplied at a rate greater than oxygen consumption), and the circulatory status and hemodynamic volume were adequate.

In 1956, an objective analysis to determine the value and limitation of transtracheal ventilation in human subjects was carried out.[15] At that time, many anesthesiologists were understandably reluctant to recommend tracheostomy in desperate situations, in the hope that they would be able to rapidly accomplish nonsurgical intubation. At the same time, many surgeons were similarly hesitant to perform an unscheduled operation, or to initiate a procedure in which they were not comfortable or experienced. Nevertheless, it was not until another 15 years that a series was reported of more than 50 patients suffering respiratory distress or cardiopulmo-

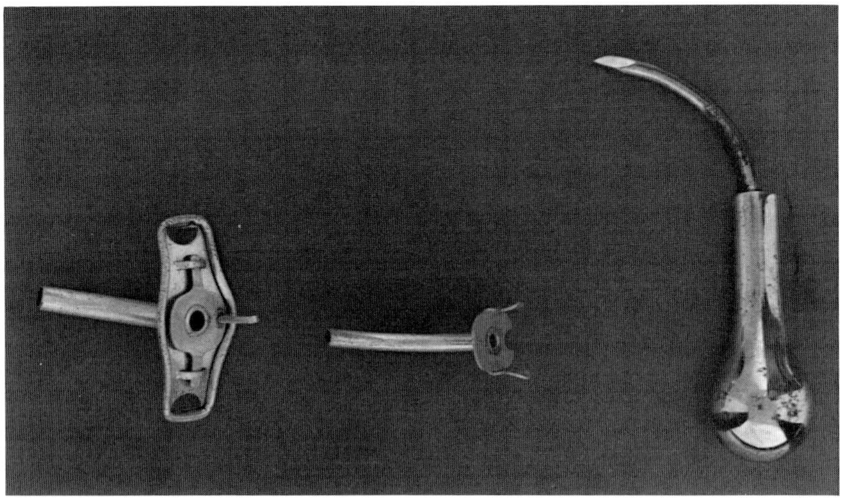

Figure 9–2 • Double concentric metal tubes with the outer tube providing a means of attachment or fixation to the neck. Note the sharp point of the bougie device.

nary arrest in whom transtracheal ventilation was used for immediate restoration of an adequate airway.[16]

Not until 1971 was it confirmed in dog models that transtracheal ventilation with an oxygen jet through a 16 gauge needle at 50 psi would supply enough force to adequately inflate the lungs and that enough flow could be produced to supply adequate ventilation for an adult patient without air entrapment.[17] These findings were confirmed in dogs and the technique was used in patients undergoing routine operations. In a series of 1500 cases, transtracheal ventilation for diagnostic and surgical procedures of the upper airways in humans was reported.[18]

In another landmark article, it was reported that transtracheal ventilation may not only have an important role in cardiopulmonary resuscitation or in ventilation under extreme circumstances but may be of particular value where partially obstructive lesions of the larynx are present.[19] It was recognized that patients who are in respiratory distress with an obstructive lesion of the larynx may have difficulty exhaling gas, which may lead to stocking of tidal volumes and bring hyperexpansion and barotrauma. It was emphasized that a dangerously high pressure may also occur with a prolonged inspiratory phase of high-pressure oxygen administration.

II. INDICATIONS

A. *Emergency Situations*

1. CANNOT-VENTILATE-BY-MASK, CANNOT-INTUBATE SITUATION

Acute upper airway obstructions that cannot be remedied in less than a few minutes by use of a face mask, oral or nasal airways, tracheal intubation, fiberoptic techniques, or even a retrograde approach using an epidural catheter must be treated with transtracheal ventilation. Such causative factors may include foreign bodies, trauma, infection, neoplasms, and laryngeal edema.

2. LACK OF TRAINED PERSONNEL AND/OR EQUIPMENT FOR CONVENTIONAL AIRWAY MANAGEMENT TECHNIQUE

When trained personnel are unavailable to rapidly secure an airway in an agitated, gasping patient, or if the proper armamentarium to perform endotracheal intubation, tracheostomy, or bronchoscopy is not immediately at hand, then institution of percutaneous transtracheal ventilation may be life-saving.

B. *Elective Situations*

1. TO FACILITATE OPERATIONS INVOLVING THE UPPER AIRWAY

There are numerous reports and recommendations for the use of the technique in planned surgical situations to avoid tracheostomy. Singh[18] reported 1500 cases of transtracheal ventilation for diagnostic and surgical procedures of the upper airways. There were 1257 cases for bronchoscopy and esophagoscopy and 135 cases for endolaryngeal surgery. Postoperative ventilatory support was carried out with this technique in 108 cases with the patients ventilated for periods of from 24 to 48 hours.

Spoerel and Greenway,[20] describing ventilation techniques during endolaryngeal surgery, similarly found adequate pulmonary ventilation with excellent conditions for microscopic surgery. Smith, Myers, and Sherman[21] reported elective transtracheal ventilation in pediatric patients undergoing surgical procedures involving the head and neck. They described the use of this technique in two pediatric patients, one undergoing an operation for laryngeal stenosis and one who had become obstructed and cyanosed in the recovery room. P_aCO_2 determinations at the end of the procedures indicated that the patients were moderately hyperventilated. Similarly, since percutaneous transtracheal jet ventilation leaves the entire airway from the vocal cords to the face accessible for surgical manipulation, it is not surprising that TTJV has been used for virtually every conceivable type of operation on these structures in adults.[22]

Finally, Wagner, Coombs, and Doyle[23] described a case where high-frequency ventilation was used with success (thus avoiding tracheostomy) in a patient with a partial upper airway obstruction caused by a hypopharyngeal foreign body with four sharp appendages.

2. TO PERMIT SAFE INTUBATION OF THE TRACHEA WITH A STANDARD ENDOTRACHEAL (ET) TUBE BY ANOTHER ROUTE (PREVENT THE CANNOT-VENTILATE-BY-MASK, CANNOT-INTUBATE SITUATION)

In situations in which an increased risk of developing a cannot-ventilate-by-mask, cannot-intubate situation can be identified, elective institution of TTJV may prevent the development of a life-threatening gas exchange problem while a more secure permanent airway is being established. Elective placement of an intravenous catheter through the cricothyroid membrane and use of TTJV are entirely compatible with a subsequent conventional oro- or nasotracheal intubation, fiberoptic-aided intubation, and retrograde intubation technique, as well as being compatible with formal tracheostomy. Indeed, one report described prophylactic TTJV that guaranteed adequate ventilation in a patient who was known to be difficult to intubate. The TTJV enabled the patient to be anesthetized, paralyzed, and intubated in a safe, nonemergent manner.[24] In another report of a 13-year-old girl with ankylosis of the temporomandibular joint secondary to a fractured mandible, TTJV was electively instituted prior to the induction of anesthesia, and the trachea was intubated with the aid of a fiberoptic bronchoscope safely and nonemergently in this well-oxygenated patient after the induction of anesthesia and paralysis.[25] Thus, it appears that TTJV can prevent the development of a life-threatening gas exchange problem in patients who are difficult to ventilate and intubate and who require general anesthesia. The technique permits uninterrupted ventilation and oxygenation while allowing the intubationist unhurried access to the patient's upper airway.

3. To Administer Respiratory Therapy

Use of the transtracheal approach in planned situations has recently been extended by Heimlich and Carr[26] in the form of a microcatheter (the Micro-trach) for use in patients with cystic fibrosis. In this patient population aggressive pulmonary toilet using a bronchoscope or specially designed endotracheal tube to wash out the bronchi has been used as an effective respiratory therapy emergency measure. Unfortunately, the procedure is dangerous and improvement is short-lived. Pulmonary lavage performed in this way requires a hospital setting, general anesthesia, and a skilled bronchoscopist and/or anesthesiologist. Even in the best of hands, the bronchial lavage procedure may terminate in the hypoxemic death of the patient, especially if the patient is a child.

The Micro-trach is a 16 gauge catheter terminating squarely at its single outlet (Fig. 9–3). The device is designed to be inserted easily with local anesthesia. The catheter is replaced at intervals varying between 1 and 6 months. Other types of in-dwelling transtracheal catheters require removal for cleaning several times a day. Their larger length, diameter, oblique tips, and side-holes predispose to mucosal injury and deposition of secretions. Indeed, mucus balls large enough to threaten airway obstruction form on such oversized catheters left in place for long periods.

Transtracheal oxygen delivery and saline instillation begin immediately after inserting the Micro-trach catheter. All patients experienced immediate relief of otherwise intractable dyspnea.[26] Oxygen administration at a rate of 0.25–3 L/min was therapeutically equivalent to 1–8 L/min delivered nasally. Over the course of the first year, a majority of the patients have continued to use the Micro-trach in preference to nasal cannulae or various forms of masks.

III. How to Do Transtracheal Ventilation

The cricothyroid membrane is palpated with the neck of the patient extended (Fig. 9–4A). Then a 12 or 14

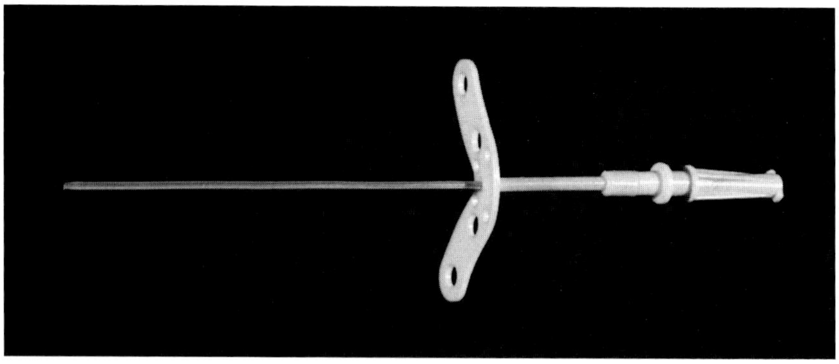

Figure 9–3 • A Heimlich Micro-trach, which is a sterile, 16 gauge (1.19-mm ID/1.65-mm OD), nontoxic microtracheal catheter made of clear, medical-grade polyethylene with a radiopaque stripe. A flange is insert-molded to the catheter to permit secure attachment.

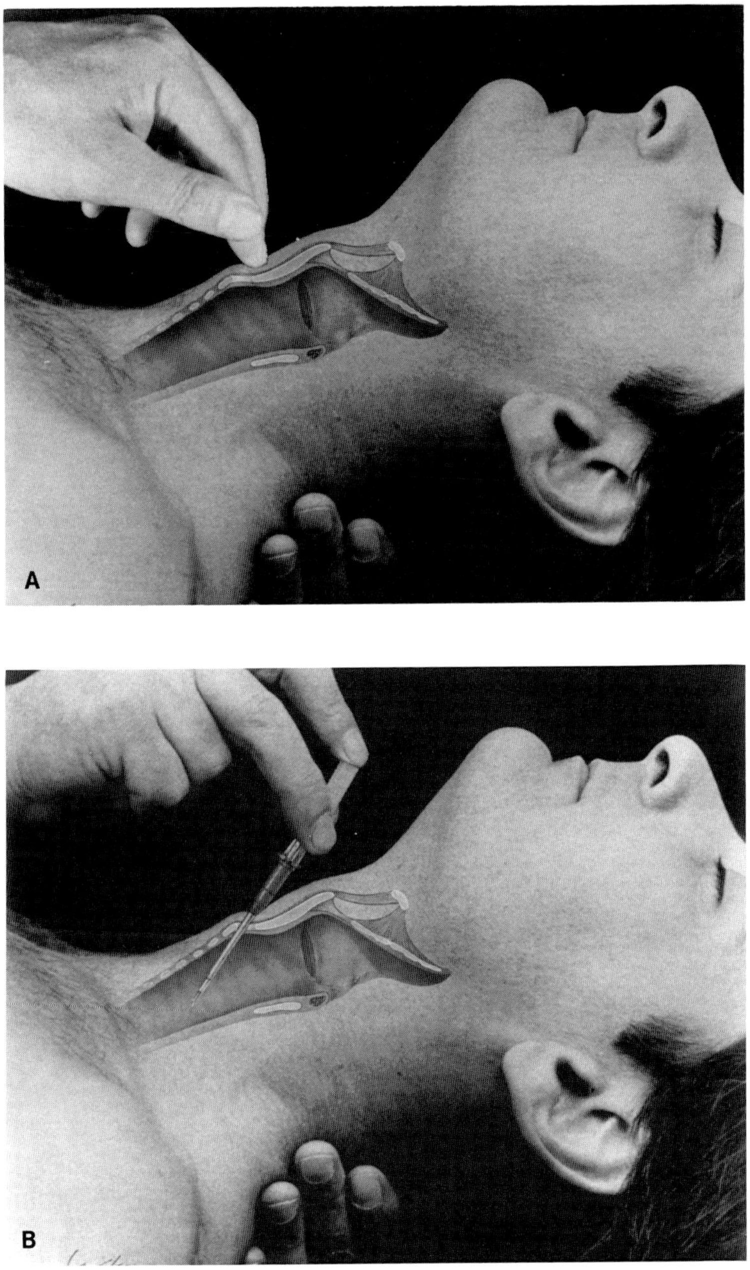

Figure 9-4 • How to insert catheter through cricothyroid membrane. (***A***) The cricothyroid membrane is palpated with the neck of the patient extended. (***B***) Then a 12 gauge or 14 gauge intravenous catheter is used at an angle of 30° caudad from the perpendicular to puncture the cricothyroid membrane.

(continued)

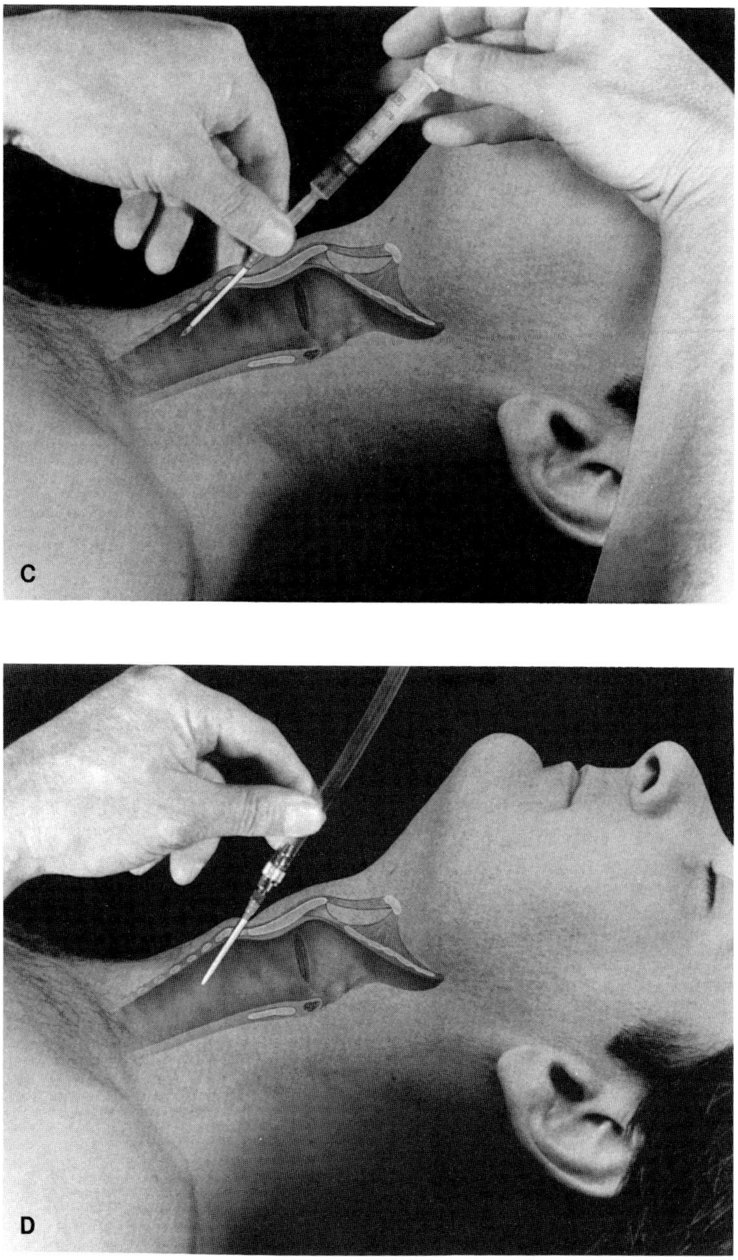

Figure 9–4 *(continued)*
(***C***) A syringe must be connected to the catheter and aspiration of air determined to verify its transtracheal location. (***D***) The needle stylet is withdrawn and the hub of the intravenous catheter is then connected to a transtracheal ventilation system.

gauge intravenous catheter with the needle pointed 30° caudad off the perpendicular is used to puncture the cricothyroid membrane (Fig. 9–4B). Then a syringe is attached to the catheter and aspiration of air indicates its transtracheal location (Fig. 9–4C). The needle stylet is withdrawn and the hub of the intravenous catheter is connected to a transtracheal ventilation system (Fig. 9–4D). During transtracheal ventilation the natural airway, which allows for the exhalation of the inspired gas, must be maintained as well as possible at all times to avoid air trapping and lung hyperexpansion.

There are two basic types of transtracheal ventilation systems: (1) a high-pressure jet injector/noncompliant tubing system (Sanders injector [blow gun] or anesthesia machine flush valve) that has a Luer lock connection to the intravenous catheter and (2) a reservoir bag/compliant tubing system (anesthesia circle system or simple resuscitation bag) that has a barrelless syringe and/or endotracheal tube adapter connection to the intravenous catheter.

A. *High-Pressure Jet Injector/Noncompliant Tubing/Luer Lock Systems*

The first type of TTJV system consists of a jet injector (blow gun) powered by regulated (Table 9–1)[27] or unregulated (Table 9–2)[27] central wall or tank (Table 9–3)[27] oxygen pressure. The great advantage of using central wall pressure to power the jet injector (provided the system is already plugged in) is the guaranteed immediate availability of a preassembled reliable, tightly jointed system to connect to the transtracheal catheter. The great advantage of regulated wall pressure is the ability to minimize barotrauma, especially in pediatric patients. The presence or absence of a regulator requires a different connection between the wall oxygen pressure source and the air hose leading to the jet injector and a moderate difference in price for the system (see Table 9–1 compared to Table 9–2). The great advantage of tank oxygen pressure is that it is mobile and can be used in anesthetizing locations that do not have a central (wall) source of high-pressure oxygen, but for this system to be effective it must be standing by or brought to these anesthetizing locations prior to the induction of anesthesia. To insure that the jet injector, which also has industrial uses, is free of an oil coating or residue, the jet injector is always soaked in acetone (which dissolves oil) after it arrives from the manufacturer. All nonthreaded connections are bonded with wire or plastic ties.

Finally, the anesthesia machine flush valve, which can, of course, be powered by either a wall or tank high-pressure oxygen source, can serve as the jet injector. The fresh gas outlet of the anesthesia machine (now an industry-wide standard 15-mm male outlet) is connected to noncompliant oxygen supply tubing by a standard 15-mm endotracheal tube adapter that fits a 4-mm ID endotracheal tube (Table 9–4).[27] The noncompliant oxygen supply tubing allows for bypass of the very compliant reservoir bag and corrugated tubing of the anesthesia circle system (see the next section). This third TTJV system is completed by connecting the oxygen supply tubing to the TTJV catheter; although this may be accomplished in many ways, our permanent TTJV sets have a bonded Luer lock/hose barb connector (no. 3, Table 9–4)[27,28] (Fig. 9–5). As a quick makeshift alternative, the TTJV catheter/oxygen supply tubing connection can be accomplished by cutting the barrel of a 1-mL syringe with a scissors and inserting the cut end of the barrel into the oxygen supply tubing and the other, uncut standard male end into the standard female intravenous catheter hub (also no. 3, Table 9–4).[27] The advantage of this system is that it can be quickly assembled from three readily available materials, is very inexpensive, and can be used wherever there is an anesthesia machine. Of course, to be effective, it must be ready to go before a cannot-ventilate-by-mask, cannot-intubate situation develops (ie, always).

B. *Reservoir Bag/Compliant Tubing/Syringe and/or Endotracheal Tube Adapter Systems*

The compliant tubing method consists of using the anesthesia machine oxygen flush valve (powered by either wall or tank oxygen) and the anesthesia circle system corrugated tubing to deliver the oxygen to the transtracheal catheter. The reservoir bag method is predictably less effective and consists of manually ventilating the patient by vigorously squeezing a self-inflating reservoir bag. If either of these two methods must be used (the compliance of both of these systems impedes effective ventilation of the lungs), the standard 15-mm elbow connector, which is at the end of both an anesthesia circle system and a self-inflating reservoir bag, can be connected to the transtracheal intravenous catheter in two ways: (1) by inserting the male end of a 15-mm endotracheal tube adapter that fits a 3-mm ID endotracheal tube directly into the standard female hub of the intravenous catheter[29–31]; (2) by inserting the male end of a plungerless 3-, 5-, or 10-mL syringe into the standard female hub of the intravenous catheter, and the male end of a 15-mm endotracheal tube adapter that fits a 7-, a 9-, and a 12-mm ID endotracheal tube, respectively, into the empty barrel of the syringe (Fig. 9–6).[31,32]

Finally, in the syringe and/or endotracheal tube method recommended by Reich and Schwartz,[33] an entire cuffed endotracheal tube (size 6.5 mm to 8.5 mm) is plugged into a 5-, 10-, or 20-mL syringe vessel. The cuff is then inflated to obtain an airtight seal (Fig. 9–7). The Luer lock connection of the syringe attaches to the transtracheal cannula and the proximal end of the endotracheal tube provides a standard 15-mm connector. This device will deliver in excess of 50 cm H_2O pressure to the transtracheal catheter when connected to a resuscitation bag or anesthesia machine.

(Text continued on p. 205)

Table 9-1 • Transtracheal Jet Ventilation Systems Using Regulated Wall O_2 Pressure.*

Transtracheal Jet Ventilation (TTJV) Systems	Component-to-Component Schematic	Part	Company	Model Number
TTJV using jet injector powered by regulated central wall O_2 pressure	Wall O_2 pressure 1.	1. Chemetron wall O_2 quick disconnect + 1/4" OD hose barb	Tri-Anim	11-01-0003
	2. O_2 hose	2. Chemetron O_2 hose	Tri-Anim	15-11-0001
	3.	3. 1/4" ID hose barb + 1/8" NPT adapter	Western Enterpr.	MH-7
	4. Regulator	4. Miniregulator gauge 0–50 psi	Bird Bird	2322 6765
	5.	5. 1/8" NPT male reducing adapter + 1/4" NPT female adapter	Western Enterpr.	MA-9
	6. Air hose	6. Air hose 25′	Lawson or Sears	81070 or 9HT16224
	7. Jet injector	7. Jet injector	Lawson or Sears	11903 or 9HT16235
	8.	8. 1/8" NPT male adapter + 1/4" ID hose barb	Western Enterpr.	MH-7
	9. O_2 tubing	9. Tygon tubing R-3603 3/8" OD, 1/4" ID	Cole-Parmer	6408-50
	10.	10. 1/4" hose barb + male luer lok	Becton-Dickinson	9067
	11. TTJV Catheter	11. Intravenous catheter with standard hub		

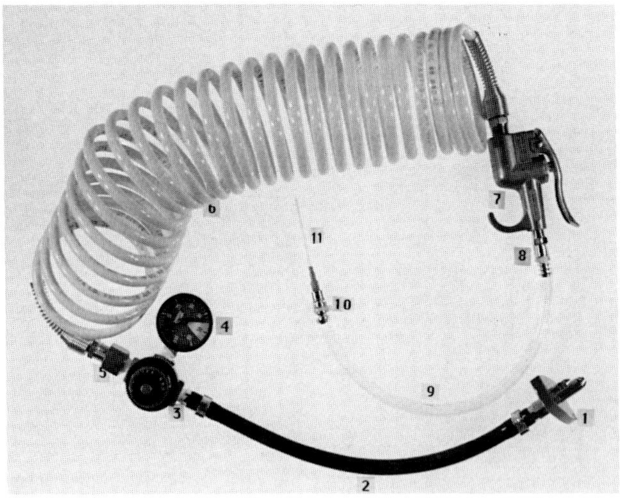

▷▷▷ = hose barb; ▨ = threaded screw connection; ▭ = male-female connection; NPT = National Pipe Thread. The parts list is the one used in our hospital.

Relevant addresses and telephone numbers of manufacturing and distributing companies for ordering parts are listed in the Appendix. Total cost = $145. Mr. Ron Rusk, personal communication.

*All nonthreaded connections should be bonded together with wire or plastic ties (see photographs). (From Benumof JL, Scheller MS. The importance of transtracheal jet ventilation in the management of the difficult airway. Anesthesiology 55:606–607, 1981; with permission.)

Table 9–2 • Transtracheal Jet Ventilation Systems Using Unregulated Wall O_2 Pressure.*

Transtracheal Jet Ventilation (TTJV) Systems	Component-to-Component Schematic	Part	Company	Model Number
TTJV using jet injector powered by unregulated central wall O_2 pressure	Wall O_2 pressure 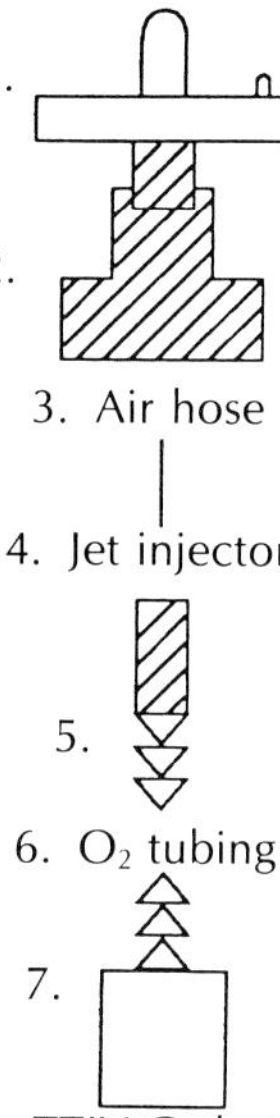 1.	1. Chemetron wall O_2 quick disconnect + ⅛″ ID NPT male adapter	Tri-Anim	11-01-0007
	2.	2. ⅛″ NPT male adapter + ¼″ reducing coupling	Lawson	5308
	3. Air hose	3. Air hose 25′	Lawson or Sears	81070 or 9HT16224
	4. Jet injector	4. Jet injector	Lawson or Sears	11903 or 9HT16235
	5.	5. ⅛″ NPT male adapter + ¼″ ID hose barb	Western Enterpr.	MH-7
	6. O_2 tubing	6. Tygon tubing R-3603 ⅜″ OD, ¼″ ID	Cole-Parmer	6408-50
	7.	7. ¼″ hose barb male luer lok	Becton-Dickinson	9067
	8. TTJV Catheter	8. Intravenous catheter with standard hub		

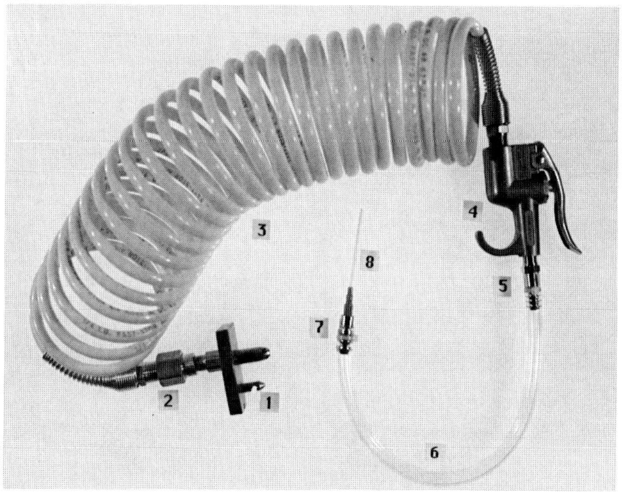

▷▷▷ = hose barb; ▨ = threaded screw connection; ▭ = male-female connection; NPT = National Pipe Thread. The parts list is the one used in our hospital.

Relevant addresses and telephone numbers of manufacturing and distributing companies for ordering parts are listed in Appendix II. Total cost = $83. Mr. Ron Rusk, personal communication.

*All nonthreaded connections should be bonded together with wire or plastic ties (see photographs). (From Benumof JL, Scheller MS. The importance of transtracheal jet ventilation in the management of the difficult airway. Anesthesiology 55:606–607, 1981; with permission.)

Table 9-3 • Transtracheal Jet Ventilation Systems Using O_2 Tank Regulator.*

Transtracheal Jet Ventilation (TTJV) Systems	Component-to-Component Schematic	Part	Company	Model Number
TTJV using jet injector powered by O_2 tank regulator	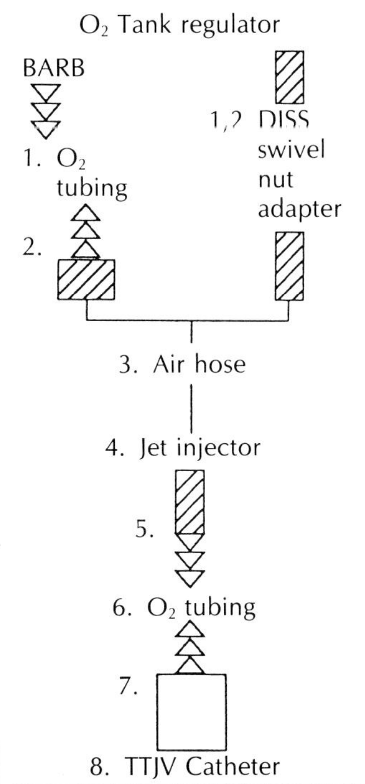	1. Tygon tubing R-3603 + ⅜″ OD, ¼″ ID	Cole-Parmer	6408-50
		2. ¼″ ID hose barb + ¼″ NPT female adapter	Western Enterpr.	MH-7
		1,2. DISS swivel nut adapter + ¼″ NPT female adapter	Western Enterpr.	M24-35
		3. Air hose 25′	Lawson or Sears	81070 or 9HT16224
		4. Jet injector	Lawson or Sears	11903 or 9HT16235
		5. ⅛″ NPT male adapter + ¼″ ID hose barb	Western Enterpr.	MH-7
		6. Tygon tubing R-3603 ⅜″ OD, ¼″ ID	Cole-Parmer	6408-50
		7. ¼″ hose barb male luer lok	Becton-Dickinson	9067
		8. Intravenous catheter with standard hub		

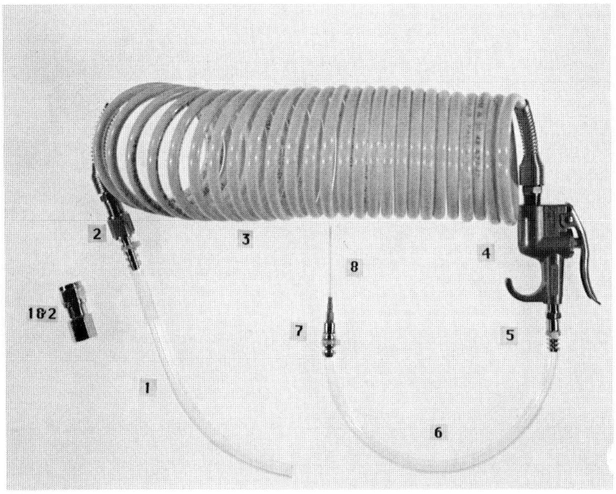

▷▷▷ = hose barb; ▨ = threaded screw connection; ▭ = male-female connection; NPT = National Pipe Thread. The parts list is the one used in our hospital.

Relevant addresses and telephone numbers of manufacturing and distributing companies for ordering parts are listed in Appendix II. Total cost = $73. Mr. Ron Rusk, personal communication.

*All nonthreaded connections should be bonded together with wire or plastic ties (see photographs). (From Benumof JL, Scheller MS. The importance of transtracheal jet ventilation in the management of the difficult airway. Anesthesiology 55:606–607, 1981; with permission.)

Table 9-4 • Transtracheal Jet Ventilation Systems Using Anesthesia Machine Fresh Gas Outlet and Flush Valve.*

Transtracheal Jet Ventilation (TTJV) Systems	Component-to-Component Schematic	Part	Company	Model Number
TTJV using anesthesia machine fresh gas outlet and flush valve	Anesthesia machine fresh gas outlet 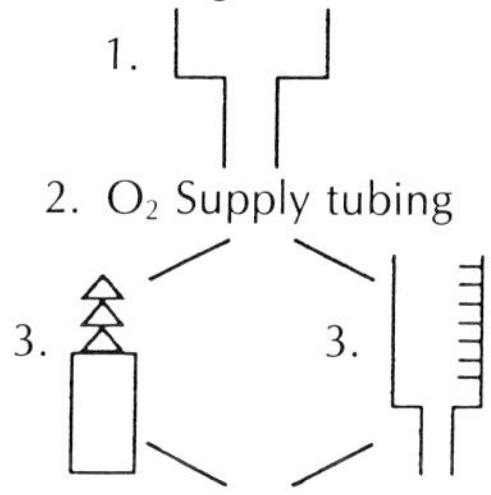 1. 2. O_2 Supply tubing 3. 3. 4. TTJV Catheter	1. 15-mm ET tube adapter for 4-mm ID ET tube	Many companies	
		2. O_2 supply tubing	Many companies	
		3. ¼″ hose barb male Luer lock or 3. cut-off 1-ml syringe	Becton-Dickinson	9067
		4. Intravenous catheter with standard hub		

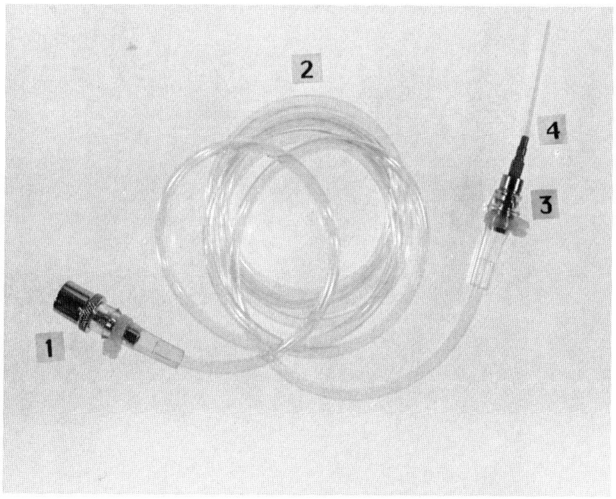

▷▷▷ = hose barb; ▨ = threaded screw connection; ▭ = male-female connection; NPT = National Pipe Thread. The parts list is the one used in our hospital.

Relevant addresses and telephone numbers of manufacturing and distributing companies for ordering parts are listed in Appendix II. Total cost = $6. Mr. Ron Rusk, personal communication.

*All nonthreaded connections should be bonded together with wire or plastic ties (see photographs). (From Benumof JL, Scheller MS. The importance of transtracheal jet ventilation in the management of the difficult airway. Anesthesiology 55:606–607, 1981; with permission.)

IV. DISCUSSION

The quickest, easiest, most efficacious solution to a cannot-ventilate-by-mask, cannot-intubate situation is TTJV through an intravenous catheter. In addition, TTJV can facilitate upper airway surgery; intubation via conventional laryngoscopy, via antegrade fiberoptic bronchoscopy, or via initial retrograde intubation; and cricothyroidotomy and tracheostomy. The mechanism of efficacy is by mass movement of gas from the jet itself, as well as by air entrainment by the Venturi principle, and healthy and critically ill patients have been successfully ventilated by this method. Exhalation occurs passively during the interval between oxygen injections through the natural airway. This is possible because obstruction in the upper airway, if present, is usually due to a valvelike effect, and not a total obstruction. At times, a jet of oxygen itself may be sufficient to cause a partially obstructing foreign body or particulate matter

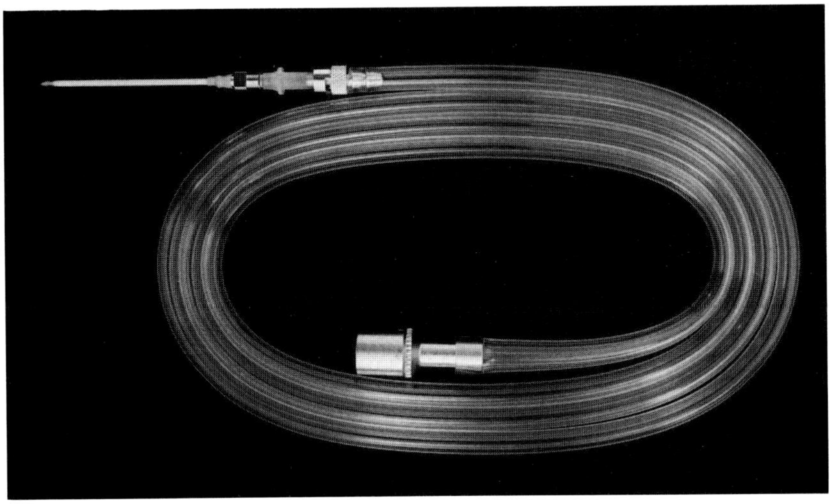

Figure 9–5 • Noncompliant tubing with an anesthesia machine adapter at one end and a Luer lock and an intravenous needle/catheter set at the other end for emergency transtracheal ventilation.

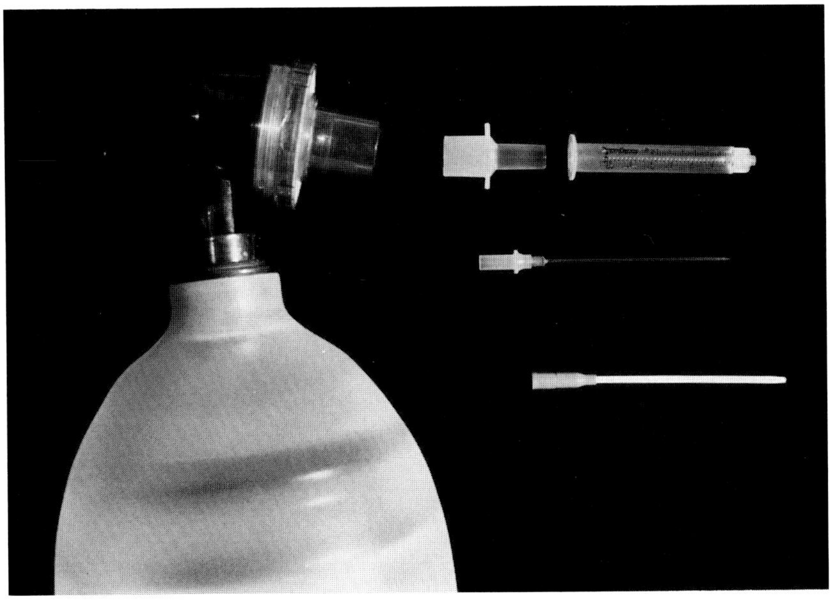

Figure 9–6 • Assembly of readily available equipment to allow a resuscitation bag to be connected to an intravenous needle and/or cannula. The adapter of an 8-mm endotracheal (ET) tube is fitted to the barrel of a 3-mL disposable plastic syringe from which the plunger has been removed.

to be expelled, particularly if from below or inferior to the offending article.

The systems of choice, in descending order of preference, are jet injector powered by regulated wall or oxygen tank pressure, jet injector powered by unregulated wall or tank oxygen pressure, and anesthesia machine flush valve using noncompliant tubing from the fresh gas outlet. A less efficacious transtracheal ventilation system consists of an anesthesia machine flush valve jetting gas to patient via the compliant tubing of the anesthesia circle system (which also contains a reservoir bag). In this instance, the very compliant reservoir bag and corrugated tubing absorbs, by distention, most of the jet from the anesthesia machine fresh gas outlet and prevents effective ventilation of the lungs. An even less efficacious system is produced by connecting a reservoir bag directly to the transtracheal catheter. In this instance, it is impossible to achieve a significant amount of ventilation through the intravenous catheter and the P_aCO_2 increases at a rate of 4 mmHg/min,[34] which is close to the rate of carbon dioxide increase of 6 mmHg/min during apneic oxygen insufflation in barbiturate-anesthetized animals.[34] Nevertheless, it should be pointed out that these two systems can still provide improved (perhaps acceptable) oxygenation.

One could argue that an indication to use a transtracheal catheter–reservoir bag system, would be in cases in which the upper airway (ie, cephalad to the cricothy-

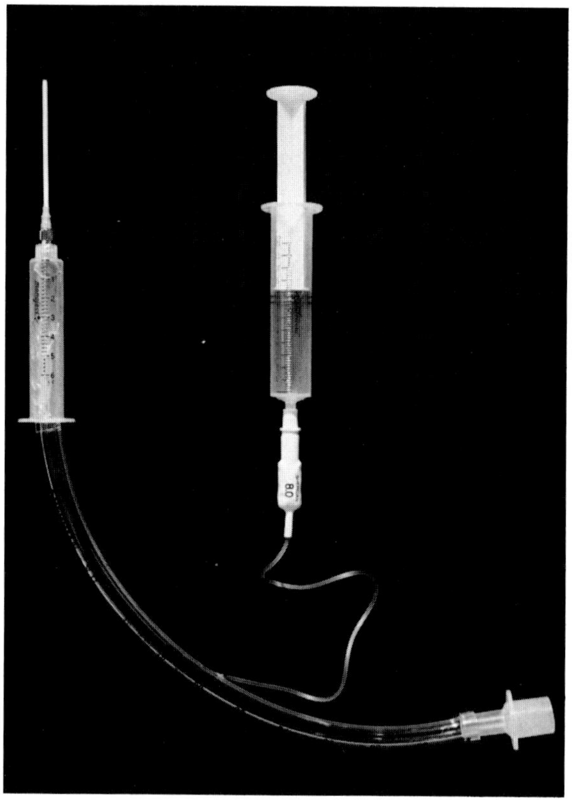

Figure 9–7 • An entire cuffed ET tube (sizes 6.5–8.5 mm) will fit into a 5-, 10-, or 20-mL syringe barrel. The cuff of the ET tube is then inflated to ensure an airtight seal prior to attaching the Luer lock connector to the transtracheal cannula.

roid membrane) was totally obstructed.[36] In cases of total upper airway obstruction, inability to expel the TTJV gas from the lungs would greatly increase the risk of barotrauma caused by gas trapping and lung hyperexpansion. With a transtracheal catheter–reservoir bag system, only small amounts of oxygen can be delivered to the alveolar space per unit time (but perhaps still sufficient to maintain a life-sustaining level of oxygenation),[35] with a significantly reduced risk of barotrauma. On the other hand, one could equally well argue that small amounts of oxygen could also be delivered to the alveolar space by true TTJV (by either jet injector or anesthesia machine flush valve with any kind of tubing) by simply using very slow respiratory rates and short jet injection times (ie, very low inspiration–expiration ratios). In any case of total upper airway obstruction, any and all percutaneous transtracheal ventilation systems used for emergency situations must be converted to a formal cricothyroidotomy or tracheostomy tube, and the patients must be well ventilated with conventional intermittent positive pressure ventilation as soon as possible.

V. COMPLICATIONS

The techniques of transtracheal ventilation described are not innocuous. As in any invasive procedure, particularly in an emergency situation and if performed by inexperienced, untrained personnel, the possible risks and complications are compounded.

Reported complications of transtracheal puncture include hemoptysis, subcutaneous emphysema, mediastinal emphysema, vagal reflexes, hypoxia, and infection.[37] Moreover, the possibility of puncture of the great vessels of the neck leading to massive hemorrhage or even perforation of the esophagus cannot be ignored. Holt et al[38] described a patient with massive hemoptysis following a transtracheal puncture that was treated by subsequent endotracheal intubation with balloon tamponade of the bleeding site; resolution of the problem occurred within 1 hour.

Even planned transtracheal ventilation for endolaryngeal surgery has not been without incident. Spoerel and Greenway[20] described massive tissue emphysema that can occur either when the jet is not fully inside the tracheal lumen or when the outflow of gas is obstructed while ventilation continues. This patient was treated with endotracheal intubation; ventilation with oxygen was maintained while needles were placed in both chest cavities to relieve bilateral pneumothorax. Since the emphysema was produced mainly by oxygen that is fairly rapidly absorbed from the tissues, the swelling receded quickly, and only minor degrees of tissue emphysema were detectable radiographically 8 hours later.

Attention to detail is imperative. Frequent and repeated aspirations are essential to verify that the tips of either needles or cannulae are correctly placed and maintained within the lumen of the trachea. Digital compression of the tissues adjacent to the puncture site for a few minutes is helpful, as is adequate muscle relaxation or concomitant use of local anesthetics in a nonparalyzed patient to minimize cough response.

In summary, we have attempted to review for the interest of health care personnel some of the different armamentaria available, and the methods of their assembly, particularly to provide emergency ventilation and oxygenation to patients who have sustained life-threatening upper airway obstructions. Most of the methods described are facilitated with equipment that is readily available, particularly to anesthesia personnel. For enhanced preparedness and increased safety for such patients, it is recommended that an "emergency setup" be maintained in a sterile manner and located in a convenient, designated area known to all personnel for use in such an emergency.

VI. Appendix

Tri-Anim Health Services, Inc.
1630 Flower Street
P.O. Box 3823
Glendale, CA 91201
(818) 545-7329

Cole-Parmer Instrument Co.
7425 North Oak Park Avenue
Chicago, IL 60648
1-800-323-4340

Western Enterprises
33672 Pin Oak Parkway
Avon Lake, OH 44012
(216) 933-2171

Lawson Products
1237 West Walnut Street
Compton, CA 90220
(213) 637-1237

Division of Becton-Dickinson & Co.
Rutherford, NJ 07070
(201) 460-2000

VII. References

1. Keenan RL, Boyan CP. Cardiac arrest due to anesthesia. JAMA 253:2373–2377, 1985.
2. Taylor G, Larson CP, Prestwich R. Unexpected cardiac arrest during anesthesia and surgery: An environmental study. JAMA 236:2758–260, 1976.
3. American Society of Anesthesiologists Committee on Professional Liability (K Posner, project director, and F Cheney, MD, chairman). Personal Communication.
4. Bolander FMF. Deaths associated with anesthesia. Br J Anaesth 47:36–40, 1975.
5. Harrison GG. Death attributable to anesthesia. Br J Anaesth 50:1041–1046, 1978.
6. Davis DA. An analysis of anesthetic mishaps from medical liability claims. Int Anesthesiol Clin 22:31–42, 1984.
7. American Heart Association. Textbook of Advanced Cardiac Life Support. Washington, DC: American Heart Association, 1987, 33–34.
8. Donegan J. Cardiopulmonary resuscitation. Chapter 61. In Miller R (ed). Anesthesia. New York, Churchill Livingstone, 1986, 21–23.
9. Holmgreen WC. Difficult intubation: Suspected. In Brady L, Smith RB (eds) Decision Making in Anesthesiology. Philadelphia, BC Decker, 1987, 16–17.
10. Holmgreen WC, Niskioka GR. Difficult intubation: Unsuspected. In Brady L, Smith RB (eds). Decision Making in Anesthesiology. Philadelphia, BC Decker, 1987, 16–17.
11. Gammage GW. Airway management. Chapter 21. In Civetta JM, Taylor RW, Kirby RR (eds). Critical Care. Philadelphia, JB Lippincott 1988, 197–199.
12. Hooke R. Experimental account: Preserving animals alive by blowing through their lungs with bellows. Philos Trans R Soc Lond 2:539–540, 1667.
13. Meltzer SJ. Continuous respiration without respiratory movements. J Exp Med 11:622–625, 1909.
14. Draper WB, Whitehead RW. Diffusion respiration in dog anesthetized by pentothal sodium. Anesthesiology 5:262–273, 1944.
15. Jacoby JJ, Hamelberg W, Ziegler CH, et al. Transtracheal resuscitation. JAMA 162:625–628, 1956.
16. Jacobs HB. Needle-catheter brings oxygen to the trachea. JAMA 222:1231–1233, 1972.
17. Spoerel WE, Narayanan PS, Singh NP. Transtracheal ventilation. Br J Anaesth 43:932–939, 1971.
18. Singh NP, Agrawal AR, Dhawan, R. Resuscitation centre for management of respiratory insufficiency cases. Indian J Chest Dis 13:99–113, 1971.
19. Smith RB, MacMillan BB, Petruscak J, Pfaeffle HH. Transtracheal ventilation for laryngoscopy. Ann Otol Rhinol Laryngol 82:347–350, 1973.
20. Spoerel WE, Greenway RE. Technique of ventilation during endolaryngeal surgery under general anesthesia. Can Anaesth Soc J 20:369–377, 1973.
21. Smith RB, Myers EN, Sherman H. Transtracheal ventilation in pediatric patients. Br J Anaesth 46:313–314, 1974.
22. Layman PR. Transtracheal ventilation in oral surgery. Ann R Coll Surg 65:318–320, 1983.
23. Wagner DJ, Coombs DW, Doyle SC. Percutaneous transtracheal ventilation for emergency dental appliance removal. Anesthesiology 62:664–666, 1985.
24. McLellan I, Gordon P, Khawaja S, Thomas A. Percutaneous transtracheal high frequency jet ventilation as an aid to difficult intubation. Can Anaesth Soc J 35:404–405, 1988.
25. Baraka A. Transtracheal jet ventilation during fiberoptic intubation under general anesthesia. Anesth Analg 65:1091–1092, 1986.
26. Heimlich HJ, Carr GC. Transtracheal catheter technique for pulmonary rehabilitation. Ann Otol Rhinol Laryngol 94:502–504, 1985.
27. Benumof JL, Scheller MS. The importance of transtracheal jet ventilation in the management of the difficult airway. Anesthesiology 71:769–778, 1989.
28. Delisser EA, Muravchick S. Emergency transtracheal ventilation. Anesthesiology 55:606–607, 1981.
29. Attia RR, Battit GE, Murphy JD. Transtracheal ventilation. JAMA 234:1152–1153, 1975.
30. Fisher JA. A "last ditch" airway. Can Anaesth Soc J 26:225–230, 1979.
31. Patel R. Systems for transtracheal ventilation. Anesthesiology 59:165, 1983.

32. Stinson TW. A simple connector for transtracheal ventilation. Anesthesiology 47:232, 1977.
33. Reich DL, Schwartz N. An easily assembled device for transtracheal oxygenation. Anesthesiology 66:437–438, 1987.
34. Thomas T, Zornow M, Scheller MS, Unger. R. The efficacy of three different modes of trans-tracheal ventilation in hypoxic hypercarbic swine. Can J Anaesth 35:S61, 1988.
35. Klain M, Smith RB. High frequency percutaneous transtracheal jet ventilation. Crit Care Med 5:280–287, 1977.
36. Cote CJ, Eavey RD, Todres D, Jones DE. Cricothyroid membrane puncture: Oxygenation and ventilation in a dog model using an intravenous catheter. Crit Care Med 16:615–619, 1988.
37. Spencer CD, Beatty HN. Complications of transtracheal aspiration. N Engl J Med 286:304–305, 1972.
38. Holt GR, Davis WE, Ailor EJ, et al. Massive airway hemorrhage after transtracheal aspiration. South Med J 71:325–327, 1978.

Chapter 10

•

Steven R. Shackford, MD

Tracheostomy and Cricothyroidotomy

OUTLINE

I. Introduction and Indications

Tracheostomy and cricothyroidotomy are surgical procedures performed to gain access to the airway. They differ from less invasive means of airway access, such as nasotracheal or orotracheal intubation, in that a tube is placed through an incision in the trachea (transtracheal intubation) rather than passed through the larynx (translaryngeal intubation). This distinction is noteworthy when considering both the indications for and the complications of surgical airway access.

Surgical procedures on the obstructed airway have been performed since antiquity,[1] but technically satisfactory procedures were not developed until the mid-1800s. Credit for the modern technique of tracheostomy is conventionally given to Jackson.[1] His technique has subsequently been described and modified by a variety of specialists, including general surgeons, neurosurgeons, plastic and reconstructive surgeons, emergency physicians, intensivists, and internists.[2-7] Such familiarity and frequent use of the procedure by multiple specialists and subspecialists should not imply that the operations for airway access are minor and can be relegated to the most junior member of the operative team. On the contrary, surgical access to the airway requires a thorough knowledge of the regional anatomy, skillful and meticulous technique, specific equipment, and optimal conditions. As Hardy[7] has stated, ''Probably no other operative procedure produces so much dramatic help if properly executed and managed, but has more potential for life threatening complications and prolonged suffering if poorly performed.'' Hardy regrettably noted that the majority of complications were due to poor surgical technique.[7] This has been noted by others,[3,8] and it is apparent that the complication rate and the number of technical errors appear to be inversely related to the skill of the surgeon and the urgency of the situation.[3,4,8,9] McGill[3] noted a complication rate of 32% when cricothyroidotomy was performed as an emergency procedure by emergency physicians in the emergency room. Despite this caveat, there will be situations in the intensive care unit (ICU) that require surgical access to the airway that must be obtained by less than a fully skilled surgeon in clearly unfavorable conditions in order to be life-saving.[2,5] In those acute situations in which the airway is lost and cannot be established by less invasive means, surgical access is indicated even if it must be performed by less skilled individuals in a less than optimal environment.

A. *Tracheostomy: Indications*

Tracheostomy (see Table 10–1 for a list of indications) was used sparingly until the mid-1950s, and then only for acute airway obstruction. The application of tracheostomy to conditions other than obstruction began when polio epidemics demonstrated a need for prolonged intubation of the airway. McClelland[9] noted a ninefold increase in the annual frequency of tracheostomy performed at his institution in the decade between 1950 and 1959. Similarly, Enfors[10] noted a sixfold increase between 1954 and 1964. Beatrous[4] noted a similar trend at Charity Hospital. At about this time orotracheal intubation had become common, but physicians were wary of the laryngeal complications of prolonged translaryngeal intubation. Significant laryngeal mucosal injury was noted as soon as 7 hours after translaryngeal intubation and moderate-sized granulomas requiring surgical removal were noted in 1% to 3% of patients with translaryngeal intubation longer than 2 days.[1] Because of the concern for laryngeal and subglottic complications, it was recommended that tracheostomy be performed routinely in all patients requiring ventilatory support for more than 4 days. However, subsequent well-done prospective studies[1,11,12] have demonstrated that prolonged translaryngeal intubation does not result in significant clinical morbidity. Most of the laryngeal injury that can be viewed via laryngotracheoscopy heals rapidly without long-term clinical sequelae. As a result of these studies, the number of tracheostomies per-

Table 10–1 • Tracheostomy: Indications

Emergency
Obstruction
Severe laryngeal trauma
Elective*
Obstruction
Sleep apnea
Orofacial injuries
Toilet/Protection
Comatose patients
Ventilation
Respiratory failure in adults and children
Prolonged Weaning
Other
Congenital airway anomalies
Major complication of OT/NT† intubation

*Contraindicated if recent sternotomy incision present.
†OT = orotracheal; NT = nasotracheal.

formed at major centers has decreased as physicians have relied on translaryngeal intubation to provide airway access in patients requiring prolonged ventilatory support. The need for tracheostomy in certain other diseases has also decreased. Diphtheria, a frequent indication for tracheostomy in the early 1900s, is now extremely rare. Flail chest injury, previously mandating tracheostomy in all cases, is being treated less often with a ventilator and rarely with a tracheostomy.[13]

Despite the reduction in the frequency of tracheostomy, there are still several indications for its use. The application of these indications to a specific patient requires judgment. The physician must individualize the approach in each patient and must consider such variables as the patient's overall clinical condition, the anticipated duration of ventilatory support, the availability of an operating room and an operating team, and the necessity for future operations that might necessitate reintubation.

1. EMERGENCY INDICATIONS

Emergency tracheostomy is rarely indicated or performed. Cricothyroidotomy (see later) and percutaneous transtracheal ventilation (see Chapter 9) have supplanted tracheostomy for emergency airway access except in the case of severe laryngeal trauma. Severe crush injuries to the larynx obscure the anatomy of the cricothyroid membrane and will invariably interfere with placement of a tube through the cricothyroid membrane. Therefore, if airway control cannot be obtained from above through the injury, emergency tracheostomy is indicated. It is imperative in the emergency situation that the tracheostomy be performed by the most skilled member of the team. Many, if not all, of the superficial landmarks will be distorted by the injury, and expeditious control of the airway will require the skills of an experienced surgeon.

2. ELECTIVE INDICATIONS

For the most part, tracheostomy has become an elective or semielective procedure done in the operating room with an endotracheal tube in place and control of the airway assured.

a. Obstructive Sleep Apnea

Tracheostomy is indicated for the treatment of severe obstructive sleep apnea in those patients with documented cardiopulmonary problems who have failed conservative measures.[14,15] In fact, obstructive sleep apnea may require a permanent tracheostomy.

b. Severe Orofacial Injuries

Tracheostomy can provide optimal guaranteed airway access for pulmonary hygiene and ventilation in patients with severe maxillofacial or oropharyngeal injuries in whom accidental nasotracheal or orotracheal extubation would be disastrous. Inadvertent endotracheal tube extubation is not rare in this situation, occurring in 13% of Stauffer's[11] patients. Major swelling of the face and neck would drastically diminish chances for successful reintubation should the endotracheal tube become dislodged. This is particularly important in the patient who has an associated head injury in whom transient hypercarbia or hypoxemia would produce significant secondary cerebral injury. Tracheostomy should be performed at the time the facial injuries are treated operatively.

c. Tracheobronchial Toilet and Airway Protection

All comatose patients are candidates for elective tracheostomy. The tracheostomy will facilitate suctioning for removal of pulmonary secretions and will diminish greatly the chances for major aspiration. However, a cuffed tracheostomy tube does not prevent aspiration. On the contrary, there is good evidence to suggest[12] that tracheostomy increases airway contamination more than translaryngeal intubation. However, major aspiration, a common problem in the comatose patient, can be greatly diminished by the cuffed tube. Tracheostomy is also much easier to care for in an institutional, chronic rehabilitation setting.

d. Ventilation

Approximately 80% of patients with respiratory failure will require mechanical ventilation for less than 2 weeks.[1,5] The 20% who require intubation for longer than 2 weeks are candidates for tracheostomy. Although it seems intuitive that prolonged endotracheal intubation increases the incidence of laryngeal complications, the exact relationship between the duration of translaryngeal intubation and the incidence and severity of laryngeal complications has not been determined.[1,9,11,12,17] Many factors appear to affect the degree of airway injury, including duration of intubation, tube size relative to larynx size, presence of infection, and amount of tube movement.[1,9,11,12,17,18] These factors should all be considered when determining both the need and the timing for tracheostomy in patients with established respiratory failure. Consequently, it seems prudent to consider tracheostomy in infected, actively moving (at least the head and neck) patients who will require intubation for longer than 14 days. Heffner[17] suggests upper airway endoscopy after 11 days. If the lesions are advanced he recommends tracheostomy at that time. However, if they are not significant, he recommends continuing with translaryngeal intubation. Others[2] recommend a more empirical approach with tracheostomy performed 2 weeks after translaryngeal intubation. Stock[2] points out the advantages of surgical airway access in the critically ill patient on the ICU: (1) improved patient comfort, (2) less chance of inadvertent extubation, (3) ease of airway suctioning, and (4) an earlier discharge from the ICU without an increase in total hospital stay. Tracheostomy also eases the weaning process in patients with respiratory failure in that it allows one to be more aggressive in removing support, since failure of a weaning technique requires not reintubation but simply reattachment of the tube to the ventilator. It has been my experience that tracheostomy is especially useful during the weaning process in debilitated, elderly patients in whom the removal of 50–75 mL of dead space decreases airway resistance and work of breathing to the point that patients wean more rapidly.

e. *Other Elective Indications*

Tracheostomy is indicated in children and neonates with congenital airway anomalies,[19] such as laryngotracheo-esophageal cleft and cervical hemangioma.

Elective tracheostomy is used in those patients who have suffered major upper airway complications of orotracheal and nasotracheal intubation, such as subglottic stenosis and maxillary or nasal sinusitis.

Tracheostomy should be avoided, if possible, in patients who have had a recent sternotomy incision. Despite meticulous attention to the stoma, all these new incisions will eventually become colonized and subclinically infected. Because of the proximity of the tracheostome to the sternotomy incision, the infection may spread from the stoma to the sternal incision with resultant wound infection, sternal dehiscence, and mediastinitis, a disastrous, life-threatening complication.

B. *Cricothyroidotomy: Indications*

Cricothyroidotomy, or "high tracheostomy" (see Table 10–2 for indications), was soundly condemned by Chevalier Jackson in 1921 because of an extremely high incidence of failed decannulation due to subglottic stenosis.[20] As a result, the procedure received little attention until 1976, when Brantigan and Grow[20] rekindled interest with their report of 655 cricothyroidotomies performed in cardiothoracic patients without a single case of subglottic stenosis. Their experience was confirmed by others,[21,22] whose combined series demonstrated an incidence of subglottic stenosis of less than 2%. A review of Jackson's data and subsequent laboratory studies have suggested that the subglottic stenosis is due not to the procedure itself, but to the condition of the larynx at the time the procedure was performed. Virtually all Jackson's patients had diphtheria, a severe inflammatory condition of the larynx. The addition of a foreign body (the tracheostomy tube) only added to the inflammatory reaction, resulting in exuberant granulation tissue and scarring with resultant subglottic stenosis. Clearly, cricothyroidotomy would be contraindicated in such conditions. Recent work[21,22] suggests that cricothyroidotomy is similarly contraindicated in patients who have had translaryngeal intubation for more than 72 hours. The posterior laryngeal inflammation associated with translaryngeal intubation of 72 hours duration would create an inflammatory condition not dissimilar to that of diphtheria. Except in emergency situations, cricothyroidotomy is also contraindicated in all prepubertal children, since the cricothyroid cartilage represents the narrowest part of a child's airway and any inflammatory tissue in that area could severely restrict air movement.

Table 10–2 • Cricothyroidotomy: Indications

Emergency
Obstruction
All except laryngeal trauma
Failed OT/NT† intubation
Elective
Toilet/protection
Comatose patients*
Ventilation
Respiratory failure in adults*

*Provided prior OT/NT intubation has been required for <72 hours and there is no major laryngeal inflammation.

†OT = orotracheal; NT = nasotracheal.

If cricothyroidotomy is needed as emergency access for airway obstruction in children, it is advisable to convert the cricothyroidotomy to a formal tracheostomy within 48–72 hours.

1. EMERGENCY INDICATIONS

Except in the case of severe laryngeal trauma, cricothyroidotomy is the procedure of choice for acute surgical airway access. It should be used in all cases in which orotracheal or nasotracheal intubation has failed to control the airway after a reasonable number of attempts.

2. ELECTIVE INDICATIONS

Cricothyroidotomy can be used for long-term airway access in comatose patients and patients with respiratory failure.[21] However, if the patient has had translaryngeal intubation for greater than 72 hours, tracheostomy should be the primary choice for surgical airway access. If a cricothyroidotomy was placed for emergency airway access in an adult without prior translaryngeal intubation, there is no need to convert it to a formal tracheostomy, since the incidence of subglottic stenosis in this situation is very low.[21]

C. *Indications: Summary and Recommendations*

Except in cases of severe laryngeal trauma, cricothyroidotomy is the primary choice for emergency surgical airway access. If the patient requires continued airway access, the cricothyroidotomy can be left in place for as long as the patient requires an airway. If the patient with translaryngeal intubation has need of prolonged mechanical ventilatory support, tracheostomy should be performed at 2 weeks. Comatose patients who show no evidence of neurologic improvement after 10 days to 2 weeks also should undergo tracheostomy for pulmonary hygiene, airway protection, and ease of placement into a rehabilitation program.

Table 10–3 • Equipment

Essential
Knife blade #11, #10
Electrocautery
Tracheal hook
Trousseau dilator
Tracheostomy tube
High Volume, high-compliance, low-pressure cuff
Cotton "twill" tape
20-mL Syringe
10-mL 1% Xylocaine without epinephrine
Optimal
Coaxial headlamp
Sterile suction catheter
Sterile lubricant
Sterile adapter for anesthesia machine

II. HOW TO DO TRACHEOSTOMY AND CRICOTHYROIDOTOMY: TECHNICAL ASPECTS

A. *Tracheostomy*

1. EQUIPMENT

As stated previously, virtually all tracheostomies are elective procedures to be performed in the operating room by a skilled surgeon with a skilled anesthesiologist in attendance, and the airway controlled prior to operation by translaryngeal intubation. Several instruments are essential, others are optimal (see Table 10–3 for a list of equipment). Good lighting and suction are essential for optimal visualization of the surgical field. The Trousseau dilator is essential for enlarging the tracheal incision so that it will accommodate the tracheostomy tube. The tracheal hook is particularly important in patients of short stature with a thick neck in whom the trachea may lie deeply in the soft tissues and may even reside behind the sternum. The tracheal hook will allow the surgeon to bring the trachea more into the operative field. The 20-mL syringe is used to check the integrity of the air cuff and pilot balloon. The sterile lubricating gel facilitates placement of the tracheostomy tube into the tracheal incision. The soft, long, sterile suction catheter can be used by the surgeon to directly suction the tracheostomy tube after placement. The sterile adapter for the anesthesia machine or ventilator can be attached to the tracheostomy tube after insertion and the connecting tubing can be handed off to the anesthesiologist to maintain field sterility. A coaxial headlight is invaluable to the operating surgeon and assistant, especially in those patients with the more dorsally placed trachea. Cotton tracheal "twill tape" is used to secure the tracheostomy tube in place.

2. Patient Positioning and Preparation

The positioning of the patient is crucial to a successful operation. The patient is placed supine on the operating table and, if possible, the neck is hyperextended by placing a rolled sheet transversely across the scapulae. Hyperextension is contraindicated in a patient with proven or suspected cervical spine injury. After hyperextension of the neck, the occiput should be placed on a soft halo sponge cushion to prevent pressure necrosis of the occipital scalp. If possible, the operating table should be placed at approximately 15° of reverse Trendelenburg position to decrease venous bleeding in the field. However, it should be noted that in this position the patient is more prone to air embolism if a major venous injury occurs and the patient is not receiving positive pressure ventilation. With the patient positioned prior to being prepped, the surgeons should carefully review the superficial landmarks of the regional anatomy, including the tip of the chin, the tip of the thyroid cartilage, the indentation of the cricothyroid membrane (just below the thyroid cartilage), and the sternal notch (Fig. 10–1A). This will be the last opportunity for the surgeon to survey this landscape and plan the procedure before prepping and draping. After prepping and draping, most of these landmarks will be obscured by drapes and it is very easy to stray from the midline structures.

I prefer a Betadine scrub and prep. I also prefer a transversely oriented tracheostomy drape that allows the surgeon wide access to the area of incision and operation, namely, the area approximately two fingerbreadths above the sternum (see Fig. 10–1B).

Tracheostomy can be performed under local or general anesthesia. When performed under local anesthesia, the skin, subcutaneous tissues, and the airway are injected with 1% Xylocaine without epinephrine, being careful not to exceed administration of 7 mg/kg and not to inject the Xylocaine directly into a vessel.

3. Operative Technique

The skin is incised transversely with the knife (Fig. 10–2A, top left panel), and the subcutaneous tissues and platysma are divided transversely with the electrocautery (see Fig. 10–2A, right panel). One must be meticulous about hemostasis in this area. Any major venous branches should be clamped and ligated with a 3-0 absorbable suture material.

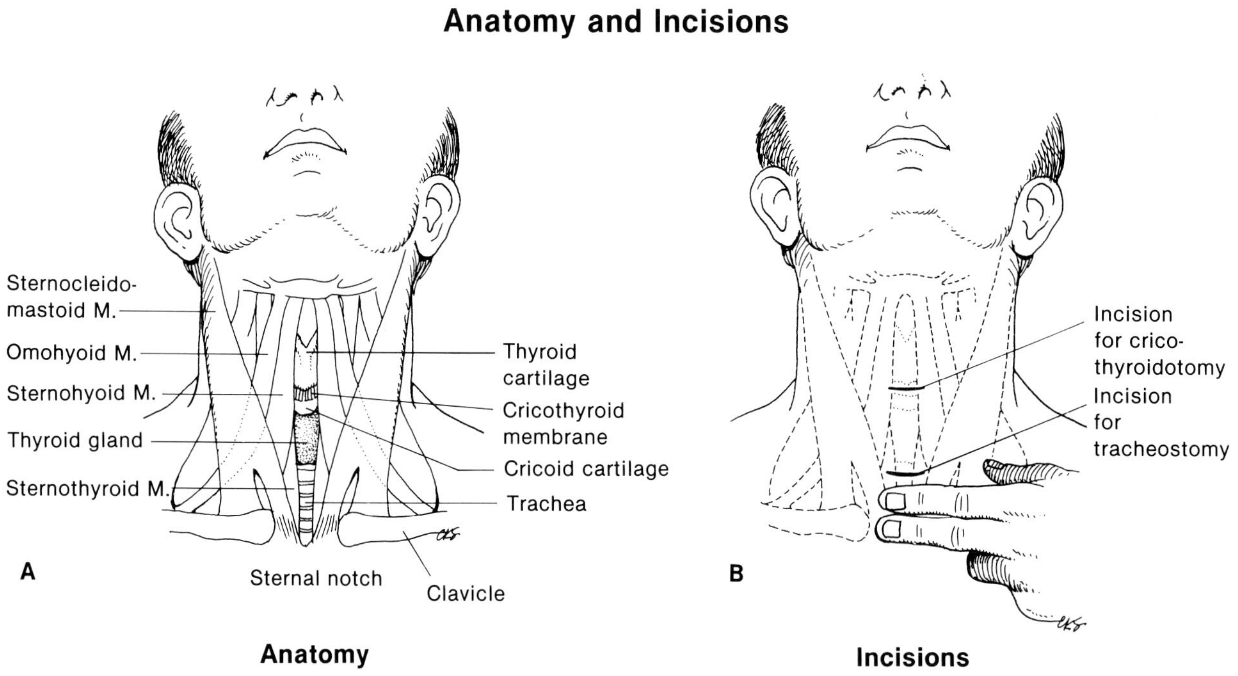

Figure 10–1 • (*A*) The relevant anatomy for tracheostomy and cricothyroidotomy. (*B*) The corresponding level of incisions for tracheostomy and cricothryoidotomy. The tracheostomy incision is made approximately two fingerbreadths above the sternum.

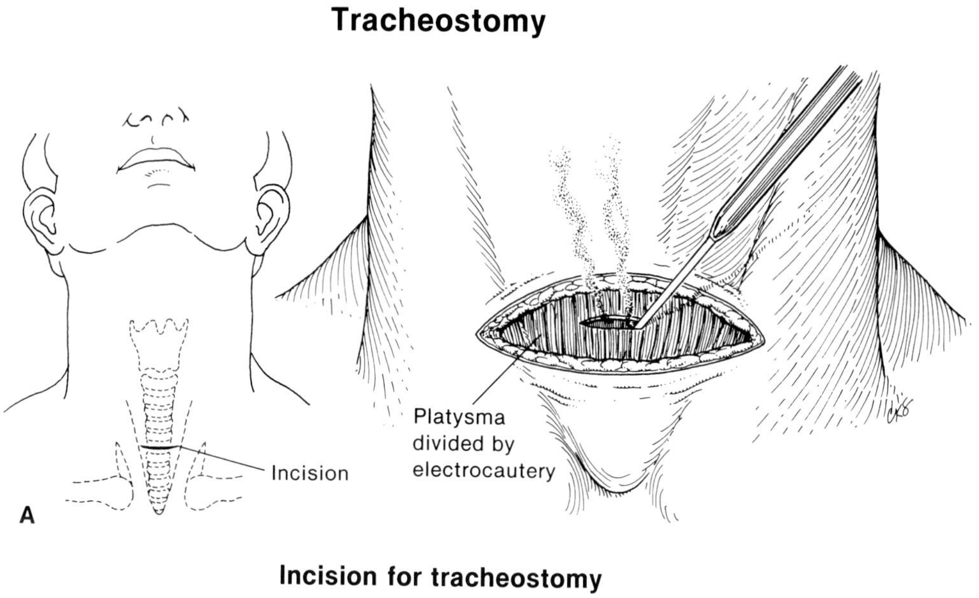

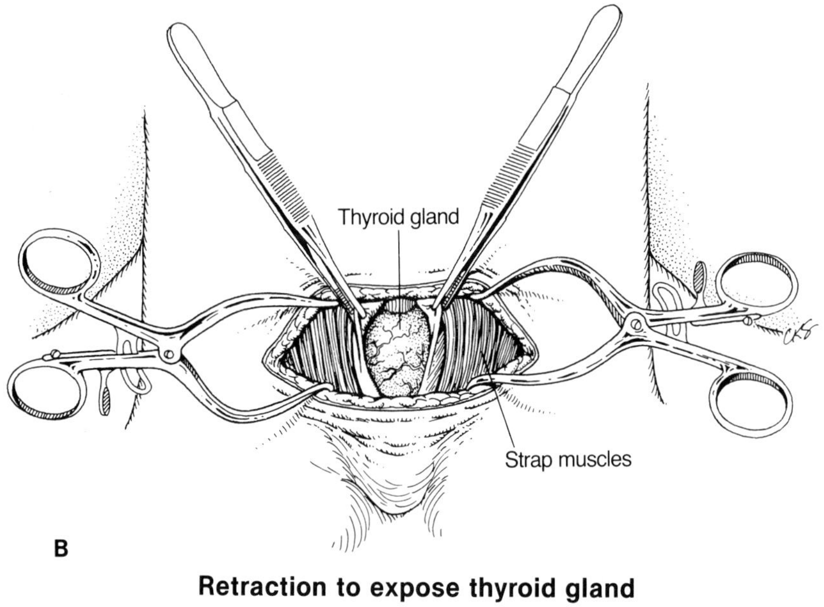

Figure 10–2 • The schematic sequence shows how to perform a tracheostomy. (***A***) The level of incision (see Fig. 10–1B) and the division of the superficial tissues by electrocautery. (***B***) Retraction and division of the strap muscles to expose the thyroid gland.
(continued)

The fascia between the strap muscles (sternohyoid, omohyoid, and sternothyroid) is divided vertically with scissors or electrocautery (see Fig. 10–2B). This is accomplished by picking up the tissue in the midline with forceps and incising this fascial layer after it has been retracted off the thyroid. One should make every effort to remain in the midline during this procedure, since the midline fascia between the strap muscles is relatively avascular (see Fig. 10–2B).

After division of this midline fascia in a vertical plane, the thyroid will be exposed (see Fig. 10–2B). In the performance of every tracheostomy, I completely divide the isthmus of the thyroid. This is done to define better the surgical anatomy of the trachea to assure that the stoma is placed between the second and third tracheal rings. Assurance that the tracheostome is placed between the second and third rings is of more than cosmetic interest, since higher placement may result in

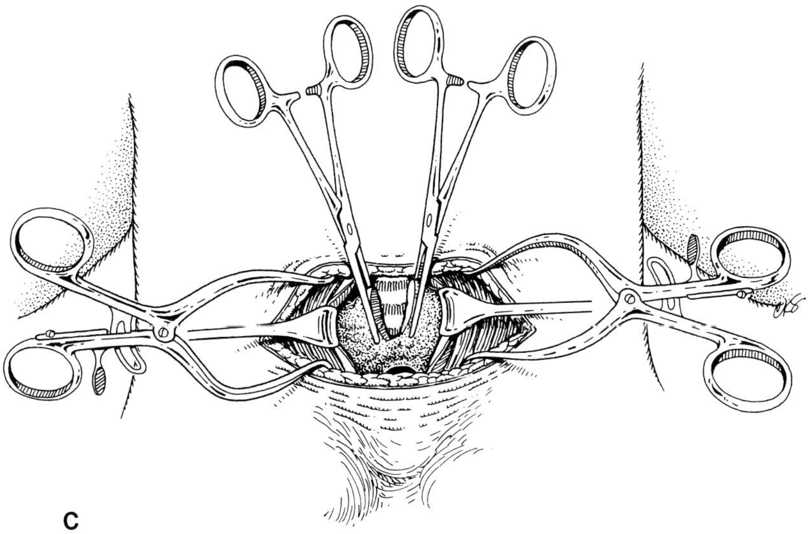

Figure 10–2 *(continued)*
(C) Clamping and division of the thyroid gland to expose the trachea.

subglottic stenosis and lower placement may result in erosion of the innominate artery, producing a tracheoinnominate artery fistula. Division of the thyroid isthmus also allows one to estimate better the circumference of the trachea in order to use an appropriately sized tracheostomy tube. Division of the thyroid isthmus should be initiated at its cephalad aspect. With blunt dissection, the superior aspect of the gland is identified and, again with blunt dissection using a cotton dissector, the thyroid isthmus is dissected from the trachea. Clamps are placed on either side of the intended area of division (see Fig. 10–2C), and the isthmus is sequentially clamped, divided, and ligated with suture ligatures of 2-0 absorbable suture material (Fig. 10–3A). One must be very meticulous about hemostasis, since the thyroid gland is quite well vascularized. With such sequential clamping, division, and ligature, the isthmus can be divided in three or four steps. With division of the thyroid, the tracheal rings are readily apparent and their relationship to the cricothyroid cartilage can be noted. The second tracheal ring is identified and marked with the electrocautery.

With the trachea thus prepared, the surgeon should select and adequately prepare and check the tracheostomy tube. Air is injected into the tracheal cuff to insure that there are no leaks. All the air is then removed from the tracheal cuff and the inner cannula is replaced with the blunt-tipped obturator. Water-soluble lubricating jelly is then applied to the tip tube to facilitate insertion into the tracheal incision at the appropriate time. The size of the tube selected depends on the size of the airway. Generally, the tracheal tube should occupy approximately three-fourths of the tracheal diameter. There is no correlation between airway size and the patient's race, age, height, or weight. However, women have a smaller larynx and a smaller trachea than men. Usually a size 8 tracheostomy tube is satisfactory for men and a 6 or 7 is satisfactory for women. However, a standard adult diagnostic fiberoptic bronchoscope will not fit through a size 7 tracheostomy tube.

After preparation of the tube, attention is again directed to the surgical field. Even if general anesthesia is used, the airway is infiltrated with 3–5 mL of 1% Xylocaine without epinephrine. This will anesthetize the airway somewhat and diminish the coughing and bucking that may occur when the airway is entered. A cruciate incision is then made with the transverse component of the incision being placed between the second and third tracheal ring (see Fig. 10–3B).

The cruciate incision is then dilated with the Trousseau dilator (see Fig. 10–3C). With the edges of the incision retracted with the dilator, the endotracheal tube (which is usually present; see indications) should be easily visualized within the depths of the tracheal incision. The anesthesiologist is then asked to deflate the endotracheal tube cuff and to slowly remove the endotracheal tube cephalad under the direct vision of the operating surgeons. When the tip of the endotracheal tube

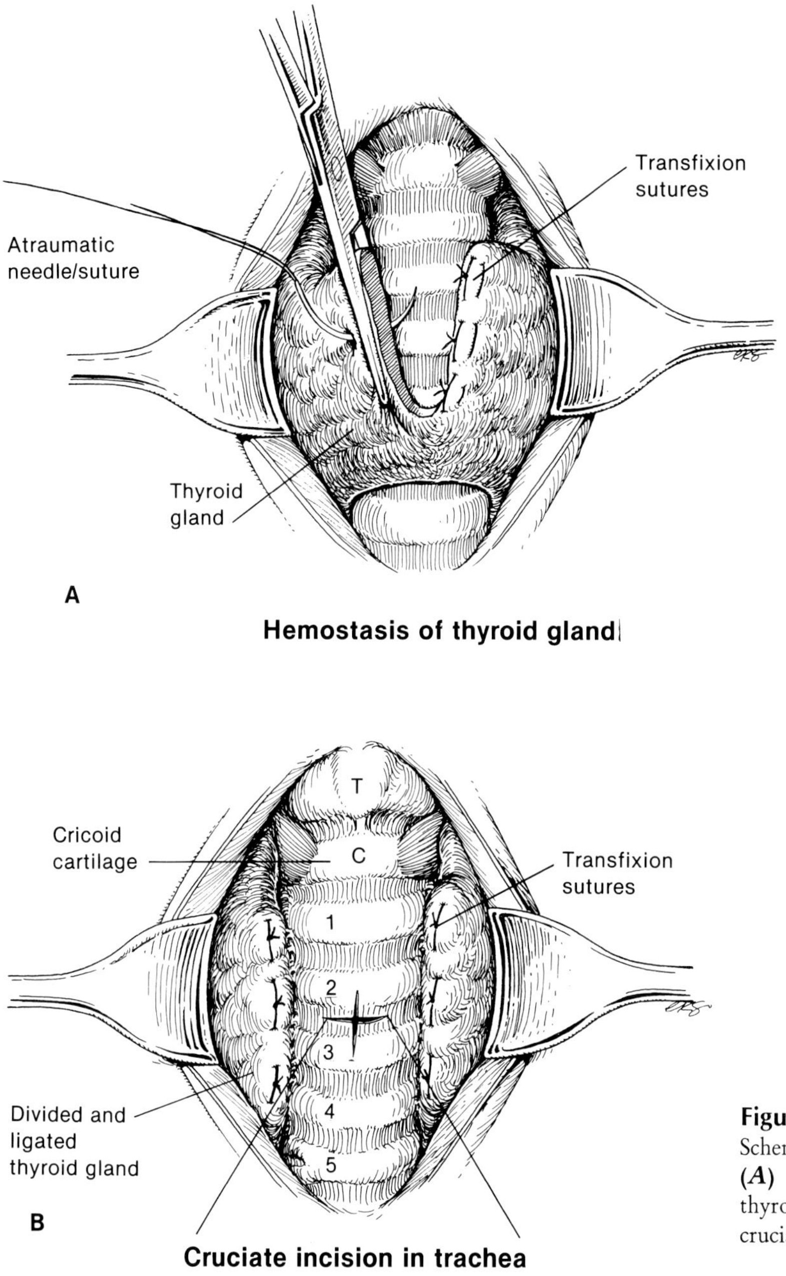

Figure 10–3 • (Continuation of Fig. 10–2. Schematic sequence of how to do a tracheostomy). **(*A*)** Suture ligation to obtain hemostasis of the thyroid gland. **(*B*)** The trachea is incised by a cruciate incision at the 2–3 tracheal ring space.
(continued)

is just barely visible in the cephalad portion of the tracheal incision, the prepared tracheostomy tube is inserted by directing the tube posteriorly at first; once the tip of the tube is safely within the tracheal incision, the tip is rotated 90° in the vertical plane, so that the tip that was initially pointed posteriorly faces caudad (see Fig. 10–3D). In an almost simultaneous movement the tube is pushed deeper into the trachea, being careful not to injure the membranous posterior wall of the trachea.

Immediately after the tube is inserted, I place a suction catheter into the lumen of the tube and aspirate through the suction catheter. The appearance of airway secretions in the suction catheter assures me that the tube has been placed safely into the airway. Next, the inner cannula is inserted into the tracheostomy tube and the adapter to the anesthesia machine is passed off to the anesthesiologist. The cuff is then inflated with a minimal occluding volume. After a satisfactory seal between

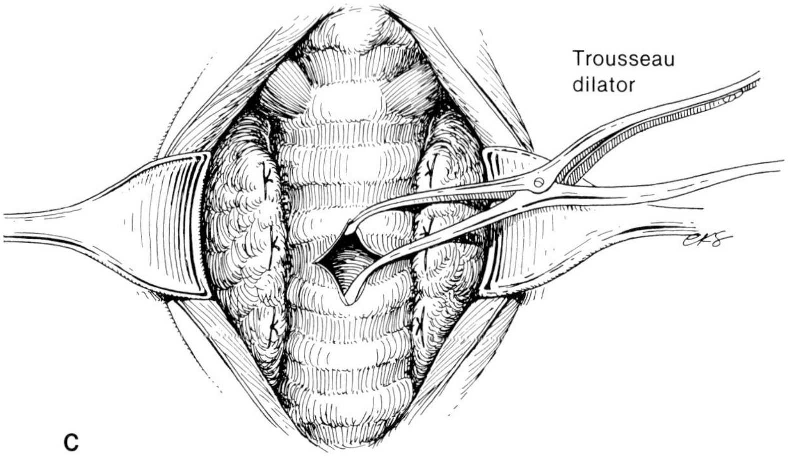

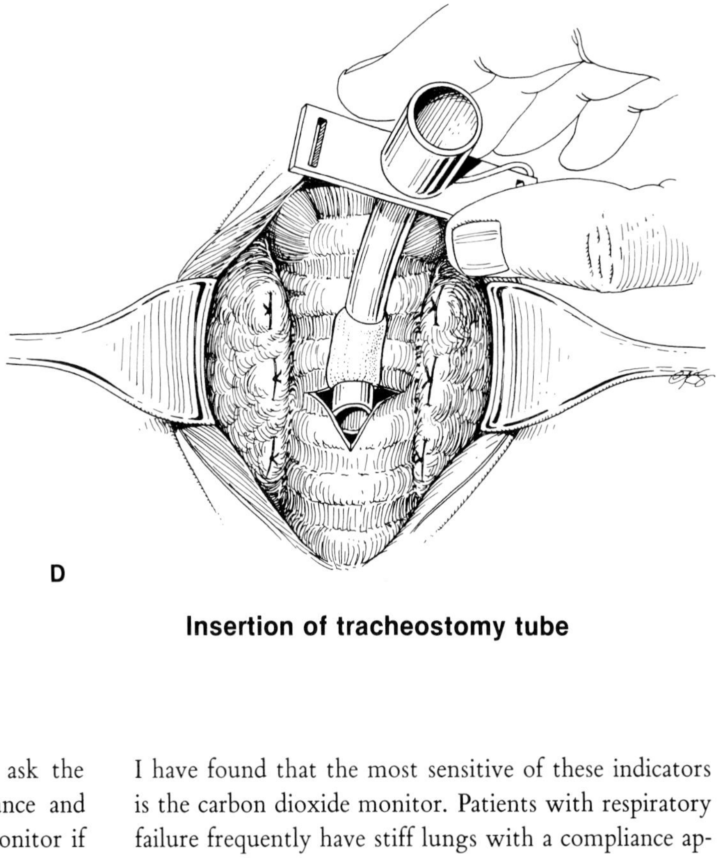

Figure 10–3 *(continued)*
(*C*) Dilation of the cruciate incision by a Trousseau dilator. **(*D*)** Insertion of the tracheostomy tube into the dilated cruciate incision.

the airway and the cuff has been obtained, I ask the anesthesiologist about the pulmonary compliance and have him or her connect the carbon dioxide monitor if this has not already been done. Ease of manual reservoir bag ventilation and the appearance of an end-tidal carbon dioxide concentration of greater than 1% assures me that I have inserted the tube correctly into the airway. It is also prudent to have an oxygen saturation monitor placed on the patient. Rapid desaturation, less than 1% carbon dioxide, and difficulties with ventilation suggest a tube malposition that must be corrected immediately. I have found that the most sensitive of these indicators is the carbon dioxide monitor. Patients with respiratory failure frequently have stiff lungs with a compliance approaching that of the subcutaneous tissues, and the anesthesiologist may not note a difference in compliance between the patient's subcutaneous tissue and the patient's lungs. If one suspects that the tube is malpositioned, it must quickly be replaced.

With the tube in satisfactory position, the tracheal incision is not sutured shut, but left open. The cotton "twill tape" is placed through both arms of the flange and then placed behind the patient's neck and tied on one side (as in Figure 10–4D).

a. Discussion

The skin incision may be placed vertically. A vertical incision is helpful to the inexperienced surgeon who may have to extend the incision, either inferiorly or superiorly, if he finds that his superficial landmarks were in error. The vertical incision heals as well as the horizontal and has the same cosmetic result.

Many authors[5,7,19,23] recommend a vertical rather than a cruciate incision in the trachea. A vertical incision is certainly acceptable in adults and preferable in children. Most authors deplore excision of a section of anterior trachea for placement of the tracheostomy tube. Webb[24] feels that excision of a piece of the anterior tracheal wall is primarily responsible for tracheal stenosis occurring at the stomal site.

B. *Cricothyroidotomy*

1. EQUIPMENT

The equipment necessary for cricothyroidotomy is similar to that needed for tracheostomy (see Table 10–3).

2. PATIENT POSITIONING AND PREPARATION

The patient is positioned, prepped, and draped in a similar fashion to tracheostomy. The important superficial landmarks for cricothyroidotomy include the tip of the thyroid cartilage and the area of the cricothyroid membrane that is the first depression or indentation that can be felt below the tip of the thyroid cartilage (see Fig. 10–4A, left panel).

3. OPERATIVE TECHNIQUE

Cricothyroidotomy can be performed under either local or general anesthesia. If performed under local anesthesia, the skin overlying the cricothyroidotomy is copiously infiltrated with 1% Xylocaine without epinephrine. A transverse incision is made in the skin (see Fig. 10–4A).

After the skin is incised, the subcutaneous tissue is dissected bluntly with a hemostat down to the level of the cricothyroid membrane (see Fig. 10–4A, right panel). The membrane is meticulously cleaned, being careful not to injure the vascular arcade that can be found in the most cephalad portion of the membrane. The membrane should be cleaned sufficiently to expose the right and left cricothyroideus muscle, which should be found laterally in the wound. A transverse incision is made in the cricothyroid membrane (see Fig. 10–4B) and the incision is dilated with a Trousseau dilator. The tube is inserted in a fashion identical to that described for tracheostomy (see Fig. 10–4C). As in tracheostomy, the same assurances must be made regarding tube placement: there is no rapid oxygen desaturation, there is an end-tidal carbon dioxide concentration of greater than 1%, and there are no major pulmonary compliance changes. The cricothyroidotomy tube is tied in as described for a tracheostomy tube (see Fig. 10–4D).

a. Discussion (Percutaneous Seldinger Technique and "Stab" Cricothyroidotomies)

There are two major variants to the procedure described for cricothyroidotomy. The first (which also applies to tracheostomy) is the percutaneously placed tube using a guide wire Seldinger technique. This has been described by Ciaglia[25] and Toye.[26] The procedure consists of locating the lumen of the trachea with a needle. Once the lumen is located, a guide wire is inserted into the trachea through the needle. The needle is removed so that the guide wire remains in place in the trachea and a skin incision is made next to the guide wire. The skin incision should be large enough to accommodate the tracheostomy tube. Dilators are then passed over the guide wire. Once the incision has been satisfactorily dilated, the cricothyroidotomy (or tracheostomy) tube is inserted.

The tube placed percutaneously is much smaller than most conventional tracheostomy tubes and therefore would prohibit the use of the bronchoscope.

The other variant of the cricothyroidotomy procedure is the "stab" cricothyroidotomy, which can be used by less experienced individuals in the performance of emergency surgical airway access. In essence, the skin incision and the incision into the cricothyroid membrane are made with a single stab. Once the incision is made, the scalpel handle is inserted fully into the wound and turned 90° to dilate the cricothyroid membrane stoma. This by itself will allow for an adequate airway if there is proximal airway obstruction. With dilation of the cricothyroidotomy with the scalpel handle, a tube can also be inserted. One must be very careful not to enter the posterior wall of the trachea with the "stab" incision.

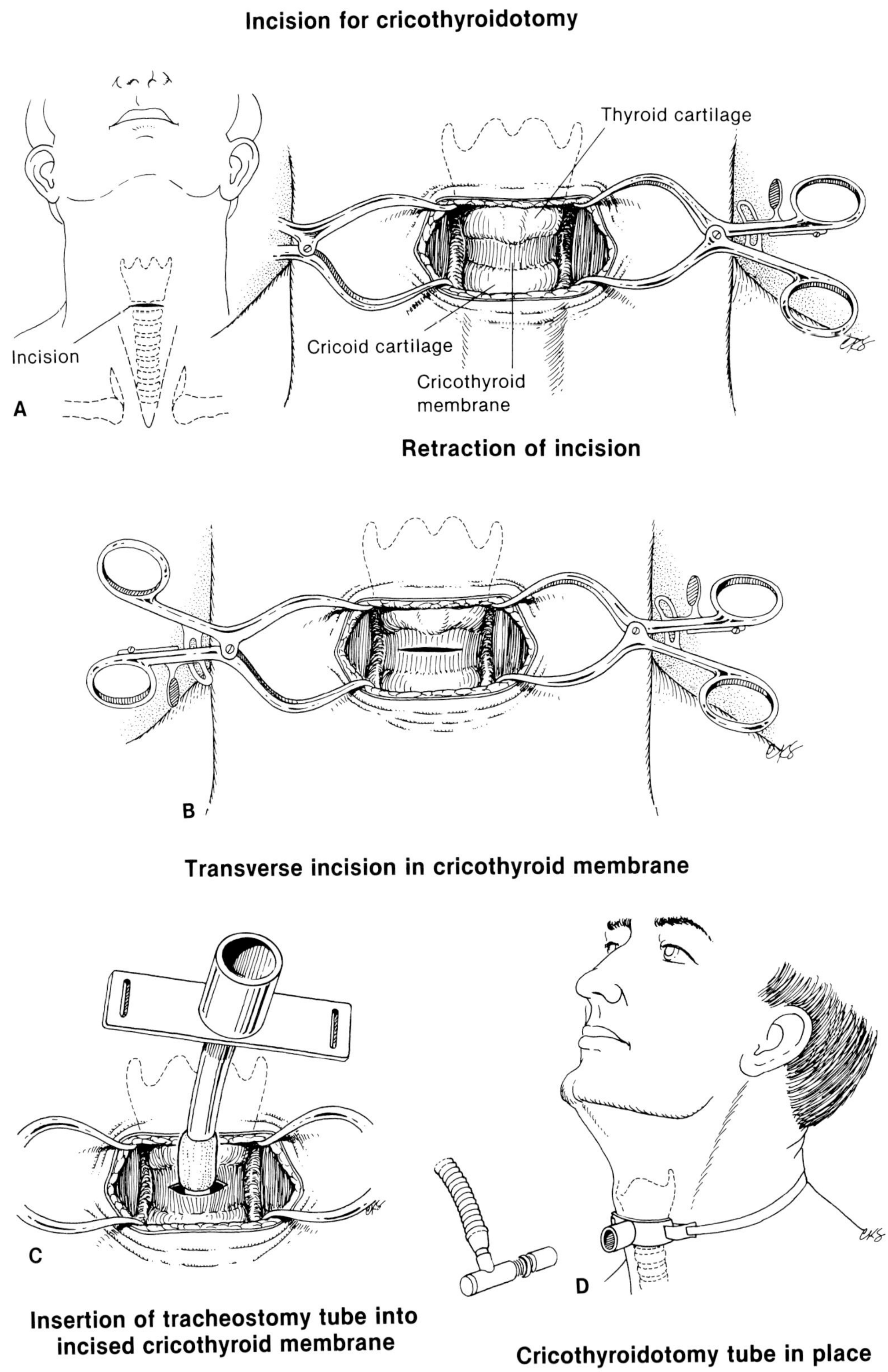

Figure 10–4 • Schematic sequence of how to do a cricothyroidotomy. (***A***) The left panel shows the level of the incision (over the cricothyroid membrane). The right panel shows the cricothryoid membrane, which has been cleaned of the retracted subcutaneous tissue. (***B***) A transverse incision in the cricothyroid membrane (which has been dilated with a Trousseau dilator). (***C***) The tracheostomy tube is then inserted into the incised cricothyroid membrane in a fashion identical to that described for a tracheostomy. (***D***) The tracheostomy tube is tied in place with umbilical tape.

III. COMPLICATIONS

Complications of tracheostomy and cricothyroidotomy are similar and will be grouped together under the general headings Intraoperative, Early Postoperative, and Late Postoperative Complications.

A. *Intraoperative Complications*

1. DEATH

The hospital mortality of patients undergoing tracheostomy is as high as 50% in some series.[1,10] This mortality is not due to the procedure itself, but to the condition of the patient. These patients are often critically ill with adult respiratory distress syndrome or multiorgan failure. The mortality rate for emergency surgical airway access is at least double that for elective airway access.[17]

2. HEMORRHAGE

Venous hemorrhage is most common and originates from communicating veins in the anterior jugular system or from the thyroid gland. Major arterial hemorrhage can come from the thyroid ima artery located near the isthmus of the thyroid. If the dissection strays from the midline, the carotid artery, jugular vein, or subclavian vessels can be injured.

3. AIR EMBOLISM

Air embolism can occur if a major vein is lacerated and intrathoracic pressure is less than ambient. This very rare complication is more likely to occur under local anesthesia with the patient breathing spontaneously.

4. PNEUMOTHORAX

Pneumothorax can occur with lateral dissection and is most frequent in children because the apical pleural dome of the child can reach as high as the area of dissection. Because of the potential for pneumothorax it is prudent to obtain a chest radiograph routinely at the completion of either cricothyroidotomy or tracheostomy.

5. OTHER COMPLICATIONS

False passage, malpositioned tube, injury to the recurrent laryngeal nerves, laceration of the posterior tracheal wall, lacerations of the esophagus, arterial and venous injury, and cardiac arrest have also been described.[4,9,18] Injury to the posterior wall of the trachea or the esophagus should be primarily repaired once it has been discovered. Esophageal repairs should be drained and the stomach prophylactically decompressed with a nasogastric tube. If air embolism occurs, the patient should be quickly placed in the left lateral decubitus Trendelenburg position. This position should prevent the air from entering the right ventricle. The air can then be aspirated through a central venous catheter.

B. *Early Postoperative Complications*

1. ATELECTASIS

Atelectasis is a frequent complication and is usually due to hypoventilation immediately after placement of the tracheostomy tube. It can be corrected by vigorous suctioning and hyperinflation in the early postoperative period.

2. HEMORRHAGE

Hemorrhage is usually due to inadequate hemostasis at the time of surgery and is often precipitated by the patient's cough. The bleeding is usually venous in nature and can usually be controlled with packing and may infrequently require a suture ligature.

3. INFECTION

Infections associated with surgical access to the airway include the following: tracheitis, tracheobronchitis, mediastinitis, pneumonia, and necrotizing soft tissue infections.[27] Tracheal, bronchial, and pulmonary infections are usually due to the increased frequency of aspiration associated with tracheostomy and cricothyroidotomy.[12] As such, the microflora of the infections includes those organisms resident in the pharynx, hypopharynx, and airway as well as those that colonize the wound and gain direct access to the airway. This combination of organisms (external colonizing plus resident ones) can set up a severe necrotizing synergistic soft tissue infection.[27]

The incidence of significant aspiration can be reduced by frequent suctioning of the pharynx and hypopharynx. The incidence of infections can also be reduced by using sterile technique when suctioning or changing the inner cannula. Snow[27] has suggested that severe soft tissue infections may be due to suture approximation of the skin and subcutaneous tissues around the tracheostome at the time of the operation. The use of prophylactic antibiotics has not been shown to decrease the incidence of infectious complications. Infections, when they occur in the airway, are thought to play a significant role in the development of late airway complications.

4. ACCIDENTAL EXTUBATION

Extubation may occur during violent coughing or during hyperflexion or hyperextension of the neck. Because the potential for this complication is greater during the immediate postoperative period, these patients should be observed for the first 48 hours in an ICU or in an intermediate care unit.

5. AIRWAY OBSTRUCTION

Obstruction is most frequently due to either blood clots or desiccated tracheobronchial secretions in the inner cannula. Accumulation of a clot can be avoided by frequent early suctioning. Desiccated secretions can be avoided by adequate humidification of the airway and frequent changing and cleaning of the inner cannula. Obstruction may also occur with malposition of the tube, resulting in apposition of the tip of the tube against the anterior tracheal wall. This can be corrected by simply repositioning the tube.

C. *Late Postoperative Complications*

1. TRACHEOESOPHAGEAL FISTULA

Tracheoesophageal fistula is a result of ischemic necrosis of the posterior tracheal wall with erosion into the esophagus. This is generally due to mechanical factors caused by tube movement, high intracuff pressures, and the presence of a nasogastric tube.[1,8] Local infection may also play a role. The signs that a tracheoesophageal fistula may be present include increased secretions in the airway, violent coughing associated with swallowing, and bile staining or tube feedings in the tracheal aspirate. Tracheoesophageal fistulas are treated surgically with closure of the esophageal and tracheal communications and interposition of a muscle flap.[28] Early removal of the nasogastric tube, reduction in tube movement, and monitoring of cuff pressure should minimize the chances of this rare complication.

2. TRACHEOINNOMINATE ARTERY FISTULA

Tracheoinnominate artery fistula occurs when the innominate artery is eroded by the tracheostomy tube, either at the stomal site[29] or at the cuff site.[30] The occurrence of transient minor bleeding (''herald'' bleed) and tracheal cannula pulsation are, according to Jones,[30] early premonitory signs of tracheoinnominate artery fistula and deserve investigation. Diagnostic procedures, including arteriography and bronchoscopy, however, have been unrewarding.[30] This disastrous complication most commonly occurs when the tracheal incision is inadvertently placed below the fourth tracheal ring. Without rapid intervention, the patient will die from exsanguination and airway obstruction. The priorities are, therefore, to maintain a patent airway and to control hemorrhage. Both priorities can be obtained with hyperinflation of the tracheostomy tube cuff if the fistula occurs at the cuff site. Hyperinflation of the cuff will occlude the innominate artery and allow suctioning of residual blood through the tracheostomy tube. If hyperinflation of the cuff does not control the hemorrhage, one must assume that the bleeding is not at the cuff site but rather at the stomal site. The tracheostomy tube should then be removed and the airway controlled with orotracheal intubation. An incision is then quickly made at the tracheostome, through which a finger is inserted and blunt dissection is carried out in a plane anterior to the trachea down to the level of the innominate artery (immediately behind the sternum). Control of the artery is then obtained by finger compression against the posterior aspect of the sternum.[29] After the airway has been controlled and hemorrhage stopped, definitive therapy must be carried out. This requires resection of the innominate artery and closure of the trachea.

3. AIRWAY COMPLICATIONS

a. *Subglottic Stenosis*

Subglottic stenosis occurs in approximately 2% of cricothyroidotomies[22] and rarely after tracheostomy. In virtually all instances it is a complication of prolonged translaryngeal intubation. It appears to be more frequent in neonates because the subglottic region is the narrowest part of the airway in the child.[31]

b. *Tracheal Stenosis*

Tracheal stenosis may occur at the stomal site or at the cuff site. When it occurs at the stomal site it is likely due to excision of a section of anterior trachea for the stoma.[24] The use of the cruciate or vertical incision has virtually eliminated stenosis at the stomal site. When it occurs at the cuff site, tracheal stenosis is the result of ischemic necrosis produced by high pressures in the cuff. The incidence of this complication has decreased in recent years because of the use of the high-volume, low-pressure cuff.[32] Use of minimal occluding volume or minimal occluding pressure to achieve a seal at the cuff during positive pressure ventilation can also be expected to reduce this complication.

Airway complications can present minutes to months after the decannulation.[17] Patients who present with exertional dyspnea after a tracheostomy are frequently misdiagnosed as having asthma or tracheobronchitis. Any patient with respiratory difficulty after tracheostomy requires evaluation of the airway. Otherson[33] suggests an especially aggressive approach in children. If the tracheostomy tube has been in place for more than 2 weeks, he advocates early bronchoscopy at the time of extubation, with local injection of steroids, systemic administration of steroids, and the use of a Portex stent for 72 hours after decannulation.

The diagnosis of tracheal stenosis can be obtained by soft tissue tomography of the neck or by magnetic resonance imaging (MRI). Laryngeal injuries can be diagnosed utilizing computed tomography scanning or MRI. Bronchoscopy with laser therapy provides a means of follow-up and treatment.

The treatment of tracheal stenosis often requires segmental resection. Subglottic stenosis and tracheal stenosis can be treated with laser therapy.[17]

4. SUMMARY

Significant morbidity has been associated with surgical access to the airway. The complication rate varies between 6% and 51%.[1,2] The high complication rate is often wrongly attributed to the procedure of tracheostomy or cricothyroidotomy when in fact complications are due to the underlying disease process for which tracheostomy is performed, or to the fact that the patient has undergone prolonged translaryngeal intubation prior to the tracheostomy or cricothyroidotomy. A well-done tracheostomy or cricothyroidotomy should be associated with no mortalities and a morbidity rate of less than 20%.

IV. REFERENCES

1. Colice GL. Prolonged intubation versus tracheostomy in the adult. J Int Care Med 2:85–102, 1987.
2. Stock MC, Woodward CG, Shapiro BA, et al. Perioperative complications of elective tracheostomy in critically ill patients. Crit Care Med 14:861–864, 1986.
3. McGill J, Clinton JE, Ruiz E. Cricothyroidotomy in the emergency department. Ann Emerg Med 11:361–364, 1982.
4. Beatrous WP. Tracheostomy: Its expanded indications and its present status. Laryngoscope 78:3–55, 1968.
5. Heffner JE, Miller KS, Sahn SA. Tracheostomy in the intensive care unit. Chest 90:269–274, 1986.
6. Miller JD, Kapp JP. Complications of tracheostomies in neurosurgical patients. Surg Neurol 22:186–188, 1985.
7. Hardy KL. Tracheostomy: Indications, technics, and tubes. A Reappraisal. Am J Surg 126:300–310, 1973.
8. Stemmer EA, Oliver C, Carey JP, Connolly JE. Fatal complications of tracheostomy. Am J Surg 131:288–290, 1976.
9. McClelland RM. Complications of tracheostomy. Br Med J 2:567–569, 1965.
10. Enfors B, Lindelof G. Tracheostomy in general surgery. Acta Chir Scand 133:217–221, 1966.
11. Stauffer JL, Olson DE, Petty TL. Complications and consequences of endotracheal intubation and tracheostomy: A prospective study of 150 critically ill adult patients. Am J Med 70:65–76, 1981.
12. Elnaggar M, Sadagopan S, Levine H, et al. Factors influencing choice between tracheostomy and prolonged translaryngeal intubation in acute respiratory failure: A prospective study. Anesth Analg 55:195–201, 1976.
13. Shackford SR. Blunt chest trauma: The intensivist's perspective. J Int Care Med 1:125–136, 1986.
14. Guilleminault C, Simmons FB, Motta J, et al. Obstructive sleep apnea syndrome and tracheostomy: Long-term follow-up experience. Arch Intern Med 141:985–988, 1981.
15. Conway WA, Victor LD, Magilligan DJ, et al. Adverse effects of tracheostomy for sleep apnea. JAMA 246:347–350, 1981.
16. Chew JY, Cantrell RW. Tracheostomy: Complications and their management. Arch Otolaryngol 96:538–545, 1972.
17. Heffner JE, Miller KS, Sahn SA. Tracheostomy in the intensive care unit, Part 2: Complications. Chest 90:430–436, 1986.
18. Kenan PD. Complications associated with tracheostomy: Prevention and treatment. Otolaryngol Clin North Am 12:807–817, 1979.
19. Tepas JJ, Heroy JH, Shermeta DW, Haller JA. Tracheostomy in neonates and small infants: Problems and pitfalls. Surgery 89:635–639, 1981.
20. Brantigan CO, Grow JB. Cricothyroidotomy: Elective use in respiratory problems requiring tracheotomy. J Thorac Cardiovasc Surg 71:72–81, 1976.
21. Sise MJ, Shackford SR, Cruickshank JC, et al. Cricothyroidotomy for long term tracheal access. Ann Surg 200:13–17, 1984.
22. Cole RR, Aguilar EA. Cricothyroidotomy versus tracheotomy: An otolaryngologist's perspective. Laryngoscope 98:131–135, 1988.
23. Dunham MC, LaMonica C. Prolonged tracheal intubation in the trauma patient. J Trauma 24:120–124, 1984.
24. Webb WR, Ozdemir IA, Ikins PM, Parker FB. Surgical management of tracheal stenosis. Ann Surg 179:819–824, 1974.
25. Ciaglia P, Firsching R, Syniec C. Elective percutaneous dilatational tracheostomy: A new simple bedside procedure. Chest 87:715–719, 1985.

26. Toye FJ, Weinstein JD. Clinical experience with percutaneous tracheostomy and cricothyroidotomy in 100 patients. J Trauma 26:1034–1040, 1986.
27. Snow N, Richardson JD, Flint LM. Management of necrotizing tracheostomy infections. J Thorac Cardiovasc Surg 82:341–344, 1981.
28. Thomas AN. Management of tracheoesophageal fistula caused by cuffed tracheal tubes. Am J Surg 124:181–189, 1972.
29. Utley JR, Singer MM, Roe BB, et al. Definitive management of innominate artery hemorrhage complicating tracheostomy. JAMA 220:577–579, 1972.
30. Jones JW, Reynolds M. Hewitt RL, Drapanas T. Tracheo-innominate artery erosion: Successful surgical management of a devastating complication. Ann Surg 184:194–204, 1976.
31. Quiney RE, Gould SJ. Subglottic stenosis: A clinicopathological study. Clin Otolaryngol 10:315–327, 1985.
32. Grillo HC, Cooper JD, Geffin B, Pontoppidan H. A low-pressure cuff for tracheostomy tubes to minimize tracheal injury: A comparative clinical trial. J Thoracic Cardiovasc Surg 62:898–906, 1971.
33. Otherson HB. Intubation injuries of the trachea in children: Management and prevention. Ann Surg 189:601–606, 1979.

Chapter 11

•

Jonathan L. Benumof, MD

Separation of the Two Lungs (with Special Emphasis on Double-Lumen Tube Intubation)

OUTLINE

I. Introduction

The complete functional separation of the two lungs is often the most important consideration for patients undergoing thoracic surgery. The procedure can occasionally be life-saving in patients with asymmetrical adult respiratory distress syndrome (ARDS) or severe unilateral lung disease. Newly introduced disposable plastic double-lumen tubes that are relatively nontraumatic and easy to insert and the advent of fiberoptic bronchoscopy, which makes location of a double-lumen tube under direct vision possible and therefore a precise, repeatable, low-risk maneuver, have greatly increased the efficacy and use of double-lumen tubes. This chapter sequentially discusses the indications for separation of the two lungs and which procedures (see later) are best for patients of various ages. Since double-lumen tube intubation is by far the most common method of lung separation, the majority of the chapter is devoted to conventional techniques of double-lumen tube insertion and determination of position, use of the fiberoptic bronchoscope to insert a double-lumen tube, and determination of precise double-lumen tube position by fiberoptic bronchoscopy. Endobronchial intubation with single-lumen tube and bronchial blockers are considered next. The discussion of lung separation focuses on the management of one-lung ventilation (to facilitate anesthesia for thoracic surgery) and differential lung ventilation (in the intensive care unit [ICU]). The chapter concludes with the complications of the various lung separation procedures.

II. Indications for Separation of the Two Lungs

There are several absolute and relative indications for separation of the two lungs during thoracic operations and in the ICU (Table 11–1).

Table 11–1 • Indications for Separation of the Two Lungs (Double-Lumen Tube Intubation) and/or One-Lung Ventilation

Absolute

1. Isolation of one lung from the other to avoid spillage or contamination
   A. Infection
   B. Massive hemorrhage
2. Control of the distribution of ventilation
   A. Bronchopleural fistula
   B. Bronchopleural cutaneous fistula
   C. Surgical opening of a major conducting airway
   D. Giant unilateral lung cyst or bulla
   E. Tracheobronchial tree disruption
3. Unilateral bronchopulmonary lavage
   A. Pulmonary alveolar proteinosis

Relative

1. Surgical exposure—high priority
   A. Thoracic aortic aneurysm
   B. Pneumonectomy
   C. Upper lobectomy
2. Surgical exposure—lower priority
   A. Middle and lower lobectomies and subsegmental resections
   B. Esophageal resection
   C. Thoracoscopy
   D. Procedures on the thoracic spine
3. Postcardiopulmonary bypass status after removal of totally occluding chronic unilateral pulmonary emboli
4. Differential lung ventilation in unilateral ARDS

A. *Absolute Indications*

Separation of the two lungs for any of the absolute indications discussed here should be considered a life-saving maneuver, because failure to separate the two lungs under any of these conditions could result in a life-threatening situation. There are three absolute indications for separating the two lungs (see Table 11–1). First, separation of one lung from the other is absolutely necessary to prevent spillage of pus or blood from an infected (abscessed) lung or a bleeding lung, respectively, to a noninvolved lung. Acute contamination of a lung with either blood or pus from the other lung usually results in severe massive (bilateral) atelectasis, pneumonia, and sepsis. Second, a number of unilateral lung problems can prevent adequate ventilation of the other noninvolved side. A large bronchopleural or bronchopleural cutaneous fistula or a surgically opened conducting airway has such a low resistance to gas flow that a tidal inspiration delivered by positive pressure will exit via the low-resistance pathway, and it will become impossible to ventilate the other, more normal lung adequately. A giant unilateral bulla or cyst may rupture if exposed to positive-pressure ventilation of a lung and result in a tension pneumothorax or pneumomediastinum. Finally, positive-pressure ventilation of a lung with a tracheobronchial tree disruption can cause dissection of gas into the pulmonary interstitial space or mediastinum, resulting in a tension pneumomediastinum. Third, separation of the two lungs is absolutely necessary to perform unilateral bronchopulmonary lavage in patients with pulmonary alveolar proteinosis (and rarely, asthma and cystic fibrosis).

The absolute indications for one-lung ventilation in pediatric patients are the same as those for adults. However, by far the most common indication for lung separation in neonates and children is the presence of infection in one lung, which could contaminate the other lung. The infections consist of lung abscess, empyema, and hydatid cysts. Lung abscess may be caused by foreign bodies, infection within true congenital lung cysts, lung sequestration, and hypoplastic lobes and may occur following pneumonia. Other absolute indications for lung separation in pediatric patients consist of infected bronchiectasis and major bronchopleural fistula.

B. *Relative Indications*

There are a large number of relative indications for separation of the two lungs, and they are for the purpose of facilitating surgical exposure by collapsing the lung in the operative hemithorax and for dealing with unilateral lung disease problems. The surgical exposure relative indications can be divided into high-priority and lower-priority categories (see Table 11–1). In the high-priority category, repair of a thoracic aortic aneurysm is usually the most important, because it requires exposure of the thoracic aorta as it runs the entire length of the left hemithorax. A pneumonectomy, especially if performed through a median sternotomy,[1] is greatly aided by the wide exposure of the lung hilum that is afforded by collapse of the operative lung. Similarly, an upper lobectomy, which is technically the most difficult lobectomy, and many mediastinal exposures may be made much easier by eliminating ventilation to the lung on the side of the procedure. The surgical items in the lower-priority category do not routinely require collapse of the lung on the operative side, but still they significantly aid surgical exposure and eliminate the need for the surgeon to handle (retract, compress, pack away) the operative lung. Severe intraoperative retraction of the lung on the operated side can traumatize the operative lung and impair gas exchange both intra-[2,3] and postoperatively.[4,5] The lower-priority items consist of middle and lower lobectomies, less extensive pulmonary resections, thoracic spinal procedures that are approached anteriorly through the chest, and esophageal surgery. However, even relatively small operations such as wedge and segmental resections benefit by double-lumen tube insertion because of the ability to alternate easily and quickly between lung collapse and inflation, which is sometimes required to better visualize lung morphology and to facilitate identification and separation of important planes and fissures. Examination of the pleural space (thoracoscopy) is considerably aided by collapse of the ipsilateral lung. An anterior or axillary approach to surgical procedures on the thoracic spine is also greatly aided by the collapse of the lung on the side of the approach. The separation of the lungs following removal of totally occluding and predominantly unilateral chronic pulmonary emboli (postcardiopulmonary bypass) can be very helpful because of the possibility of massive transudation of hemorrhagic fluid across the alveolar capillary membrane in the region of the lung supplied by the previously occluded vessel (reperfusion of a previously and chronically nonperfused vascular bed). Should significant and predominantly unilateral postthromboembolectomy post-cardiopulmonary bypass pulmonary edema occur, the patient should be returned to cardiopulmonary bypass, and a double-lumen endotracheal tube should be inserted so that differential lung ventilation may be used. Finally, unilateral or asymmetrical ARDS can be another strong relative indication for double-lumen tube intubation (to administer differential lung ventilation).

C. *Indications for the Various Methods of Lung Separation (Double-Lumen Tube Intubation, Bronchial Blocker, Endobronchial Intubation with a Single-Lumen Tube)*

Double-lumen endotracheal tubes have become the technique of choice for most cases of lung separation in adults and older children (older than 10 years of age) and will be discussed here in great detail. Bronchial blockers and endobronchial tubes are not often used today and are only briefly described at the end of the chapter. Double-lumen tubes are favored over bronchial blockers and endobronchial tubes for lung separation for many reasons. First, double-lumen tubes are relatively easily placed by even inexperienced anesthesiologists, whereas a much higher degree of skill is required to position bronchial blockers and endobronchial tubes correctly. Second, double-lumen tubes allow easy, repeated, and rapid conversion from two-lung ventilation to one-lung ventilation and vice versa at any time during surgery, whereas bronchial blockers and endobronchial tubes preclude two-lung ventilation. Third, double-lumen tubes allow for suctioning of both lungs, whereas bronchial blockers and endobronchial tubes preclude suctioning of the collapsed lung. Fourth, double-lumen tubes allow continuous positive airway pressure (CPAP) to be applied to the nonventilated lung, whereas with bronchial blockers and endobronchial tubes no ventilatory maneuvers can be used on the lung under operation. Rarely, in adult patients with unilateral hemoptysis and in adult patients who cannot be taken off a ventilator for even a minute, bronchial blockers, endobronchial intubation, or both may be the procedure of choice for lung separation.

The smallest double-lumen tube manufactured is 28 French (9 mm outer diameter [OD]) and cannot be used in children less than 10–12 years of age. Consequently, the procedure of choice for lung separation in children between the ages of 2 and 10 years is endobronchial intubation with a cuffed single-lumen tube and/or use of bronchial blocker. The smallest cuffed single-lumen tube manufactured is 5 mm and cannot be used in children less than 1 or 2 years of age. Uncuffed single-lumen endobronchial tubes cannot be relied on to effectively separate the lungs for two reasons: first, uncuffed tubes may permit spillage from a contaminated lung to an unsoiled lung; second, uncuffed tubes may not remain stationary within the very short mainstem bronchus. (It is difficult to prevent either upper lobe obstruction or decannulation of the mainstem bronchus.) Consequently, the procedure of choice for lung separation for neonates through 1- to 2-year-olds is use of a bronchial blocker.

III. How to Separate the Two Lungs

A. *Double-Lumen Tube Intubation*

1. Left- and Right-Sided Double-Lumen Endotracheal Tubes

Double-lumen tubes are essentially two catheters bonded together and each lumen is intended to ventilate one of the two lungs. Double-lumen tubes are made as left- and right-sided tubes. A left-sided tube means that the left lung catheter is placed into the left mainstem bronchus, whereas the right lung catheter ends in the trachea. Therefore, for the left-sided tube, the left lung catheter is longer than the right lung catheter (Fig. 11–1). A right-sided tube means that the right lung catheter is placed into the right mainstem bronchus, whereas the left lung catheter ends in the trachea; therefore, for a right-sided tube, the right lung catheter is longer than the left lung catheter (see Fig. 11–1). All the double-lumen tubes have a proximal cuff for the trachea and a distal cuff for a mainstem bronchus; the endobronchial cuff causes separation and sealing off of the two lungs from each other, and the tracheal cuff causes separation and sealing off of the lungs from the environ-

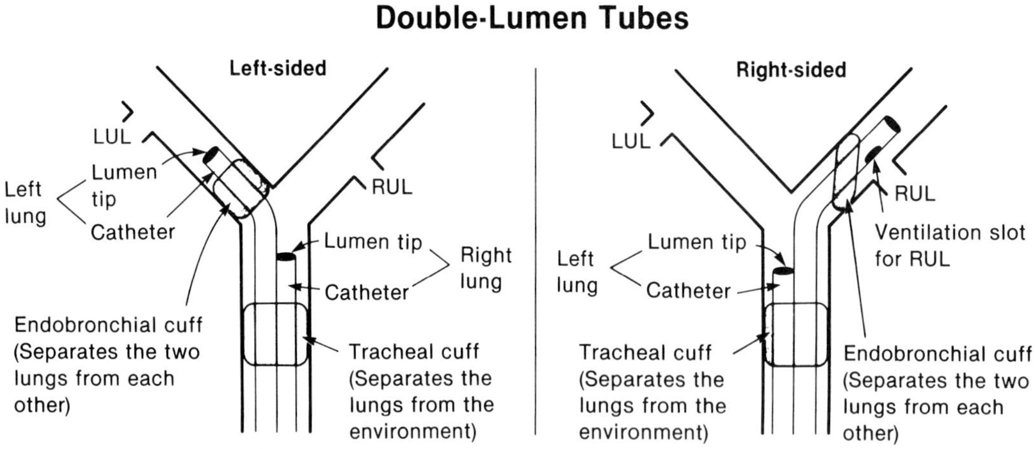

Figure 11–1 • This schematic diagram depicts the essential features and parts of right-sided and left-sided double-lumen tubes. (*RUL = right upper lobe; LUL = left upper lobe.*) (Reproduced with permission from Benumof JL. Anesthesia for Thoracic Surgery. Philadelphia, WB Saunders, 1987, Fig. 9–3, p. 227.)

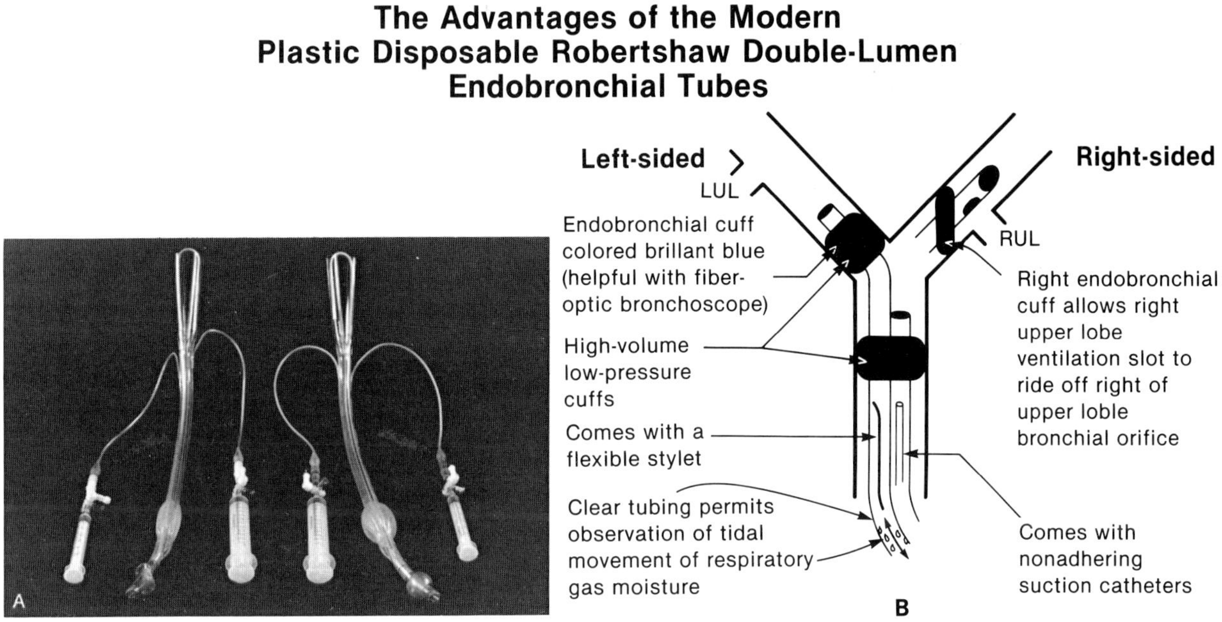

Figure 11–2 • (***A***) Photograph of left-sided and right-sided disposable Robertshaw double-lumen tubes. (***B***) Schematic diagram depicts the advantages of left-sided and right-sided modern plastic disposable Robertshaw double-lumen endobronchial tubes. Both lumens of the left-sided double-lumen tube are shown, whereas only the distal endobronchial lumen of the right-sided double-lumen tube is shown. (Reproduced with permission from Benumof JL. Anesthesia for Thoracic Surgery. Philadelphia, WB Saunders, 1987, Fig. 9–7, p. 231.)

ment. The part of the right lung catheter of the right-sided double-lumen tube that is in the right mainstem bronchus must be slotted to allow for ventilation of the right upper lobe because the right mainstem bronchus is too short to accommodate both the right endobronchial cuff and the very tip of the right lumen (see Fig. 11–1). All the double-lumen endotracheal tubes have two curves that lie in planes approximately 90° apart from one another. The two curves are designed to facilitate placement of the distal catheter tip into the appropriate mainstem bronchus.

a. *The Modern, Plastic, Disposable Robertshaw Double-Lumen Endotracheal Tube*

The Robertshaw-type tube (lumina are D-shaped, lie side by side, and therefore provide the largest possible lumina in order to decrease airway resistance and facilitate removal of secretions) is now made of a clear, nontoxic, tissue-implantable plastic (denoted by the marking Z-79) and is disposable (Fig. 11–2). The tubes are made (by the Mallinkrodt, Rusch, and Sheridan Companies) in sizes 41, 39, 37, 35, and 28 French (internal diameter of each lumen is approximately 6.5, 6.0, 5.5, 5.0, and 4.5 mm, respectively). These tubes are relatively easy to insert and have appropriate end-of-lumen and cuff arrangements that minimize lobar obstruction. The endobronchial cuff is colored brilliant blue, which is a very important feature for recognition of proper tube position when using a fiberoptic bronchoscope. The ends of both lumina have a black radiopaque line, which is an essential recognition marker when viewing a chest radiograph. The tubes have high-volume, low-pressure tracheal and endobronchial cuffs. The National Catheter Corporation (Mallinkrodt) tube has a slanted, dough-nut-shaped endobronchial cuff on the right-sided double-lumen tube that allows the right upper lobe ventilation slot to ride off (away from) the right upper lobe orifice, which minimizes the chance of right upper lobe obstruction by the tube. The clear tubing is helpful because it permits continuous observation of the tidal movement of respiratory moisture as well as observation of secretions from each lung. The tubes are packaged with malleable stylets and are relatively easy to insert and to position. These tubes have large internal- to external-diameter ratios and therefore allow suctioning to be done relatively easily. They are packaged with their own nonadhering suction catheters. The large internal-to external-diameter ratio also provides a relatively low resistance to ventilation. For these reasons the Robertshaw-type tubes are now considered by far the double-lumen endotracheal tube of choice by most anesthesiologists.

A left-sided double-lumen endotracheal tube should be used for right thoracotomies requiring collapse of the right lung and ventilation of the left lung (Fig. 11–3). A left- or right-sided tube may be used for left thoracotomies requiring collapse of the left lung and ventilation of the right lung (see Fig. 11–3). However, since the right upper lobe ventilation slot of a right-sided tube has to be closely apposed to the right upper lobe orifice for unobstructed right upper lobe ventilation to occur, and since there is considerable anatomic variation in the exact position of the right upper lobe orifice—and therefore length of the right mainstem bronchus—the margin of safety in positioning a right-sided double-lumen tube is much less than the margin of safety in positioning a left-sided double-lumen tube.[6–8] In other words, use of a right-sided tube for left lung collapse has a much higher risk of inadequate right upper lobe ventilation compared to inadequate left upper lobe ventilation when using a left-sided double-lumen tube for right or left lung collapse.[6–8] For this reason, a left-sided tube is preferable for most cases requiring one-lung ventilation. If clamping of the left mainstem bronchus is necessary, the tube can be withdrawn at that time into the trachea (this requires a modicum of communication between surgeon and anesthesiologist) and then used in the same manner as a single-lumen endotracheal tube (ventilate the right lung with both lumina) (see Fig. 11–3). Contraindications to use of a left-sided double-lumen tube are carinal and proximal left mainstem bronchial lesions that could be traumatized by the passage of a left-sided tube. These lesions include strictures, endoluminal tumors, tracheobronchial disruptions, and compression of the airway by an external mass. The largest tube that can comfortably pass the glottis should be used, since a relatively small double-lumen tube may require excessive cuff volume for an endobronchial cuff seal to be obtained (see the discussion of endobronchial cuff problems in Section III.A.4 and Fig. 11–9) and may cause difficulty with suctioning secretions.

In summary, the new plastic disposable Robertshaw-type double-lumen tubes are by far the most com-

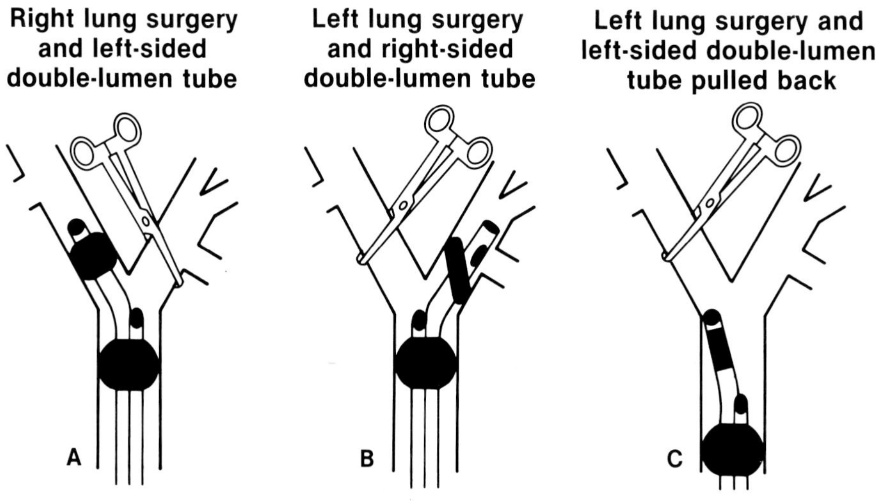

Figure 11–3 • Use of left-sided and right-sided double-lumen tubes for left and right lung surgery (as indicated by the clamp). When surgery is going to be performed on the right lung, a left-sided double-lumen tube should be used. (***A***). When surgery is going to be performed on the left lung, a right-sided double-lumen tube can be used (***B***). However, because of uncertainty as to the alignment of the right upper lobe ventilation slot to the right upper lobe orifice, a left-sided double-lumen tube can also be used for left lung surgery (***C***). If the left lung surgery requires a clamp to be placed high on the left mainstem bronchus, the left endobronchial cuff should be deflated, the left-sided double-lumen tube pulled back into the trachea, and the right lung ventilated through both of the lumens (use the double-lumen tube as a single-lumen tube). (Reproduced with permission from Benumof JL. Anesthesia for Thoracic Surgery. Philadelphia, WB Saunders, 1987, Fig. 9–8, p. 232.)

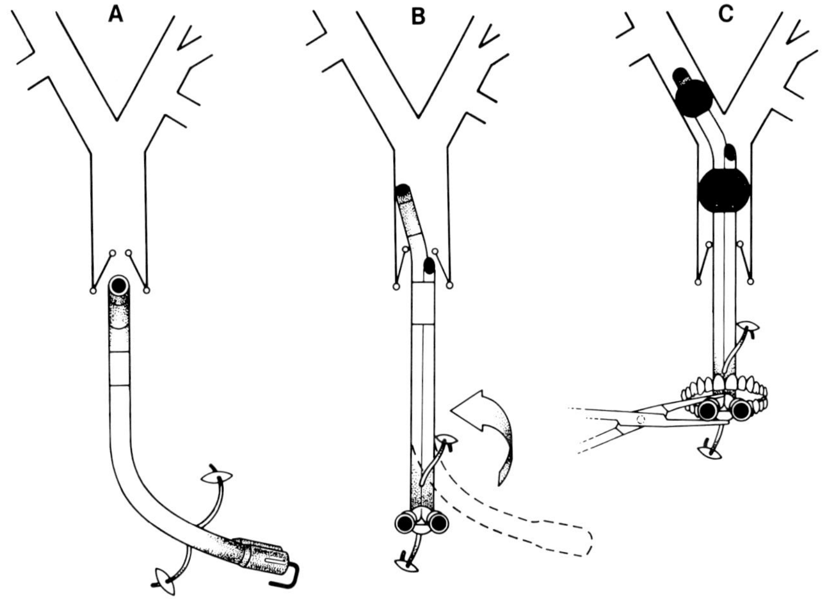

Figure 11–4 • This schematic diagram depicts the passage of the left-sided double-lumen tube in a supine patient. (***A***) The tube is held with the distal curvature concave anteriorly and the proximal curve concave to the right and in a plane parallel to the floor. The tube is then inserted through the vocal cords until the left cuff passes the vocal cords. The stylet is then removed. (***B***) The tube is rotated 90° counterclockwise so that the distal curvature is concave anteriorly and the proximal curvature is concave to the left and in a plane parallel to the floor. (***C***) The tube is inserted until either a moderate resistance to further passage is encountered or the end of the common molding of the two lumina is at the teeth. Both cuffs are then inflated, and both lungs are ventilated. Finally, one side is clamped while the other side is ventilated and vice versa (see text for further explanation). (Reproduced with permission from Benumof JL. Anesthesia for Thoracic Surgery. Philadelphia, WB Saunders, 1987, Fig. 9–9, p. 233.)

monly used double-lumen tubes. Since a right-sided tube incurs the risk of inadequate right upper lobe ventilation, left-sided tubes are used far more commonly than right-sided tubes. Consequently, the rest of this chapter will emphasize the insertion and location of the left-sided Robertshaw-type double-lumen tube.

2. The Conventional Double-Lumen Tube Intubation Procedure

Prior to intubation with a double-lumen endotracheal tube, both cuffs and lumen connections are checked. A 3-mL syringe should be placed on the end of the bronchial cuff pilot tube, since proper bronchial cuff inflation rarely requires more than 1–2 mL of air; a 10-mL syringe should be placed on the tracheal cuff pilot tube. Since the high-volume, low-pressure cuffs can be easily torn by teeth, the distal tube and cuffs are coated with a lubricating ointment (preferably containing a local anesthetic) to minimize this possibility. (The lubricant allows the cuffs to slide by the teeth more easily.) If a less than optimal view of the larynx is anticipated, the stylet that comes packaged with the tube is lubricated, inserted into the left lumen, and appropriately curved. The patient is then anesthetized and paralyzed. A curved open-phalanged blade (Macintosh) (see Chapter 6) is usually preferred for laryngoscopy, since it approximates the curvature of the tube and therefore provides the largest possible area through which to pass the tube. However, a straight (Miller) blade may be a better choice in patients with overriding teeth or an excessively anterior larynx.

The Robertshaw double-lumen tube is passed with the distal curvature initially concave anteriorly (Fig. 11–4A). After the tube tip passes the larynx, and while anterior force on the laryngoscope is continued, the stylet (if used) is removed and the tube is carefully rotated 90° (so that the distal curve is now concave toward the appropriate side and the proximal curve is concave anteriorly) to allow endobronchial intubation on the appropriate side (Fig. 11–4B). Continued anterior force by the laryngoscope during tube rotation prevents hypopharyngeal structures from falling in around the tube and interfering with a free 90° distal tube tip rotation. Failure to obtain close to a 90° rotation of the distal tube tip, while the proximal end does rotate 90°, will cause a kink or a twist in the shaft of the tube and/or prevent the distal end of the lumen from lying free in the mainstem bronchus (ie, not up against the bronchial wall). After rotation, the tube is advanced until most of it is inserted (the proximal end of the common or two-lumen binding mold should be near or at the level of the teeth [usually at the 28-cm mark] in a normal-sized person) or moderate resistance to further passage is encountered, indicating that the tube tip has been firmly seated in a mainstem bronchus (Fig. 11–4C). Double-lumen endotracheal tubes may also be passed successfully via tracheostomy, although it should be remembered that the tracheal cuff may be at the tracheal stoma or lie partly outside the trachea in this situation.[9,10]

Once the tube tip is thought to be in an endobronchial position, the following checklist is carried out to insure proper functioning of the tube. Inflate the tracheal and endobronchial cuffs until moderate tension is palpated in the external pilot balloons (the endobronchial cuff should not require more than 2–3 mL of air), deliver several positive-pressure ventilations and auscultate and observe the chest bilaterally to determine that the trachea, rather than the esophagus, has been intubated and that both lungs are being ventilated (see Fig. 11–4C). In addition to seeing the tube go through the vocal cords, correct intubation position is checked by feeling and observing the anesthesia reservoir bag to make sure it has the appropriate compliance and movement, maintaining normal pulse oximetry and end-tidal carbon dioxide values, and perhaps palpating the tracheal cuff in the neck. If only unilateral breath sounds or chest movement are present, it is likely that both of the lumina of the tube have entered a mainstem bronchus. (If both of the lumina enter the left mainstem bronchus, the findings may mimic an esophageal intubation and vice versa.) In this situation, quickly deflate the cuffs, withdraw the tube 1–2 cm at a time, inflate the cuffs, and reassess ventilation until bilateral breath sounds are heard. If bilateral breath sounds are not heard and the tube has been withdrawn a significant amount, the entire procedure must be repeated, beginning with establishing the airway and oxygen ventilation via mask, laryngoscopy, and reinsertion of the double-lumen tube through the vocal cords. If bilateral breath sounds are present, then one side is clamped, and breath sounds and chest movement should disappear on the ipsilateral side and remain on the contralateral side. Next, the clamped side should be unclamped and the breath sounds and chest movement should reappear on that side. During unilateral clamping, the breath sounds on the ventilated side should be compared with and calibrated against unilateral chest wall movements and the inspiratory disappearance and expiratory appearance of respiratory gas moisture in the clear tubing of the ventilated side (Fig. 11–5). In addition, the compliance of the lung should be gauged by using hand ventilation. The unilateral clamping and unclamping should then be repeated on the opposite side to assure adequate lung separation and cuff seal.

In summary, when double-lumen endotracheal tube position is correct, the breath sounds are normal and follow the expected unilateral pattern with unilat-

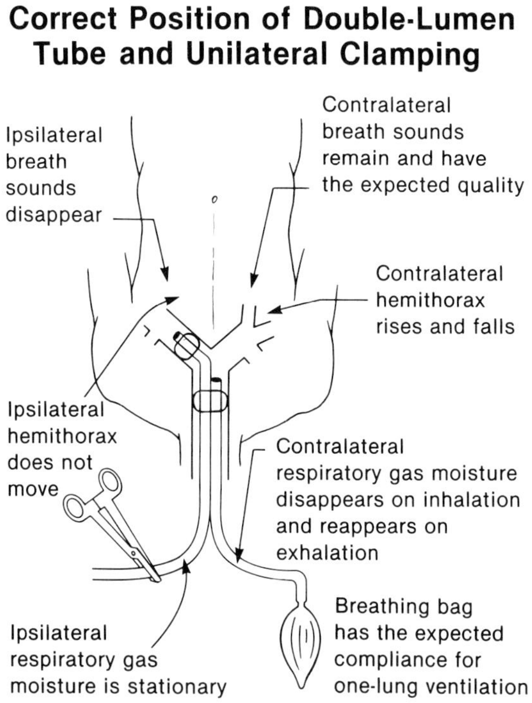

Figure 11–5 • This schematic diagram shows the results of unilateral clamping when the double-lumen tube is in the correct position. (Reproduced with permission from Benumof JL. Anesthesia for Thoracic Surgery. Philadelphia, WB Saunders, 1987, Fig. 9–10, p. 234.)

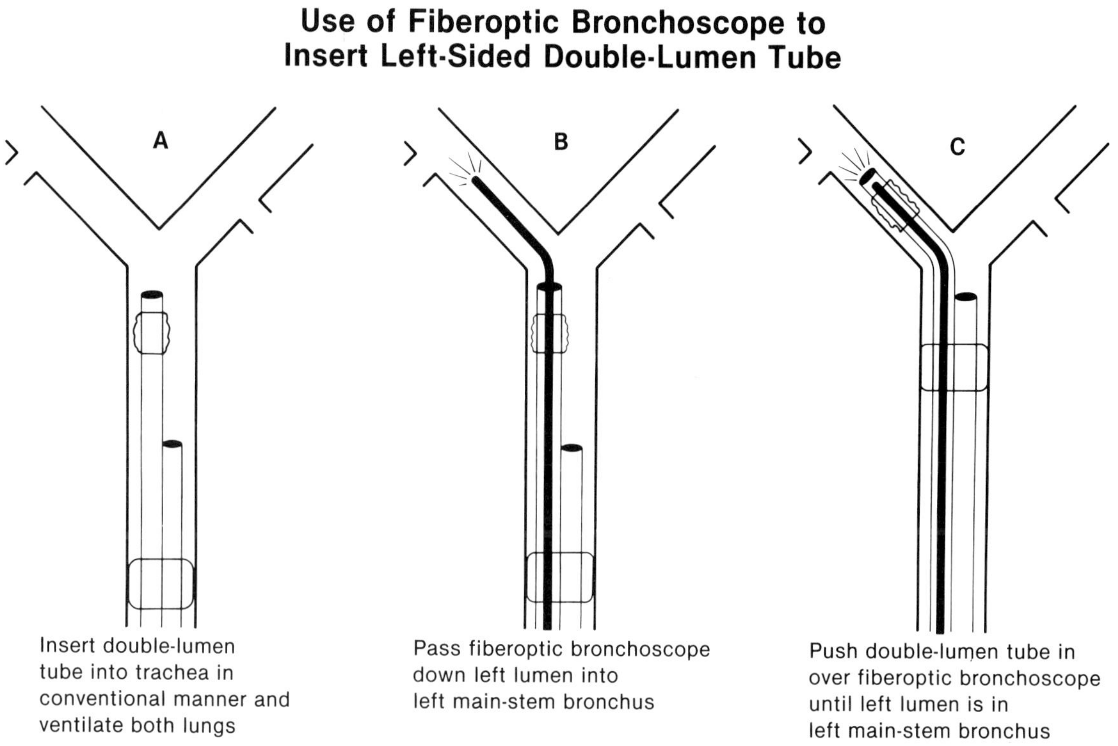

Figure 11–6 • This schematic diagram portrays use of the fiberoptic bronchoscope to insert a left-sided double-lumen tube. The double-lumen tube can be put into the trachea in a conventional manner, and both lungs can be ventilated by both lumens (***A***). The fiberoptic bronchoscope may be inserted into the left lumen of the double-lumen tube through a self-sealing diaphragm in the elbow connector to the left lumen; this allows continued positive pressure ventilation of both lungs through the right lumen without creating a leak. After the fiberoptic bronchoscope has been passed into the left mainstem bronchus (***B***), it is used as a stylet for the aftercoming left lumen (***C***). The fiberoptic bronchoscope is then withdrawn. Final precise positioning of the double-lumen tube is performed with a fiberoptic bronchoscope in the right lumen (see Fig. 12–7). (Reproduced with permission from Benumof JL. Anesthesia for Thoracic Surgery. Philadelphia, WB Saunders, 1987, Fig. 9–13, p. 237.)

eral clamping, the chest rises and falls in accordance with the breath sounds, the ventilated lung feels reasonably compliant, no leaks are present, and respiratory gas moisture appears and disappears with each tidal ventilation (see Fig. 11-5). Conversely, when the double-lumen endotracheal tube is malpositioned any or all of the following may occur: the breath sounds are poor and correlate poorly with unilateral clamping, the chest movements do not follow the expected pattern, the ventilated lung feels noncompliant, leaks are present, or the respiratory gas moisture in the clear tubing is relatively stationary. It is very important to realize, however, that even if the double-lumen tube appears by clinical signs to be properly positioned, subsequent fiberoptic bronchoscopy may reveal a clinically significant incidence of malpositioning.[6-8,11]

The solution to any uncertainty as to the exact position of the double-lumen tube is to determine the position by use of fiberoptic bronchoscopy (see Section III.A.4, "Use of Fiberoptic Bronchoscope to Determine Precise Double-Lumen Tube Position").

3. USE OF FIBEROPTIC BRONCHOSCOPE TO INSERT THE BRONCHIAL LUMEN OF A DOUBLE-LUMEN TUBE INTO A MAIN-STEM BRONCHUS

The insertion of the bronchial lumen of a double-lumen tube into the appropriate mainstem bronchus may be aided by the use of a fiberoptic bronchoscope (Fig. 11-6). The double-lumen tube is first placed in the trachea in a conventional manner (laryngoscopy, manual tube insertion) until the tracheal cuff just passes the vocal cords, the tracheal cuff is inflated, and both lungs are ventilated with both lumina (use the double-lumen tube as if it were a single-lumen tube). A pediatric fiberoptic bronchoscope can then be inserted into the bronchial lumen through a self-sealing diaphragm in the elbow connector to the bronchial lumen (which permits continued positive pressure ventilation through that lumen around the fiberoptic bronchoscope) and passed into the appropriate mainstem bronchus. The tracheal cuff is then deflated and the bronchial lumen is passed over the fiberoptic bronchoscope stylet into the appropriate mainstem bronchus. The fiberoptic bronchoscope is then withdrawn from the bronchial lumen and passed down the tracheal lumen to determine the precise double-lumen tube position (see Section III.A.4).

Alternatively, once the double-lumen tube is in the trachea, the fiberoptic bronchoscope can be inserted into the tracheal lumen through a self-sealing diaphragm in the elbow connector to the tracheal lumen (which permits continued positive pressure ventilation through that lumen around the fiberoptic bronchoscope) and passed just proximal to the tracheal carina. While the carina and the two mainstem bronchial orifices are in view, the double-lumen tube can be advanced and the degree of lateral rotation adjusted so that the left lumen enters the left mainstem bronchus. Final precise posi-

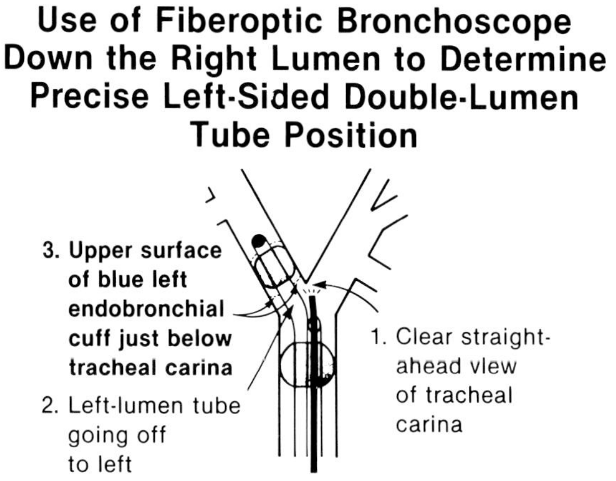

Figure 11–7 • This schematic diagram portrays use of the fiberoptic bronchoscope down the right lumen to determine precise left-sided double-lumen tube position. The endoscopist should see a clear straight-ahead view of the tracheal carina, the left lumen going off into the left mainstem bronchus, and most important (*in bold print*), the upper surface of the blue left endobronchial cuff just below the tracheal carina. (Reproduced with permission from Benumof JL. Anesthesia for Thoracic Surgery. Philadelphia, WB Saunders, 1987, Fig. 9–14, p. 238.)

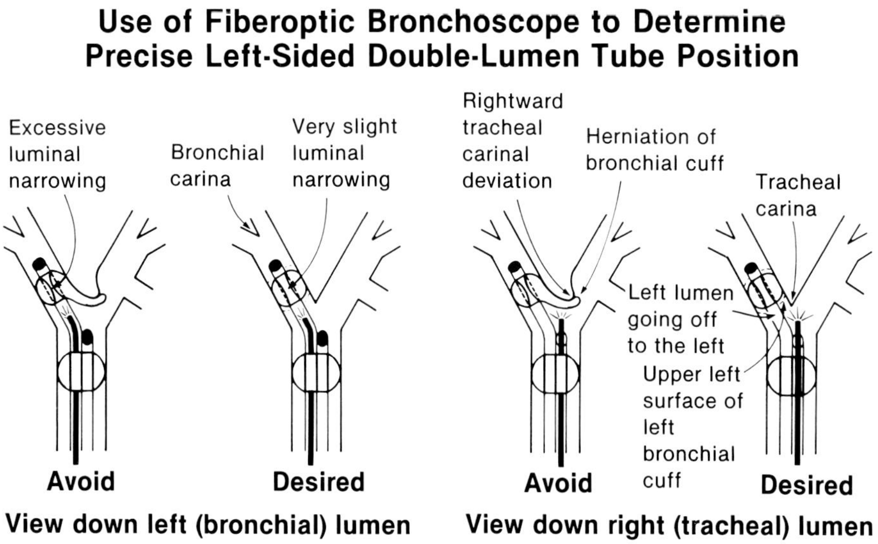

Figure 11–8 • This schematic diagram depicts the complete fiberoptic bronchoscopy picture of left-sided double-lumen tubes (both the desired view and the view to be avoided from both of the lumens). When the bronchoscope is passed down the right lumen of the left-sided tube, the endoscopist should see a clear straight-ahead view of the tracheal carina and the upper surface of the blue left endobronchial cuff just below the tracheal carina. Excessive pressure in the endobronchial cuff, as manifested by tracheal carinal deviation to the right and herniation of the endobronchial cuff over the carina, should be avoided. When the bronchoscope is passed down the left lumen of the left-sided tube, the endoscopist should see a very slight left luminal narrowing and a clear straight-ahead view of the bronchial carina off in the distance. Excessive left luminal narrowing should be avoided. (Reproduced with permission from Benumof JL. Anesthesia for Thoracic Surgery. Philadelphia, WB Saunders, 1987, Fig. 9–15, p. 239.)

tioning (see Section III.A.4) can be done with the fiberoptic bronchoscope remaining in the tracheal lumen.

4. Use of Fiberoptic Bronchoscope to Determine Precise Double-Lumen Tube Position

As noted previously, even when a double-lumen tube is thought to be in proper position based on clinical signs, subsequent fiberoptic bronchoscopy will reveal a 48% incidence of malpositioning.[11] Indeed, when the position of the double-lumen tube is checked only by clinical signs, 25% of the time there will be intraoperative problems with either deflating the nondependent lung, ventilating the dependent lung, or completely separating the two lungs.[12] The exact position of a left-sided double-lumen endotracheal tube can be ascertained at any time, in less than a minute, by simply passing a pediatric fiberoptic bronchoscope through the tracheal lumen of the double-lumen tube. It is rarely necessary to also have to pass the fiberoptic bronchoscope down the left endobronchial lumen. With reference to a left-sided double-lumen tube, looking down the right (tracheal) lumen the endoscopist should see a clear straight-ahead view of the tracheal carina, the left lumen going off to the left, and the upper surface of the left endobronchial balloon just below the tracheal carina (Figs. 11–7 and 11–8). (The importance of seeing the upper surface of the left endobronchial cuff below the tracheal carina will be emphasized in the following section.) It is important that the volume of air used to fill the left endobronchial left cuff does not cause the endobronchial cuff to herniate over the tracheal carina or cause the tracheal carina to deviate to the right (Figs. 11–8 and 11–9). Both cuff herniation and carinal deviation can be readily appreciated looking down the tracheal lumen. Looking down the left lumen (which is sometimes done when inserting a left-sided double-lumen tube with a fiberoptic bronchoscope and in all cases of bronchopulmonary lavage in which perfect tube position and tight cuff seal are extremely critical), the endoscopist should see a very slight narrowing of the left lumen (due to endobronchial cuff pressure) as well as the bronchial carina distal to the end of the tube (see Fig. 11–8). The endoscopist should not see excessive left luminal narrowing (due to excessive left cuff pressure) (see Fig. 11–9). Thus, aside from gross malposition, important undesirable findings on endoscopy are related to excessive left cuff inflation and pressure and consist of cuff herniation over the tracheal carina, deviation to the right (both of which may block the right mainstem bronchial orifice and impair right lung ventilation), and excessive left lumen constriction (invagination), which may impair left lung ventilation (see Fig. 11–9).[13] In addition, when an inappropriately undersized tube is used, the large endobronchial cuff volume required for endobronchial cuff seal tends to force the entire double-lumen tube cephalad, making a functional bronchial seal more difficult.[14]

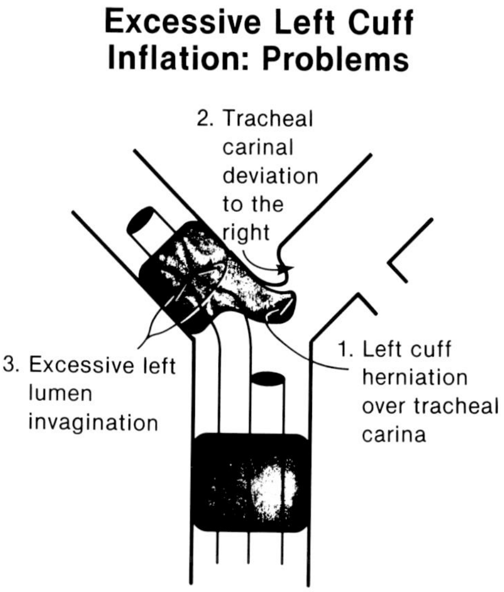

Figure 11–9 • Excessive inflation of the left cuff of a left-sided double-lumen tube can cause impaired ventilation of both the right and left lungs. Right lung ventilation may be impaired by left cuff herniation over the tracheal carina (caused by excessive left cuff volume) and by tracheal carinal deviation to the right (caused by excessive left cuff pressure). Left lung ventilation may be impaired by invagination of the left lumen caused by excessive left cuff pressure. (Reproduced with permission from Benumof JL. Anesthesia for Thoracic Surgery. Philadelphia, WB Saunders, 1987, Fig. 9–16, p. 239.)

With reference to a right-sided double-lumen tube, looking down the left (tracheal) lumen, the endoscopist should see a clear straight-ahead view of the tracheal carina, with the right lumen going off to the right (Fig. 11–10A). The upper surface of the right endobronchial balloon may not be visible below the tracheal carina. Looking down the right lumen, the endoscopist should see a very slight narrowing of the right lumen as well as the right middle and lower lobe bronchial carina distal to the end of the tube. Most important, the endoscopist should locate the right upper lobe ventilation slot and be able to look directly into the right upper lobe orifice through the right upper lobe ventilation slot by simply flexing the tip of the fiberoptic bronchoscope

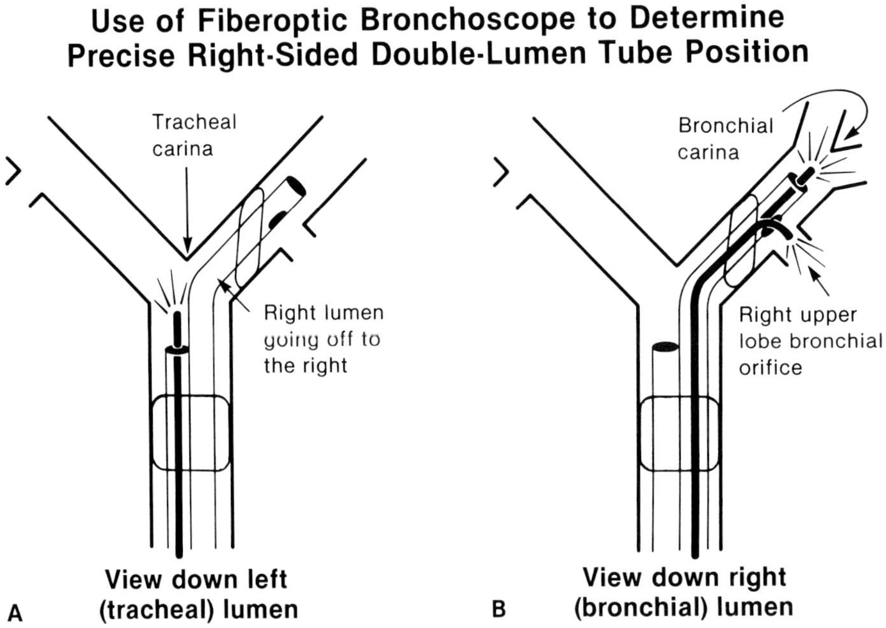

Figure 11–10 • This schematic diagram portrays use of a fiberoptic bronchoscope to determine precise right-sided double-lumen tube position. (***A***) When the fiberoptic bronchoscope is passed down the left (tracheal) lumen, the endoscopist should see a clear straight-ahead view of the tracheal carina and the right lumen going off into the right mainstem bronchus. (***B***) When the fiberoptic bronchoscope is passed down the right (bronchial) lumen, the endoscopist should see the bronchial carina off in the distance. When the fiberoptic bronchoscope is flexed cephalad and passed through the right–upper-lobe ventilation slot, the right–upper-lobe bronchial orifice should be visualized. (Reproduced with permission from Benumof JL. Anesthesia for Thoracic Surgery. Philadelphia, WB Saunders, 1987, Fig. 9–17, p. 240.)

superiorly (Fig. 11–10B). There should be no overriding of the right upper lobe ventilation slot on the bronchial mucosa, and the bronchial mucosa should not be covering any of the right upper lobe ventilation slot. The fact that there is little room for error in aligning the right upper lobe ventilation slot with the right upper lobe makes left-sided double-lumen tubes the tube of choice in a large majority of instances.

a. Relationship of Fiberoptic Bronchoscope Size to Double-Lumen Tube Size

Table 11–2 summarizes the various fiberoptic bronchoscope–double-lumen tube size relationships. (See also the comments on Table 11–3 in Section III.A.7.) The clear plastic disposable right- and left-sided double-lumen endotracheal tubes are manufactured in five sizes: 28, 35, 37, 39, and 41 French. A 5.6-mm OD diagnostic fiberoptic bronchoscope will not pass down the lumina of any size of double-lumen tube. A 4.9-mm external diameter fiberoptic bronchoscope passes easily through the lumina of the 41 French tube, moderately easily with lubrication through the 39 French tube, causes a tight fit that needs a liberal amount of lubrication and a strong pushing force to pass through the 37 French tube, and does not pass through the lumen of the 35 French tube. A silicon-based fluid (such as is made by the American Cystoscope Co.) is the best lubricant for a fiberoptic bronchoscope because it does not dry out or crust and does not interfere with the view even if it coats the tip of the bronchoscope. Fortunately, in view of using a 4.9-mm OD fiberoptic bronchoscope, a tube 37 French or larger can be used in almost all adult women and a tube 39 French or larger can be used in almost all adult men. A 3.6–4.2-mm OD (pediatric) fiberoptic bronchoscope passes easily through the lumina of all sizes of double-lumen endotracheal tubes and, because the bronchoscope has an increased amount of space, the maneuverability of the tip of the bronchoscope is greatly increased. Therefore, the 3.6–4.2-mm OD bronchoscope is obviously the bronchoscope of choice for double-lumen tubes. Several companies (Olympus, Machida, Pen-

Table 11-2 • Relationship of Fiberoptic Bronchoscope Size to Double-Lumen Tube Size

Fiberoptic Bronchoscope: Outside Diameter (mm)	Double-Lumen Tube Size (French)	Fit of Fiberoptic Bronchoscope Inside Double-Lumen Tube
5.6	All sizes	Does not fit
	41	Easy passage
	39	Moderately easy passage
4.9	37	Tight fit, needs lubricant,* Hard push
	35	Does not fit
3.6–4.2	All Sizes	Easy passage

*Lubricant recommended is a silicon-based fluid made by the American Cystoscope Company.

tax) presently manufacture 4.9 and 3.6–4.2-mm OD fiberoptic bronchoscopes that are of adequate length and have a suction channel.

5. USE OF CHEST RADIOGRAPH TO DETERMINE DOUBLE-LUMEN TUBE POSITION

The chest radiograph can be used to determine double-lumen tube position. The usefulness of a chest radiograph may be greater than conventional unilateral auscultation and clamping in some patients, but it is always less precise than fiberoptic bronchoscopy. To use the chest radiograph, the double-lumen tube must have radiopaque markers at the end of the right and left lumina. The key to discerning double-lumen tube position on the chest radiograph is seeing where the marker at the end of the tracheal lumen is in relation to the tracheal carina. The end of the tracheal lumen marker must be above the tracheal carina; however, this does not guarantee correct position because this technique may not reveal a subtle obstruction of an upper lobe. If the tracheal carina cannot be seen (which is often the case with a portable anterior–posterior film), then the chest radiograph method of determining double-lumen tube position is not usable. Furthermore, the chest radiographic method is time-consuming (for film transport, film development), costly, and awkward to perform and may dislodge the tube. (The cassettes are often difficult to place under the operating room table and may require movement of the patient.)

6. QUANTITATIVE DETERMINATION OF CUFF SEAL PRESSURE HOLD

The use of fiberoptic bronchoscopy to determine double-lumen tube position does not provide evidence or a guarantee that the two lungs are functionally separated (ie, against a fluid and/or air pressure gradient). There are times, such as during unilateral pulmonary lavage, when the anesthesiologist must be absolutely certain that functional separation has been achieved. Complete separation of the two lungs by the left endobronchial cuff can be demonstrated in a left-sided tube by clamping the connecting tube to the right lung proximal to the right suction port and attaching a small tube (ie, intravenous extension tubing) to the open right suction port (by appropriate adapters) (Fig. 11–11). The free end of this tube is submerged in a beaker of water. When the left lung is statically inflated to any pressure considered necessary and the left endobronchial cuff is not sealed, air will enter the left lung as well as escape out from around the unsealed left cuff, travel up the right lumen to the small connecting tube, and bubble through the beaker of water (Fig. 11–11B). If the left endobronchial cuff is sealed, no bubbles should be observed passing through the beaker of water (Fig. 11–11A). Following demonstration of functional lung separation, the right connecting tube is unclamped, the right suction port is closed, and ventilation to both lungs is resumed. To test for lung separation with the pressure gradient across the endobronchial balloon reversed, the left airway connecting tube is clamped proximal to the left suction port, the left suction port is opened to the beaker of water via the small tube, the right lung is statically inflated to any desired pressure, and the absence or presence of air bubbles in the beaker of water is noted. It should be remembered that even though the left endobronchial cuff may be adequately sealed, during these maneuvers compression of the nonventilated lung by the ventilated lung (via movement of the mediastinum) may initially cause some small amount of bubbling in the beaker, which will cease with repeated inflation of the ventilated lung (no bubbles should be seen following several inflations).[13,14] The absence of airflow from the nonventilated lung suction port is a very simple but sensitive indicator of functional separation of the two lungs.

7. RELATIVE CONTRAINDICATIONS TO USE OF DOUBLE-LUMEN ENDOTRACHEAL TUBES

There are several situations in which lung separation by a double-lumen tube may be relatively contraindicated

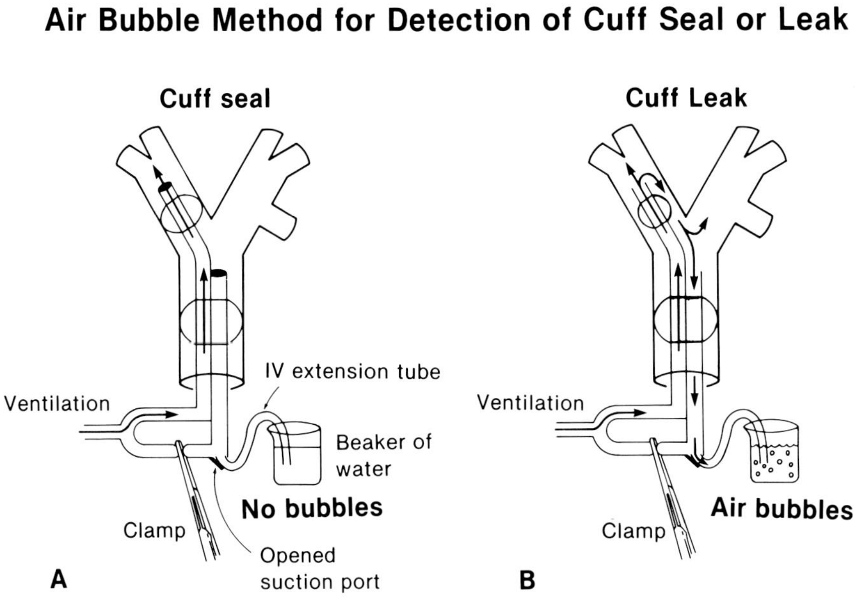

Figure 11–11 • This schematic diagram shows the air bubble detection method for checking adequacy of the seal of the left endobronchial cuff of a left-sided double-lumen tube. When the left lung is selectively ventilated or exposed to any desired distending pressure and the left cuff is adequately sealed, no air will escape around the left cuff and out the open right suction port. Thus, no bubbles will be observed passing through the beaker of water (***A***). When the left lung is ventilated or exposed to any desired distending pressure and the left endobronchial cuff is not adequately sealed, air will escape around the left cuff and out the open right suction port. Thus, air bubbles will be observed passing through the beaker of water (***B***). (Reproduced with permission from Benumof JL. Anesthesia for Thoracic Surgery. Philadelphia, WB Saunders, 1987, Fig. 9–28, p. 251.)

because insertion of the double-lumen tube is either difficult or dangerous (Table 11–3). These situations include patients who have a full stomach (risk of aspiration), patients who have a lesion (airway stricture,[15] endoluminal tumor) that is present somewhere along the pathway of the double-lumen tube and thus could be traumatized, small patients in whom a 28 French tube is too large to fit comfortably through the larynx, patients whose upper airway anatomy precludes safe insertion of the tube (recessed jaw, prominent teeth, bull neck, anterior larynx), critically ill patients who have a single-lumen tube already in place and will not tolerate being taken off mechanical ventilation and positive end-expiratory pressure (PEEP) (even for the short time of 1 minute), and patients having some combination of all these problems. Under these circumstances, it is still possible to separate the lungs safely and adequately by using a single-lumen tube and fiberoptic bronchoscopic placement of a bronchial blocker or by fiberoptic bronchoscopic placement of a single-lumen tube in a mainstem bronchus.

B. *Bronchial Blockers (with Single-Lumen Endotracheal Tubes)*

Lung separation can be effectively achieved with the use of a single-lumen tube and a bronchoscopically (rigid or fiberoptic) placed bronchial blocker (Fig. 11–12). This is the lung separation procedure of choice in neonates to age 1 and is a method sometimes used in children aged 1–10 years. Bronchial blockers are the lung separation

Table 11–3 • Relative Contraindications to Use of Double-Lumen Tube

1. Presence of lesion along double-lumen tube pathway
2. Difficult/impossible conventional direct vision intubation
3. Critically ill patients with single-lumen tube *in situ* who cannot tolerate even a short period off mechanical ventilation
4. Full stomach/high risk of aspiration
5. Some combination of the preceding

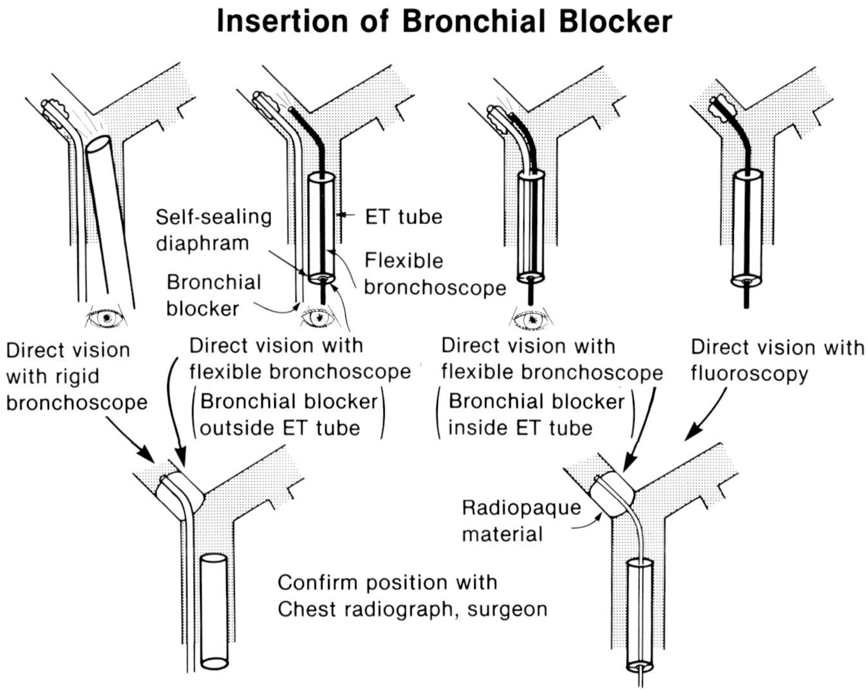

Figure 11–12 • Insertion of a bronchial blocker may be accomplished by a number of methods, depending on the age of the patient and the size of the endotracheal (ET) tube that can be used. In older children and adults the sequence shown by going from the second-to-the-left upper panel to the left lower panel is used. (Reproduced with permission from Benumof JL. Anesthesia for Thoracic Surgery. Philadelphia, WB Saunders, 1987, Fig. 17-7, p. 425.)

procedure of choice in neonates to age 1 because single-lumen endobronchial tubes must be uncuffed for this age group and therefore cannot guarantee a seal of the bronchus or nonmovement of the tip of the tube past an upper lobe or out of the mainstem bronchus. Bronchial blockers that are balloon-tipped luminal catheters have the advantage of allowing suctioning and injection of oxygen down the central lumen. The Fogarty catheter comes with a stylet in place, so that it is possible to place a curvature at the distal tip. Bronchial blockers have the disadvantage of sometimes requiring rigid bronchoscopy for placement, and because they have high-pressure, spherically inflating balloons, there is a tendency for them to back out of the bronchus into the trachea (see the following).

For bronchial blockade in very small children (neonates to age 1 or those 10 kg or less), a 3 French Fogarty embolectomy catheter with a balloon capacity of 0.5 mL or a Swan-Ganz catheter (1-mL balloon) should be used.[16] A fully inflated 0.5-mL balloon has a length of 10 mm and a width of 7.5 mm. When the patient is sufficiently deeply anesthetized, the tracheobronchial tree can be sprayed with local anesthetic, and either a rigid (3.2–3.6-mm OD) or a fiberoptic (2.7–3.6-mm OD)[16,17] bronchoscope is passed into the appropriate mainstem bronchus (see Fig. 11–12). Under direct vision the Fogarty embolectomy catheter can be placed in the appropriate mainstem bronchus, and the Fogarty catheter is inflated with 0.5 mL of sterile normal saline. If a rigid bronchoscope is used, the patient can be ventilated via the side-arm. The bronchoscope is then removed and the patient is ventilated and oxygenated. A single-lumen tube (3.5–4.5-mm OD) is then placed in the trachea. The bronchial blocker may also be guided into place with fluoroscopy (see Fig. 11–12).[18]

Alternatively, and if the patient is large enough, a single-lumen tube (4.5–6.0-mm OD) may be placed first and connected to an elbow adapter with a self-sealing diaphragm (see Fig. 11–12). The pediatric fiberoptic bronchoscope (3.2–3.6-mm OD) is then passed through the self-sealing diaphragm and identifies the carina. Then, depending on the size of the endotracheal tube used, the Fogarty embolectomy catheter can be passed alongside or within the endotracheal tube (also through the self-sealing diaphragm) into the proper mainstem bronchial position (see Fig. 11–12). The stylet allows the operator to twirl the proximal end of the bronchial blocker in the fingertips until the curved distal tip locates in the desired mainstem bronchus. The self-sealing diaphragm in the elbow connector permits uninterrupted positive pressure ventilation around the fiberoptic bronchoscope and bronchial blocker.

The position of the single-lumen endotracheal tube and bronchial blocker should be confirmed with a chest radiograph. The bronchial blocker can be readily appreciated on chest radiograph if a radiopaque material is instilled into the blocking balloon.

In older children and adults, the bronchial blocker most often used is a Fogarty occlusion (embolectomy) catheter with a 3-mL balloon.[19] If no endotracheal tube is in place, the operator exposes the larynx and places a single-lumen tube with a high-volume cuff in the trachea. The Fogarty catheter is then placed alongside the single-lumen tube. A fiberoptic bronchoscope is passed down to the end of the single-lumen tube through a self-sealing diaphragm in the elbow connector (which permits continued positive-pressure ventilation around the fiberoptic bronchoscope) and the Fogarty catheter is visualized below the tip of the single-lumen tube. The proximal end of the bronchial blocker is then twirled in the fingertips until the distal tip locates in the desired mainstem bronchus. The catheter balloon is then inflated under direct visualization, and the fiberoptic bronchoscope is withdrawn through the self-sealing diaphragm.

The bronchial blocker technique for older children and adults has been modified so that the bronchial blocker can be passed along with (at the same time as) the single-lumen endotracheal tube.[20,21] With this commercial modification (Univent, Fuji Systems Corporation, Tokyo, Japan), the bronchial blocker is housed in a small channel bored through the anterior wall of the endotracheal tube, which allows the bronchial blocker to be transmitted to the distal trachea by the endotracheal tube. The bronchial blocker is then visualized by the fiberoptic bronchoscope and is manipulated into the desired mainstem bronchus as previously described although the original authors inappropriately recommend doing this blindly (ie, turning the concavity of the single-lumen tube toward the appropriate mainstem bronchus, advancing the bronchial blocker distally, and inflating the balloon without visualization of the location of the balloon). Finally, other balloon-tipped luminal catheters (such as a Magill- or Foley-type catheter) may be used as bronchial blockers.

C. *Endobronchial Intubation with Single-Lumen Tubes*

In children and adults presenting with hemoptysis, endobronchial intubation with a single-lumen tube is often the easiest, quickest way of effectively separating the two lungs, especially if the left lung is bleeding. If the left lung is bleeding, one can simply take an uncut single-lumen endotracheal tube and advance it inward until moderate resistance is felt (Fig. 11–13A).[22] In the vast majority of patients the single-lumen tube will locate in

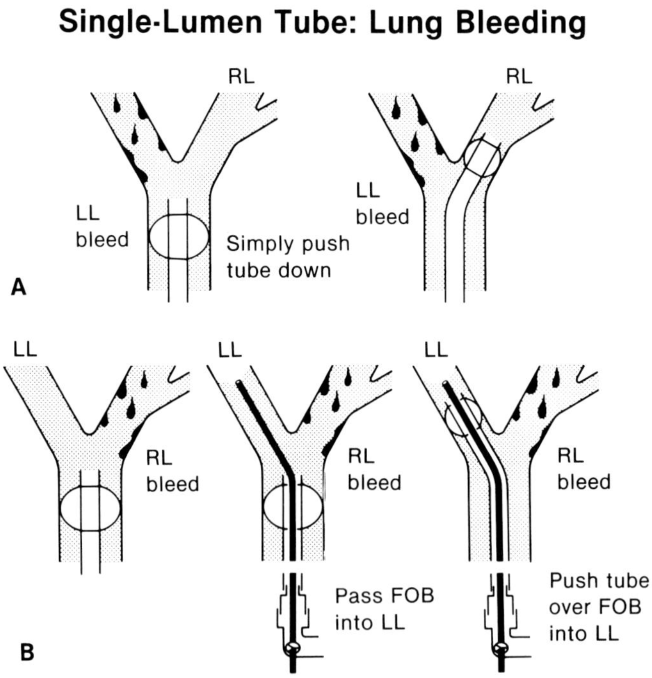

Figure 11–13 • This figure shows how to separate the two lungs with a single-lumen tube in the presence of massive lung bleeding. When the left lung is bleeding (***A***) an uncut single-lumen tube may simply be inserted its full length, and in the vast majority of cases, it will enter the right mainstem bronchus, thereby effectively sealing off the right lung from the left lung. However, one can expect that the cuff of the single-lumen tube will obstruct the right upper lobe. When the right lung is bleeding (***B***), a fiberoptic bronchoscope, which is jacketed on its proximal end with an endotracheal (ET) tube, can be passed through a self-sealing diaphragm in the elbow connector to the ET tube (which allows continued positive pressure breathing) and, if a moment's view of the tracheal carina can be obtained, passed into the left mainstem bronchus. Using the fiberoptic bronchoscope as a stylet, the ET tube can be passed over the fiberoptic bronchoscope into the left mainstem bronchus. The fiberoptic bronchoscope is then withdrawn. (*LL = left lung; RL = right lung; FOB = fiberoptic bronchoscope.*) (Reproduced with permission from Benumof JL. Anesthesia for Thoracic Surgery. Philadelphia, WB Saunders, 1987, Fig. 9–30, p. 257.)

the right mainstem bronchus, thereby blocking off the bleeding left lung and allowing for selective ventilation of just the right lung. Under these circumstances it is very possible that the right upper lobe bronchus will be blocked off as well, resulting in ventilation of just the right middle and lower lobes, and a high risk of significant hypoxemia. Nevertheless, the procedure can be immediately life saving, and after several ventilations the tube can be carefully withdrawn in an attempt to hear breath sounds over the entire right hemithorax.

If the right lung is bleeding and the situation is life threatening, blind left mainstem intubation with a single-lumen tube should be attempted first, since a 92% success rate in 4–5 seconds has recently been reported.[22] The head should be rotated to the right, and the single-lumen tube should be rotated 180° (the concavity of the tube will be facing posteriorly rather than anteriorly). After initial left mainstem bronchus intubation, the tube should be slowly withdrawn until breath sounds are heard over the entire left hemithorax.

If the right lung is bleeding and the situation is not life threatening and/or left lung catheterization cannot be achieved blindly, a fiberoptic bronchoscope can be passed through a self-sealing diaphragm in the single-lumen tube elbow connector and directed into the left mainstem bronchus. Persistent large soft catheter suctioning of the carinal area through the single-lumen tube prior to use of the fiberoptic bronchoscope and suctioning through the fiberoptic bronchoscope may be required to visualize the tracheal carina (Fig. 11–13B). The single-lumen tube can then be passed over the fiberoptic bronchoscope into the left mainstem bronchus, thereby sealing off the bleeding right lung and allowing for selective ventilation of the left lung. Passing the fiberoptic bronchoscope through a self-sealing diaphragm allows for the continuance of positive-pressure ventilation and PEEP around the bronchoscope. However, it should be realized that visualization of the carina may not be possible when the bleeding is copious and that the only hope for the patient may lie in blind left mainstem intubation (see earlier) and/or rapid thoracotomy, and control of bleeding from within the chest. In addition, under these very adverse conditions in adults and children over 10 years of age, conventional passage of a double-lumen tube may more rapidly and effectively separate the two lungs than trying to visualize anatomy with a fiberoptic bronchoscope. Other alternatives, such as use of curved stylets[23,24] and fluoroscopy,[18] are not ordinarily readily available.

Following any method of insertion, the position of the mainstem bronchial endotracheal tube should be further confirmed by chest radiograph. With either mainstem bronchial intubation, the surgeon can further check the position of the tube at the time of thoracotomy.

D. *Bronchial Blocker Plus Endobronchial Intubation*

To more securely guarantee lung separation, a bronchial blocker can be used in conjunction with mainstem bronchial intubation.[17] A bronchial blocker must first be placed under bronchoscopic (either rigid or fiberoptic; see earlier) or fluoroscopic control (see Fig. 11–12) and the mainstem bronchial intubation must be placed under fiberoptic bronchoscopic control, fluoroscopic control, or both (see Fig. 11–13). When the bronchial blocker is used with a mainstem bronchial intubation, a curved stylet is relatively contraindicated because if the single-lumen endotracheal tube enters the mainstem bronchus in which the bronchial blocker sits, ventilation will not be possible and the tube may cause malpositioning of the bronchial blocker. Finally, the position of the bronchial balloon and mainstem bronchial ventilating catheter should be confirmed with a chest radiograph preoperatively and by the surgeon intraoperatively, as described earlier.

IV. Discussion of Separation of the Two Lungs: Management of Lung Separation

The lungs are separated either to facilitate thoracic surgery by instituting one-lung ventilation or to treat asymmetrical or unilateral adult respiratory distress syndrome by instituting differential lung ventilation. The management of these two situations is very different, and this discussion will outline these procedures.

A. *Management of One-Lung Ventilation (to Facilitate Anesthesia for Thoracic Surgery)*

Anesthesia for thoracic surgery is most commonly performed with the patient in the lateral decubitus position, with the nondependent hemithorax comprising the operative field. When one-lung ventilation is employed, the nondependent lung is the nonventilated and collapsed (atelectatic) lung, and the dependent lung is the ventilated lung. The section first considers the usual management of one-lung ventilation in terms of the most appropriate inspired oxygen concentration, tidal volume, and respiratory rate that should be used (Table 11–4) and then considers several specialized techniques for management of one-lung ventilation.

1. Initial Ventilator Settings

Although the theoretical possibilities of absorption atelectasis and oxygen toxicity exist, the benefits of ventilating the dependent lung with 100% oxygen, in terms of increasing the P_aO_2 from arrhythmogenic and life-threatening levels to safer levels, far exceeds these remote risks. The dependent lung should be ventilated with a tidal volume of 10 mL/kg. Use of a tidal volume much less than 10 mL/kg might promote dependent lung atelectasis. Use of a tidal volume much greater than 10 mL/kg might excessively increase dependent lung airway pressure and vascular resistance[25] and thereby increase nondependent lung blood flow. The respiratory rate should be set so that the P_aCO_2 remains at 40 mmHg. Since a dependent lung tidal volume of 10 mL/kg represents a 20% decrease from the usual two-lung tidal volume of 12 mL/kg, the respiratory rate usually needs to be increased by 20% to 30% in order to maintain carbon dioxide hemostasis. No dependent lung PEEP should be used initially, because of concern about unnecessarily increasing dependent lung vascular resistance and shunting blood flow up to the nonventilated nondependent lung.

Table 11–4 • Initial Conventional Ventilatory Management of One-Lung Anesthesia

1. Maintain two-lung ventilation as long as possible.
2. Begin one-lung ventilation with tidal volume of 10 mL/kg.
3. Adjust the respiratory rate so that P_aCO_2 = 40 mmHg.
4. Use F_IO_2 = 1.0.
5. Monitor arterial PO_2 and PCO_2 frequently and continuously.

2. Dependent Lung PEEP

The effect of dependent lung PEEP on arterial oxygenation during one-lung ventilation is a trade-off between the positive effect of increasing dependent lung functional residual capacity and ventilation–perfusion ratio and the negative effect of increasing dependent lung vascular resistance and shunting blood flow to the nonventilated lung. Thus, the various one-lung ventilation PEEP studies have involved patients who have had an increase,[25–27] no change,[26,27,29] or a decrease[25,27,30,31] in oxygenation. Although in none of these studies was a dose (ventilated lung PEEP)–response (P_aO_2, Q_s/Q_t value) relationship described, it seems reasonable to postulate on the basis of these results that the therapeutic margin of using PEEP to just the ventilated lung to increase P_aO_2 during one-lung ventilation is quite narrow. PEEP to just the dependent ventilated lung may be delivered by the same anesthesia machine apparatus that is ordinarily used to deliver PEEP to the whole lung. Other studies have shown that high tidal volumes,[32] variations in the inspiratory–expiratory ratio,[28] and intermittent manual hyperventilation of the lower lung[28] are not beneficial in increasing P_aO_2 during one-lung ventilation.

3. Nondependent Lung CPAP

Positive pressure can be selectively and statically applied to just the nonventilated nondependent lung. Since under these conditions the nonventilated lung is only slightly but constantly distended by oxygen, an appropriate term for this ventilatory arrangement is nonventilated-lung continuous positive airway pressure (CPAP). The constant distention of the nondependent lung by CPAP, which is proportional to the amount of CPAP, greatly decreases the shunt through the nondependent lung (Fig. 11–14); even if the nondependent lung CPAP causes some diversion of blood flow away from the nondependent lung, this diverted blood flow can participate in gas exchange in the ventilated dependent lung.

In all patients in all clinical studies to date, 5–10 cm H_2O of nondependent lung CPAP has significantly increased P_aO_2 during one-lung ventilation.[31,33–38] It should be concluded that the single most efficacious maneuver to increase P_aO_2 during one-lung ventilation is to apply 5–10 cm H_2O to the nondependent lung. In my experience, low levels of nonventilated CPAP have corrected severe hypoxemia (P_aO_2 of less than 50

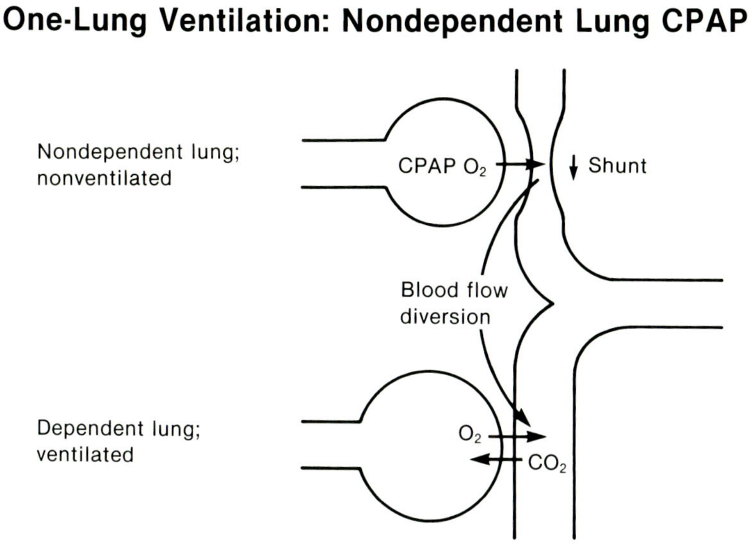

Figure 11–14 • Selective continuous positive airway pressure (CPAP) to the nonventilated nondependent lung (static distension without tidal movement) allows this lung to participate in oxygen uptake and markedly decreases the shunt through the nonventilated nondependent lung. Even if the nonventilated, nondependent lung CPAP causes blood flow diversion to the ventilated dependent lung, the diverted flow still can participate in oxygen uptake and CO_2 elimination in the ventilated dependent lung. Usually 5–10 mL H_2O of nondependent lung CPAP is all that is clinically needed, and this amount of CPAP does not cause any significant surgical interference. (Reproduced with permission from Benumof JL. Anesthesia for Thoracic Surgery. Philadelphia, WB Saunders, 1987, Fig. 11–6, p. 278.)

mmHg) more than 90% of the time, provided the double-lumen tube was correctly positioned. However, the nondependent lung CPAP must be applied during the deflation phase of a large tidal volume so that the deflating lung can lock into a CPAP level with uniform expansion and avoid the need to overcome critical opening pressures.

Several selective nondependent lung CPAP systems that are easy to assemble have been recently described.[29,36–38] All these nondependent lung CPAP systems have three features in common (Fig. 11–15). First, there must be a source of oxygen to flow into the nonventilated lung. Second, there must be some sort of restrictive mechanism (hand-screw valve, pop-off valve, weight-loaded valve) to prevent the egress of oxygen from the nonventilated lung so that the nonventilated lung may become distended. Thus, a free-flowing pressurized source of oxygen flows into a lung, but the es-

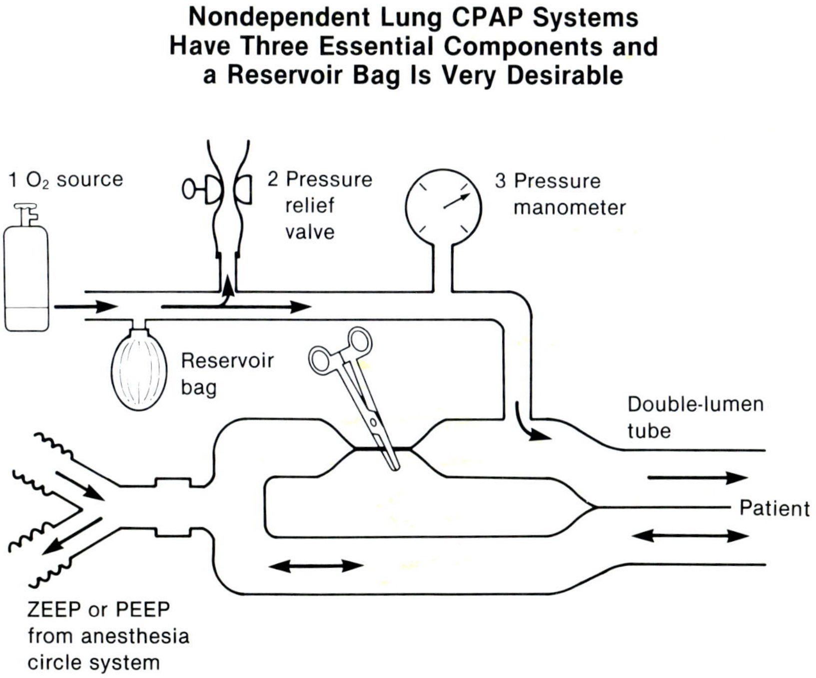

Figure 11–15 • The three essential components of a nondependent lung continuous positive airway pressure (CPAP) system consist of (*1*) an oxygen source, (*2*) a pressure relief valve, and (*3*) a pressure manometer to measure the CPAP. The CPAP is created by the free flow of oxygen into the lung vs. the restricted outflow of oxygen from the lung by the pressure relief valve. *(ZEEP = zero end-expiratory pressure.)* It is also highly desirable to have a reservoir bag in the system because it allows the anesthesiologist also to ventilate the collapsed lung when coordinated with the surgeon's activities, and the amount of distention of the reservoir bag reflects the amount of lung distention. (Reproduced with permission from Benumof JL. Anesthesia for Thoracic Surgery. Philadelphia, WB Saunders, 1987, Fig. 11–7, p. 279.)

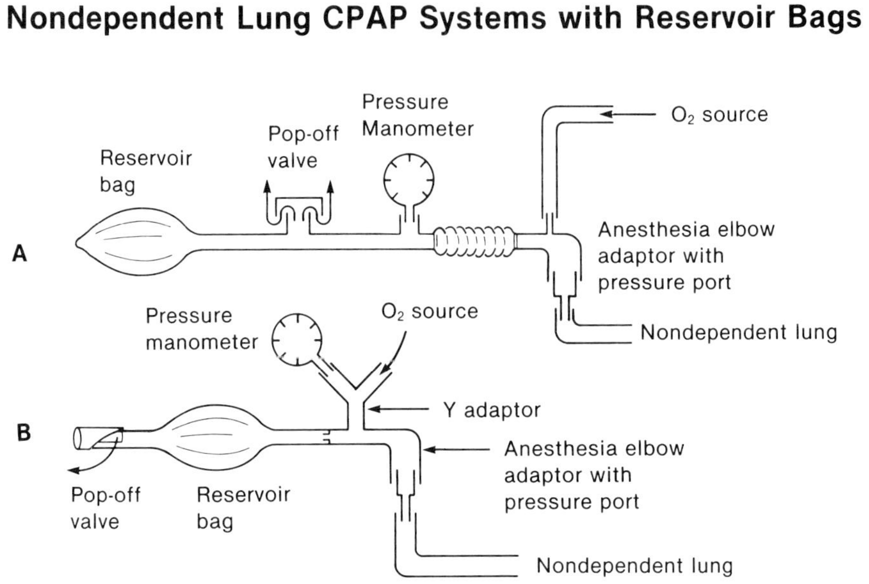

Figure 11–16 • This schematic diagram shows two (***A*** and ***B***) nondependent-lung continuous positive airway pressure (CPAP) systems with reservoir bags. Both of these systems contain an oxygen source, some type of pressure relief valve, and a pressure manometer to measure the CPAP. The presence of a reservoir bag allows for intermittent positive pressure breathing and sighing, if desired. The author uses both systems. (Reproduced with permission from Benumof JL. Anesthesia for Thoracic Surgery. Philadelphia, WB Saunders, 1987, Fig. 11–8, p. 280.)

cape of the oxygen is restricted; the unrestricted flow in and the restricted flow out creates a constant distending pressure. Third, the distending pressure must be measured by a manometer. In practice it is simplest to keep the restrictive mechanism constant and adjust the distending pressure with a relatively fine sensitivity by changing the oxygen flow rate. If the nondependent lung CPAP system has a reservoir bag included, which is very strongly recommended, the nondependent lung may also be ventilated with intermittent positive pressure whenever desired (Fig. 11–16). This is very important because it is often possible, by looking at the operative field, to coordinate small tidal volume ventilation to the operative lung with what the surgeon is doing, as well as intermittently sigh the operative lung, without interfering with the performance of surgery.

4. Differential Lung PEEP, CPAP

In theory, and from the preceding considerations, it appears that the ideal way to improve oxygenation during one-lung ventilation is to apply differential lung CPAP/PEEP (Fig. 11–17). In this situation, the ventilated (dependent) lung is given PEEP in the usual conventional

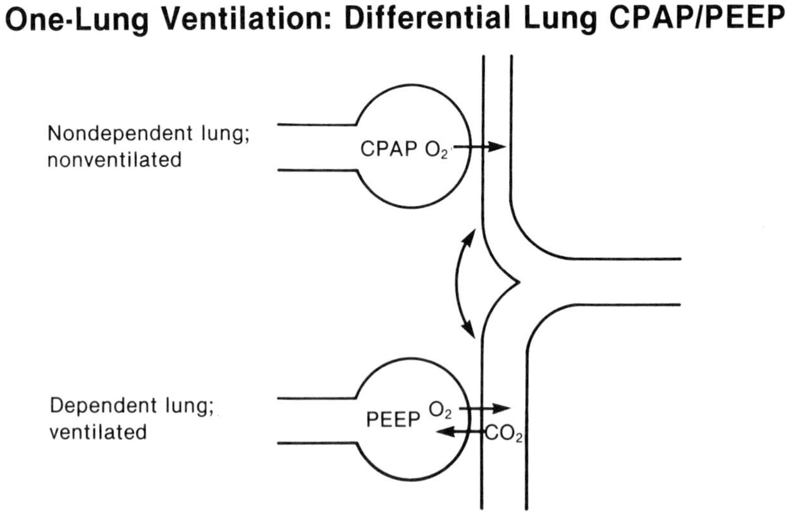

Figure 11–17 • Differential lung continuous positive airway pressure (CPAP)/positive end-expiratory pressure (PEEP) during one-lung ventilation allows for the whole lung to participate in oxygen uptake and markedly reduces the shunt during one-lung ventilation. With differential lung CPAP/PEEP, the distribution of blood flow is not critically important because the whole lung can participate in oxygen uptake. (Reproduced with permission from Benumof JL. Anesthesia for Thoracic Surgery. Philadelphia, WB Saunders, 1987, Fig. 11–10, p. 282.)

manner in an effort to improve ventilated lung volume and ventilation–perfusion relationships. Simultaneously, the nonventilated (nondependent) lung receives CPAP in an attempt to improve oxygenation of the blood perfusing this lung. Therefore, with differential lung PEEP or PEEP/CPAP, it does not matter where the blood flow goes nearly as much as during simple one-lung ventilation, since wherever it goes (to either ventilated or nonventilated lung), it has at least some chance to participate in gas exchange with alveoli that are expanded with oxygen.

Differential lung PEEP/CPAP should begin with the application of 5–10 cm H_2O CPAP to the nondependent lung (Fig. 11–18). Nondependent lung CPAP should be applied during the deflation phase of a large tidal volume breath in order to overcome critical opening pressures in the atelectatic lung. If oxygenation does not improve with nondependent lung CPAP (which it does in the large majority of cases), 5–10 cm H_2O of PEEP to the ventilated dependent lung should then be applied. If dependent lung PEEP does not improve oxygenation, nondependent lung CPAP should be increased to 10–15 cm H_2O while the dependent lung is maintained at 5–10 cm H_2O of CPAP. If arterial oxygenation is still not satisfactory, then the nondependent lung CPAP level should be matched with an equal amount of dependent lung PEEP. In this way, a differential lung CPAP/PEEP search for the maximum compliance and a minimum right-to-left transpulmonary shunt is done in an attempt to find the optimal end-expiratory pressure for each lung and the patient as a whole.

B. *Management of Differential Lung Ventilation (in the Intensive Care Unit)*

There are now multiple reports of significant increases in oxygenation obtained with the application of differential lung ventilation and positive end-expiratory pressure (either PEEP/PEEP, PEEP/CPAP, or CPAP/CPAP) through double-lumen endotracheal tubes to patients in the ICU with acute respiratory failure due to predominantly unilateral lung disease.[39–50] In all cases, conventional two-lung therapy (mechanical ventilation, PEEP, CPAP) was administered via a standard single-lumen tube and either failed to improve or actually decreased oxygenation.

The main criterion for initiating differential lung ventilation in patients with unilateral lung disease is an increase in shunt and a decrease in arterial oxygen tension caused by PEEP to all the lung[51,52]; presumably, the PEEP causes further distention of only the normal lung, and there is continued failure to expand the diseased areas of lung. The distention of normal lung increases normal lung pulmonary vascular resistance, causing a diversion of blood flow away from the normal lung to the hypoxic lung. Of course, the chest radiograph must show severe unilateral asymmetric lung disease. An additional specific indication for initiation of differential lung ventilation, which is independent of the PEEP-induced shunting issue, is the presence of a bronchopleural fistula that prevents positive pressure ventilation because of loss of tidal volume through the fistula.

There are several methods for demonstrating a PEEP-induced increase in shunt with unilateral lung disease. First and most common, shunt can be measured before and after the application of PEEP. Second, pulmonary angiograms, which provide a qualitative measure of regional lung blood flow, can be obtained via a pulmonary artery catheter injection.[53] Third, lung perfusion scans, which provide a quantitative measure of regional blood flow, can be performed with radioisotopes.[54]

The specific management of differential lung ventilation and PEEP for the patient with unilateral lung disease is as follows. Since it may be necessary to deter-

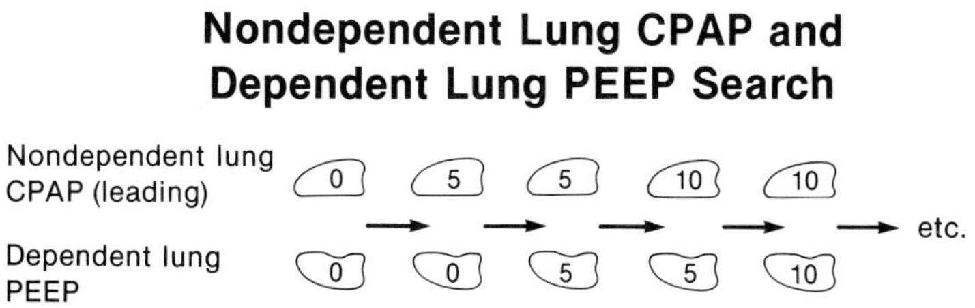

Figure 11–18 • A search for optimal nondependent-lung continuous positive airway pressure (CPAP) and dependent-lung positive end-expiratory pressure (PEEP) is performed by leading with nondependent-lung CPAP and following with dependent-lung PEEP. Leading with nondependent-lung CPAP removes the deleterious arterial oxygenation blood flow diversion effects of dependent-lung PEEP. (Reproduced with permission from Benumof JL. Anesthesia for Thoracic Surgery. Philadelphia, WB Saunders, 1987, Fig. 11–13, p. 285.)

mine the position of the double-lumen tube with precision at any time (eg, following any significant patient movement), a fiberoptic bronchoscope should be at bedside. The more diseased lung should be placed in a nondependent position. The compliance of each lung should then be measured separately. The amount of PEEP applied to lung should initially be inversely proportional to the compliance of each lung. For example, if one lung has one-third the compliance of the other lung, then it would be reasonable to initially apply 15 cm H_2O to the diseased lung and 5 cm H_2O to the nondiseased lung. The tidal volume to each lung should be equal; equal tidal volumes will, of course, result in different peak inspiratory pressures. The application of PEEP inversely proportional to lung compliance and use of equal tidal volumes has most often resulted in equal functional residual capacities and blood flows to each lung. Poorer results have been obtained with ventilator settings resulting in equal end-tidal carbon dioxide concentrations or equal airway pressures.[55]

It was originally thought that the two lungs would have to be ventilated synchronously because asynchronous differential lung ventilation would cause mediastinal movements that would impair cardiovascular performance. However, experimental and clinical experience has not supported this hypothesis, and the two lungs do not have to be ventilated synchronously.[56,57] In fact, some studies suggest that asynchronous or alternating differential lung ventilation actually improves compliance of each lung because one lung does not have to compete with the other during inspiration for space within the thorax.[56,57] When the two lungs have achieved an equal compliance and the chest radiograph has improved, the double-lumen tube should be switched to a single-lumen tube, and treatment should proceed as described in Chapter 6.

V. Complications of Lung Separation Procedures

A. *Double-Lumen Tube Intubation*

An impediment to arterial oxygenation is inherent in the use of double-lumen endotracheal tubes for one-lung anesthesia; in addition, the tubes themselves are occasionally the cause of other serious complications (Table 11-5). The first three of the complications in Table 11-5 are self-explanatory. The fourth, suturing of a double-lumen tube to an intrathoracic structure, has been a cause of death.[58] The possibility of a suture through the endotracheal tube should be considered whenever excessive resistance to extubation is encountered; the consideration of this complication may warrant reexploration of the chest. The possibility of this complication occurring during pneumonectomy should be minimized if an opposite-sided double-lumen endotracheal tube is used or if the double-lumen endotracheal tube is withdrawn into the trachea just before the bronchus is clamped.

Table 11-5 • Complications of Double-Lumen Tubes

1. Malpositioning
2. Tracheobronchial tree disruption
3. Traumatic laryngitis
4. Suturing of double-lumen tube to intrathoracic structure

In a series of approximately 2700 thoracic procedures in which a red rubber Carlens tube was used, five cases of traumatic tracheobronchial rupture were discovered.[59] In three cases the rupture was noted intraoperatively, and in the other two it was discovered early in the postoperative period. All patients underwent successful direct repair of the injuries. The authors suggested that factors leading to this injury included the use of inappropriately sized double-lumen tubes, tube malpositioning, and rapid and excessive inflation of tube cuffs (Table 11-6). These reports emphasize that postoperative bronchoscopy should be performed to rule out

Table 11-6 • Endobronchial Cuff Considerations to Minimize Tracheobronchial Wall Damage (Disruption)

1. Be particularly cautious in patients with bronchial wall abnormalities.
2. Pick an appropriately sized tube.
3. Be certain tube is not malpositioned.*
4. Avoid overinflation of endobronchial cuff.*
5. Deflate endobronchial cuff during turning.
6. Inflate endobronchial cuff slowly.
7. Inflate endobronchial cuff with inspired gases.
8. Do not allow tube to move during turning.*

*Most important considerations.

the diagnosis of tracheobronchial rupture when an unexplained serious pneumothorax or pneumomediastinum persists after thoracotomy.

Bronchial rupture has also occurred with the use of the red rubber Robertshaw double-lumen endotracheal tube. An intraoperative diagnosis of bronchial rupture was made by the detection of mediastinal bubbles and subsequent direct inspection of the left bronchus; intraoperative repair resulted in an uneventful recovery.[60] The authors suggest that this complication can be avoided by proper selection of tube size, deflation of the endobronchial cuff prior to turning to the lateral decubitus position, and checking the integrity of the previously intubated bronchus at the time of testing the bronchial stump for leaks (see Table 11–6). Obviously, great care must be taken when moving the patient from the supine to the lateral decubitus position to prevent tube movement, which can cause not only tube malposition, but also tracheobronchial tree damage (see Table 11–5).

Bronchial rupture has also occurred with the use of the red rubber White double-lumen tube.[61] In this case of right mainstem bronchial rupture, nitrous oxide diffusion into the right endobronchial cuff causing excessive right endobronchial cuff volumes was felt to be the cause. The authors therefore recommend that the cuffs be inflated with a sample of the inspired mixture of gases rather than with room air, or that cuff pressures be monitored, so that variation in cuff pressure can be observed and corrected (see Table 11–6). As a simple method of monitoring cuff pressures and dealing with excessive cuff volumes and pressures, the tension in the pilot balloons to the cuffs can be periodically palpated and gas removed from the cuffs if the tension appears to be increasing (by the same standard of practice as with single-lumen tubes) (see Table 11–6). The authors also noted that bronchial rupture is more likely to occur in patients with congenital abnormalities of the bronchus; weakness of the bronchial wall caused by infiltration of tumor, by infection, or by poor-quality tissues (sepsis, alcoholism, drug abuse); and distortion of the bronchial tree by enlarged mediastinal lymph glands or extrabronchial tumors (see Table 11–6). In addition, the authors felt that the bevel of the tube or carinal hook can dissect underneath the mucosa. Finally, the authors correctly warned of the dangers of advancing the stylet beyond the vocal cords and of using force to advance the tube further whenever resistance is encountered.

A common thought in the preceding reports is that excessive air volume and pressure in the bronchial balloon may be a major factor in the genesis of tracheobronchial tree tears following double-lumen tube insertion. Consequently, this complication was the logical inspiration for the development of clear plastic, tissue-implantable double-lumen tubes with high-volume, low-pressure cuffs (as it was the earlier inspiration for single-lumen tubes). Indeed, when the tracheobronchial tree is inspected with a fiberoptic bronchoscope after double-lumen tube insertion, much less mucosal damage is caused by the tissue-implantable, low-pressure cuffed tubes than with the red rubber, high-pressure cuffed tubes.[62] Despite these expected findings, tracheobronchial tree disruption has also occurred following the use of the tissue-implantable, low-pressure cuffed double-lumen tubes,[63,64] and the precautions listed in Table 11–6 must be considered even with the modern double-lumen tubes.

B. *Bronchial Blockers*

The problem with a bronchial blocker is its propensity to back out of the mainstem bronchus, especially when surgical manipulation of the hilum is performed. The backing out of a mainstem bronchial blocker into the trachea can be catastrophic for two reasons. First, if the bronchial blocker was being used to seal off a fluid (blood or pus) in one lung, then loss of the seal between the two lungs may cause both lungs to become contaminated with the fluid. Second, the trachea will be at least partially, if not totally, obstructed by the blocker, and ventilation will be greatly impaired. Therefore, bronchial blockage requires that the anesthesiologist continuously and intensively monitor the compliance and breath sounds of the ventilated lung. Because of these potentially catastrophic problems, bronchial blockers are rarely used for elective procedures for adults today.[65] Other disadvantages of bronchial blockage compared with double-lumen endotracheal tube lung separation include the inability to suction or ventilate the lung distal to the blocker, increased placement time, and the definite need for a fiberoptic or rigid bronchoscope.

C. *Endobronchial Intubation with a Single-Lumen Tube*

Endobronchial single-lumen tubes have the same complications as double-lumen tubes. In addition, in view of their mode of placement in urgent situations (hemoptysis) and the use of cuffed tubes in children with short mainstem bronchi, the incidence of upper lobe obstruction is probably much higher than with double-lumen tubes. Finally, endobronchial single-lumen tubes do not allow suctioning or ventilation of the bypassed lung and may require use of a fiberoptic bronchoscope (for left lung intubation).

VI. References

1. Urschel HC Jr, Razzuk MA. Median sternotomy as a standard approach for pulmonary resection. Ann Thorac Surg 41:130–134, 1986.
2. Anderson HW, Benumof JL. Intrapulmonary shunting during one-lung ventilation and surgical manipulation. Anesthesiology 55:A377, 1981.
3. Thomson DF, Campbell D. Changes in arterial oxygen tension during one-lung anesthesia. Br J Anaesth 45:611–616, 1973.
4. Boysen PG. Pulmonary resection and postoperative pulmonary function. Chest 77:718–719, 1980.
5. Boysen PG, Block AG, Moulder PV. Relationship between preoperative pulmonary function tests and complications after thoracotomy. Surg Obstet Gynecol 152:813–815, 1981.
6. Benumof JL, Partridge B, Salvatierra C, Keating J. Margin of safety in positioning modern double-lumen tubes. Anesthesiology 67:729–738, 1987.
7. McKenna MJ, Wilson RS, Botelho RJ. Right upper lobe obstruction with right-sided double-lumen endobronchial tubes: A comparison of two tube types. J Cardiothorac Anesth 2:734–740, 1988.
8. Benumof JL. Improving the design and function of double-lumen tubes. J Cardiothorac Anesth 2:729–733, 1988.
9. Simpson PM. Tracheal intubation with a Robertshaw tube via a tracheostomy. Br J Anaesth 48:373–375, 1976.
10. Seed RF, Wedley JR. Tracheal intubation with a Robertshaw tube via a tracheostomy (letter). Br J Anaesth 49:639, 1977.
11. Smith G, Hirsch N, Ehrenwerth J. Sight and sound: Can double-lumen endotracheal tubes be placed accurately without fiberoptic bronchoscopy? Anaesth Analg 65:S1–S170, 1986.
12. Read RC, Frenchiday CD, Eason CN. Prospective study of the Robertshaw endobronchial catheter in thoracic surgery. Ann Thorac Surg 24:156, 1977.
13. Alfery DD, Benumof JL, Spragg RG. Anesthesia for bronchopulmonary lavage. In Kaplan, J (ed). Thoracic Anesthesia. New York, Churchill-Livingstone, 1982, 403–419.
14. Spragg RG, Benumof JL, Alfery DD. New methods for performance of unilateral lung lavage. Anesthesiology 57:535–538, 1982.
15. Cohen JA, Denisco RA, Richards TS, et al. Hazardous placement of a Robertshaw-type endobronchial tube. Anesth Analg 65:100–101, 1986.
16. Vale R. Selective bronchial blocking in a small child. Br J Anaesth 41:453–454, 1969.
17. Rao CC, Krishna G, Grosfeld JL, et al. One lung pediatric anesthesia. Anesth Analg 60:450, 1981.
18. Cay DL, Csenderits LE, Lines V, et al. Selective bronchial blocking in children. Anaesth Intensive Care 3:117, 1975.
19. Ginsberg RJ. New technique for one lung anesthesia using an endobronchial blocker. J Thorac Cardiovasc Surg 82:542–546, 1981.
20. Inoue H, Shohtsu A, Ogawa J, et al. New device for one lung anesthesia: Endotracheal tube with moveable blocker. J Thorac Cardiovasc Surg 83:940–941, 1982.
21. Kamaya H, Krishna PR. New endotracheal tube (Univent tube) for selective blockade of one lung. Anesthesiology 63:342–343, 1985.
22. Kubota H, Kubota Y, Toyoda Y, et al. Selective blind endobronchial intubation in children and adults. Anesthesiology 67:587–589, 1987.
23. Kubota Y, Magaribuchi T, Toyoda Y, et al. Selective bronchial suctioning in the adult using a curved-tipped catheter with a guide mark. Crit Care Med 10:767–769, 1982.
24. Kubota Y, Toyoda Y, Kubota H, et al. Selective bronchial suctioning in infants and children. Crit Care Med 14:902–903, 1986.
25. Kerr JH. Physiological aspects of one lung (endobronchial) anesthesia. Int Anesth Clin 10:61–78, 1972.
26. Katz JA, Laverne RG, Fairley HB, Thomas AN. Pulmonary oxygen exchange during endobronchial anesthesia: Effects of tidal volume and PEEP. Anesthesiology 56:164–171, 1982.
27. Cohen E, Thys DM, Eisenkraft JB, Kaplan JA. PEEP during one-lung anesthesia improves oxygenation in patients with low arterial P_aO_2. Anesth Analg 64:201, 1985.
28. Khanam T, Branthwaite MA. Arterial oxygenation during one-lung anesthesia. Part 2. Anaesthesia 23:280–290, 1973.
29. Aalto-Setala M, Heinonen J, Salorinne Y. Cardiorespiratory function during thoracic anesthesia: Comparison of two-lung ventilation and one-lung ventilation with and without PEEP. Acta Anaesthesiol Scand 19:287–295, 1975.
30. Tarhan S, Lundborg RO. Effects of increased expiratory pressure on blood gas tensions and pulmonary shunting during thoracotomy with use of the Carlens catheter. Can Anaesth Soc J 17:4–11, 1970.
31. Capan LM, Turndorf H, Chandrakant P, et al. Optimization of arterial oxygenation during one-lung anesthesia. Anesth Analg 59:847–851, 1980.
32. Khanom T, Branthwaite MA. Arterial oxygenation during one-lung anesthesia. Part 1: A study in man. Anaesthesia 28:132–138, 1973.
33. Eisenkraft JB, Thys DM, Cohen E, Kaplan JA. Hemodynamic effects of CPAP and PEEP during one-lung anesthesia with isoflurane. Anesthesiology 61:A520, 1984.
34. Cohen E, Thys DM, Eisenkraft JB, et al. Effect of CPAP and PEEP during one-lung anesthesia: Left versus right thoracotomies. Anesthesiology 63:A564, 1985.
35. Merridew CG, Jones RDM. Nondependent lung CPAP (5 cm H_2O) with oxygen during ketamine, halothane, or isoflurane anesthesia and one-lung ventilation. Anesthesiology 63:A567, 1985.
36. Thiagarajah S, Job C, Rao A. A device for applying CPAP to the nonventilated upper lung during one lung ventilation. I. Anesthesiology 60:253–254, 1984.
37. Hannenberg AA, Satwicz PR, Pienes RS Jr, O'Brien JC. A device for applying CPAP to the nonventilated upper lung during one lung ventilation. II. Anesthesiology 60:254–255, 1984.
38. Brown DL, Davis RS. A simple device for oxygen insufflation with continuous positive airway pressure during one-lung ventilation. Anesthesiology 61:481–482, 1984.
39. Powner DJ, Eross B, Grenvik A. Differential lung ventilation with PEEP in the treatment of unilateral lung ventilation. Crit Care Med 5:170–172, 1977.

40. Gallagher TJ, Banner MJ, Smith RA. A simplified method of independent lung ventilation. Crit Care Med 8:396–398, 1980.
41. Glass DD, Tonnesen AD, Gabel JC, Arens JF. Therapy of unilateral pulmonary insufficiency with a double-lumen endotracheal tube. Crit Care Med 4:323–326, 1976.
42. Trew F, Warren BR, Potter WA. Differential lung ventilation in man. Crit Care Med 4:112, 1976.
43. Benjaminsson E, Klain N. Intraoperative dual-mode independent lung ventilation of a patient with bronchopleural fistula. Anesth Analg 60:118–119, 1981.
44. Rafferty TD, Palma J, Motoyama, EK, Schachter N, Ciarcia F. Management of a bronchopleural fistula with differential lung ventilation and positive end-expiratory pressure. Respir Care 25:654–657, 1980.
45. Rivara D, Bourgaim L, Rieuf P, et al. Differential ventilation in unilateral lung disease: Effects of respiratory mechanics and gas exchange. Intensive Care Med 5:189–191, 1979.
46. Ray C, Carlon GC, Miodownik S, Glodiner PL. A method of synchronizing two MA-1 ventilators for independent lung ventilation. Crit Care Med 6:99, 1978.
47. Parish JM, Gracey DR, Southorn PA, et al. Differential mechanical ventilation in respiratory failure due to severe unilateral lung disease. Mayo Clin Proc 59:822, 1984.
48. Murray JF. Treatment of acute total atelectasis: Use of a double-lumen tube. Anaesthesia 40:158–162, 1985.
49. Stow PJ, Grant I. Asynchronous independent lung ventilation: Its use in the treatment of acute unilateral lung disease. Anaesthesia 40:163–166, 1985.
50. Hillman KM, Barber JD. Asynchronous independent lung ventilation (AILV). Crit Care Med 8:390–395, 1980.
51. Carlon GC, Ray C Jr, Klein R, et al. Criteria for selective positive end-expiratory pressure and independent synchronized ventilation of each lung. Chest 74:501–507, 1978.
52. Hedenstierna G, Baehrendtz S, Frostell C, et al. Differential ventilation in acute respiratory failure. Indications and outcome. Bull Eur Physiopathol Respir 21:281–285, 1985.
53. Carlon GC, Kahn R, Howland WS, et al. Acute life-threatening ventilation-perfusion inequality: An indication for independent lung ventilation. Crit Care Med 6:380–383, 1978.
54. Kanarek DJ, Shannon DC. Adverse effect of positive end-expiratory pressure on pulmonary perfusion and oxygenation. Am Rev Respir Dis 112:457–459, 1975.
55. East TD, Pace NL, Westenskow DR, et al. Differential ventilation with unilateral PEEP following unilateral hydrochloric acid aspiration in the dog. Acta Anaesthesiol Scand 27:356–360, 1983.
56. Muneyuki M, Konishi K, Horiguchi R, et al. Effects of alternating lung ventilation on cardiopulmonary function in dogs. Anesthesiology 58:353–356, 1983.
57. Hameroff SR, Caukins JM, Waterson CK, et al. High-frequency alternating lung ventilation. Anesthesiology 54:237–239, 1981.
58. Dryden GE. Circulatory collapse after pneumonectomy (an unusual complication from the use of a Carlens catheter): Case report. Anesth Analg 56:451, 1977.
59. Guernelli N, Bragaglia RB, Briccoli A, et al. Tracheobronchial ruptures due to cuffed Carlens tubes. Ann Thorac Surg 28:66, 1979.
60. Heiser M, Steinberg JJ, MacVaugh H, et al. Bronchial rupture, a complication of use of the Robertshaw double-lumen tube. Anesthesiology 51:88, 1979.
61. Foster JNG, Lau OJ, Alimo EB. Ruptures bronchus following endobronchial intubation. Br J Anaesth 55:687–688, 1983.
62. Clapham MCC, Vaughan RS. Bronchial intubation. A comparison between polyvinyl chloride and red rubber double lumen tubes. Anaesthesia 40:1111–1114, 1985.
63. Wagner DL, Gammage GW, Wong ML. Tracheal rupture following the insertion of a disposable double-lumen endotracheal tube. Anesthesiology 63:698–700, 1985.
64. Burton NA, Fall SM, Lyons T, Graeber GM. Rupture of the left mainstem bronchus with a polyvinylchloride double-lumen tube. Chest 83:928–929, 1983.
65. Pappin JC. The current practice of endobronchial intubation. Anaesthesia 34:57–64, 1979.

Chapter 12

•

Joanne Zupan, MD

Fiberoptic Bronchoscopy in Anesthesia and Critical Care

OUTLINE

I. INTRODUCTION

The flexible fiberoptic bronchoscope (FOB) has become an important tool in the practice of anesthesia and critical care. In particular, it has greatly enhanced the ability of the anesthesiologist to evaluate and manage the airway.

A multitude of diagnostic and therapeutic procedures may be performed with a bronchoscope.[1] These applications require rigorous, supervised training; the prerequisites for certification as a fully trained bronchoscopist are clearly defined by the American College of Chest Physicians. Minimal acceptable training includes 50 cases done under direct supervision, at least 25 of which are diagnostic. Because most anesthesiologists do not meet these requirements, the emphasis of this chapter will be on applications of flexible bronchoscopy in airway management, which are within the realm of anesthesia training. For further discussion of the use of flexible bronchoscopy in the practice of pulmonology, the reader is referred to several reviews.[2–7]

A. *Design and Construction of the Fiberoptic Bronchoscope*

The flexible FOB has several components. It has at least two fiberoptic light bundles, one to transmit light and another to transmit an image back to the viewer. Most bronchoscopes contain a working channel for suction and passage of instruments such as brushes and forceps. Other details of construction, such as length, bending radius of the tip, number of fiber bundles, and immersibility in water, affect the cost and versatility of the instrument. For purposes of evaluation and management of the adult airway, a bronchoscope with an outer diameter (OD) of 5 mm and a suction channel of 2 to 2.2 mm is usually suitable. This can be placed in endotracheal tubes with as small as 6 mm internal diameter (ID). Many bronchoscopes will accommodate a teaching head, camera, or video recorder as well. Several types of light sources are available; they vary in cost and quality, but most are suitable for the anesthesiologist's purposes. Of particular importance is the outer diameter (OD) of the scope. Larger FOBs typically have the advantage of a larger suction channel, or more fiber bundles, or both. However, larger scopes are more difficult to pass through endotrachial tubes (ETs) and small airways. The resistance to airflow through an airway of fixed diameter is inversely proportional to the fourth power of its radius. A bronchoscope effectively decreases the internal diameter of the ET it occupies. The larger the scope, the smaller the effective internal diameter of the ET (Fig. 12–1).[8] Thus, a small increase in OD of a bronchoscope can produce a substantial increase in airway resistance with a consequent increase in the work of breathing and a requirement for higher airway pressure or flow if positive pressure ventilation is being provided.[8–10]

II. Indications for Fiberoptic Bronchoscopy

A number of uses for the bronchoscope in the practice of anesthesia and critical care have been described (Table 12–1). Fiberoptic endotracheal intubation is indicated in patients in whom direct laryngoscopy or blind intubation is expected to be difficult or impossible.[11–13] Such patients include those with mouth contractures (eg, burns), arthritis of the temporomandibular joint or cervical spine,[14,15] maxillofacial trauma, airway compromise (eg, tumor, edema, hematoma), anatomic abnormalities (eg, acromegaly, micrognathia, congenital anomalies), previous airway surgery, a fixed cervical spine (eg, halo, previous fusion), morbid obesity, or myopathy. Bronchoscopic intubation is also indicated in patients in whom neck extension is to be avoided (eg, patients with cervical radiculopathies, unstable cervical spines, or vertebrobasilar insufficiency). The FOB may be used routinely (ie, in the absence of the expectation of airway difficulty) to facilitate awake intubation (eg, prior to awake prone positioning in patients with spine injuries).

Obstruction of airways by secretions or mucus plugs is a common indication for therapeutic pulmonary toilet via the bronchoscope.[16,17] Successful reexpansion

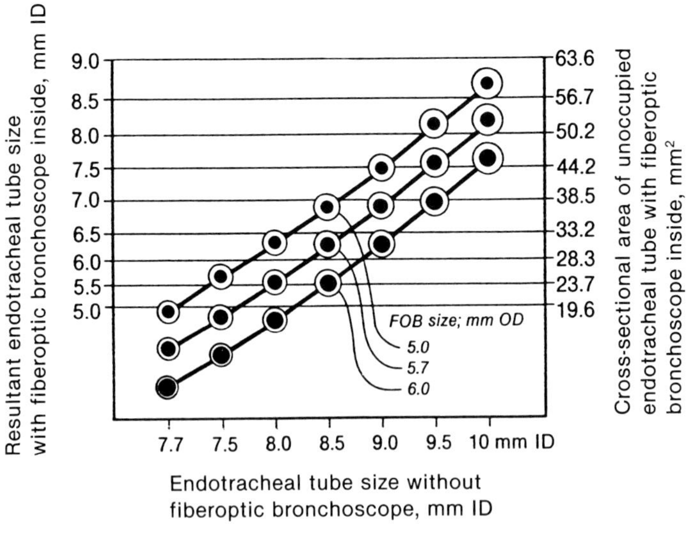

Figure 12–1 • This diagram relates the size of an endotracheal (ET) tube without an indwelling fiberoptic bronchoscope (x axis) to the resultant functional size that the endotracheal tube would have with an indwelling fiberoptic bronchoscope (left-hand y axis). Bronchoscopes of three different outside diameters are shown: 5.0, 5.7, and 6.0 mm. The remaining cross-sectional area of endotracheal tube (in mm) that is responsible for the resultant functional size is shown on the right-hand y axis. (Reproduced with permission from Benumof JL. Anesthesia for Thoracic Surgery. Philadelphia, WB Saunders, 1987, pp. 241–243.)

Table 12-1 • Clinical Applications of Fiberoptic Bronchoscopy

Endotracheal intubation
Awake: oral, nasal
Anesthetized: oral, nasal
Pulmonary toilet
Foreign body removal
Evaluation of airway trauma or burns
Verification of endotracheal tube position
Double-lumen
Single-lumen
Endobronchial intubation
Evaluation of endotracheal tube obstruction
Endotracheal tube change
Tracheal extubation

of atelectatic lobes by selective application of positive pressure via the bronchoscope has been described.[18] Bronchoscopy is valuable in both diagnosis and treatment of aspiration of gastric contents, teeth, or foreign bodies.[19-21]

Indications for diagnostic bronchoscopy include pneumothorax and wounds that possibly involve the airway (to rule out airway rupture or laceration).[17] Localization and occlusion of bronchopleural fistulas via a bronchoscope has been reported.[22] Diagnostic bronchoscopy should be performed in patients with inhalation injuries, including those with a history of a close facial burn, cough productive of sooty material, hoarseness, stridor, singed nasal hairs, or increased carbon monoxide level. Early bronchoscopy following inhalation injury provides diagnostically and prognostically useful information with respect to extent of airway injury and need for tracheal intubation.[23-25]

The bronchoscope is used to verify position of both single- and double-lumen ETs,[26,27] to perform deliberate endobronchial intubation, to evaluate airway obstruction,[28] to change an ET,[29-31] and to evaluate and resecure (if necessary) the airway at the time of extubation.[32]

III. How to Clinically Use Fiberoptic Bronchoscopy

A. *Equipment Preparation and Care*

Preparation of equipment for bronchoscopy is simple. The FOB is connected to the light source. The scope is usually held so that the greater degree of bending radius is downward, ie, toward the operator. The suction tubing is connected; the pedal to activate the suction is positioned where it can be comfortably reached. The focus is adjusted, and attachments such as teaching head or camera are connected. The insertion tube is lubricated with a silicon-based fluid. Ancillary airway equipment, including nasal trumpets, oral airways, oxygen and anesthesia masks, laryngoscopes, and ETs should be readily available. Masks and oral airways modified to facilitate bronchoscopic endotracheal intubation are useful aids.[31,33,34]

The FOB must be decontaminated and disinfected following each use, regardless of patient diagnosis. Iatrogenic infection following airway instrumentation with contaminated bronchoscopes has been reported to occur with several pathogens including *Pseudomonas*, *M. tuberculosis*, and *Bacillus* and *Serratia* species.[35-37] No cases of viral transmission have been reported.

The most important infection control measure is thorough cleaning of the bronchoscope. The exterior of the instrument as well as its working channel should be cleaned with a detergent (eg, hexachlorophene) immediately following each patient contact to remove secretions and debris before they dry. Proteinaceous material may support the growth of microorganisms and inhibit the action of the disinfectant. After cleaning, disinfection is achieved by soaking the instrument in 2% glutaraldehyde for 10 to 30 minutes. It is then rinsed with either 70% alcohol or water. Alcohol is a potent mycobactericide but may damage the instrument if it is immersed or kept in contact for more than a few minutes.

Contamination of bronchoscopes with *M. tuberculosis* or human immunodeficiency virus (HIV) is reduced by more than 99% by cleaning with detergent. When these cleaned instruments are then disinfected in 2% alkaline glutaraldehyde, all detectable antigens from these organisms are removed.[35]

B. *Patient Preparation and Monitoring*

1. Monitoring

Whether in the operating room or intensive care unit (ICU), the patient will be prepared and monitored similarly for most applications. Routine operating room monitors, including pulse oximeter, blood pressure cuff, and electrocardiograph (ECG), should be applied.

2. PREMEDICATION

Patients should not be fed for at least 8 hours prior to elective bronchoscopy to minimize the risk of vomiting and aspiration of gastric contents. A vagolytic agent, usually atropine or glycopyrrolate, is administered prior to the procedure for several reasons. Both agents cause an increase in heart rate,[38] and are thought to prevent a vagally mediated bradycardia in response to airway manipulation.[39] Both produce bronchodilatation and decreased airway resistance,[38] and may attenuate bronchospasm when it occurs. Vital capacity, forced expiratory volume in 1 second (FEV_1), and expiratory flow rate are all increased.[39,40] The increase in anatomic dead space attributable to atropine[41] may require an increase in minute ventilation to maintain normocapnea, but it is extremely rare for this to be clinically important. Both are excellent drying agents. Patients with a history of reactive airway disease may be premedicated with inhaled bronchodilators, intravenous steroids, or aminophylline. Patients may be sedated with a benzodiazepine or narcotic to improve patient comfort and acceptance, but this must be done cautiously to avoid significant respiratory depression. Sedation is frequently unnecessary when the airway has been well prepared with topical anesthetic.

3. SUPPLEMENTAL OXYGEN

Supplemental oxygen should always be administered. Arterial hypoxemia during bronchoscopy has been well documented, with an average decrease in P_aO_2 of 20–30 mmHg in patients breathing room air. Baseline P_aO_2 may not be reached for several hours postbronchoscopy.[42] Cardiac arrhythmias frequently occur during periods of hypoxemia.[43] Supplemental oxygen can be conveniently delivered via nasal cannulae or a face mask with a hole in one side to permit easy passage of the bronchoscope.

4. TOPICAL AIRWAY ANESTHESIA

Adequate airway anesthesia is essential for optimal patient acceptance and working conditions. Local anesthetic is sprayed through an atomizer into the nostrils (if a nasal approach is to be used) and oropharynx. The airway is prepared for nasotracheal intubation as follows. A vasoconstrictor is applied to decrease mucosal swelling and prevent bleeding. The patient may be asked to inhale oxymetazolone or neosynephrine 0.25% nosedrops, or epinephrine may be added to the atomized local anesthetic. Either tetracaine 0.45% with epinephrine 1:80,000 to a total tetracaine dose of 2 mg/kg, or lidocaine 1%–2% to a maximal dose of 7 mg/kg may be used topically. Alternatively, nasal pledgets soaked in 4% cocaine may be used for both vasoconstriction and anesthesia. Atomized local anesthetic is applied to the nostril and oropharynx. A flow of 8–10 L of oxygen per minute is delivered through tubing connected to the atomizer, with a hole cut in the tubing near the connection to the atomizer. When this hole is occluded, local anesthetic will be sprayed through the atomizer tip (Fig. 12–2). The larger nostril is then serially dilated with rubber nasal trumpets (26–34 Fr) lubricated with 2% lidocaine jelly.

For orotracheal intubation, the oropharynx is sprayed with atomized local anesthetic as described above. The patient is encouraged to breathe deeply so that the anesthetic is carried into the larynx and trachea.

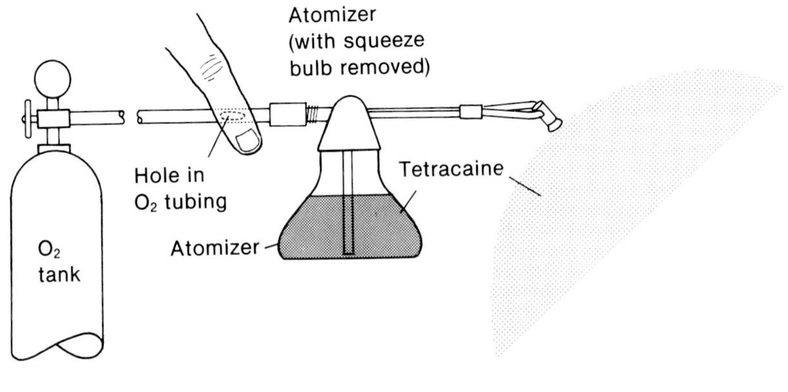

Figure 12–2 • This schematic diagram shows the system for creating a fine mist of local anesthetic. Oxygen tubing is connected to an oxygen tank. A hole is cut in the oxygen tubing near the nebulization chamber. When oxygen is flowing in the tubing and a finger is placed over the hole, a fine mist from the nebulization chamber results. The size and velocity of the spray of mist is proportional to the oxygen flow rate. (Reproduced with permission from Benumof JL. Anesthesia for Thoracic Surgery. Philadelphia, WB Saunders, 1987, pp. 241–243.)

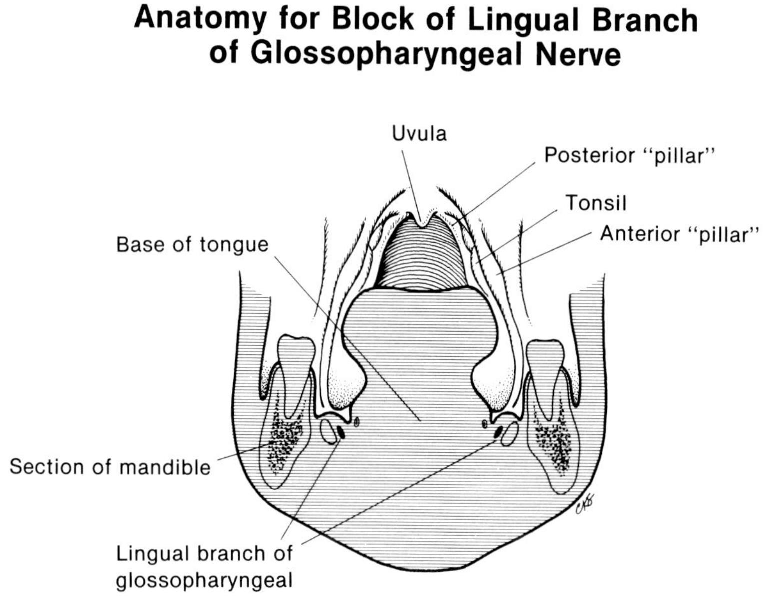

Figure 12–3 • Coronal section through the mouth at the level of the anterior tonsillar pillar. The glossopharyngeal nerve is blocked by injecting 1–2 mL of local anesthetic at the base of the tongue where it meets the anterior tonsillar pillar. The needle should be directed slightly laterally and posteriorly at a 45° angle to the floor of the mouth while aspirating.

5. Supplemental Nerve Blocks

Anesthesia for either approach (oral or nasal) may be supplemented with glossopharyngeal nerve block at the base of the tongue, superior laryngeal nerve block, or transtracheal spraying of local anesthetic.

The glossopharyngeal nerve carries the sensory innervation of the pharynx, tonsils, and posterior third of the tongue.[44,45] It is blocked by retracting the tongue laterally and identifying the anterior tonsillar pillar. A 25 gauge needle is inserted into the anterior tonsillar pillar near the base of the tongue and advanced slightly laterally and posteriorly at a 45° angle to the floor of the mouth while aspirating. If air is aspirated, the needle has passed through the glossopalatal arch into the posterior pharynx and should be pulled back. If neither air nor blood is aspirated, 2 mL of 1% lidocaine are injected bilaterally (Fig. 12–3).

The internal branch of the superior laryngeal nerve supplies the sensory innervation of the epiglottis, aryepiglottic folds, and mucus membranes of the larynx down to the false cords. It is blocked by palpating the greater cornu of the hyoid bone near the tip. A 25 gauge needle is inserted just inferiorly and medially, and 2–3 mL of 1% lidocaine are injected superficially (Fig. 12–4). The block is performed bilaterally.[46,47]

Transtracheal spray of 2–4 mL of 1% lidocaine will anesthetize the upper larynx. The cricothyroid membrane is punctured with a 25 gauge needle at 90° to the skin, and the needle is advanced until air is aspirated from the trachea. The local anesthetic is then injected.[46]

If the patient's trachea is already intubated, local anesthetic may be injected directly into the airway via the ET prior to diagnostic or therapeutic bronchoscopy.

C. *Fiberoptic Endotracheal Intubation Techniques*

The FOB facilitates endotracheal intubation by both oral and nasal routes in the awake or anesthetized patient. Excellent working conditions can be achieved in a mildly sedated patient with a well-topicalized airway. General anesthesia with or without topical anesthesia is more commonly employed in the pediatric population.

1. Nasotracheal Intubation

a. Awake Patient

For awake nasotracheal intubation, the airway is topicalized as described above. The ET may be immersed in warm sterile water for a few minutes to make it softer and more pliable. The cuff is inflated, checked for leakage, and deflated; the ET is then lubricated with a silicone-based fluid or lidocaine jelly. The 15-mm connector is removed, and the tube is threaded over the bronchoscope (Fig. 12–5). The operator stands on the

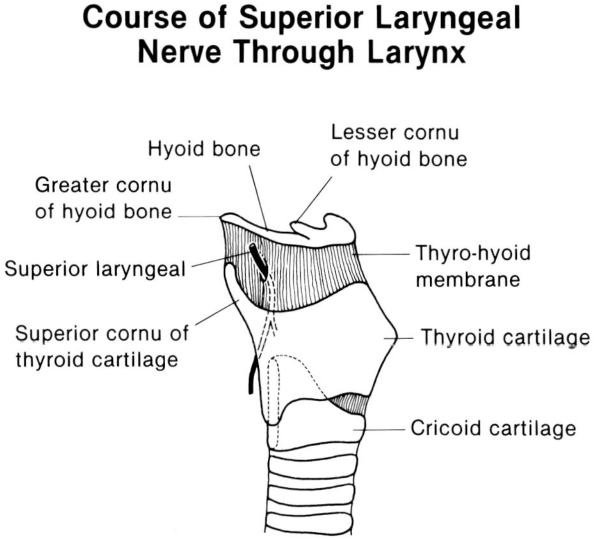

Figure 12–4 • Important landmarks for block of the internal branch of the superior laryngeal nerve. The nerve pierces the thyrohyoid membrane between the superior cornu of the thyroid cartilage and the greater cornu of the hyoid bone. Block of this nerve will produce anesthesia of the epiglottis, aryepiglottic folds, and mucus membranes of the larynx down to the false cords.

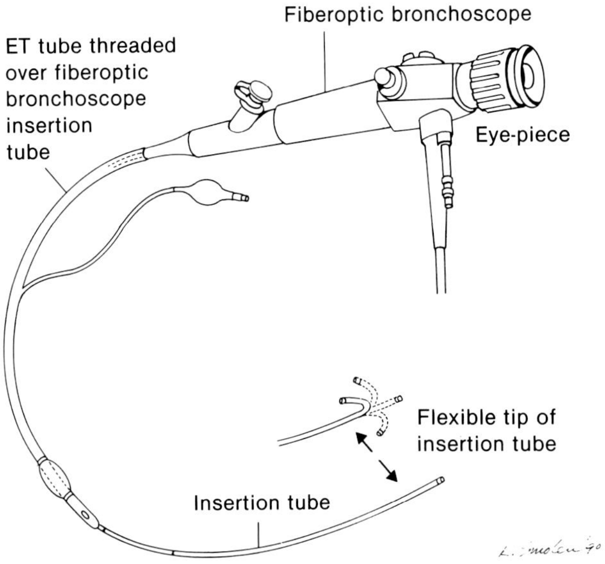

Figure 12–5 • The endotracheal (ET) tube is ensleeved over the insertion tube of the bronchoscope. The 15-mm connector has been removed, and the endotracheal tube is secured to the body of the scope with a piece of tape. The distal end of the insertion tube is lubricated with a silicon-based fluid, and the cuff of the endotracheal tube is deflated.

patient's right side and facing him. The FOB is placed through the fenestration in the oxygen mask and into the patient's larger nostril (usually determined by asking the patient through which nostril it is easier to breathe). The insertion tube is oriented such that the greater degree of bending radius is downward. Slight tension is maintained between the body of the bronchoscope and the hand controlling the insertion tube, so that rotational movements or changes in angulation of the body are more readily translated to the working end of the insertion tube (Fig 12–6). When suction is necessary, the FOB should be advanced and pulled back 1–2 cm several times during the course of suctioning. This will remove secretions more effectively than when the FOB is held stationary, and is less traumatic to mucosa than continued negative pressure applied to a small surface area.

The tip of the FOB is advanced along the floor of the nasal passage. This keeps the turbinates in view, and the lumen of the passage is easily identified (it is black). If the lumen is lost to view, the scope should be slowly pulled back until it is reidentified, then advanced with a slight change in rotation or tip angulation (usually downward) to keep the lumen in view. It is usually possible to pass the FOB through the nasal passage with the tip in neutral position (ie, unbent) until the nasopharynx is reached. At this point, the tip is bent downward while advancing around the curve from the posterior nasopharynx into the oropharynx. The epiglottis will now come into view. The scope is advanced to the cords, usually with the tip in neutral position. The vallecula, piriform fossa, or esophagus may be entered; if so, the scope is withdrawn until the posterior pharynx is identified, then advanced. Once again, a slight modification of rotation or tip bending is usually all that is needed to bring the cords back into view and advance to them. The cords are examined for mobility and presence of lessons. Five to ten mL local anesthetic are sprayed onto the cords through the suction channel, producing anesthesia within a few seconds. The FOB is then passed through the cords and advanced into the trachea (Fig. 12–7). The ET is gently advanced over the insertion tube until its tip is 2–3 cm above the carina. The scope is then removed; the 15-mm adapter is connected to the ET, and the patient is ventilated with oxygen. The ET is secured in position. Anesthesia may then be induced.

An alternative approach is to place the ET blindly through the nasal passage until its tip is in the pharynx, and then advance the FOB through it until the cords

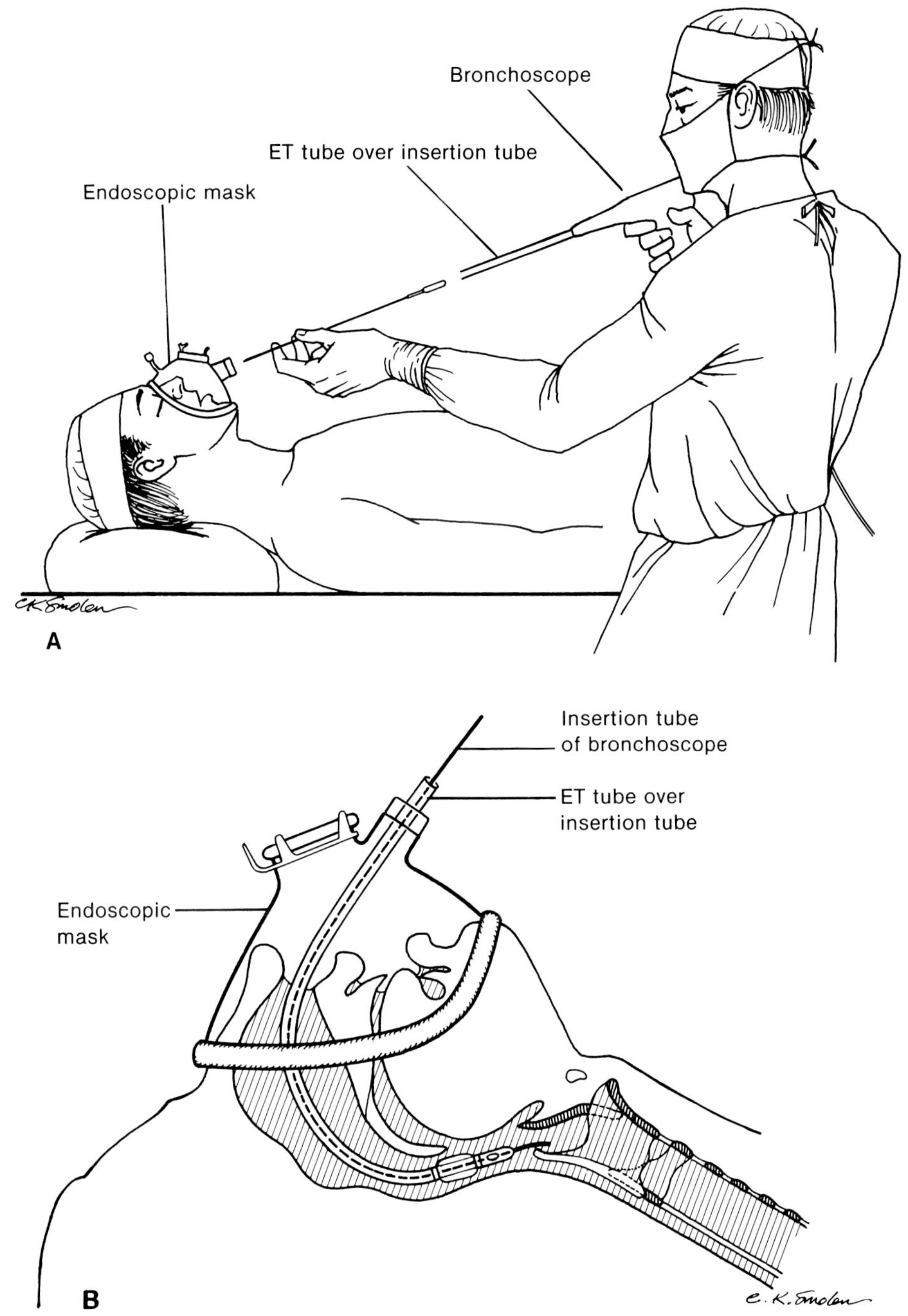

Figure 12–6 • (***A***) Tension is maintained between the body of the bronchoscope in the right hand and the insertion tube in the left hand, so that rotational movements in the body will be translated to the distal end of the scope. (***B***) When bronchoscopy is being performed in a patient who is already intubated, an elbow adapter fitted with a rubber diaphragm is placed in the ventilator circuit. The bronchoscope is passed through the diaphragm, which will prevent leakage of gas from the circuit so that positive-pressure ventilation may be continued during the procedure.

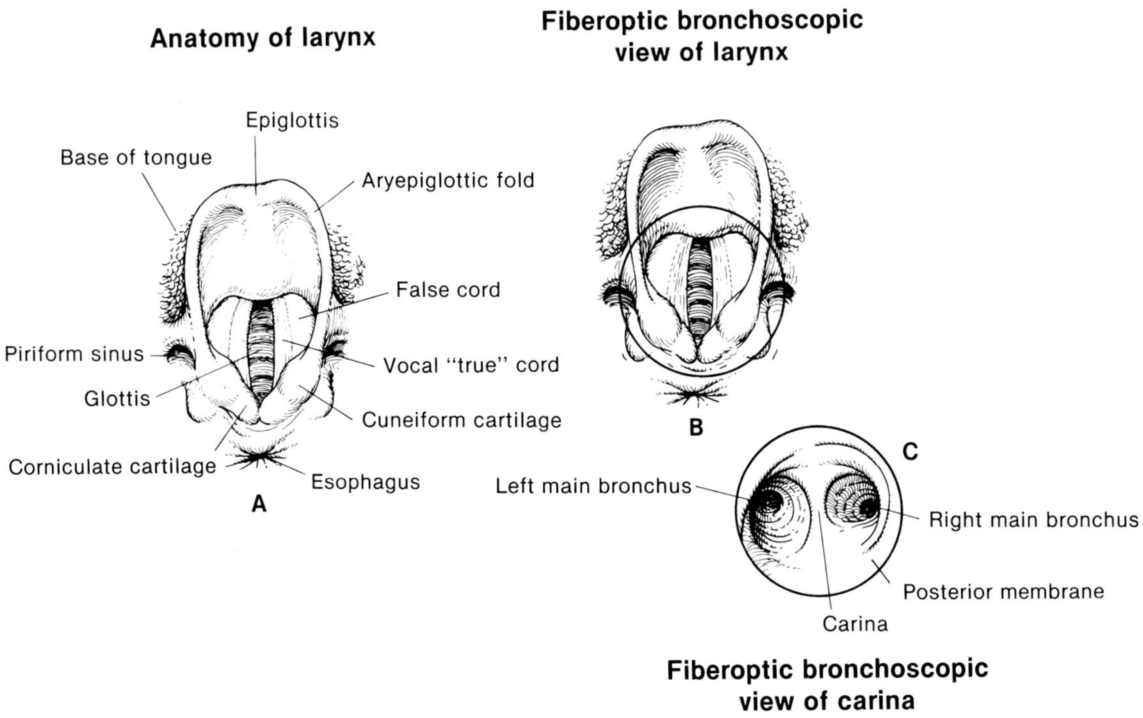

Figure 12–7 • (***A***) View of laryngeal structures that can be visualized through the bronchoscope includes epiglottis, base of tongue, false vocal cords, true vocal cords, glottic inlet, aryepiglottic folds, corniculate and cuneiform cartilages. (***B***) The true field of view is smaller than shown in ***A*** (ie, it is usually not possible to see all of these structures simultaneously at close range. It is usually possible to obtain a view similar to that enclosed in the circle). (***C***) After passage through the vocal cords, the bronchoscope is advanced until the tracheal carina comes into view. The tracheal cartilages are C-shaped. The posterior wall of the trachea is membranous and contains no cartilage. It appears as a flat surface without rings.

are identified. The remainder of the procedure is carried out as above. This is less technically demanding than the above approach. However, prior passage of the FOB by the first method will dilate the nasal lumen somewhat, and permits identification of nasal lesions such as polyps or tumor.

b. Anesthetized Patient

The approach to nasotracheal intubation under general anesthesia is similar. The airway should be topicalized and the nostril dilated in the same manner. Intravenous, inhalational, or combined general anesthesia is induced, with spontaneous ventilation of 100% oxygen maintained. Neuromuscular blockade is obviously avoided in patients in whom difficulty with airway management is anticipated. When the patient is well oxygenated and adequately anesthetized, the anesthesia mask is removed completely or is placed over the patient's mouth. Nasal intubation then proceeds as previously described. Anesthesia may be supplemented with intravenous agents, if necessary, during the procedure. If oxyhemoglobin desaturation occurs, the scope should be withdrawn and mask ventilation with 100% oxygen resumed until oxygenation improves before the procedure is again attempted.

2. Orotracheal Intubation

a. Awake Patient

The airway is topicalized as described previously for orotracheal intubation, and mask oxygen is provided. To prevent the patient from biting the insertion tube, either a hollow bite block or an intubating airway should be placed in the mouth (Fig. 12–8A). The latter will protect the bronchoscope, prevent airway obstruction by holding the tongue out of the pharynx, and will guide the scope over the base of the tongue and close to the glottic inlet. The ET is prepared as described for nasal

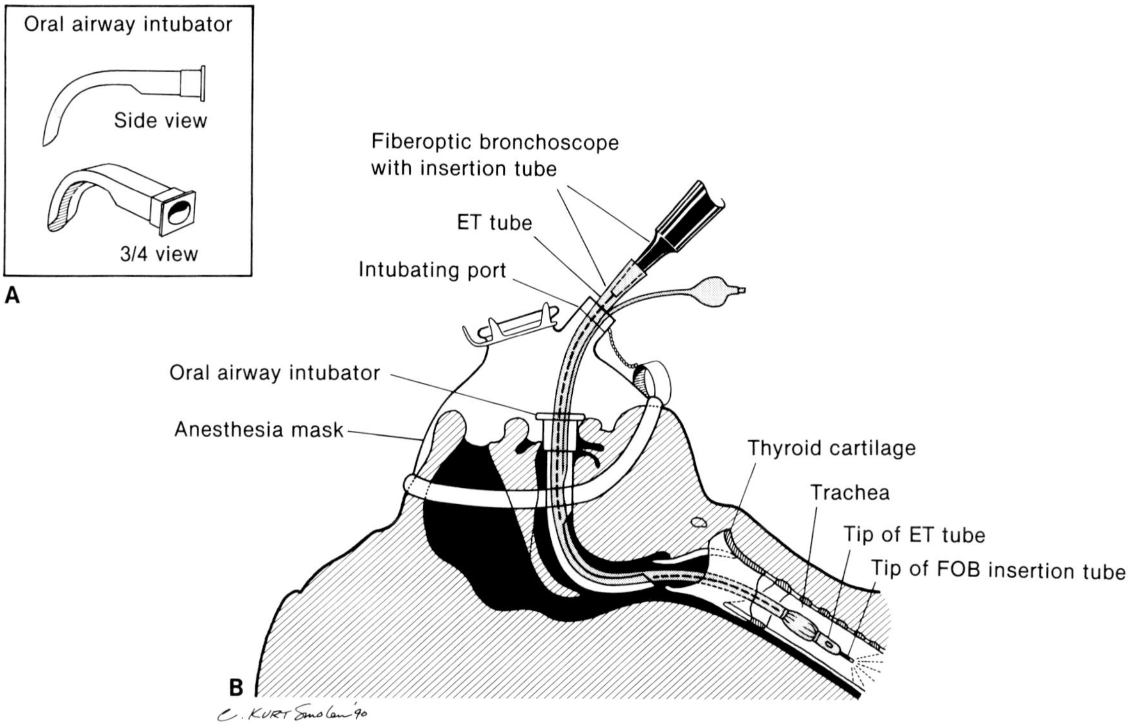

Figure 12–8 • (***A***) The oral airway intubator has a channel large enough to pass an 8.0-mm endotracheal (ET) tube. It curves over the posterior aspect of the tongue, and will guide the bronchoscope close to the glottic inlet. A hollow bite block may also be used to protect the bronchoscope, but offers less control of the instrument in the oropharynx. (***B***) Cutaway view of oral bronchoscopic intubation through the anesthesia mask. The scope passes via the mask port through the intubating oral airway and then into the trachea. The endotracheal tube (previously ensleeved over the bronchoscope) is then advanced into the trachea. The bronchoscope is withdrawn; the endotracheal tube is grasped near the patient's mouth, and the anesthesia mask is removed, with care not to pull back the endotracheal tube in the process.

intubation and is threaded over the FOB. The bronchoscope is advanced through the airway until the cords come into view, and 5–10 mL of local anesthetic are applied to the cords through the suction channel. The bronchoscope is then advanced into the trachea, and the ET is threaded over it and positioned 2–3 cm above the carina. The scope is removed, the 15-mm adapter is connected, and oxygen delivered via the anesthesia circuit. The intubating airway may also be removed before reconnecting the 15-mm adapter (Fig. 12–8B).

b. Anesthetized Patient

Orotracheal intubation under general anesthesia is performed in a similar manner, with the patient spontaneously breathing 100% oxygen. An anesthesia mask with an intubating port fitted with a fenestrated diaphragm has been designed to allow ongoing delivery of 100% oxygen and inhaled anesthetic during the procedure.[34] The bronchoscope is placed through the diaphragm and into the oral airway (see Fig. 12–8B); the mask fit over the patient's face is maintained continually in the usual manner. When the bronchoscope is well into the trachea, the ET is threaded over it through the diaphragm on the mask port. After the ET has been positioned appropriately, the bronchoscope is withdrawn. The ET is then grasped close to the patient's mouth, and the mask is removed. The remainder of the procedure is as described above.

D. Verification of Endotracheal Tube Position

1. SINGLE-LUMEN ENDOTRACHEAL TUBE PLACEMENT

The position of both single- and double-lumen ETs may be verified bronchoscopically. The tip of the single-lumen ET should be 2–3 cm above the carina in adults. In women this corresponds to a depth of insertion of 19–20 cm at the incisors for an oral ET, or 25–26 cm at the naris for a nasal ET; in men these distances are 20–22 cm or 26–28 cm, respectively.

It is important to note that the ET cuff is usually palpable in the suprasternal notch when the depth of insertion is correct. In addition, the distance from ET tip to carina is usually easily determined on chest radiograph. Because correct ET position is so readily verified by these methods, we do not advocate bronchoscopy solely for this purpose. However, when bronchoscopy is performed for other indications, the ET may be correctly positioned during the procedure. The patient's head is held in neutral position, and the tip of the bronchoscope is placed at the carina. The scope is then pulled back 2–3 cm. The ET is repositioned so that its tip is seen through the bronchoscope to be at the same level as the FOB tip, and secured.

2. Double-Lumen Endotracheal Tube Placement

Precise positioning of double-lumen ETs (DLETT) may be achieved with the FOB (see also Chapter 11). The indications for separation of the lungs via DLETT, and the criteria for selection of left- or right-sided DLETTs are discussed at length by Benumof[48] and will not be recapitulated here.

A DLETT possesses two lumina: one designated as tracheal, which will open into the distal trachea when the ET is properly positioned; and the other designated as bronchial, which is placed in a mainstem bronchus. The bronchial portion of a left-sided DLETT (Fig. 12–9A) is placed into the left mainstem bronchus, while the bronchial portion of a right-sided DLETT (Fig. 12–10A) is placed into the right mainstem bronchus.

If a DLETT is inserted too deeply, it is possible for the bronchial portion to occlude the upper lobe bronchus on that side, or for the tracheal lumen to be too close to the carina. If the DLETT is not inserted deeply enough, the bronchial cuff may be placed in the trachea. When this occurs, flow from the tracheal lumen will be obstructed by the bronchial cuff; the opposite lung may or may not be ventilated, depending on the depth of insertion of the bronchial lumen; and separation of the lungs is not achieved. This is of particular concern when a right-sided DLETT is used because the right mainstem bronchus is quite short, with an average distance from tracheal carina to right upper lobe (RUL) bronchus of 21 ± 7 mm in adult women and 23 ± 7 mm in adult men. The left mainstem bronchus is somewhat longer, 45 ± 7 mm in women and 50 ± 7 mm in men.[48] Because the margin for error in correct positioning is so

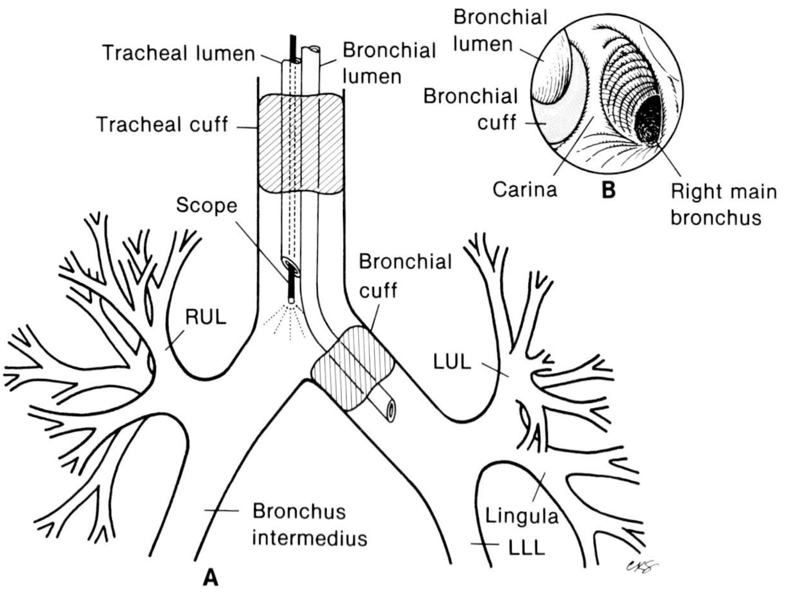

Figure 12–9 • (***A***) Schematic cutaway of a left-sided double-lumen tube in place, with the bronchoscope passed through the tracheal lumen to verify position of the bronchial portion. The tracheal lumen is usually 2–3 cm above the carina. The upper surface of the bronchial cuff is just at the level of the carina. The bronchial lumen opens proximal to the left upper lobe bronchus. (***B***) View through the tracheal lumen of a left-sided double-lumen tube in proper position. The bronchial portion can be seen entering the left main-stem bronchus, with the upper surface of the bronchial cuff just at the level of the carina. The right-main-steam bronchus is unobstructed.

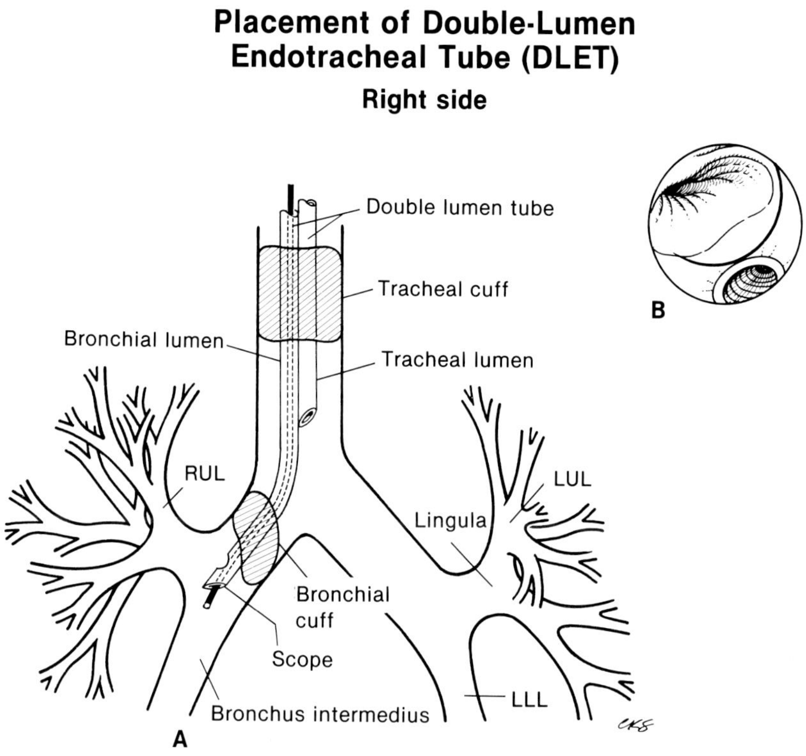

Figure 12–10 • (***A***) Right-sided double-lumen endotracheal (ET) tube in proper position. The tracheal lumen is usually 2–3 cm above the carina. The upper surface of the bronchial cuff is just at the level of the carina. The ventilation slot is positioned at the orifice of the right upper lobe bronchus. The bronchial lumen opens proximal to the right middle lobe bronchus. (***B***) Bronchoscopic view through the ventilation slot of a right-sided double-lumen tube in correct position. The right upper lobe bronchus appears as a crescent. The distal opening of the bronchial lumen lies beyond the ventilation slot.

small, the FOB should be used to verify correct position of the DLETT. The upper lobe bronchi, tracheal carina, and bronchial cuff may all be clearly identified.

The patient should receive 100% oxygen. Local anesthetic may be applied directly to the airway through the bronchoscope if needed. One lumen of the DLETT will be occupied by the FOB while the other lumen will provide ventilation to only one lung. Thus, tidal volume, gas flow rate, inspiratory–expiratory ratio, and respiratory rate should be adjusted appropriately for one-lung ventilation during the examination.

First, the tracheal lumen is clamped proximally so that all of the ventilation is delivered to one lung via the bronchial lumen. The FOB is inserted into the tracheal lumen through the elbow adapter, which contains a capped port. The tracheal carina will come into view, and the bronchial portion of the DLETT should be seen occupying the appropriate mainstem bronchus. If the DLETT has been inserted to an adequate depth, the blue bronchial cuff will be seen in the mainstem bronchus just below the carina (see Fig. 12–9B). If the ET has not been placed deeply enough, the blue bronchial cuff will be seen to override the carina, occupying part of the distal trachea and possibly obstructing part of the opposite mainstem bronchus. If this is the case, both the bronchial and tracheal cuffs should be deflated, the ET advanced until the bronchial cuff is below the carina, and both reinflated. If the ET has been inserted too deeply, the bronchial cuff may be lost to view, and the tip of the tracheal lumen will be too close to the carina (< 1–2 cm). In this case, both cuffs are deflated and the ET is pulled back until the bronchial cuff is just below the carina. Both cuffs are then reinflated.

The bronchoscope is next passed through the bronchial lumen to rule out obstruction of the upper lobe bronchus. The tracheal lumen is unclamped to permit ventilation to the opposite lung, and the bronchial lumen is then clamped proximally. The scope is passed via the port in the elbow adapter down the bronchial lumen. The bronchial lumen of a left-sided DLETT has a typical circumferential cuff and a bevelled tip, through which the FOB is passed. The first division of the left mainstem bronchus divides into the left upper lobe (LUL) and lingular bronchi at a carina that looks much like the tracheal carina. These two bronchi each bifurcate again into segmental bronchi. Once the LUL bronchus has been identified beyond the tip of the bronchial lumen, the DLETT should be secured with note made of the centimeter mark at the incisors.

A right-sided DLETT has a ventilation slot for the RUL in the side of the bronchial lumen that resembles a Murphy eye. The bronchial cuff is placed at an angle above and below this slot, and the bevelled tip lies just beyond the cuff (see Fig. 12–10A). When the tube is correctly positioned, the ventilation slot will lie at the origin of the RUL bronchus. When the RUL bronchus is viewed en face, its trifurcation into apical, anterior, and posterior segments is clearly seen; no other segment of the bronchial tree has this anatomy (Fig. 12–11). However, because of the narrow diameter of the ventilation slot and the acute angle of the RUL bronchus, it is very difficult to maneuver the tip of the ROB through the ventilation slot and into the RUL bronchus to achieve this view (Fig. 12–12). It is possible to identify the takeoff of the RUL bronchus, which will appear as a crescent when seen through the ventilation slot (see Fig. 12–10B). The diameter of the slot is about the same as that of the RUL bronchus; hence, it must be precisely positioned just at the level of the bronchus to ensure ventilation to the RUL. The FOB may then be passed through the distal tip of the bronchial lumen to view the right middle lobe bronchus. When proper position has been verified, the ET should be carefully secured, both lumina unclamped, and ventilator settings readjusted appropriately for two-lung ventilation.

Fiberoptic Bronchoscopic View of Right Upper Lobe Bronchi (normal)

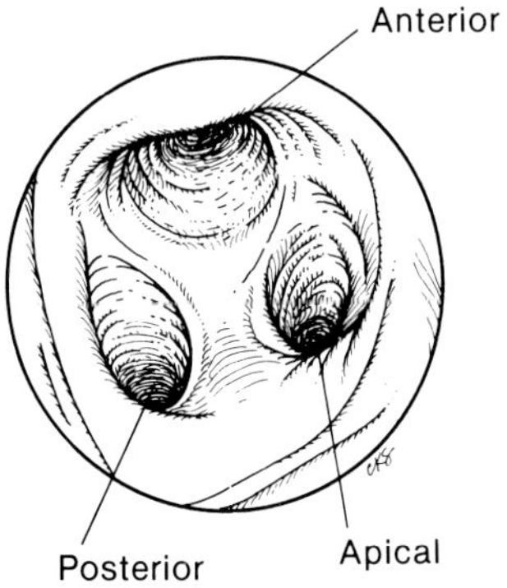

Figure 12–11 • Normal bronchoscopic view of the right upper lobe bronchus. The apical, anterior, and posterior segments form a trifurcation. No other portion of the bronchial tree possesses this anatomy.

E. Endotracheal Tube Change

A problem frequently encountered in the ICU is the need to change an ET (see also Chapter 8). Indications include damage to the cuff producing a persistent leak, the need for an ET of different ID, and the need to relocate the ET (eg, change oral to nasal or vice versa). This may be quite hazardous in patients in whom laryngoscopy is difficult or impossible, or in patients with marginal pulmonary reserve. In this circumstance, the bronchoscope is useful both for direct visual inspection of the airway and to insure quick access to the trachea after the original ET is removed.

The procedures described below are designed to provide the greatest possible assurance of access to the trachea following removal of the original ET. This assurance rests on placement of a stent (either the bronchoscope itself or an ET changer) into the trachea prior to removal of the in situ ET. When the new ET is threaded over this stent, the only path it should follow is into the trachea. However, in rare circumstances it may not be possible to advance the new ET over the stent due to swelling and obstruction of the glottic inlet. In this emergent situation, the anesthesiologist must be prepared for either percutaneous intravenous catheter cricothyrotomy and jet ventilation (see Chapter 9), or tracheostomy (see Chapter 10). Thus, appropriate equipment and personnel for these procedures (including a surgeon, if emergency tracheostomy is anticipated) should be available at the bedside while the ET is being changed in patients with significant laryngeal swelling.

The patient should be ventilated with 100% oxygen for 5–10 minutes prior to and during the procedure. The airway is topicalized appropriately and a pulse oximeter is applied. The new ET is ensleeved over the insertion tube of the bronchoscope after removal of the 15-mm adapter (see Fig. 12–5). The scope is placed in the nose or mouth and advanced to the glottis. In the absence of glottic edema, it is usually possible to advance the scope into the trachea through the anterior commissure, just above the ET in situ (see Chapter 8). As the scope is advanced, the cuff should be deflated so that the scope may be placed well into the trachea. The ET in situ is then removed, and the new ET advanced over the bronchoscope into the trachea. Note that the airway is secure at all times, and that the ET in situ is not

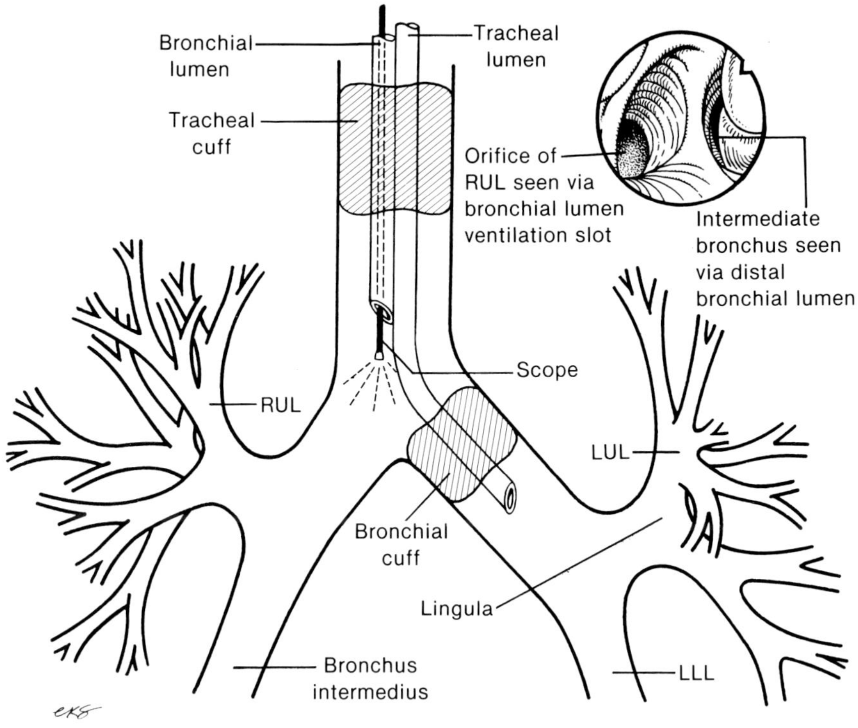

Figure 12–12 • Right-sided double-lumen endotracheal tube shown next to a cast of an adult trachea. The ventilation slot lies just at the orifice of the right upper lobe bronchus. The tip of the scope is positioned at the ventilation slot. It is too large to flex through the slot to obtain an en-face view of the right upper lobe bronchus. Consequently, this bronchus will appear as a crescent when the slot is correctly positioned at its orifice.

removed until the bronchoscope is well into the trachea, ensuring the ability to place the new ET over the bronchoscope, which acts as a stent.

In patients with laryngeal edema, it may be impossible to advance the bronchoscope into the trachea beside the ET in situ due to swelling around the glottic inlet. If the ET is removed and the bronchoscope then advanced into the trachea, the airway will be unsecured at least momentarily, with no certainty of the ability to reintubate the trachea. Edematous laryngeal structures may quickly obscure the glottic inlet, making it difficult to advance the bronchoscope after removing the ET. A stent placed into the trachea through the ET in situ will assure access to the airway during the time between removal of the ET and placement of the scope and new ET. If, following removal of the tube, it is not possible to advance the bronchoscope past the cords, the original ET is threaded over the stent back into the trachea.

The patient is preoxygenated, and the bronchoscope ensleeved with the new ET is positioned at the glottic inlet. A semirigid ET changer is placed into the ET in situ and advanced far enough so that its tip is 2–3 cm beyond the tip of the ET (ie, well into the trachea). The centimeter markings on the tube changer enable the correct depth to be reached. An assistant deflates the cuff and pulls back the ET over the tube changer, taking care not to pull back the tube changer as well. The bronchoscopist next advances the scope into the trachea. The tube changer may then be removed, and the new ET is threaded over the scope to the correct depth and secured. If difficulty is encountered in advancing the scope, the original ET should be threaded back over the tube changer into the trachea. Note that the patient will remain unventilated from the time the tube changer is inserted until the new ET is placed. Ventilation with 100% oxygen should be resumed as soon as the new tube is inserted.

F. *Tracheal Extubation*

A similar rationale to assure tracheal access is employed when extubation is planned in patients in whom concern exists about airway patency following extubation (eg, in patients with airway edema or extrinsic airway compression). The bronchoscope is first passed either orally or nasally to examine the larynx and surrounding structures for evidence of potential airway obstruction. If obstruction appears unlikely, extubation may then be attempted. The patient is preoxygenated, and an oxygen mask placed on the face to provide oxygen immediately upon withdrawal of the ET. The bronchoscope is advanced through the ET into the trachea. The cuff is deflated, and the ET is pulled back over the scope and out of the larynx. If the patient develops stridor or obstruction, the tube may be threaded back over the scope. If the airway remains patent after 2–3 minutes, the bronchoscope is withdrawn and the larynx and surrounding structures inspected on the way out. Swollen airway tissues may mold themselves to the shape of the ET, so that the glottic inlet is initially patent following extubation. However, the edematous tissue may expand further to compromise the airway minutes or hours following extubation. Thus, if it appears that airway edema is still present at the time of extubation, it is prudent to electively reintubate the patient while the airway is still readily accessible.

IV. Complications

Complications of bronchoscopy include those attributable to sedation, airway topicalization, and the procedure itself. Studies of several large patient cohorts appear in the pulmonary literature. These were patients presenting for diagnostic or therapeutic bronchoscopy and typically had underlying known or suspected pulmonary or airway pathology; they were not necessarily surgical patients, and most did not undergo endotracheal intubation. However, it is instructive to review these reports and to cautiously extrapolate their findings to potential complications of bronchoscopy in anesthesia because of the substantial overlap in patient preparation and bronchoscopic technique in both groups.

Two large retrospective studies[49,50] based on responses to questionnaires reported a very low incidence of complications from bronchoscopy. In the first,[49] major complications occurred in 0.08% and death in 0.01% of a cohort of 24,251 patients. Half of the complications were attributed to adverse reactions to local anesthesia (seizure, respiratory arrest, methemoglobinemia) or to premedication (respiratory depression), while the remaining half were related to bronchoscopy itself and included bronchospasm, respiratory compromise, syncope, dysrhythmias, and pneumonia. Of four deaths reported, one was due to anesthesia, two to the procedure itself, and one to an unspecified ancillary procedure. Most complications described in this study were considered to have been preventable. The importance of providing supplemental oxygen and of avoiding oversedation was emphasized.

The second study,[50] examining a cohort of approximately 48,000 patients, reported severe reactions to anesthesia in 0.09%, to sedative medication in 0.04%, life-threatening cardiovascular complications in 0.06%, and life-threatening airway complications in 0.11%. Death occurred in 0.025% of patients; causes included cardiac arrest in six patients, myocardial infarction in four, and massive hemorrhage from tumor in two. All patients who died had at least one of four underlying illnesses, including cardiovascular disease, severe chronic obstructive pulmonary disease (COPD), pneumonia, or cancer. Hypoxemia was proven or suspected in nearly half the deaths, while sedation was thought to contribute in 25% and topical anesthetic in 17%.

A prospective study of 908 patients[51] followed this early work, and reported higher rates of mortality (0.1%) and major complications (1.7%), including respiratory arrest, pneumonia, pneumothorax, and airway obstruction. The only patients found to be predisposed to complications were those with a history of hemoptysis; these patients had an increased risk of bleeding as a result of the procedure itself. Minor reactions occurred in 6.5% of patients and included vasovagal reactions, fever, dysrhythmias, bleeding, mild airway obstruction, nausea and vomiting, pneumothorax (<20%), ECG abnormalities, psychotic reaction, and aphonia.

The occurrence of hypoxemia during bronchoscopy is now well recognized.[8,42,43,52,53] In one study of "good risk" patients with an average room-air P_aO_2 of 81 mmHg, a decline in P_aO_2 of 20 mmHg during transnasal bronchoscopy with spontaneous ventilation was noted and persisted for 1 to 4 hours postbronchoscopy.[42] Lindholm et al[8] documented a decline in P_aO_2 from 128 mmHg prebronchoscopy to 94 mmHg during the procedure in spontaneously breathing, critically ill patients receiving supplemental oxygen; P_aO_2 increased to 142 mmHg 15 minutes after bronchoscopy. Interestingly, they noted an increase in P_aO_2 from 106 mmHg at baseline to 118 mmHg during bronchoscopy in intubated patients who were mechanically ventilated during bronchoscopy. This increase was attributed to positive end-expiratory pressure (PEEP) created by the presence of the bronchoscope in the ET and to the removal of mucus plugs and secretions prior to arterial blood gas sampling during the procedure. Several studies of cardiac rhythm changes during bronchoscopy[43,52,53] document similar declines in P_aO_2 or oxyhemoglobin saturation during and following bronchoscopy.

A number of cardiac rhythm disturbances during bronchoscopy have been described.[43,52–54] Shrader and Lakshminarian[53] monitored the ECG for 1 hour before, during, and after bronchoscopy in 70 patients receiving 2L/min supplemental oxygen and 2% lidocaine for airway topicalization. They defined major arrhythmias as those having the potential to cause hemodynamic compromise, including sinus bradycardia less than 40 beats per minute (bpm), atrial fibrillation with ventricular rate more than 120 bpm, supraventricular tachycardia more than 140 bpm, premature ventricular contractions more than 50/hr, and any other ventricular arrhythmia. All others were considered minor. Minor arrhythmias occurred in 49% of patients prior to and 70% during bronchoscopy; major arrhythmias in 7% and 11%, respectively, with no change or worsening of arrhythmia during the procedure in those in whom it was previously present. Patients with risk factors including coronary artery disease, abnormal ECG, cardiac medication, COPD, theophylline therapy, or age above 60 years exhibited no increased risk of occurrence or worsening of arrhythmia during bronchoscopy. Atropine premedication and respiratory alkalosis were also found to present no increased risk. Venous lidocaine levels varied widely but were no different between groups having major or minor arrhythmias. Hypoxemia (P_aO_2 <60 mmHg) was the only factor that significantly correlated with the development of a major arrhythmia. All arrhythmias were self-limited and none required treatment.

Elguindi et al[52] monitored the ECG for 12 hours before, during, and 12 hours after bronchoscopy in 26 patients premedicated with atropine and topicalized with lidocaine. Supplemental oxygen was not given. Major and minor arrhythmias were defined in the same manner as in the previously described study (excluding atrial fibrillation). Those authors noted a striking decrease in the incidence of both major and minor arrhythmias during bronchoscopy, except sinus tachycardia, which increased markedly. Three factors were thought to account for this decrease, including a longer monitoring period to establish a more accurate baseline of arrhythmia occurrence, low incidence of hypoxemia, and a high dose of lidocaine (resulting in a mean peak plasma level of 5.0 μg/ml), which may have exerted a protective effect. As in other studies, a decline in P_aO_2 during bronchoscopy was also noted.

Katz et al[43] prospectively examined rhythm changes in 50 patients undergoing ECG monitoring for 2.5 hours before, during, and 4 hours after bronchoscopy, as well as ear oximetry for a slightly shorter period. Patients with a baseline P_aO_2 less than 80 mmHg received supplemental oxygen, two thirds of all patients were premedicated with atropine, and lidocaine was used for airway topicalization. Major arrhythmias (atrial, ventricular, or both) occurred in 40% of patients; half of these were ventricular and were most common during passage of the bronchoscope through the vocal cords. Arrhythmias occurred most frequently during periods of maximal oxygen desaturation. Seventy percent of ventricular and 50% of atrial arrhythmias occurred in close temporal relationship to maximal heart rate; maximal heart rate and maximal oxygen desaturation often occurred simultaneously. Two patients who were not pretreated with atropine developed Wenckebach block. Patients with a preexisting conduction disturbance exhibited no increased risk of arrhythmia or worsening conduction abnormality. No correlation was noted between frequency of arrhythmias and age, sex, prior medication, premedication, or medical history of cardiac or pulmonary disorders. None of the arrhythmias had clinically important sequelae such as hypotension.

Most reported complications of bronchoscopic airway management involve mechanical rather than physiologic problems. Ovassapian[55] reported three cases in which the bronchoscope could not be removed from the ET following bronchoscopic nasal intubation. Nichols and Zornow[56] reported inability to advance a nasotracheal tube past the vocal cords over a bronchoscope. In all cases, the bronchoscope and ET were removed as a unit, and the insertion tube of the scope was noted to have passed through the Murphy eye rather than the distal opening of the ET. These authors recommended that the ET be threaded over the insertion tube prior to placing it in the airway to avoid this complication.

Moorthy and Dierdorf[57] attempted nasal fiberoptic intubation in a child with craniofacial dysostosis. They placed the insertion tube in the trachea, threaded an ET over it, withdrew the scope with difficulty, and found that the ET was in the esophagus. They concluded that as the ET was being advanced, it was bending the insertion tube and pulling it into the esophagus, even though the tip of the scope remained in the trachea. Successful intubation was performed by elevating the patient's head and pressing on her larynx to achieve a more favorable alignment of the nasopharynx and larynx.

Siegel and Coleprate[58] reported inability to withdraw a bronchoscope through an ET following diagnostic bronchoscopy. The ET and scope were withdrawn as a unit. The tip of the bronchoscope had intussuscepted into the covering sleeve of the insertion tube so that the sleeve had buckled out and occluded the ET.

All of these reports emphasize the importance of withdrawing the bronchoscope and ET from the patient as a unit if resistance is met while either attempting to advance the ET or to remove the bronchoscope.

Ovassapian et al[11] reported causes of difficulty or failure of fiberoptic nasotracheal intubation in 423 patients. Narrow nasal passages made placement of a nasotracheal tube impossible in ten patients. Five failures occurred in the remaining patients; one due to a posterior pharyngeal tumor, one due to inability to visualize the larynx, and three due to inability to advance the ET over the insertion tube into the trachea. About 10% of the procedures were considered difficult due to distorted airway anatomy or presence of secretions. These authors note that if a cervical or oropharyngeal mass has distorted the airway, exposure of the larynx is usually easier via the nostril on the side opposite the mass; while if distortion of the airway is due to contraction of soft tissues, laryngeal exposure is usually easier via the nostril on the same side.

V. Discussion

A. *Physiologic Effects of Bronchoscopy and Intubation*

Bronchoscopy and intubation produce important changes in hemodynamics, pulmonary mechanics, and gas exchange. These changes have been examined during both diagnostic/therapeutic bronchoscopy alone, and during fiberoptic-assisted tracheal intubation. These studies are summarized in Table 12–2. Several important points deserve emphasis.

First, specific stages in both bronchoscopy and intubation are more physiologically stressful than others. Increases in heart rate, blood pressure, and pulmonary capillary wedge pressure are greatest during placement of an ET in a nostril, during passage of an ET or bronchoscope through the vocal cords, and during suctioning. As noted earlier,[43] passage through the vocal cords also elicits the highest frequency of major cardiac rhythm disturbances.

Second, pulmonary mechanics are significantly affected by bronchoscopy. Lindholm et al[8] and Matsushima et al[59] noted substantial changes in airway resistance, tracheal pressure, and PEEP during bronchoscopy. Bronchoscopy produces a decline in vital capacity

Table 12–2 • Hemodynamic Changes During Fiberoptic Bronchoscopy and Fiberoptic-Assisted Tracheal Intubation

Reference	n	Blood Pressure	Heart Rate
Lindholm et al[8]	55		
Lundgren et al[60]	10	Greatest increase during passage through larynx, application of anesthetic to trachea, and suctioning	Increases during same three periods
Sutherland and Williams[71]	20	Systolic BP unchanged from baseline during topicalization and intubation	Increases only during intubation (about 10%)
Ovassapian et al[72]	200	Greatest increase during passage of ET* in nostril (10 mmHg > baseline); lesser increase with placement of ET in trachea (6 mmHg > baseline)	Maximal increase when ET placed in trachea (mean, 14 bpm)

bpm = beats per minute; ET = endotracheal tube; PC = pulmonary capillary.

as well as inspiratory and expiratory flow rates; intubation causes a greater decrease, and bronchoscopy via an ET in spontaneously breathing patients causes a still further decline in vital capacity, FEV_1, and inspiratory flow. A 5.2-mm bronchoscope in the adult trachea produces about a twofold increase in airway resistance; intubation, about threefold; and a 5.2-mm bronchoscope in an 8.0-mm ET produces an 11-fold increase in airway resistance.[59] This emphasizes the potential for a substantial increase in work of breathing for spontaneously breathing patients. The presence of a bronchoscope in an ET during positive pressure ventilation causes an increase in both peak ventilator pressure and true tracheal pressure, produces PEEP, and decreases delivered tidal volume. The risk of barotrauma and hypoventilation may be increased under these circumstances.

Third, suctioning in the airway is not a benign intervention. It may produce an increase in blood pressure, heart rate, cardiac output, and pulmonary capillary wedge pressure. Tidal volume decreases as gas is removed from the airway, and lung volume may decrease to below functional residual capacity. The P_aO_2 falls as a result. Ischemic ECG changes have been noted in some patients during suctioning and hypoxemia.[60]

These observations suggest that the physiologic stresses of bronchoscopy and fiberoptic intubation may be minimized by relatively simple measures. Supplemental oxygen should always be given. Time and patience should be allotted for adequate airway topicalization. Suction should be applied judiciously and for short periods of time. Bronchoscopy in intubated patients should be accomplished as quickly as possible; rest periods should be given every 2–3 minutes to allow a return to normal ventilation and lower airway pressure.

B. *Local Anesthetics*

Adequate airway topicalization is essential to produce good working conditions, insure patient comfort, and minimize hemodynamic responses to airway instrumentation. A number of investigators have studied airway topicalization with lidocaine delivered by various means, including gargling, atomization, nebulization, and direct bolus application to the airway. Total drug dose, route of administration, blood levels, time to peak level, and adequacy of topicalization were evaluated in most of these studies, which are summarized in Table 12–3.

A striking feature of all these studies is the consistent demonstration of blood levels well below the toxic range (5 μg/ml) at drug doses shown to approach the toxic limit when delivered by other routes, such as intercostal or epidural.[61] In doses from 170 to 540 mg, peak venous blood levels ranged from 0.42 μg/ml[62] to 4.0 μg/ml.[63] Patterson et al[62] recorded a peak level of 18.2

Cardiac Output	PC Wedge Pressure	Sedation	Procedure
Increases to 150% during suctioning		Not stated	Diagnostic or therapeutic bronchoscopy in critically ill patients
	Increases during same three periods	Morphine	Routine diagnostic bronchoscopy
		Fentanyl, diazepam	Awake intubation
		Diazepam and/or morphine	Awake intubation

Table 12–3 • Drug Dose, Route of Administration, and Mean Peak Blood Levels of Local Anesthetics Delivered by Various Routes for Airway Topicalization

Reference	n	Drug Dose	Route*
Berger et al[64]	18 patients 21 volunteers	1682 mg (L)	G, A, N
Kirkpatrick et al[69]	10	400 mg (L)	N
Smith et al[63]	18	325 mg (L)	A (URT); B (LRT)
Karvonen et al[68]	15	400 mg (L)	N
Gomez et al[65]	29	180–400 mg (L)	B (LRT)
Gove et al[67]	52	540 mg (L) 450 mg (L)	B N
Patterson et al[62]	21	170–380 mg (L)	B
Sutherland and Williams[71]	20	300–540 mg (L)	N, G, B
McBurney et al[70]	10	118 mg (L) 200 mg (L) 17 mg (Bu) 25 mg (Bu)	A (URT)[†] B (LRT) A (URT) B (LRT)

A = atomized; B = direct bolus application to mucosa through suction channel of bronchoscope; Bu = bupivacaine; G = gargled; L = lidocaine; LRT = lower respiratory tract, ie, vocal cords and/or tracheobronchial tree; N = nebulized; URT = upper respiratory tract (ie, nasal passages, nasopharynx, and oropharynx to level above vocal cords).

*Drug was administered to all patients in each study by all routes listed except by McBurney et al (see below).

[†]One group of patients received atomized lidocaine in the URT and bolused bupivacaine in the LRT; the other group received atomized bupivacaine in the URT and bolused lidocaine in the LRT.

μg/ml following a dose of 360 mg in a patient with lung carcinoma and liver metastases; he showed no symptoms of lidocaine toxicity. A later study[63] failed to demonstrate increased blood lidocaine levels in bronchoscopy patients with liver metastases and/or elevated transaminases compared to controls. Berger et al[64] delivered a large total dose of lidocaine (mean =1682 mg) according to a standardized protocol of gargling, atomization, and nebulization, and found a mean peak level of only 3.0 μg/ml in patients and 1.5 μg/ml in healthy young volunteers. Gomez et al[65] gave 180–400 mg of lidocaine by direct bolus application to the tracheobronchial tree. Using an assumed value for volume of distribution and multiple blood level determinations, they calculated that 21%–61% of the total dose is absorbed when delivered by this route.

Several explanations are suggested for the occurrence of low blood levels following large lidocaine doses. When the drug is nebulized, some of it is exhaled and lost to the atmosphere. Some drug will also be lost when secretions are suctioned. Drug that is swallowed and absorbed from the gut undergoes extensive first-pass hepatic metabolism, and very little unchanged drug will enter the systemic circulation.[66] Drug may also be absorbed more slowly when applied topically compared to other routes, such as intercostal, producing lower peak

Peak Level (μg/mL)	Time to peak (min)	Remarks	Conditions
3.0 (patients) 1.5 (volunteers)	30	Mean patient age, 62; mean volunteer age, 27	Minimal/no cough in 80%
0.52	20	Healthy volunteers	No bronchoscopies done
1.89 (liver disease) 2.60 (no liver disease)	30	Highest peak = 4.0 in patient without liver disease; peak correlates with age and total bolus dose	Not stated
1.39 (arterial) 1.07 (venous)	10	Arterial = venous after 30 min	Good in all
1.21 ± 0.64	36	21%–61% of total dose absorbed	Not stated
1.44 ± 0.8 1.01 ± 0.6	60 (single measurement)		15% of N group required supplemental boluses
0.42–2.32 18.2 (liver disease)	5–30	High peak in patient with liver metastases; asymptomatic	Not stated
0.6 ± 0.3 1.6 (highest)	28	No changes in blood pressure or heart rate during topicalization and intubation	No or minimal discomfort; awake intubation
0.66 ± 0.18 1.54 ± 1.20 0.27 ± 0.18 0.27 ± 0.06	38 (L, URT) 33 (L, LRT) 33 (Bu, URT) 27 (Bu, LRT)	1 drug (L or Bu) applied to URT, other to LRT in each patient; greater absorption of L from URT than LRT when corrected for dose	Good in all

levels and a longer half-life. This is supported by the consistent finding that peak levels occur about 30 minutes after the start of topicalization, compared to about 15 minutes when local anesthetic is given as an intercostal or epidural injection.[61]

Working conditions and patient acceptance were good in the majority of patients following airway topicalization by all of the methods described. It is to be emphasized that "tincture of time" is central to the success of airway anesthesia. Adequate time and patience are required to achieve solid anesthesia, patient comfort, and hemodynamic stability for a procedure as potentially stressful and stimulating as airway instrumentation.

IV. REFERENCES

1. Sokolowski M Jr, Burgher LW, Jones FL Jr, Patterson JR, et al. Guidelines for fiberoptic bronchoscopy in adults. Am Rev Respir Dis 136:1066, 1987.
2. VanGundy K, Boylen CT. Fiberoptic bronchoscopy: Indications, complications, contraindications. Postgrad Med 83:289–294, 1988.
3. Zavala DC. Bronchoscopy, lung biopsy and other procedures. In Murray JF, Nadel JA (eds). Textbook of Respiratory Medicine. Philadelphia, WB Saunders, 1988. 562–596
4. Fulkerson WJ. Fiberoptic bronchoscopy. New England J Med 311:511–515, 1984.
5. Sanderson DR. Bronchoscopy. Br Med Bull 42:244–248, 1986.
6. Mitchell DM, Emerson CJ, Collyer J, Collins JV. Fiberoptic bronchoscopy: Ten years on. Br Med J 281:360–363, 1980.

7. Denneny JC, Keane WM, Atkins JP. Fiberoptic bronchoscopy: Review of 1,000 cases. Ear Nose and Throat Journal 62:65–83, 1983.
8. Lindholm CE, Ollman B, Snyder JV, Millen EG, et al. Cardiorespiratory effects of flexible fiberoptic bronchoscopy in critically ill patients. Chest 74:362–368, 1978.
9. Baier H, Begin R, Sackner MA. Effect of airway diameter, suction catheters, and the bronchofiberscope on airflow in endotracheal and tracheostomy tubes. Heart Lung 5:235–238, 1976.
10. Bolder PM, Heal TEJ, Bolder AR, Beatty PCW, et al. The extra work of breathing through adult endotracheal tubes. Anesth Analg 65:853–859, 1986.
11. Ovassapian A, Yelich SJ, Dykes MHM, Brunner EE. Fiberoptic nasotracheal intubation—Incidence and causes of failure. Anesth Analg 62:692–695, 1983.
12. Raj P, Forestner J, Watson TD, Morris RE, et al. Technics for fiberoptic laryngoscopy in anesthesia. Anesth Analg 53:708–714, 1974.
13. Shulman MS, Brodsky JB, Levesque PR. Fiberoptic bronchoscopy for tracheal and endobronchial intubation with a double-lumen tube. Can J Anaesth 34:172–173, 1987.
14. Messeter KH, Pettersson KI. Endotracheal intubation with the fiber-optic bronchoscope. Anaesthesia 35:294–298, 1980.
15. Keenan MA, Stiles CM, Kaufman RL. Acquired laryngeal deviation associated with cervical spine disease in erosive polyarticular arthritis. Anesthesiology 58:445–449, 1983.
16. Barrett CR Jr, Vecchione JJ, Loomis Bell AL Jr. Flexible fiberoptic bronchoscopy for airway management during acute respiratory failure. Am Rev Respir Dis 109:429–434, 1974.
17. Snow N, Lucas AE. Bronchoscopy in the critically ill surgical patient. Am Surg 50:441–445, 1984.
18. Harada K, Mutsuda T, Saoyama N, Taniki T, et al. Re-expansion of refractory atelectasis using a bronchofiberscope with a balloon cuff. Chest 84:725–728, 1983.
19. Clark PT, Williams TJ, Teichtahl H, Bowes G, et al. Removal of proximal and peripheral endobronchial foreign bodies with the flexible fiberoptic bronchoscope. Anaesth Intensive Care 17:205–208, 1989.
20. Campinos L, Duval G, Couturier M, Brage J, et al. The value of early fiberoptic bronchoscopy after aspiration of gastric contents. Br J Anaesth 55:1103–1105, 1983.
21. Wolfe JE, Bone RC, Ruth WE. Diagnosis of gastric aspiration by fiberoptic bronchoscopy. Chest 70:458–459, 1976.
22. Regel G, Sturm JA, Neumann C, Schueler S, et al. Occlusion of bronchopleural fistula after lung injury—A new treatment by bronchoscopy. J Trauma 29:223–226, 1989.
23. Wanner A, Cutchavaree A. Early recognition of upper airway obstruction following smoke inhalation. Am Rev Respir Dis 108:1421–1423, 1973.
24. Schneider W, Berger A, Mailander P, Tempka A. Diagnostic and therapeutic possibilities for fiberoptic bronchoscopy in inhalation injury. Burns Incl Therm Inj 14:53–57, 1988.
25. Clark CJ, Reid WH, Telfer ABM, Campbell D. Respiratory injury in the burned patient: The role of flexible bronchoscopy. Anaesthesia 38:35–39, 1983.
26. O'Brien D, Curran J, Conroy J, Bouchier-Hays D. Fiber-optic assessment of tracheal tube position. A comparison of tracheal tube position as estimated by fiber-optic bronchoscopy and by chest X-ray. Anaesthesia 40:73–76, 1985.
27. Moyers J, Gregory GA. Use of fiberoptic bronchoscopy to reposition an endotracheal tube intraoperatively. Anesthesiology 43: 685, 1975.
28. Baranowski AP. Unusual tracheal tube obstruction leading to an unusual bronchoscopic technique (letter). Anaesthesia 44:359–360, 1989.
29. Lee KC, Weedman D, Peters WJ. Innovations in burn care. J Burn Care Rehabil 7:348–350, 1986.
30. Rosenbaum SH, Rosenbaum LM, Cole RP, Askanazi J, et al. Use of the flexible fiberoptic bronchoscope to change endotracheal tube in critically ill patients. Anesthesiology 54:169–170, 1981.
31. Ovassapian A, Dykes MHM. The role of fiber-optic endoscopy in airway management. Semin Anesth 6:93–104, 1987.
32. Younker D, Clark R, Coveler L. Fiberoptic endobronchial intubation for resection of an anterior mediastinal mass. Anesthesiology 70:144–146, 1989.
33. Patil V, Stehling LC, Zauder HL, Koch JP. Mechanical aids for fiberoptic endoscopy. Anesthesiology 57:69–70, 1982.
34. Rogers SN, Benumof JL. New and easy techniques for fiberoptic endoscopy-aided tracheal intubation. Anesthesiology 59:569–572, 1983.
35. Hanson PJV, Collins JV. AIDS, aprons, and elbow grease: Preventing the nosocomial spread of human immunodeficiency virus and associated organisms. Thorax 44:778–783, 1989.
36. Hanson PJV, Jeffries DJ, Batten JC, Collins JV. Infection control revisited: Dilemma facing today's bronchoscopists. Br Med J 297:185–187, 1988.
37. Wheeler PW, Lancaster D, Kaiser AB. Bronchopulmonary cross-colonization and infection related to mycobacterial contamination of suction valves of bronchoscopes. J Infect Dis 159:954–958, 1989.
38. Gal TJ, Suratt PM. Atropine and glycopyrrolate effects on lung mechanics in normal man. Anesth Analg 60:85–90, 1981.
39. Belen J, Neuhaus A, Markowitz D, Rotman HH. Modification of the effect of fiberoptic bronchoscopy on pulmonary mechanics. Chest 79:516-519, 1981.
40. Zavala DC, Godsey K, Bedell GN. The response to atropine sulfate given by aerosol and intramuscular routes to patients undergoing fiberoptic bronchoscopy. Chest 79:512–515, 1981.
41. Severinghaus JW, Stupfel M. Respiratory dead space increase following atropine in man, and atropine, vagal or ganglionic blockade and hypothermia in dogs. J Appl Physiol 8:81–87, 1955.
42. Albertini RE, Harrell JH II, Kurihara N, Moser KM. Arterial hypoxemia induced by fiberoptic bronchoscopy. JAMA 230:1666–1667, 1974.
43. Katz AS, Michelson EL, Stawicki J, Holford FD. Cardiac arrhythmias: Frequency during fiberoptic bronchoscopy and correlation with hypoxemia. Arch Intern Med 141:603–606, 1981.
44. Barton S, Williams JD. Glossopharyngeal nerve block. Arch Otolaryngol 93:186–188, 1971.
45. Calcaterra TC, House J. Local anesthesia for suspension microlaryngoscopy. Ann Otol Rhinol Laryngol 85:71–73, 1976.
46. Murphy, TM. Somatic blockade. In Cousins MJ, Bridenbaugh PO (eds). Neural Blockade in Clinical Anesthesia and Management of Pain. Philadelphia, JB Lippincott, 1980, 418–419.
47. Gotta AW, Sullivan CA. Anaesthesia of the upper airway using topical anaesthetic and superior laryngeal nerve block. Br J Anaesth 53:1055–1057, 1981.
48. Benumof JL. Anesthesia for Thoracic Surgery. Philadelphia, WB Saunders, 1987, 241–243.
49. Credle WF Jr, Smiddy JF, Elliott RC. Complications of fiberoptic bronchoscopy. Am Rev Respir Dis 109:67–72, 1974.
50. Surratt PM, Smiddy JF, Gruber B. Deaths and complications associated with fiberoptic bronchoscopy. Chest 69:747–751, 1976.
51. Pereira W Jr, Kovnat DM, Snider GL. A prospective cooperative study of complications following flexible fiberoptic bronchoscopy. Chest 73:813–816, 1978.
52. Elguindi AS, Harrison GN, Abdulla AM, Chaudhary BA, et al.

Cardiac rhythm disturbances during fiberoptic bronchoscopy: A prospective study. J Thorac Cardiovasc Surg 77:557–561, 1979.
53. Shrader DL, Lakshminarayan S. The effect of fiberoptic bronchoscopy on cardiac rhythm. Chest 73:821–824, 1978.
54. Borgeat A, Chiolero R, Mosimann B, Freeman J. Accelerated idioventricular rhythm during flexible fiberoptic bronchoscopy. Crit Care Med 15:274–275, 1978.
55. Ovassapian A. Failure to withdraw flexible fiberoptic laryngoscope after nasotracheal intubation (letter). Anesthesiology 63:124–125, 1985.
56. Nichols KP, Zornow M. A potential complication of fiberoptic intubation (letter). Anesthesiology 70:562–563, 1989.
57. Moorthy SS, Dierdorf SF. An unusual difficulty in fiberoptic intubation (letter). Anesthesiology 63:229, 1985.
58. Siegel M, Coleprate P. Complication of fiberoptic bronchoscope (letter). Anesthesiology 61:214–215, 1984.
59. Matsushima Y, Jones RL, King EG, Moysa G, et al. Alterations in pulmonary mechanics and gas exchange during routine fiberoptic bronchoscopy. Chest 86:184–188, 1984.
60. Lundgren R, Haggmark S, Reiz S. Hemodynamic effects of flexible fiberoptic bronchoscopy performed under topical anesthesia. Chest 82:295–299, 1982.
61. Scott DB, Jebson PJR, Braid DP, Ortengren B, et al. Factors affecting plasma levels of lignocaine and prilocaine. Br J Anaesth 44:1040–1048, 1972.
62. Patterson JR, Blaschke TF, Hunt K Jr, Meffin PJ. Lidocaine blood concentrations during fiberoptic bronchoscopy. Am Rev Respir Dis 112:53–57, 1975.
63. Smith MJ, Dhillon DP, Hayler AM, Holt DW, et al. Is fiberoptic bronchoscopy in patients with lung cancer and hepatic metastases potentially dangerous? Br J Dis Chest 79:368–373, 1985.
64. Berger R, McConnell JW, Phillips B, Overman TL. Safety and efficacy of using high-dose topical and nebulized anesthesia to obtain endobronchial cultures. Chest 95:299–303, 1989.
65. Gomez F, Barrueco M, Lanao JM, Vicente MT, et al. Serum lidocaine levels in patients undergoing fibrobronchoscopy. Ther Drug Monit 5:201–203, 1983.
66. Thomson PD, Melmon KL, Richardson JA, Cohn K, et al: Lidocaine pharmacokinetics in advanced heart failure, liver disease and renal failure in humans. Ann Intern Med 78:499–508, 1973.
67. Gove RI, Wiggins J, Stableforth DE. A study of the use of ultrasonically nebulized lignocaine for local anesthesia during fiberoptic bronchoscopy. Br J Dis Chest 79:49–59, 1985.
68. Karvonen S, Jokinen K, Karvonen P, Hollmen A. Arterial and venous blood lidocaine concentrations after local anaesthesia of the respiratory tract using an ultrasonic nebulizer. Acta Anaesthesiol Scand 20:156–159, 1976.
69. Kirkpatrick MB, Sanders RV, Bass JB Jr. Physiologic effects and serum lidocaine concentrations after inhalation of lidocaine from a compressed gas-powered jet nebulizer. Am Rev Respir Dis 136:447–449, 1987.
70. McBurney A, Jones DA, Stanley PJ, Ward JW. Absorption of lignocaine and bupivacaine from the respiratory tract during fiberoptic bronchoscopy. Br J Clin Pharmacol 17:61–66, 1984.
71. Sutherland AD, Williams RT. Cardiovascular responses and lidocaine absorption in fiberoptic-assisted awake intubation. Anesth Analg 65:389–391, 1986.
72. Ovassapian A, Yelich SJ, Dykes MHM, Brunner EE. Blood pressure and heart rate changes during awake fiberoptic nasotracheal intubation. Anesth Analg 62:951–954, 1983.

Chapter 13

•

T. James Gallagher, MD, FCCM

Ventilatory Techniques

OUTLINE

Mechanical ventilation supports alveolar ventilation and thereby removes carbon dioxide from the body. Mechanical ventilatory support also usually improves ventilation-to-perfusion relationships and therefore also supports oxygenation. There are many ways to accomplish these two goals, and although all the techniques discussed in this chapter can work well, some techniques work better than others in some patients, and some techniques allow a very smooth transition to weaning from mechanical ventilation. This chapter discusses the various modes of the indications and contraindications, the procedures for using each mode, weaning from the mode, and the complications of the mode.

I. Continuous Positive Airway Pressure (CPAP)

A. *Description*

Continuous positive airway pressures (CPAP) can best be described by consideration of a patient breathing spontaneously and not requiring mechanical ventilation. In these circumstances the patient initiates spontaneous respiration at an airway pressure above baseline. This corresponds to the designated level of CPAP (Fig. 13–1). During each spontaneous inspiratory effort the baseline airway pressure decreases toward 0 cm H_2O, or ambient pressure. However, it never quite reaches that baseline. The greater the inspiratory effort or force, the greater the decrease in the airway pressure toward ambient pressure. At end-exhalation the pressure returns to the baseline. This back pressure in the lung results in the recruitment and reexpansion of hypoventilated or collapsed alveoli. The resulting improvement in lung volume (functional residual capacity) leads to improved matching of ventilation to perfusion and ultimately enhanced oxygenation, as evidenced by increased P_aO_2.

Continuous positive airway pressure often uses a demand valve as part of the system (Fig. 13–2). Adjusting the demand valve pressurization just slightly less than the level of CPAP means that a minimal inspiratory effort will lower the airway pressure below the pressurization level of the demand valve. At that instant the valve rapidly opens and gas flows at a high delivery rate into the patient's lungs during the remainder of the spontaneous effort. To encourage a greater inspiratory effort, the system can be pressurized at a pressure much less than the CPAP level. The patient must then lower the airway pressure during the inspiratory effort to slightly less than the demand valve pressurization level before any gas flow takes place. The work of breathing increases during these circumstances.

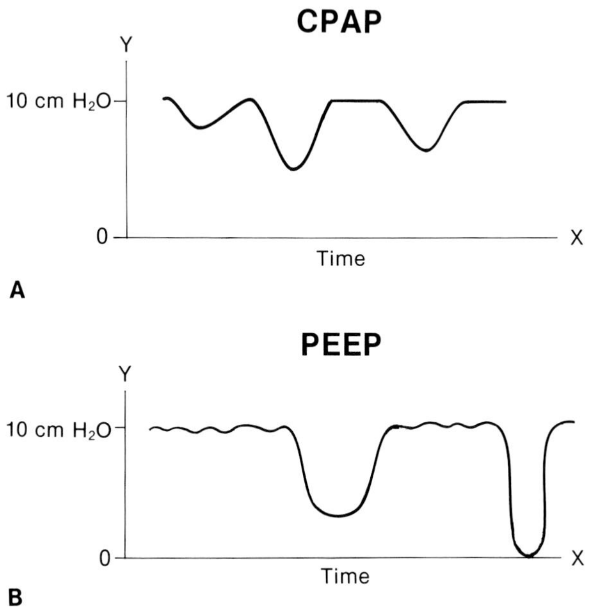

Figure 13–1 • (***A***) Spontaneous breathing with CPAP. Each breath represents a different inspiratory effort. During all phases of the respiratory cycle the airway pressure remains positive. (***B***) This spontaneous breath represents PEEP. The second inspiratory effort reaches ambient pressure. The airway pressure remains positive only at end exhalation.

Continuous positive airway pressure can be combined with mechanical ventilatory support. Under these circumstances after the delivery of each positive-pressure breath, the baseline pressure does not return to ambient, but remains at some elevated level predetermined or selected by the clinician. In this system, a low gas flow, usually 20 L/min, and at the same F_IO_2 at which the ventilator breath is provided to the patient on an uninterrupted basis. During spontaneous breathing in conjunction with a ventilator, the patient may receive CPAP through either an endotracheal or tracheostomy tube. Likewise, a tight-fitting face mask may also be utilized to deliver CPAP without a mechanical ventilator.

B. *Indications*

CPAP usually improves oxygenation in patients with any degree of hypoxemia. Hypoxemia may develop be-

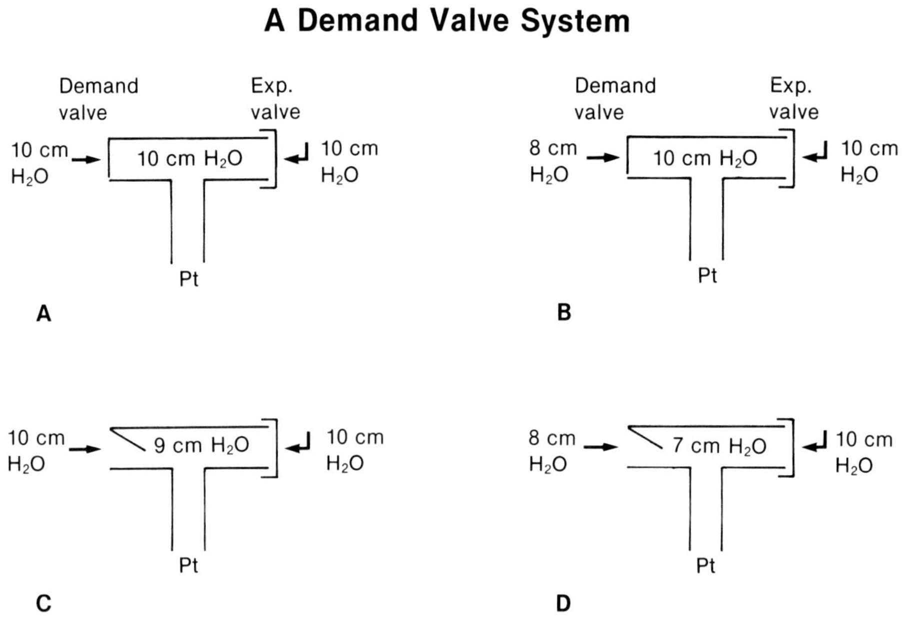

Figure 13–2 • Figure schematic of how a demand valve system works. (***A***) A demand valve. The expiratory valve pressurizes the airway and the system at 10 cm H_2O. This represents CPAP. The demand valve remains closed. To open the exhalation valve the patient must develop an airway pressure during exhalation less than 10 cm H_2O. (***B***) The patient initiates a spontaneous effort. When the airway pressure drops below that of the pressurized demand valve (10 cm H_2O), the demand valve opens and delivers gas flow to the patient. (***C***) The demand valve is less sensitive now set to 8 cm H_2O. (***D***) The patient must generate a greater inspiratory effort to decrease the airway pressure to 7 cm H_2O or less. At that point the demand valve opens and delivers flow to the patient.

cause of decreased lung volume, secondary to intraabdominal or intrathoracic surgical procedures, hypoventilation, or other factors. Severe forms of respiratory failure include the adult respiratory distress syndrome (ARDS), which involves accumulation of fluid in both interstitial and interalveolar spaces of the lung.[1] The fluid accumulation results in a loss of lung volume, low ventilation to perfusion areas, and atelectasis, which in turn causes severe hypoxemia. CPAP works best as a mechanism to maintain sufficient back pressure in the lung to prevent alveolar collapse and loss of lung volume.[2] Ordinarily, the pressures required to expand collapsed or partially collapsed alveoli are higher than the level of CPAP that then keeps them open. Therefore, this method works best when coupled with mechanical positive-pressure breaths that develop much higher airway pressures. Usually, the pressures developed with the mechanical breath are of sufficient magnitude to overcome the alveolar opening airway pressures and restore lung volume. When coupled with CPAP, this method provides sufficient pressure to maintain the expansion.

C. *Contraindications*

CPAP has limited efficacy in a number of different patients or situations. First, the use of CPAP in spontaneously breathing patients or those with a CPAP mask requires cooperation.[3,4] Second, ordinarily patients with carbon dioxide retention will not respond with simple face mask CPAP therapy. Third, those patients with previous gastric surgery or distention may swallow air and cause gastric overdistention with possible disruption of suture lines. Fourth, almost all patients do not tolerate face mask CPAP levels in excess of 12–15 cm H_2O. The high pressures become uncomfortable despite the various types of masks available.

Finally, patients with chronic lung disease who require mechanical ventilation may need little, if any, CPAP. Respiratory failure in these patients usually represents carbon dioxide retention, not loss of functional residual capacity (FRC). However, a few chronic lung disease patients may develop mild or severe hypoxemia secondary to loss of their usual lung volume or FRC.

Under these circumstances modest amounts of CPAP may be beneficial in restoring adequate oxygenation in these patients.

D. How to Use CPAP

Most clinicians consider a minimal level or baseline of CPAP to be 5 cm H_2O. This practice can be traced back to earlier continuous-flow systems that always resulted in some small level of CPAP. Since the introduction of demand valves, this small level of CPAP does not necessarily occur; however, many clinicians have remained with 5 cm H_2O as a baseline level.

To select the appropriate level of CPAP the clinician must first decide on a consistent endpoint for oxygenation. Several have been proposed and used over the years. These include a saturation of 90% coupled with and F_IO_2 below 0.5,[5] or maximal compliance, and optimal oxygen delivery.[6] The optimal oxygen delivery parameter takes into account the frequent association of CPAP with a reduction in cardiac output. Often end points have included reduction of intrapulmonary shunt or venous admixture (Q_s/Q_t) to levels of 15% to 20%. This level of shunting is consistent with the definition as to when the onset of respiratory distress syndrome occurs.[7] When shunt cannot be measured because of absence of a pulmonary artery catheter, P_aO_2/F_IO_2 ratios can be used.[8] Acceptable P_aO_2/F_IO_2 levels usually include values above 250. While not commonly used today, arterial oxygen gradient $(A-aDO_2)$ below 350 mmHg on F_IO_2 equal to 1.0 was an acceptable end point. Currently, because F_IO_2 of 1.0 may cause increased shunt and loss of lung volume, the $(A-aDO_2)$ on F_IO_2 of 1.0 is not often used.[9] We have also proposed use of the gradient between end-tidal carbon dioxide ($ETco_2$) and P_aCO_2 as an acceptable end point.[10] The increased gradient coincides with an expansion of an alveolar dead space, secondary to overdistention. This can be a useful method, especially when the severity of lung disease prevents shunt reduction to levels of 15% to 20%.

After end point selection, incrementally increase CPAP in 3–5-cm H_2O increments. Any expected changes in blood gas or other circulatory parameters should occur within the first 5 minutes after the change has been made.[11] Therefore, we either follow the patient with arterial blood gas determination or monitor oxygen saturation with pulse oximetry, and vital signs are frequently taken. The changes are incrementally made until the appropriate end point has been reached. Once the end point has been reached, the level of CPAP should be maintained for a minimum of 6–24 hours. The actual duration of maintenance of the end point level of CPAP should be proportional to the level of underlying disease. The more involved or sicker the lung, the longer that particular level of CPAP will be maintained. Obviously, the patient should be clinically stable in terms of cardiovascular and other functions before one begins to change (either increase or decrease) the level of CPAP. Decreases in cardiac output caused by CPAP can usually be offset by intravascular volume expansion.

E. Weaning from CPAP

Weaning should take place in exactly the same manner in which CPAP was titrated upward. That requires pressure reduction in 3–5-cm H_2O increments. The blood gases should remain essentially unchanged during the weaning process. After approximately 20 minutes, data analysis should reveal the full effect of the CPAP decrease. The rapidity of the weaning will depend on the clinical circumstances. Those patients who required high CPAP levels because of very diseased lungs will progress more slowly than those who had less disease involvement. Ordinarily, we reduce the level of CPAP by a maximum of one-third of the original level during the first 24 hours of weaning. With attempts to wean faster, so-called overshoot occurs. Blood gases deteriorate and require reinstitution of CPAP, perhaps to the original levels, but certainly higher than those immediately preceding the blood gas deterioration. Weaning from CPAP levels of less than 15 cm H_2O can often proceed in a rather expeditious manner and be accomplished within 24–36 hours. Most important, the clinician should always gauge the patient's response to decreasing CPAP levels with measurement of the clinical parameters outlined earlier. Any deterioration of blood gas exchange requires the restoration of CPAP until the previously defined parameters are again met.

F. Complications

CPAP may have a number of undesirable effects. First, high levels of CPAP may result in an excessive increase in the expiratory work of breathing. As CPAP increases lung volume, the patient shifts upward on the pressure

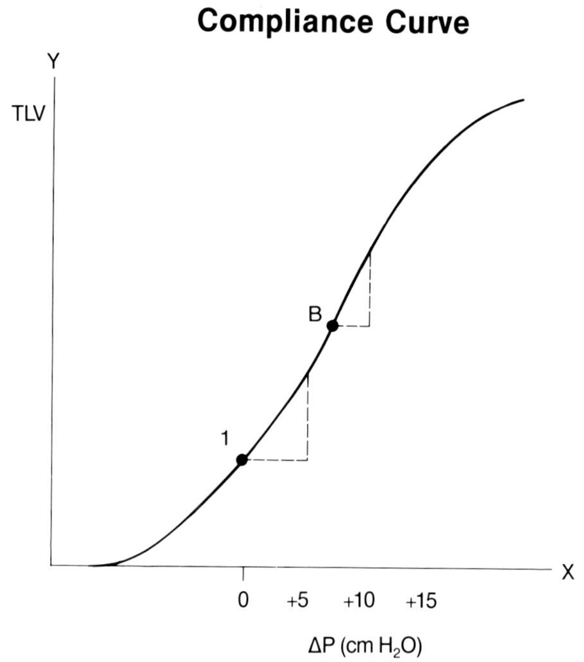

Figure 13–3 • The effect of CPAP on tidal volume and lung compliance. Point 1 represents a lung volume in a patient with respiratory failure. A large transpulmonary pressure gradient is necessary to deliver a tidal volume to the patient. The application of 7.5 cm H_2O CPAP increases lung volume to point 2. At point 2, a much smaller change in transpulmonary pressure delivers the same tidal volume.

volume curve (Fig. 13–3). However, as lung volume increases, alveolar dead space may increase. Clinically, the added alveolar dead space causes an elevated P_aCO_2. Second, marked overdistention also increases significantly the expiratory work of breathing. Patients, if awake and cooperative, will complain of an uncomfortable feeling and difficulty in breathing, especially exhalation.

Third, excessive CPAP also decreases cardiac output. Two major mechanisms for CPAP-induced decrease in cardiac output include a decreased venous return to the right side of the heart, as well as right ventricular failure due to increased pulmonary vascular resistance (see later). However, in upward of 90% of cases, cardiac output reductions represent a decrease in venous return, secondary to relative or true hypovolemia. The elevated airway pressures are transmitted across the pulmonary parenchyma to the intrathoracic space, which diminishes venous return. The greater the degree of lung compliance, the greater the transmission of airway pressures and interference with venous return and cardiac output. With appropriate titration of CPAP as previously described (intravascular volume expansion as necessary), little interference of venous return develops. A small number of patients experience right ventricular failure secondary to the elevated airway pressure.[12,13] Transmission of the airway pressures to the pulmonary vascular bed causes an elevated pulmonary vascular resistance. The cardiac response includes right ventricular dilatation, which is limited by the surrounding pericardium. Elevation of right ventricular pressure follows. Ultimately, when right ventricular pressure equals or exceeds left ventricular pressure, the intraventricular septum shifts into the left ventricular outflow tract. Left ventricular stroke volume then diminishes.

Fourth, CPAP can cause pulmonary barotrauma, including pneumothorax and pneumomediastinum. However, this problem primarily relates to the high peak airway pressures developed during positive-pressure mechanical ventilation as well as to the number of mechanical breaths delivered rather than directly due to the level of CPAP.[14] Nevertheless, since CPAP increases the baseline pressure, CPAP must also ultimately increase the peak inflation pressure developed during delivery of positive-pressure breaths.

Finally, too low a CPAP level will cause a deterioration in gas exchange. Pathophysiologic changes include a loss of lung volume, compliance, and a worsening of ventilation-to-perfusion relationships. At times this loss of compliance may elevate the work of breathing and may be coupled with an excessive respiratory rate. Under these circumstances spontaneous respiratory rate increases represent the loss in lung volume, increased work of breathing, and hypoxemia. Respiratory rate and minute ventilation increase in an attempt to minimize the work of breathing but still maintain oxygenation and carbon dioxide elimination. Often oxygenation cannot be successfully maintained because of inability to generate a great enough transthoracic pressure to ventilate the recollapsed alveoli.

II. INTERMITTENT MANDATORY VENTILATION (IMV)

A. *Description*

Intermittent mandatory ventilation (IMV) involves the delivery of a set number of predetermined positive-pressure breaths coupled with spontaneous breathing between the positive-pressure breaths (Fig. 13–4). The

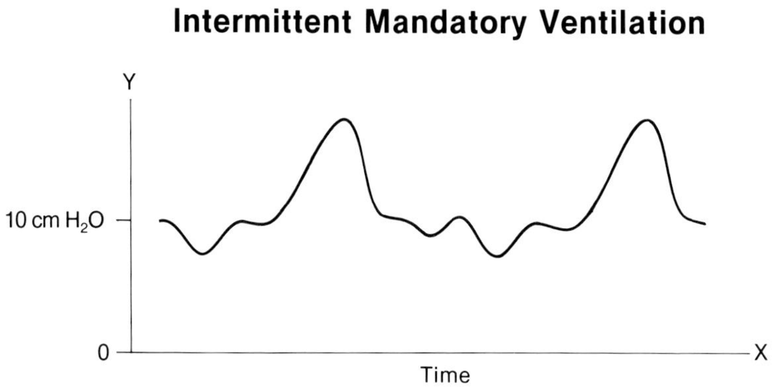

Figure 13–4 • Intermittent mandatory ventilation. The baseline pressure is 10 cm H_2O. Mandated positive-pressure breaths are delivered at predetermined intervals. Between mechanical positive-pressure breaths, spontaneous respiratory efforts of varying duration and intensity occur.

tidal volume is preselected for the mechanical breaths. A number of various mechanisms to deliver the tidal volume may be used. For some machines this involves simple selection of tidal volume, whereas in other machines it involves control of inspiratory time and flow rate.

Intermittent mandatory ventilation incorporates a circuitry that permits spontaneous respiration between breaths from the mechanical ventilator. These spontaneous breaths are undertaken with a minimal increase in work of breathing and usually are not associated with any asynchrony with the mechanical ventilator. Synchronized IMV (SIMV) assures that the mechanical breath will not be delivered at a time the patient initiates a spontaneous breath.[15,16] This sensing mechanism, used on some mechanical ventilators, prevents breath stacking, which develops if a positive-pressure tidal volume is delivered at the same time a patient initiates a spontaneous effort. Clinical studies have indicated that SIMV is not necessary under most situations. It appears that the patient develops a degree of synchrony with the system. The combination of mechanical breaths with spontaneous breathing results in a decrease in the number of mechanical breaths required compared to most other forms of ventilation. Selection of the appropriate mechanical rate with intermittent mandatory ventilation is based on physiologic parameters. These include the spontaneous respiratory rate, $PaCO_2$, and pH.

B. *Indications*

There are several indications for IMV. First, the method (the number of mandatory breaths) can potentially provide the exact need of the patient to achieve adequate alveolar ventilation. Second, IMV, by allowing spontaneous ventilation, is particularly helpful when high levels of continuous positive airway pressure, or CPAP, are employed. Third, the decreased number of mechanical breaths compared with either assist-control or controlled mechanical ventilation may result in less barotrauma. Factors causing IMV to result in less barotrauma include the reduction in number of positive-pressure breaths and reduced required mean airway pressure.[17] Fourth, the comparative decrease in the number of mechanical breaths improves cardiovascular function, probably because of the minimization of mean airway pressure. The spontaneous respiration associated with IMV causes a decrease in intrathoracic pressure, which then promotes venous return. The increase in venous return supports the cardiac output, particularly with high levels of CPAP.

Fifth, intermittent mandatory ventilation preserves the function of the muscles of respiration. Since patients can and do breathe spontaneously, the possibility of disuse atrophy greatly diminishes. Maintenance of normal respiration enhances the ability to later wean the patients, particularly if long-term mechanical ventilatory support becomes necessary.

Finally, intermittent mandatory ventilation also provides the best matching of ventilation to perfusion[18,19]; the reason for this requires explanation in detail. At end-exhalation the dependent alveoli are less expanded than those in the nondependent portions of the lung. Both the weight of the lung and the column of blood present in the lung contribute to alveolar compression in dependent areas. The compression of the dependent alveoli places them on a more favorable portion of the pressure–volume curve. Less distending pressure (the difference between intrathoracic and airway pressure) is required to open the dependent units than those already maximally expanded and commonly found in the nondependent portions. Thus, during spontaneous breathing, gas distributes itself primarily to the dependent portions of the lung. Likewise, the pulmonary circulation as a low-pressure system (mean pressure 15 ≈ mmHg) also flows primarily to the dependent lung portions. Thus, during spontaneous breathing the increased ventilation to the dependent lung matches the increased perfusion to the dependent lung and results in the best matching of ventilation to perfusion.

With the patient supine during positive-pressure ventilation these ventilation-to-perfusion relationships no longer hold, because with controlled mechanical ventilation the diaphragm moves passively secondary to changes generated by the positive-pressure ventilation. Most of this motion occurs in the anterior or nondependent portion; the smaller part of the motion occurs in the posterior or dependent portion.[20] The reason for this distribution of diaphragmatic motion is that the abdominal contents including the liver and spleen resist the motion of the posterior portions of the diaphragm. The resistance to motion in the posterior portion provides for preferential expansion of the nondependent portions of the lung. Therefore, during mechanical ventilation maldistribution of gas takes place, with most of the gas flowing primarily to the nondependent portions of the lung. Since blood flows primarily to the dependent parts of the lung, the preferential ventilation of the nondependent lung results in mismatching of ventilation to perfusion. When individuals are ventilated with small tidal volumes (4–6 mL / kg) that distribute primarily to nondependent lung, eventual hypoventilation and atelectasis ensue. Compared to spontaneous ventilation, larger tidal volumes must be delivered to overcome this maldistribution of ventilation and perfusion. Currently, we ventilate with tidal volumes of 12–15 mL / kg.[21] The large tidal volume provides a "spillover" effect to ventilate the previously nonventilated dependent portions. Intermittent mandatory ventilation minimizes the situation, since it promotes spontaneous breathing and limits the number of positive-pressure breaths required. As a result, it may have a greater influence on matching ventilation to perfusion.

C. *Contraindications*

There are a few times when spontaneous breathing is neither desirable nor helpful. These circumstances include the need to hyperventilate a patient with closed head injury and an increased intracranial pressure. In very unstable patients with a high metabolic rate, low cardiac output, or both, any spontaneous ventilation may contribute to an undesirable increase in oxygen consumption. Outside of these specialized situations, the use of intermittent mandatory ventilation or a ventilator capable of allowing for spontaneous ventilation between mechanical breaths (without causing asynchrony) can be used.

D. *How to Use IMV*

In using IMV (see also Chapter 6), the clinician must first select a tidal volume. As indicated previously, large tidal volumes are necessary. This ordinarily means 10–15 mL / kg. The appropriate ventilator rate should maintain a normal P_aCO_2 and pH coupled with a spontaneous respiratory rate of less than 30/min. This implies that adequate alveolar ventilation has been achieved without causing the patient an excessive amount of work to breathe. In the absence of a significant elevation of metabolic rate, 8 mechanical breaths/min will ordinarily result in a normal P_aCO_2 and pH. Since the carbon dioxide dissociation curve is a straight line, changes in minute ventilation are inversely reflected by changes in arterial P_aCO_2. A 25% increase in minute ventilation will reduce the arterial P_aCO_2 by the same amount.

If it is necessary to reduce P_aCO_2 (assuming one started with a tidal volume of 10–15 mg/kg and a respiratory rate of 8/min), the clinician can increase either the mechanical ventilator rate or the tidal volume. In my opinion, the tidal volume should first be altered. Moderate increases in tidal volume usually result in a minimal increase in peak and mean airway pressure and do not expose the lung to an increased number of breaths, with the resultant risk of barotrauma. Increases in tidal volume that result in a small increase in peak inflation pressure ($<$6–7 cm H_2O) are appropriate. A larger increase in peak inflation may reflect a shift in the compliance curve up and to the right, indicating lung overexpansion. In this case an increase in the ventilator rate will be necessary to further reduce P_aCO_2.

If the P_aCO_2 remains higher than expected for the degree of minute ventilation, several technical factors must be accounted for. First, the tidal volume delivered may be inappropriate. The clinician cannot rely on the delivered tidal volume from the ventilator as an indication of what the patient actually received. A significant portion of tidal volume may be lost in the ventilator circuitry because of its compliance. Using the corrugated disposable tubing, 3 mL of tidal volume will be lost per 1 cm H_2O of airway pressure. The only accurate way to determine tidal volume is to measure the exhaled volume at the airway (with a spirometer). Attempts to measure the tidal volume at the exhalation valve will erroneously include the volume originally lost within the circuitry itself. System leaks can also develop and account for loss of tidal volume.

Second, in the case of a bronchopleural fistula, significant volume can be lost via the chest tubes. Third, the clinician should also search for physiologic causes of increased carbon dioxide levels, such as elevated metabolic rate, sepsis, fever, agitation, and shivering. At times, inappropriate nutritional support can contribute to an increase in metabolic rate.[22,23] This ordinarily occurs with excessive infusion of glucose calories. The individual of average size can usually accommodate 30–40 cal/kg per 24 hours. Finally, other factors responsible for inadequate ventilation and an increase in P_aCO_2 include pneumothorax, right mainstem intubation, and ventilator failure. With a low IMV mechanical ventilator rate, patient apnea can result in hypercapnia.

E. *Weaning from IMV*

During IMV, commencement of the weaning process does not necessarily require measurement of mechanical parameters such as compliance, V_d/V_t ratios, or vital capacity. (See also Chapter 6 for a discussion of weaning from IMV.) Time and countless trials have demonstrated that following specific physiologic parameters will provide sufficient information to proceed. These parameters include a spontaneous respiratory rate of less than 30/min, P_aCO_2 of 38–42 mmHg, and pH above 7.35. The mechanical factors only become important preweaning factors when patients are not allowed to breathe during mechanical ventilation and therefore the clinician has no indication of the patient's breathing ability.

Reductions in the IMV rate should be made as 1–2 breaths/min changes. Usually, one change per hour implies satisfactory progress. For an unstable patient the number of changes per unit time may be much less frequent. The clinician should test blood gas levels or follow pulse oximetry end-tidal CO_2 within 15–20 minutes after reduction in the IMV rate. By that time patients should have stabilized. One can also follow noninvasive parameters such as end-tidal carbon dioxide and pulse oximetry. However, since we are most interested in alveolar ventilation, pulse oximetry will not be as helpful to monitor the weaning process. Conversely, expired carbon dioxide and the spontaneous respiratory rate provide more useful information. Patients who have only been ventilated a short time, such as overnight, or who have had only mild respiratory insufficiency may be ready for extubation when the IMV is 2/min. This presumes all the described weaning parameters (spontaneous respiratory rate <30/min, P_aCO_2 38–42 mmHg, and pH >7.35) are still met. It also presumes adequate oxygenation with an F_IO_2 <0.5 and CPAP $\leq$ 5 cm H_2O. Obviously, there should be no question of the patient's ability to maintain an airway after extubation. Patients who have required long-term ventilation or have had severe respiratory impairment may require additional observation at an IMV of zero prior to extubation. These patients may still have a degree of pulmonary instability that does not manifest itself until the IMV breaths have all been removed.

F. *Complications*

If the mechanical ventilator rate is too slow to help supply the required minute ventilation, the patient's spontaneous respiratory efforts will increase in an attempt to maintain adequate alveolar ventilation. This will significantly increase both the work of breathing and oxygen consumption and can harm the patient. Too rapid a ventilator rate will increase mean airway pressure. As a consequence, cardiac output may decrease secondary to the decrease in venous return previously mentioned. Also the risk of pulmonary barotrauma increases in conjunction with the elevated mechanical ventilator rate. Generally, a rapid ventilator rate also results in hyperventilation and a respiratory alkalosis and the alkalosis can precipitate cardiac arrhythmias. These may be particularly likely to occur in the immediate postoperative patient, who may also experience hypothermia and hypokalemia. The respiratory alkalosis also causes a shift of the oxyhemoglobin disassociation curve to the left, which decreases oxygen availability to the peripheral sites.

Since IMV often assumes patient contribution to minute ventilation, any sudden or unexpected decrease in patients' spontaneous respiratory rate may result in hypoventilation. When demand valves are used they must be able to respond rapidly enough to supply sufficient gas flow during spontaneous ventilation. A valve that requires significant inspiratory effort to open may excessively increase the work of breathing. Likewise, in-

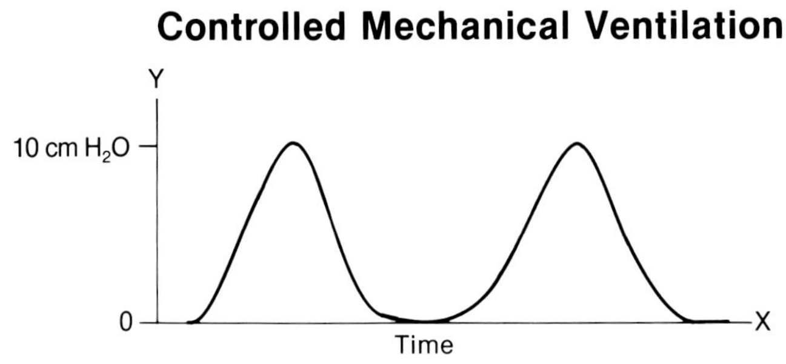

Figure 13–5 • Controlled mechanical ventilation. The only ventilation that occurs is when a positive-pressure breath is delivered to the patient. At the end of inspiration the airway pressure returns to ambient.

adequate flow in a continuous-flow system can also increase the work of breathing.

III. CONTROLLED MECHANICAL VENTILATION (CMV)

A. *Description*

Controlled mechanical ventilation (CMV) involves delivery of a programmed or previously selected tidal volume (Figs. 13–5, 13–6). Controlled ventilation provides all the respiratory support via these tidal volume breaths. The clinician selects the interval between breaths or the number of breaths per minute delivered to the patient. This concept does not provide or permit spontaneous breathing between mechanical ventilator breaths. Controlled mechanical ventilation may be delivered with or without CPAP therapy.

B. *Indications*

Compared to IMV, controlled mechanical ventilation generally results in higher mean airway pressures and in an increase in the number of mechanical breaths per time interval delivered to the patient. Since the tidal volume of the mechanical breath delivered to the patient is similar to that during IMV, one can expect essentially the same peak inflation pressures with either method.

In general, controlled mechanical ventilation can be used whenever mechanical ventilatory support is required.

When patients cannot or are not permitted to breathe spontaneously, controlled mechanical ventilation remains the method of choice. Examples include the paralyzed patient undergoing anesthesia and surgery or those influenced by drugs or injury. It can be especially helpful to hyperventilate patients, as in the case of a closed head injury with increased intracranial pressure. Central apnea may also result secondary to drug overdose or central nervous system damage such as closed head injury.

C. *Contraindications*

Controlled mechanical ventilation has no absolute contraindications. However, whenever the physician wants to assess the patient's spontaneous breathing efforts, controlled mechanical ventilation makes this process difficult. Relative contraindications include the necessity of minimizing the effect of mechanical ventilation on

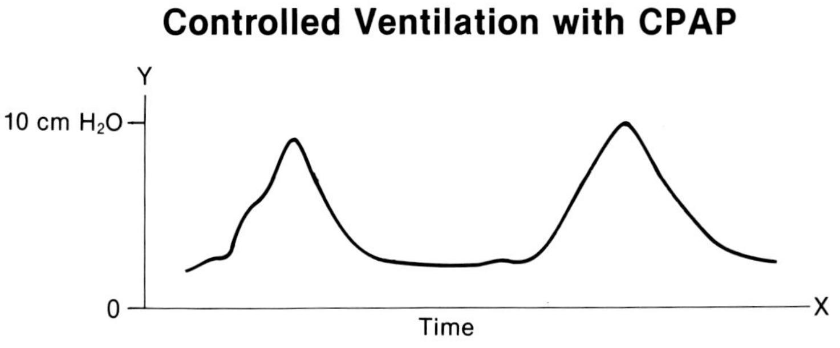

Figure 13–6 • Controlled mechanical ventilation with CPAP. Again no spontaneous breathing takes place. However, at the end of each mechanical breath the airway pressure returns to a level above the ambient pressure.

cardiovascular performance. Agitated patients may "fight" the ventilator, and this asynchrony usually results from attempts to breathe spontaneously. Under these circumstances the patient may require paralysis or transition to another form of ventilation such as IMV.

D. How to Use CMV

Tidal volume selection with CMV proceeds in exactly the same manner as with IMV. This involves the use of large tidal volumes in a range of 10–15 mL/kg. Use of that tidal volume coupled with a mechanical rate of approximately 8/min and normal metabolic demands usually results in a P_aCO_2 in the range of 38–42 mmHg. Dependent on the desired eventual P_aCO_2, the mechanical rate can be adjusted accordingly. Again, patients may be monitored with end-tidal carbon dioxide as previously described in the IMV section. The patient is generally maintained at the appropriate ventilator rate until weaning commences.

As previously indicated, patient attempts to breathe spontaneously in this system may result in "bucking" or "fighting" the ventilator because no air enters the thorax with the spontaneous efforts and this feeling unsettles the patient. Paralysis can accomplish this; hyperventilation with removal of the respiratory drive secondary to the hypocapnic alkalosis can also be effective.

E. Weaning from CMV

During CMV weaning usually does not proceed until all systems are stable and all problems are resolved. This includes resolution of the underlying pulmonary problems as evidenced by blood gas changes, radiographs, and pulmonary mechanics, including compliance. Clearly, the patient should have stable cardiovascular function, as evidenced by lack of major fluctuations in blood pressure and no arrhythmias. There is no requirement for pressor support for blood pressure.

Since the patient does not breathe during CMV, this function must be assessed prior to commencing the weaning process. In addition to the previously listed parameters, other pulmonary mechanics require testing. Transitioning the patient to a T-tube system (Blow-by) with a continuous flow of at least 20 L/min enables the weaning evaluation to take place. Generally, to insure safety while on the T-tube the F_IO_2 is maintained at 1.0 (at least initially). Various mechanical tests assess the patient's readiness for weaning. Negative inspiratory force (NIF) should exceed 25 cm H_2O. Patients must demonstrate a spontaneous tidal volume of at least 4–6 mL/kg. Vital capacity should equal or exceed 10 mL/kg.

Once lung mechanics tests and clinical evaluation indicate readiness, weaning can proceed. Generally, the patient is changed gradually to the T-tube and continuously observed for the initial short period, usually 5–10 minutes. At the end of this initial trial the patient should be reattached to the mechanical ventilator and CMV reinstituted. During the T-tube observations, end-tidal carbon dioxide can be monitored, as can oxygen saturation and vital signs. After a sufficient rest period on CMV, the patient can again be placed on the T-tube, this time for a longer period. This process continues with breathing through a T-tube for progressively longer times and alternating with shorter durations of mechanical ventilation. With relatively normal lungs the entire process can conclude in 4–6 hours.

Patients recovering from severe respiratory distress or with previous underlying lung disease may take much longer to wean, perhaps 24 hours or more. For extremely ill or previously debilitated patients, weaning may involve intermittent periods of time back on CMV. This might include the patient breathing through a T-tube during the daytime, but ventilation with CMV during sleep. Over time, the amount of ventilator sleep time is gradually reduced until the patient is able to support all breathing requirements through spontaneous efforts. After successful transition to permanent T-tube circuitry, extubation can occur. After extubation the patient should be continually assessed and the clinician assured that the patient can maintain the airway.

In a few patients endotracheal intubation is accomplished with a narrow-diameter tube. During CMV this presents no particular problems for the patient. However, during weaning with a T-tube, the work of breathing may be significantly increased secondary to the increased resistance of the narrow tube. In adult males this generally occurs with tubes smaller than 7 mm ID. For women resistance significantly increases to tubes with an internal diameter below 6 mm. In these situations the patient may be allowed to spend a minimum time on T-tube prior to extubation. In fact, some patients who have had a small-diameter tube *in situ* during T-tube weaning actually breathe with greater ease and improved blood gases and vital signs after extubation, probably because of the lowered airway resistance and work of breathing.

F. *Complications*

The major potential complication of CMV is cardiovascular depression. Patients suffering from this complication also have a propensity to "fight" the respirator if allowed to breathe spontaneously. This may result in lack of coordination and difficulty in maintaining adequate gas exchange. In addition, the thrashing patient movement can cause high inflation pressures with each mechanical breath.

Study of available literature indicates that the major factors associated with pulmonary barotrauma include the ventilator rate and tidal volume as well as the peak inflation pressure.[14,24,25] Because of design, CMV results in the highest number of mechanical breaths per minute. The peak inflation pressures developed during CMV are at least the equal of those during IMV or assist-controlled ventilation. Therefore, at least two of the major factors promoting barotrauma are most prominent during CMV. The clinician should, at the very least, have a high index of suspicion and carefully observe the patient for signs or symptoms of barotrauma. These symptoms may vary and can include all the following: elevated P_aCO_2, decreased P_aO_2, elevated peak inflation pressure, decreased chest movement on the involved side, hyperresonance on the affected side, subcutaneous air, evidence of pneumothorax, or pneumomediastinum on chest radiograph.

IV. ASSISTED AND ASSIST-CONTROL VENTILATION

A. *Description*

Assisted ventilation permits the patient to make spontaneous respiratory efforts. The spontaneous respiratory effort triggers the mechanical ventilator then to deliver a preprogrammed tidal volume to the patient (Fig. 13–7). The triggering mechanism can vary in sensitivity, resulting in a greater or lesser inspiratory effort on the part of the patient. In the event that the patient does not breathe at all, no mechanical breaths are delivered to the patient.

Assisted ventilation is often combined with controlled ventilation to provide the assist-control mode of mechanical ventilation (Figs. 13–8, 13–9). In addition to the assisted breaths, the patient receives a number of breaths with the same tidal volume as the assist breath but at a preselected interval. The control aspect of the assist-control mode insures some degree of ventilation irrespective of any patient apnea.

The number of assisted breaths delivered depends on the patient's spontaneous rate. It is not unusual for patients to breathe at such a rapid rate that hypocapnia develops, which in turn leads to apnea. As P_aCO_2 rises during the apneic period, the respiratory centers are

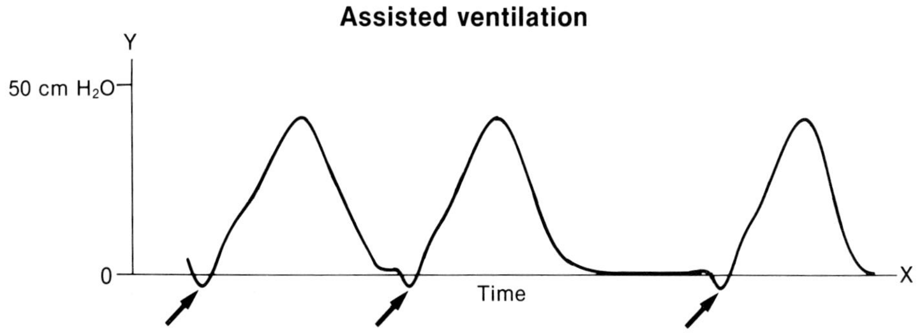

Figure 13–7 • Assisted ventilation. Each spontaneous inspiratory effort (*arrows*) is denoted by a slight deflection of the airway pressure below ambient. This in turn triggers the ventilator to deliver a predetermined tidal volume. Each assisted breath delivers the same tidal volume and should result in approximately the same peak airway pressure. The frequency of these positive-pressure breaths is determined by the patient's own spontaneous respiratory efforts.

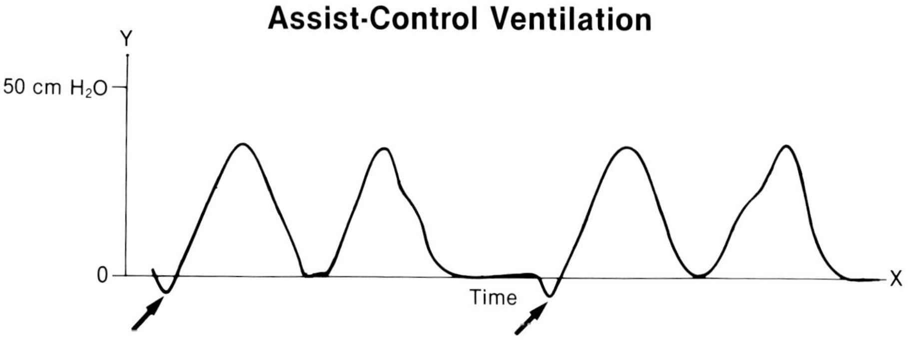

Figure 13–8 • Assist-control ventilation. In this schematic the first and third breaths (*arrows*) represent assisted ventilation as previously described. Each of these breaths is followed by a mandated breath. These mandated breaths are not triggered by a spontaneous respiratory effort, but are delivered at predetermined intervals.

again triggered and the patient initiates spontaneous efforts. Thus, spontaneous breathing in the assist mode may be cyclic.

B. *Indications*

Indications for assisted ventilation and assist-control ventilation assume the patient can initiate spontaneous respiratory efforts. The clinician expects that despite spontaneous respiratory efforts, the mechanical ventilator will be responsible for the entire minute ventilation. One benefit of assisted or assist-control ventilation is the preservation of the patient's own inspiratory efforts and muscles of respiration. However, since these inspiratory efforts do not actually participate in gas delivery to the patient, the amount of work done by the inspiratory muscles remains minimal and contributes little, if anything, to minute ventilation.[26] Most clinicians combine both forms and use assist-control ventilation rather than assisted ventilation alone.

C. *Contraindications*

Contraindications to assisted ventilation are apneic patients or conditions that induce apnea. These include central nervous system involvement as well as paralysis, either induced or as a result of trauma. Various sedatives or narcotics may also cause apnea or severe hypoventilation secondary to alteration of respiratory drive. Assisted ventilation may be inadvisable under these circumstances. The clinician may want to consider assist-control ventilation instead.

D. *How to Use Assist-Control Ventilation*

The clinician must choose the tidal volume to be delivered with each assisted breath. This tidal volume should be chosen in the same way as for CMV and IMV and should equal 10–15 mL/kg. The actual number of assisted breaths delivered per minute will be determined by the patient's spontaneous efforts.

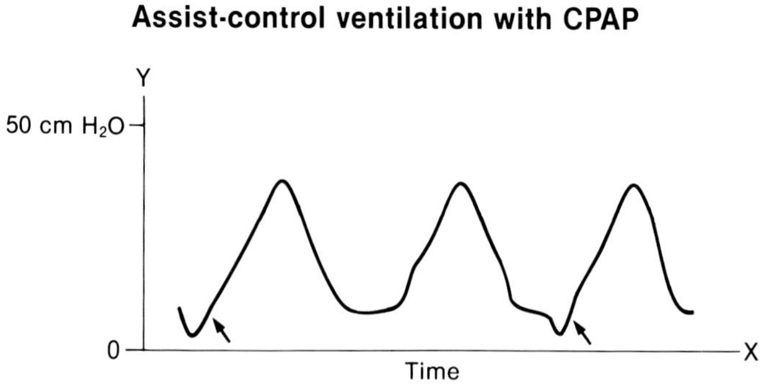

Figure 13–9 • Assist-control ventilation with CPAP. After each mechanical breath the airway pressure returns to a level above the baseline. With an assisted breath (*arrows*) the airway pressure has a slight negative deflection from baseline but does not reach ambient levels.

With a rapid, spontaneous rate the clinician may want to slow the patient's respiratory rate with sedation and/or narcotics. Also the introduction of controlled breaths will increase minute ventilation, reduce P_aCO_2, and often slow the patient's own spontaneous rate. Since the patient's respiratory rate can determine the overall minute ventilation and the respiratory rate may vary from time to time, there may be variations in the final P_aCO_2 and pH. Therefore, the clinician must accept a wider range for these values rather than the more narrow ranges used with CMV and IMV.

The clinician may also choose to adjust the ventilator sensitivity. The more sensitive the machine, the less inspiratory effort required to trigger delivery of the next breath and the greater the increased minute ventilation. Reduced sensitivity requires a greater inspiratory effort and may result in a decreased number of assisted breaths delivered per unit of time.

E. *Weaning from Assist-Control Ventilation*

Weaning from assisted or assist-control ventilation employs the same mechanical parameters as CMV does. Obviously, the patient should demonstrate cardiovascular stability and have resolved all the pulmonary indications that resulted in mechanical ventilation. If the patient is on assist-control mode, the controlled breaths are weaned first. As the number of controlled breaths is reduced, the patient can be followed by monitoring vital signs, blood gases, and end-tidal carbon dioxide. The controlled breaths should be weaned in a fashion similar to that described for IMV. A significant elevation in the patient's spontaneous rate following the weaning of the controlled breaths may indicate intolerance for further weaning efforts. To wean from assisted ventilation one technique involves progressively reducing sensitivity of the trigger mechanism. Others recommend transition to a T-tube circuit, as described for CMV. Since patients only initiate an inspiratory effort during assisted ventilation but do not actually ventilate themselves, introduction of a T-tube circuit for progressively longer periods of time will give the best indication of how rapidly weaning can progress.

F. *Complications*

Over the years manufacturers have had difficulty developing an adequate sensitivity control. On the one hand, if the sensitivity of the mechanical ventilator trigger mechanism is increased, the number of assisted breaths will increase. In some instances the mere movement of the patient, even without a clear inspiratory effort, can trigger the machine, and hyperventilation then ensues. On the other hand, a very insensitive trigger device can increase the work of breathing, reduce the number of assisted breaths delivered, and result in severe hypoventilation. This may also induce the patient to "buck" or "fight" the ventilator.

Because all the breaths delivered with assisted or assist-control ventilation are positive-pressure breaths, high mean airway pressures, with their attendant complications, can develop. In fact, this mode of ventilation may result in the highest mean airway pressures due to the combination of assisted and control breaths the patient receives (stacking of one breath on top of the other). However, studies to date have not indicated an overall higher incidence of pulmonary barotrauma with assisted or assist-control ventilation.

V. HIGH-FREQUENCY JET VENTILATION (HFJV)

A. *Description*

High-frequency jet ventilation (HFJV) uses small tidal volumes and rapid ventilator rates (Figs. 13–10, 13–11). Although the tidal volume has been previously characterized as being less than the dead space, the tidal volume may actually exceed the anatomic dead space in adults.[27,28] High-frequency jet ventilation operates at rates between 150 and 400/min. Compared to other mechanical ventilator techniques, the combination of small tidal volume and rapid respiratory rates results in a lowered mean airway pressure. High-frequency jet ventilation may be used in combination with CPAP.

Also contrary to all other types of mechanical ventilators, jet ventilators can operate with drive pressures less than the conventional 47–52 psig. Reduction of the drive pressure decreases flow from the machine and therefore ultimately tidal volume.

In contrast to other ventilators, the HFJV circuitry is also different. The tubing has less compliance and smaller diameter; both of these characteristics reduce gas loss into the circuitry itself. On reaching the airway the gas passes through an elongated orifice usually located at the proximal airway and about 2 in long (the

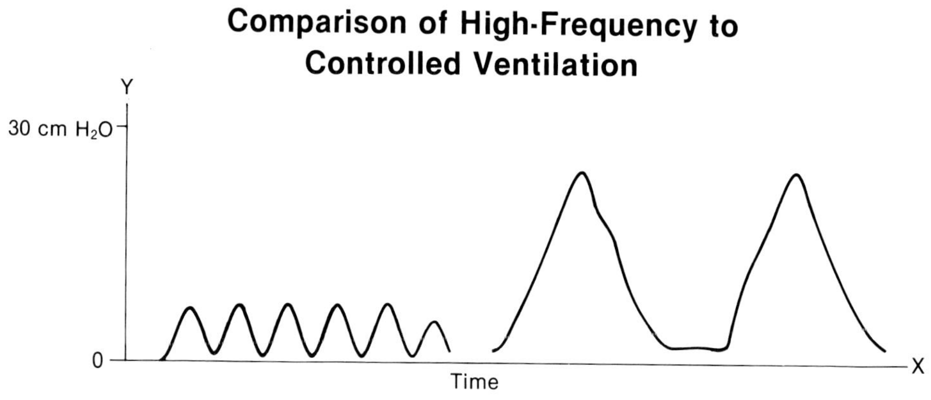

Figure 13–10 • Comparison of high-frequency jet ventilation to controlled mechanical ventilation. Note the reduction in airway pressure with high-frequency jet ventilation. The area under the curve can in effect represent tidal volume, which is also significantly reduced when compared to controlled ventilation.

injector). The smaller diameter of this orifice causes an acceleration or jetting of the gases as they are delivered into the airway and the endotracheal tube. The accelerated gas flow through the jet injector develops a surrounding area of negative pressure. A second parallel flow of gas (20 L / min) can be entrained by the negative pressure (Bernoulli effect). The entrained gas usually passes through a humidifier and helps to improve overall humidification.

Development of HFJV has been hampered by an inability to deliver adequate humidification. In addition to humidifying the entrained flow, efforts now include aerosolization of saline drops delivered directly in front of the injector. The resultant particles are of variable size and may or may not actually increase humidification. Without strict control of flow rate of the saline drops (< 20 mL / hr), airway overhydration can easily develop.

The small tidal volumes and rapid flow rate during HFJV are compatible with normal spontaneous breathing. In fact, except if hyperventilation does develop, spontaneous breathing is characteristic of this ventilation mode.

While ordinarily connected to an endotracheal tube, a high-frequency jet circuit can be altered to other delivery systems. This includes a needle introduced into the trachea via cricothyrotomy (see Chapter 9). High-frequency jet ventilation has been administered via a small-diameter tubing placed through the larynx for translaryngeal and other types of surgical procedures.[29] This is especially important when airway space is at a premium. The high-frequency ventilator can also be attached to a ventilating or fiberoptic bronchoscope.

B. *Indications*

Contrary to previous speculation and enthusiasm for the technique, HFJV appears to work best only in specialized circumstances. These include ventilation during fiberoptic bronchoscopy and airway procedures.[30] The ability to use HFJV with small tubes such as a feeding

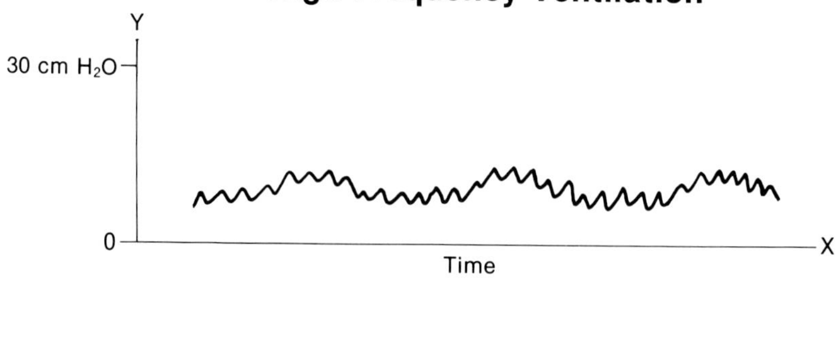

Figure 13–11 • High-frequency ventilation. The varying pattern of the baseline indicates the patient's own spontaneous efforts during high-frequency jet ventilation. In this example a small level of CPAP has been applied so that the airway pressure does not return to ambient.

tube introduced into the airway can insure adequate ventilation during various laryngeal procedures.

High-frequency jet ventilation has also been helpful in the treatment of bronchopleural fistula.[31] Bronchopleural fistula often results in gas loss from the lung via an *in situ* chest tube during a large tidal volume positive-pressure breath. During the acute and resolution phases of the illness, HFJV, with its attendant lower airway pressures, may reduce gas loss through the lung. The lower pressures also promote a healing environment for the fistula.

With its ability to deliver a high minute ventilation, HFJV may help reduce intracranial pressure. It does not appear to be any more beneficial for treatment of patients with ARDS. In fact, to obtain adequate gas exchange in patients with ARDS, the same mean airway pressures developed during conventional ventilation are required.[32] Although HFJV does reduce the peak inflation pressure, it can still reduce cardiac output.

C. *How to Use HFJV*

To initiate HFJV, first choose a drive pressure for the machine. With compliant lungs, a 30-psig drive pressure will deliver adequate flow and tidal volume. As compliance deteriorates, drive pressure must increase. At the same compliance and rate the higher the drive pressure, the larger is the tidal volume and the greater the reduction in P_aCO_2. A rate of 100–150/min will provide adequate oxygenation and carbon dioxide elimination in most patients. At times, higher rates may be necessary to further reduce P_aCO_2. The rate must be coupled with an inspiratory time of 30% to 50% of the entire inspiratory–expiratory cycle. The greater the inspiratory time, the larger the tidal volume delivered.[33] High inspiratory times coupled with high rates may cause air trapping and thereby prevent airway pressure from returning to baseline (and result in inadvertent CPAP).

Monitoring during HFJV should be carried out as with other forms of ventilation. However, the rapid respiratory rates during HFJV do not allow accurate measurement of expired carbon dioxide. CPAP may be added as necessary to restore oxygenation. In general, with HFJV, ventilator rate, percent inspiratory time, and drive pressure control P_aCO_2, whereas CPAP and F_IO_2 control oxygenation. One must remember that CPAP, rate, and drive pressure all contribute to mean airway pressure, which then affects oxygenation and circulatory status.

D. *Weaning from HFJV*

To wean the patient from HFJV some degree of resolution of the disease processes should have occurred. There are no clearcut means to successfully wean all patients from HFJV. One method progressively reduces the drive pressure. Decreasing drive pressure decreases tidal volume but still permits an adequate gas flow to support spontaneous breathing. When drive pressure has been successfully reduced to low levels, perhaps 15 psig, the patient should either be extubated or changed gradually to conventional ventilation. Another method of weaning from HFJV progressively decreases the ventilator rate. When the rate reaches 80/min, patients can usually be successfully changed to conventional ventilation with larger tidal volumes at rates of approximately 15–20/min. If HFJV has been used for the specialized situations previously mentioned, the patient can be converted to conventional ventilation when the disease process has been significantly resolved.

E. *Complications*

Inadequate humidity is a major complications with HFJV. The humidification systems for HFJV have been described earlier. At best these humidification systems are only marginally successful. When HFJV persists for prolonged periods, special attention must be paid to humidification. In addition, a number of patients may fail on HFJV. This often results because of poor lung and chest wall compliance, coupled with a large body habitus. Not surprisingly, then, many HFJV failures have involved patients with ARDS. Thus, it appears that high inflation pressures and an elevated mean airway pressure as well as increased CPAP may be necessary not only to reexpand some alveoli but to keep them expanded, even with HFJV. Finally, as previously mentioned, a short expiratory time coupled with a rapid rate may result in inadvertent CPAP.

VI. PRESSURE SUPPORT VENTILATION (PSV)

A. *Description*

Pressure support ventilation (PSV) combines spontaneous breathing with delivery of positive-pressure breaths

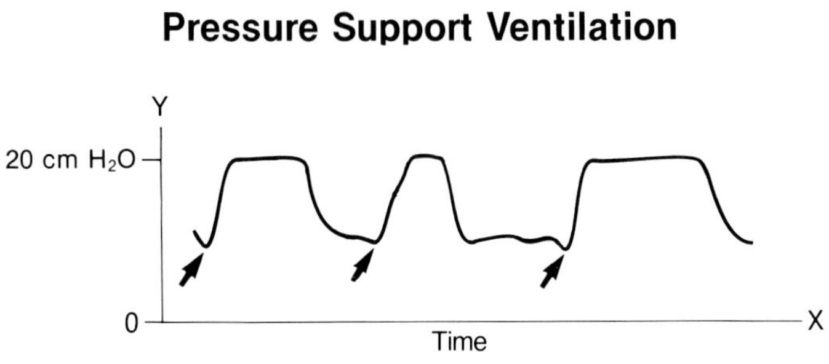

Figure 13–12 • Pressure support ventilation with CPAP. The baseline pressure is elevated above ambient. These three breaths all represent a pressure support mode of ventilation. Initial negative deflection (*arrows*) is followed by a rapid rise in pressure to a predetermined level, here 20 cm H_2O. However, the duration of each breath varies upon the patient's own efforts.

(Fig. 13–12). Unlike the spontaneous breathing during intermittent mandatory ventilation, which reduces mean airway pressure, each spontaneous breath with pressure support causes development of positive-pressure that actually increases the mean airway pressure.[34,35] This type of dual ventilation with each breath requires a microprocessor-controlled ventilator. One selects an airway pressure at some level above the baseline pressure (ambient or some elevated CPAP or PEEP level). With the initiation of a spontaneous effort, the ventilator senses the negative deflection in airway pressure. The machine then delivers an inspiratory flow with a sufficient rate to develop an airway pressure equal to the preselected level above baseline. The tidal volume results from the pressure support level selected as well as inspiratory time. The very high flow rate associated with this mode significantly reduces the inspiratory work of breathing. Ordinarily, this corresponds to a 25% decrease in the inspiratory effort. The duration of the inspiratory pressure support breath depends on the patient's own spontaneous effort. During delivery the ventilator continues to sense any negative deflections in airway pressure and adjusts the flow rate to maintain the desired pressure above baseline. Each ventilator uses its own algorithm to detect the end of inspiration. This mode can be combined with conventional positive-pressure breaths, as in controlled or intermittent mandatory ventilation (Fig. 13–13). The mandated breaths are delivered at a predetermined tidal volume and frequency.

B. *Indications*

Pressure support ventilation works best as a method to reduce the inspiratory work of breathing. Clinical indications of increased work of breathing include a rapid respiratory rate (>30/min) or an inspiratory effort that causes a large negative deflection of airway pressure. Other indirect indications of increased work of breathing include agitation, tachypnea, hypertension, and tachycardia. Pressure support ventilation helps synchronize the patient's spontaneous efforts with the mechanical ventilator. Since the method contributes to an overall increase in mean airway pressure, it may have some positive impact on oxygenation.

C. *How to Use PSV*

With pure pressure support the clinician selects a level of pressure support above the baseline pressure that results in a decrease of the inspiratory effort, as well as a

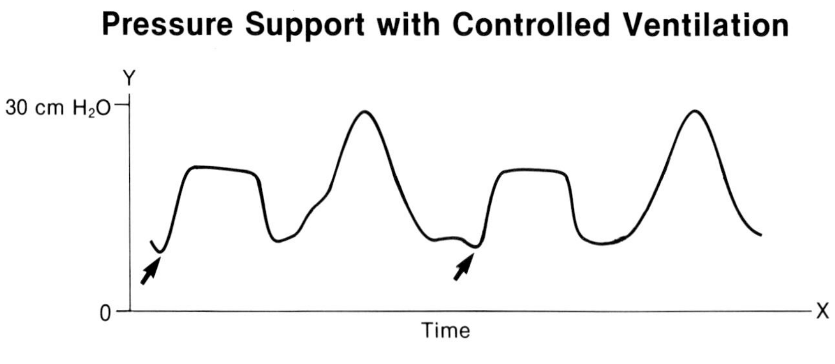

Figure 13–13 • Pressure support ventilation with predetermined positive pressure breaths. After each pressure support breath (*arrows*) a mandated positive pressure breath is delivered. The mandated positive pressure breaths occur at predetermined intervals. Baseline pressures are elevated above ambient.

decrease in respiratory rate. When these parameters are met one should also note less agitation and less "fighting" of the ventilator. Often vital signs return to more normal values. In the usual postoperative patient a pressure support level of 10 cm H_2O will minimize the inspiratory work. If the patient experiences tachypnea or increased dyspnea, a higher pressure support level may be needed.

If the clinician wishes to reduce P_aCO_2, the pressure support level should be increased. If inspiratory time remains constant, minute ventilation will increase as the pressure support level increases. More often, one combines preselected positive-pressure breaths in combination with spontaneous positive-pressure–supported breaths. The tidal volume of the preselected or mandated breath should be identical to the other modes of ventilation previously described (10–15 mL/kg). With pressure support the rate selected for the mandated breaths should be between 6 and 10/min.

Improvement in arterial oxygenation will depend on the inspired F_IO_2 and the level of CPAP. CPAP should be titrated as previously described. Ordinarily, the level of pressure support will vary between 5 and 30 cm H_2O. The end point includes adequate blood gas exchange and a calm patient exhibiting minimal signs of inspiratory breathing work, as previously described. Monitoring can proceed as it ordinarily does with the other forms of mechanical ventilation, such as IMV and CMV.

D. *Weaning from PSV*

Weaning with pressure support ventilation consists initially of a reduction in the level of pressure support. We usually accomplish this in 5-cm H_2O increments and permit the patient to stabilize for 1–2 hours before decreasing the pressure support level further. As with the other ventilatory modes, the number of changes made over a time period will depend on the original severity of the patient's illness. The longer and more severe the pulmonary involvement, the fewer the interventions made in any time period. As the level of pressure support decreases, the parameters monitored should change minimally. At pressure support levels of 5 cm H_2O or less, the mode can be discontinued. Since the patient has been breathing spontaneously, the usual transition would be to a low level of intermittent mandatory ventilation. Some clinicians elect to maintain the patient on low levels of pressure support and extubate from the low-level pressure support mode. To accomplish this latter weaning technique, the mandated positive-pressure breaths (if present) must also be eliminated. The mandated positive-pressure breaths should be weaned from the patient in exactly the same manner as previously described for IMV.

E. *Complications*

Major complications with pressure support ventilation relate to airway pressure. The mode, as opposed to intermittent mandatory ventilation, increases mean airway pressure. The usual complications can then be expected. These include cardiovascular depression and pulmonary barotrauma. To some degree there may be a mismatch of ventilation to perfusion.

Since PSV minimizes the inspiratory work of breathing, respiratory muscle atrophy may develop. The degree of atrophy may be proportional to the duration of the mechanical support.[36-39] Other factors contributing to respiratory muscle fatigue and failure include the patient's premorbid physical condition and nutritional status.

Excessive pressure support levels cause hyperventilation. Hyperventilation and the resultant hypocapnia reduce respiratory drive. The patient may then cycle between hyper- and hypoventilation. The attendant changes in pH and the complications due to respiratory alkalosis, as previously mentioned, can ensue.

VII. INDEPENDENT LUNG VENTILATION (ILV)

A. *Description*

Independent lung ventilation (ILV) consists of different tidal volumes, different levels of CPAP, and possibly different mechanical ventilator rates to each lung. (See also Chapter 12 for a discussion of ILV.) The technique requires isolation of each lung field with a double-lumen endotracheal tube. Initially, it seemed that the technique required synchronized ventilators to insure simultaneous delivery of separate tidal volumes to each lung field. Subsequent research has demonstrated that ventilation of each lung may be out of phase by as much as 90° without any detrimental effects on cardiovascular or pulmonary performance.[40]

B. Indications

Independent lung ventilation works best for unilateral lung disease.[41,42] Examples include contusion, aspiration, interstitial pneumonia, or severe atelectasis. Almost all these conditions require some increase in airway pressure both to ventilate and to recruit lung volume in the affected lung. As such, utilizing a single ventilator and a conventional single-lumen endotracheal tube may actually increase the amount of ventilation–perfusion mismatch. The reason for increased ventilation–perfusion mismatch under these circumstances (unilateral lung disease, single-lumen tube) is that the gas delivered into the airway by positive pressure will take the path of least resistance and go to the healthy, noninvolved, more compliant lung. The overexpanded healthy lung may have an increased vascular resistance and decreased perfusion. Thus, pulmonary blood flow will be directed away from the best-ventilated areas to the involved disease segments and significant ventilation perfusion mismatch will ensue.

Isolation of each lung with the double-lumen tube permits specific tidal volumes with appropriate airway pressures to be delivered to each lung. The involved lung ordinarily requires higher pressures both to expand and to maintain the lung at near-normal functional residual capacity. Maintenance of lung expansion can usually be accomplished by individual CPAP titration to each lung field.

Double-lumen tubes can also be used for lung surgery. After isolation of each lung field, the operated side can be collapsed to facilitate the procedure. Following the procedure, continuation of the double-lumen tube may prevent delivery of high pressures to the operated side with possible disruption of suture lines.

Significant hemoptysis may also require the use of a double-lumen tube. The tube essentially isolates each lung and prevents spillage of blood into the nonbleeding lung. While both bleeding complications and surgery may require independent ventilation more often than not, it must be understood that these procedures require isolation of the involved side with ventilation essentially directed to the noninvolved lung.

C. How to Use ILV

Each lung must be isolated by placement of a double-lumen endotracheal tube. Most clinicians use left-sided double-lumen tubes with the tip of the tube being located just distal to the carina in the left mainstem bronchus (see Chapter 12). A right-sided double-lumen tube runs the high risk of occlusion to the takeoff to the right upper lobe.[43,44] Several tubes have been available to preclude this right-sided problem, but none have worked exceptionally well. In my opinion, the only time a right-sided tube should be used is for surgery on the left lung or when it is impossible to enter the left mainstem bronchus.

Independent lung ventilation requires two ventilators, which can be synchronized so that tidal volumes are delivered at the same time and for the same duration. Specialized electronic devices for this task are available from the manufacturers. However, as mentioned earlier, this does not appear to be necessary, but the clinician should avoid having the ventilators continually 180° out of phase, since this may cause excessive mediastinal movement and impair circulatory function. Specially designed ventilators have been developed that allow the use of essentially one machine but that can direct independent and totally controlled tidal volumes to each lung field.[45]

Ordinarily, the right lung receives 60% of the total delivered tidal volume. However, under conditions requiring reexpansion of an individual lung, tidal volume to one side may be altered so as to develop an adequate peak inflation pressure to expand the affected side. CPAP should be titrated independently and ordinarily will be higher on the involved or affected side.

To improve P_aO_2 the clinician should first attempt to increase the level of CPAP to the affected lung. Titration to the preselected end point has been previously described. To titrate P_aCO_2 both tidal volumes and mechanical ventilator rate should be adjusted. Under conditions of severe atelectasis, larger tidal volumes may be required to develop airway pressures sufficient to reexpand the affected lung.

A carinal hook on the double-lumen tube aids in placement, particularly if used for long-term ventilation (see Chapter 11). These double-lumen tubes are placed essentially like any other endotracheal tube. To facilitate passage through the larynx the carinal hook should be in the anterior position; once the carinal hook is past the cords, the tube is rotated 180° so that the carinal hook faces in a posterior direction. The tube is then rotated another 90° to aid in appropriate endotracheal intubation (see Chapter 12). Most double-lumen tubes have an attachment that allows ventilation of each lumen with a single ventilator, air-mask-bag unit (AMBU), or other self-inflating type of bag. A fiberoptic bronchoscope passed through one lumen can help determine tube position. Once in place the endobronchial and tracheal cuffs are inflated. Care should be taken not to overinflate the endobronchial cuff that functions more as a low-volume, high-pressure seal. Each lumen should be occluded during ventilation of the other lumen with the self-inflating bag or ventilator and the chest auscultated. With proper placement the clinician will only hear breath sounds on the nonoccluded side. Chest movement should also only occur on the nonoccluded side. Double-lumen tubes without a carinal hook are especially prone to migrate distally. Since these are most often left-sided endobronchial tubes, the movement results in occlusion of the left upper lobe and of the right lumen against the carina. When tubes are kept in place for several days in nonsedated, nonparalyzed patients, continual close observation, especially with periodic fiberoptic bronchoscope checks, will help detect any tube movement.

D. *Weaning from ILV*

Continuous positive airway pressure levels should be weaned in exactly the same manner as previously indicated. When the affected side has a CPAP of less than 10 cm H_2O and peak inflation pressures below 60 cm H_2O, independent lung ventilation may no longer be required. To test this hypothesis, attach the adapter that permits ventilation to both lung fields from the same source. Both lungs can then be ventilated with one total tidal volume and the same CPAP level (as one would with a single-lumen tube). Maintenance of blood gas exchange indicates that independent ventilation can be safely discontinued. At this point the double-lumen tube can be removed and replaced with a single-lumen tube and ventilation can be carried out in normal fashion.

E. *Complications*

As previously indicated, a double-lumen tube can migrate further into either the right or left mainstem bronchus. (See also Chapter 12 for a discussion of ILV complications.) On placement the tube may become twisted and occlude one lumen or both lumina. This can easily be diagnosed by insertion of a fiberoptic bronchoscope. Some clinicians prefer to place a tube with a fiberoptic bronchoscope already in one lumen, usually the one destined for location above the carina. This allows direct visualization and insurance of appropriate placement.

The relatively narrow lumina of the double-lumen tube can cause significant problems, including difficult suctioning. Attempts to breathe spontaneously through these narrow lumina may result in both increased resistance and increased work of breathing.

Totally asynchronous independent ventilation may result in a pendulumlike movement of the mediastinum with resultant cardiac compromise. Although ventilators do not necessarily need to be synchronized, they should not be completely or 180° out of phase with one another.

VIII. AIRWAY PRESSURE RELEASE VENTILATION (APRV)

A. *Description*

Airway pressure release ventilation (APRV) does not use delivery of positive-pressure breaths to the airway.[46] Instead it relies on intermittently releasing and reducing a constant static position pressure to the airway. In effect, it develops into bimodal CPAP. Therefore, the method is very much like spontaneous respirations between two levels of CPAP. Both the amount of decrease in the airway pressure and its duration can be controlled and varied. The greater the decrease in pressure and the greater the frequency, the further the reduction in P_aCO_2. Spontaneous breathing can certainly occur with this system. The basic supposition behind APRV is that respiratory failure, as evidenced by hypoxemia, results secondary to loss of lung volume.[47] Therefore, establishment of a constant positive airway presure should ultimately restore lung volume and improve gas exchange.[48,49] The pressure is intermittently reduced, with concomitant loss of lung volume. The longer the reduction in airway pressure, the more likely that it will cause a reduction in oxygenation. Major benefits of airway pressure release ventilation include a reduced mean airway pressure and peak inflation pressure.

B. *Indications*

Airway pressure release ventilation works best for mild to moderate cases of ARDS. In more severe cases very high airway pressures may be necessary to recruit and reexpand partially or completely collapsed alveoli. The major benefits of APRV are explained by the theory of airway pressure reduction.

At this writing the technique remains experimental. In the author's experience it appears to work best in cases of moderate lung disease. It seems an ideal treatment when the likelihood of barotrauma remains high.

C. *How to Use APRV*

As with other methods, the clinician must select appropriate end points for both oxygenation and carbon dioxide elimination. The F_IO_2 and the CPAP level are titrated until the desired improvement in gas exchange occurs. With this mode of ventilation the CPAP level also determines the amount of carbon dioxide removal. Airway pressure release ventilation usually entails starting at some arbitrary level of pressure, ordinarily 10 cm H_2O or higher. Pressure should then be increased in 3–5-cm H_2O increments. Oxygenation is not adequate. Carbon dioxide elimination results from both the frequency and degree of pressure reduction from a given CPAP level. In our own clinical practice we have found that pressure reduction frequencies of 6–10/min appear adequate for most situations. The loss of lung volume mimics the changes observed during active patient exhalation. The airway reduction can be to either ambient pressure or slightly above, such as 5 cm H_2O. Duration will vary between 1 and 3 seconds. Again these factors must be balanced, since they all contribute to a decrease in mean airway pressure and may ultimately affect oxygenation. Maintenance at the suitable end point should be conducted as described for other methods of ventilation.

D. *Weaning from APRV*

To date, minimal clinical experience exists with APRV. Therefore, well-defined criteria for weaning or elimination have not been developed. In general, one should reduce pressure support ultimately to approximately 10 cm H_2O or less. It appears that pressure reduction in 3–5-cm H_2O increments works well. As carbon dioxide elimination improves, the frequency of airway pressure reduction can be diminished.

E. *Complications*

A number of patients cannot be adequately oxygenated with pressure support ventilation. They either require exceedingly high levels or, alternatively, require high peak inflation pressures as developed with positive-pressure breaths from the mechanical ventilator. Patients who are already tachypneic may not reduce respiratory rate once changed gradually to APRV. They may require support with delivery of positive-pressure breaths.

IX. Minute Mandatory Ventilation (MMV)

A. *Description*

Mechanical ventilation using minute mandatory ventilation (MMV) aims to insure that the patient receives a minimum minute ventilation.[50] The minute ventilation includes both spontaneous and mechanical breaths. The minute ventilation may be composed of any combination of spontaneous rate and tidal volume and mechanical ventilator rate and tidal volume. With the use of microprocessors the machine monitors the patient's spontaneous efforts. Whenever the rate and tidal volume indicate a failure to meet the programmed minute ventilation, the ventilator begins to deliver the positive-pressure breaths. These breaths are delivered at a predetermined frequency and tidal volume until the minute ventilation demands are met.

B. *Indications*

For patients with a variable respiratory pattern or in whom apnea or hypoventilation is a risk, MMV insures maintenance of the total minute ventilation. This is unlike IMV, in which a decrease in the patient's spontaneous efforts results in an overall decrease in minute ventilation and potential development of hypercapnia.

C. *How to Use MMV*

The physician must first determine the minute ventilation necessary to result in a desired pH and P_aCO_2.

Next, the maximum mechanical ventilator rate required to deliver the minute ventilation must be determined. The ventilator will then monitor the patient's spontaneous efforts. Often the ventilator will not account for small volumes that only ventilate dead space. Therefore, the spontaneous efforts must be of sufficient volume to be sensed and counted by the machine. When spontaneous ventilation drops below the minimal level, the ventilator cycles and delivers positive-pressure breaths. With a preselected tidal volume, the number of positive-pressure breaths delivered will be based on both the discrepancy between the patient's own spontaneous efforts and the preselected desired minute volume.

D. *Weaning from MMV*

It appears easiest to wean patients from minute mandatory ventilation by decreasing the desired minute volume. This has the effect of insuring that more work will be continually performed by the patient with less reliance on the ventilator. One may also elect to incrementally decrease the number of positive-pressure breaths as the delivered minute volume requirements are decreased.

E. *Complications*

The variable number of positive-pressure breaths that may be delivered on a minute-to-minute basis may have an effect on blood return and cardiac output. Of course, hypovolemia accentuates the situation. If the ventilator fails to calculate minute ventilation accurately, this may result in an alteration of the ultimate minute volume received by the patient. Patients may actually hypoventilate if the ventilator counts small tidal volume breaths, which in effect only contribute to dead space ventilation and not necessarily carbon dioxide removal. The ventilator must have an accurate and reliable method of apnea detection.

X. REFERENCES

1. Teplitz C. The core pathobiology and integrated medical science of adult acute respiratory insufficiency. Surg Clin North Am 56:109–1133, 1976.
2. Layon AJ, Banner MJ, Jaeger MJ, et al. Continuous positive airway pressure and expiratory positive airway pressure increase functional residual capacity equivalently. Chest 89:517–521, 1986.
3. Dehaven CB, Hurst JM, Branson RD. Post extubation hypoxemia treated with continuous positive airway pressure by masks. Crit Care Med 13:46–48, 1985.
4. Smith RA, Kirby RR, Gooding JM. Continuous positive airway pressure (CPAP) by face mask. Crit Care Med 8:483–485, 1980.
5. Nelson LD, Civetta JM, Hudson-Civetta J. Titrating positive-end expiratory pressure therapy in patients with early moderate arterial hypoxemia. Crit Care Med 15:14–19, 1987.
6. Suter P, Fairly HB, Isenberg MD. Optimum end expiratory airway pressure in patients with acute pulmonary failure. N Engl J Med 292:284, 1975.
7. Gallagher TJ, Civetta JM, Kirby RR. Terminology update: Optimal PEEP. Crit Care Med 6:323–326, 1978.
8. Horovitz JA, Carrico CJ, Shires GT. Pulmonary response to major injury. Arch Surg 108:349, 1974.
9. Suter PM, Fairley HB, Schlobohn RM. Shunt, lung volume and perfusion during short periods of ventilation with oxygen. Anesthesiology 43:617–726, 1975.
10. Murray IP, Modell JH, Gallagher TJ, et al. Titration of PEEP by arterial minus end-tidal carbon dioxide gradient. Chest 85:100–104, 1984.
11. DeCampo T, Civetta JM. The effect of short term discontinuation of high level PEEP in patients with acute respiratory failure. Crit Care Med 7:47–49, 1979.
12. Dhainaut JF, Devaux JY, Monsallier JF, et al. Mechanisms of decreased left ventricular preload during continuous positive-pressure ventilation in ARDS. Chest 90:74–80, 1986.
13. Jardin F, Farcot JC, Boisant L, et al. Influence of positive end expiratory pressure on left ventricular performance. N Engl J Med 304:387–392, 1981.
14. Peterson GW, Baier H. Incidence of pulmonary barotrauma in a medical ICU. Crit Care Med 11:67–69, 1983.
15. Heenan TJ, Downs JB, Douglas ME. Intermittent mandatory ventilation: Is synchronization important? Chest 77:598, 1980.
16. Hasten RW, Downs JB, Heenan TJ. A comparison of synchronized and non-synchronized intermittent mandatory ventilation. Respir Care 25:554, 1980.
17. Primiano FP, Chatburn RL, Lough MD. Mean airway pressure. Crit Care Med 10:378–383, 1982.
18. Wolf G, Brunner J, Grandel E. Gas exchange during mechanical ventilation and spontaneous breathing: Intermittent mandatory ventilation after open heart surgery. Chest 90:11–17, 1986.
19. Downs JB, Douglas ME, Stanfelippo PM, et al. Ventilatory pattern, intrapleural pressure and cardiac output. Anesth Analg 56:88–96, 1975.
20. Froese AB, Bryan AC. Effects of anesthesia and paralysis on diaphragmatic mechanism in man. Anesthesiology 44:247–255, 1974.
21. Kacmarek RM, Venegas J. Mechanical ventilatory rates and tidal volumes. Respir Care 32:466–478, 1987.
22. Askanazi J. Rosenbaum SH, Hyman Al, et al. Respiratory changes induced by the large glucose loads of parenteral nutrition. JAMA 243:1444–1447, 1980.
23. Askanazi J, Nordenstrom J, Rosenbaum SH, et al. Nutrition for the patient with respiratory failure: Glucose vs fat. Anesthesiology 54:373–377, 1981.
24. Caldwell EJ, Powell RD Jr, Mullooly JP. Interstitial emphysema: A study of physiologic factors involved in experimental induction of the lesion. Am Rev Respir Dis 101:516–525, 1970.

25. Mathru M, Rao TLK, Venus B. Ventilator induced barotrauma in controlled mechanical ventilation versus intermittent mandatory ventilation. Crit Care Med 11:359–361, 1983.
26. Marini JJ, Capps JS, Culver BH. The inspiratory work of breathing during assisted mechanical ventilation. Chest 87:612–618, 1985.
27. Gallagher TJ. High frequency ventilation. Med Clin North Am 67:633–643, 1983.
28. McCulloch PR, Froese AB. High frequency ventilation. Anesth Clin North Am 5:873–891, 1987.
29. Klain M, Keszler H. High frequency jet ventilation. Surg Clin North Am 65:917–930, 1985.
30. Gallagher RC, Banner MJ, Modell JM. Comparison of delivery systems for high frequency jet ventilation. Crit Care Med 13:313, 1985.
31. Carlon G, Ray C, Klain M, et al. High frequency positive pressure ventilation in management of a patient with bronchopleural fistula. Anesthesiology 52:160–162, 1980.
32. Gallagher TJ, Banner MJ. High frequency positive pressure ventilation for oleic acid induced lung injury. Crit Care Med 8:232, 1980.
33. Banner MJ, Gallagher TJ, Caruthers-Banner T. Determining ideal frequency and inspiratory time for high frequency jet ventilation in dogs, abstracted. Anesth Analg 62:249, 1983.
34. MacIntyre N. Pressure support ventilation: Effects of ventilatory reflexes and ventilatory muscle workloads. Respir Care 32:447–457, 1987.
35. MacIntyre N. New modalities of ventilation: Pressure support ventilation. In Stoelting RK (ed). Advances in Anesthesia. Chicago, Year Book Medical Publishers, 1989, 6:219–230.
36. Roussos C, Macklem PT. The respiratory muscles. N Engl J Med 307:786–796, 1982.
37. Roussos C. Function and fatigue of respiratory muscles. Chest 88:1245–1325, 1985.
38. Mal H, Armengaud MH, Aubier M. Clinical importance of inspiratory muscle fatigue in acutely ill patients. J Crit Care 3:267–274, 1988,
39. Rochester DF, Arora NS. Respiratory Muscle Failure. Med Clin North Am 67:573–597, 1983.
40. Pace WL, East TD, Westenskow, et al. Differential lung ventilation after unilateral hydrochloric acid aspiration in the dog. Crit Care Med 11:17–20, 1983.
41. Carlon GC, Kahn R, Howland WS. Acute life threatening ventilation-perfusion inequity: An indication for independent lung ventilation. Crit Care Med 6:380–383, 1978.
42. Carlon GC, Ray C, Klein R, et al. Criteria for selective positive end-expiratory pressure and independent synchronized ventilation of each lung. Chest 74:501–507, 1978.
43. Benumof JL. Editorial: Improving the design and function of double lumen tubes. J Cardiothorac Anesth 2:729–733, 1988.
44. McKenna MJ, Wilson RS, Botelbo. Right upper lobe obstruction with right sided double lumen endotracheal tubes: A comparison of two tube types. J Cardiothorac Anesth 2:734–740, 1988.
45. Gallagher TJ, Banner MJ, Smith RA. A simplified method of independent lung ventilation. Crit Care Med 8:396–399, 1980.
46. Downs JB, Stock MC. Editorial: Airway pressure release ventilation: A new concept in ventilatory support. Crit Care Med 15–459, 1987.
47. Rasanen J, Downs JB. New techniques of positive pressure ventilation. Anesth Clin North Am 3:893–900, 1987.
48. Stock MC, Downs JB. Airway pressure release ventilation. A new approach to ventilatory support during acute lung injury. Respir Care 32:517, 1987.
49. Stock MC, Downs JB, Frolicher DA. Airway pressure release ventilation. Crit Care Med 15:462–478, 1987.
50. Havlett AM, Platt AS, Terry VG. Mandatory minute volume: A new concept in weaning from mechanical ventilation. Anesthesia 32:163–169, 1977.

Chapter 14

David V. Feliciano, MD

Thoracentesis

OUTLINE

I. Introduction and Indications

Thoracentesis, or the introduction of a needle into the pleural space, is a commonly performed clinical maneuver with numerous indications. Diagnostic indications include the removal of pleural fluid for analysis or use of the Cope needle to obtain a biopsy of the parietal pleura. Therapeutic indications include the aspiration of a pneumothorax or pleural fluid to allow for reexpansion of a collapsed lung.

A. *Diagnosis—Removal of Pleural Fluid*

Pleural fluid collections under 400–500 mL may not be evident on clinical examination or a chest radiograph because the fluid is distributed throughout the costophrenic sinuses when the patient is upright. Hence, pleural fluid collections that can be diagnosed are usually of substantial size and are amenable to thoracentesis.

When the removal of pleural fluid is the indication for thoracentesis, careful localization of the effusion is mandatory. Physical examination using percussion is the single most accurate maneuver for obtaining this information. Dullness at the upper edge of the fluid with the level curving higher in the axilla than medially (S curve of Ellis); flatness over the area of effusion, especially in the axilla; and loss of the normal change in the lower border of lung resonance with respiration (Litten's sign) have all proved to be useful in many patients. Radiographic examination by anteroposterior, lateral, and oblique views is also done and may be diagnostic in certain patients when physical examination is not; however, the level of the diaphragm on the affected side is obscured in many patients.

B. Diagnosis—Pleural Biopsy

Either primary (mesothelioma) or secondary (metastases most commonly from carcinoma of lung, breast, pancreas, or stomach) pleural tumors may be diagnosed by the use of a Cope needle. The technique is similar to that described later for thoracentesis, except that the Cope grooved needle is inserted through a hollow needle to allow for pleural biopsy prior to removal.

Table 14–1 • Equipment for Thoracentesis

Antiseptic solution and drapes
1% Xylocaine
25 gauge needle, 22 gauge needle, 10-mL syringe
18 gauge needle, 50-mL syringe, hemostat
Three-way stopcock, rubber tubing, sterile basin
Specimen collection tubes

Modified from Fisher JC. Clinical Procedures. Baltimore, Williams & Wilkins, 1970, 115.

C. Therapy—Aspiration of a Pneumothorax

Aspiration of a "small" (10% to 15%) pneumothorax is often advocated as an alternative to tube thoracostomy. Although this technique may be useful in some patients, it can lead to certain problems. First, the commonly diagnosed 10% to 15% pneumothorax on an anteroposterior chest radiograph is in reality a 36% decrease in lung volume based on the volume formula for a cylinder (pleural cavity or lung)—$\pi r^2 h$. In most centers, a 50% collapse of the lung, if known, would be primarily treated with a tube thoracostomy rather than thoracentesis. Second, a commonly recognized complication of thoracentesis is the creation of a pneumothorax, which might be more severe than the original noted in the patient. Should thoracentesis for evacuation of a pneumothorax be chosen, the removal of 1000 mL of air without resolution of the pneumothorax would usually indicate that a tube thoracostomy is still necessary.

D. Therapy—Aspiration of Pleural Fluid

Pleural effusions may be serous, hemorrhagic, purulent, or chylous. In the patient with compromised respiration and a moderate-sized (500–1000 mL) pleural effusion, thoracentesis will allow for reexpansion of the compressed lung and improvements in both ventilation and oxygenation. Should the pleural effusion be hemorrhagic secondary to recent thoracic trauma, thoracentesis with aspiration of the blood may preclude the need for a thoracostomy tube. Many authorities suggest, however, that the removal of 500–1000 mL of blood after trauma mandates the insertion of a thoracostomy tube to monitor the rate of further bleeding. Also, aspiration of more than 1500 mL of any of the other types of pleural effusions may result in well-recognized complications (to be discussed).

In patients with infectious pleural effusions, aspiration of purulent material has obvious diagnostic and therapeutic benefits. Thoracentesis may be the only therapy required in patients with exudative empyemas and thin pus with a pH of more than 7.2, glucose of more than 40 mg %, and an LDH of less than 1000 IU/L.[1]

II. PERFORMING THORACENTESIS

A. Equipment

The equipment for performing a thoracentesis is listed in Table 14–1.

B. Positioning and Anatomic Considerations

Once the equipment is available, the patient is positioned for either an anterior or posterior thoracentesis. An anterior thoracentesis is indicated for a pneumothorax, and the patient's upper trunk is maintained at 75 degrees to 90 degrees above the horizontal plane. Aspiration is performed in the middle of the second or third intercostal space in the midclavicular line of such a patient (Fig. 14–1). It is helpful to remember that the second interspace is at the same level as the sternal prominence or angle of Louis. The middle of the interspace is chosen, as there are two neurovascular bundles in each intercostal space anterior to the midaxillary line (Fig. 14–2).[2] A posterior thoracentesis is indicated for drainage of a pleural effusion, and the patient is asked to sit on the side of the bed with the feet resting on a stool. The patient then leans slightly forward while resting his arms on an elevated bedside table (Fig. 14–3). Percussion of the thorax along with a review of the chest radio-

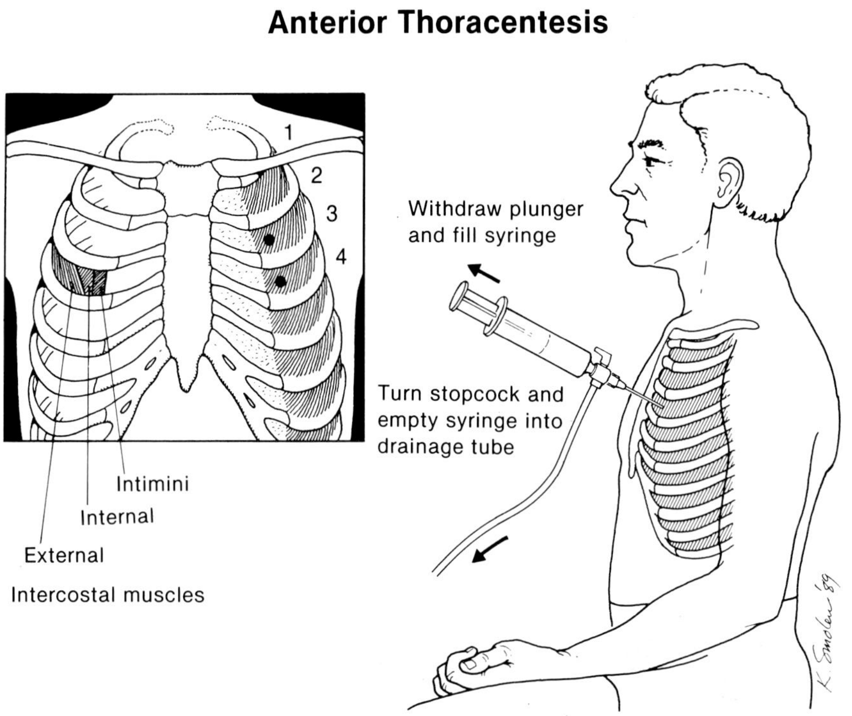

Figure 14–1 • Anterior thoracentesis to drain a pneumothorax is performed through the second or third intercostal space in the midclavicular line with the patient in the upright position.

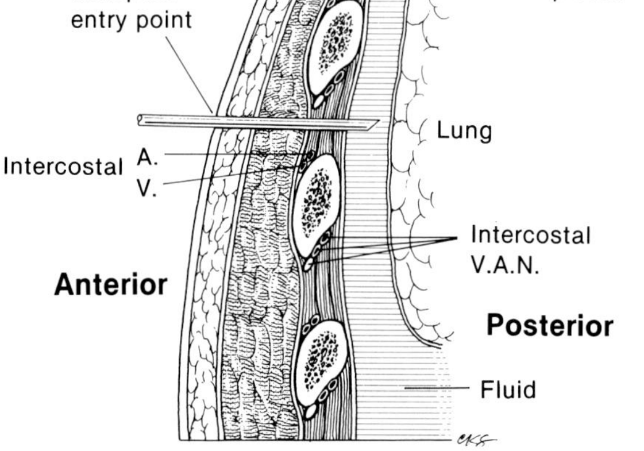

Figure 14–2 • Anterior thoracentesis is performed through the middle of the interspace as there are two neurovascular bundles in each intercostal space. One bundle lies posteriocaudad to the rib and one lies anteriocephalad to the rib.

graphs will determine which posterior or lateral interspace should be aspirated. A frequently used safety rule for thoracentesis at any site is that a needle should never be inserted below the fifth rib in the midclavicular line, the seventh rib in the midaxillary line, or the ninth rib in the scapular line.[2] At each of these sites the costophrenic angle lies three interspaces below and damage to the diaphragm or intraabdominal structures is minimized by following the rule. To aid in localizing the appropriate posterior interspace, it is also helpful to remember that the inferior tip of the scapula overlies the seventh rib or interspace. As there is only one neurovascular bundle at the inferior edge of each rib posterior to the midaxillary line, a posterolateral or posterior thoracentesis is performed at the inferior aspect of the *interspace* that is chosen (Fig. 14–4).

C. *Technique*

After preparation of the skin and draping with sterile towels, the skin at the site chosen for the thoracentesis is anesthetized with 1% Xylocaine injected with a 25

Posterior Thoracentesis

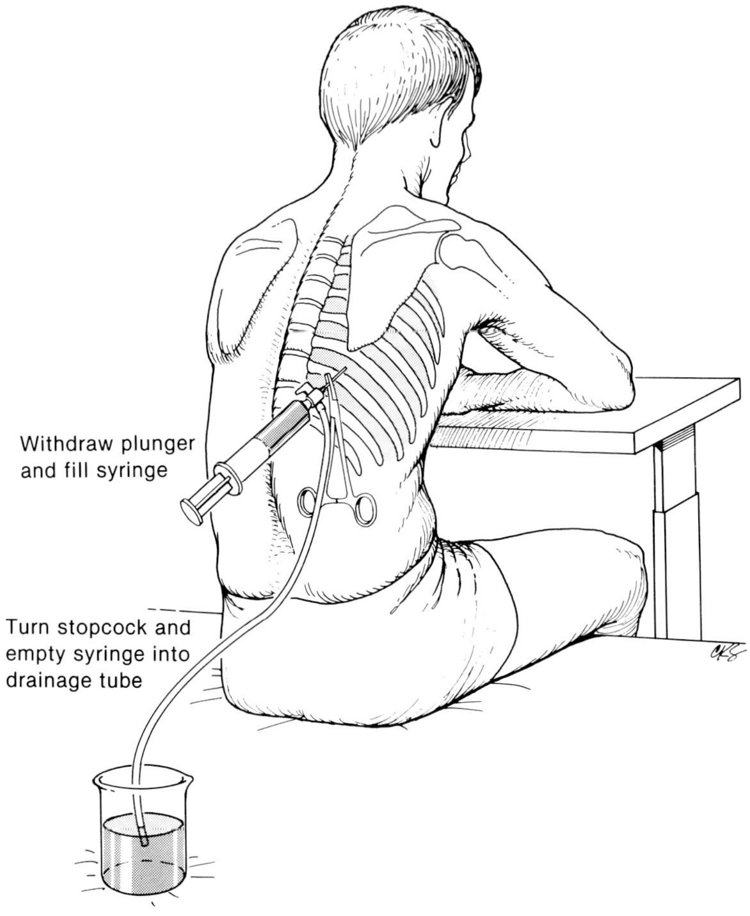

Figure 14–3 • Posterior thoracentesis to drain a pleural effusion is performed through an intercostal space above the ninth rib with the patient in the upright position.

Posterior Thoracentesis

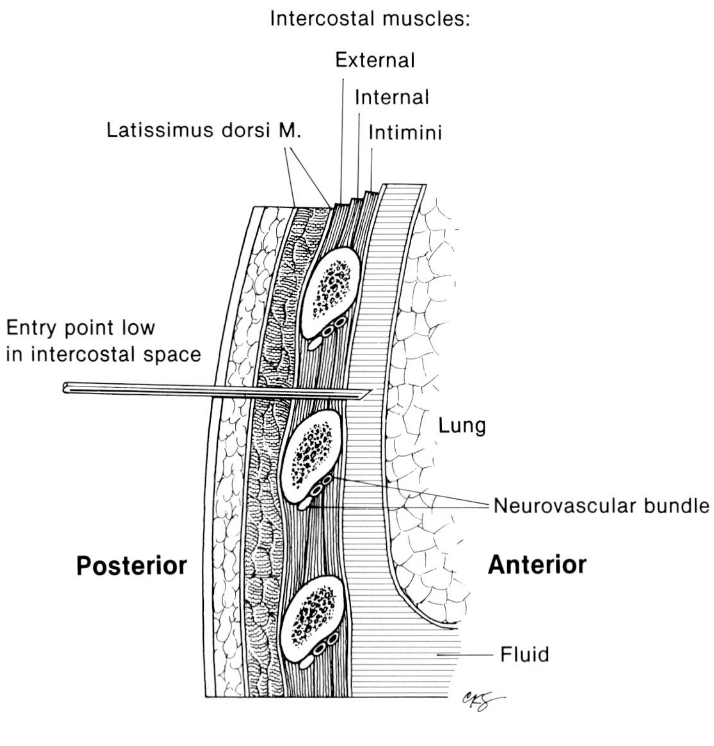

Figure 14–4 • Posterior thoracentesis is performed at the inferior aspect of the interspace as there is only one neurovascular bundle at the inferior edge of each rib.

gauge needle. A 22 gauge needle is then substituted, and 2–3 mL of the Xylocaine is injected into the subcutaneous tissue and intercostal muscles as the needle is slowly advanced to the pleural cavity. Entrance into the pleural cavity is usually distinct, and either air or fluid will be aspirated into the syringe by maintaining back pressure. To document the proper depth of insertion, a hemostat is placed on the 22 gauge needle at the level of the skin prior to removal. An 18 gauge needle is then applied to a 50-mL syringe with a three-way stopcock at its tip, and the needle is marked with a hemostat at the same level as was noted on the 22 gauge needle. The 18 gauge needle is advanced into the pleural cavity until the attached hemostat abuts the skin (Fig. 14–5). At this point, the rubber tubing is attached to the three-way stopcock and fluid (or air) is removed in 50-mL aliquots into a sterile basin (see Fig. 14–3). Classically, the aspirated fluid has been sent for a leukocyte count with differential, glucose, amylase, and pH measurements; cell block for tumor cytology; and cultures for aerobes, anaerobes, fungi, and acid-fast bacilli. As previously noted, suggested limits of aspiration (technique terminated or thoracostomy tube inserted) include 500–1000 mL of blood, 1000 mL of air, or 1500 mL of any other effusion.[3–5]

If the pleura is thickened and the 22 gauge needle does not penetrate the pleural cavity, it is acceptable to switch to the 18 gauge needle and 50-mL syringe for pleural penetration. A hemostat is once again applied to the 18 gauge needle at the level of the skin once the pleura is penetrated so as to prevent damage to the underlying lung.

A comprehensive analysis of effusions is beyond the scope of this chapter, but a brief overview may be worthwhile for the reader. It is generally accepted that transudates are clear yellow or blood-tinged, have a specific gravity of less than 1.016 and a protein content of less than 3 g %, and are due to systemic diseases such as congestive heart failure, renal failure, or cirrhosis. In contrast, exudates are clear yellow with increased cells, blood-tinged, chylous, or purulent; have a specific gravity of more than 1.016 and a protein content more than 3 g %; and are due to diseases in the pleural cavities.

As previously noted, multiple laboratory tests and cultures are routinely performed in patients with pleural effusions that may only be transudates rather than exudates. Light et al[6] have suggested and Peterman et al[7] have confirmed that a limited thoracentesis with preliminary analysis of the protein and lactate dehydrogenase (LDH) levels as compared to those in the patient's se-

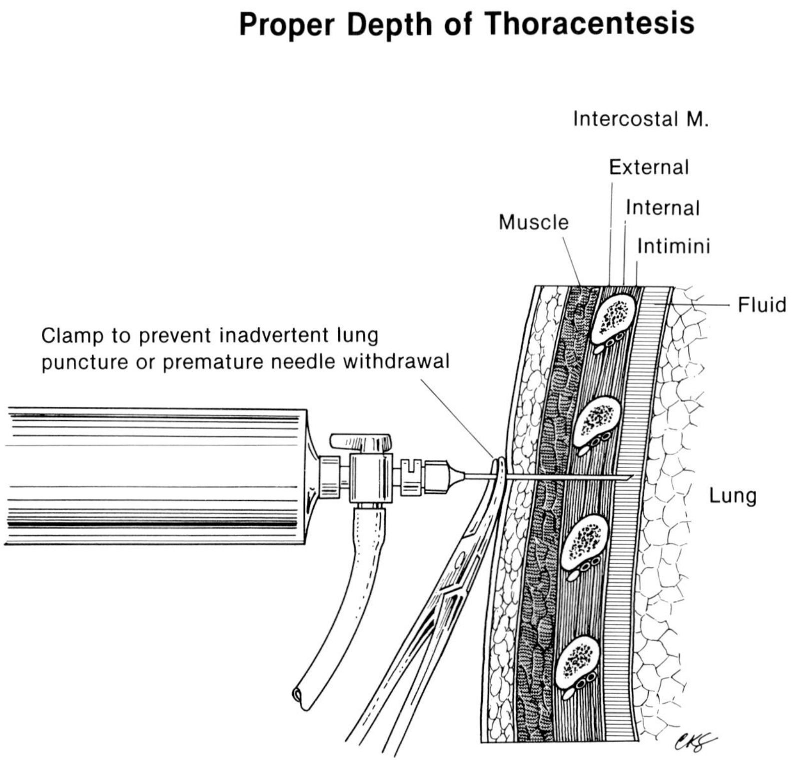

Figure 14–5 • Hemostat applied to thoracentesis needle prevents further penetration that might injure the lung. The proper length of needle tip to hemostat is determined first by inserting a 22 gauge identifying needle into the pleural space.

rum may eliminate the need for further tests in patients with transudates. The finding of a pleural fluid protein–serum protein ratio of more than 0.5, a pleural fluid LDH–serum ratio of more than 0.6, or a pleural fluid LDH level greater than two-thirds of the upper limit of normal for serum LDH was found only in patients with exudates with few exceptions in both studies.[6,7] Therefore, a patient with a transudate on preliminary analysis of the protein and LDH levels would not need all the tests routinely ordered.

III. COMPLICATIONS

A. *Pneumothorax*

Puncture of the lung during thoracentesis is the most likely cause of pneumothorax. Should the patient cough following puncture of the lung, more air will be forced into the pleural cavity. If a pneumothorax is suspected during the performance of the thoracentesis, aspiration of the air may be the only therapy that is required. A persistent pneumothorax or tension pneumothorax documented on a postthoracentesis physical examination or chest radiograph is treated with insertion of a thoracostomy tube.

B. *Hemorrhage*

Hemorrhage is usually due to injury to an intercostal vessel or the lung, although intraabdominal hemorrhage may occur if a paracentesis rather than a thoracentesis is performed. Once again, aspiration of the pleural blood can be performed during the thoracentesis if the complication is recognized. Continuing intrapleural hemorrhage documented on a postthoracentesis physical examination or chest radiograph is treated with insertion of a thoracostomy tube or, on rare occasions, an emergency thoracotomy.

C. *Pleural Shock*

Pleural shock refers to a sudden syncopal episode or cardiac arrest during the thoracentesis. It is thought to be secondary to an air embolism to the left side of the heart resulting from simultaneous penetration of a bronchus or alveolus and a pulmonary vein by the thoracentesis needle.[8] The treatment for syncope coupled with coughing is to turn the patient on his right side with his lower extremities elevated. This maneuver will trap the embolized air in the left ventricle and prevent it from entering the coronary or cerebral vessels. The treatment for a patient who suffers a cardiac arrest is the standard cardiopulmonary resuscitation with external cardiac compression.

D. *Unilateral Pulmonary Edema*

Unilateral pulmonary edema after aspiration of a large volume of pleural air or effusion that has been present for a prolonged period of time has been reported many times since the original description by Carlson et al in 1959.[9] The basic pathophysiology is thought to be loss of autoregulation of the pulmonary circulation in a collapsed lobe or entire lung secondary to anoxia. A sudden removal of all the offending air or fluid around the collapsed lobe or lung then leads to a rapid increase in pulmonary blood flow and resultant unilobar or unilateral pulmonary edema.[10] A deficiency of surfactant in a chronically collapsed lung may also be a factor as the higher negative pressures necessary to expand such a lung may cause transcapillary leakage of fluid.

To avoid this complication, thoracentesis with aspiration of pleural air or fluid around a chronically collapsed lobe or lung should be restricted to removal of 1000–1500 mL at one time.[10,11] Also, pleural drainage via a thoracostomy tube without suction may be indicated in high-risk patients.

Unilateral pulmonary edema is treated with respiratory support as indicated and usually resolves within hours to days. Deaths have been reported in patients who developed acute respiratory failure necessitating prolonged support on a ventilator.

E. *Empyema*

Empyema may result when a thoracentesis needle enters an infected lung and contamination of the pleural cavity itself occurs. Reexpansion of the injured lung may prevent this complication, but appropriate antibiotics based on a Gram stain and culture of the contaminated effusion should be started. Established empyema is treated with appropriate antibiotics and thoracentesis, tube thoracostomy, or surgical drainage, depending on the type.

IV. References

1. Takaro T, Scott SM. The pleura and empyema. In Sabiston DC Jr (ed). Textbook of Surgery. Philadelphia, WB Saunders, 1986, 2029.
2. Fisher JC. Thoracentesis. In Fisher JC (ed). Clinical Procedures. Baltimore, Williams & Wilkins, 1970, 115–116.
3. Takaro T, Scott SM. The pleura and empyema. In Sabiston DC Jr (ed). Textbook of Surgery. Philadelphia, WB Saunders, 1986, 2023.
4. Fisher JC. Thoracentesis. In Fisher JC (ed). Clinical Procedures. Baltimore, Williams & Wilkins, 1970, 119.
5. Rutherford RB, Campbell DN. Thoracic injuries. In Zuidema GD, Rutherford RB, Ballinger WF (eds). The Management of Trauma. Philadelphia, WB Saunders, 1985, 419.
6. Light RW, MacGregor MI, Luchsinger PC, et al. Pleural effusions: The diagnostic separation of transudates and exudates. Ann Int Med 77:507–513, 1972.
7. Peterman TA, Speicher CE. Evaluating pleural effusions: A two-stage laboratory approach. JAMA 252:1051–1053, 1984.
8. Webb WR. Postoperative pulmonary complications. Including complications of bronchoscopy. In Artz CP, Hardy, JD (eds). Management of Surgical Complications. Philadelphia, WB Saunders, 1975, 105.
9. Carlson RI, Classen KL, Gollan F, et al. Pulmonary edema following the rapid reexpansion of a totally collapsed lung due to a pneumothorax: A clinical and experimental study. Surg Forum 9:367–371, 1959.
10. Murphy K, Tomlanovich MC. Unilateral pulmonary edema after drainage of a spontaneous pneumothorax: Case report and review of the world literature. J Emer Med 1:29–36, 1983.
11. Trapnell DH, Thurston JGB. Unilateral pulmonary oedema after pleural aspiration. Lancet 1:1367–1369, 1970.

Chapter 15

David V. Feliciano, MD

Tube Thoracostomy

OUTLINE

I. INTRODUCTION AND INDICATIONS

Tube thoracostomy refers to the insertion of a large-bore plastic drainage tube into the pleural cavity. First performed in 1875 for patients with empyema, tube thoracostomy is now routinely used in the therapy of patients with a variety of acute or chronic intrapleural problems. Suggested indications include the drainage of a closed, open, or tension pneumothorax *or* of a pleural effusion from any cause to allow for reexpansion of a collapsed lung.

A. *Drainage of a Pneumothorax*

A patient who has suffered either compressive trauma or direct puncture of a lung by a fractured rib in a motor vehicle accident may develop a closed pneumothorax. As previously noted, the "10% to 15% pneumothorax" diagnosed on routine anteroposterior chest radiographs after trauma reflects a 36% collapse of the ipsilateral lung. Also, although such a pneumothorax may remain stable if the pulmonary rupture is small, the leak can persist and eventually create a tension pneumothorax on the affected side. For these reasons, tube thoracostomy remains the safest and quickest way to drain a closed pneumothorax.

An open pneumothorax refers to a defect in the thoracic wall that allows air to move in and out of the pleural cavity rather than through the tracheobronchial tree. On rare occasions, the chest wall defect will act as a one-way valve and a tension pneumothorax will result. Once the defect in the thoracic wall has been temporarily sealed in the field or emergency room, the most expedient way to drain the large pneumothorax that is present is by inserting a thoracostomy tube.

A tension pneumothorax is one in which there is rapid progression with complete collapse of the ipsilateral lung, deviation of the mediastinum with secondary compromise of venous return through the vena cavae, and, finally, compression of the contralateral pleural cavity and lung. This entity is rarely seen in the emergency department because most victims will succumb at the scene of injury or during transit. It occurs most commonly in patients with acute respiratory failure aggravated by hospital-acquired pneumonia during prolonged periods of ventilatory support. The onset is acute and is characterized by an agitated patient with sudden hypotension and, often, cyanosis. A rapid examination of the chest should document the absence of breath sounds on the affected side. Deviation of the trachea away from the affected side is uncommon. An emergency chest radiograph is indicated in such a patient but is almost never available quickly enough to be reviewed before therapy is instituted. Hence, the diagnosis in the traumatized patient in the emergency department or ventilated patient in the intensive care unit is made on clinical grounds in most instances. Should the patient be on the verge of a cardiopulmonary arrest, an emergency thoracentesis is performed in any convenient location on the affected side using an 18 gauge needle and a glass barrel syringe. Rapid resolution of the patient's symptoms following the release of air via the thoracentesis confirms the diagnosis, and a thoracostomy tube can then be inserted in a more controlled fashion for definitive treatment.

Table 15-1 • Equipment for Tube Thoracostomy

Antiseptic solution and drapes
1% Xylocaine
25 gauge needle, 22 gauge needle, 10 mL syringe
#10 scalpel blade, Kelly clamp, #32-#36 thoracostomy tube
Collection bottle, underwater seal bottle, suction control bottle, or commercial unit including all three
Plastic connectors, plastic tubing
Gauze pads, adhesive tape

Modified from Fisher JC. Clinical Procedures. Baltimore, Williams & Wilkins 1970, 126.

B. *Removal of Pleural Fluid*

Pleural fluid collections that cannot be satisfactorily evacuated by repeated thoracenteses are best treated by insertion of a thoracostomy tube. Also, massive pleural fluid collections (more than 2000 mL) suggested by physical examination and chest radiographs should be treated in a similar fashion without a preliminary thoracentesis. This is especially true when the effusion is actually a hemothorax secondary to acute thoracic trauma, a loculated empyema that is creating a septic state, or a recurrent malignant effusion secondary to pleural metastases.

II. Performing Tube Thoracostomy

A. *Equipment*

The equipment to perform a tube thoracostomy is listed in Table 15-1.

B. *Positioning and Anatomic Considerations*

Once the equipment is available, the patient is positioned for either an anterior or posterior tube thoracostomy. An anterior tube thoracostomy is favored in some centers as the site for insertion in a patient with a pneumothorax. As with thoracentesis (see Chapter 14), the patient is maintained in an upright position as the tube is inserted in the second intercostal space in the midclavicular line. There are several problems with this location for tube thoracostomy. The first is that the large bulk of the pectoralis major muscle through which the tube must be inserted makes the procedure a difficult one for the patient and a short-fingered physician. The second is that the fixed nature of the anterior costochondral junctions and ribs does not allow for the insertion of any tube of significant size through the second intercostal space. Finally, an anterior thoracostomy tube is painful for the patient after insertion and restricts coughing and ambulation.

For the reasons listed earlier and to promote continuity of in-hospital therapeutic services, tube thoracostomy for pneumothoraces, hemothoraces, and nonloculated effusions is most commonly performed at the same location in all patients—that is, the fourth or fifth intercostal space anterior to or at the midaxillary line. This location is readily accessible in a patient in either an upright or a supine position. Also, as the site of insertion is posterior to the lateral border of the pectoralis major muscle, there is less need for blunt dissection through soft tissues before the pleural cavity is entered. Finally, this site is lateral to the nipple, a helpful anatomic landmark for young house officers.

The ideal position for the patient about to undergo a tube thoracostomy in the recommended location is a sitting one with the patient's upper trunk maintained at 75° to 90° above the horizontal plane. In truth, the vast majority of patients who undergo the procedure, particularly in the emergency department, are in the supine position. This is done because of comfort, unavailability of flexible resuscitation room tables, and hemodynamic instability. The major problem created by this position is that the diaphragm may actually reach the third intercostal space in the traumatized patient with a massive hemoperitoneum. Therefore, the physician must assess each patient individually and use a higher location for a lateral thoracostomy site when the condition and position of the patient warrant it.

As with a thoracentesis, the entrance into the pleural cavity should be just above the fifth or sixth rib when the thoracostomy tube is inserted at the midaxillary line. This will avoid the intercostal neurovascular bundle at the lower border of the upper rib.

One consideration in picking a site for a thoracostomy tube is to avoid a previous site or old thoracostomy scar. Adhesions between the underlying lung and the parietal pleura should be expected at such a site and avoided to avert damage to the lung during insertion.

C. *Size of Thoracostomy Tube*

The proper size of a thoracostomy tube depends on the condition for which the tube is to be inserted, the severity of the condition, and the patient's size. Pneumothoraces are readily drained with 24–32 French thoracostomy tubes in adults. Sizes below 24 French have a tendency to occlude or kink, particularly if inserted in the anterior second interspace, and are best avoided in adults.

Hemothoraces or thick empyemas are best drained with 36 French thoracostomy tubes in adults. Despite the greater difficulty in insertion, a more rapid evacuation of the effusion and less of a tendency to occlude make these large tubes the best choice. In the small adult patient with an effusion, a 32 French thoracostomy tube is an alternative.

D. *Technique of Insertion*

After preparation of the skin and draping with sterile towels, the interspace chosen for the insertion site of the thoracostomy tube is marked with an impression from the blunt end of the knife handle. The actual skin incision is made approximately 1 inch inferior to this, so that the thoracostomy tube will have an oblique tract as it passes through the thoracic wall. This, of course, decreases the risk of transmission of infection from the skin incision into the pleural cavity. Also, it diminishes the chance of creating a pneumothorax on removal of the tube, as the oblique tract will collapse rapidly.

The skin at the site chosen for the insertion is anesthetized with 1% Xylocaine injected with a 25 gauge needle over a 2–3-cm transverse line. A 22 gauge needle is then substituted, and 3–5 mL of 1% Xylocaine is injected along the oblique tract and into the area of periosteum of the rib that the tube will pass over (Fig. 15–1).

A transverse skin incision is made with the scalpel at the area previously anesthetized. When the subcutaneous tissue is visible, the operator uses a Kelly clamp to gently spread these soft tissues until the upper border of the chosen rib is reached. Excessive spreading beyond the diameter of the thoracostomy tube to be inserted will lead to the complication of subcutaneous emphysema after insertion. Further spreading is performed in a medial direction through the intercostal muscles (Fig. 15–2). Finally, the tip of the clamp is closed and the parietal pleura is penetrated by directing the clamp in a posterosuperior direction away from the mediastinum. A sudden rush of air, blood, or pleural fluid documents that the pleural cavity has been entered. The clamp is quickly removed, and the operator's index finger is inserted through the oblique tract into the pleural cavity. A "finger thoracotomy" is performed in all directions as far as the index finger can reach (Fig. 15–3). Although this is a painful maneuver for the patient, much valuable information may result. The presence of pleural adhesions that cannot be separated by the operator's finger means that only a short thoracostomy tube can be inserted or that another site for insertion should be chosen. If the operator cannot palpate the lung, heart, or

Tube Thoracostomy

Local anesthetic infiltration

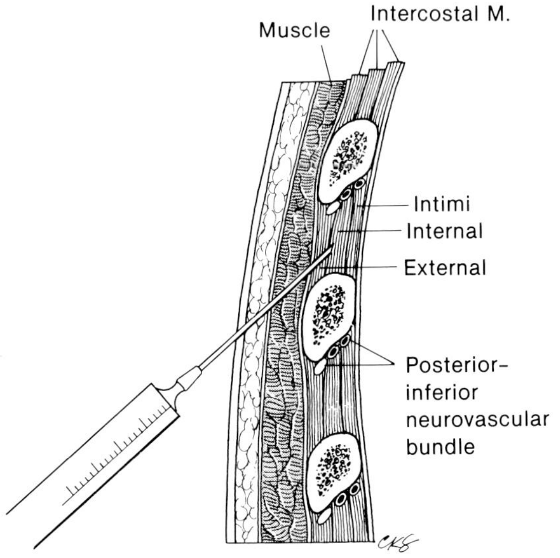

Figure 15–1 • Local anesthetic is applied to oblique tract and periosteum of lower rib before insertion of a thoracostomy tube. The transverse skin incision and point of entry are below the interspace in question.

Tube Thoracostomy

Blunt dissection

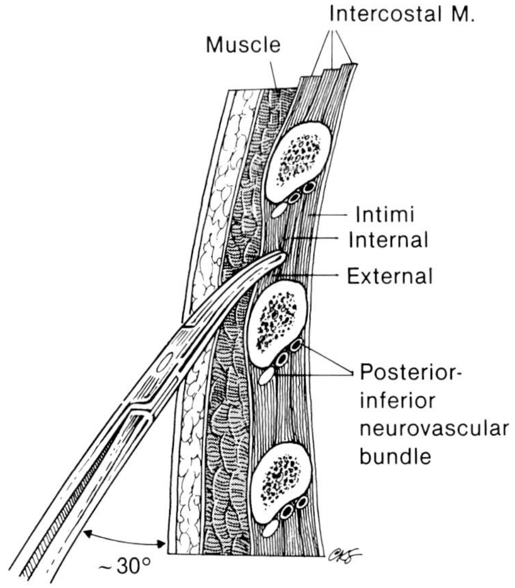

Figure 15–2 • Blunt dissection through the subcutaneous tissues and intercostal muscles is performed with a Kelly clamp.

Finger Thoracotomy

Temporary insertion of finger

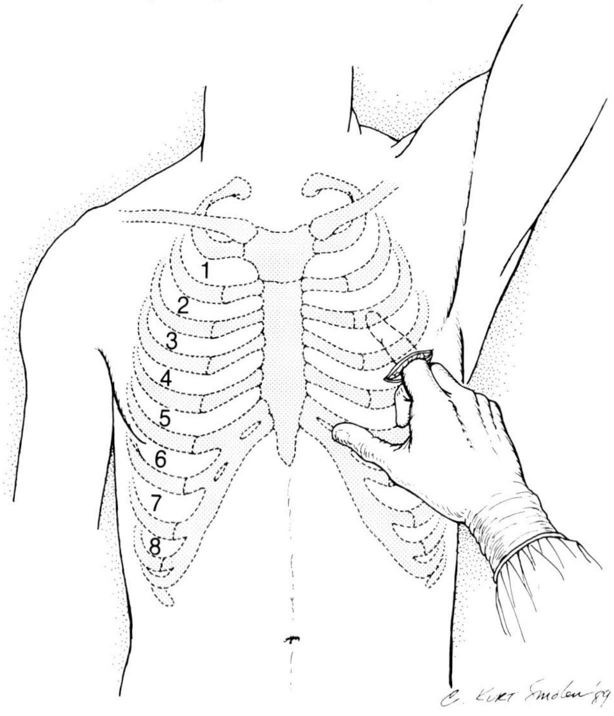

Figure 15–3 • Finger thoracotomy is performed prior to insertion of the thoracostomy tube.

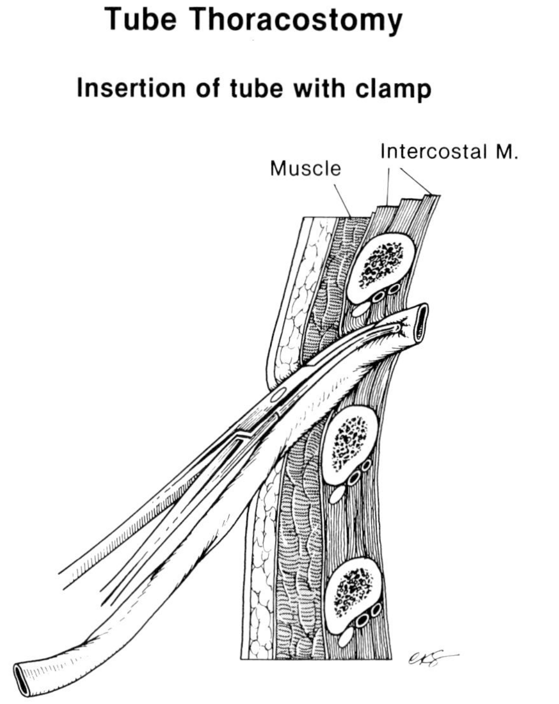

Figure 15–4 • The thoracostomy tube is carried into the pleural cavity in the jaws of a Kelly clamp.

diaphragm, the tract may still be only in the subcutaneous tissue rather than in the pleural cavity. If the spleen or liver is palpable inferiorly, the operator has entered the peritoneal cavity rather than the pleural cavity. Finally, a palpable defect in the diaphragm inferiorly or the mediastinum medially after a penetrating thoracic wound would mandate emergent laparotomy or thoracotomy, respectively, in many trauma centers.[1]

After the operator's finger is removed, the tip of the thoracostomy tube that is clamped at its connecting end is grasped with a Kelly clamp. Both are bluntly advanced through the previously created oblique tract (Fig. 15–4). An intrapleural position is documented by "fogging" of the tube as the patient breathes. In patients with hemothoraces or mobile effusions, the tube should be directed posteriorly to allow for rapid evacuation of the fluid while the patient is supine (Fig. 15–5). The tube is advanced until it meets resistance from the apex of the pleural cavity or mediastinum or until the last hole of the tube is clearly within the pleural cavity.

The alternative technique of insertion using a trochar or stylet will not be discussed. Numerous reports of injuries to the lung, heart, liver, and spleen strongly suggest that this is not a safe approach.

Fixation of the tube is most secure when a purse-string suture is placed around the skin entrance site, pulled up snugly, wrapped around the tube in opposite directions, and finally tied with a surgeon's knot and bow (Fig. 15–6A–C). This will allow for simple loosening of the knot on the tube at the time chosen for removal and for use of the purse-string suture to seal the skin site after removal. The major objection to this approach is that necrosis of the skin at the entrance site frequently results after the purse-string suture is tightened. This may lead to an infection at the site, as well as being painful for the patient. An alternative approach is to place one suture through one side (or two sutures

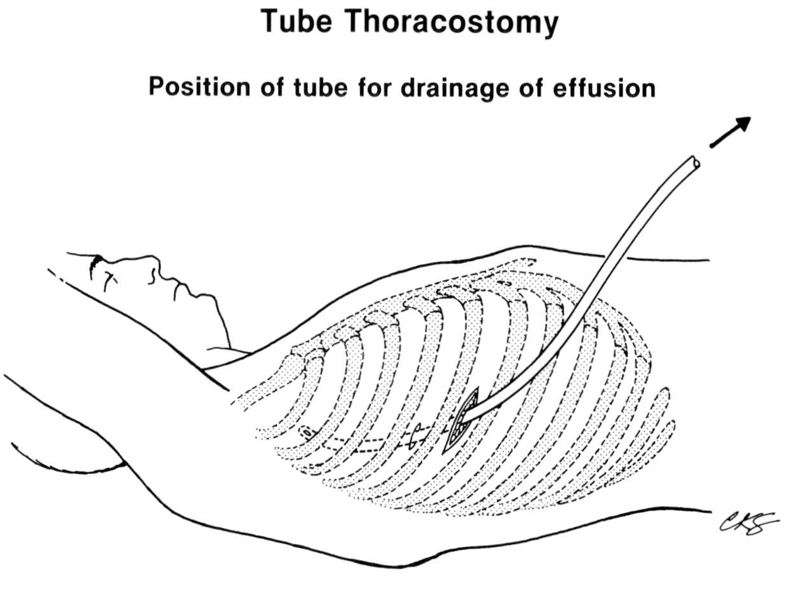

Figure 15–5 • The thoracostomy tube is directed posteriorly and superiorly in patients with pleural effusions including hemothoraces.

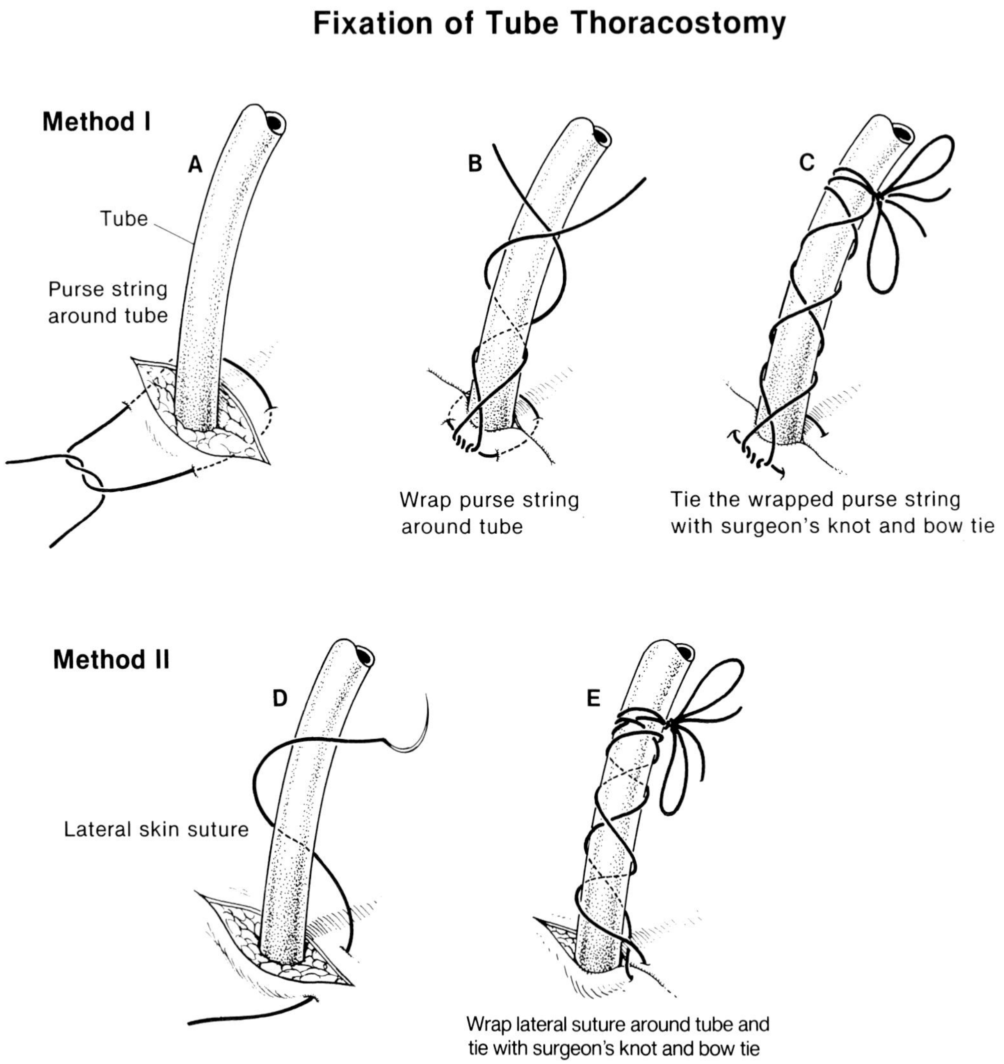

Figure 15–6 • Two separate techniques (method I [*A–C*] and method II [*D–E*]) for fixing a thoracostomy tube to the skin. (See text for full explanation.)

through both sides) of the skin incision lateral to the thoracostomy tube. Either this loop is snugged up modestly or one knot throw is placed before looping the tube and tying with a surgeon's knot and bow as described earlier (Fig. 15–6D–E).

Finally, a chest radiograph is performed to document an appropriate position for the tube.

E. Drainage and Collecting Systems

Most hospitals now use a commercial variant of the standard three-bottle system (Fig. 15–7). The first bottle closest to the patient is a *collection* or *trap bottle* for evacuated blood or other pleural effusions. In the commercial systems it is metered so that the volume and rate of efflux can be measured. This bottle is airtight, and air from a pneumothorax is simply sucked into a second bottle, where it bubbles out of a tube with a tip placed 2–3 cm under a water level—hence, the name *underwater seal.* Underwater seal is the fundamental principle that must be understood by the physician performing a tube thoracostomy. Basically, the presence of one tube in the system with its tip under water means that the patient can never suck air from the room back into the pleural cavity, no matter how vigorous his or her inspiratory

Three-Bottle Drainage and Collection System

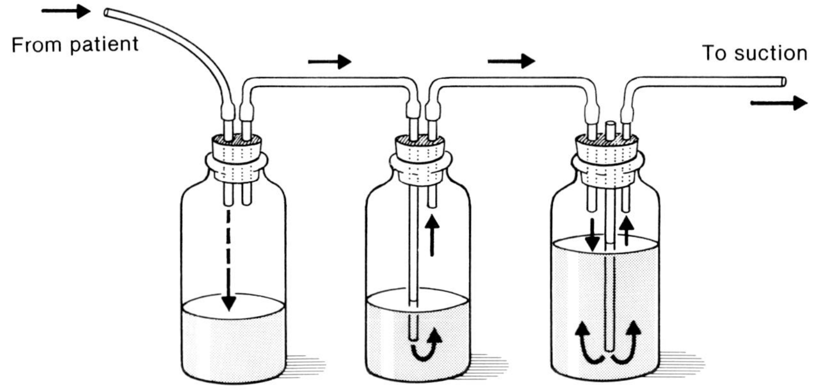

Figure 15–7 • Standard three-bottle drainage and collection system. (See text for full explanation of the function of each bottle.)

efforts are. The third bottle in the system is known as the *suction control.* This bottle has airtight connections to the underwater seal and the suction machine; however, it also includes a hollow central column open to the air with its opposite tip placed 10–20 cm under the water level in the bottle. As soon as the suction pressure in the system is numerically greater than the number of centimeters that the open column is under the level of water, air is sucked into the system from the room no matter what negative pressure is exerted by the suction machine. Therefore, the system is maintained at a safety level or suction control whenever there is continuous bubbling of air in the water level of the third bottle. Finally, a suction machine is usually attached to the system to hasten the removal of the air or pleural fluid that is present and to allow for rapid reexpansion of the collapsed lung.

F. *Role of Antibiotic Prophylaxis*

Antibiotic prophylaxis for the presence of a thoracostomy tube remains controversial. Grover et al[2] found a lower incidence of radiographic pneumonia, fevers, and positive pleural and wound cultures when antibiotic prophylaxis with clindamycin phosphate was used. Similar findings were subsequently documented by Stone et al[3] using cefamandole and LoCurto et al[4] using cefoxitin. In contrast, Mandal et al,[5] using doxycycline, and LeBlanc et al,[6] using cephapirin, noted no differences in infection between treated and untreated groups.

Although the data are unclear, primarily based on the modest size of the series mentioned, most trauma centers and thoracic and cardiovascular surgeons use a combination of intravenous and oral antibiotics until all thoracostomy tubes are removed.

G. *Technique for Removal of a Thoracostomy Tube*

As a general rule, a thoracostomy tube inserted to drain a pneumothorax is removed when the pneumothorax has cleared. Also, there should be no detectable air leak bubbling into the underwater seal bottle off suction when the patient coughs or performs a Valsalva maneuver. In many centers, a fully expanded lung on a chest radiograph and the absence of an air leak while on suction will prompt the removal of suction from the drainage system. If the lung remains expanded on a chest radiograph after 24 hours off suction and there is still no air leak as the patient coughs or strains, the tube can be safely removed in almost all patients. As a further precaution against premature removal of the tube, some centers will clamp the thoracostomy tube next to the patient for 24 more hours before the tube is removed. This is similar to removal but allows for reopening the system with ease should the need arise.

A thoracostomy tube inserted to drain a pleural effusion is removed when the effusion is completely evacuated, when the tube is occluded, or when total drainage is less than 50 mL/day for consecutive days.

Should both an anterior tube for a pneumothorax and a posterior tube for a hemothorax be present and neither be necessary, only one is removed on a given day. Some surgeons choose to first pull the tube that was less indicated at the time of insertion.

Because of the smaller number of medical, nursing, and radiograph personnel in the hospital after 3 P.M., thoracostomy tubes should be removed only during morning hours. Vaseline gauge and 8-inch-long strips of 1- or 2-inch-wide adhesive tape, along with a suture removal set, should be available at the patient's bedside when the thoracostomy tube is to be removed. The dressing is removed, the suture with a bow is untied and unwound off the tube, and the two ends are pulled up tight with the left hand, which is resting on the tract of the tube under the skin. The patient is instructed to inspire slowly and deeply and then to expire slowly and deeply ("deep breath in, deep breath out"). As the end of expiration approaches, the operator twists the tube with the right hand to dislodge the adherent lung. He or she then rapidly removes the tube with the right hand while compressing the oblique tract *and* holding the skin suture with the left hand. The suture is pulled very tight and a knot is completed, followed by the application of Vaseline gauze and the adhesive tape. Should there be no suture present or should it break during loosening or tying, the operator's left hand maintains pressure on the tract as the right hand applies the Vaseline gauze and adhesive tape to the skin site.

The alternative approach for removal is to complete it while the patient performs a Valsalva maneuver. In the author's experience, the pain of removal often prompts a quick inspiration in the midst of this maneuver. This increases the negative intrapleural pressure (makes it more negative) and may create a recurrent pneumothorax.

III. COMPLICATIONS

A. *Hemorrhage*

As with a thoracentesis, injury to an intercostal vessel or the lung may occur with an improper technique of insertion. The rate of bleeding should be monitored, with emergency thoracotomy reserved for patients with continuous arterial hemorrhage (more than 100–200 mL blood/hour for approximately 4 hours) after the original pneumothorax or hemothorax is cleared.

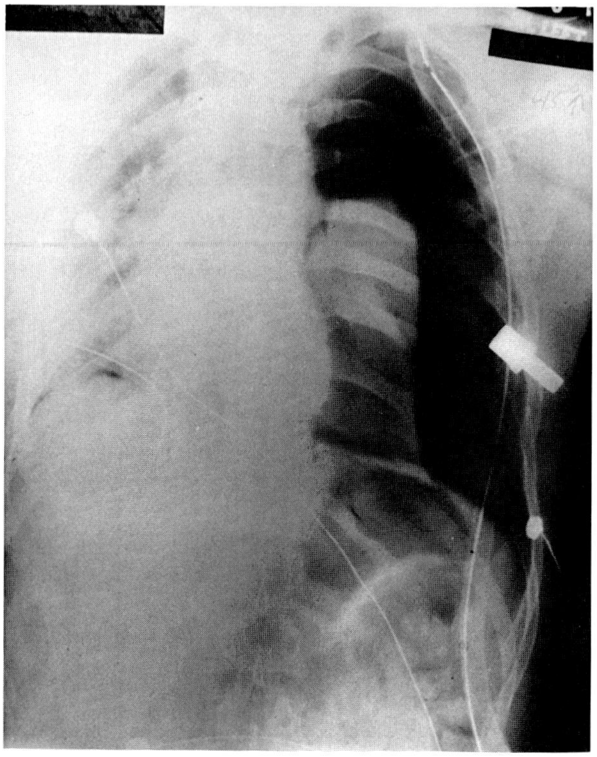

Figure 15-8 • Extrapleural placement of a left thoracostomy tube in a patient with a tension pneumothorax.

B. *Injury to the Lung and Other Intrathoracic Structures*

Failure to free pleural adhesions to the lung may lead to intraparenchymal placement of a thoracostomy tube. As previously noted, this can be prevented by avoiding old thoracostomy and thoracotomy sites and by using finger thoracotomy to free adhesions before inserting the tube.

Erosion of the tip of a thoracostomy tube into structures such as the mediastinum or extrapleural subclavian vessels has been reported but is extraordinarily rare.

C. *Extrapleural Position of the Tube*

An intrapleural position of the tube is confirmed by the evacuation of air, blood, or effusion as the pleura is penetrated, by palpation of the lung during finger thoracotomy, by "fogging" of the tube after insertion before suction is attached, and by the postinsertion chest radiograph. Failure to follow these guidelines may lead to extrapleural (Fig. 15-8) or intraabdominal (Fig. 15-9)

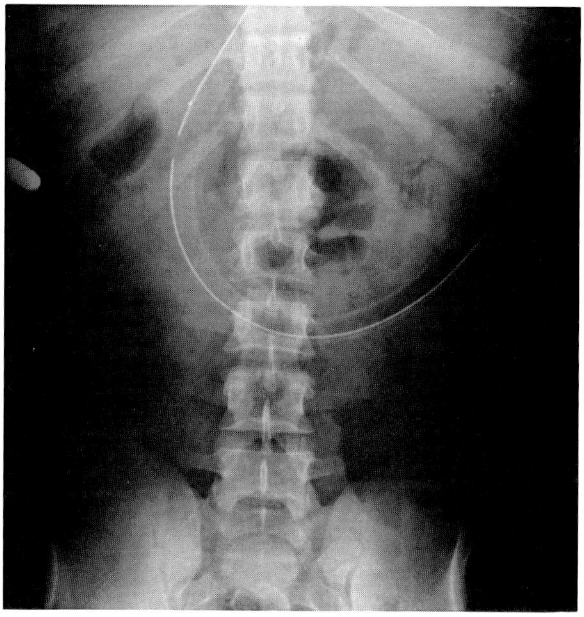

Figure 15-9 • Intraabdominal placement of an intended left thoracostomy tube caused rupture of the spleen.

placement, which may be lethal. Extrapleural or intraabdominal placement has occurred in 1% to 1.8% of patients in major trauma centers in recent years.[7,8]

D. *Subcutaneous Emphysema*

Subcutaneous emphysema results when the tract created is much larger than the diameter of the tube that is inserted, when the last hole of the tube is outside the pleural cavity, or when a large air leak from a bronchus or pulmonary rupture is present. The first two of these are readily preventable; the third is not.

This complication is painful for the patient and distressing to medical personnel and the patient's family. But it is self-limited and does not threaten the patient's life. Maneuvers such as aspiration of the ''inflated'' scrotum are unrewarding and meddlesome.

E. *Failure to Drain a Pneumothorax*

Failure to drain a pneumothorax is due to a large air leak from a bronchus or pulmonary rupture or to a mucus plug in the chest tube. Large air leaks are best treated with the insertion of extra thoracostomy tubes *after* bronchoscopy has ruled out the presence of a ruptured bronchus.

F. *Persistent Air Leak*

The most common causes of a persistent air leak are the presence of the last hole of the thoracostomy tube outside the pleural cavity and a loose connection in the drainage system outside the chest. If neither is present and the lung is expanded while on suction, one option is to decrease the suction pressure applied to the system to allow for healing of the pulmonary rupture.

G. *Pneumothorax After Removal of the Tube*

The problem of recurrent pneumothorax should occur infrequently if all the preceding precautions are followed. When this complication does occur, it is usually a reflection of physician impatience, careless technique, or poor lung compliance from the original injury.[9] In one recent study, recurrent pneumothoraces occurred after removal of the thoracostomy tube in 24% of patients with blunt trauma and in 23% of patients with penetrating trauma![10]

H. *Infection*

The incidence of empyema after insertion of a thoracostomy tube is approximately 2% to 4%, with a higher incidence always reported in patients after blunt as compared to penetrating trauma.[2,10] A higher incidence than this reflects prolonged delays between injury and insertion of a thoracostomy tube, unsterile technique of insertion, various nosocomial factors in the intensive care unit, and possible failure to use prophylactic antibiotics.

IV. REFERENCES

1. Feliciano DV, Cruse PA, Mattox KH, et al. Delayed diagnosis of injuries to the diaphragm after penetrating wounds. J Trauma 28:1135–1144, 1988.
2. Grover El, Richardson JD, Fewel JG, et al. Prophylactic antibiotics in the treatment of penetrating chest wounds. A prospective double-blind study. J Thorac Cardiovasc Surg 74:528–536, 1977.

3. Stone HH, Symbas PN, Hooper CA. Cefamandole for prophylaxis against infection in closed tube thoracostomy. J Trauma 21:975–977, 1981.
4. LoCurto JL Jr, Tischler CD, Swan KG, et al. Tube thoracostomy and trauma—antibiotics or not. J Trauma 26:1067–1072, 1986.
5. Mandal AK, Montano J, Thadepalli H. Prophylactic antibiotics and no antibiotics compared in penetrating chest trauma. J Trauma 25:639–643, 1985.
6. LeBlanc KA, Tucker WY. Prophylactic antibiotics and closed tube thoracostomy. Surg Gynecol Obstet 160:259–263, 1985.
7. Millikan JS, Moore EE, Steiner E, et al. Complications of tube thoracostomy for acute trauma. Am J Surg 140:738–741, 1980.
8. Daly RC, Mucha P, Pairolero PC, et al. The risk of percutaneous chest tube thoracostomy for blunt thoracic trauma. Ann Emer Med 14:865–870, 1985.
9. Levitsky S, Annable CA, Thomas PA. The management of empyema after thoracic wounding: Observation on 25 Vietnam casualties. J Thorac Cardiovasc Surg 59:630–634, 1970.
10. Helling TS, Gyles NR III, Eisenstein CL, et al. Complications following blunt and penetrating injuries in 216 victims of chest trauma requiring tube thoracostomy. J Trauma 29:1367–1370, 1989.

Section III

Cardiovascular Procedures

Chapter 16

C. F. Ward, MD

Peripheral Intravenous Access

OUTLINE

I. INTRODUCTION

A. *History*

Teflon™ intravenous catheters and intravenous fluids are so ubiquitous in hospitals now that it is difficult to recall that they did not appear along with the plans to build the hospital. Attempting to reconstruct the why and how of intravenous therapy from a 1990 vantage started off to be a substantial task until I discovered a delightful presentation of the entire business by M. T. Jenkins.[1] The following background information is based in large measure on Jenkins's work.

The year 1628, the date of Harvey's publication concerning blood and circulation, marks the starting point for a rational approach to injecting anything into the vascular compartment. However, the first recorded transfusion occurred in 1492 (a year generally remembered in the United States for other reasons), when Pope

Innocent VIII received a blood transfusion from three boys. All four participants eventually expired, which cooled interest in the subject substantially. It was not mentioned again until 1628, interestingly not by Harvey but by De Colle of Padua. In 1656, Christopher Wren injected opium into dogs using a quill attached to a small bladder. One year later, he tried the technique on a man. In 1667, Elsholtz proposed that the injecting of substances into veins be called ''The New Clyster,'' or the art of the enema applied to veins by injecting through a syringe and needle. Strangely, following this whirl of activity, things fell silent until 1831, when O'Shaughnessy suggested the injection of ''highly-oxygenized salts'' into the jugular vein via a tube of gold or ivory, ''free of air.'' Lewins and then Latta, in separate letters the same year, reported on fluid resuscitation of cholera patients with substantial amounts (eg, 23 lb) of salt solution over 7 hours or so. These lessons were forgotten, and two decades later, when the next cholera epidemic occurred, intravenous hydration was ignored. In fact, this concept was not resurrected until 1874, when Fagge employed fluid therapy for diabetic coma. About this time, the syringe was introduced into practice, although it is not clear today just how this came about. Wood, Rynd, Pravaz, and Luer all contributed, but none seems to be *the* actual contributor. Lister established the concept of antisepsis in 1875, and Bernard introduced the idea of homeostasis in 1879. In 1891, Matas reported on his success with intravenous saline solution with 19 patients from Charity Hospital in New Orleans, which established this therapy as acceptable by the turn of the century. This advance is interesting to look back on, for Matas actually reported that 12 out of 19 patients died, although the immediate effect from saline was ''good.''

Although this appears to be a substantial package of information, during the first two decades of the twentieth century there seems to be little mention of fluid therapy in conjunction with surgery and anesthesia, even though it was well known that urine formation decreased when patients underwent surgery.

Landsteiner unlocked the mystery of blood types in 1900, but this hardly caused an immediate therapeutic revolution. In 1918, Robertson, an American army surgeon, discovered that citrate could preserve blood in an icebox for 1 week; however, blood transfusion still did not enter clinical practice in a substantial way until after the recognition of the Rh factor and the end of World War II. In fact, World War I was a war of salt; World War II, one of plasma; and Korea, finally, a war of blood. Given the current concern about HIV infection, it may be that, war excepted, the frequency of blood transfusion will decline.

The 1940s was a confusing period, filled with concerns about fever and pyrogens from rubber tubing and with admonitions from the University of Michigan Surgery Department—and one of its apostles in Texas, Carl Moyer—to limit saline solution strongly in the first 72 hours after surgery. In the summer of 1950, Moyer made an abrupt about-face and began to advocate very liberal saline administration. His recommendations were somewhat tempered by his pupil Shires, who introduced the idea of the ''third space'' in 1959. Modern fluid therapy basically dates to the concepts introduced by Moyer and Shires during this decade.

The subject of mechanical venous access was moderately popular in the 1930s. At the time it involved surgical cut-downs for the insertion of fairly large-bore silver- or gold-plated cannulae. Evolution of cannulae since that time has largely been influenced, first by metallurgy, allowing for smaller thin-walled disposable needles (stainless steel—silver and gold do not go in the trash) and then by organic chemistry, which perfected polymerization and gave us plastics. By 1948, polyethylene tubing was being used for pediatric intravenous therapy and complication rates for adult plastic catheters, of the type inserted through a large-bore needle, were well known in the mid-1950s. In the same year that Moyer reversed his position on postoperative fluids, the ''Rochester plastic needle'' was described in *Anesthesiology*[2] by its creator, David Massa. This was the first plastic catheter-over-the-needle design of the sort that now seems so commonplace, but this original model consisted of three, rather than two, separate pieces: a stylet, a plastic cannula, and an independent cannula hub, which was in fact a 3/8-inch-long 16 gauge needle that was forcefully inserted into the plastic cannula. This provided for Murphy-style accidents, wherein the plastic cannula could surreptitiously detach from the hub and vanish somewhere into the circulation. The answer to this, a decade or so later, came from the combined efforts of David S. Sheridan and Ralph D. Alley, MD, who gave birth to the catheter with integral connector.

Indwelling needles were passé in adult practice by the mid-1960s. Along the way, the nomenclature changed, and *cannula* fell out of favor, to be replaced by *catheter.* During the 1970s, neonatology created new, increasingly minute, patients, but eventually technology caught up even there and by the early 1980s, Teflon™ 24 gauge catheter-over-the-needle designs were equal to the task posed by the 2-lb infant. This removed the last bastion of the steel needle, the traditional pediatric "butterfly," when it was finally made clear that the reason needles caused a lower incidence of phlebitis was that they never stayed in a vein long enough to cause that problem.

The engineering progress in the past two decades, as exemplified by elimination of toxic tin stabilizers from medical polyvinylchloride in 1968, can be estimated by the decline during the 1980s in major interest in catheter-induced phlebitis, at least in peripheral veins. In comparison, during the 1960s, the reported incidence of this problem was about 50% for catheters left in place for 24 hours or longer.[3] This is not to say that available materials are perfect, or that progress should just stop where it is. However, we may well have reached the point where the irritation due to the catheter is lost in the background noise caused by the spectrum of drugs and fluids infused into peripheral vessels. Current concerns are largely about catheter-related sepsis, which is a complicated relationship among a vascular foreign body, stagnant blood, and bacterial contamination that does not seem easily solved solely by altering the construction of the foreign body.

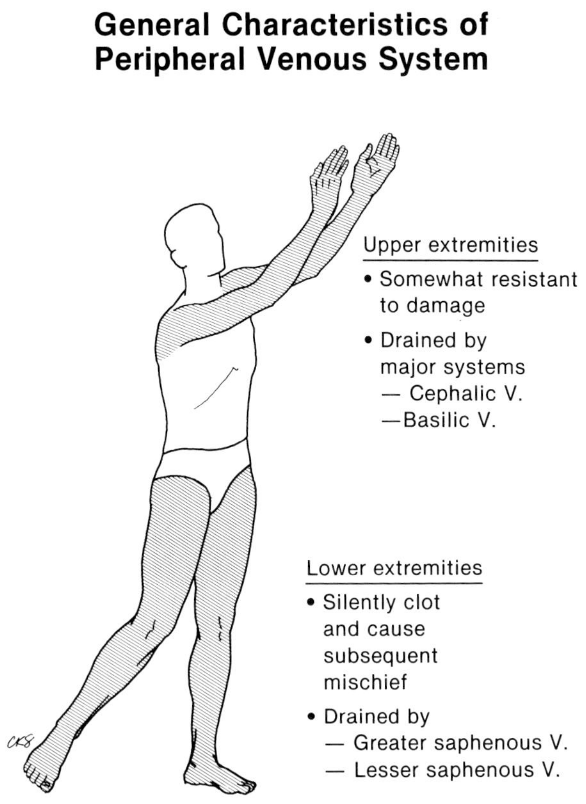

Figure 16–1 • There are two general anatomic subdivisions of the peripheral venous system. The upper-extremity system is somewhat resistant to damage, whereas the lower-extremity system has a propensity to thrombosis, phlebitis, and embolism. The upper extremities are drained by the cephalic and basilic veins, whereas the lower extremities are drained by the greater and lesser saphenous veins.

B. *Anatomy of Peripheral Veins*

1. UPPER-EXTREMITY VEINS

A minimal exposure to surgical patients and their postoperative complications quickly demonstrates that there are two anatomic subdivisions of peripheral veins (Fig. 16–1): upper-extremity veins (Fig. 16–2), which seem somewhat resistant to damage, and lower-extremity veins, which clot silently and cause great subsequent mischief (eg, phlebitis, embolism). The predictability of superficial venous anatomy also fits these categories. The upper extremity is drained by two major systems, the cephalic and the basilic, but the topography presented by these two systems is quite variable. In general, the basilic begins on the ulnar side of the forearm, often first becoming prominently visible on the dorsum of the hand halfway between the metacarpal–phalangeal joint of the ring finger and the wrist. The cephalic vein originates on the radial side of the forearm, often achieving prominence just distal to the anatomic "snuff box" at the base of the thumb. These two systems often communicate at the wrist level but remain moderately distinct until the shoulder joint is reached. At elbow level, a median vein from the forearm joins the median cubital vein, which in turn obliquely connects the two systems just superficial to the bicipital aponeurosis. This aponeurosis separates the brachial artery and its companion, the median nerve, from the superficial venous anatomy. In the middle of the upper arm, the basilic vein enters the deep fascia and follows the brachial artery into the axilla. Leaving the elbow, the cephalic vein travels up the lateral bicipital furrow, pierces the deltopectoral triangle, and joins the axillary vein. All the veins in the upper extremity are liberally equipped with unidirectional valves, a fact clearly demonstrated in 1628 by Harvey's drawings.

2. LOWER-EXTREMITY VEINS

The lower extremity demonstrates much less obvious venous drainage. The great saphenous vein begins at the medial side of the dorsal venous arch of the foot and

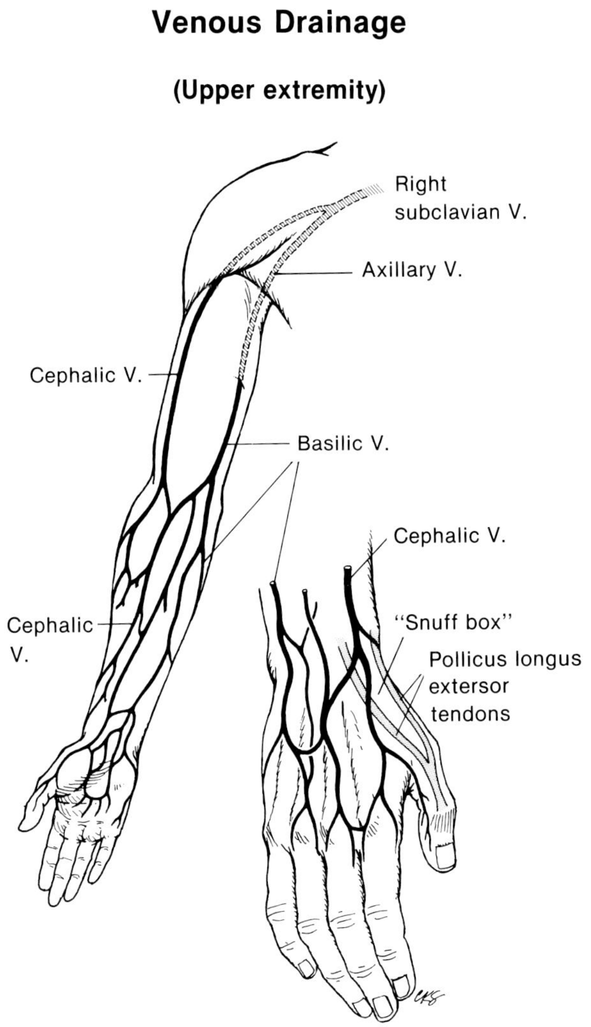

Figure 16–2 • Schematic diagram of the details of the cephalic and basilic venous drainage systems of the upper extremities. The cephalic vein originates on the radial side of the forearm just distal to the anatomic "snuff box" at the base of the thumb. The two systems often communicate at the wrist and elbow levels but remain moderately distinct until the shoulder joint is reached.

passes a few centimeters in front of the medial malleolus, following which it parallels the medial border of the tibia to the knee in the subcutaneous fat. By description, this vein should be fairly visible, but in fact this is rarely the case above the ankle. The short saphenous vein originates from the lateral portion of the dorsal arch, then passes below and then behind the lateral malleolus, following which it pierces the fascia and is generally no longer visible. The known propensity for lower-extremity veins to form clots, which in turn may migrate centripetally, makes both these systems far less desirable for elective fluid administration in adults. The situation in children often comes down to using whatever is available, but only for short periods, thus making it more likely that lower-extremity veins will be cannulated. On occasion, however, lower-extremity veins are used as infusion sites for a prolonged period in a seriously ill child, and even then thrombosis and central embolization are rare. The reasons are not clear but may be related to the fact that children's veins have not been subjected to gravitational assault for multiple decades as adult veins have, and to children's fairly high cardiac index.

3. Relation to Peripheral Arteries

Prior to the routine use of plastic catheters, it was common to induce anesthesia with an intravenous barbiturate directly injected via an intravascular needle mated directly to a syringe. From this technique there developed a literature concerning anomalous arterial tributaries, most of which were inadvertently discovered using thiopental as an active destructive biologic marker.[4] In the contemporary era of injection only into free-flowing infusions, this may seem irrelevant, but it is still possible to enter and infuse into one of these small arteries, given proper enthusiasm, reduced systemic blood pressure, and pressurized fluid administration.

Both the radial and ulnar arteries are vulnerable. The radial can be mistakenly entered just deep to the cephalic vein origin because a small aberrant branch of the artery crosses the "snuff box" quite superficially in about 1% of the population.[5] This is of more than passing interest, for at this location one can often find a very robust virgin vein that is ideal for a 14 gauge catheter. The ulnar artery may originate above the cubital fossa and travel a superficial course down the arm as far as the wrist. This ulnar artery variant is responsible for the majority of unintended arterial cannulations reported in the past. At the elbow itself, a misdirected catheter may enter an unusually superficial brachial artery, although it should be rare for this to go undetected because pressure in this proximal vessel, absent shock, should make arterial trespass fairly obvious. Probably of greater concern is the possibility of transfixing the median nerve, which lies nearby, should access be attempted in an unresponsive patient.

Experience gained from arterial monitoring gives insight as to why lower-extremity arteries have rarely been entered by mistake during attempts at venous access. Both the dorsalis pedis and posterior tibial arteries

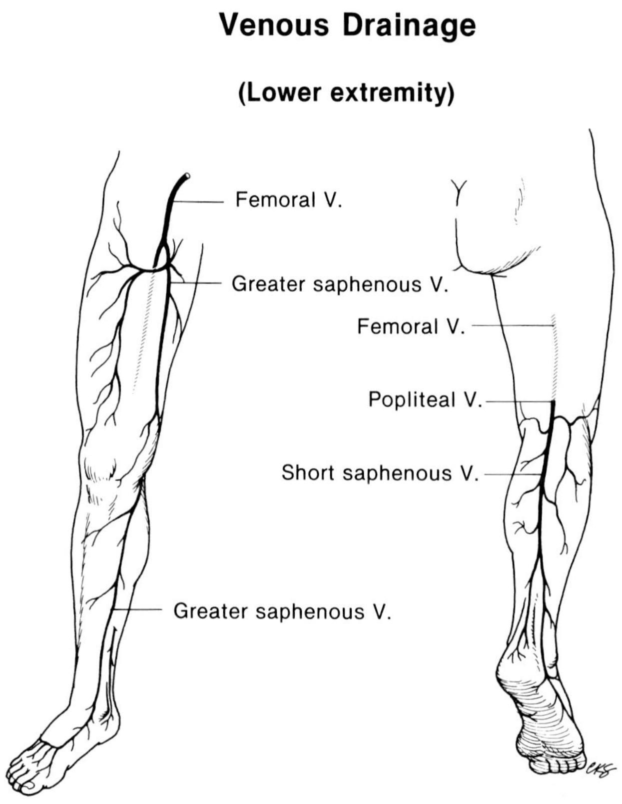

Figure 16–3 • Schematic diagram of the details of the venous drainage system of the lower extremity. The great saphenous vein begins at the medial side of the foot, passes a few centimeters in front of the medial malleolus, and then parallels the medial border of the tibia to the knee in the subcutaneous tissue. The short saphenous vein originates from the lateral portion of the foot, passes below and behind the lateral mallelus, and then becomes a deep vein and is no longer visible.

are subfascial and lie beneath virgin sensitive skin, unlike the hand's environmentally toughened epidermis. Direct injection into the veins of the foot has therefore never been popular, while cannulation for infusion has generally been reserved for the pediatric population. Theoretically, it is possible to enter a lower-extremity artery during attempted venous cannulation, but the diminutive arterial size seems to make this relatively uncommon—on occasion, even when the artery is the actual target (Fig. 16–3).

II. How to Obtain Peripheral Venous Access

A. *Increasing the Visibility and/or Size of a Peripheral Vein*

1. Temperature and Sympathetic Nervous System Influences

The ease with which blood pressure can be measured has long provoked a fixation with the arterial side of the circulation. This is true despite the fact that 60% of blood volume normally resides in the venous circulation, which is in turn quite well supplied with outflow from the sympathetic nervous system. Peripheral access to a vein must transit the skin one way or the other, and this large organ, with its function as waterproof upholstery, can markedly interfere with finding a vein to cannulate. Blood flow to the skin is subject to tremendous variability (from 0% to 30% of cardiac output), largely in response to temperature considerations and autonomic nervous system activity. Often a first interaction with any patient in a hospital, after the insurance forms, is to rapidly uncover as much skin as possible, preferably in a 18°C room with rapidly circulating air, and then, while clutching a plastic-sheathed railroad spike, to share wonderment with the patient at the paucity of visible veins in the upper extremities. How much of a role the sympathetic nervous system plays in this vanishing act can only be surmised, but reports[6] of peripheral venospasm do appear from time to time and one certainly develops the impression that premedicated, or less terrified, patients seem to have more visible veins. Application of a venous tourniquet rarely seems to influence this situation to the desired degree, nor does allowing the extremity to hang dependent.

On the other hand, application of heat can seduce invisible veins into reappearing, and I make it a habit to find warm blankets (Fig. 16–4A). prior to searching for a tourniquet and starting the rub-and-pat ritual (Fig. 16–4B) in an attempt to unravel the mystery of just how blood *does* invisibly exit the upper extremity. Recently, a very sophisticated chemical heat source has become available to aid in warming extremities for this task, but a calorie is a calorie, so the source probably does not matter—in conscious patients. For unresponsive patients, an overzealous pursuit of local heating, especially if it involves an active device that gets warmer with time, might cause harm.

2. Usual Tourniquet Method to Enlarge Veins

In modern terminology, the device is a tourniquet, from the French word meaning "to turn" (Fig. 16–4C). Three hundred and fifty years ago the arm was tied off as for bloodletting. No matter, the result is the same—to trap blood distally and cause veins to engorge. In the United States, rubber surgical drains are commonly used to accomplish this task, and in this age of complex devices it is refreshing to stumble on something in medicine so obviously simple that it does not have an instruction manual. There are a few simple hints that come with experience, even for this item with no moving parts. First, it is important to place the tourniquet relatively close to the potential puncture site. Allowing trapped blood too many options for hiding is of little benefit if many of the choices are not visible. On occasion, when nothing seems even about to become visible, a blood pressure cuff can be placed very proximally and inflated to suprasystolic levels for some minutes and then deflated to take advantage of potential reactive hyperemia. Second, pay some attention to the mass of the limb and the patient's probable mean blood pressure. It is

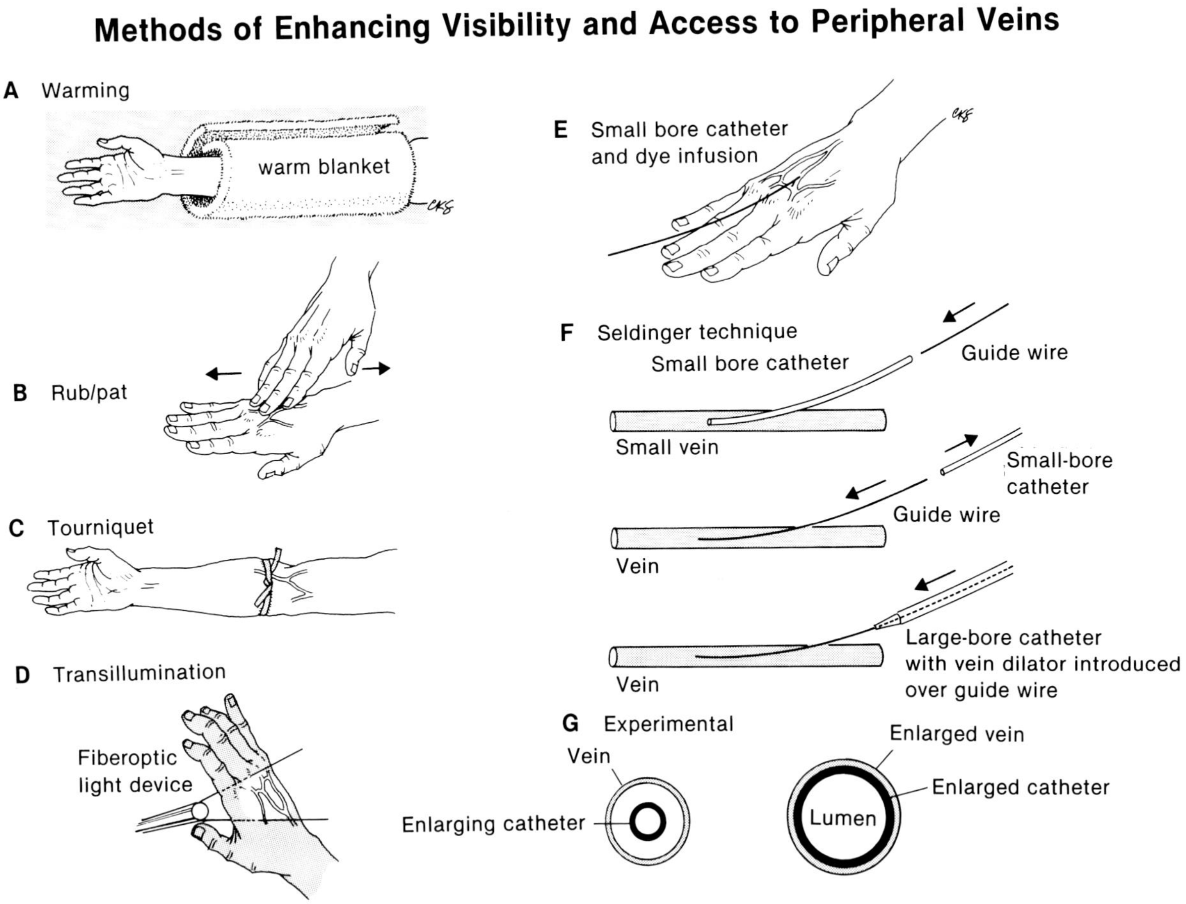

Figure 16–4 • Schematic diagram of numerous methods for enhancing the visibility and access to peripheral veins. (See text for full explanation of subsections *A–G*.)

surprisingly easy, given a small arm and low blood pressure, to diminish or even eliminate arterial inflow to an extremity if the tourniquet is applied with particular zeal. The give-away that this has happened is that the arm, in lightly pigmented patients, turns pale instead of dusky. When in doubt, check the peripheral pulse. Remember that it only takes about 40 mm of pressure to completely eliminate venous outflow from an extremity. Finally, if using a surgical drain, ask the patient to externally rotate his or her arms into the so-called anatomic position and then place the tourniquet so that the tuck-under portion is over the medial aspect of the arm. This last step matters little in women, but men will appreciate the absence of the usual depilation, because there is almost no hair on this side of the arm, even in very hairy men. This also keeps the "tail" of the tourniquet off the puncture site, where a variation of Murphy's law often causes it to lie.

After the tourniquet has been applied, ask the patient to open and close the fist, as though compressing an imaginary rubber ball in exercise, to increase blood flow to the extremity while allowing, if feasible, the extremity to hang dependent and enlist gravity in the process. During the actual puncture, asking the patient to hold a clenched fist may form an unyielding support of muscle against which to trap an elusive vessel.

It is only human nature to rotate the forearm through 180° and ignore the fact that the ulna remains in contact with the mattress during this exercise. When all else fails, a delightful discovery can be made by flexing the elbow 90° and looking for the vein that is frequently hiding along this aspect of the arm. Placing the catheter in this vein may require some agility, but the size of the vessel usually makes this worthwhile.

3. UNUSUAL NONINVASIVE AIDS TO MAKE SMALLER VEINS BECOME LARGER VEINS

The veinless arm eventually bedevils all those involved in starting IVs. The large numbers of operators and events mandates that there will be an effusion of ideas about how best to solve the problem. The number also suggests that no one answer always works. The following is a list of possibly helpful alternatives.

a. Fiberoptic Transillumination of the Hand

Fiberoptic transillumination of the hand is an old technique in pediatric patients but works in adults as well (Fig. 16–4D).[7] In the absence of some special dedicated device for this purpose, the use of a fiberoptic light source, addition of heat shield, and insertion of a red filter represent a start toward this capability. Unfortunately, each light source will have its own power range, so it will then be necessary to determine safe limits of skin contact at full, or reduced, power for each final product. It is suggested that the creator of each device use his or her own forearm as a test bed. There is now available a commercial light source, called a Landry Vein Light™, that appears to transilluminate veins by projecting light from both sides of a suspected location. The device itself has some resemblance to a modernistic redesign of a beetle, and evaluation of the effectiveness is currently not available.

b. Reverse Esmarch's Wrap of the Arm

Reverse Esmarch's wrap of the arm, proximally to distally, drives blood from the proximal to the distal direction, thus engorging distal veins.

c. Local Application of Nitroglycerin Ointment to the Skin[8]

Local application of nitroglycerin ointment to the skin overlying the proposed insertion site requires time, minimally 15 minutes, to be effective. Once the local effect has been achieved, the drug should be removed from the skin. Possible, as yet unreported, side effects would be those associated with nitrate therapy.

d. Combination Approach

For the patient with peripheral edema, conventional wrap with an Esmarch's bandage, in conjunction with direct pressure over the intended puncture site, to transiently eliminate tissue fluid[9,10] may reveal a vein "protected" from prior assault, as well as one supported by increased tissue turgor.

e. Proper Oblique Lighting

Insure that ambient light is used to advantage. Direct, bright overhead illumination destroys shadows and thus eliminates the third dimension, depth. Oblique lighting can be used to enhance shadows and thereby create this useful parameter. "Helpers" will go to some lengths to defeat this idea if allowed to do so.

4. Unusual Invasive Aids to Make Small Veins Become Larger Veins

a. *Use of a Small-Bore Catheter, Fluid and Dye Infusion*

A distressing combination of events often seems to present a patient, generally obese, with a need for a 16 gauge catheter but with only 20 gauge veins. The novice will try to force the issue at the outset. This most reliably produces a 16 gauge electrolyte-filled tumor. A better idea is to insert the small-bore catheter and then follow this with 50–100 mL of sterile body-temperature saline containing a small amount of methylene blue dye (Fig. 16–4e).[11] One then examines the rest of the arm distal to the tourniquet for distended blue veins. Obviously, the dye technique is most useful in patients with little or no natural pigmentation.

b. *Use of Seldinger Technique to Exchange a Small-Bore Catheter for a Large-Bore Catheter*

If nothing becomes visible after infusion of warm dye-filled fluid, some judgment is called for. One option is to leave the small-bore catheter as is and hydrate and warm the patient, with the intent to return for another examination later. The concept of venospasm once again floats to the surface, for it often seems that infusion rate improves with time in this situation. Newtonian fluids can flow quite freely through fairly small-bore catheters, especially with pressure augmentation. On the other hand, if a prominent non-Newtonian fluid, blood, must be infused, it may be better to insert a guide wire through the small-bore catheter, remove it, and insert a larger catheter down the wire into the vein (Fig. 16–4F). In fact, a commercially available product (Rapid Infusion Catheter Exchange Set; Arrow International, Inc.; Reading, PA) has been designed to facilitate this exchange. However, removing the sole venous access catheter does take courage, and common sense dictates that if the anatomic site in question has never, in the operator's experience, accepted a catheter larger than 18 gauge in any patient, then trying to thread in a 6 French device in this situation seems ill advised.

c. *Use of Catheters that Enlarge While in Vivo*

A fascinating advance in the technology of catheter construction has recently appeared in the form of a polyurethane hydrogel (Aquavene®) that undergoes swelling with hydration such that the available cross-sectional area of the catheter increases, with resultant effective improvement in flow of 25% in vivo (Fig. 16–4G). For those not willing to struggle with calculations, this results in a 20 gauge catheter with flow equal to or better than an 18 gauge standard catheter. Obviously there is no such thing as a free lunch, and these catheters cost more. However, for a small-vein–large-flow equation, they may well be worth the premium (Streamline®, Menlo Care; Palo Alto, CA).

5. Final Choice of Insertion Site Considerations

If a multitude of access sites is available, then fate has indeed been kind. The site chosen for the infusion must not only be reasonable for the operator and the patient but must also avoid future conflict. Such conflict may be quite obvious, as in avoiding an extremity where surgery is planned, or it may be less clear, as in avoiding an extremity that is usually compressed or folded during a surgical procedure so that flow is mechanically impeded. In general, an ideal site might be in the forearm of the nondominant arm, but important additional factors to consider are the following: (1) operative/injured site; (2) prior extremity surgery, especially vascular access; (3) recent intravenous insertion; (4) patient position during surgery; (5) central cavity or extensive torso surgery resulting in extremity edema; (6) patient preference; (7) prior extremity trauma, especially burns; (8) neurologic abnormalities leading to increased or decreased sensation, or muscle spasm, in an extremity; (9) proximal venous stasis or thrombosis between the extremity and the central circulation; (10) mechanical impediment to central venous flow, such as markedly elevated abdominal pressure or a Military antishock trouser (MAST) suit; and (11) surgical interruption of venous drainage, either by ligation or removal. Note that these are listed as factors, not contraindications. Given urgent circumstances, the only factors that preclude venous access in any given site are technical inability or the dominant impression that local or proximal anatomy will make such an attempt at best useless and at worst harmful. The latter situation may seem quite improbable, but a pressure transfusion of 500 mL of blood through a nonvenous infiltrated catheter is so unattractive as to be easily remembered as an example. Finally, a puncture site removed from a joint line will prevent the tip of the catheter from crossing the joint, which in turn decreases the stress to the catheter and to the proximal vein when the joint is exercised by patient motion. Decreased catheter and proximal vein stress probably greatly diminish the risk of catheter perforation of the vein.

B. *Inserting the Catheter*

1. Skin Preparation

Once a likely target has been selected, the course of the vein should be thoroughly prepared, proximally to distally, with alcohol. The proximal to distal preparation not only cleans the skin but may further engorge the vessel in question. Obviously, other solutions can be used, but they should not decrease visibility or lubricate the skin. Current infection concerns suggest that one should perform this step, and those that follow, while wearing gloves to protect all involved.

A word here about natural sweaters. Male patients often have increased body hair distributed about the forearms. Finding a vein beneath this coverage is often like looking for tree roots in a grass-filled yard. Then, even following identification of a suitable target, precise delineation of the vein course remains doubtful. This seems a reasonable time to resort to mini-shaving to better see the vein and to improve the foundation for the follow-on adhesive dressing. However, before unsheathing the razor, be reasonably certain of site suitability. Most men do not mind some shaving, but most do not want their sweater sleeves to appear moth-eaten.

2. Local Anesthesia/Precatheter Skin Penetration

If the catheter is large (>20 gauge) and the patient is responsive, then local anesthesia should be used just prior to skin penetration. If the catheter is quite small or the patient is unresponsive, topical anesthesia can be bypassed. However, if local anesthesia is not used, then the issue of a prior skin puncture with a needle may arise. I include such a puncture as part of the ritual for inserting very-small-bore catheters or for penetrating seemingly weathered skin with larger catheters, knowing full well that actually proving the effectiveness of the step is problematic at best. The insertion site must be chosen with precision. As patients age, tissue turgor decreases and vessels "roll" away from needles (Fig. 16–5). An insertion site at a junction of tributaries can avoid this mobility issue. However, even this technique can prove troublesome when tissue resistance is very

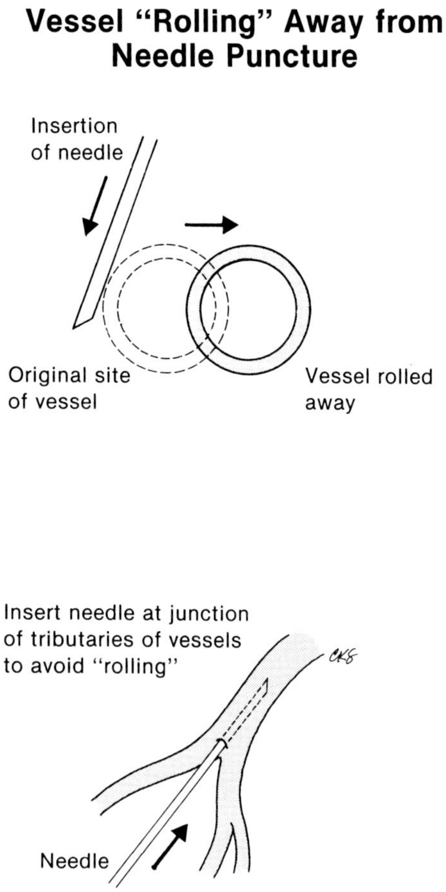

Figure 16–5 • Vessels may roll away from an approaching needle (*upper panel*). This problem increases with age because tissue turgor decreases. Insertion of the needle at a junction of venous tributaries minimizes the chance that the vessel can roll away from the approaching needle (*lower panel*).

low, for the junction site may withdraw from the slow advance of the stylet, only to abruptly spring distally, when the stylet penetrates the vein wall, just enough to penetrate the opposite vessel wall in one smooth, epithet-filled move. To circumvent this, align the catheter with the longitudinal axis of the proximal vein so that the lunge is directed more or less up the lumen (see Fig. 16–5). I prefer to "tunnel" the catheter a centimeter or so prior to venipuncture to establish the correct plane of advance and perhaps to place a bacterial barrier of normal skin between the skin hole and vein entry (Fig. 16–6). With or without this step, anticipate that resistance to advance of the catheter will be proportional to catheter size, inversely proportional to the patient's age, and nonexistent for patients taking corticosteroids.

Current research into transdermal drug delivery[12,13] raises the possibility that it may soon be possible

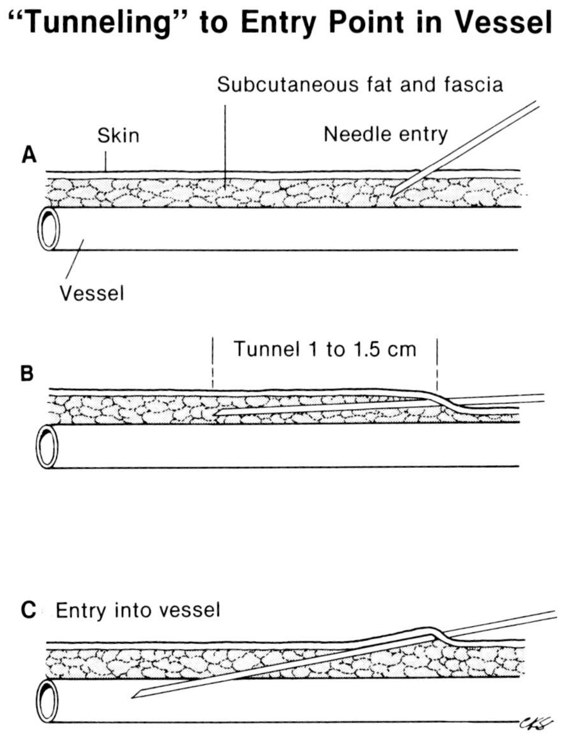

Figure 16–6 • If the entry point of the needle is 1.0–1.5 cm away from the intended site of vessel puncture, the correct plane of advance of the needle can be better established and the subcutaneous tunnel may place a barrier to bacterial infection. (***A***) shows puncture of the needle through the skin. (***B***) shows the correct plane of advancement being established through the subcutaneous tunnel. (***C***) shows entry of the needle into the vessel.

to completely eliminate injecting local anesthetic into the skin prior to catheter insertion (Fig. 16–7). For most situations, this would represent a small comfort improvement for the average patient, but for some it would be truly an anxiety-reducing step and would absolutely eliminate one more opportunity for operators to stick themselves with used needles. This idea has created substantial interest, as one might imagine, in pediatrics, but those with children will instantly realize that anxiety-free catheter insertion will not be achieved without some form of prior experience. To expect a 5-year-old to gaze indifferently at the insertion of 30-mm nail into his hand while an obviously lying strange adult says, "It won't hurt"—and restrains his arm—is reasonable only for those who also expect that the phrase "act your age" will paradoxically result in instantaneous adult behavior. Furthermore, at the moment, transcutaneous anesthesia requires much more time than does a quick subcutaneous injection. The discomfort of the subcutaneous injection seems related to rapid injection rate and the substance injected.[14] The patient perceives a small needle prick, followed by a short-lived, modestly intense burning sensation when lidocaine is used. I have tried, with varying results, substituting bacteriostatic saline with benzyl alcohol for lidocaine. Others have recommended buffering the acidic lidocaine with bicarbonate[15] to decrease the burning sensation, or using other solutions. In an extreme situation, a topical anesthetic spray can be applied to the skin prior to injection. However, this not only cools the local area but is usually unnecessary. In fact, most adult patients tolerate the injection with relative impunity—particularly if their last catheter was inserted without any anesthesia whatsoever— thereby serving as a significant benchmark of cutaneous sensitivity.

3. CATHETER PREPARATION

After skin preparation, the selected catheter should be removed from the package and inspected. Unless the op-

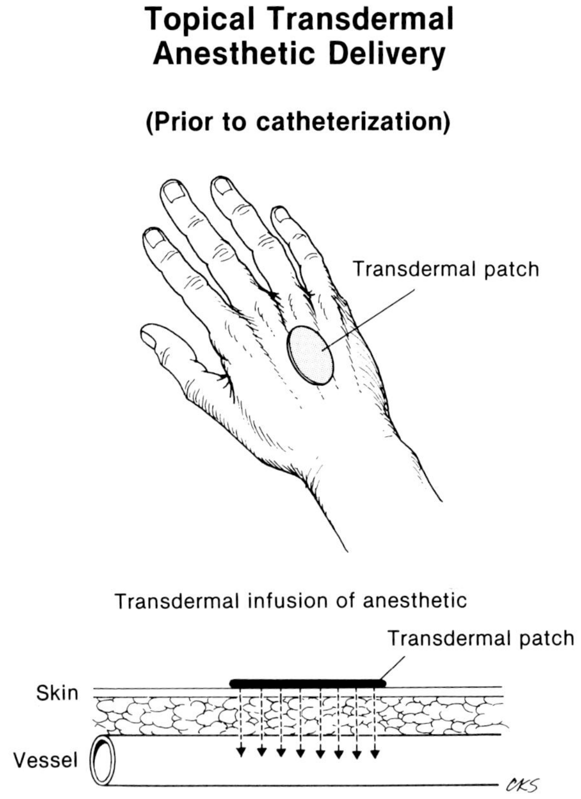

Figure 16–7 • Schematic diagram of the application of a patch of local anesthetic to the skin (*upper panel*). Transdermal infusion of the anesthetic through the tissue resulting in local anesthesia (*lower panel*).

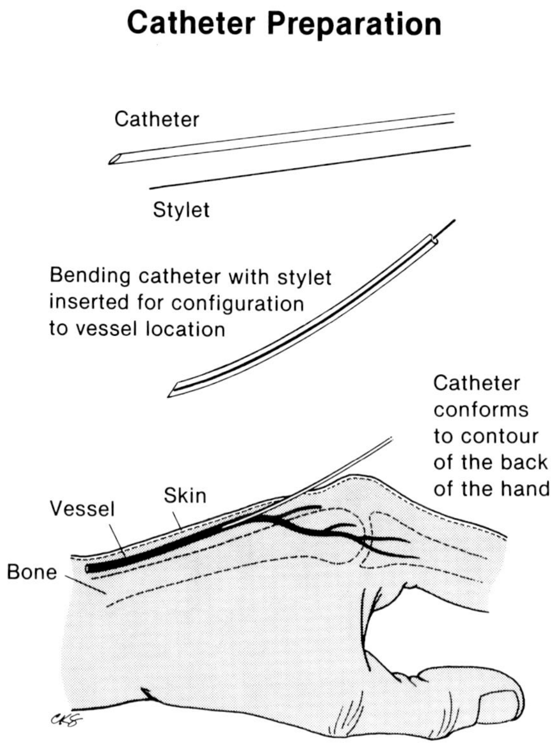

Figure 16–8 • Occasionally the intravenous catheter and stylet will need bending (*upper panel*) to configure the needle and catheter to the contour of the surface anatomy of the area of the vein in question (*lower panel*).

erator has a dark sense of humor or the patient is blind, holding a large-bore catheter-over-the-needle device in the air for all to see is not recommended. If the device is intact, it is useful to rotate the catheter about the stylet and slide it up and down a few millimeters to insure smooth advance postinsertion. In some anatomically awkward situations, the straight design of the device will prove troublesome and one can use the catheter sheath to put a gentle bend or curve on the stylet prior to use[16] (Fig. 16–8). Usually, the need for this is obvious once insertion is attempted. However, a not-so-obvious situation occurs when cannulating a hand vein directly in line with a prominent metacarpal–phalangeal joint, usually of the ring finger, where the vein can be easily entered but the knuckle prevents passage of the connecting hub over the joint and extensor tendon.

4. INSERTING THE CATHETER

The catheter is now finally inserted in the skin, initially at an acute angle for penetration. Once the catheter is inserted, the distal end is oriented to a plane parallel to the epidermis and directed toward the target site. Crucial to this process is distal countertraction with the operator's other hand, just sufficient to tense the skin against the catheter but not so great as to collapse the veins. With both older needles and catheters, vein entry could be easily felt, much like the "click" of fascial penetration with axillary block or lumbar puncture. As needles have gotten sharper and catheter walls thinner, this has been lost to some degree. The resulting sense is one of smooth, painless advance, with the appearance of blood continually flowing back through the stylet hub until the stylet plug is reached. This forces insertion to be somewhat slower, as the blood return may lag behind vein entry by as much as 5 seconds when the smallest catheters are being inserted. In any case, once the vein has been entered and blood return noted, the catheter should be advanced forward while the stylet is held immobile. Then both should be advanced as a unit, catheter tip first, further into the vein. If the stylet was bent to accommodate the local anatomy, it can be anticipated that advancement of the catheter off the stylet will be somewhat more difficult. Following complete insertion, I pin the catheter hub to the skin with an index finger while proximally occluding the vein just beyond the catheter tip with the ring finger of the same hand, thus holding the catheter immobile and preventing messy blood back-flow onto the patient as the stylet is pulled back. The infusion should be firmly connected to the catheter once the stylet has been removed. For those wearing gloves, a sterile adhesive, clear plastic occlusive dressing is applied, because handling tape with gloves generally succeeds only in making the patient lose all faith in one's motor skills and may result in removing the catheter in the process.

During the insertion process, events do not always go exactly as planned. The catheter can be advanced to just the correct spot but no vein entry may be achieved. Catheters come in varying lengths, from roughly 14 mm to 50 mm or so, and it is important to pay some attention to how much catheter remains outside the patient during pursuit of an errant vein. If 25% or less is visible, it is generally better to withdraw and try again. The epitome of frustration is to finally gain vascular access, only to realize that the catheter hub is already dimpling the skin and only the stylet is in the vein. Unfortunately, while catheters can grow in diameter, they cannot grow in length, and there is no solution to this frustrating situation, other than quickly trying to find a guide wire small enough to pass through the stylet and at least save the vein for cannulation if a longer catheter can be produced. If this situation occurs, insert the guide wire, release the tourniquet, raise the arm to decrease hydraulic pressure, and put pressure over the puncture site while awaiting an opportunity to reuse the vein (via the guide wire).

It seems improbable that a vein could be entered without any visible indication of blood return, but it happens surprisingly often, and this situation can be sometimes rescued by very slowly withdrawing the catheter, often with the stylet at least partially removed, and looking for a dark shadow moving down the plastic tube, coincident with the partial collapse of the distended vein just proximal to the catheter. When this is observed, the catheter can often be inserted up the vein using a rapid rotary (clockwise–counterclockwise) oscillation of the catheter hub to ''help'' the process. If the stylet has been removed, gloves are essential for this, as blood will inevitably escape the catheter onto the operator's hands. The probability that this withdrawal technique will work can sometimes be estimated by moving the catheter laterally left and right about 20° prior to withdrawal, and observing the vein thought to have been transfixed. If the entire vein seems to twist when the catheter moves, there seems to be, in my experience, a higher incidence of unrecognized vein entry during insertion. If only a small portion of the vein moves, it is more likely that a through-and-through transfixion has occurred. The withdrawal technique may still work, but it is less likely.

5. Trouble-Shooting Inserted Catheters

On occasion, the intravenous catheter insertion process breaks down at the advancement stage, where the patient reports pain. The catheter has most likely penetrated the opposite vein wall. I leave the tourniquet on unless an obvious hematoma develops and attach a syringe containing a few milliliters of saline to the catheter. A minute injection will either confirm or eliminate correct placement without distorting the local anatomy. If the catheter is misplaced, withdraw it very slowly with gentle aspiration of the syringe until blood flows back in the syringe and then reattempt advancement of the catheter while aspirating very gently. A variant of this problem is the ''positional'' catheter, which usually means imprecisely ''I know that this is a good catheter because I placed it, but it only flows well when the patient has carpopedal spasm.'' This situation is attributed to various unproven anatomic entities, most commonly a venous valve. Often flow will markedly improve when the catheter is withdrawn a few millimeters. It seems best to apply the clear sterile dressing, allow the infusion to flow (warm fluids are best), and return a bit later to first examine the site for electrolyte tumors and then possibly reattempt catheter advancement. This works often enough to make it worth the time, but the catheter must obviously remain sterile for this to be a justifiable option.

While all eyes are on the completion of this process, it is all too easy to lose track of the bloody stylet, usually casually sitting nearby. This spear represents a hazard to the patient and the operator and must be disposed of without injury to either. This process can be aided by placing the empty catheter sheath where the stylet can be reinserted with one hand after catheter insertion. Unless this is planned in advance, the sheath will inevitably end up behind the operator and under a blanket where it will not be found until patient discharge. A recent new product has been introduced that seems to eliminate this potential hazard. Time will tell whether the success rate of insertion remains as high with this shrouded stylet design.

III. Discussion and Complications

The vast majority of patients who are treated in an in-hospital setting and virtually all patients undergoing surgery require that peripheral venous access be obtained. Ordinarily, this is accomplished easily by simply putting a tourniquet on an upper extremity and choosing an appropriately sized vein for the intended catheter size. However, on occasion one may need to increase the visibility and size of the intended target by using a variety of noninvasive or invasive methods. The noninvasive methods consist of warming the extremity, decreasing sympathetic tone, fiberoptic illumination, reverse Esmarch's wrap, local application of nitroglycerin ointment, and use of proper oblique lighting. The invasive methods consist of fluid and dye infusion through a small-bore catheter, use of a Seldinger technique to exchange a small-bore with a large-bore catheter, and use of catheters that actually enlarge once they are in vivo. With all attempts to obtain peripheral venous access, proper technique with regard to insertion site selection, skin preparation, use of local anesthesia, and a skin hole, putting a bend in the catheter and ''saving'' a possible "failed" attempt may be of paramount importance. Most complications of obtaining peripheral venous access, such as transsecting a vein (interstitial fluid extravasation, hematoma), arterial infusion, peripheral nerve (median nerve) infusion, thrombosis and thromboembolism, and infection, can be avoided by strict attention to these proper techniques. Failure to obtain peripheral venous access in a patient who requires *some* venous access may result in the need to obtain central venous access (see Chapter 18), to do a venous cut-down (see Chapter 20), or in urgent and pediatric cases to initiate an interosseous infusion (see Chapter 17).

IV. REFERENCES

1. Jenkins MT. History of sequestered edema associated with surgical operations and trauma. In Brown, BR (ed). Fluid and Blood Therapy in Anesthesia. Philadelphia, FA Davis, 1983.
2. Massa DJ. A plastic needle. Anesthesiology, 772–773.
3. Cheney FW, Lincoln JR. Phlebitis from plastic intravenous catheters. Anesthesiology 25:650–652, 1964.
4. Stone HH, Donnelly CC. The accidental intra-arterial injection of thiopental. Anesthesiology 22:995–1006, 1961.
5. McCormack LJ, Cauldwell EW, Arvon BJ. Brachial and antebrachial arterial patterns. Surg Gynecol Obstet 96:43–54, 1953.
6. Cunningham E, Korbon GA. Venospasm preventing peripheral venous access. Anesthesiology 59:141–142, 1983.
7. Bellotti GA, Bedford RF, Arnold WP. Fiberoptic transillumination for intravenous cannulation under general anesthesia. Anesth Analg 60:348–51, 1981.
8. Moore PL. Nitroglycerine improves venous cannulation. Anesthesiology 64:533, 1986.
9. O'Driscoll SW, Reid SR. Inserting large-bore peripheral intravenous catheters in grossly edematous patients. Crit Care Med 14:259, 1986.
10. Owens JJ. Pitting edema and intravenous access. Anesth Analg 67:1020–1021, 1988.
11. McCrory J. Facilitation of wide bore cannula insertion. Anaesthesia 40:612, 1985.
12. Gesztes A, Mezei M. Topical anesthesia of the skin by liposome-encapsulated tetracaine. Anesth Analg 67:1079–1081, 1988.
13. McCafferty DF, Wolfson AD, Boston V. In vivo assessment of percutaneous local anaesthetic preparations. Br J Anaesth 62:17–12, 1989.
14. Morris R, McKay W, Mushlin P. Comparison of pain associated with intradermal and subcutaneous infiltration with various local anesthetic solutions. Anesth Analg 66:1180–1182, 1987.
15. McKay W, Morris R, Mushlin P. Sodium bicarbonate attenuates pain on skin infiltration with lidocaine, with or without epinephrine. Anesth Analg 66:572–574, 1987.
16. Petty WC. A simple technique for inserting catheters intravenously in difficult anatomic areas. Anesthesiology 39:555–556, 1973.

Chapter 17

•

Jonathan L. Benumof, MD

Intraosseous Infusion

OUTLINE

I. INTRODUCTION

The treatment of life-threatening emergencies with life-saving drugs and fluids requires rapid access to the venous circulation. Establishing venous access in patients who are near death by directly cannulating a vein often requires a considerable amount of skill; even in the best hands, the procedure can sometimes be frustratingly difficult and time consuming. Alternative methods of administering vital fluids or drugs have been suggested and include subcutaneous, intramuscular, intraperitoneal, intracardiac, endotracheal, and intraosseous injections. The subcutaneous, intramuscular, and intraperitoneal routes cause unacceptable delay in uptake by the venous circulation, and intracardiac injections involve much additional risk. The intraosseous route of injection can be quickly, safely, and reliably established and permits rapid venous uptake of drugs and fluids; consequently, it is a viable alternative to direct intravenous cannulation and is quite suitable when used in emergency resuscitation.

Tocantins first described the administration of fluids into the general circulation by way of the bone marrow in 1940.[1] At the time, parenteral therapy in general was relatively new, and intravenous techniques in particular were still in their infancy. Tocantins's animal and human studies suggested that the uptake kinetics of fluids or drugs injected into the marrow cavity were very similar to the uptake kinetics of intravenously injected materials.[1-4] Very shortly thereafter, Papper and Rovenstine used intramedullary infusions of fluids and drugs (such as thiopental sodium) and found that the method worked "as rapidly and as easily as by intravenous injection."[5,6] The intramedullary technique quickly became popular for use in pediatric patients, in whom it could be especially troublesome to establish and maintain intravenous cannulae; numerous case studies attested to the safety and utility of the procedure.[7-12] Some authors even advocated routine use of the intramedullary route in place of intravenous therapy.[11] A much more recent report describes the successful use of intraosseous infusion under emergency circumstances in 15 patients without complications.[13]

II. INDICATIONS

Intraosseous infusion is indicated in emergency situations when life-saving fluids or drugs must be rapidly introduced into the circulation and intravenous cannulation is either too difficult or too time-consuming to perform. Patients, particularly pediatric ones, in whom this potentially life-saving procedure might be most useful include those suffering from cardiac arrest, shock, widespread burns, and massive trauma. Other patients in whom intravenous cannulation might be exceedingly difficult and who are, therefore, candidates for this procedure include severely obese individuals and patients with peripheral edema, a history of intravenous drug abuse, or prolonged prior intravenous therapy. It should be stressed that intramedullary infusion is an emergency resuscitative procedure that should be replaced by more conventional intravenous therapy when the clinical situation becomes less urgent and intravenous access can be obtained.

One recent study has appropriately emphasized the back-up nature of this procedure and determined the incidence of real need for intraosseous infusion during pediatric cardiopulmonary resuscitation when an intravenous infusion could not be established, even though a well-conceived protocol was followed.[14] The protocol involved use of a specified sequence of measures; the protocol reduced cardiopulmonary resuscitation intravenous access time from a mean of 10.0 minutes (range, 2–40 minutes when no protocol was used) to a mean of 4.5 minutes (range, 2–10 minutes when the protocol was followed). The protocol (Fig. 17–1) began with a 1.5-minute attempt to insert a catheter into a peripheral vein percutaneously. This technique was abandoned in favor of more invasive methods if it was unsuccessful after 1.5 minutes. If sufficient personnel were available, peripheral intravenous attempts were continued along with the other measures. Between 1.5 and 5 minutes of the resuscitation, simultaneous efforts were made to insert a femoral vein catheter percutaneously, as well as to perform a cutdown on the saphenous vein just anterior and superior to the medial malleolus at the contralateral ankle. If intravenous access had not been achieved by the fifth minute of the resuscitation, a needle was placed in the bone marrow 1–3 cm below the tibial tuberosity while other attempts at intravenous catheterization continued. All techniques were performed by standard methods.[15–18]

The techniques used to achieve initial intravenous access in these pediatric patients undergoing cardiopul-

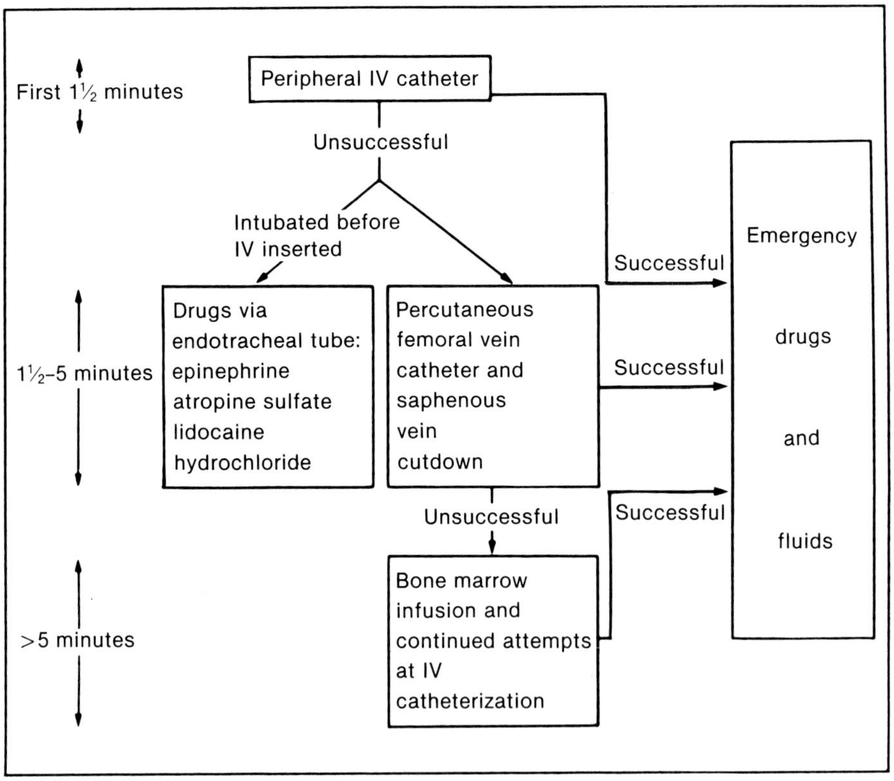

Figure 17–1 • Protocol for emergency intravenous (IV) access during pediatric resuscitations. (From Kanter RK, Zimmerman JJ, Strauss RH, Stoeckel KA: Pediatric emergency intravenous access. Am J Dis Child 140:132–134, 1986; with permission.)

monary resuscitation are shown in Table 17–1.[14] Intraosseous infusion was the first intravenous access route in a very significant 13% of patients. Intravenous access was ultimately successfully achieved in 36 (95%) of 38 resuscitations; in the two patients in whom direct intravenous access could not be obtained, intraosseous infusion remained the sole intravenous access route. Because compliance with the protocol was associated with significantly more rapid intravenous access, it may be inferred that more aggressive use of all available techniques per protocol would reduce unnecessary delays. The ability to place a needle in the bone marrow rapidly with a high degree of success suggests that this method should be more readily employed when other measures fail during the first 5 minutes of resuscitation.

Contraindications to this procedure are few, especially in urgent situations, when the alternative may be death. The only absolute contraindication is gross infection at the intended site of puncture. Generalized sepsis is a relative contraindication in view of the possibility of seeding infection into bone, but again this must be weighed against the need for life-saving therapy.

III. HOW TO INITIATE AN INTRAOSSEOUS INFUSION

A. *Equipment*

A minimum of equipment is required for this technique. A large-bore (approximately 16 gauge) metal needle with a stylet that is sturdy enough for passage through bony cortex will work. Needles used routinely by hematologists for bone marrow aspiration or biopsy are ideal. They include the short Rosenthal or Osgood needles (16 gauge × 1 5/16 inches) (left panel, Fig. 17–2) and the larger, Silverman-type biopsy needle used without the split inner cannula (10 gauge × 3 inches), all of which are available from Becton-Dickinson. (Rutherford, NJ). A special sternal bone marrow infusion needle with a trephine-type inner cannula is also available from Becton-Dickinson (right panel, Fig. 17–2), but its use may be time consuming and is not necessary for this procedure. In desperate situations, the sturdiest needle that is immediately available should be used.

Standard phlebotomy and intravenous needles are unsatisfactory for adults. These needles tend to bend on penetration of the adult bony cortex. However, in children less than 18 months of age, standard phlebotomy needles (16 gauge or larger diameter) or 18 to 20 gauge spinal needles may be used for intraosseous infusion because the cortices of the bones of these children are much softer and, therefore, more penetrable. We recommend that the physician intent on using this technique obtain marrow needles and have them kept in readily available sterile set-ups. A 5- or 10-mL syringe should be available to confirm placement by aspiration and to flush the needle, plus a smaller syringe and needle for administering local anesthesia, if necessary.

Table 17–1 • Technique Used to Achieve Initial Intravenous Access in Pediatric Patients Who Required Cardiopulmonary Resuscitation[14]

	No. of Patients (%)
Peripheral vein, first 1.5 minutes	7 (18)
Peripheral vein, after 1.5 minutes	8 (21)
Femoral vessel (percutaneous)	7 (18)
Cutdown	7 (18)
Bone marrow	5 (13)
Umbilical vein	2 (5)
Unsuccessful	2 (5)

B. *Site Preference*

Any marrow-containing cavity is a potential site for infusion. Many locations have been used successfully, including the sternum, the greater trochanter, the distal femur, the tibial tuberosity, the medial and lateral malleoli, and the os calcis. The sternum was initially the most popular site in adults, because it is easily accessible. In addition, its thin cortex and abundant marrow make insertion easy. However, sternal puncture may also produce a number of serious complications. The proximity of the underlying pleura and great vessels is a potential cause of disaster (tension pneumothorax and vascular rupture). Additionally, a sternal needle may interfere with effective chest compression during cardiopulmonary resuscitation. A less dangerous and usually more easily accessible site is the tibial (medial) malleolus (Fig. 17–3). The cortex of the bone and the overlying tissue are both thin. Used frequently for intraosseous venography,[19,20] it is now the site of choice in adults. In children under 6 years of age and in infants, the locations

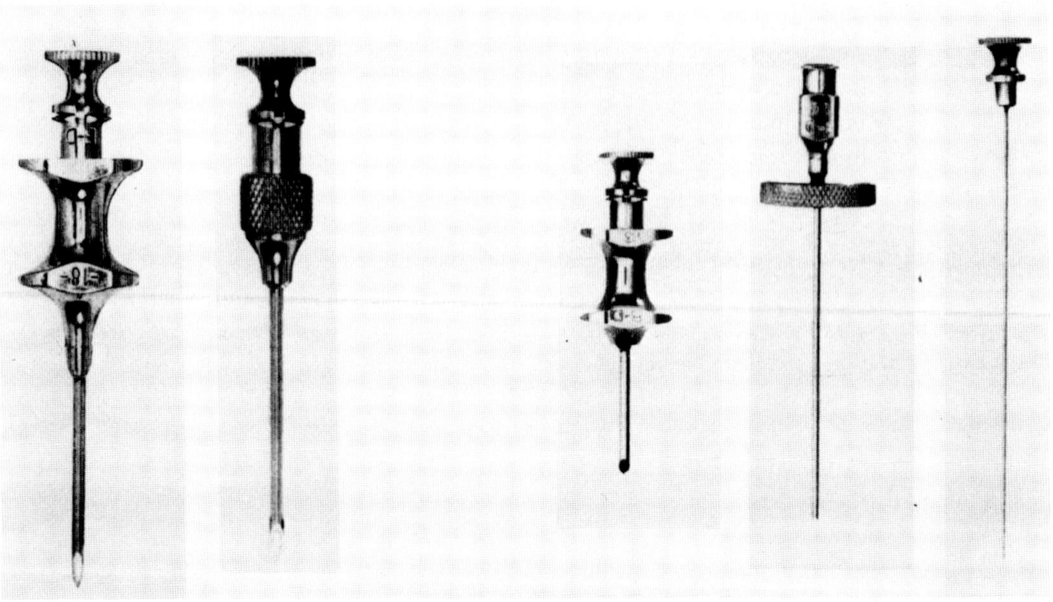

Figure 17–2 • Needles used for bone marrow infusion. *Left panel:* The Rosenthal and Osgood bone marrow aspiration needles with stylets. *Right panel:* The special sternal bone marrow infusion needle with its trephine-type inner cannula and stylet. The short needle is placed into the periosteum, and the trephine inner cannula is used to drill through the cortex. The short needle is then pushed through the hole into the marrow cavity.

of choice are the proximal tibia and, far less commonly, the distal femur. The proximal tibia is selected because it has a broad, flat surface with a thin layer of skin covering the bone (Fig. 17–4). After 6 years of age, the proximal tibia becomes much thicker and harder to penetrate. The distal femur is a large bone in which to insert a needle, but because of the overlying muscles and fat, it is sometimes difficult to palpate bony landmarks. With all bones in all children, care should be taken to avoid the epiphyseal plates.

C. *The Procedure*

Under most circumstances, this procedure should be performed simply and expeditiously. The skin at the site of puncture is wiped with alcohol. The skin and the periosteum may be anesthetized with lidocaine, although in obtunded or moribund patients this is not necessary.

In adults, a site approximately 2 cm proximal to the tip of the medial malleolus is selected, with the

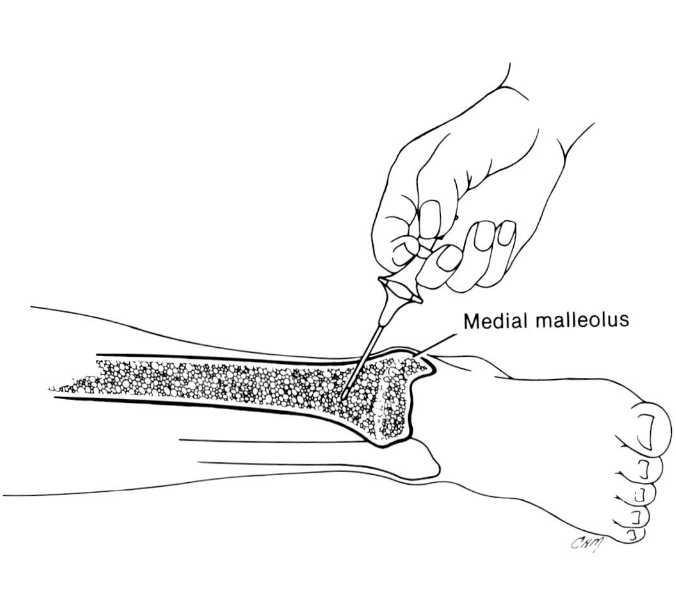

Figure 17–3 • A diagrammatic representation of intramedullary needle placement in the tibial malleolus of an adult. The needle is placed 2–3 cm proximal to the medial malleolus and is directed slightly cephalad. Confirmation of intramedullary placement is obtained by aspiration of blood or marrow with a syringe.

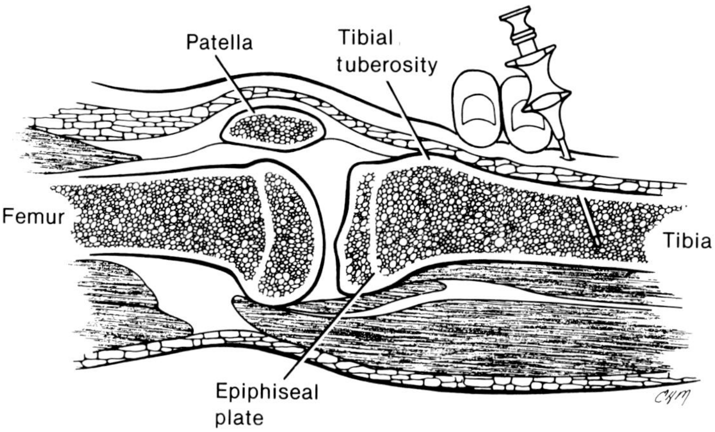

Figure 17–4 • A diagrammatic representation of intramedullary needle placement in infants and children. A point 2 cm (two fingerbreadths) below the tibial tuberosity is selected. The needle is directed distally to avoid the epiphyseal growth plate.

needle directed slightly cephalad (see Fig. 17–3). Firm pressure and a back-and-forth rotary motion are used to push the needle through the skin and the bony cortex. Entrance into the marrow cavity is indicated by a loss of resistance.

In infants and children, the proximal tibia should be used. The point of entry on the flat anteromedial surface of the tibia is the intersection between a vertical line halfway between the tibial tuberosity and medial border of the tibia and a horizontal line 2 cm below the cartilaginous tibial tubercle. The needle should be directed slightly distally (between 0° to 30° from the perpendicular), away from the epiphyseal line, and with the bevel pointing away from the joint space (see Fig. 17–4). A back-and-forth rotary motion is applied until there is a slight decrease in resistance, indicating that the cortex of the bone has been punctured. The needle usually does not need to be advanced further.

Once a loss of resistance is felt, the needle will feel firmly fixed by the bone at this point and will sustain an erect posture without support, and removal of the stylet will usually allow free flow of blood from the needle. One obtains confirmation of position by freely aspirating blood or marrow contents into the syringe. Aspiration may be uncomfortable for the awake patient. The syringe should be flushed with fluid, and a continuous infusion should be begun or the stylet replaced before clotting can occur. Standard intravenous tubing is used to connect the marrow needle to the intravenous bag or bottle. Although gravity drainage may suffice for many infusions, pressurized infusions (by use of a blood pump or a syringe and stopcock system) may be needed during resuscitation to increase the flow rate. The needle should be fixed by the bone firmly enough to remain secure with only a sterile dressing. Intraosseous infusions should be discontinued as soon as venous access has been established.

The distance from the skin through the cortex is rarely more than 1 centimeter in an infant or child, and penetration to this depth is usually adequate. One of the most common mistakes is to advance the needle through the opposite side of the bone (Fig. 17–5B). This can best be avoided by holding the needle in the palm of the hand with the index finger approximately 1 centimeter from the bevel of the needle to avoid pushing it past this mark. Another method is to use a needle with a preset plastic depth indicator on the shaft. If a standard hypodermic or phlebotomy needle was used (no stylet) and it is thought to be obstructed by bone (not embedded in either the distal or proximal cortex sides of the marrow space), then introducing a smaller hypodermic needle into the intraosseous needle will clear the intraosseous needle.

Occasionally one may encounter difficulty in penetrating the cortex or aspirating marrow (Fig. 17–5A). If penetration is difficult, another site, such as the lateral malleolus or the more proximal tibia, should be chosen. Rarely, if the needle does not fit snugly into the cortex (Fig. 17–5C) or if a previous cortical puncture site is nearby (Fig. 17–5D), fluid may escape out of the medullary cavity and infiltrate surrounding tissue. This is remedied by firm external pressure over the bone at the leak site or by replacement of the needle at another site. In other rare cases, as with cardiac arrest or when using an 18 or 20 gauge needle, it may be difficult to aspirate marrow contents. In these cases, if the needle is firmly in place, indicating it has penetrated the cortex, 2 or 3 mL of sterile saline solution may be infused slowly while

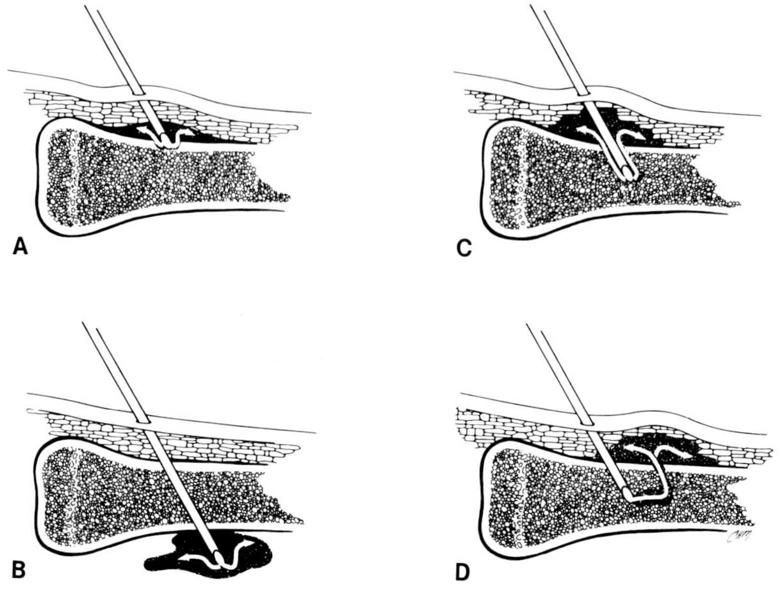

Figure 17–5 • A schematic diagram of possible problems encountered with intraosseous infusions. (***A***) Incomplete penetration of the boney cortex. (***B***) Penetration of the posterior cortex. (***C***) Fluid escaping around the needle through the puncture site. (***D***) Fluid leaking through a nearby previous cortical puncture site.

palpating the limb for extravasation. When fluid is infused by syringe or a hand-pump squeeze chamber, there is normally a slight resistance similar to that felt when filling a balloon with fluid. If significant resistance is met, the bevel of the needle may not have penetrated the cortex or may be lodged against the opposite cortex. If extravasation occurs, the needle should be withdrawn and the bone not used as a site for further infusion.

IV. Discussion

The ability of the bone marrow to accept an infusion of fluids and drugs with subsequent effects like those of an intravenous injection has been well documented. The explanation for the apparent "intravenous injection" is found in anatomic and radiographic studies that demonstrate a rich venous drainage from the bone marrow.[19–21] The marrow of long bones contains a spacious network of venous sinusoids that drain into large central medullary venous channels and then, by way of nutrient or emissary veins, into the systemic venous system (Fig. 17–6).[21] Radiopaque dye, even when injected forcefully into the marrow, rarely spreads more than a few centimeters before rapidly entering the venous circulation.[19] In essence, the bone marrow is a noncollapsible vein.

A review of the literature reveals that a number of fluids, including blood, plasma, saline, and dextrose solutions, have been infused into the bone marrow of adults, children, and even premature infants.[1–12] Infusions have been carried out for various lengths of time and at various flow rates, sometimes resulting in a very large volume of infused fluid (more than 42 L).[13] In sheep, normal saline could be infused at an average rate of 2400 mL/hour through a 13 gauge intramedullary needle under an infusion pressure of 300 mmHg.[22] Average flow rates of 600 mL/hour were achieved by gravity infusion. Flow rates of 11 mL/min with gravity, and 24 mL/min with 300 mmHg pressure have been demonstrated in hypovolemic puppies with a 20

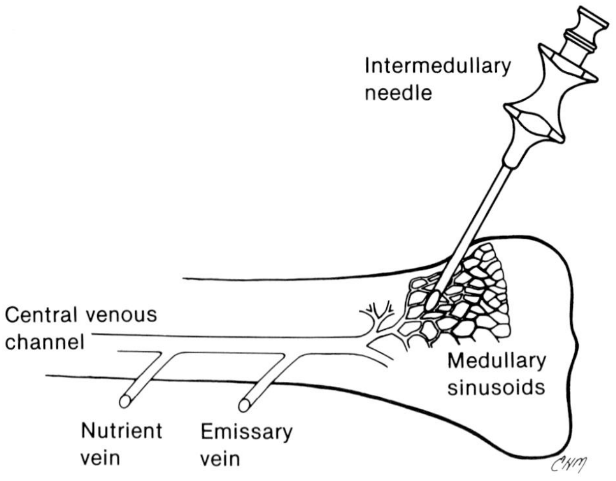

Figure 17–6 • A schematic diagram illustrating the venous drainage from the marrow of a long bone with an intramedullary needle in place.

gauge needle.[23] Similar flow rates can be achieved in humans.[7,24]

Intraosseously infused tracer substances and vasoactive drugs produce effects nearly identical to those of an intravenous injection. In an infant, the hemodynamic response to tibial tuberosity dopamine and dobutamine infusion was immediate.[25] In sheep, the hemodynamic response to intramedullary epinephrine and ephedrine is as rapid as after intravenous injection.[22] Indocyanine green dye injected into the medullary cavity of a dog, also in ventricular fibrillation but receiving internal cardiac massage, can reach the left atrium in less than 15 seconds during internal cardiac massage (Rogers and Benumof, unpublished data). Congo red injected into the tibia of the rabbit appears in the right ventricle within 10 seconds.[2] Other investigators have compared the intraosseus and intravenous injection of drugs and demonstrated that they result in similar blood levels.[26,27] Intraosseous infusion is also effective with closed-chest cardiac massage. Blood pH increases more after intraosseous sodium bicarbonate infusion than with sodium bicarbonate injected intravenously in animals during cardiopulmonary resuscitation.[28] Serum levels of drugs administered by the intraosseous route tend to be elevated longer than when administered intravenously, indicating that there may be a depot effect in the marrow cavity. This effect is minor and should not change the dose of the drug. Drugs should be given in the same dose as with the intravenous route; fluids are given at the same rate. One method to improve the transport of drugs from the marrow cavity is to follow the drug injection with a 10-mL injection of saline solution. This is particularly useful in case of cardiac arrest, when external chest compressions are used to circulate blood. The saline may force the drug out of the marrow cavity into the venous system of the legs, where it can be transported to the central circulation.[28]

V. COMPLICATIONS

The reported complication rate is low and consists mainly of minor incidents. The most common problem is the inability to enter the marrow cavity. Either the cavity is not penetrated or, more commonly, the needle is accidentally forced through the opposite side of the bone. Extravasation of fluid around the puncture site is a minor but frequently reported problem. This is most commonly seen with pressure infusion or long-term use of intraosseous infusion. If the extravasated fluid is crystalloid, this is usually no problem. If it is sodium bicarbonate or another potentially cytotoxic agent, the infusion should be stopped or slowed to minimize the extravasation and pressure should be applied to the site. Extravasation may occur at any site where there has been a break in the cortex. For this reason, intraosseous infusion is not recommended in a bone that is fractured or has holes in the cortex from unsuccessful attempts.

A few cases of osteomyelitis secondary to intraosseous infusions have been reported.[29] In most of these cases, sepsis combined with difficulty in needle placement or prolonged infusion probably contributed to the complication. Papper reported the postoperative death of a patient who received a sternal bone marrow infusion intraoperatively.[5] Postmortem examination revealed 2 L of 5% dextrose in the pleural spaces (an example of the dangers of sternal puncture). The much-feared complication of fat embolization has not been reported, even with pressurized high-volume infusions.[29,30] The reason for the lack of this complication in children is that the pediatric bone marrow is relatively fat free. Similarly, damage to the epiphyseal plate is another concern, although there has never been a reported case caused by intraosseous infusion.

VI. REFERENCES

1. Tocantins LM. Rapid absorption of substances injected into the bone marrow. Proc Soc Exp Biol Med 45:292, 1940.
2. Tocantins LM, O'Neill JF. Infusion of blood and other fluids into the circulation via the bone marrow. Proc Soc Exp Biol Med 45:782, 1940.
3. Tocantins LM, O'Neill JF. Infusions of blood and other fluids into the general circulation via the bone marrow. Surg Gynecol Obstet 73:281, 1941.
4. Tocantins LM, O'Neill JF, Jones HW. Infusions of blood and other fluids via the bone marrow. JAMA 117:1229, 1941.
5. Papper EM. The bone marrow route for injecting fluid and drugs into the general circulation. Anesthesiology 3:307, 1942.
6. Papper EM, Rovenstine EA. Utility of marrow cavity of sternum for parenteral fluid therapy. War Medicine 2:177, 1942.
7. Arbeiter HI, Greengard J. Tibial bone marrow infusions in infancy. J Pediatr 25:1, 1944.
8. Behr G. Bone-marrow infusions for infants. Lancet 2:472, 1944.
9. Dowd EA, Pysell JE. Massive intramedullary infusions. JAMA 120:1212, 1942.
10. Reisman HA, Tansky IA. Bone marrow as alternate route of transfusion in pediatrics. Am J Dis Child 68:253, 1944.
11. Meola F. Bone marrow infusions as routine procedures in children. J Pediatr 25:13, 1944.

12. Elston JT, Jaynes RV, Kaump DH, Irwin WA. Intraosseous infusion in infants. Am J Clin Pathol 17:143, 1947.
13. Valdes MM. Intraosseous fluid administration in emergencies. Lancet i:1235, 1977.
14. Kanter RK, Zimmerman JJ, Strauss RH, Stoeckel KA. Pediatric emergency intravenous access. Am J Dis Child 140:132–134, 1986.
15. Randolph J. Technique for insertion of plastic catheter into saphenous vein. Pediatrics 24:631–637, 1959.
16. Swanson RS. Emergency intravenous access through the femoral vein. Ann Emerg Med 13:244–247, 1984.
17. Berg RA. Emergency infusion of catecholamines into bone marrow. Am J Dis Child 138:810–811, 1984.
18. Chameides L, Melker R, Raye JR, et al. Resuscitation of infants and children. In McIntyre KM, Lewis AJ (eds). Textbook of Advanced Cardiac Life Support. Dallas, American Heart Association, 1983, 255–272.
19. Begg AC. Intraosseous venography of the lower limb and pelvis. Br J Radiol 27:218, 1954.
20. Kwaan JHM, Jones RN, Connolly JE. Simplified technique for the management of refractory varicose ulcers. Surgery 80:743, 1976.
21. Root WS. The flow of blood through bones and joints. In Hamilton WF (ed). Handbook of Physiology. Vol. 2. Baltimore, Williams & Wilkins, 1966, 1651–1655.
22. Shoor PM, Berryhill RE, Benumof JL. Intraosseous infusion: Pressure-flow relationship in pharmacokinetics. J Trauma 19:772, 1979.
23. Hodge D, Delgado-Paredes C, Fleischer G. Intraosseous infusion flow rates in hypovolemic "pediatric" dogs. Ann Emerg Med 16:305–307, 1987.
24. Iserson KV, Criss E. Intraosseous infusions: A usable technique. Am J Emerg Med 4:540–542, 1986.
25. Berg RA. Emergency infusion of catecholamine into bone marrow. Am J Dis Child 138:810–811, 1987.
26. Prete MR, Hannan CJ, Burkle FM. Plasma atropine concentrations via the intravenous, endotracheal and intraosseous routes of administration. Ann Emerg Med 15:195, 1986.
27. Spivey WH, Unger HD, Lathers DM, et al. Intraosseous diazepam suppression of pentylenetetrazol-induced epileptogenic activity in pigs. Ann Emerg Med 16:156–159, 1987.
28. Spivey WH, Lathers CM, Malone DR, et al. Comparison of intraosseous, central, and peripheral routes of sodium bicarbonate administration during CPR in pigs. Ann Emerg Med 14:1135–1140, 1985.
29. O'Neill JF. Complications of intraosseous therapy. Ann Surg 2:266, 1945.
30. Bisgard JD, Baker C. Experimental fat embolism. Am J Surg 47:466, 1940.

Chapter 18

Frederick G. Mihm, MD
Myer H. Rosenthal, MD

Central Venous Catheterization

OUTLINE

I. Introduction

Although considerable attention was directed toward the importance of right atrial pressure monitoring during the latter half of the nineteenth century in experimental laboratory environments, it was not until the 1950s and 1960s that the application of the principles governing the adequacy of cardiac function led to the monitoring of central venous pressure (CVP) as an indicator of intravascular volume, preload, and cardiac performance.[1-3] Also at this time, however, the shortcomings of this monitoring technique became evident as investigators realized that assessment of right heart filling pressure often provided erroneous data regarding the more frequently occurring left heart dysfunction.[4,5] Such knowledge soon led to the common practice of pulmonary artery catheterization to monitor left ventricular filling pressure.

Table 18-1 • Indications for Central Venous Catheterization

Monitoring
Transvenous pacemaker placement
Parenteral nutrition
Drug administration
Lack of peripheral venous access
Rapid fluid resuscitation
Aspiration for venous air embolism
Emergency dialysis

Common to both left and right heart filling pressure assessment is the need for central venous access. The past 30 years have witnessed a dramatic, if not excessive, increase in central venous cannulation as peripheral access from the femoral, basilic, and cephalic veins has been superseded by more central routes, notably subclavian and internal jugular veins. Advantages of more direct access, which is unencumbered by valves, angles, long catheter length, and greater patency in low volume states, has caused these newer approaches to nearly totally replace the use of peripheral veins. However, the risks of pneumothorax and arterial laceration with hemorrhage are far greater using these central approaches. Increased orientation toward doing procedures, and a multitude of perceived indications by acute care medical personnel, have made central venous access one of the most common procedures performed in the hospital setting.

II. INDICATIONS

Indications for central venous access are listed in Table 18–1.[6] It is immediately obvious that monitoring of cardiac preload certainly does not account for all the central venous catheterizations performed. Indeed, if one totals those catheterizations done for volume, drug, and nutritional infusions, they would likely account for a significant majority. All of the indications for central venous access listed in Table 18–1 except the last two can be discussed under the headings of monitoring (different functions and types) and infusions (different types).

A. *Monitoring*

Central venous access is required or preferred for a number of monitoring functions. Frank, Starling, and later others described the relationship of preload as right atrial pressure to ventricular output.[7] Later McMichael expanded this concept to a family of curves relating preload to ventricular output with varying myocardial contractility.[8] Figure 18–1 shows these relationships. Whereas preload is an indication of ventricular end-diastolic fiber length, it is the end-diastolic volume that defines preload. For monitoring purposes the end-diastolic pressure correlate of this volume is used. Thus, central venous pressure—being almost equal to right atrial pressure, which in turn approximates right ventricular end-diastolic pressure—becomes the monitor of right heart preload in the absence of tricuspid outflow obstruction. The limitation of CVP assessment for cardiac preload was identified by Sarnoff and Berglund in pointing to the discrepancy in preload evaluation of the right and left sides of the heart.[9] Inherent differences in compliance due to the different thicknesses of the two ventricular walls are shown in Fig. 18–2, and the effects of this on the Starling relationship for the normal heart in Fig. 18–3. Awareness of the impact of the difference in the slope of these two curves is vital in evaluating the impact of increased filling pressure on ventricular output (stroke volume) for the two ventricles. A further consideration involves selective heart failure of the right or left side altering the preload to ventricular output relationship individually, which is far more common than in combination. These differences led to the now common practice of flow-directed pulmonary artery catheterization to assess left-sided preload (see Chapter 21). This technique has now been adapted to measure not only left heart filling pressures but also CVP, cardiac output, mixed venous oxygen saturation, and the inclusion of

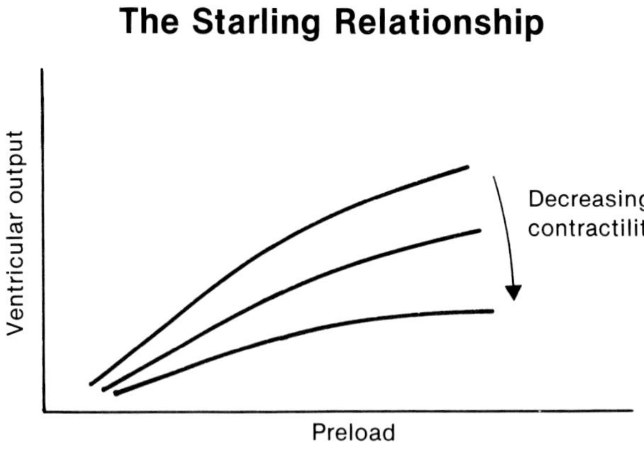

Figure 18–1 • The Starling relationship of preload to ventricular output, demonstrating the effect of altered contractility.

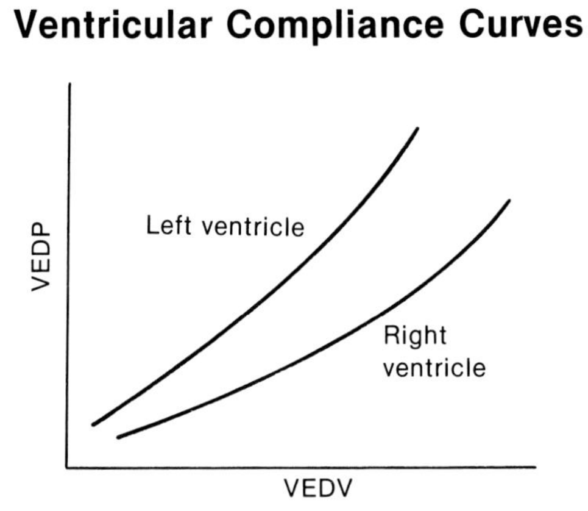

Figure 18–2 • Compliance curves relating ventricular end-diastolic volume (*VEDV*) to ventricular end-diastolic pressure (*VEDP*).

atrial and ventricular pacing. Experimental evaluations are presently underway for the eventual monitoring of electrolytes and other substances (eg, lactic acid) with adapted pulmonary artery catheters. Further monitoring options requiring central venous access include the need for systemic vascular resistance determination, as shown in the equation below:

$$SVR = \frac{MAP - CVP}{CO} \times 80$$

and for the placement of intracardiac electrocardiographic (ECG) leads for identification, differentiation, and treatment of dysrhythmias.

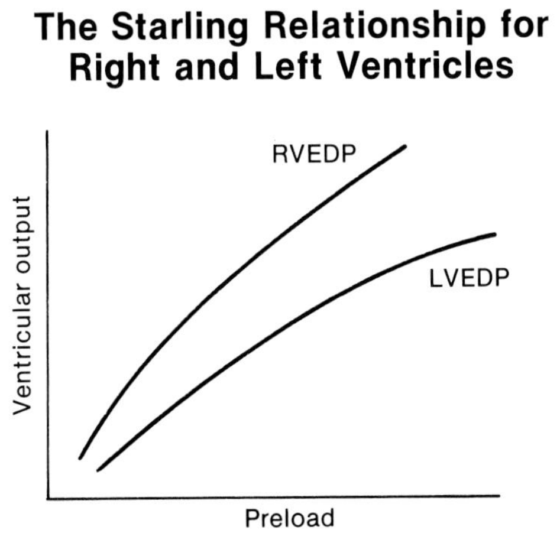

Figure 18–3 • The Starling relationship of preload to ventricular output for the two sides of the heart, using right ventricular end-diastolic pressure (*RVEDP*) and left ventricular end-diastolic pressure (*LVEDP*) as estimates of right and left ventricular preload, respectively.

Earlier CVP monitoring commonly used water-filled manometers and assessed CVP in centimeters of water (cmH_2O) with normal values of 6 to 12. Recently, greater use of electric transducers has provided for improved accuracy in assessing mean pressure as compared to higher readings using the water manometer. Transduced measurement of CVP is read as millimeters of mercury (mmHg) with a normal range of 5 to 10. Further advantages include greater speed and interpretation of waveforms. For example, examination of the central venous waveform as shown in Fig. 18–4 can assist in assessing tricuspid valvular competency as well as interpreting the value of the CVP in the face of altered "a" or "cv" waves, relating to valvular stenosis or insufficiency.

B. Infusions

Central venous access is preferred and often required for large-volume infusions, hyperosmolal nutritional support, potent vasoactive drug administration, and the infusion of a variety of medications and solutions whose potential for irritation and inflammation would result in phlebitis if smaller veins with less intrinsic dilution capability were to be selected. The risk of severe ischemia due to the administration of medications with vasoconstrictor activity requires the use of large-diameter veins with high blood flow. These agents include norepinephrine, epinephrine, dopamine, phenylephrine, metaraminol, and vasopressin. Sclerosis of veins appears to be related to the osmolality of the solution infused. Those with higher osmolality should be administered into more central veins, whose large diameter permits increased dilution. Examples of such solutions include 8.4% sodium bicarbonate (2000 mOsm/L), 10% calcium chloride (2096 mOsm/L), 50% dextrose (2525 mOsm/L), and 2 mEq/mL potassium chloride (4000 mOsm/L). Solutions prepared for hyperalimentation also are likely to be hyperosmolar, the degree greatly dependent on the dextrose concentration. A solution of 4.25% crystalline amino acids with 25% dextrose will have an osmolality of 1675 mOsm/L, while a similar amino acid solution mixed with 10% dextrose will be 925 mOsm/L. It is advisable to restrict peripheral infusions to those solutions with osmolality less than 400 to 450 mOsm/L to minimize the risk of severe sclerosis and phlebitis.

Central venous catheterization is also necessary when peripheral venous access is unavailable. This may

Central Venous Pressure Tracings

Normal

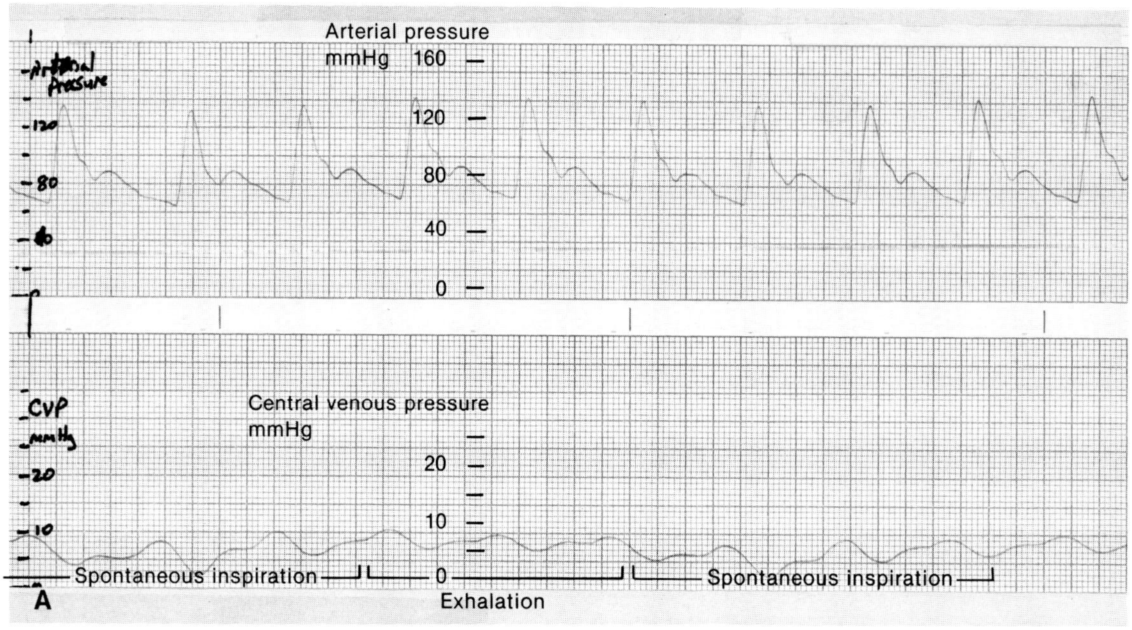

Tricuspid regurgitation

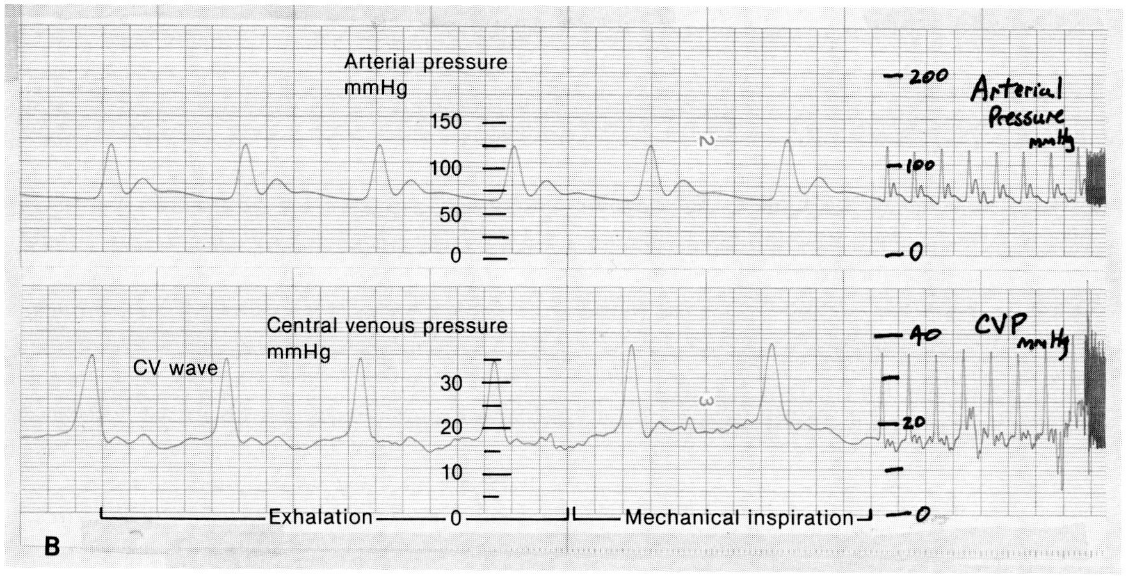

Figure 18–4 • Central venous and systemic arterial pressure tracings in a normal patient and a patient with tricuspid insufficiency. (***A***) Normal patient has both a normal central venous pressure waveform (ie, no pathologic a or cv wave greater than 5 mmHg above the baseline) and a normal mean central venous pressure (*CVP*). This patient is quietly breathing spontaneously, and during inspiration the CVP tracing falls slightly. Measured in exhalation, the correct mean CVP is 7–8 mmHg. (***B***) Patient with both an abnormal pressure waveform and an abnormally elevated CVP. This patient is anesthetized, paralyzed, and receiving positive pressure ventilation without PEEP. The effect of intermittent transmitted positive airway pressure is demonstrated by the modest rise of the waveform during inspiration, as indicated. The tracing is abnormal because of a pathologic 34 mmHg cv wave seen to appear at the onset of ventricular systole. The mean CVP is 15 mmHg if the cv wave is ignored, as it should be to assess ventricular filling pressure in diastole. (Compare this cv wave from tricuspid regurgitation to the pathologic cv wave seen with mitral regurgitation in Fig. 21–12. The cv wave of mitral regurgitation is delayed in appearance compared to the cv wave of tricuspid regurgitation, because the pulmonary artery catheter is some distance from the left atrium while the central venous catheter is very close to the right atrium.)

apply to clinically stable patients who, because of their anatomy (eg, obesity), long-term hospitalization, or burns, have simply "run out" of accessible peripheral veins. In emergencies, patients may present in shock, needing immediate fluid resuscitation. Central venous access has proven useful in these situations for rapid fluid administration as well.[10,11]

C. *Aspiration for Venous Air Embolism*

Central venous catheters are useful therapeutically to treat venous air embolism if it occurs during various neurosurgical, orthopedic, or cardiovascular procedures, or as a result of a disconnection of the central venous catheter. Air aspiration from the catheter not only provides specific confirmation of the diagnosis, but may be crucial in preventing or relieving right ventricular outflow obstruction. Early aspiration of air via the catheter may also minimize the likelihood of right ventricular strain and elevated right atrial pressures that encourage the chances for paradoxical air embolism through a probe-patent foramen ovale.[12]

D. *Emergency Dialysis*

Large-bore double-lumen catheters placed traditionally in the subclavian or femoral veins provide immediate vascular access for patients requiring temporary or emergent hemodialysis or ultrafiltration.[13] Successful experience with this technique has virtually eliminated the need for arteriovenous fistulas (eg, Scribner shunt) where long-term dialysis is not anticipated.

III. How to Do Central Venous Catherization of the Central Venous Access Sites

A. *Localization*

Standard insertion sites for placement of a central venous catheter include internal and external jugular, subclavian, femoral, and basilic veins (Fig. 18–5). These are the same sites from which venous access can be achieved for pulmonary artery catheterization. Factors such as anatomy, systemic or major organ dysfunction such as a coagulopathy, or severe local problems such as edema,

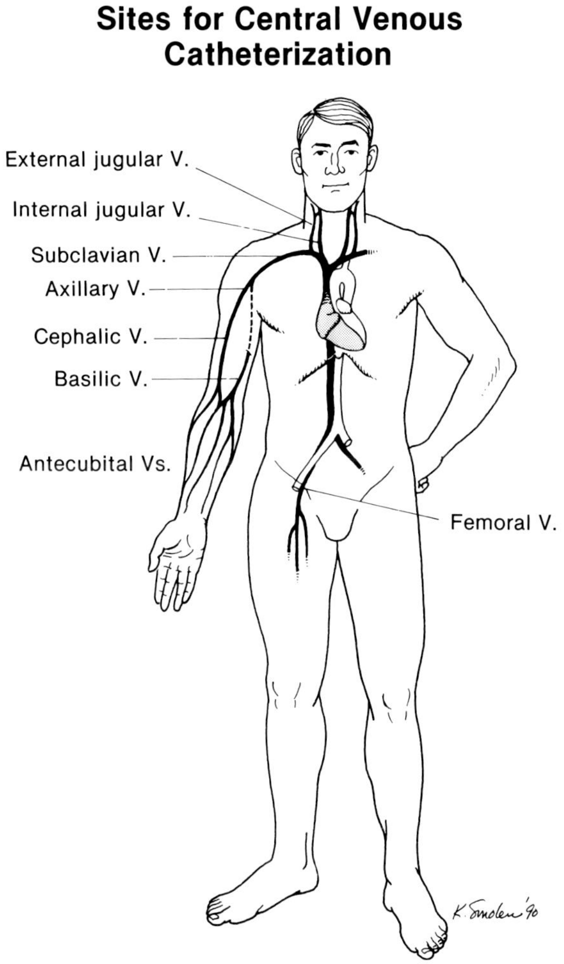

Figure 18–5 • Possible sites for percutaneous central venous access.

skin abrasions, rashes, or infection, dictate the safest site to use for central venous catheterization. For example, patients with respiratory insufficiency or increased intracranial pressure who will not tolerate the Trendelenberg position may be better catheterized using veins that do not require this position (basilic, femoral). For further example, in the presence of a known or suspected coagulapathy, the subclavian vein is less desirable as a catheterization site because any bleeding complication is not visible or controllable by direct compression, as it would be from the other possible sites. Good clinical judgment must be used to choose the most appropriate site for each patient.

1. Internal Jugular Vein

The internal jugular vein lies in the carotid sheath; as it descends the neck towards the clavicle, it changes from a position behind the carotid to a lateral and then an anterolateral position as it passes under the sternocleidomastoid muscle[14] (Fig. 18–6). Its anatomic orientation is remarkably consistent and not altered by prior carotid artery surgery.[15] The internal jugular vein is the most popular site for central venous catheterization. Depending on the needle orientation, the vein can be entered by taking a direction away from both the carotid artery and the pleural space. It is therefore no surprise that the complication rate of arterial puncture and pneumothorax is lower than when a subclavian site is used. It has also been shown to be safe in small children and infants,[16] and also in the presence of a coagulopathy.[17] The right internal jugular vein is the most convenient side because of closeness to the heart; it allows a "straight shot" at the right ventricle (RV), it is slightly larger than the left, the dome of the pleura is lower on the right, and the thoracic duct is on the left.[14] The left internal jugular vein is a good alternative, but provides a slightly more tortuous route for a catheter to traverse to enter the superior vena cava.

2. External Jugular Vein

The external jugular vein drains the superficial veins of the face and around the ear and travels down the side of the neck to eventually join the subclavian vein (see Fig. 18–6). This site is frequently not considered for central venous or PA catheterization, but can be used quite satisfactorily in most patients with a success rate of more than 85% to 95% with either type of catheter.[18–20] This site has also been used successfully in small children.[16] Concerns about valves at the external jugular–subclavian junction, lateral displacement of the catheter into the arm, or existence of a venous plexus are not warranted.[20] This access provides an excellent site for patients with severe coagulopathies, because any bleeding can be easily controlled.

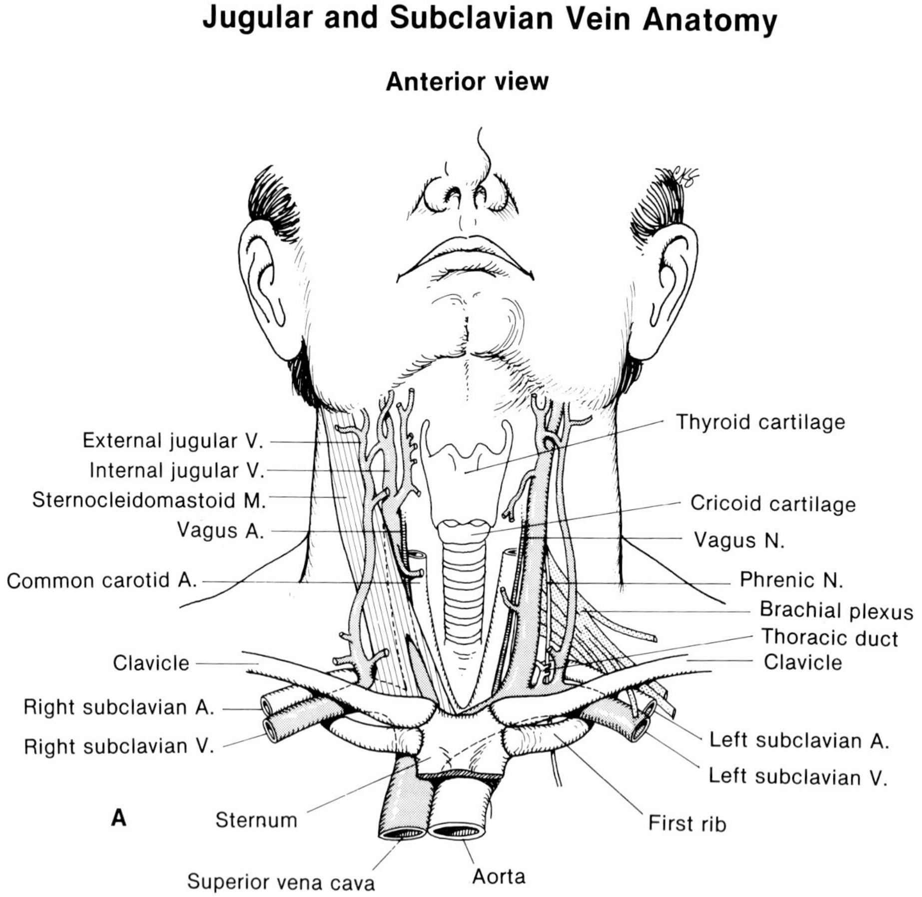

Figure 18–6 • The anatomy of the jugular and subclavian veins. (***A***) Anteroposterior view.

(continued)

3. SUBCLAVIAN VEIN

The subclavian vein is a large central vein of 1–2 cm in diameter running from the axillary vein to the internal jugular vein, which it joins to become the innominate vein (see Fig. 18–6). Behind and slightly above it lies the subclavian artery.[14] The vein maintains a fixed position because it is supported by fibrous tissue that is attached to the first rib, clavicle, and subclavius muscle; for this reason its size may be less affected by hypovolemic states than other venous sites. The catheter can be fixed and dressed on a flat part of the chest wall, thereby decreasing the risk of infection and improving comfort, both factors that may be important when long-term catheterization or total parenteral nutrition is considered. Care should be taken if this site is chosen in patients receiving mechanical ventilation plus PEEP or in patients with chronic obstructive pulmonary disease (COPD) and associated bullous emphysema in the upper lobes of the lung. The right side is preferred to avoid possible thoracic duct injury, which is admittedly rare. Massive hemorrhage may result from subclavian vein puncture in the presence of a coagulopathy (sepsis, hepatic or renal failure); therefore, other sites should be used in these situations. Although initial experience was positive in using this vein for catheterization of infants and small children,[21] subsequent experience suggests a higher complication rate in this age group compared to other sites.[22]

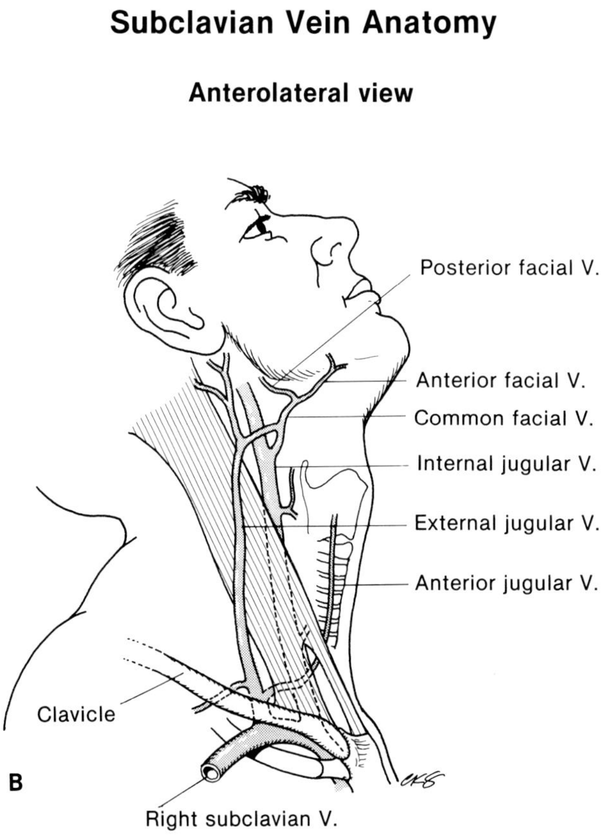

Figure 18–6 *(continued)*
(***B***) Anterolateral view.

4. ANTECUBITAL VEINS

The antecubital veins travel from the antecubital fossa to the axilla, where they eventually join the axillary vein and gain access to the central circulation (Fig. 18–7). An antecubital vein is a viable alternative site when other sites cannot be or have already been used. It is also a good choice in patients with respiratory distress. Central venous catheterization via all arm veins fails in 20% to 40% of attempts because the catheter cannot be negotiated through the axilla;[23] this success rate is significantly worse compared to other sites. However, successful placement via the basilic vein is significantly better (75%–100%) than cephalic vein (55%–80%) catheterizations.[23] Using this location for central venous catheterization presents a unique problem in that arm movement abduction can cause up to 9 cm of catheter movement.[24]

5. FEMORAL VEINS

The femoral veins are the largest veins of the legs and are easily located below the inguinal ligament just beside the femoral artery (Fig. 18–8). This site is also excellent for rapid establishment of venous access for fluid resuscitation of patients in shock, and can be placed even when femoral arterial pulsations are weak or absent.[10,11,25] The femoral veins are an excellent choice for patients in respiratory distress. The main disadvantage to this technique is the increased risk of infection associated with the problem of maintaining sterility at groin venous access sites. This site is not safe in patients with deep venous thrombosis in the lower extremities, or who need long-term catheterization for total parenteral nutrition.

B. Equipment

The materials necessary for percutaneous central venous catheterization vary slightly depending on the sites cho-

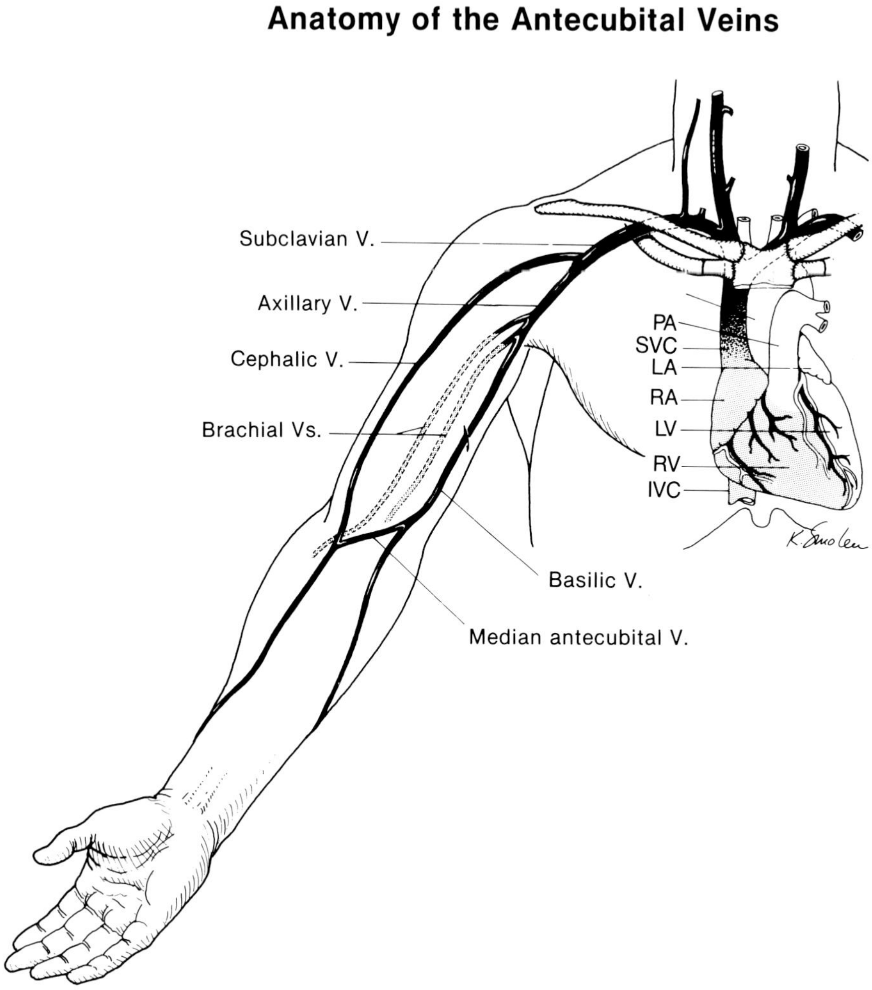

Figure 18–7 • Antecubital vein anatomy and connection to central veins. The basilic vein takes a smoother course through the axilla and into the axillary vein than the cephalic, making it the perferred arm vein for percutaneous catheterization. The brachial veins travel deep to the basilic and are in either side of the brachial artery. These veins are accessible by cutdown if needed.

sen, ie, those veins close to the heart (internal and external jugular, subclavian veins) vs. those veins at some distance from the heart (basilic, femoral veins) (Table 18–2). For the jugular and subclavian veins the Seldinger technique is preferred.[26] This technique permits placement over a guide wire of a catheter that is larger than the needle used to enter the vessel (Fig. 18–9). Besides the standard single-lumen central venous catheter, there are a variety of double- and triple-lumen catheters available that provide extra lumina so that drug infusions, hyperalimentation, and central venous pressure monitoring can be performed simultaneously. There are also special, large-bore, double-lumen catheters for dialysis and introducers for subsequent placement of a pulmonary artery catheter (Fig. 18–10). Although the Seldinger technique could also be used in the femoral and basilic veins, the length of catheter necessary to reach the superior or inferior vena cava would necessitate a guide wire of greater than 100 cm, which can be cumbersome but has been used.[23] The risks of using a larger needle (14–17 gauge) are not a great concern in these peripheral sites; therefore, the traditional catheter-through-the-needle technique is employed. There are several different catheter designs available (Fig. 18–11). There are insufficient comparison studies to conclude that one design is better than another.[27]

C. *Insertion of the Central Venous Catheter*

As with any procedure, prior to central venous catheterization, inform your patient, check vital signs, and assess for anxiety. Reassure and/or sedate and administer oxygen as indicated.

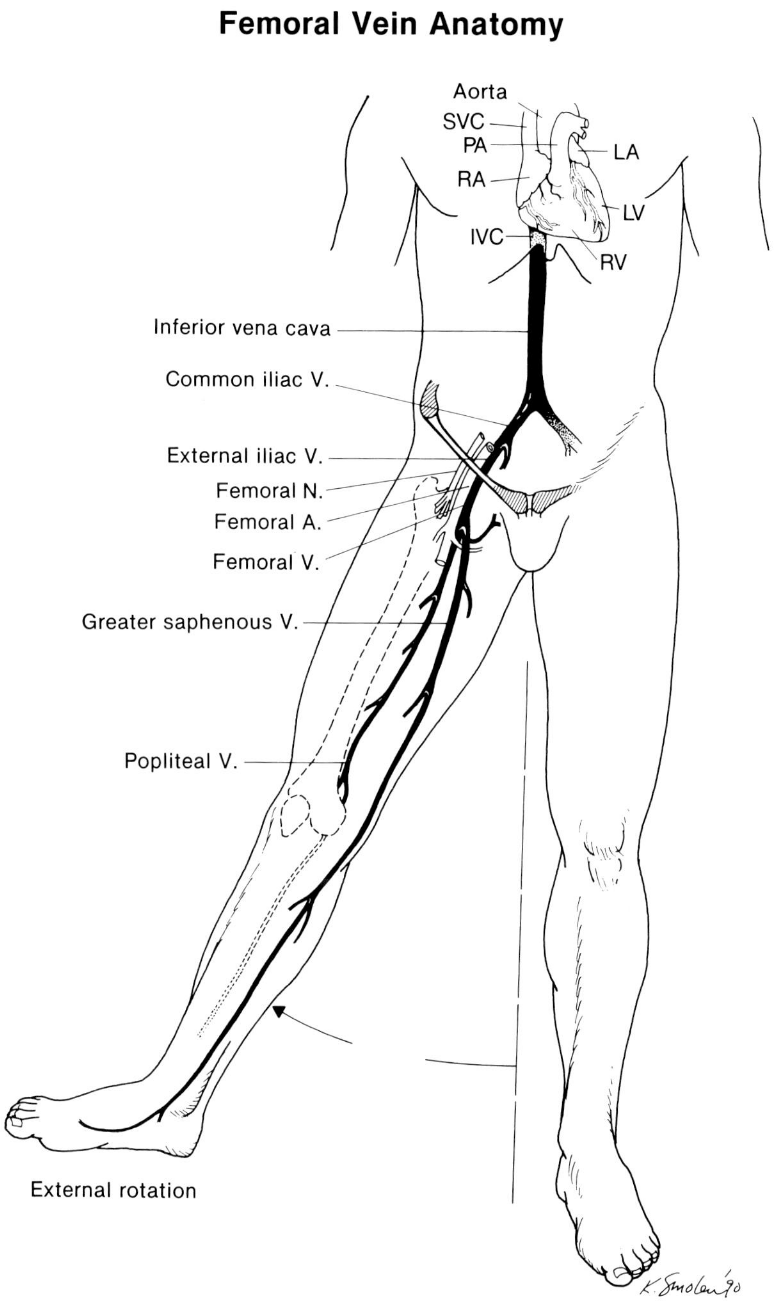

Figure 18–8 • Femoral vein anatomy.

1. Internal Jugular Vein Catheterization

Remove any pillows from behind the head and have the patient turn his or her head away from the side to be used. Supplemental oxygen administration is almost always indicated to support arterial oxygenation and is also a good way to avoid rebreathing of carbon dioxide if the patient's face is to be covered with drapes. The area of insertion should be prepared and draped so that the clavicle, sternal notch, and external jugular vein are visible (Fig. 18–12). Generous exposure of the insertion area will maximize use of superficial landmarks. In addition, exposure of the external jugular vein provides immediate access to this vessel if the internal jugular vein cannot be cannulated. The subclavian vein is also accessible with no need to redrape.

Identify the triangle made by the sternal and clavicular bellies of the sternocleidomastoid muscle and the

Table 18–2 • Equipment for Central Venous Catheterization*

General	
Betadine prep solution 3 Drapes 4 4×4 gauze 5 mL 2% Xylocaine 25 Gauge needle for local anesthetic 3-0 Suture on a straight needle	
Jugular or Subclavian Veins	**Femoral or Antecubital Veins**
Two 5 mL syringes 22 gauge "finder" needle 18 gauge thin-wall needle 0.035 in with "J" 16 gauge 20–30 cm central venous catheter	One 5 mL syringe 16–18 gauge 50–70 cm central venous catheter

*Standard adult-size needles and catheters are listed.

clavicle. There are differences of opinion as to the most appropriate approach to the internal jugular vein in terms of highest success rate and degree of safety. No less than 13 different techniques have been published in the literature[16,28-38] (Fig. 18–13). We prefer the approach that enters the skin more medial than the other "high triangle" approaches, meaning an entry on the lateral edge of the sternal belly of the sternocleidomastoid muscle.[16] The actual point of entry along the lateral edge of this muscle can be easily determined by identifying the fibers from either the opposite clavicular head of the muscle or the level of the cricoid cartilage. From this point of entry, the needle is directed away from the carotid artery and out over the first rib toward the nipple (Fig. 18–14). Other approaches that start lateral to the internal jugular vein require the needle to be directed back at the carotid artery with the expectation of entering the jugular vein first. These are less safe techniques.

Place local anesthetic as a skin wheal high in the triangle (see Fig. 18–14) and infiltrate the subcutaneous tissue with a further 3–5 mL. If there is any question about the adequacy of the analgesic, be generous with the local anesthetic and allow adequate time for it to diffuse and take effect. While the local anesthetic is diffusing, place the patient in the Trendelenburg position. Release the two 5-mL syringe plungers so they do not stick, and attach the 22 gauge finder needle and 18 gauge thinwall needle. Be careful not to jam the thinwall needle too tightly onto its syringe, because once the vein is entered this syringe must be removed in order to pass the guide wire. Have the thinwall needle, syringe, and guide wire within convenient reach so that all attention can be given to the field with minimal distractions.

Place your free hand on the patient's head just above the triangle to remind the patient to keep his or her head still and to provide rest and stability for the syringe as it enters the skin (see Fig. 18–14). Enter the skin with the finder needle while applying slight negative pressure on the syringe plunger. Do not apply too much negative pressure in the syringe because this can cause the vein to collapse when the needle enters it. The finder needle must be passed in a straight line (do not

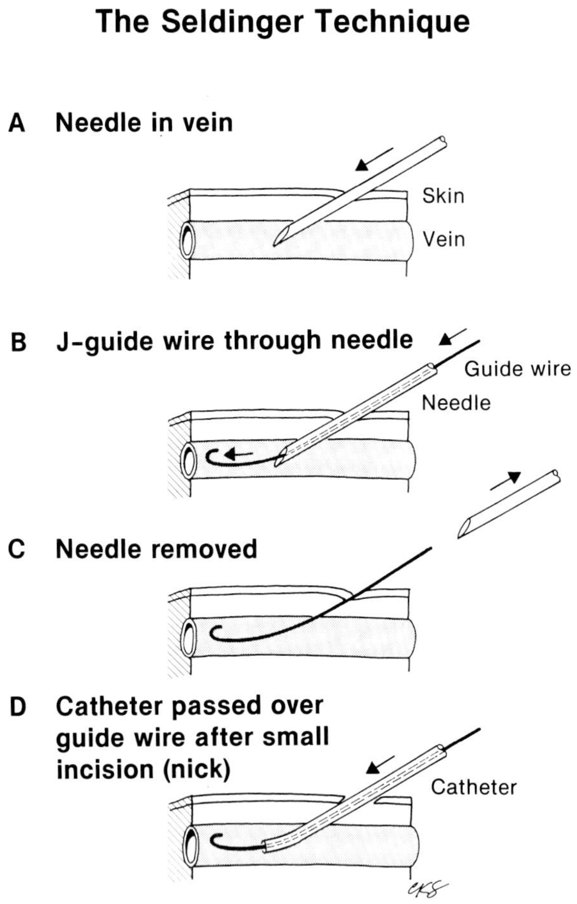

Figure 18–9 • The Seldinger technique for vascular cannulation. (***A***) Step 1: thinwall, narrow-gauge needle placed in vessel. (***B***) Step 2: J-tipped guidewire passed through needle. (***C***) Step 3: needle removed. (***D***) Step 4: catheter passed over guidewire into vessel.

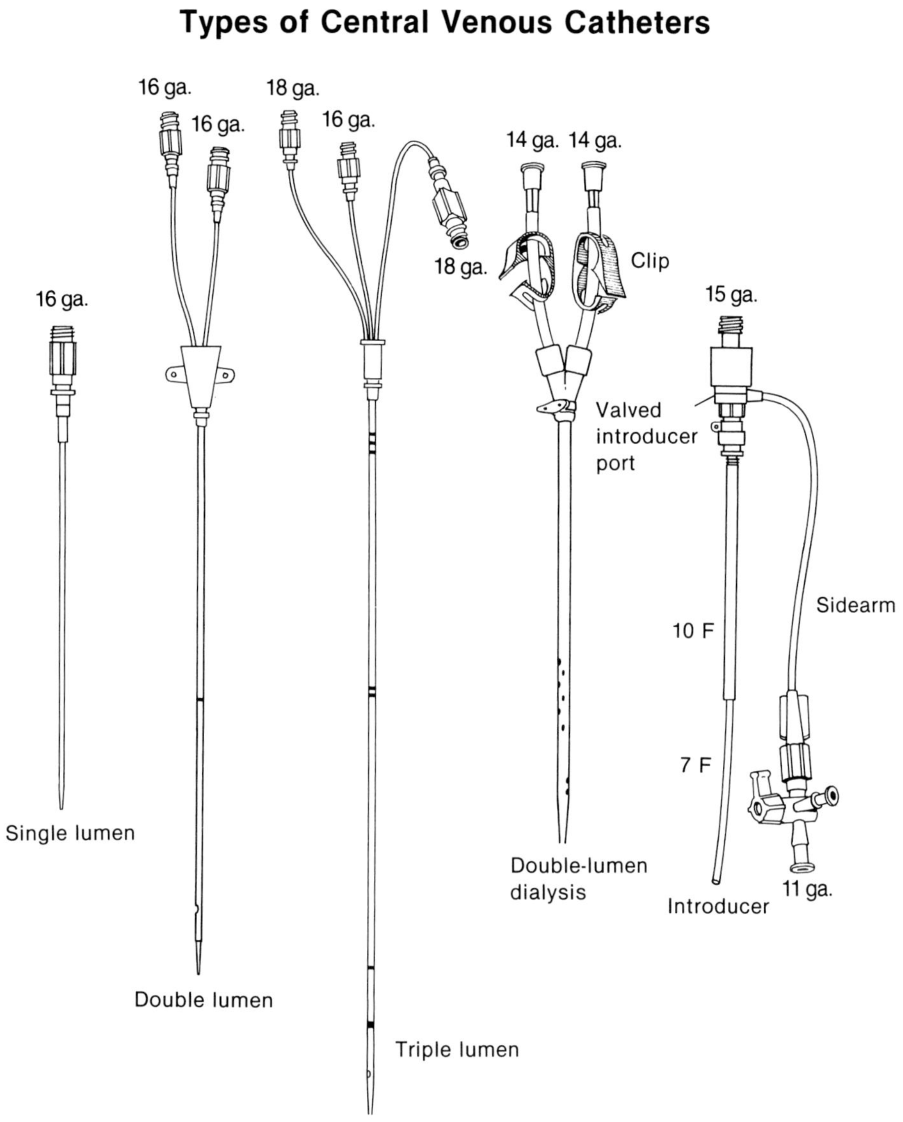

External size				
5 F	7 F	7 F	11 F	10 F/7 F
Length				
6–10 in	8 in	12 in	6 in	4 in/8 in

Figure 18–10 • Various types of central venous catheters in standard adult sizes. The usual, single-lumen 16 gauge catheter is satisfactory for many applications; however, the double- and triple-lumen catheters provide separate lumens for drug infusions, hyperalimentation, and continuous CVP monitoring. The large 11 French double-lumen dialysis catheter is obviously ideal for hemodialysis, if needed, but also is an excellent large-bore catheter for rapid-volume resuscitation. The 10 French introducer can also serve well as a rapid infusion line, and will also accept another central venous catheter through its valved top port, as shown. If the 7 French catheter is removed, this introducer will allow rapid placement of a pulmonary artery catheter when the situation requires it. If rapid infusion is needed, both the 7 French catheter and the sidearm can be removed and one intravenous line connected directly to the introducer.

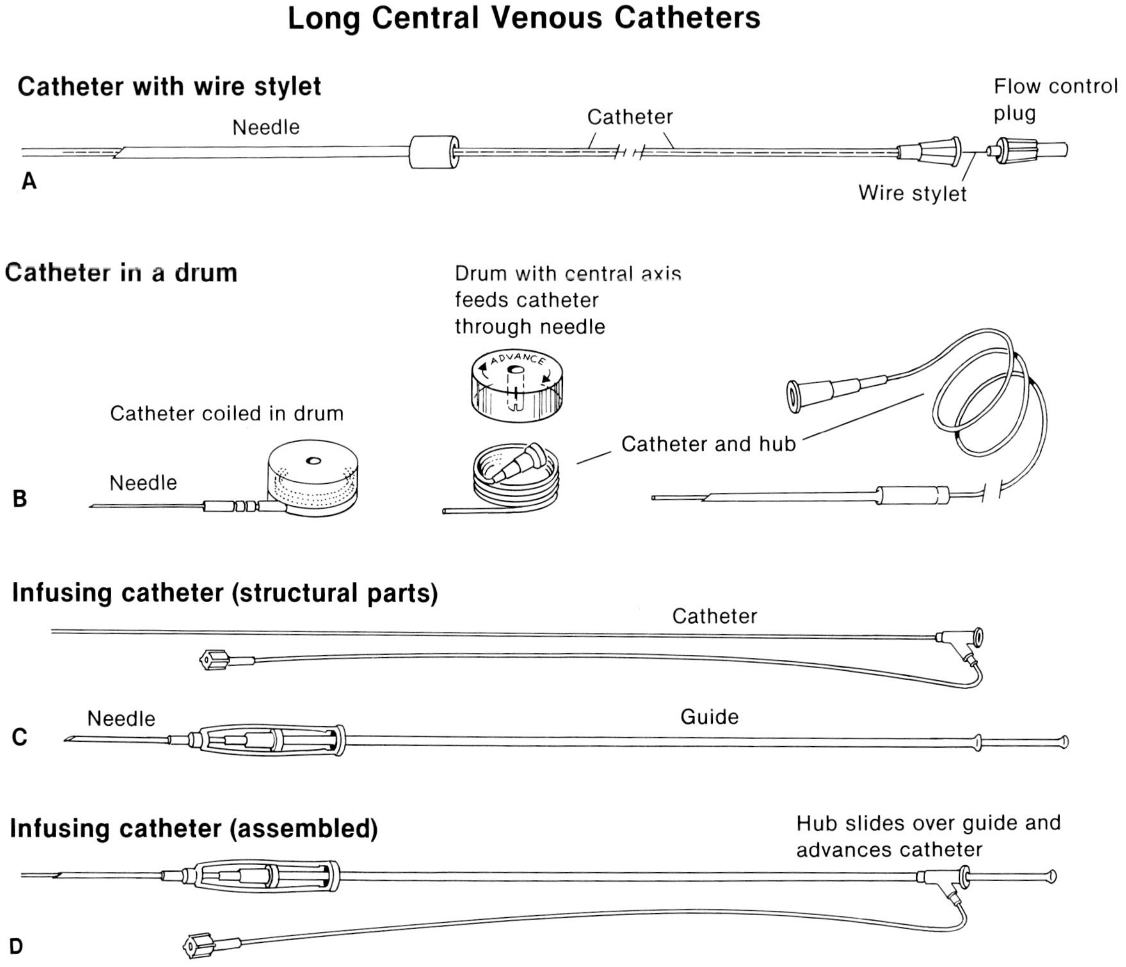

Figure 18–11 • Three types of long (21–28 in) central venous catheters that can be advanced to the vena cava from either the antecubital or the femoral veins. All these catheters are through-the-needle types and are available in various diameters. The standard adult size uses a 14 gauge needle to puncture the vein, through which a 16 gauge catheter is passed. (***A***) The standard catheter is provided with a stiff wire stylet that may or may not help advancement of the catheter. This equipment does allow the operator to easily disconnect the needle from the catheter so that the vein (antecubital or femoral) can be punctured using a syringe on the needle. After the vein is entered, then the syringe can be removed and the catheter passed. (***B***) The catheter coiled in a drum provides a long catheter in a convenient container. After entry into the vein, the catheter is advanced by rotating the drum. This catheter can be separated from its needle for a needle–syringe venous puncture just like the standard catheter. (***C*** and ***D***) The infusing catheter allows infusion of an intravenous solution after vein has been entered and during advancement of the catheter. The infused fluid may dilate the venous lumen ahead of the catheter and thereby enhance catheter passage past valves and tortuous paths of arm veins. This catheter cannot be separated from its needle, like the other two catheters.

zigzag) at a 45° angle with the skin and in the direction of the nipple (see Fig. 18–15). If there is no blood return indicating entry into the vessel, pull back slowly (maintaining slight negative pressure in the syringe), because blood aspiration on needle withdrawal is common. If no blood is obtained, pull the needle back to just beneath the skin and redirect slightly more medially. Check for needle patency after every two to three passes. If the vessel cannot be located with repeated probes, move lower in the triangle and try again or use the external jugular vein.

When blood is aspirated, observe carefully both the orientation and the depth of the finder needle (see Fig. 18–15), then remove the needle, lay it down, pick

Draping for Internal Jugular Cannulation

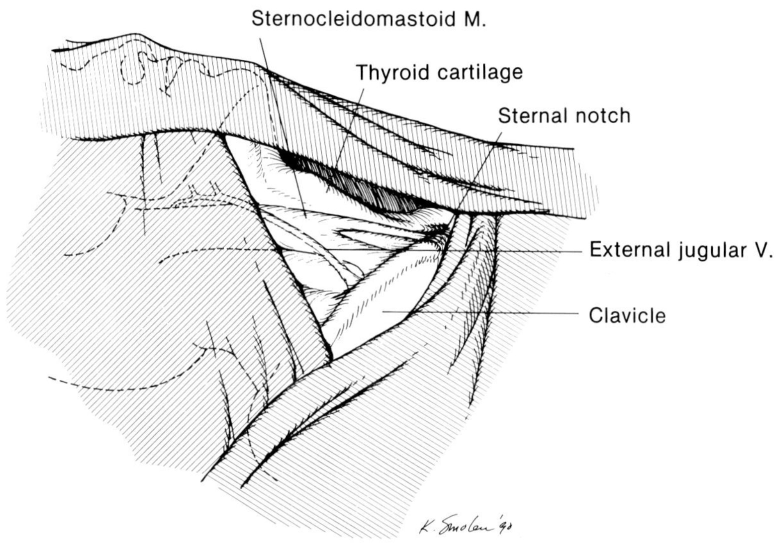

Figure 18–12 • Draping for internal jugular cannulation. Wide exposure prevents loss of valuable visual anatomic landmarks. With this draping procedure, both the external jugular and subclavian veins are also adequately exposed, thus avoiding unnecessary delays if they need to be used.

up the thinwall needle and syringe, and repeat the needle location of the jugular vein. Keep your hand on the field to remind the patient to keep his or her head still and to remind you where you are going! Remember that the thinwall needle is longer than the finder needle. When blood is reaspirated through the thinwall needle, the syringe can be tilted slightly downward to orient the needle in the direction of the vein and encourage proper passage of the guide wire toward the heart (Fig. 18–16).

When the thinwall needle has been oriented correctly, secure and hold the needle perfectly still, disconnect the syringe, and pass the guide wire through the thinwall needle.

The guide wire should pass through the thinwall needle without resistance and no force should be used. If it does not pass easily, withdraw the guide wire and recheck for free aspiration of blood. Reposition the needle if necessary to obtain freer aspiration of blood and attempt to repass the guide wire. When the guide wire does pass without resistance, be careful not to pass the guide wire too far beyond 20–25 cm and thereby cause cardiac dysrhythmias.

Remove the thinwall needle and pass the central venous access catheter over the wire. Do not introduce the catheter into the skin unless the guide wire extends outside the proximal end of the catheter. If the catheter is 14 gauge or larger, it is usually necessary to make a small skin incision (nick) for the catheter to pass through the skin. However, it is usually unnecessary to make a skin nick if the catheter is 16 gauge or smaller, and one should avoid making a skin nick if possible because risk of infection may be increased if the skin entry site is much larger than the catheter.

While the guide wire is in the catheter, secure the catheter with a suture so that the catheter cannot be moved, yet the guide wire is still mobile within the catheter. Avoid making the skin knot so tight that skin necrosis occurs, and the catheter knot so tight that the catheter lumen is pinched off. A guide wire that moves freely confirms that the suture has not compressed the catheter lumen.

Remove the guide wire and attach the catheter to an intravenous fluid administration set. Demonstrate easy aspiration of blood from the catheter before any fluid administration. Apply bacteriocidal ointment (eg, povidine-iodine) and a sterile nonocclusive dressing, which should be changed once a day. Obtain a chest radiograph to confirm proper location of the tip of the central venous catheter in the superior vena cava above the level of the carina. The tip of the catheter must not be left in the right atrium or right ventricle because it may precipitate arrhythmias in these locations. The radiograph also rules out immediate complications such as a pneumo- or hemothorax.

The other techniques of central venous access will be described only as they differ significantly from internal jugular catheterization.

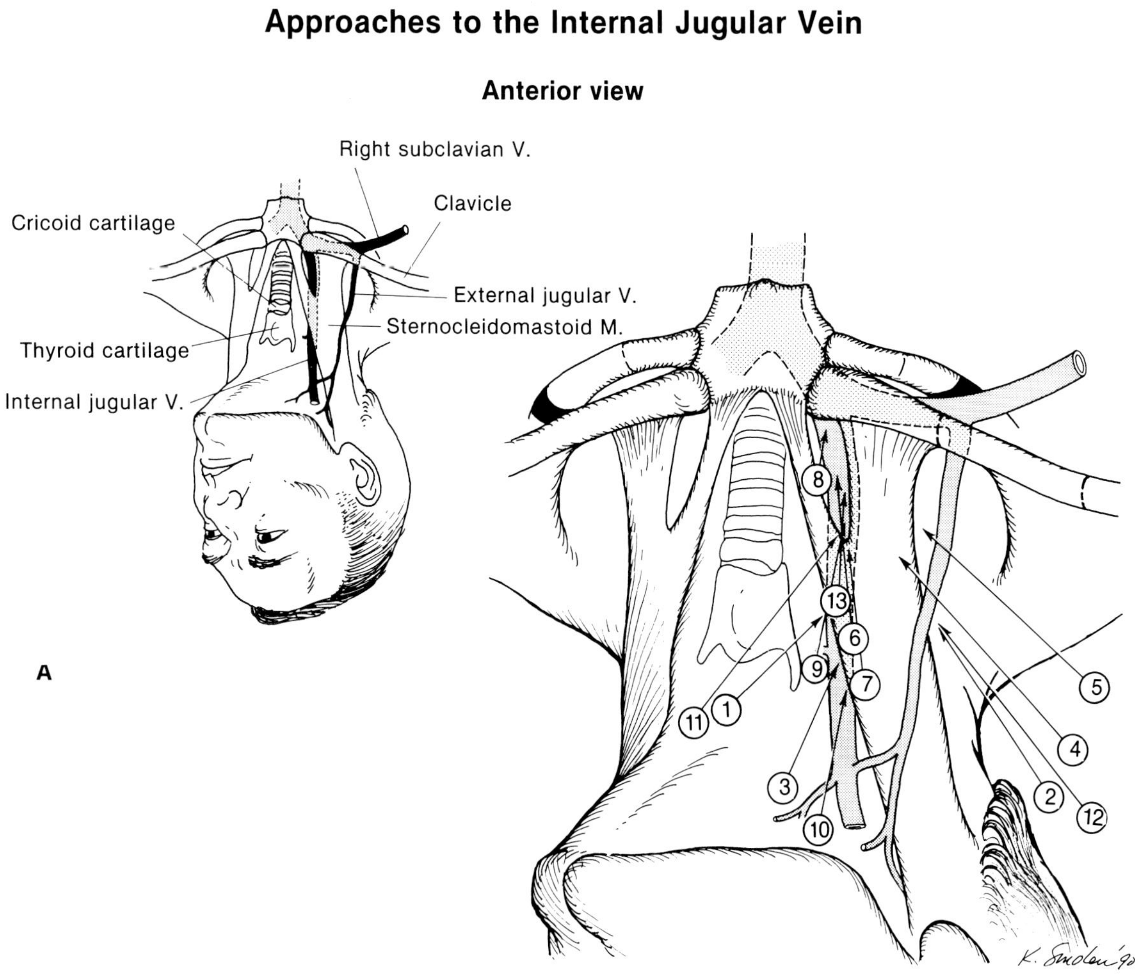

Figure 18–13 • Thirteen approaches to the internal jugular vein that are documented in the literature. (***A***) Anterior view.

(continued)

2. External Jugular Vein

The patient should be prepared and draped as for the internal jugular vein procedure (see Fig. 18–12). The patient should be placed in the Trendelenburg position and the vein identified. The exact location of the vein is variable; direct visualization of the path of this vessel is crucial. Some pressure exerted by fingers placed at the base of the neck will help obstruct and engorge the vein for better visualization. If this procedure dramatically improves identification and engorgement of the vein, either place the patient in steeper Trendelenburg position, or have an assistant exert pressure during needle localization of the vein. A skin wheal with local anesthetic should be placed in the neck directly over the vessel. Note that deep infiltration is not necessary because this vessel is very superficial.

While applying some traction to the skin, enter the skin with the 18 gauge thinwall needle. Note that the finder needle is not necessary for this procedure because the vein is already visually "found." Apply a minimal negative pressure to the syringe to achieve blood return without collapsing the vein (Fig. 18–17). The vessel should be entered at a 30° angle to the skin, and one should be careful not to angle the needle so low (<30°) that the vessel is not entered until the needle is near the base of the neck. It is important to enter the vessel in the straight portion of the vein along the middle third of the neck before it disappears and curves into the base of the neck. If this is accomplished, there will

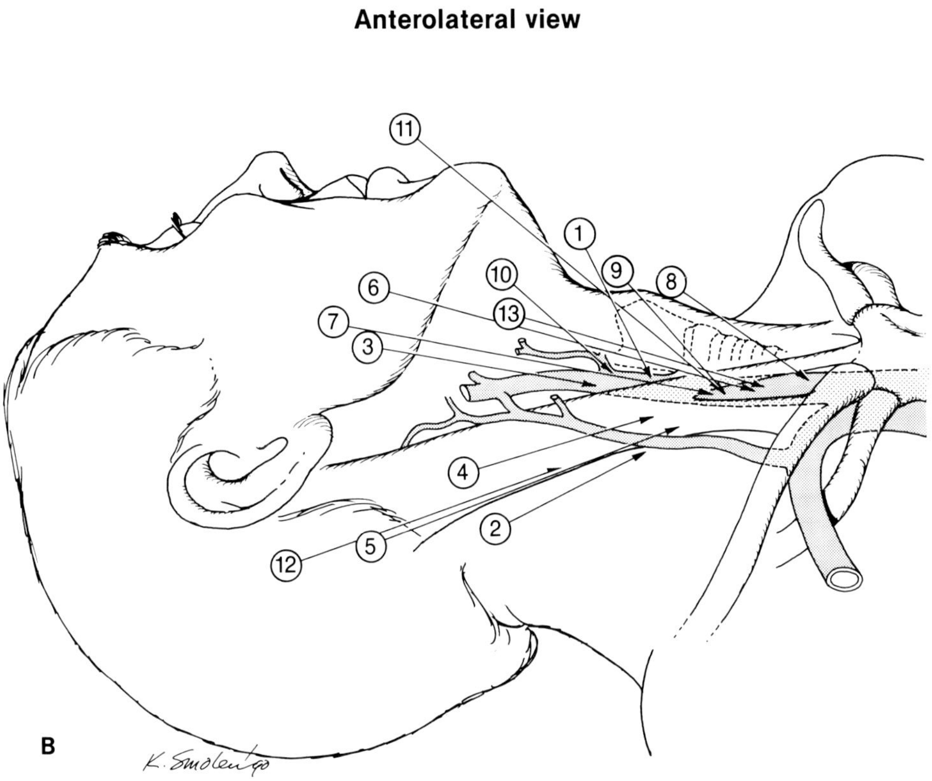

Figure 18–3 *(continued)*

(***B***) Anterolateral view. The various descriptions to the numbered approaches are given: (*1*) Needle enters medial border of sternocleidomastoid (*SCM*) at level of the thyroid cartilage and directed laterally under the posterior border of the muscle. (*2*) Needle enters just above junction of external jugular vein and lateral border of SCM muscle and is directed under the muscle toward the sternal notch. (*3*) Needle enters on medial border of SCM halfway along its course and is directed under the muscle toward the junction of the middle and medial thirds of the clavicle. (*4*) Needle enters 3 fingerbreadths above clavicle and 1 cm medial to SCM lateral border and is directed parallel to anterior muscle border at 30° to skin. (*5*) Needle enters 2 fingerbreadths above the clavicle at the outer border of the SCM muscle and directed toward the sternal notch. (*6*) Needle enters in middle of SCM triangle and is directed parallel to midline at 30° to skin. (7) Needle enters at apex of SCM triangle and is directed parallel to midline at 30° to skin. (*8*) Needle enters just above the clavicular ''notch'' (0.25–1 cm lateral to sternal end) and directed parallel to the midline at a 30°–40° angle to the skin. (*9*) Needle enters below apex of SCM triangle and is directed slightly lateral to midline at 30°–40° to the skin. (*10*) Needle enters at point where internal jugular vein is best palpated and directed slightly lateral to midline at 30°–40° to the skin. (*11*) Needle enters at apex of SCM triangle and is directed laterally toward the ipsilateral nipple at 45° to the skin. (*12*) Needle enters at midpoint of lateral edge of SCM muscle and is directed at the sternal notch. (*13*) Needle enters 3 cm lateral to midsternal line and 2–3 cm above clavicle and is directed in a caudad direction.

Suggested Approach to Internal Jugular Vein

Anterolateral view

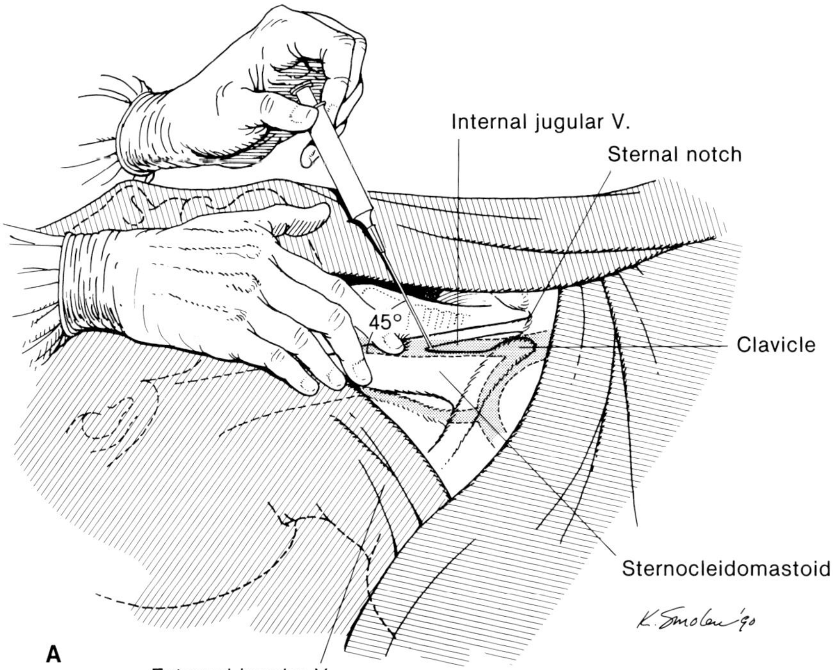

A

Anterior view

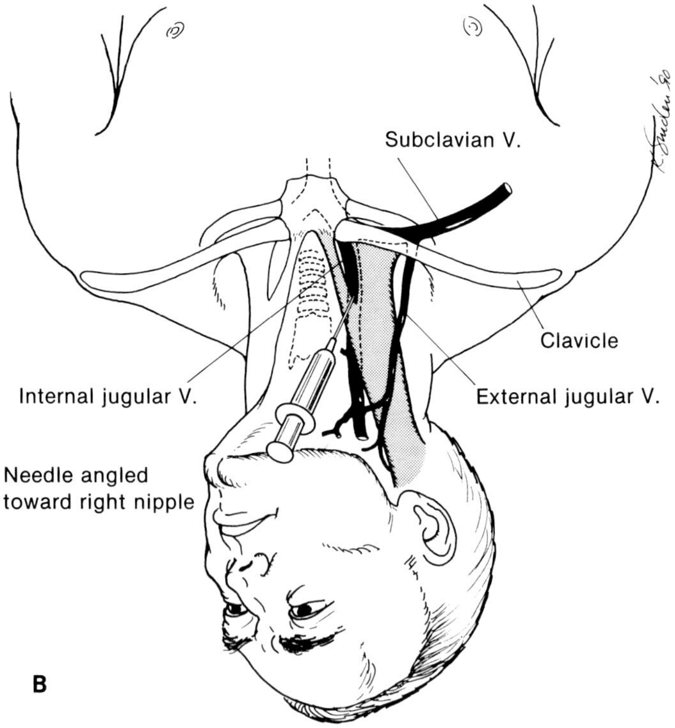

B

Figure 18–14 • One approach to locating the internal jugular vein. (***A***) Anterolateral view. (***B***) Anterior view.

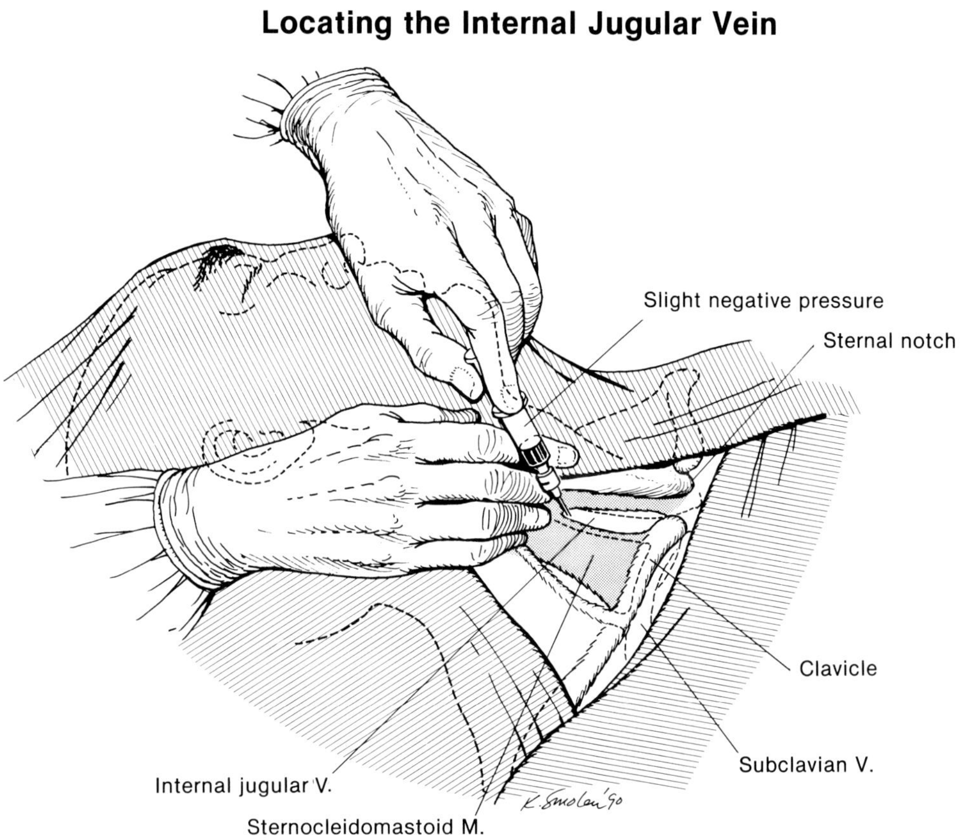

Figure 18–15 • The finder needle locates the internal jugular vein from a high triangle approach.

be more freedom in manipulating the guide wire so that the curves of the vessel can be negotiated without worrying about pulling the guide wire back out of the vessel.

Once the vessel is entered and easy blood return is confirmed, *carefully* fix the position of the needle with the other hand *without* releasing the skin traction used for entering the vein (Fig. 18–18). Holding the traction is important because it is extremely easy to displace the needle out of the vein at this point in the procedure.

Remove the syringe and pass the guide wire with the "J" end in first (see Fig. 18–18). Cannulation of the external jugular vein frequently requires manipulation of the guide wire and therefore takes special advantage of the "J" design (allows tight curves to be negotiated by the wire). If there is resistance to initial passage of the guide wire as it exits the tip of the needle, *do not* use any force. The needle tip is almost always no longer in the vessel lumen and must be repositioned. After free blood return is reestablished, pass the guide wire again. If the guide wire passes easily until it reaches the normal curvature of the vessel as it takes its path to join the subclavian vein, and then hangs up, pull back the guide wire and try to pass again.

The normal anatomy of the external jugular vein may be difficult to negotiate, but do not give up too early (see Fig. 18–6). If repassing the guide wire does not work, be sure the guide wire is withdrawn sufficiently to give it a chance to take a new direction. If the vein has been entered high in the neck, the guide wire can be withdrawn until the "J" end can be seen or palpated in the base of the neck. The guide wire can also be twisted until the "J" flips and changes its orientation in the vessel. Other manuevers that may be effective include turning the head toward the side of cannulation, using a steeper Trendelenburg position, having the patient perform a Valsalva manuever,[19] changing the position of the shoulder (down first, then up),[39] and deep palpation in the base of the neck to direct the guide wire more medially as it is being passed. These efforts are almost always worth the effort and often lead to success-

(Text continued on p. 358)

Positioning Thinwall Needle and Placement of Guide Wire into Internal Jugular Vein

Thinwall needle in vessel

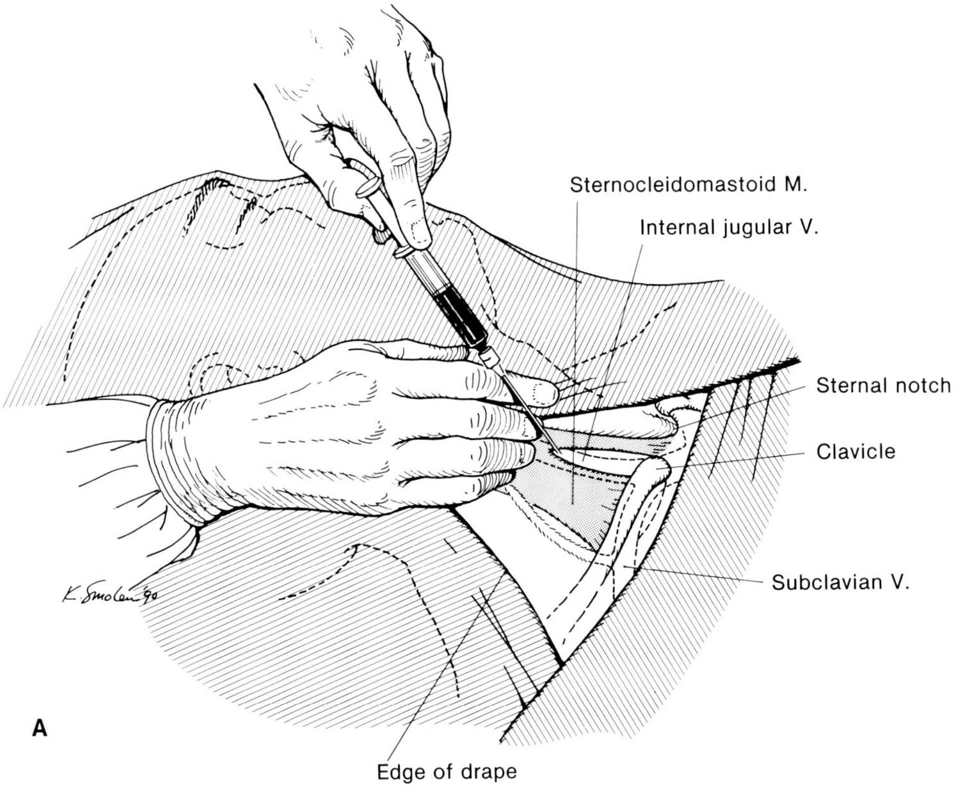

Figure 18–16 • (***A***) The thinwall needle has been passed in the same direction as the finder needle. Note that the hand in the field has not changed position to maintain orientation between the two needle passes. (***B***) The thinwall needle is tilted down to orient it to the direction of the internal jugular vein so that the guide wire will pass toward the heart rather than up to the head. (***C***) Guide wire passage. The guide wire should pass through the needle and into the vessel with virtually no resistance. No force should be used.

Needle tilted down

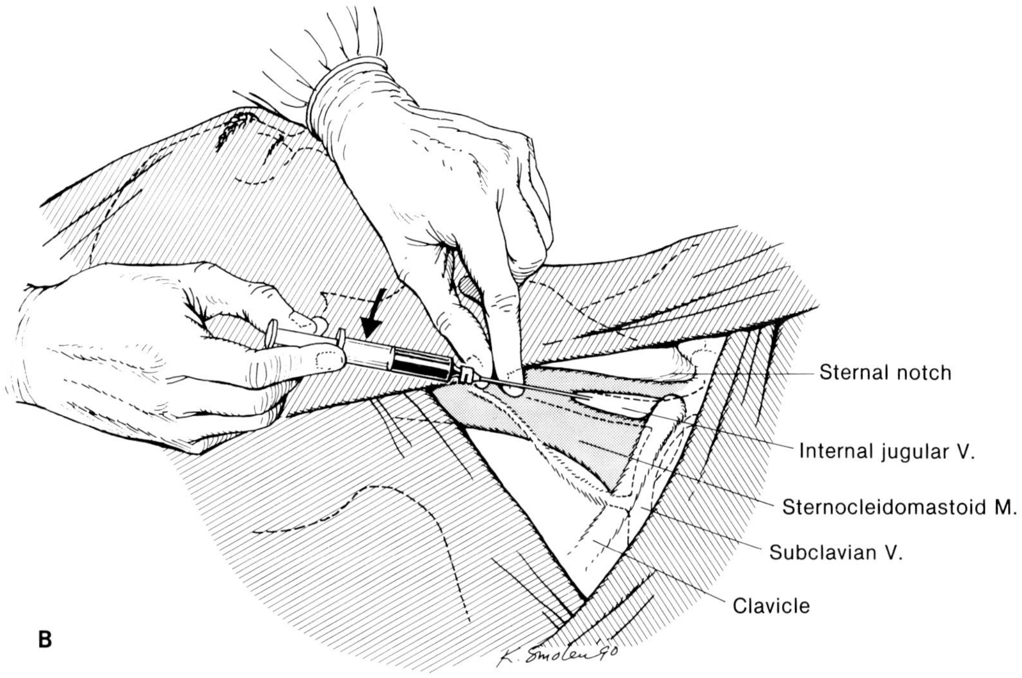

B

Guide wire passed

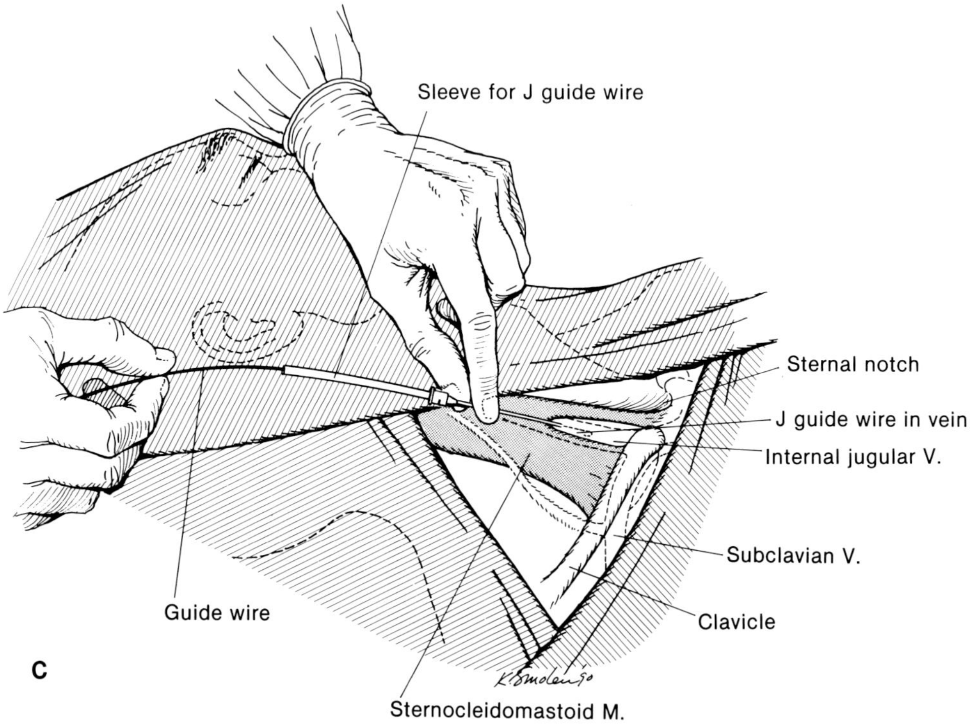

C

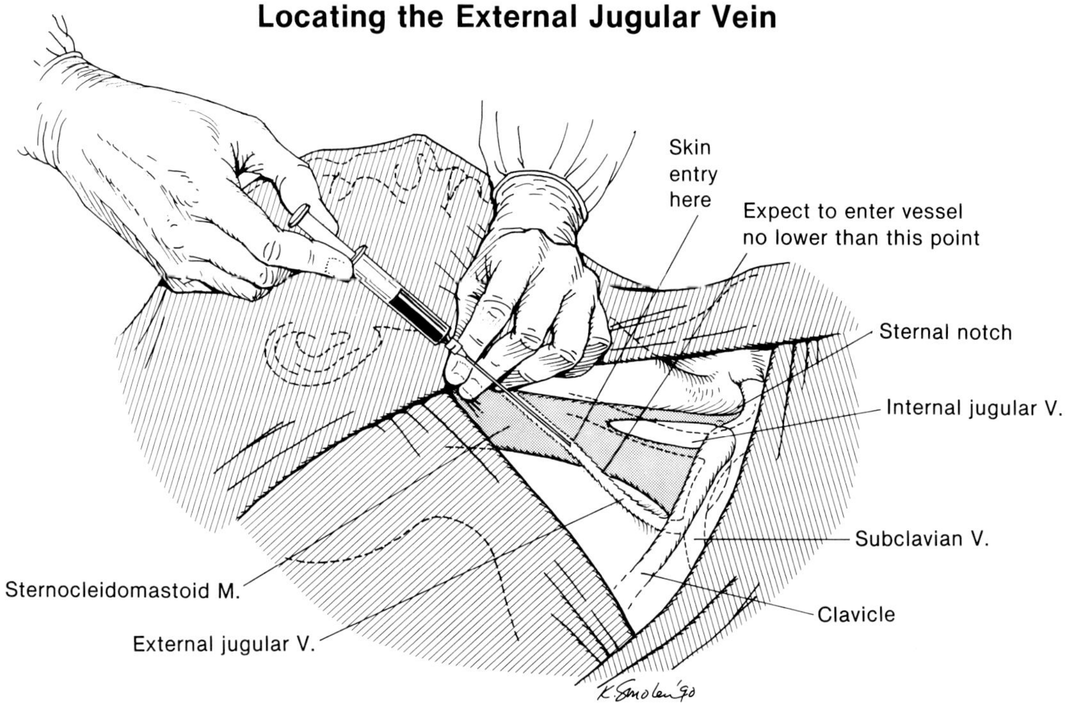

Figure 18–17 • Needle puncture of the external jugular vein. Enter the vein as high in the neck as possible, so that guide wire can be manipulated to negotiate the terminal course of the vein without risking inadvertent removal of the guide wire.

ful passage of the guide wire. An occasional patient may have an external jugular vein that ends in a venous plexus just above the clavicle, which will prevent successful catheter passage.[18]

3. Subclavian Vein Catheterization

The patient should be placed in the Trendelenburg position with the arm pulled straight down against the insertion side. Some authors also recommend a pillow be placed under the vertebral column to allow the patient's shoulder to fall back, minimizing interference by the humeral head. The patient should be prepared and draped as described for the internal jugular technique, being sure to expose the sternal notch and an area 2 inches below the clavicle (see Fig. 18–6).

There are at least seven approaches to the subclavian vein [2,21,40-46](Fig. 18–19). A popular approach is infraclavicular, using a more lateral entry site.[45] This approach is farthest away from the pleural space, and minimizes the possibility of getting lost in the bony morass of the junction of the clavicle, first rib, and sternum. Administer local anesthetic wheal at the entry site, located 2 cm below the junction of the middle and distal third of the clavicle. Use the finder needle to infiltrate deeply to the undersurface of the clavicle. However, it is important to note that the finder needle is not long enough to reach the subclavian vein in most patients.

The thinwall needle should be directed immediately under the clavicle to a point about 2 cm behind the sternal notch by placing the index finger of the free hand in the sternal notch to that depth (Fig. 18–20). To hug the undersurface of the clavicle, it is usually safer to "walk off" the lower aspect of this bone. Continuous slight negative pressure should be maintained in the syringe and the rapid return of blood will indicate entry

(Text continued on p. 362)

Figure 18–18 • After entry into the external jugular vein, the needle must be firmly fixed in position as shown without letting up on skin traction used for needle puncture. The syringe can then be removed (***A***) and the guidewire passed (***B***).

Fixing Needle Position in the External Jugular Vein

Fix needle position

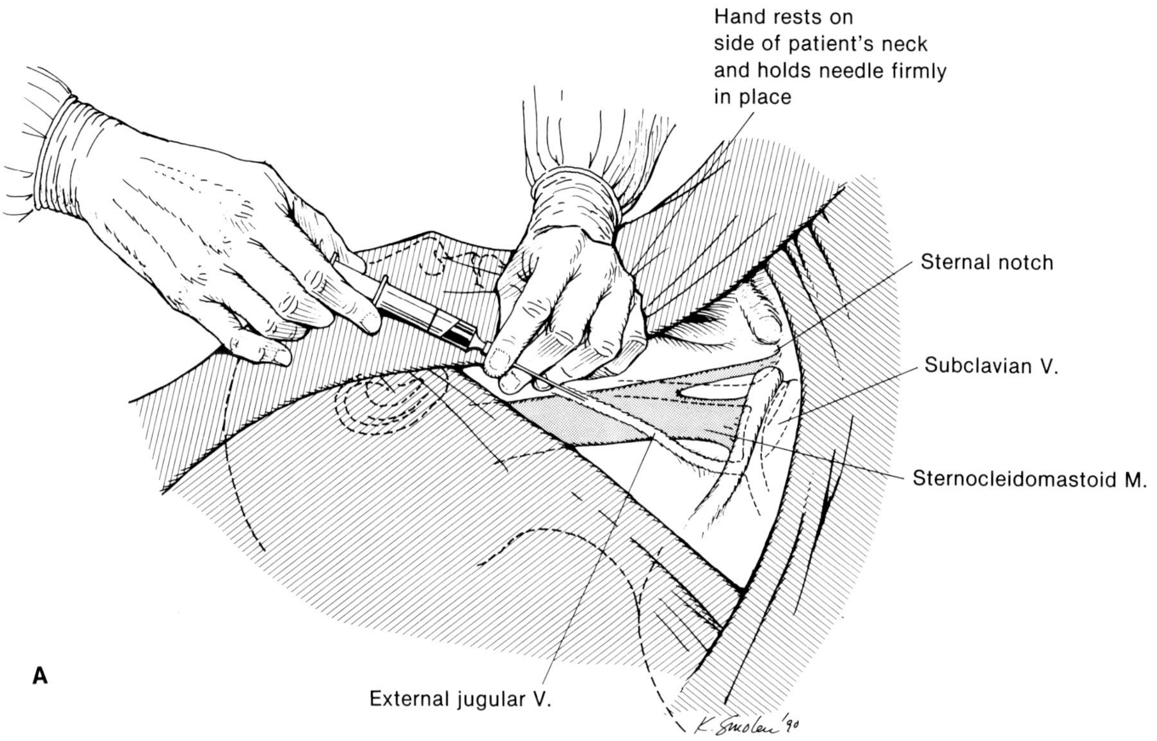

Passing guide wire

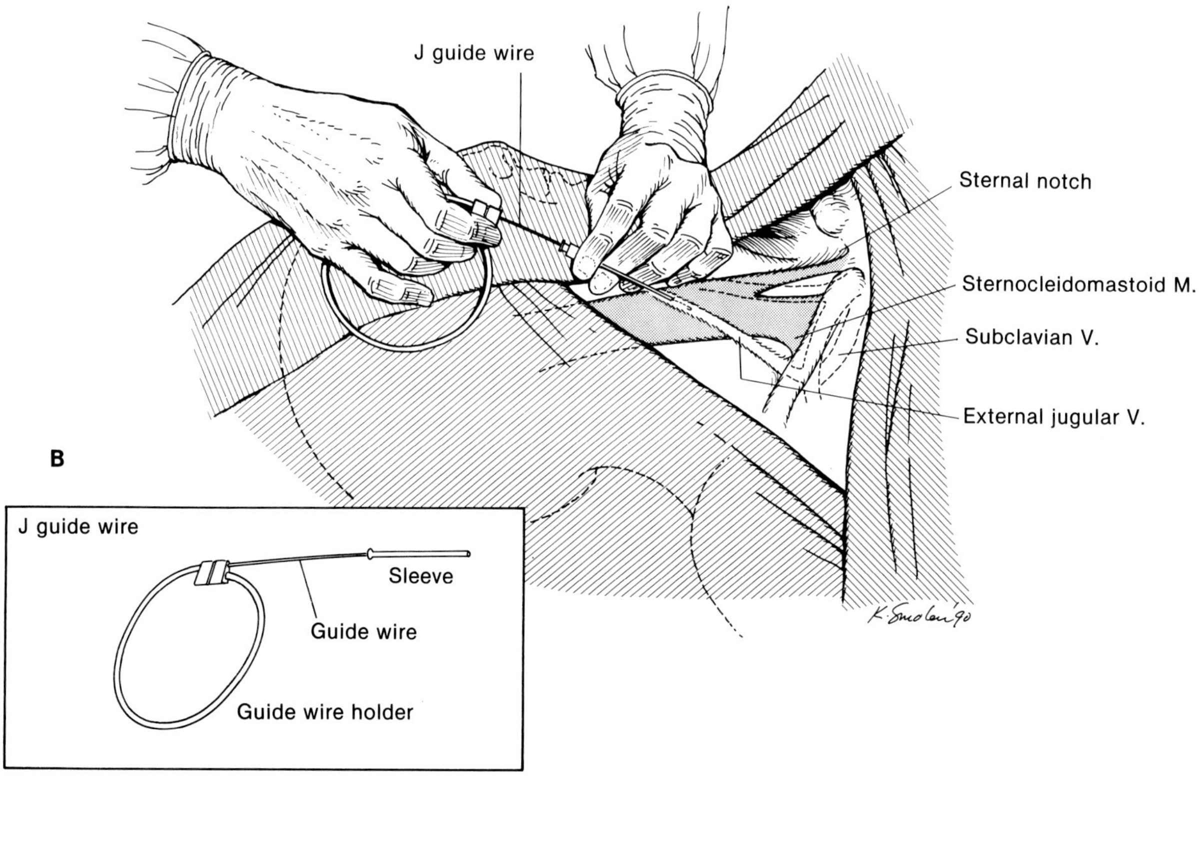

Seven Approaches to the Subclavian Vein

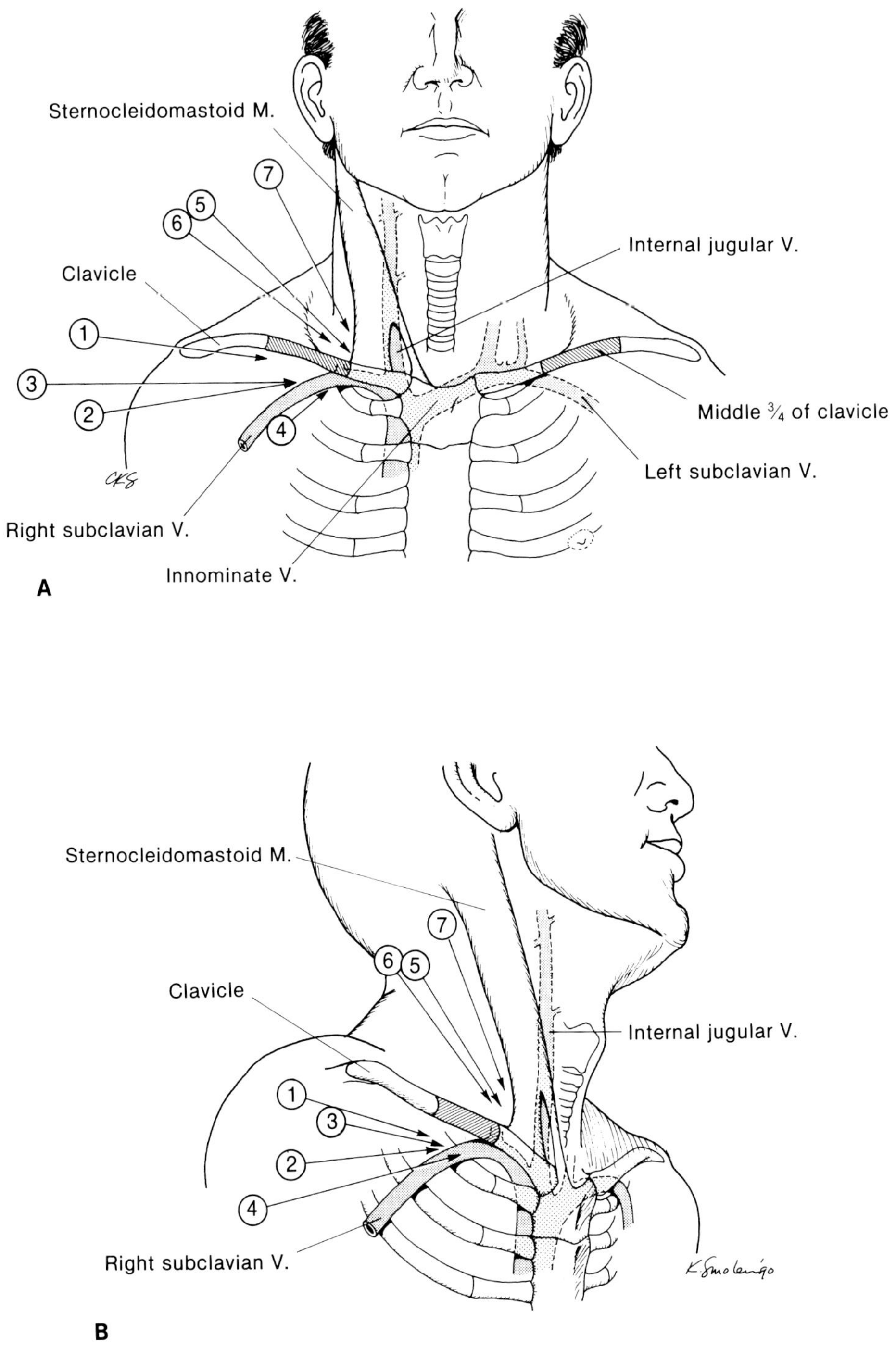

Figure 18–19 • Seven approaches to the subclavian vein that are documented in the literature. From the literature the various descriptions of the numbered approaches are given: (*1*) The needle enters lateral to midclavicular line beneath clavicle and is directed toward tip of finger in sternal notch.[93] (*2*) The needle enters just beneath midclavicle medially and is directed a little superiorly toward the triangle formed by the sternal and clavicular attachments of the sternocleidomastoid (SCM) muscle.[12] (*3*) The needle enters under midclavicle parallel to back and is directed toward finger placed in sternal notch.[83] (*4*) The needle walks off clavicle and is then redirected superiorly at the small triangle formed by the clavicle and the two heads of the sternocleidomastoid muscle.[4] (*5*) The needle enters at clavisternomastoid angle and is directed at 45° to sagittal and 15° forward of the coronal plane.[91] The needle bisects angle of sternocleidomastoid muscle and clavicle, 10° in front of coronal plane and is directed at the submanubrial area at the level of the angle of Louis.[92] (*6*) The needle enters 1 cm lateral to sternocleidomastoid and 1 centimeter above clavicle and is directed 10°–15° ahead of frontal plane (upward) toward centralateral nipple.[9] (*7*) The needle enters 2–3 cm above clavicle along lateral edge of sternocleidomastoid, and is directed 35° from sagittal, slightly ahead of frontal plane. Needle enters vein 1–2 cm lateral from sternoclavicular articulation.[44]

Locating the Subclavian Vein

Anterior view

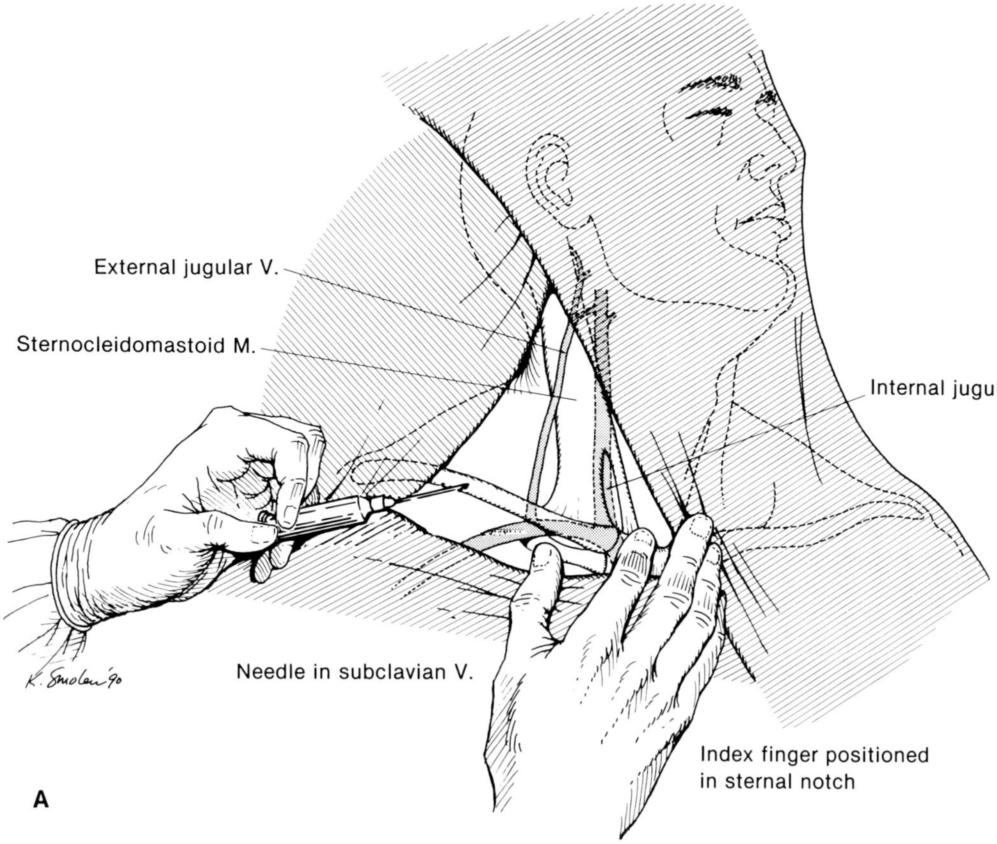

Anterolateral view

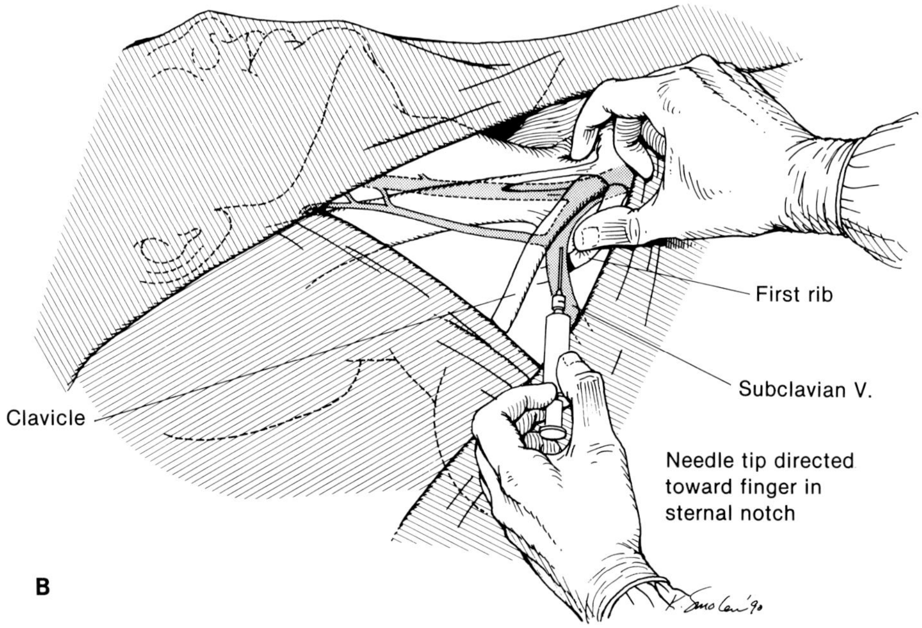

Figure 18–20 • One approach to the subclavian vein. The thinwall needle is directed under the clavicle slightly posterior and slightly cephalad toward a point 2 cm behind the sternal notch (tip of index finger in the notch).

into the vein. Once the vein has been entered, the needle should be fixed with the free hand, the syringe removed, and the guide wire passed. If the guide wire passes with a "metal-on-metal" noise, stop passing, withdraw the guide wire slowly, and check blood return again. If the blood return is satisfactory, rotate the needle 180° and try to pass the guide wire again. Once the guide wire passes successfully, the catheter should be passed over the wire; continue the steps outlined in the internal jugular vein technique.

4. Antecubital Vein Catheterization

The basilic vein is located in the medial aspect of the antecubital fossa and travels along the inner aspect of the arm, eventually joining the underlying deep brachial veins, together forming the axillary vein in the axilla.[47] The median antecubital vein in most patients travels diagonally across the antecubital fossa to join the basilic vein. The cephalic vein is located in the lateral aspect of the antecubital fossa and travels superficially up the lateral aspect of the arm, and normally turns sharply as it goes under the clavicle to join the axillary vein[48] (see Fig. 18–7).

Arm vein anatomy is extremely variable, especially the cephalic vein, which may terminate or decrease in size, or even terminate in the external jugular vein.[48] Of the two veins, the cephalic is more likely to make a sharp angle along its course (see Fig. 18–7).[49] It is therefore no surprise that some series report less than a 50% success rate with cephalic vein catheterization attempts.[48] The basilic vein (or median antecubital vein to access the basilic vein) is clearly the preferred site if an arm vein is to be used.[23]

There are three ways to perform percutaneous central venous catheterization from the basilic vein with a long catheter (50–70 cm). One way is to directly puncture the vessel with a large-bore needle through which the catheter is passed (see catheters in Fig. 18–11). A second method uses a standard introducer (used primarily for passing pulmonary artery catheters), which can be placed in this vein using the Seldinger technique. A long central venous catheter can then be passed through the valved part of the introducer. A third method also employs the Seldinger technique but uses a long (150 cm) guide wire with a J-tip to negotiate the entire path to the axillary vein, over which the catheter is passed.[23]

The first method is simple and may be a faster technique. The second technique, using the introducer, provides the flexibility of rapidly changing the central venous catheter for a pulmonary artery catheter if it is needed, because it can be passed through the introducer that is already in place. The last technique, using the long J-tip, is cumbersome but may increase the likelihood of successful central venous catheter placement. The first technique will be described.

A tourniquet should be placed high on the arm to engorge the basilic vein. The arm should be positioned in 30° abduction and full external rotation, and prepared and draped (Fig. 18–21). Local anesthetic wheal should be placed just over the vessel, and the "long-arm" catheter taken out of the package and the insertion needle exposed. Before puncturing the vessel, be sure that the catheter passes easily through the needle and is completely withdrawn into the needle; also, make an approximate estimate of the catheter length needed to reach the superior vena cava by holding the catheter above the patient.

The needle should then enter the vessel and blood return into catheter should be noted. The catheter should be passed a few centimeters and the tourniquet released. At this point the "Intrafuser"-type central venous catheter can be attached to an intravenous fluid administration set and fluid infused to aid further passage (see Fig. 18–11). If the catheter hangs up in the axilla, withdraw several centimeters and pass again. If the catheter still fails to pass, consider the following maneuvers: abducting the arm to 90° from the side of the body, and/or administering a fluid bolus or 50 mg Xylocaine through the catheter before passage to relieve spasm of small veins. After placement of the catheter, withdraw the needle from the skin, place it in the protective plastic holder, and secure the catheter with a suture.

5. Femoral Vein Catheterization

The femoral vein is cannulated just below the inguinal ligament and just medial to the femoral artery, which are usually two very easy landmarks to identify (see Fig. 18–8). There are several catheter options when cannulating the femoral vein for central venous access. If central venous pressure monitoring is not needed, then a standard short central venous catheter can be placed using the Seldinger technique as previously described. If vascular access for dialysis is needed, the large double-lumen dialysis catheters are placed just like standard short central venous catheters and provide a means for dialysis or

Basilic Vein Catheterization

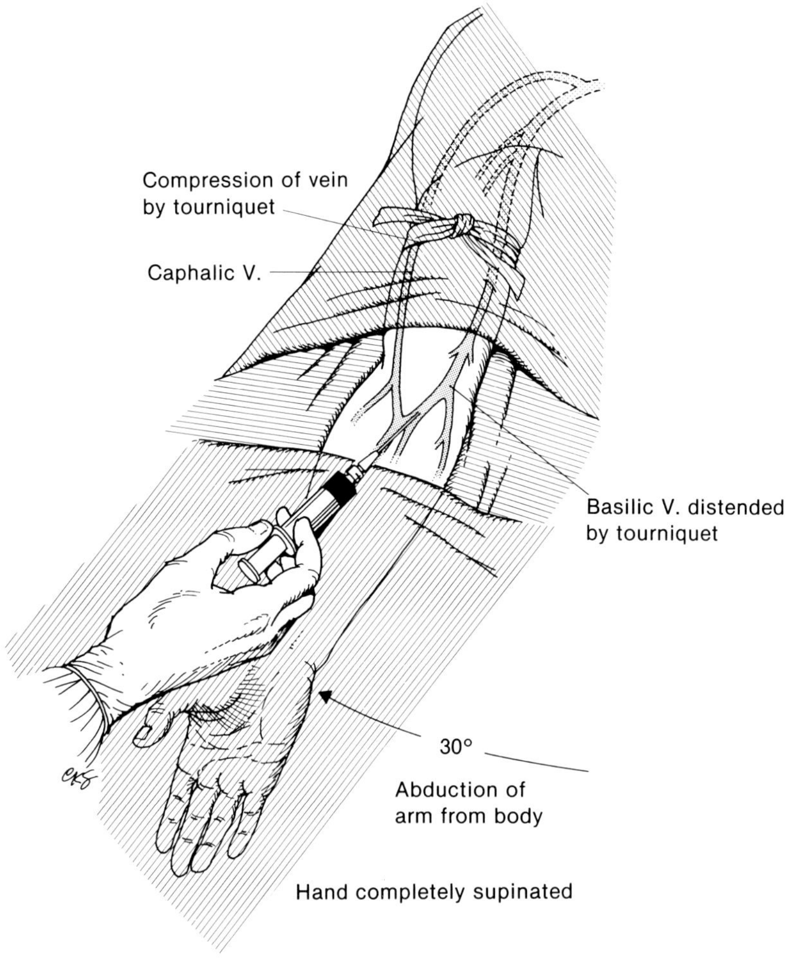

Figure 18–21 • Percutaneous catheterization of the basilic vein is shown using a through-the-needle long central venous catheter with stylet (see Fig. 18–8). Once the vein is entered with the 14 gauge needle, the 16 gauge catheter can be advanced inside the needle. After partial advancement, the tourniquet must be removed to continue passing the catheter into the superior vena cava.

rapid volume administration, but again without central venous pressure monitoring (see Fig. 18–10).

For central venous pressure monitoring, a long catheter, like that used for the basilic vein, can be used; its direct placement is described below. Alternatively, just as with the basilic vein, an 8.0–8.5 French introducer could be placed first by the Seldinger technique, and then a long CVP catheter could be passed through the introducer. As with the basilic vein, the introducer allows a pulmonary artery catheter to placed without insertion difficulty at any time.

The leg on the side to be used should be positioned in full external rotation and 30° abduction, and the area prepared and draped (see Fig. 18–8). Some authors also recommend placing a pillow under the buttocks.[50]

A local anesthetic wheal and deep infiltration should be placed 3 cm below the inguinal ligament and 1 centimeter medial to the femoral artery pulsation. The needle on the long central venous catheter should be exposed and catheter movement within the needle checked. The catheter should be detached from the needle and the needle attached to a 10-mL syringe. Using a syringe to puncture the vein, thus allowing aspiration of blood to confirm needle position, is desirable because a tourniquet cannot be used to increase venous pressure in the femoral vein (as can be done with the antecubital veins).

The skin should be entered at 45° with the needle directed cephalad toward the opposite ear (Fig. 18–22). If a pillow is used under the buttocks, use a lower angle of 30°. If the vein is not entered, withdraw the needle and try again. If the patient moves suddenly during needle insertion, the femoral nerve has probably been contacted and the needle should be redirected more medially. If the femoral artery is entered, the needle should be redirected more medially, but first pressure should be held on the puncture site to avoid a hematoma that may distort the anatomy and make vein catheterization more difficult. Once the blood vessel is entered, fix the position of the needle, remove the syringe, and pass the catheter through the needle. After placement, withdraw the needle from the skin, place it within the protective plastic holder, and secure the catheter to the skin with a suture.

Cutdown methods provide a viable alternative to percutaneous techniques when the latter have been tried

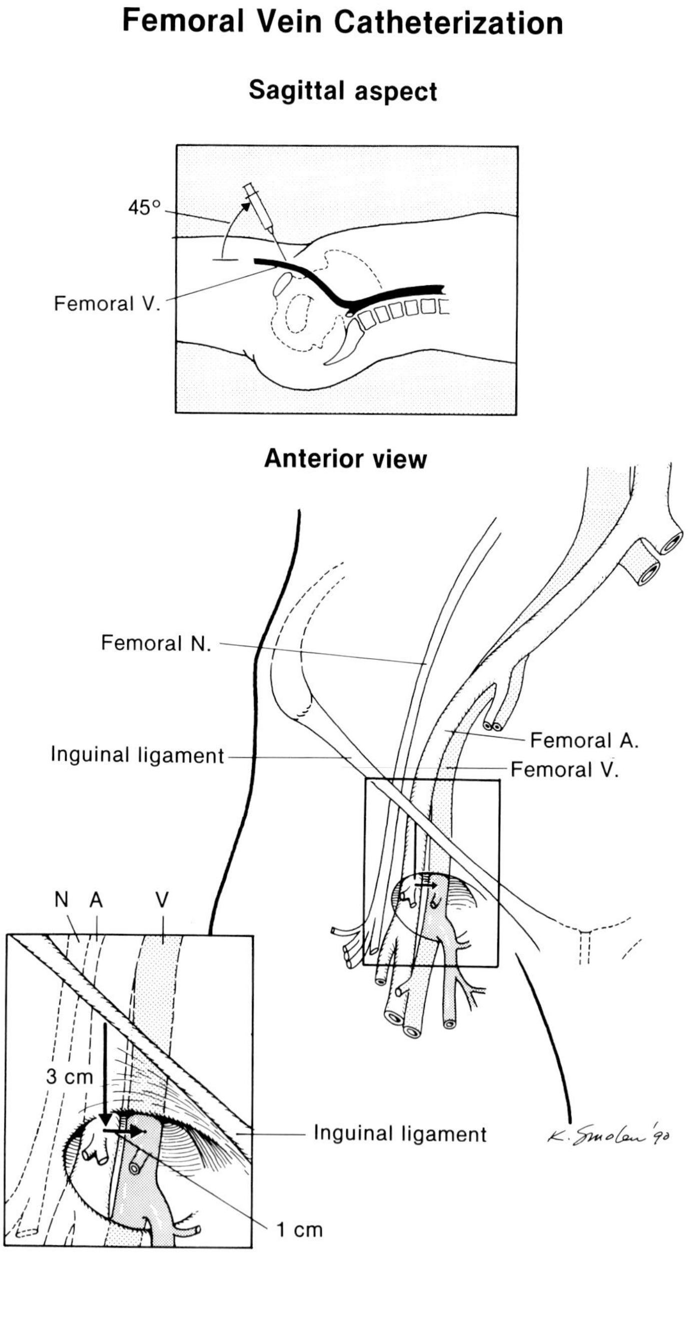

Figure 18–22 • Femoral vein catheterization. The leg should be positioned in external rotation and 30° abduction. The skin is entered at a 45° angle 3 cm below the inguinal ligament and 1 cm medial to the maximal femoral artery pulsation.

and failed or when severe coagulopathics, anatomic deformities, local edema, or other factors contraindicate percutaneous attempts. Cutdown techniques will be discussed in Chapter 20.

IV. COMPLICATIONS

The majority of common complications associated with central venous catheterization are iatrogenic and therefore preventable (Table 18–3). Inadequate teaching and supervision of catheterization techniques are related to many complications that occur during placement.[51] The very unusual complications associated with central venous catheterization will not be emphasized in this chapter but are listed in Table 18–4.[52] Some data suggest that patients who are unconscious and mechanically ventilated have 50% fewer complications caused by physicians learning central venous catheterization if they are properly supervised by experienced physicians.[53] Clinical teachers may do well to more carefully select ''teaching situations'' in the best interests of their patients.

A. *Pneumothorax*

Pneumothorax is one of the most serious and potentially life-threatening complications of central venous catheterizations.[54] This complication occurs predominantly with subclavian vein techniques, but can occur much less commonly with internal jugular approaches.[55] The higher incidence with the subclavian vein technique is understandable, because the parietal pleura is in direct contact with the posterior inferior side of the subclavian vein as it passes from the first rib to join the innominate vein.[56] The incidence varies from 0% to 6% and varies more with the experience of the operator rather than with other factors.[51,54] Fatal bilateral pneumothoraces have occurred as a result of making attempts at both subclavian veins before confirming the absence of a pneumothorax on the first side used.[54] It should be appreciated that respiratory distress from a pneumothorax may not develop for hours or days after catheterization.[54]

Table 18–3 • Central Venous Catheterization Complications

Pneumothorax	Infection
Vascular/cardiac perforation	Nerve injury
Air embolism	Thoracic duct injury
Thrombosis	Catheter knotting
Arrhythmias	Misinterpretation

Table 18–4 • Unusual Complications of Central Venous Catheterization

Clavicular osteomyelitis
Fistulas—arteriovenous, bronchocaval
Tracheal perforation
Cervical artery laceration and pseudoaneurysm
Aortic puncture
Aortic dissection
Ascites
Hydrocephalus

There are several things that can be done to minimize the incidence of pneumothorax.[25] First, central venous catheterization by operators with fewer than 25 previous procedures should be supervised. Second, subclavian catheterization should be avoided in high-risk patients such as those with COPD, bullous disease, or apical blebs; patients on positive pressure or ventilation with high PEEP; and patients with even moderate risk, such as the obese and those with musculoskeletal abnormalities. Finally, one should avoid repeated probing for the vein if it is not located on first or second pass.

If the patient develops respiratory distress during the procedure, stop the procedure immediately and assess the patient for a possible pneumothorax. Under these circumstances, always administer 100% oxygen. However, it is important to remember that the patient may be in respiratory distress for other reasons, such as air embolism, fluid overload, atelectasis or respiratory fatigue from prolonged Trendelenberg position, stress-induced myocardial ischemia with left ventricular failure, etc. Assess for pneumothorax by observing an immediate chest radiograph, chest wall movement, hyperresonance to percussion, and decreased breath sound over the hemithorax in question. Tension pneumothorax should be presumed to be present if the patient has the above findings plus hypotension that cannot be readily explained. To relieve the tension, the patient only needs a small needle or catheter placed into the pleural space on the side.[55] A chest tube can be placed later under less duress.

B. Vascular/Cardiac Perforation

Of the serious complications associated with central venous catheters, none are as insidious as the various events associated with vascular or cardiac perforation.

1. Hematoma

Hematoma formation during central venous catheterization is frequently due to inadvertent arterial puncture. A hematoma from carotid puncture can lead to upper airway obstruction in a rare patient.[57] The incidence of both carotid or subclavian artery puncture is low in recent large series of internal jugular and subclavian vein catheterizations, with an incidence of 2.8% (260 in 9024)[20,57,58] and 0.9% (113 in 13,086),[59] respectively. Rapid airway control (intubation) and blood pressure control are crucial in the immediate care of this complication if significant respiratory distress develops. Bleeding from subclavian artery puncture can result in massive hematoma formation and bleeding from the skin site or hemothorax development. An occasional series reports a fatality secondary to bleeding,[20,60] which should punctuate the need to assess carefully and quickly the extent of blood loss in any patient developing a hematoma after central venous access. Most hematomas, however, can be managed conservatively and will resolve. An unusual patient may develop a chronic hematoma requiring surgical resection.[61]

2. Cardiac Tamponade

Cardiac tamponade is a rare yet devastating complication of central venous catheters. The 70% mortality reported in 1986 reflects the problem in delayed diagnosis because other diagnoses are entertained (eg, pulmonary embolism or myocardial infarction.[62]) The perforation is presumably gradual, which explains why the pericardial cavity fills with intravenous fluid rather than blood in 70% of the cases.[62] Once perforation has occurred, tamponade physiology will develop quickly because only 100–300 mL is potentially fatal in adults, while as little as 8–50 mL can be fatal in children.[62] The usual signs and symptoms include chest or epigastric pain, nausea, dyspnea, tachycardia, hypotension, and distant heart sound.[63] Pulsus paradoxus and low voltage on the ECG may not always be present.[62] Patients developing these symptoms on a nonmonitored ward may not be identified until they have a cardiac arrest. The association of these signs and symptoms or even the cardiac arrest with the central venous catheter is missed because the majority of cases of tamponade present greater than 24 hours after placement.[62,64] Misdiagnosis of this condition is reported to be 73%.[64] Cardiac tamponade should be suspected in any patient with a central venous catheter who has an unexplained cardiac arrest, particularly if he or she appears to be in electromechanical dissociation and responds poorly to closed chest compression. It is important to verify in all cardiac arrests that a central venous catheter has good blood return before giving resuscitative drugs through that catheter, or else the situation may be made worse.

It is not a coincidence that in 80% of tamponade events the central venous catheters have been placed in antecubital or subclavian veins.[62] Arm adduction causes an average of 2–3 cm advancement of the catheter.[24] Flexion at the elbow and crossing the arm over the chest can cause equal additive amounts of advancement.[65] In some patients, over 9 cm of movement has been observed.[24] All this catheter migration could easily push the catheter tip into the heart. Significant advancement of catheters placed via jugular veins is also possible by neck flexion.[66,67]

With subclavian-placed catheters, tamponade has developed in patients whose catheter tips abut the superior vena wall (below the pericardial reflections).[64] Catheters placed via the left internal or external jugular veins also can be found in this position after initial placement.[68,69]

An additional concern is the wide acceptance of the central venous catheter tip in the right atrium or a casual attitude about the correct position of the catheter on chest radiograph.[63,70] Other than for short-term placement during surgical procedures where the risk of venous air embolism from the surgical field is significant, there is no reason to leave a catheter tip in or near the right atrium, particularly with the understanding that catheter movement occurs with changes in body position.[63] A position above the level of the carina will assure catheter tip location in the superior vena cava. Even if the catheter does not move significantly, perforation of the superior vena cava can cause tamponade because the pericardial reflections continue up to the level innominate vein.[71]

There are several ways to minimize the likelihood of cardiac tamponade. First, verify the catheter tip location 1–2 cm above the level of the carina on chest radiograph. Indeed, an even more conservative approach that has been suggested is to position the catheter tip no lower than 2 cm below the inferior border of the end of the clavicles.[72]

Second, reposition the catheter if the tip appears to abut a vessel wall. Third, require regular (every 12 hours) documentation of blood return from a central venous catheter. Finally, for central venous catheters placed via antecubital veins, chest radiographs for catheter position should be taken with the arm in full adduction and arm movement limited.

3. HYDROMEDIASTINUM AND HYDROTHORAX

Hydromediastinum and hydrothorax may occur right after attempted placement of a central venous catheter, but if the catheter is not a blood vessel it should be obvious by the absence of blood return, venous pressure waveforms, and chest radiograph. These complications generally occur later as the catheter, which was once intraluminal, erodes through the vessel wall above the pericardial reflections either into the mediastinum or pleural space. Hydromediastinum can present with the same tamponade physiology as pericardial fluid collection.[71] Attempts at pericardiocentesis in this situation may successfully drain the mediastinum.[71]

Hydrothorax usually presents as an asymptomatic chest radiograph finding but can cause significant hypoxemia or even hypotension if a tension hydrothorax develops.[69] The misdiagnosis of congestive heart failure is often made in a patient with hydromediastinum and/or hydrothorax because of a prominent mediastinum and hazy lung fields. Dye can be placed through the catheter with a follow-up radiograph if there is any question as to the location of the catheter, and may be important to do diagnostically before the catheter is arbitrarily removed.[64] The decision to perform thoracentesis or mediastinal fluid aspiration will be based on the severity of the patient's clinical condition.

4. HEMOTHORAX

Hemothorax is a well-recognized but not a common complication of subclavian and more rarely internal jugular catheterization.[52] A number of series, however, including one of 13,000 subclavian vein catheterizations, report no hemothoraces.[5,20,27,40,41,59,73] When it does occur, it usually is the result of laceration of the subclavian vein or artery. Fluid resuscitation, blood transfusion, and chest drainage are important parts of successful treatment of this complication. If the patient can be stabilized, the extent the vascular injuries can be investigated by angiography, with surgical repair performed as indicated by the angiography.[52]

C. *Air Embolism*

Venous air embolism is a complication of central venous catheterization that may occur for several reasons. The tragedy of many early reports of air embolism is that the majority of these events occurred simply because of disconnections.[74] Disconnections still occur today, but much less often because Luer lock connectors are routinely used. Patients can also suck air through a catheter tract after removal of a central venous catheter.[75]

The patient is at risk of air embolism during placement of a central venous catheter, particularly if there is respiratory distress or anxiety resulting in marked tachypnea. If a large catheter is to be placed (eg, an 8.0 French introducer or hemodialysis catheter) the risks are increased further. If these catheters are placed in the jugular or subclavian veins, sufficient air can be embolized in one inspiration so that a cardiac arrest will result.

Paradoxical air embolism has also been reported to result in focal neurologic deficits. It is presumed that these patients have either arteriovenous communications across their lung or a probe-patent foramen ovale that opens during right heart air embolization because right atrial pressure exceeds left atrial pressure.[76]

The occurrence of air embolism can be minimized by observing several principles. First, the Trendelenburg position should be used for subclavian or jugular veins. Second, patients who are in marked respiratory distress often will not tolerate the Trendelenburg procedure and therefore are not good candidates for internal jugular or subclavian vein approaches. Alternate venous access sites should be considered in these patients. Third, open lumina of needles and catheters should be covered during placement; ie, cover the needle lumen while getting the guide wire, and cover the catheter lumen or leave the guide wire in the catheter while getting the connecting tubing. Fourth, during passage of multilumen catheters, the other lumina not negotiated by the guide wire should be occluded. Fifth, all connections should be secured with Luer lock mechanisms only. Finally, after removal of the catheter, occlude the insertion hole with ointment and massage the skin over the site to help obliterate the subcutaneous tract. If air embolism occurs, prompt therapy should be initiated as described in Chapter 19 on pulmonary artery catheterization.

D. Thrombosis

All of the materials that are used to make central venous catheters are thrombogenic. It is therefore no surprise to find studies showing a 90% incidence of some degree of venous thrombosis in patients receiving long-term hyperalimentation through central venous catheters.[77] For catheters used short-term, the incidence of mural thrombi has been reported to be 30%, but is over 80% when large hemodialysis catheters are used and may be 100% when central venous catheters are placed from the arm.[78,79] Catheter movement associated with arm movement may be a significant cause of endothelial damage and stimulus for thrombosis when catheters are placed in antecubital veins.[79] In spite of this high incidence of thrombosis, the incidence of valvular thrombi or pulmonary embolism is very low.[78,79] The incidence of asymptomatic thrombosis of the superior vena cava or a major tributary is not low in some studies (20%–70%),[73,80] but clinically symptomatic complete superior vena caval occlusion is rare.[81] Pulmonary emboli are detected postmortem in patients with central venous catheters, but these are rarely clinically significant. Patients with symptomatic thrombosis should be considered for anticoagulant therapy with heparin or even thrombolytic therapy.[81] A rare patient may require surgical removal of the thrombus.

There is little that can be done to minimize catheter-induced thrombosis. Important points to remember are to minimize the length of time central venous catheters are used, restrict arm movement of patients with antecubital vein catheters, and reposition catheter tips that abut vessel walls.

E. Dysrhythmias

Dysrhythmias commonly occur during central venous catheterization because of direct myocardial stimulation by the guide wire or a catheter that has been advanced too far. These dysrhythmias immediately resolve when the catheter or guide wire is withdrawn slightly. Central venous catheters placed via arm veins can migrate into the heart with arm movement (abduction and arm across chest) and cause serious ventricular dysrhythmias.[24,82] Anesthesiologists who are in the habit of placing central venous catheters before surgery and not checking the catheter position by chest radiograph until after surgery are at greater risk of causing this complication. Continuous ECG monitoring and immediate access to antiarrhythmic agents and cardioversion equipment should be routine during catheterization.

Several things can be done to minimize the occurrence of dysrhythmias. First, be careful not to pass the guide wire too deeply in small patients, particularly when the right internal jugular or subclavian veins are used. Second, estimate distances from the insertion site to the vena cava in every patient before catheterization. Third, be aware of potential catheter movement when the patient's body position is changed, especially with catheters placed via antecubital veins. Finally, continuously monitor central venous pressure to detect a right ventricular pressure trace on a catheter that migrates, perhaps before it causes dysrhthymias. If unexplained dysrhythmias occur, check the position of the central venous catheter by observing the pressure waveform. If there is any question, withdraw the catheter 2–3 cm.

Dysrhythmias also can occur because of direct carotid sinus stimulation by palpation during the procedure. Techniques that encourage carotid "retraction"[30] are potentially dangerous in older patients.

F. Infection

Infectious complications from central venous catheters are a serious problem about which we still have incomplete information. In no area of central venous catheterization there are more differences in opinion and practice, particularly regarding routine precautions to be taken to avoid catheter-induced infection (septicemia, endocarditis). Routine protocols for skin preparation, suturing technique, dressing, dressing change interval, and stopcock care vary widely from hospital to hospital and often from physician to physician.

Central venous catheters are said to have been colonized if, on removal, semiquantitative culture (a count of colony-forming units on a blood agar plate after the catheter tip is rolled across it)[83] demonstrates more than 15 colony-forming units. By this technique, catheter colonization occurs with an incidence of 15% to 30%, with coagulase-negative staphylococci and *Staphylococcus aureus* being the two most common organisms.[83-86] These organisms usually do not cause or relate to systemic infection. Gram-negative bacilli (Pseudomonas, Enterobacter, Serratia, Klebsiella, etc) and fungi (Candida species) are much less often cultured from catheters, but are much more likely to be related to systemic evidence of infection (ie, positive blood culture for the same organism).[83-86] When these culture results (positive blood and catheter culture for the same organism) are found in a patient with no evidence for another nidus of infection, it is presumed to demonstrate catheter-caused bacteremia/septicemia.[83] Catheter-caused sepsis occurs with an incidence of 3% to 8%.[83-86] Because critically ill patients may have many possible causes of infection, it is important to rule out the central venous catheter as a possible source. The semiquantitative culture technique is a reasonable test because its predictive value is 99% if the catheter culture is negative.[84] For more rapid feedback, a Gram stain of the catheter tip will predict fairly well whether or not the culture results will be positive.[86]

Certain types of catheters seem more prone to infection than others. A single-lumen central venous catheter placed exclusively for hyperalimentation and maintained carefully can remain in patients for weeks without causing infection locally or systemically.[87] Conversely, large-bore hemodialysis catheters and triple-lumen central venous catheters have a much higher incidence of infection compared with a standard, single-lumen catheter.[87] There appear to be two mechanisms of catheter contamination, one of which is internal, via stopcocks and contaminated infusions, as suggested by these data; and the other, which is external, by skin contamination, suggested by other studies.[83,88]

There is a clear association of catheter colonization and catheter-caused sepsis. The routine changing of all catheters every 3 to 5 days is based on studies that show that 3 to 5 days is within the window of time before catheter-caused sepsis will occur in some patients.[83,89] This practice may put patients at greater risk of complications from repeated venous access at new sites than from possible infection. In this regard, the practice of changing catheters over guide wires is commonly employed to check the catheter for signs of colonization or association with sepsis without exposing the patient to unnecessary risk. If the catheter culture is negative, the catheter in the same site is left in place unless local evidence of inflammation or infection occurs.[85] If the catheter culture is positive, the issue is less clear, but most authorities recommend removing the new catheter that has been placed in the old site, even without any systemic evidence of infection.[83,85,87] New techniques to reduce infectious complications have recently been proposed. One method used a silver-impregnated cuff imbedded under the skin and demonstrated 65% and 70% reductions in catheter colonization and catheter-caused sepsis, respectively.[83] Another technique used an iodophor-impregnated sterile film through which venous cannulation was accomplished; catheter colonization was dramatically reduced.[88]

The following are recommended to minimize infectious complications from central venous catheterization. First, daily reexamine the need for continued central venous access and remove catheters expeditiously. Second, examine the insertion site daily; remove the catheter and establish a new site if local inflammation or drainage is observed. Third, change the catheter over the guide wire every 4 to 5 days and culture the tip semiquantitatively. Fourth, if the catheter culture is positive, remove the catheter and find a new site. Fifth, if the catheter culture is negative, leave the new line in the old site. The recommendation for catheter changes every 4 to 5 days is not necessary with single lumen catheters used exclusively for hyperalimentation.[89]

If a patient develops signs of infection without obvious source, all central venous catheters are suspect and should be cultured and changed over a guide wire. If cultures are negative and the patient does not respond to empiric antibiotic therapy, consider arbitrarily removing existing catheters and establishing new sites based on the relative risks of establishing new venous access in that patient.

G. *Nerve Injury*

A number of peripheral nerve injuries have occurred during central venous catheterization (Table 18–5). They occur almost exclusively with subclavian and internal jugular vein attempts, and usually are the result of probing too deeply or in the wrong direction while trying to locate one of these veins. The various neurologic deficits include sensory-motor loss to upper extremity, paralyzed diaphragm, Horner's syndrome, hoarseness,

Table 18–5 • Nerves Injured During Central Venous Catheterization

Brachial plexus
Phrenic nerve
Cervical sympathetic trunk
Recurrent laryngeal
Vagus

etc; they may be caused by compression from a hematoma and usually resolve without specific therapy.[16,17,73] However, if the nerves have been lacerated or transected by the probing needle, regeneration may take months to recover, if it ever does.[73,90]

H. *Thoracic Duct Injury*

The upper part of the thoracic duct ascends in front of the prevertebral fascia to the level of the seventh cervical vertebra, then arches over the dome of the left lung lateral to the left internal jugular vein and joins the subclavian vein at the internal jugular–subclavian angle.[91] There is some anatomic variability. The thoracic duct is most vulnerable to the supraclavicular approach to the subclavian vein with a reported 1% incidence of injury (6 out of a series of 600 catheterizations).[42] Most thoracic duct punctures are successfully managed by simply removing the catheter and applying compression.[42] Some cases will result in chylothorax, which may require surgery to ligate the injured vessel.[92] Thoracic duct injury can be minimized by avoiding supraclavicular approaches to the left subclavian vein and by using right-sided over left-sided jugular and subclavian veins when possible.

I. *Catheter Knotting*

Central venous catheter looping and knotting are possible if the catheter is overmanipulated or forcibly advanced.[93] Knotting of the guide wire has also been reported.[94] The first clue to this complication may be the inability to withdraw the catheter. It is important to not forcibly try to remove the catheter, as this may only tighten the loop or knot. While the knot or loop is loose an interventional radiologist may still be able to retrieve the catheter without having to resort to surgery.

J. *Misinterpretation*

There are a number of causes that lead to incorrect central venous pressure (CVP) measurements (Table 18–6). Patients should be horizontal for all measurements, unless there is a good reason to establish a new position from which to follow changes in CVP measurements. The zero reference for measurements must be identified and, most important, kept constant between repeated CVP measurements. A most convenient zero point is 3–5 cm below the angle of Louis. Partial or complete catheter obstruction from catheter pinching or twisting, partially closed stopcocks, a tight suture ligature, blood clots, drug precipitation, or vessel wall apposition occur frequently and are easily handled if recognized. It should be obvious that fluid infusions should not be administered through the central catheter while CVP measurements are made.[14]

Table 18–6 • Causes of CVP Misinterpretation

Patient not horizontal
Incorrect zero reference
Aberrant catheter location
Fluid infusion during measurement
Transmitted airway and transpulmonary pressures
Pathologic cv waveforms

The remaining causes of CVP misinterpretation are more subtle and are not related to a malfunction of the CVP monitoring system, yet may result in dramatically erroneous estimates of CVP. To avoid most respiratory-induced artifacts, CVP values should be read during exhalation (see Fig. 18–4). However, patients with elevated thoracic pressures during exhalation from transmitted transpulmonary or transdiaphragmatic pressures may have grossly overestimated CVP measurements. These same artifacts may perturb pulmonary artery pressure measurements and are discussed more completely in Chapter 22 on PA catheterization. Because there is no simple way to subtract out the artifact that results in overestimation of CVP in these cases, it is important to recognize those patients in whom these artifacts are likely to occur. This includes patients in respiratory distress who are using accessory muscles of exhalation (eg, asthmatic, bronchospastic COPD, and cardiac asthma patients), as well as patients who perform the Valsalva maneuver, grunt or groan in pain, or breathe with pursed lips; those with upper airway obstruction; and those with a pneumothorax or hydrothorax under some tension.[5] Only the trend in the artifactually high CVP values uniformly observed in these patients should be used to guide medical care.

Patients with tricuspid regurgitation present another problem of interpretation because of the presence of pathologic cv waves on the central venous pressure tracing (see Fig. 18–4). The usual practice to estimate mean central venous pressure will grossly overestimate right ventricular filling pressures unless the cv wave is ignored. This situation is analogous to estimating left ventricular filling pressures in patients with mitral regurgitation who have large cv waves on their pulmonary artery occlusion pressure tracing. In either case, because the cv wave is reflecting ventricular pressures in systole, they must be ignored when trying to estimate end-diastolic ventricular pressures.

V. REFERENCES

1. Aubanine R. L'injection intraveineuse sous-claviculaire: Advantages et technique. Presse Med 60:1456–1460, 1952.
2. Wilson JN, Grow JB, Demong CV, Prevedel AE, et al. Central venous pressure in optimal blood volume maintenance. Arch Surg 85:563–578, 1962.
3. Stahl MM. Resuscitation in trauma: The value of central venous pressure monitoring. J Trauma 5:200–211, 1965.
4. Brisman R, Parks LC, Benson DW. Pitfalls in the clinical use of central venous pressure. Arch Surg 95:902–907, 1967.
5. James PM, Myers RT. Central venous pressure monitoring: Misinterpretation, abuses, indications and a new technique. Ann Surg 175:693–700, 1972.
6. Linos DA, Mucha P, Van Heerden JA. Subclavian vein: A golden route. Mayo Clin Proc 55:315–321, 1980.
7. Starling EH. The Linacre Lecture on the Law of the Heart. London, Longmans, Green and Co., 1918.
8. McMichael J. Dynamics of heart failure. Br Med J 2:525–529, 1952.
9. Sarnoff SJ, Berglund E. Ventricular function. I. Starling's law of the heart studied by means of simultaneous right and left ventricular function curves in the dog. Circulation 9:706–718, 1954.
10. Swanson RS, Uhlig PN, Gross PL, McCabe CJ. Emergency intravenous access through the femoral vein. Ann Emerg Med 13:244–247, 1984.
11. Arrighi DA, Farrell MB, Mucha P, Ilstrup DM, et al. Prospective, randomized trial of rapid venous access for patients in hypovolemic shock. Ann Emerg Med 18:927–930, 1989.
12. Cucchiara RF, Nugent M, Seward JB, Messick JM. Air embolism in upright neurosurgical patients: Detection and localization by two-dimensional transesophageal echocardiography. Anesthesiology 60:353–355, 1984.
13. Kjellstrand CM, Merino GE, Mauer SM, Casali R, et al. Complications of percutaneous femoral vein catheterizations for hemodialysis. Clin Nephrol 4:37–40, 1975.
14. Stenzel JP, Green TP, Fuhrman BP, Carlson PE, et al. Percutaneous femoral venous catheterizations: A prospective study of complications. J Pediatr 114:411–415, 1989.
15. Horrow JC, Metz S, Thickman D, Frederic MVV. Prior carotid surgery does not affect the reliability of landmarks for location of the internal jugular vein. Anesth Analg 66:452–456, 1987.
16. Prince SR, Sullivan RL, Hackel A. Percutaneous catheterization of the internal jugular vein in infants and children. Anesthesiology 44:170–174, 1976.
17. Goldfarb G, Lebreg D. Percutaneous cannulation of the internal jugular vein in patients with coagulopathies: An experience based on 1000 attempts. Anesthesiology 56:321–323, 1982.
18. Blitt CD, Wright WA, Petty WC, Webster TA. Central venous catheterization via the external jugular vein: A technique employing the J-wire. JAMA 229:817–818, 1974.
19. Giesy J. External jugular vein access to central venous system. JAMA 219:1216–1217, 1972.
20. Schwartz AJ, Jobes DR, Levy WJ, Paterys L, et al. Intrathoracic vascular catheterization via the external jugular vein. Anesthesiology 56:400–402, 1982.
21. Morgan WW, Harkins GA. Percutaneous introduction of long-term indwelling venous catheters in infants. J Pediatr Surg 7:538–541, 1972.
22. Groff DB, Ahmed N. Subclavian vein catheterization in the infant. J Pediatr Surg 9:171–174, 1974.
23. Smith SL, Albin MS, Ritter RR, Bunegin L. CVP catheter placement from the antecubital veins using a J wire catheter guide. Anesthesiology 60:238–240, 1984.
24. Kalso E, Rosenberg PH, Veorialho M, Pietila K. How much do arm movements displace cubital central venous catheters? Acta Anaesth Scand 26:354–356, 1982.
25. Getzen LC, Pollak EW. Short-term femoral vein catheterization: A safe alternative venous access? Am J Surg 138:875–878, 1979.
26. Seldinger SI. Catheter replacement of the needle in percutaneous arteriography. Acta Radiol 39:368–376, 1953.
27. Ng WS, Rosen M. Positioning central venous catheters through the basilic vein: A comparison of catheters. Br J Anaesth 45:1211–1214, 1973.
28. Boulanger M, Delva E, Maille JG, Paiement B. Une nouvelle voie d'abord de la veine jugulaire interne. Can Anaesth Soc J 23:609–615, 1976.
29. Brinkman AJ, Costley DO. Internal jugular puncture. JAMA 223:182–183, 1973.
30. Mostert JW, Lenny GM, Murphy GP. Safe placement of central venous catheter internal jugular veins. Arch Surg 101:431–432, 1970.
31. Civetta JM, Gabel JC. Flow directed-pulmonary artery catheterization in surgical patients: Indications and medications of technic. Ann Surg 176:753–756, 1972.
32. Jernigan WR, Gardner WC, Mahr MM, Milburn JL. Use of the internal jugular vein for placement of central venous catheter. Surg Gynecol Obstet 130:520–524, 1970.
33. Daily PO, Griepp RB, Shumway NE. Percutaneous internal jugular vein cannulation. Arch Surg 101:534–536, 1970.
34. Vaughan RW, Weygandt GR. Reliable percutaneous central venous pressure measurement. Anesth Analg 52:709–716, 1973.
35. Rao TLK, Wong AY, Salem MR. A new approach to percutaneous catheterization of the internal jugular vein. Anesthesiology 46:362–367, 1977.
36. English ICW, Frew RM, Zaki M. Percutaneous catheterization of the internal jugular vein. Anaesthesia 24:521–531, 1969.
37. Hall DMB, Geebhuysen J. Percutaneous catheterization of the internal jugular vein in infants and children. J Pediatr Surg 12:719–722, 1977.
38. Hermosura B, Vanags L, Dickey MW. Measurement of pressure during intravenous therapy. JAMA 195:181, 1966.
39. Rams JJ, Daicoff GR, Moulder PV. A simple method for central venous pressure measurements. Arch Surg 92:886, 1966.
40. Magil RA, DeLaurentis DA, Rosemond GP. The intraclavicular venipuncture. Arch Surg 95:320–324, 1967.
41. Dronen S, Thompson B, Nowak R, Tomlanovich M. Subclavian vein catheterization during cardiopulmonary resuscitation. JAMA 247:3227–3230, 1982.
42. Haapaniemi L, Slatis P. Supraclavicular catheterization of the supior vena cava. Acta Anaesth Scand 18:12–22, 1974.

43. Yoffa D. Supraclavicular subclavian venipuncture and catheterization. Lancet ii:614–616, 1965.
44. James PM, Myers RT. Central venous pressure monitoring: Complications and a new technique. Am Surg 39:75–81, 1973.
45. Tofield JJ. A safer technique of percutaneous catheterization of the subclavian vein. Surg Gynecol Obstet 128:1069, 1969.
46. Longerbeum JK, Vannix R, Wagner W, Jorgenson E. Central venous pressure monitoring. Am J Surg 110:220–230, 1965.
47. Kwn KB, Gorfine S, Berman M, Ibesti TJ, et al. Percutaneous catheterization of the basilic vein for central venous access. Surg Gynecol Obstet 159:287–288, 1984.
48. Webre DR, Arens JF. Use of cephalic and basilic veins for introduction of central venous catheters. Anesthesiology 38:389–392, 1973.
49. Guilde RE, Malinak LR, McMullen FF, Turell OJ, et al. Percutaneous subclavian catheterization of the right heart and pulmonary arteries. Am Heart J 70:481–485, 1965.
50. Duffy BJ. The clinical use of polyethylene tubing for intravenous therapy. Ann Surg 130:929–930, 1949.
51. Bernard RW, Stahl WM. Subclavian vein catheterizations: A prospective study. Noninfectious complications. Ann Surg 173:184–190, 1971.
52. McGoon MD, Benedetto PW, Greene BM. Complications of percutaneous central venous catheterization: A report of two cases and review of the literature. Johns Hopkins Med J 145: 1–6, 1979.
53. Sznaijder JI, Zveibil FR, Bitterman H, Weiner P, et al. Central vein catheterization: Failure and complication rates by three percutaneous approaches. Arch Intern Med 146:259–261, 1986.
54. Maggs PR, Schwaber JR. Fatal bilateral pneumothoraces complicating subclavian vein catheterization. Chest 71:552–553, 1977.
55. Cook TL, Dueker CW. Tension pneumothorax following internal jugular cumulation and general anesthesia. Anesthesiology 45:554–555, 1976.
56. Knoop R, Dailey RH. Central venous cannulation and pressure monitoring. J. Amer Coll Emerg Phys 6:358–366, 1977.
57. Shah KB, Rao TLK, Laughlin S, El-Ets AA. A review of pulmonary artery catheterization in 6,245 patients. Anesthesiology 61:271–275, 1984.
58. Damen J, Bolton D. A prospective analysis of 1400 pulmonary artery catheterizations in patients undergoing cardiac surgery. Acta Anaesth Scand 30:386–392, 1986.
59. Eerola R, Laukinen L, Laukinen S. Analysis of 13800 subclavian vein catheterizations. Acta Anaesth Scand 29:193–197, 1985.
60. Groff DB, Ahmed N. Subclavian vein catheterization in the infant. J Pediatr Surg 9:171–174, 1974.
61. Brown CS, Wallace CT. Chronic hematoma - a complication of percutaneous catheterization of the internal jugular vein. Anesthesiology 45:368–369, 1976.
62. Aldridge HE, Jay AWL. Central venous catheters and heart perforation. Can Med Assoc J 135:1082–1084, 1986.
63. Karnanchow PN. Cardiac tamponade from central venous catheterization. Can Med Assoc J 135:1145–1147, 1986.
64. Ellis LN, Vogel SB, Copeland EM. Central venous catheter vascular erosions. Ann Surg 209:475–478, 1989.
65. VanDijk B, Bakker PM. Appraisal of the dislocation of central venous catheter tips using subclavian and arm veins. Anaesthetist 26:138–140, 1977.
66. Lingefelter AL, Guskiewicz RA, Munson ES. Displacement of right atrial and endotracheal catheters with neck flexion. Anesth Analg 57:371–373, 1978.
67. Fisher GW, Scherz RG. Neck vein catheters and pericardial tamponade. Pediatrics 52:868–871, 1973.
68. Iberti TJ, Katz LB, Reiner MA, Brownie T, et al. Hydrothorax as a late complication of central venous indwelling catheters. Surgery 94:842–846, 1983.
69. Ghani GA, Berry AJ. Right hydrothorax after left external jugular vein catheterization. Anesthesiology 58:93–94, 1983.
70. Jay AWL, Aldridge HE. Perforation of the heart or vena cava by central venous catheters inserted for monitoring or infusion therapy. Can Med Assoc J 135:1143–1144, 1986.
71. Sheep RE, Guiney WB. Fatal cardiac tamponade: Occurrence with other complications after left internal jugular vein catheterization. JAMA 248:1632–1635, 1982.
72. Greenwall MJ, Blewitt RW, McMahon MJ. Cardiac tamponade and central venous catheters. Br Med J 2.595–597, 1975.
73. Ryan JA, Abel RM, Abbott WM, Hopkins CC, et al. Catheter complications in total parenteral nutrition: A prospective study of 200 consecutive patients. N Engl J Med 290:757–761, 1974.
74. Peters JL, Armstrong R. Air embolism occurring as a complication of central venous catheterization. Ann Surg 187:375–378, 1978.
75. Paskin DL, Hoffman WS, Tuddenham WJ. A new complication of subclavian vein catheterization. Ann Surg 179:266–268, 1974.
76. Furuya H, Okumura F. Detection of paradoxical air embolism by transesophageal echocardiography. Anesthesiology 50:374–377, 1984.
77. Jeejeebhoy KN, Langer B, Tsallus GT, Chu RC, et al. Total parenteral nutrition at home: Studies in patients surviving four months to five years. Gastroenterology 71:543–593, 1976.
78. Ducatman BS, McMichan JC, Edwards WB. Catheter-induced lesions of the right side of the heart: A prospective study of 141 autopsies. JAMA 253:791–795, 1985.
79. Bennegard K, Curelasu I, Gustavsson B, Linder LE, et al. Material thrombogenecity in central venous catheterization. Acta Anaesth Scand 26:112–120, 1982.
80. Torosian MH, Meranze S, Mullen JL, McLean G. Central venous access with occlusive superior central venous thrombosis. Ann Surg 203:30–33, 1986.
81. Rubenstein M, Creger WP. Successful streptokinase therapy for catheter-induced subclavian vein thrombosis. Arch Intern Med 140:1370–1371, 1980.
82. Kasten GW, Ownes E, Kennedy D. Ventricular tachycardia resulting from central venous catheter tip migration due to arm position changes: Report of two cases. Anesthesiology 62:185–187, 1985.
83. Maki DG, Cobb L, Garman JK, Shapiro JM, et al. An attachable silver-impregnated cuff for prevention of infection with central venous catheters: A prospective randomized multicenter trial. Am J Med 85:307–314, 1988.
84. Collignon PJ, Soni N, Pearson IY, Woods WP, et al. Is semiquantitative culture of central vein catheter tips useful in the diagnosis of catheter-associated bacteremia? J Clin Microbiol 14:532–535, 1986.
85. Armstrong CW, Mayhall CG, Miller KB, Newsome HH, et al. Prospective study of catheter placement and other risk factors for infection of hyperalimentation catheters. J Infect Dis 154:808–816, 1986.
86. Cooper GL, Hopkins CC. Rapid diagnosis of intravascular catheter-associated infection by direct gram staining of catheter segments. N Engl J Med 312:1142–1147, 1985.
87. Hilton E, Haslett TM, Borenstein MT, Tucci V, et al. Central catheter infections. Single versus triple lumen catheters: Influence of guide wire on infection rates when used for replacement of catheters. Am J Med 84:667–672, 1988.

88. Levy HH, Nagle DM, Curling PE, Waller JL, et al. Contamination reduction during central venous catheterization. Crit Care Med 16:165–167, 1988.
89. Wilson GL, McGregor PJ, Thompson GR. Long-term complications of intravascular cannulation. Problems in Critical Care 2:296–305, 1988.
90. Drachler DH, Koephke GH, Weg JG. Phrenic nerve injury from subclavian vein catheterization. JAMA 236:2880–2881, 1976.
91. Majek M, Maltinsky J, Kadlic T. Inadvertent thoracic duct catheterization during transjugular central venous cannulation: A case report. Acta Anaesth Scand 21:320–323, 1977.
92. Khalil KG, Parker FB, Mukherjee N. Thoracic duct injury: A complication of jugular vein catheterization. JAMA 221:908–910, 1972.
93. Handsworth JL. An uncommon complication of central venous catheterization. Anaesth Intensive Care 9:67–69, 1981.
94. Wang P, Einarsson E. A complication of subclavian vein catheterization: Extravascular knotting of a guide wire. Acta Anaesthes Scand 31:187–188, 1987.

Chapter 19

Neal H. Cohen, MD, MPH, FCCM
Claire M. Brett, MD

Arterial Catheterization

OUTLINE

I. INTRODUCTION

Arterial catheterization facilitates care of the patient in the operating room and intensive care unit by providing continuous access to the arterial circulation. This access allows for continuous blood pressure monitoring, blood gas analysis, and other blood sampling. The widespread use of this procedure attests to its clinical value.

II. INDICATIONS

Arterial catheterization provides continuous monitoring of arterial blood pressure and easy access for arterial blood sampling. In the operating room, monitoring of arterial blood pressure using an intraarterial catheter is useful for a wide variety of clinical situations. The technique is useful for patients undergoing major surgical procedures, particularly cardiac surgery requiring cardiopulmonary bypass, major vascular surgery, and other procedures for which compression of the great vessels or hemodynamic instability is anticipated. Continuous blood pressure monitoring is also commonly employed for neurosurgical procedures, particularly when maneuvers to control intracranial pressure are required. For patients requiring deliberate hypothermia or hypotension as part of anesthetic management, continuous monitoring of arterial blood pressure through an indwelling arterial catheter is essential. Direct arterial pressure monitoring is also useful for patients undergoing surgical

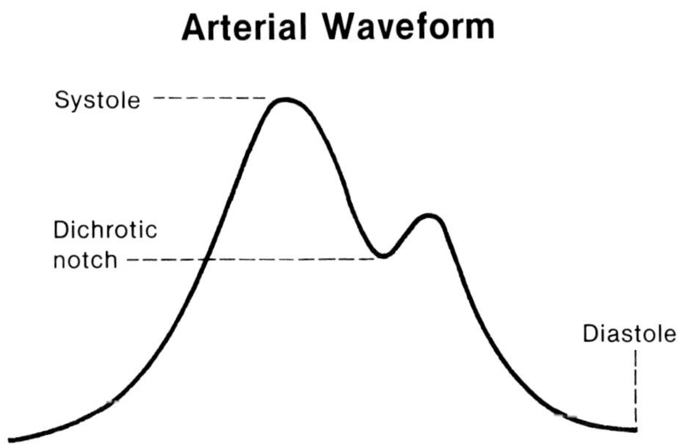

Figure 19–1 • Schematic representation of the arterial pressure waveform.

procedures for which significant fluid shifts or blood loss can be anticipated, including patients suffering extensive trauma. Direct blood pressure monitoring is also occasionally necessary when the blood pressure cannot be obtained noninvasively; for example, for the obese patient or the patient who has burns of the extremities.

Similar indications for continuous arterial blood pressure monitoring apply to the intensive care environment. For patients who are hemodynamically unstable or require pharmacologic manipulation of blood pressure or myocardial performance, direct and continuous monitoring of the arterial blood pressure provides immediate feedback about the appropriateness of therapeutic maneuvers. For patients who require cardiopulmonary resuscitation, availability of direct measurement of arterial pressure is useful to confirm the adequacy of resuscitative maneuvers, particularly when the catheter was in place prior to the cardiopulmonary arrest. Placement during resuscitation is difficult. Continuous monitoring of arterial blood pressure is also useful for the patient with cardiac dysrhythmias, allowing direct assessment of the hemodynamic significance of the dysrhythmias.

Continuous monitoring of the arterial pressure can provide the clinician with a great deal of information about the performance of the cardiovascular system and the adequacy of blood flow. Interpretation of the information requires that the clinician understand what is being monitored and the determinants of the information displayed. Peripheral arteries have higher systolic and lower diastolic pressures than values simultaneously obtained in the aorta.[1] The magnitude of the discrepancy is dependent on the extent of peripheral vasodilation (which will enhance the systolic pressure) or vasoconstriction (which tends to dampen the arterial pressure measurement). In addition to providing continuous monitoring of systolic and diastolic pressures, the arterial pressure monitoring system presents the clinician with a visual display of the arterial pressure waveform. By interpreting the components of the waveform (Fig. 19–1), the clinician can indirectly assess myocardial performance, vascular resistance, and intravascular volume.

For example, myocardial contractility can be assessed by evaluating the upstroke of the arterial pressure waveform as a reflection of left ventricular dP/dt, except in patients with aortic stenosis. Left ventricular stroke volume is reflected in the area under the arterial pressure waveform from the beginning of the upstroke to the dicrotic notch (closure of the aortic valve). As the stroke volume increases, the area increases. Because the area under the pressure waveform is directly related to stroke volume, the arterial waveform also reflects intravascular blood volume. Beat-to-beat changes in the waveform occur due to the effects of pleural pressure. The systolic blood pressure can vary considerably during the respiratory cycle, particularly when the patient is hypovolemic. When blood volume is adequate, minimal changes in systolic blood pressure occur during respiration. Systemic vascular resistance affects the position of the dicrotic notch of the arterial waveform. When the systemic vascular resistance falls, the dicrotic notch is lower. For patients receiving vasodilators, such as nitroprusside, the dicrotic notch may be as low as the diastolic blood pressure.

Arterial catheterization facilitates repetitive blood sampling. Arterial blood gas analysis is commonly used to assure adequacy of ventilation and oxygenation in the operating room and intensive care unit. Repeated blood gas analysis is useful during airway and thoracic surgical procedures and to assure adequacy of gas exchange for patients with pulmonary dysfunction. It is also useful to assess the adequacy of hyperventilation therapy for patients with increased intracranial pressure.

Arterial catheterization will also be necessary for placement of intravascular blood gas monitoring probes as they become commercially available. A recent study by Shapiro et al documents the reliability of continuously measured PaO_2, $PaCO_2$, and pH in patients with spinal cord injury requiring mechanical ventilatory support.[2]

Patients with severe metabolic abnormalities can also most effectively be monitored with frequent blood samples to evaluate acid-base and electrolyte status. Although frequent blood samples can be obtained from a central venous catheter, arterial catheters provide access for additional information, including arterial blood gases and hemodynamic monitoring. In general, arterial catheterization should not be performed to provide access for blood sampling alone, unless venous access is unavailable. When frequent arterial blood sampling or hemodynamic monitoring is also required, arterial catheterization is indicated. Arterial catheterization is useful when managing patients with diabetic ketoacidosis, patients requiring osmotherapy for increased intracranial pressure, and patients requiring anticoagulant therapy, such as those undergoing cardiopulmonary bypass or requiring heparin anticoagulation for pulmonary thromboembolism.

III. How to Do Arterial Catheterization: Techniques and Procedures

Arterial catheterization is most frequently accomplished using a peripheral arterial site. The vessel is usually catheterized percutaneously, although a cutdown technique can also be used. After access to the arterial system is obtained, the catheter is connected to a transducer and fluid-filled tubing to provide the interface between the catheter and monitor.

A. *Monitoring System*

Monitoring blood pressure through an arterial cannula requires connection to a pressure transducer. The transducer is an electromechanical device, converting the mechanical motion of the fluid in the tubing connected to the artery into electrical signals. Most transducers include a diaphragm that forms the base of a fluid-filled plastic dome and is connected to a mechanical coupling tube and stopcock. The mechanical movement of the diaphragm is converted into an electrical signal by a sensing element such as a strain gauge. By calibrating the electrical signal to the mechanical force, blood pressure is determined. The signal obtained from the transducer is transmitted to a display (monitor). Usually an analog signal reflecting arterial pressure will be displayed on an oscilloscope. The analog signal can also be converted to a digital display, providing numeric representation of systolic, diastolic, and mean arterial blood pressures. Recorders are also commonly used to provide permanent records of hemodynamic data.

To maintain patency of the arterial catheter, a heparinized flush solution is usually used, providing a continuous flow of the heparin-containing fluid through the catheter.[3–5] Recently, the need for heparin in the flush solutions has been questioned,[6] although most centers continue to add heparin (0.5–1.0 units/mL) to the solution to reduce the likelihood of catheter clotting. A number of flush devices are commercially available. Most of the devices provide a continuous flow of fluid at 3–4 mL/hour when pressurized to 300 mmHg. For the newborn, a mechanical infusion pump is often used to provide continuous flushing of the catheter, while preventing accidental infusion of large volumes of fluid.[7] Stopcocks are included in the setup to allow aspiration of blood for laboratory analysis and for calibration of the pressure transducer.

B. *Catheterization Techniques*

A number of techniques are used to catheterize the arterial circulation. After selecting the site, it should be stabilized to facilitate catheterization without patient movement. If the patient is awake and able to sense pain, a local anesthetic such as lidocaine should be used to provide local anesthesia. The site should be cleaned using a povidone-iodine solution. Drapes should be placed to isolate the area from potential contamination. The inserter should wear gloves and maintain appropriate sterile techniques. Prior to cannulation, all equipment necessary to connect the arterial catheter to the monitoring system should be available and appropriately set up.

The percutaneous technique is most commonly used for monitoring the patient in the operating room or intensive care unit. For the percutaneous approach a catheter-over-the-needle (eg, Angiocath®) system is used.[8] A nontapered Teflon or polyurethane catheter should be used. Prior to placement of the arterial catheter-needle assembly through the skin, a small skin incision should be made with the tip of a slightly larger needle to prevent a skin plug from occluding the arterial needle and catheter assembly, which would prevent identification of arterial puncture. The artery is transfixed between two fingers to stabilize and identify the course of the artery. The needle and catheter are advanced through the skin at approximately a 30° angle to the skin and parallel its course. After puncturing the artery and obtaining pulsatile blood flow, the catheter is advanced over the needle into the artery. The needle is

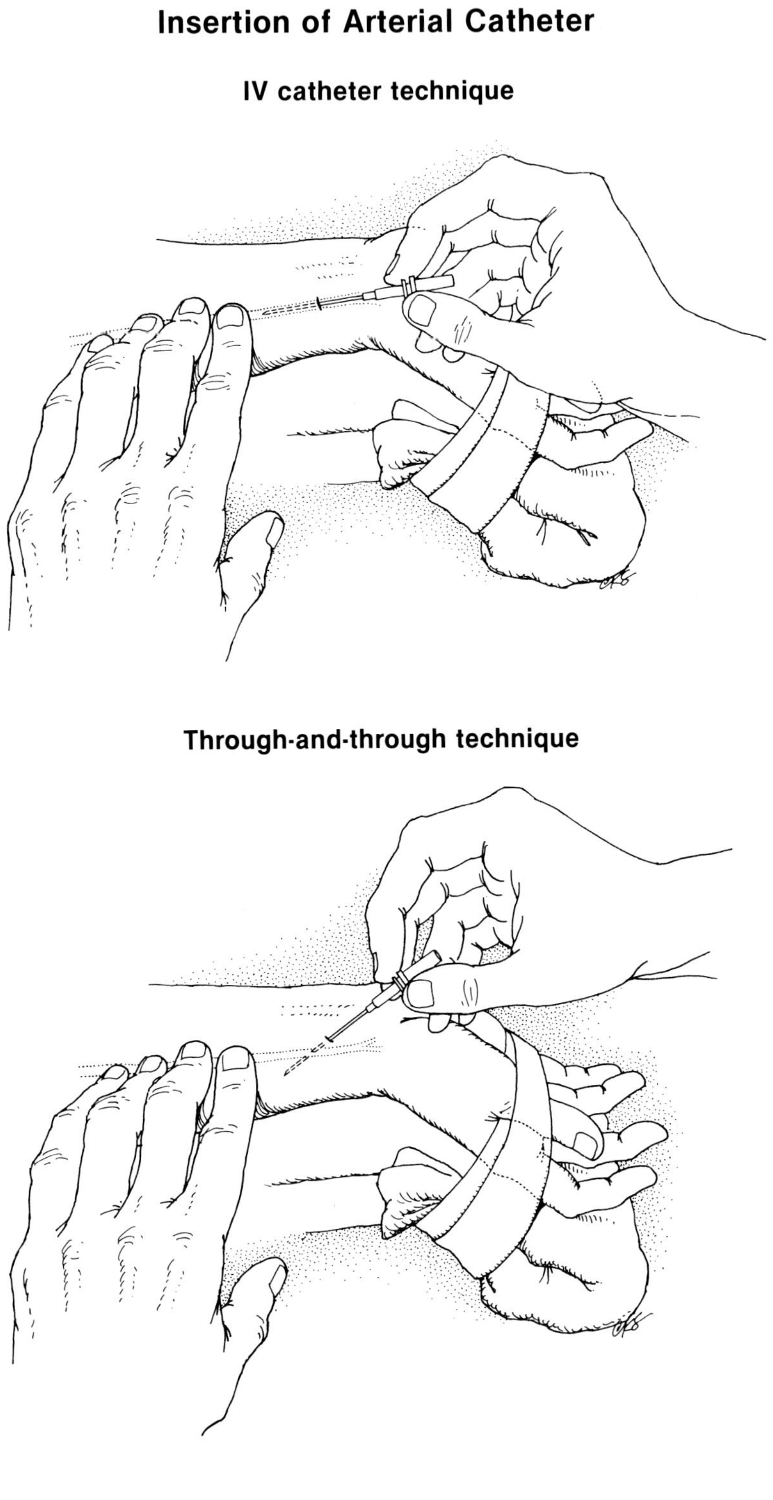

Figure 19–2 • Two approaches to cannulation of the radial artery. *Top panel:* Direct cannulation of the artery in a manner similar to cannulation of a vein. *Lower panel:* Transvascular puncture of the artery (see text).

removed and the catheter connected to the monitoring system (Fig. 19–2, top panel). The artery can also be percutaneously cannulated by advancing the needle through the back wall of the artery (Fig. 19–2, bottom panel). The needle catheter is slowly withdrawn until arterial blood flows back through the catheter-needle assembly, confirming that the catheter lies within the artery. The catheter is then advanced into the artery. Alternatively, the needle-catheter assembly can be advanced through the back wall of the artery, the needle completely removed, the catheter withdrawn until pulsatile flow occurs, and then the catheter advanced into the artery. If the catheter does not thread into the artery at this point, the catheter should be withdrawn until pulsatile flow occurs once again and then a Seldinger technique should be used (pass a guide wire through the catheter and then the catheter over the guide wire [see below]).

Arterial catheterization can also be accomplished using a cutdown approach.[79] This approach requires a transverse incision over the skin, allowing exposure and mobilization of the artery. The artery is usually exposed over 1–2 cm of its length. A ligature is placed at the distal exposed site of the artery, usually using a 2-0 silk suture. A suture may also be placed around the artery proximally, to insure control of the vessel and allow stabilization of the catheter after cannulation. After the artery has been mobilized and stabilized, the catheter needle can be used to puncture the artery and advance the catheter into the vessel. Alternatively, an incision can be made in the artery and the catheter passed directly through the incision without puncturing the vessel directly with the needle.

For some arterial sites, the Seldinger technique is preferred.[10] For the Seldinger technique, the artery is punctured percutaneously with a needle. After obtaining pulsatile arterial flow, a guide wire is passed through the needle to insure communication with the artery. The needle is removed over the wire. The catheter used for monitoring is threaded over the wire into the vessel. After removal of the wire from the catheter, the catheter is connected to the monitoring system.

C. *Catheterization Sites*

Any peripheral arterial site can be used for catheterization. The sites commonly used for monitoring in the operating room or intensive care unit include the radial, ulnar, brachial, axillary, dorsalis, pedis, posterior tibial, femoral, and superficial temporal arteries. For the newborn requiring arterial blood pressure monitoring or access for blood sampling, the umbilical artery is often catheterized shortly after birth.

The choice of a site for arterial catheterization depends on the purpose for which the catheter is placed, the anticipated duration of catheterization, ease of access during anesthesia, surgery, or intensive care, and adequacy of collateral blood flow. The arteries should be large enough to accurately reflect systemic blood pressure. The site should have sufficient collateral blood flow to prevent ischemia to tissues distal to the site of catheterization. When used for monitoring during cardiac or thoracic surgery, the site should be selected carefully so that flow will not be compromised during the surgical procedure. In addition, the preferred site for upper extremity cannulation is the nondominant arm unless contraindicated for other reasons.

For the pediatric patient, the presence of a patent ductus arteriosus must be considered when selecting a site for arterial catheterization. If the catheter is placed in a vessel arising distal to the ductus arteriosus, measured oxygen tension will be lower than that of blood perfusing the brain (and therefore the retina) and can be misinterpreted as reflecting retinal arterial PO_2. Catheterization of a vessel originating proximal to the patent ductus arteriosus will allow access to monitoring the P_aO_2 being delivered to the brain and titrating oxygen delivery and ventilatory support appropriately.

1. RADIAL ARTERY

The radial artery is most commonly used for arterial catheterization in the operating room and intensive care unit. The vessel is easily accessible (Fig. 19–3A) and usually has good collateral blood flow through the superficial palmar arch from the ulnar artery, assuring perfusion to the hand (Fig. 19–3E). Prior to catheterization, adequacy of collateral blood flow should be evaluated.[11-14] If the digits are cold or ischemic, catheterization of the radial artery is contraindicated. Although collateral flow through the ulnar artery is usually adequate,[15] Mozersky et al[13] demonstrated that 12% of adults evaluated did not have adequate collateral circulation of the hand. Because of the concerns about ischemia after placement of a radial artery, many investigators recommend performance of the Allen's test.[16] The original Allen's test evaluated flow from both the radial and ulnar artery, occluding one vessel at a time. More commonly, a modification of the Allen's test is recommended.[17] For the modified Allen's test, the radial and ulnar arteries are compressed. The patient's fist is clenched until it blanches. The patient then relaxes the hand. Pressure on the ulnar artery is released. The skin should promptly become hyperemic, indicating that ulnar collateral flow is adequate. The Allen's test, while recommended, has not been demonstrated to reduce the risk of digit ischemia or complications of radial artery catheterization. Slogoff et

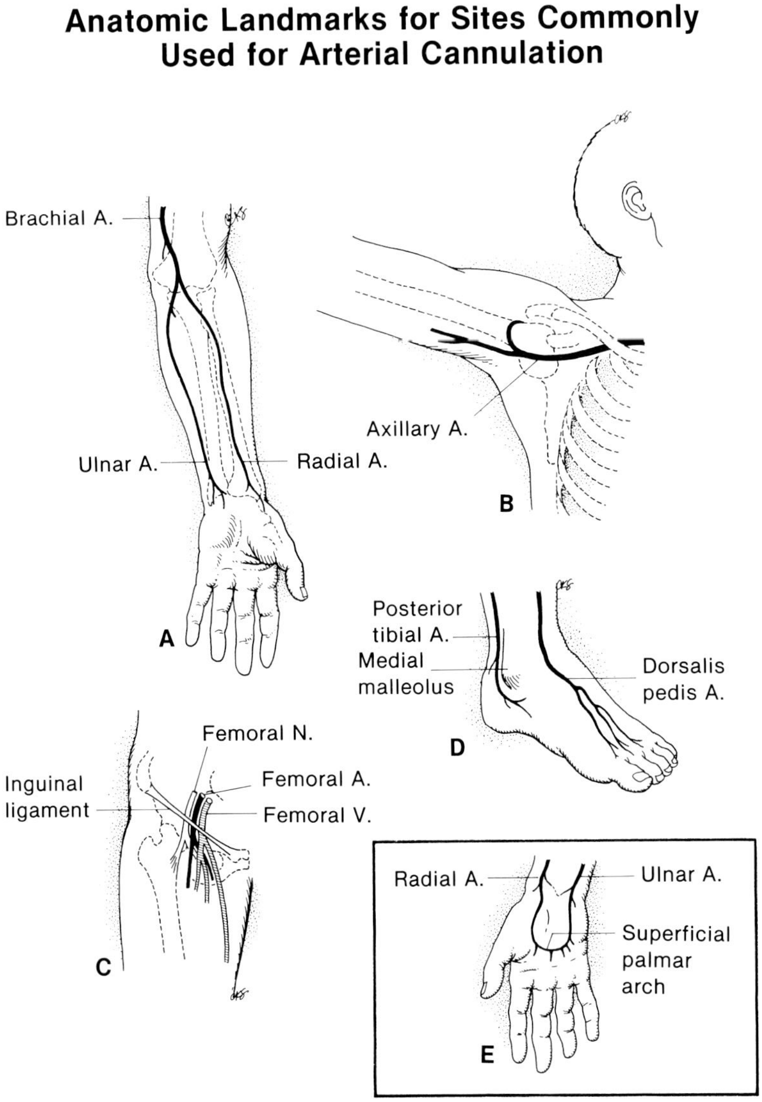

Figure 19–3 • Anatomic landmarks for sites commonly used for artery cannulation. (***A***) Arterial supply of the arm and hand. (***B***) Axillary artery. (***C***) Femoral artery. (***D***) Arterial supply of the foot. (***E***) Arterial supply of the wrist and palm.

al[18] demonstrated that the Allen's test was not predictive of ischemic damage after cannulation, and they could not demonstrate that an abnormal Allen's test increased the risk of complications after radial arterial catheterization. Other investigators have suggested use of strain-gauge plethysmography to insure adequacy of collateral flow to the hand before radial artery catheterization[19] or Doppler plethysmography.[20] None of the methods used to assess adequacy of collateral flow to the hand through the superficial palmar arch can definitively predict digit ischemia. After cannulation, perfusion to the hand must be closely monitored. If any question about impaired perfusion arises, the catheter must be removed.

Cannulation of the radial artery is usually performed percutaneously. The arm is stabilized on a short arm board. The wrist is hyperextended over a roll of gauze (see Fig. 19–2). After the catheter has been placed, it must be well secured with either tape or suture (3-0 or 4-0 silk suture) to prevent accidental dislodging. The wrist must be stabilized while the catheter is in place to prevent kinking or fracture of the catheter with flexion of the wrist. The site should be covered with a sterile dressing and should be observed frequently for signs of infection.

A 20 gauge catheter is most commonly used for cannulation of the radial artery in the adult. For the pediatric patient a 20, 22, or 24 gauge catheter is used, depending on the age and size of the patient. The catheter used for radial artery cannulation should be Teflon-coated polyurethane and nontapered. Tapered catheters and polyvinylchloride catheters cause a much higher incidence of thrombosis and should be avoided.[8]

2. ULNAR ARTERY

The ulnar artery can also be used for arterial catheterization (see Fig. 19–3A). The technique for catheterization of the ulnar artery is similar to the technique for the radial artery. The wrist is stabilized using an arm board. The vessel is most commonly cannulated percutaneously, although the cutdown technique can also be used.

Prior to cannulation of the ulnar artery, similar precautions about flow to the hand must be addressed. If multiple attempts at cannulation of the radial artery have been unsuccessful, the ipsilateral ulnar artery should not be catheterized unless adequate flow through the radial artery has been documented.

3. BRACHIAL ARTERY

The brachial artery is easily palpated medial to the biceps tendon and lateral to the median nerve and is therefore accessible for cannulation. Below the antecubital fossa, the brachial artery divides into the radial artery and the ulnar artery (see Fig. 19–3A). Because the brachial artery is the sole source of flow to the lower arm and hand, thrombosis of the brachial artery could be catastrophic. Despite this potential complication, the brachial artery has been used successfully in a large number of adult patients with no evidence of distal ischemia.[21–23]

When cannulating a brachial artery, the elbow must be stabilized to prevent flexion of the arm. An 18 gauge catheter is most often used for catheterization of the brachial artery.

4. AXILLARY ARTERY

The axillary artery should be considered as a potential site for catheterization, particularly in the unstable patient for whom monitoring central arterial pressure is essential.[24,25] The axillary artery is a continuation of the subclavian artery where it exits the neck at the lateral border of the first rib (Fig. 19–3B). The axillary artery is encased in the axillary sheath with the axillary vein and brachial plexus. Because of extensive collateral flow, ischemic complications are rare even when the artery is thrombosed.[26,27] The proximal location of the axillary artery and its size insure that even when the patient is hemodynamically unstable with marked peripheral vasoconstriction, blood pressure can continue to be accurately monitored.

Prior to cannulation of the axillary artery, the patient's arm should be hyperabducted and externally rotated. The site should be shaved and appropriately sterilized. The vessel should be catheterized as high as possible within the axilla. Either a catheter-over-the-needle percutaneous technique or a Seldinger technique can be used for cannulation of the axillary artery.

5. DORSALIS PEDIS AND POSTERIOR TIBIAL ARTERIES

Both the dorsalis pedis and posterior tibial arteries are superficial and easily palpated (Fig. 19–3D). Because the foot has extensive collateral flow, similar to the flow provided through the palmar arch of the hand, cannulation of either vessel is safe.[28,29] The dorsalis pedis artery is absent in approximately 12% of the population.[30] Despite the safety of cannulation of the dorsalis pedis and posterior tibial arteries, flow to the foot should be evaluated prior to cannulation. Techniques similar to the Allen's test or Doppler plethysmography have been described. The studies using these techniques have not confirmed that they will prevent foot ischemia after cannulation. If perfusion to the foot is satisfactory prior to cannulation, the vessels can probably be catheterized safely. Foot perfusion must be evaluated closely after catheterization, although this may vary due to vasoconstriction in the hemodynamically unstable patient and not be due to site of catheterization.

A 20 gauge catheter is most commonly used for catheterization of the dorsalis pedis or posterior tibial arteries. The technique is similar to catheterization of arteries of the wrist.

6. FEMORAL ARTERY

The femoral artery originates below the inguinal ligament as a continuation of the external iliac artery (Fig. 19–3C). The femoral artery passes through the midpoint of a line drawn between the superior iliac spine and the symphysis pubis. The femoral nerve is lateral to the femoral artery and the femoral vein is medial to the femoral artery within the femoral sheath.

The femoral artery is easily palpated below the inguinal ligament. The vessel can be cannulated using a percutaneous technique with a catheter-over-the-needle or Seldinger guide wire method. Prior to cannulation, the groin should be shaved and sterilized. Sterile barriers should be placed around the site of catheterization to prevent contamination. If the Seldinger technique is used,[31] direct cannulation of the vessel can be achieved and a guide wire inserted through the needle after obtaining free flow of blood. Alternatively, the guide needle or arterial needle-catheter assembly can be advanced through the back wall of the artery and then slowly withdrawn until free arterial flow is obtained. When free arterial flow is obtained, the guide wire can then be advanced through the guide needle, or arterial needle or arterial catheter (arterial needle removed). When advancing the wire, no resistance to passage should be elicited. If resistance is noted during insertion of the wire, the wire and needle should be removed together to prevent dissection of the vessel and knotting or dislodging of a portion of the wire. Once the wire is within the vessel lumen, a catheter is placed over the wire, the wire removed, and the catheter connected to the monitoring system.

If a catheter-over-the-needle technique is used, the catheter should be advanced over the needle once free flow of blood is obtained. After passage of the catheter into the vessel, the catheter should be secured with suture. The site should be sterilely dressed.

7. Superficial Temporal Artery

The superficial temporal artery has been used as a site to obtain arterial blood gas samples and for cannulation for arterial monitoring. The use of this site is *not* recommended for routine monitoring because of a high incidence of central nervous system complications.[32–34]

D. *Arterial Catheterization for Pediatric Patients*

Arterial catheterization of the pediatric patient carries all of the risks associated with catheterization of the adult plus those complications associated with catheterization of small vessels. Catheterization is more difficult because the vessels are small and frequently distal flow is prevented after cannulation.[35] The recommended sites for catheterization of the pediatric patient include the radial artery,[5] posterior tibial artery,[36] dorsalis pedis artery, and axillary artery.[36A] A variety of techniques have been described to facilitate catheterization of peripheral arteries in small children, including use of a fiberoptic light source[37] and Doppler flow probe.[20] More proximal vessels such as the brachial and femoral arteries are not recommended sites for catheterization, although the femoral artery has been used successfully with no higher incidence of complications than are caused by radial artery catheters in children beyond the neonatal period.[38]

Percutaneous catheterization of peripheral arteries in the newborn can be difficult. To obtain access to the arterial circulation, a cutdown technique is sometimes required for catheterization of the radial, posterior tibial, or dorsalis pedis arteries. When access to the central arterial circulation is required, umbilical artery catheterization is usually performed.[39–41] The catheter is inserted into the umbilical artery under sterile technique. The catheter can usually be inserted directly into one of the umbilical arteries, particularly if cannulation is attempted shortly after birth. If the catheter cannot be inserted directly, a cutdown procedure may be necessary.[42]

Most complications from umbilical arterial lines are secondary to vascular injury because of thrombus

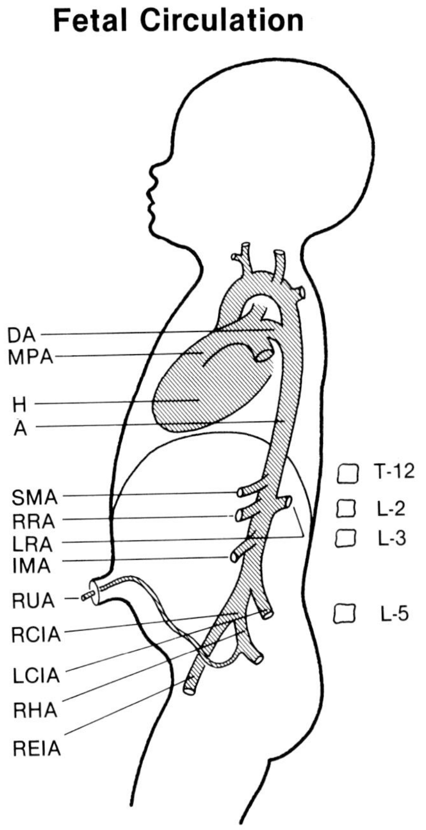

Figure 19–4 • Diagram of the newborn arterial system and its relationship to the spine. *DA* = ductus arterious; *MPA* = main pulmonary artery, *H* = heart; *A* = aorta; *SMA* = superior mesenteric artery; *RRA* = right renal artery; *LRA* = left renal artery; *IMA* = inferior mesenteric artery; *RUA* = right umbilical artery; *RCIA* = right common iliac artery; *LCIA* = left common iliac artery; *RHA* = right hypogastric artery; *REIA* = right external iliac artery.

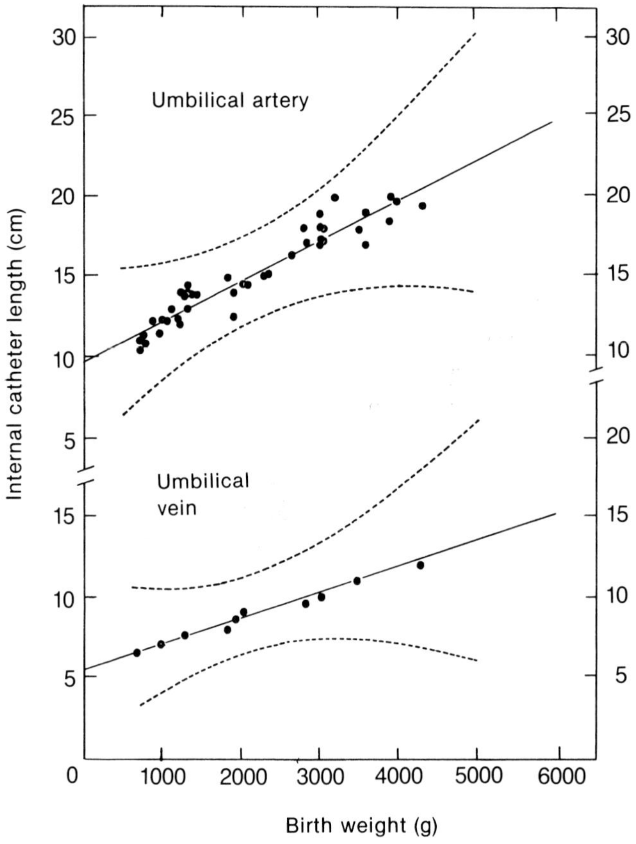

Figure 19–5 • Estimates of insertional length of umbilical catheters (umbilical artery catheter tip inserted between T-6 and T-10; umbilical vein catheter tip inserted above diaphragm in inferior vena cava near or in right atrium) based on birth weight (BW) (95% confidence intervals). Modified estimating equations using MW are as follows: umbilical artery length = 2.5 • BW + 5.6 (*bottom*), where BW is measured in kilograms and length in centimeters.

formation, embolus, or trauma (perforation). The catheter will usually pass into the descending aorta, but can go to other locations that are dangerous. For example, the catheter can pass into the carotid artery through the ductus arteriosus and, possibly, into the pulmonary artery, or down the opposite iliac artery.

The depth to which to insert the umbilical artery catheter must be carefully determined to prevent complications associated with improper placement (Fig. 19–4). There is still disagreement about the ideal positioning of the tip of an umbilical arterial catheter. Some experts favor the midthoracic aorta.[44] This position places the catheter tip above the origin of all major arterial branches and in an area of high blood flow. Shukla recently defined estimates of insertional length of umbilical catheters based on birth weight (Fig. 19–5),[45] recommending that the catheter be advanced 3 times birth weight plus 9 cm, to place the catheter high in the aorta. Other techniques have also been described, including adding the distance between the infant's xiphoid process and pubis to the distance between the pubis and the midumbilicus.[46] Other experts recommend placing the catheter in the lower aorta (T-3), but here the blood flow is lower. In either case, the catheter position must be verified by radiographs. The more severe complications (renal hypertension, necrotizing enterocolitis, paraplegia) are uncommon but tend to occur with the catheter in the high position. Less severe complications are more common and occur when the catheter is in the lower position (vascular spasm with reversible ischemia to the legs). An indwelling cannula in a peripheral artery is often safer, and an umbilical arterial catheter should be removed as soon as possible, or at the first sign of a complication.

IV. COMPLICATIONS

Catheterization of the arterial circulation must be carried out with a knowledge of the benefits to be obtained and the inherent risks. Although large numbers of arterial catheters are used in operating rooms and intensive care units without sequelae, arterial catheterization is associated with a number of complications. The major complications are ischemia and infection. Ischemia with a distal tissue necrosis can occur as a result of thrombosis, embolism, or vasospasm. Other complications include hemorrhage with hematoma, aneurysm, arteriovenous fistula, and peripheral nerve damage.

A. *Thrombosis*

Thrombosis occurs due to placement of a foreign body within the arterial lumen. The longer the catheter is in place, the greater the likelihood of thrombosis. The incidence of thrombosis increases greatly for radial artery catheters left in place for longer than 48 to 72 hours.[47,48] Catheterization of larger vessels, such as femoral arteries, has a lower incidence of thrombosis. Femoral artery catheters left in place for as long as 2 weeks have not been associated with thromboses.[49,50] Catheter size relative to vessel area is a primary determinant of intravascular thrombosis. The larger the catheter size, the higher the incidence of thrombosis.[51-53] A 20 gauge catheter is associated with the lowest incidence of thrombosis of the radial artery.[51-53] Thrombosis formation is also highest with tapered catheters; using nontapered Teflon catheters results in the lowest incidence of thrombosis.[51,53] Thrombosis formation may also occur more commonly in patients who are hemodynamically unstable, require vasopressors, or have severe peripheral vascular disease, diabetes mellitus, Raynaud's disease, or vasculitis.[54,55]

The use of continuous flush devices has also reduced the incidence of thrombosis. Prior to routine use of continuous flush devices, intermittent flushing of the catheter with heparinized saline was used to maintain catheter patency. The intermittent flushing was associated with a high incidence of thrombosis and short catheter life.[3,56,57]

Intraarterial thrombosis evaluated by Doppler scan or angiography after radial artery catheterization has been reported to be as high as 50%.[11,14,27,48] The incidence of distal ischemia associated with the local thrombosis at the site of cannulation is, however, relatively rare.[58] When thrombosis occurs at the site of catheterization, recanalization frequently occurs, although it may take several months.[11,14] The incidence of thrombosis after cannulation of other vessels is variable. Although reports of complications due to thrombosis of the dorsalis pedis or posterior tibial arteries are rare, the incidence of thrombosis has been reported to be as high as 7%.[29] The incidence of thrombosis after cannulation of more proximal vessels is low if the catheter size is small and the catheter does not totally occlude the vessel. Thrombosis of the femoral artery is common in patients with severe peripheral vascular disease and following repeated unsuccessful attempts at catheterization of the artery.[59] Thrombosis after brachial artery catheterization is extremely rare.[21,22] However, in a study of 25 patients who had catheterization with an 18 gauge polyethylene catheter, the incidence of vascular abnormalities noted by angiography was high.[23] Fourteen of the 25 subjects had absent peripheral pulses and vascular abnormalities noted after removal of the catheter. This study was performed prior to use of continuous flush devices. As a result, the incidence of thrombosis and subsequent ischemia after brachial artery catheterization may be as low as that described by Barnes et al.[21]

B. *Embolism*

The thrombi that form at the tip of the catheter can embolize. In addition, air or particulate matter introduced into the monitoring system can be embolized at the time of flushing of the arterial catheter.[60] The use of continuous flush devices minimizes the risk of thromboembolism, because the frequency of intermittent flushing is reduced.[3,52,57]

Flushing the arterial catheter with solution under high pressure can cause retrograde emboli. Flushing a radial artery catheter can cause retrograde flow of fluid to the carotid artery, increasing the risk of embolization to the cerebral circulation.[61] Prior to flushing an arterial catheter, blood should be withdrawn from the stopcock to insure that no air or clot will be flushed into the arterial circulation.

Thrombi formed at the end of an arterial catheter can also embolize peripherally. Emboli from a femoral artery catheter can produce ischemia and necrosis of the lower leg and foot; emboli from a radial artery catheter can cause gangrene of the hand or forearm.[62]

As a result of embolization or thrombosis, ischemia of distal tissue can occur. Necrosis of overlying skin has been reported[63,64] as well as gangrene of the extremity.[65] When an arterial catheter is in place, the site and skin distal to the site should be evaluated for signs of blanching or ischemia, indicating the need to replace or permanently remove the catheter. Similarly, when the waveform from the catheter is damped or sampling becomes difficult, the catheter should be removed, because of the high likelihood that thrombus has formed at the end of the catheter and vascular integrity will be compromised.[55]

C. *Hemorrhage and Hematoma*

Catheterization of the arterial circulation can result in significant bleeding. If the catheter becomes disconnected from the monitoring system, the patient can lose a large amount of blood in a very short time. In addition, particularly for patients with a bleeding diathesis, bleeding around the site of catheterization can occur. Placement of Gelfoam ® absorbable gelatin over the site often helps stop bleeding from around the catheter insertion site. The incidence of bleeding is highest after cutdown, particularly in small children with little subcutaneous tissue to seal the catheterization site. In the intensive care unit, patients with a bleeding diathesis (for example, disseminated intravascular coagulation [DIC]) and patients receiving anticoagulants may bleed from the puncture site.

A hematoma can form around the catheter insertion site. Hematoma formation occurs most commonly after multiple attempts at cannulation or after removal of the catheter. Application of pressure for 10 minutes after catheter removal will reduce the likelihood of hematoma formation.[11,55,66]

D. *Infection*

Indwelling arterial catheters impose a significant risk of infection, particularly in the critically ill patient. For patients who undergo arterial catheterization for surgery, the risk of infection is extremely low. With proper technique, no catheters placed for surgery alone should become infected.

In the critically ill patient, the risk of infection is greater.[67,68] The greatest risk appears to be after prolonged catheter placement of over 4 days.[69] Catheters inserted by cutdown have a higher incidence of infection than those inserted percutaneously. Inflammation around the catheter insertion site is also associated with an increased incidence of catheter-related infection. To prevent the risk of catheter-associated septicemia, some investigators recommend that catheter sites be rotated every 4 days, if clinically feasible. Because of the impaired access in the critically ill patient, especially the pediatric patient, routine catheter replacement may not be possible.[70] Catheter sites should be investigated daily for signs of inflammation or other clinical evidence of sepsis. Any signs of infection warrant prompt removal of the catheter, culturing of the catheter tip,[71] and appropriate antibiotic administration.

E. *Aneurysm and Arteriovenous Fistula*

Aneurysms and pseudoaneurysms have occurred after cannulation of the radial and femoral arteries.[72,73] Soderstrom[72] identified six patients who developed infected false femoral artery aneurysms secondary to arterial catheterization. The aneurysms all resulted in systemic septicemia. The aneurysms required surgical resection combined with antibiotic therapy to eliminate the septic focus.[74] Arteriovenous fistulae between the femoral artery and vein have also occurred, particularly after cannulation for cardiac catheterization and angiography.[66,75]

F. *Neurologic Complications*

Neurologic complications can occur as a result of arterial catheterization or immobilization. When immobilizing the arm or hand of a patient who will be anesthetized or who is unresponsive in the intensive care unit, care must be taken to insure that nerves are not compressed by arm boards and tape. During cannulation of the axillary artery, direct injury can occur to the brachial plexus. In addition, a hematoma of the axillary sheath can result in nerve compression and injury.[24] Neurologic complications have also been reported after brachial artery catheterization. Bleeding, hematoma, and abscess can cause median nerve neuropathy or Volkmann's contracture.[67,76,77] Catheterization of the axillary and brachial arteries should be avoided in patients receiving anticoagulant therapy or with bleeding diatheses.

G. *Complications of Umbilical Artery Catheterization*

Umbilical artery catheterization is associated with a number of the same complications as other sites of cannulation. Bleeding can occur as a result of disconnected stopcocks. Air embolism has been reported due to air injection. Thrombotic complications have been noted after umbilical artery catheterization.[78,79] Goetzman et al reported a 24% incidence of thrombotic complications noted at aortography in 98 newborn infants who underwent umbilical artery catheterization.[78] The incidence of thrombosis is highest when small catheters are used.[80] The smaller catheters (3.5 French) are, however, generally used only for smaller infants, so that the size of the child may dictate the frequency of thrombosis. The use of heparinized solutions and continuous flush systems reduces the incidence of thrombosis[80–82] or its sequelae.

Positioning of the umbilical artery catheter has also been implicated in an increased incidence of thrombosis. Mokrohisky et al found that 91% of infants with the umbilical artery tip at L-3 to L-4 had evidence of thrombosis.[46] The incidence of thrombosis was considerably lower in the group of infants whose catheter tip was between T-7 and T-8. Other studies do not find the same relationship between thrombotic complications and catheter position.[78,79]

A number of additional complications are associated with umbilical artery catheterization. Some of the complications occur during catheterization, including rupture of the umbilical artery[83] and bladder injury.[84–86] Additional complications include late thromboses[87,88] and neurologic sequelae, including paraplegia,[89] which may be due to embolization of thrombi to the spinal cord vascular supply.[90] Associated with aortic thrombosis is renal hypertension, intestinal necrosis, paraplegia, and peripheral gangrene.[79,87,88] Ischemic sequelae of umbilical artery catheterization have also been reported long after removal of the umbilical artery catheter.[91] Aortoiliac aneurysms[92–95] and umbilical artery abscesses[96] have also occurred following umbilical artery catheterization. Refractory hypoglycemia has been reported in two infants who had umbilical artery catheters in place. The cause of the hypoglycemia has been ascribed to iatrogenic hyperinsulinism due to malposition of the umbilical artery catheter.[97,98]

V. Discussion

Arterial catheterization has become a common practice in the operating room and intensive care unit to facilitate patient care and provide easy access for monitoring and blood sampling. Techniques for catheterization of the arterial system are relatively easy and the equipment for monitoring straightforward. As a result, arterial catheterization has become so commonplace that physicians forget the potential costs imposed by its use. When clinically appropriate to monitor blood pressure and hemodynamics or to provide access for frequent blood sampling, arterial catheterization is justified. When used for the convenience of the physician or nurse, arterial catheterization cannot be justified.

The site selected for arterial catheterization is dependent on the patient's anatomy and pathophysiology, and on the skill and experience of the person performing the catheterization. For most adults, radial artery catheterization is preferred. Perfusion is easily assessed, the vessel is readily accessible, and the technique straightforward. The site can be monitored and assessment of adequacy of perfusion performed as part of routine care. When radial artery catheterization is impossible due to inadequate collateral flow or impaired perfusion, axillary or femoral artery catheterization should be considered. When concerns about central arterial blood pressure are paramount, for example, immediately after cardiopulmonary bypass[99,100] or in patients with marked peripheral vasoconstriction, the axillary or femoral artery will provide more reliable hemodynamic information.[101–103]

For the infant requiring arterial blood pressure monitoring, peripheral sites can often be used. Catheterization of the radial, posterior tibial, or dorsalis pedis arteries can usually be accomplished either percutaneously or by cutdown. For the asphyxiated newborn, umbilical artery catheterization may be necessary. Under these circumstances, the risks of umbilical artery catheterization are outweighed by the need to appropriately monitor blood pressure and laboratory data.

VI. References

1. Kroeker EJ, Wood EH. Comparison of simultaneously recorded central and peripheral pressure pulses during rest, exercise and titled position in man. Circ Res 3:623-623, 1955.
2. Shapiro BA, Cane RD, Chomka CM, Gehrich JL. Evaluation of a new intra-arterial blood gas system in dogs. Crit Care Med 15:361, 1987.
3. Gardner RM, Bond EL, Clark JS. Safety and efficacy of continuous flush systems for arterial and pulmonary catheters. Ann Thorac Surg 23:534–538, 1977.
4. Oh T, Opie NJ, Davis NJ. Continuous flush system for radial artery cannulation. Anaesthesia and Intensive Care 4:29–32, 1976.
5. Sellden H, Nilsson K, Larsson LE, Ekstrom-Jodal B. Radial arterial catheters in children and neonates: A prospective study. Crit Care Med 15:1106–1109, 1987.
6. Hook ML, Reuling J, Luettgen ML, Norris SO, et al. Comparison of the patency of arterial lines maintained with heparinized and nonheparinized infusions. Heart Lung 16:693–699, 1987.
7. Galvis AG, Donahoo JS, White JJ. An improved technique for

prolonged arterial catheterization in infants and children. Crit Care Med 4:166–169, 1976.

8. Bedford RF. Percutaneous radial-artery cannulation- Increased safety using Teflon catheters. Anesthesiology 42:219–222, 1975.
9. Hayes MF, Morello DC, Rosenbaum RW, Matsumoto T. Radial artery catheterization by cutdown technique. Crit Care Med 1:51–152, 1973.
10. Seldinger SI. Catheter replacement of the needle in percutaneous arteriography: A new technique. Acta Radiol 39:368–376, 1953.
11. Bedford RF, Wollman H. Complications of percutaneous radial-artery cannulation. An objective prospective study in man. Anesthesiology 38:228–236, 1973.
12. Brodsky J. A simple method to determine patency of the ulnar artery intraoperatively prior to radial-artery cannulation. Anesthesiology 42:626–627, 1975.
13. Mozersky DJ, Buckley CJ, Hagood CO Jr, Capps WF Jr, et al. Ultrasonic evaluation of the palmar circulation. Am J Surg 126:810–812, 1973.
14. Palm T. Evaluation of peripheral arterial pressure in the thumb following radial artery cannulation. Br J Anaesth 49:819–824, 1977.
15. Husum B, Palm T. Arterial dominance in the hand. Br J Anaesth 50:913–915, 1978.
16. Allen EV. Thromboangitis obliterans: Methods of diagnosis of chronic occlusive arterial lesions distal to the wrist with illustrated cases. Am J Med Sci 178:237–244, 1929.
17. Ghandi SK, Reynolds AC. A modification of Allen's test to detect abherrant ulnar collateral circulation. Anesthesiology 59:147–148, 1983.
18. Slogoff S, Keats AS, Arlund C. On the safety of radial artery cannulation. Anesthesiology 59:42–47, 1983.
19. Husum B, Palm T. Before cannulation of the radial artery: Collateral arterial supply evaluated by strain-gauge plethysmography. Acta Anaesth Scand 24:412–414, 1980.
20. Morrayu JP, Brandford HG, Barnes LF, Oh SM, et al. Doppler-assisted radial artery cannulation in infants and children. Anesth Analg 63:346–348, 1984.
21. Barnes RW, Foster EJ, Jansen GA, Boutros AR. Safety of brachial artery catheters as monitors in the intensive care unit— Prospective evaluation with the Doppler ultrasonic velocity detector. Anesthesiology 44:260–264, 1976.
22. Barnes RW, Petersen JL, Krugmire BB Jr, Strandness DE Jr. Complications of brachial artery catheterization: Prospective evaluation with the Doppler ultrasound detector. Chest 66:363–367, 1974.
23. Lipchik EO, Sugimoto H. Percutaneous brachial artery catheterization. Radiology 160:842–843, 1986.
24. Adler DC, Bryan-Brown CW. Use of the axillary artery for intravascular monitoring. Crit Care Med 1:148–150, 1970.
25. Bryan-Brown CW, Kwun KB, Limb PD, Pia RLG, et al. The axillary artery catheter. Heart Lung 12:492–497, 1983.
26. DeAngelis J. Axillary artery monitoring. Crit Care Med 4:205–206, 1976.
27. Gardner RM, Schwartz R, Wong HC, Burke JP. Percutaneous indwelling radial-artery catheters for monitoring and cardiovascular function. Prospective study of the risk of thrombosis and infection. N Engl J Med 290:1227–1231, 1974.
28. Johnstone RE, Greenhow E. Catheterization of the dorsalis pedis artery. Anesthesiology 39:654–655, 1973.
29. Youngberg JA, Miller ED. Evaluation of percutaneous cannulation of the dorsalis pedis artery. Anesthesiology 44:80–83, 1976.
30. Barnhorst DA, Barner HB. Prevalence of congenitally absent pedal pulses. N Engl J Med 278:264–265, 1968.
31. Colvin MP, Curran JP, O'Shea PJ. Femoral artery pressure monitoring: Use of Seldinger technique. Anaesthesia 32:451–455, 1977.
32. Bull MJ, Schreiner RL, Garg BP, Hutton NM, et al. Neurologic complications following temporal artery catheterization. J Pediatr 96:1071–1073, 1980.
33. Prian GW, Wright GB, Rumach CM, O'Meara OP. Apparent cerebral embolism after temporal artery catheterization. J Pediatr 93:115–118, 1978.
34. Simmons MA, Levine RI, Lubchenco CO, Guggenheim MA. Warning: Serious sequelae of temporal artery catheterization. J Pediatr 92:284, 1978.
35. Heinonen K, Kuusela T. Peripheral artery catheters in very low birth-weight neonates. Acta Paediatr Scand 71:323–324, 1982.
36. Spahr R, MacDonald HM, Holzman IR. Catheterization of the posterior tibial artery in the neonate. Am J Dis Child 133:945–946, 1979.
36A. Greenwald BM, Notterman DA, DeBruin WJ, McCready M. Percutaneous axillary artery catheterization in critically ill infants and children. J Ped; 117:442–444, 1990.
37. Cole FS, Todres ID, Shannon DC. Technique for percutaneous cannulation of the radial artery in the newborn infant. J Pediatr 92:105–107, 1978.
38. Glenzki JA, Beynan FM, Brady J. A prospective evaluation of femoral artery monitoring in pediatric patients. Anesthesiology 66:227–229, 1987.
39. Symansky MR, Fox HA. Umbilical vessel catheterization: Indications, management and evaluation of the technique. J Pediatr 80:820–826, 1972.
40. Cole AFD, Rolbin SH. A technique for rapid catheterization of the umbilical artery. Anesthesiology 53:254–255, 1980.
41. Hashimoto T, Togari H, Yura J. Umbilical artery cutdown: An improved procedure for reinsertion. Br J Surg 72:194, 1985.
42. Clark JM, Jung AL. Umbilical artery catheterization by a cutdown procedure. Pediatrics 59:1036–1040, 1977.
43. Dunn PM. Localization of the umbilical catheter by post-mortem measurement. Arch Dis Child 41:69–75, 1966.
44. Mokrohisky ST, Levine RL, Blumhagen JD, Wesenberg RL, et al. Low positioning of umbilical-artery catheters increases associated complications in newborn infants. N Engl J Med 299:561–564, 1978.
45. Shukla H, Ferrara A. Rapid estimation of insertional length of umbilical catheters in newborns. Am J Dis Child 140:786–788, 1986.
46. Rubin BK, McRobert E, O'Neill MB. An alternate technique to determine umbilical arterial catheter length. Clin Pediatr 25:407–408, 1986.
47. Bedford RF. Long-term radial artery cannulation: Effects on subsequent vessel function. Crit Care Med 6:64–67, 1978.
48. Downs JB, Chapman RL Jr, Hawkins IF Jr. Prolonged radial artery catheterization. An evaluation of heparinized catheters and continuous irrigation. Arch Surg 108:671–673, 1974.
49. Ersoz CJ, Hedden M, Lain L. Prolonged femoral arterial catheterization for intensive care. Anesth Analg 49:160–164, 1970.
50. Russell JA, Joel M, Hudson RJ, Mangano DT, et al. Prospective evaluation of radial and femoral artery catheterization sites in critically ill adults. Crit Care Med 11:936–939, 1983.
51. Bedford RF. Radial arterial function following percutaneous cannulation with 18- and 20-gauge catheters. Anesthesiology 47:37–39, 1977.
52. Downs JB, Rackstein AD, Klein EF Jr, Hawkins IF Jr. Hazards of radial-artery catheterization. Anesthesiology 38:283–286, 1973.
53. Davis FM. Radial artery cannulation: Influence of catheter size and material on arterial occlusion. Anaesthesia and Intensive Care 6:49–53, 1978.

54. Arthurs GJ. Digital ischaemia following radial artery cannulation. Anaesthesia and Intensive Care 6:54–55, 1978.
55. Mandel MA, Dauchot PJ. Radial artery cannulation in 1,000 patients: Precautions and complications. J Hand Surg 2:482–485, 1977.
56. Cederholm I, Sorenson J, Carlsson C. Thrombosis following percutaneous radial artery cannulation. Acta Anaesthesiol Scand 30:227–230, 1986.
57. Shinebourne E, Pfitzner J. Continuous flushing device for indwelling arterial and venous cannulae. Br J Hosp Med (suppl) 9:64–66, 1973.
58. Berardis JM, Knight P, Grossi RJ, Ferraro L, et al. Delayed, distant arterial injury after brachial artery catheterization. Angiology 35:380–382, 1984.
59. Sessler CN, Alford P. Arterial occlusion after femoral artery cannulation. Crit Care Med 14:520–521, 1986.
60. Chang C, Dughi J, Shitabata P, Johnson G, et al. Air embolism and the radial arterial line. Crit Care Med 16:141–143, 1988.
61. Lowenstein E, Little JW, Lo HH. Prevention of cerebral embolization from flushing radial artery cannulae. N Engl J Med 285:1414–1415, 1971.
62. Katz AM, Birnbaum M, Moylan J, Pellett J. Gangrene of the hand and forearm: A complication of radial artery cannulation. Crit Care Med 2:270–272, 1974.
63. Johnson RW. A complication of radial artery cannulation. Anesthesiology 40:598–600, 1974.
64. Wyatt R, Glares I, Cooper DJ. Proximal skin necrosis after radial-artery cannulation. Lancet i:1135-1138, 1974.
65. Johnson FE, Sumner DS, Strandness DE. Extremity necrosis caused by indwelling arterial catheters. Am J Surg 131:375–379, 1976.
66. Christian CM, Naraghi M. A complication of femoral arterial cannulation in a patient undergoing cardiopulmonary bypass. Anesthesiology 49:436–437, 1978.
67. Lindsay SL, Kerridge R, Collett BJ. Abscess following cannulation of the radial artery. Anaesthesia 42:654–657, 1987.
68. Stamm WE, Colella JJ, Anderson RL, Dixon RE. Indwelling arterial catheters as a source of nosocomial bacteremia. N Engl J Med 292:1099–1102, 1975.
69. Band JD, Maki DG. Infections caused by arterial catheters used for hemodynamic monitoring. Am J Med 67:735–741, 1979.
70. Thomas F, Burke JP, Parker J, Orme FJ Jr, et al. The risk of infection related to radial vs femoral sites for arterial catheterization. Crit Care Med 11:807–812, 1983.
71. Maki DG, Weise CE, Sarafin HW. A semiquantitative culture method for identifying intravenous catheter-related infection. N Engl J Med 296:1305–1309, 1977.
72. Soderstrom CA, Wasserman DH, Ranson KJ, Caplan ES, et al. Infected false femoral artery aneurysms secondary to monitoring catheters. J Cardiovasc Surg 24:63–68, 1983.
73. Wolf S, Mangano DT. Pseudoaneurysm, a late complication of radial-artery catheterization. Anesthesiology 52:80–81, 1980.
74. Bolasny BL, Killen DA. Surgical management of arterial injuries secondary to angiography. Ann Surg 174:962–964, 1971.
75. Shah A, Gnoj J, Fisher VJ. Complications of selective coronary arteriography by the Judkins technique and their prevention. Am Heart J 90:353–359, 1975.
76. Macon WL IV, Futrell JW. Median nerve neuropathy after percutaneous puncture of the brachial artery in patients receiving anticoagulants. N Engl J Med 288:1396, 1973.
77. Marshall G, Edelstein G, Hirshman CA. Median nerve compression following radial artery puncture. Anesth Analg 59:953–954, 1980.
78. Goetzman BW, Stadalnik RC, Bogren HG, Blankenship WJ, et al. Thrombotic complications of umbilical artery catheters: A clinical and radiographic study. Pediatrics 56:374–379, 1975.
79. Vailas GN, Brouillette RT, Scott JP, Shkolnik A, et al. Neonatal aortic thrombosis. J Pediatr 109:101–108, 1986.
80. Bosque E, Weaver L. Continuous vs intermittent heparin infusion of umbilical artery catheters in the newborn infant. J Pediatr 108:141–143, 1986.
81. Horgan MJ, Bartoletti A, Polansky S, Peters JC, et al. Effect of heparin infusates in umbilical arterial catheters on frequency of thrombotic complications. J Pediatr 111:774–778, 1987.
82. Rajani K, Goetzman BW, Wennberg RP, Turner E, et al. Effect of heparinization on fluids infused through an umbilical artery catheter on catheter patency and frequency of complications. Pediatrics 63:552–556, 1979.
83. Sasidharan P. Umbilical arterial rupture: A major complication of catheterization. Indiana Med 78:34–35, 1985.
84. Dmochowski RR, Crandell SS, Corriere JN Jr. Bladder injury and uroascietes from umbilical artery catheterization. Pediatrics 77:421–422, 1986.
85. Kaufman JM, Pai S, Austin TL, Macpherson RI. Neonatal bladder injury occurring after umbilical artery catheterization by cutdown. JAMA 250:2968–2970, 1983.
86. Mata JA, Livne PM, Gibbons MD. Urinary ascites: Complications of umbilical artery catheterization. Urology 30:375–377, 1987.
87. Marsh JL, King W, Barrett C, Fongalsrud EW. Serious complications after umbilical artery catheterization for neonatal monitoring. Arch Surg 110:1203–1208, 1975.
88. Saia OS, Rubaltelli FF, D'Elia R, Marigo A, et al. Clinical and aortographic assessment of the complications of arterial catheterization. Eur J Pediatr 128:169–179, 1978.
89. Fok TF, Ha MH, Leung KW, Wong W. Sciatic nerve palsy complicating umbilical arterial catheterization. Eur J Pediatr 145:308–309, 1986.
90. Krishnamoorthy KS, Fernandez RJ, Todres ID, DeLong GR. Paraplegia associated with umbilical artery catheterization in the newborn. Pediatrics 58:443–445, 1976.
91. Bergqvist D, Bergentz SE, Hermansson G, Lundberg HO, et al. Late ischaemic sequelae after umbilical artery catheterization. Br J Surg 74:628–629, 1987.
92. Drucker DEM, Greenfield LJ, Ehrlich F, Salzberg AM. Aortoiliac aneurysms following umbilical artery catheterization. J Pediatr Surg 21:725–730, 1986.
93. Lally KP, Sherman NJ. Iliac artery pseudoaneurysm following umbilical artery catheterization. Surgery 101:636–638, 1987.
94. Shandall AA, Leopald PW, Shah DM, Largent JA, et al. Vischeral aortic aneurysm in a 4 1/2-year-old child: An unusual complication of umbilical artery catheterization. Surgery 100:928–931, 1986.
95. Thompson TR, Tilleli J, Johnson DE, Britt W, et al. Umbilical artery catheterization complicated by mycotic aortic aneurysm in neonates. Adv Pediatr 27:275–318, 1980.
96. Mares AJ, Siplovich L. Obliterated umbilical artery abscess simulating a strangulated umbilical hernia: A late complication of neonatal umbilical artery catheterization. Isr J Med Sci 20:1197–1198, 1984.
97. Malik M, Wilson DP. Umbilical artery catheterization: A potential cause of refractory hypoglycemia. Clin Pediatr 26:181–182, 1987.
98. Urbach J, Kaplan M, Blondheim O, Hirsch HJ. Neonatal hypoglycemia related to umbilical artery catheter malposition. J Pediatr 106:825–826, 1985.
99. Mohr R, Lavee J, Goor DA. Inaccuracy of radial artery pressure

measurement after cardiac operations. J Thorac Cardiovasc Surg 94:286–290, 1987.

100. Stern DH, Gerson JI, Allen FB, Parker FB. Can we trust the direct radial artery pressure immediately following cardiopulmonary bypass? Anesthesiology 62:557–561, 1985.

101. Gurman GM, Kriemerman S. Cannulation of big arteries in critically ill patients. Crit Care Med 13:217–220, 1985.

102. Soderstrom CA, Wasserman DH, Dunham CM, Caplan ES, et al. Superiority of the femoral artery for monitoring: A prospective study. Am J Surg 144:309–320, 1982.

103. Thomas F, Burke JP, Parker J, Orme JF, et al. The risk of infection related to radial vs femoral sites for arterial catheterization. Crit Care Med 11:807–811, 1983.

Chapter 20

Robert C. Mackersie, MD

Venous and Arterial Cutdown

OUTLINE

I. INTRODUCTION

The term cutdown refers to the process by which a vein or an artery (usually peripheral) is exposed through an incision and cannulated under direct vision. This is in contrast to most percutaneous (and therefore relatively "blind") methods for venous and arterial cannulation. Because of the sophistication of techniques and materials available for percutaneous venous cannulation (such as Seldinger wire kits), the need for cutdown cannulation performed in the nonemergent setting has decreased over the years. In situations where immediate, secure, large-bore venous cannulation is desirable (such as life-threatening injury and hypovolemic shock), and in situations where percutaneous peripheral or central access is either contraindicated or impossible to achieve, the cutdown continues to have application. Patients who are candidates for cutdown venous cannulation frequently have sustained multisystem trauma and are hemodynamically unstable, or are hospitalized in the intensive care unit with severe associated underlying illness. In most cases, cutdowns are performed outside of the operating room environment in either the critical care unit or the emergency department; in addition, they are often performed by nonsurgeons under less than optimal conditions. Careful attention to aseptic technique and an orderly stepwise approach to the procedure is necessary to ensure a high success rate and minimal chance of complications.

II. INDICATIONS

Venous cannulation is one of the most frequently performed basic procedures and is indicated for the administration of blood, fluid, or drugs via an intravenous route. The placement of central venous or pulmonary artery monitoring lines, pacemakers, and hemodialysis catheters may also be placed via venous cutdown. In the majority of cases, venous access for monitoring or therapeutic intervention can be accomplished using percutaneous methods. In cases where percutaneous access is not feasible (local injury, massive edema) or is contraindicated (severe coagulopathy), a cutdown may be indicated. Percutaneous central venous access via jugular, subclavian, or femoral approach may be difficult in patients with profound hypovolemia. Under such circumstances, for persons adept at the procedure, large-bore venous cutdown provides the most rapid, secure form of venous access for massive volume infusion. Cutdown venous access may also occasionally be required for the pediatric age groups in cases where central venous access (such as for cardiac surgery) is essential but technically very difficult.

Arterial cutdowns, although performed less commonly, are indicated in cases where arterial monitoring is required and unobtainable using percutaneous methods.

III. How to Do the Procedure

A. *Venous Cutdown*

Venous cutdown may be performed on any vein but is generally confined to easily accessible, superficial veins. The site of cutdown should be selected in accordance with the indication and desired use of the catheter. The most common sites for venous cutdown are the cephalic, basilic, and median antecubital veins in the upper extremity (Fig. 20–1A–B), and the greater saphenous vein in the leg (Fig. 20–2A–B). Occasionally, external jugular veins in the neck are appropriate for cutdowns for purposes of hyperalimentation, or the prolonged need for drug administration. Central access for monitoring or hyperalimentation, if obtained by cutdown, is generally done so via the upper extremity.

The basilic vein, because of its less acute angle with the subclavian vein, is a preferred site of cutdown in the arm (see Fig. 20–1). The most common site for basilic vein cutdown is located approximately two fingerbreadths cephalad and two fingerbreadths anterior to the medial epicondyle in the humerus. Frequently, the vein can either be seen or palpated in thin patients, making site selection a relatively simple matter. The basilic vein in this location, however, lies near the brachial vein artery and the median nerve. In order to avoid injuries to these deeper structures, the dissection should never extend below the level of the muscular fascia. Other sites for venous cutdown in the upper extremity include the proximal cephalic vein, which is used frequently for the placement of long-term indwelling central venous catheters (eg, Broviac, Hickman), and the distal cephalic vein.[1]

The most desirable site for saphenous venous cutdown is at the ankle. The vein is generally located approximately two fingerbreadths cephalad and two fingerbreadths anterior to the center of the medial malleolus. Alternatively, the vein may also be located approximately at a point midway between the prominence of the malleolus and the spine of the tibia. In many instances, the vein can be palpated and identified precisely, making reliance on other landmarks unnecessary (Figs. 20–2A, 20–3A).

The proximal saphenous vein may also be used in the event of severe lower extremity injuries. The proximal vein is located by making a transverse incision directly inferior to the pubic tubercle, at approximately the junction of the scrotal and labial folds in the thigh[2,3] (see Fig. 20–2).

The majority of cutdowns involve superficial veins; the principles of preparation, dissection, and cannulation are essentially the same. The technical details will be discussed and illustrated specifically for the distal saphenous vein cutdown. Cutdowns involving veins deep to the superficial fascia (internal jugular, proximal cephalic, etc) require more sophisticated skills and are best performed in the operating room environment. Discussion of these techniques is beyond the scope of this text.

Surgical masks and caps should always be worn. The skin is prepped widely with a 10% providone iodine solution and drapes are widely applied to isolate the surgical field (Fig. 20–3B–C). The use of local anesthetic (usually 3–5 mL 1% lidocaine) is desirable if time and circumstance permit.

A 2- to 3-cm transverse incision is made over the vein (Fig. 20–3D). The incision is carried down through the skin and well into the subcutaneous fat. It is often advantageous, particularly when using the saphenous vein, to carry an incision down through the overlying connective tissue, to the level of the anterior vein surface. The saphenous vein at the ankle is usually adherent to the fascial layer. Any superficial, smaller vein encoun-

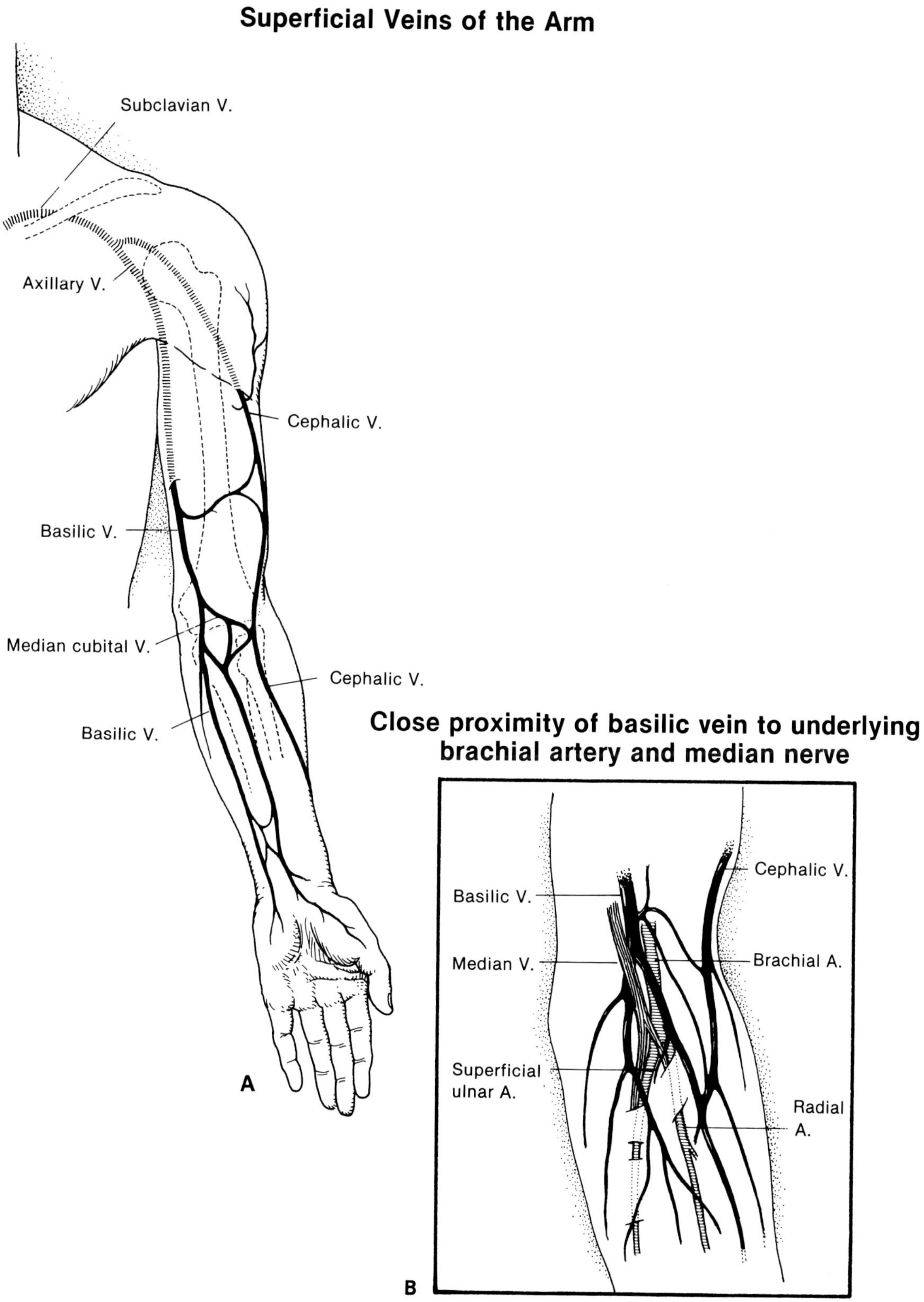

Figure 20–1 • Basilic and cephalic veins are the largest, most accessible sites for cutdown cannulation in the upper extremity.

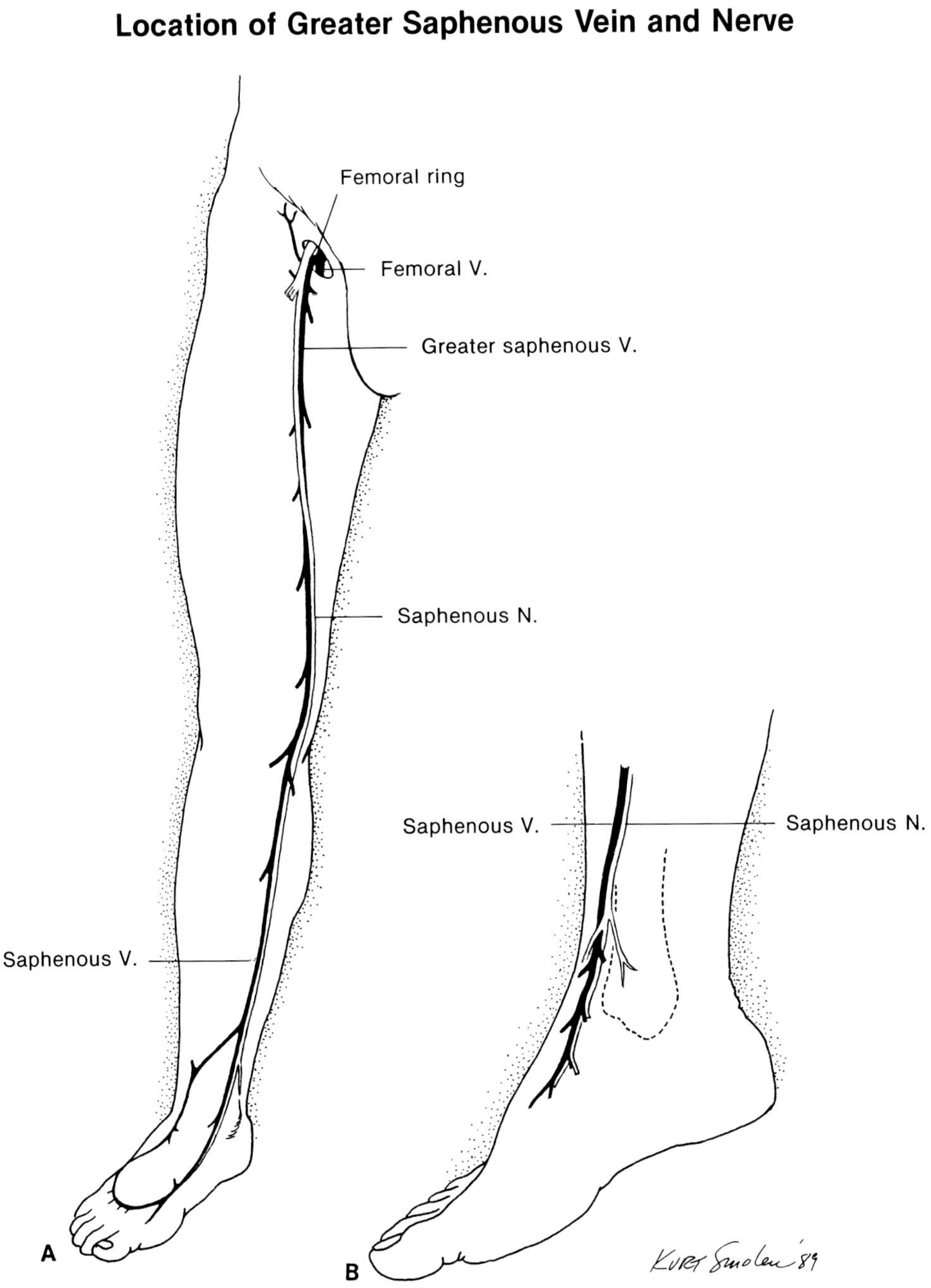

Figure 20–2 • The greater saphenous vein is the preferred site for cutdown cannulation in the lower extremity. ***(A)*** Cutdown may be performed at any point along the greater saphenous vein if necessary. ***(B)*** The distal saphenous vein is the preferred site for cutdown.

tered in the dissection should be disregarded, because cannulation of these veins is usually difficult.

The vein is dissected out using a Kelly clamp (hemostat). This maneuver involves placing the clamp with the tips pointed down, and spreading the tissue apart. When the vein is identified, it is dissected from the overlying connective tissue by placing the clamp in contact with the tissue surrounding the vein and spreading alternately on either side. It may be necessary to repeat this simple but important maneuver several times before the vein is dissected free (see Fig. 20–3D). A great

(Text continued on p. 398)

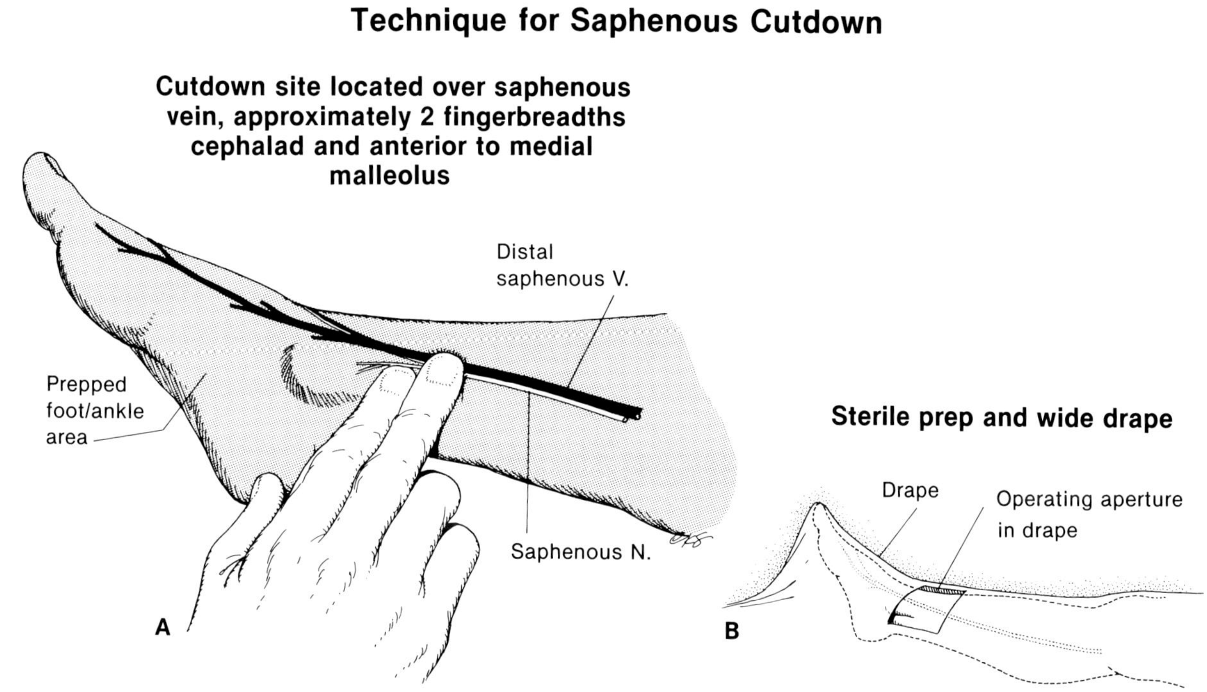

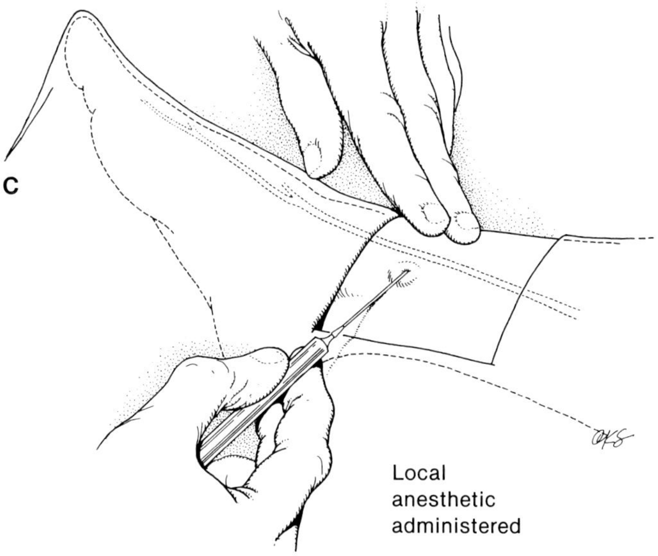

Figure 20-3 • Technique for saphenous cutdown involves localization, isolation, distal ligation, venotomy, and cannulation—manuevers common to all cutdowns performed on superficial veins.

(continued)

2-3 cm transverse incision made over vein site

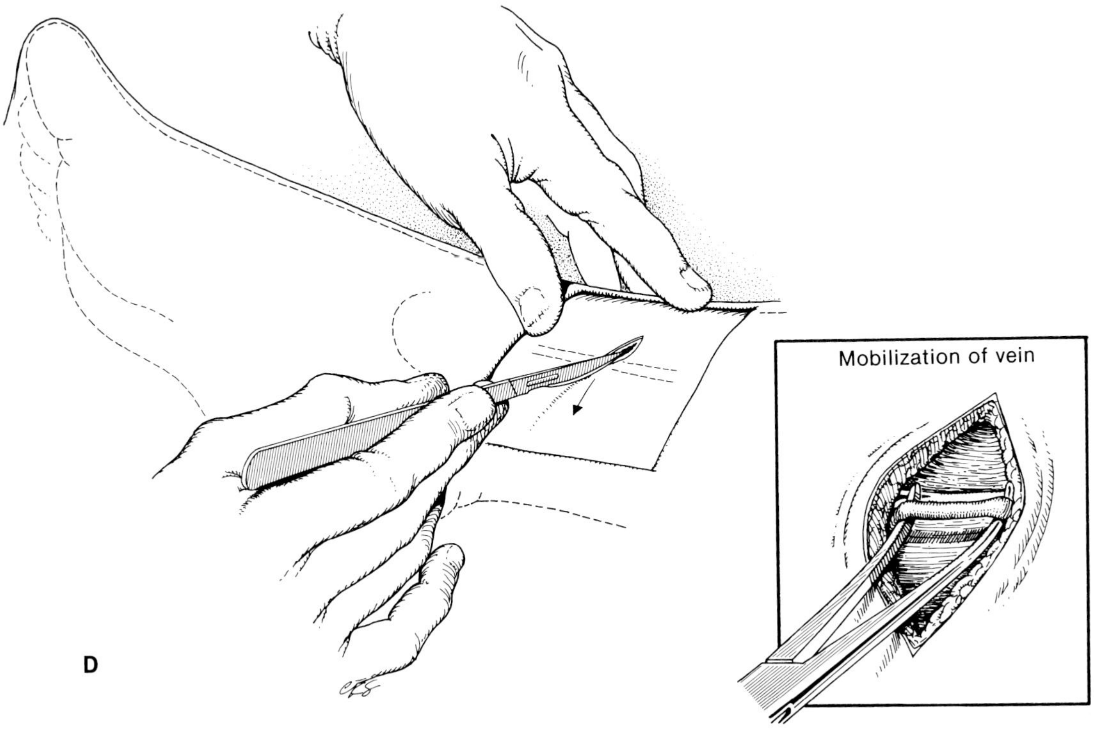

D

Vein immobilized with distal (ligated) and proximal (not ligated) ligatures

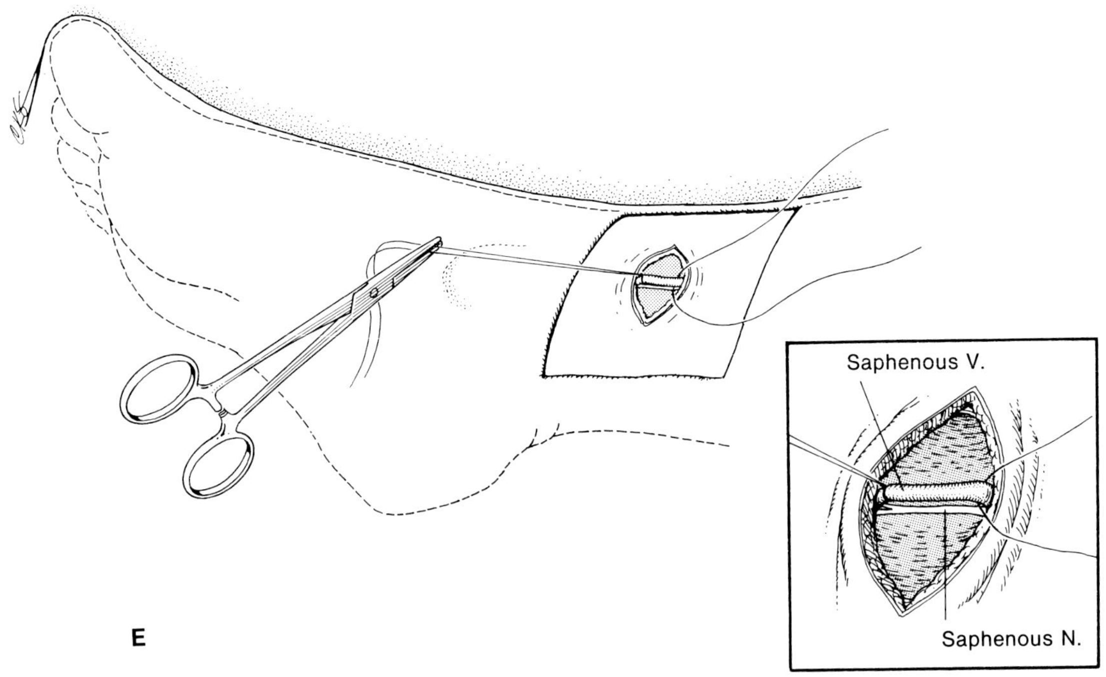

E

Figure 20-3 *(continued)*

Venotomy made while vein securely held with forceps

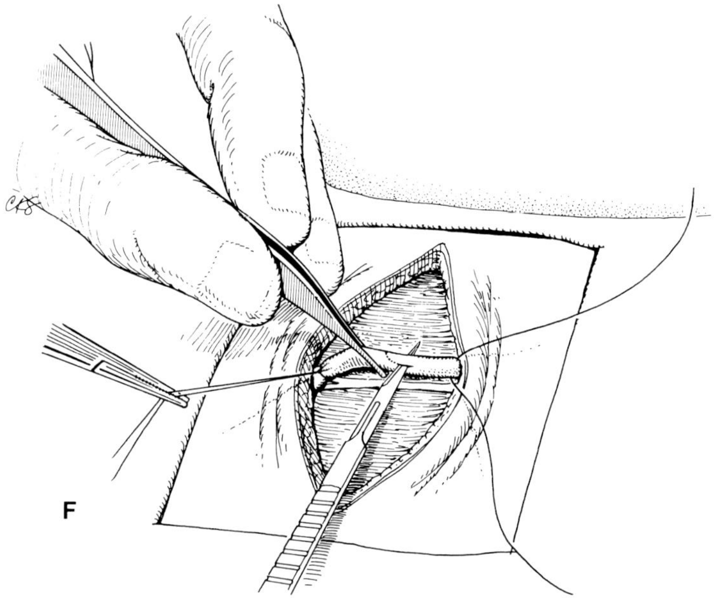

Insertion of K-50 catheter into vein using vein pick

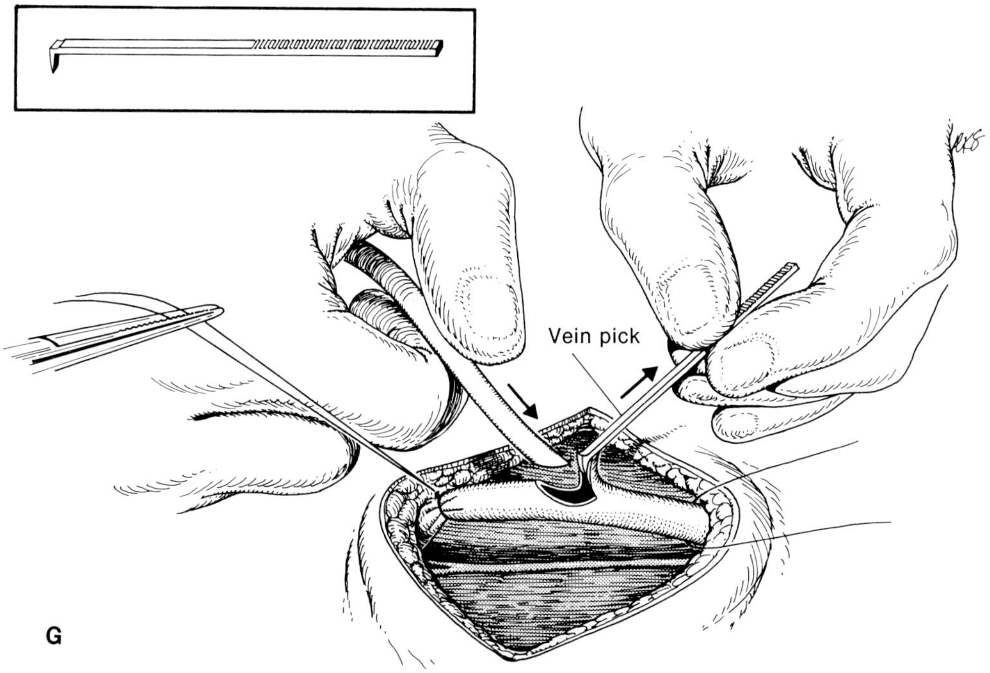

Figure 20–3 *(continued)*

deal of care should be given to avoiding injury to the greater saphenous nerve during the dissection (Fig. 20–3E).

Once the vein is dissected free, the clamp is passed underneath it and then spread vigorously to isolate approximately a 1- to 2-cm portion of vein (see Fig. 20–3D). The distal greater saphenous vein has a particularly thick, muscular coat; it is very difficult to injure the vein by spreading too vigorously. It is a common mistake to dissect out a length of vein that is too short to allow easy cannulation.

With the vein exposed, a distal tie of either 3-0 silk or 3-0 Vicryl is passed and the distal end of the vein ligated. A hemostat is then placed on the suture to stabilize the vein and provide countertraction for subsequent cannulation (see Fig. 20–3E). A proximal tie is passed under the vein as well and left untied. A transverse venotomy is made using either a No. 11 blade scalpel or a pair of fine Metzenbaum scissors (Fig. 20–3F). One of the key steps in this maneuver is stabilization of the vein between a pair of smooth forceps with the opposite hand while the venotomy is being made (see Fig. 20–3F). A common mistake at this point is to perform an inadequate venotomy. Approximately 50% of the vein should be divided to facilitate cannulation. With traction stabilization produced by the distal tie and hemostat, a vein pick is used to retract the upper portion of the venotomy, and a short (5–6 cm) portion of K-50 tubing (or equivalent large-bore catheter) that has been cut on a bevel is then inserted into the vein (Fig. 20–3G). It is generally easier to insert this large-bore tubing, which is often close to the size of the vein, with the bevel down (see Fig. 20–3G). If no vein pick is available, then a small hemostat may be used instead.

Once the catheter has been inserted up to its full length into the vein, the proximal tie around the catheter and the vein is secured in place and the intravenous tubing connected (Fig. 20–4A–B). If time permits, the cutdown incision is closed using a running 3-0 nylon suture, and the hub of the cutdown catheter is secured in position using a similar stitch (Fig. 20–5). When cutdowns are being performed for volume resuscitation, the need for diagnosis and treatment of other injuries often does not allow the time for meticulous incision closure. Under these circumstances, the wound may be dressed, left open, and wrapped using a rolled gauze sponge (Fig. 20–6A–C) to be closed at a later time (usually within 6 to 8 hours).

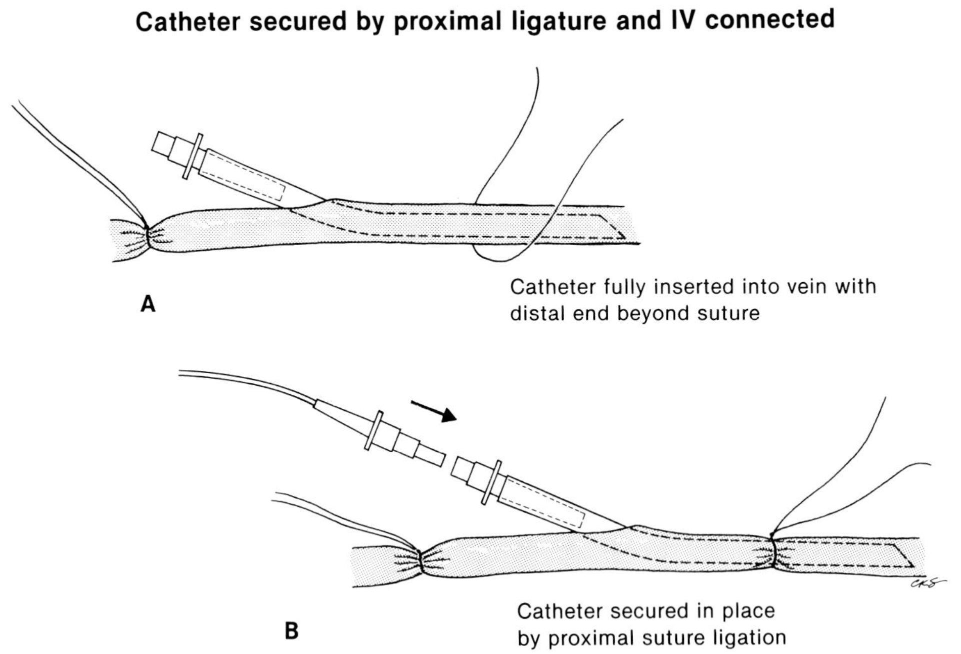

Figure 20–4 • Cannulation is performed using a short piece of K-50 IV connecting tubing (or equivalent IV catheter). ***(A)*** The catheter is fully inserted into the vein with the distal end beyond the suture. ***(B)*** The catheter is secured in place by proximal suture ligation.

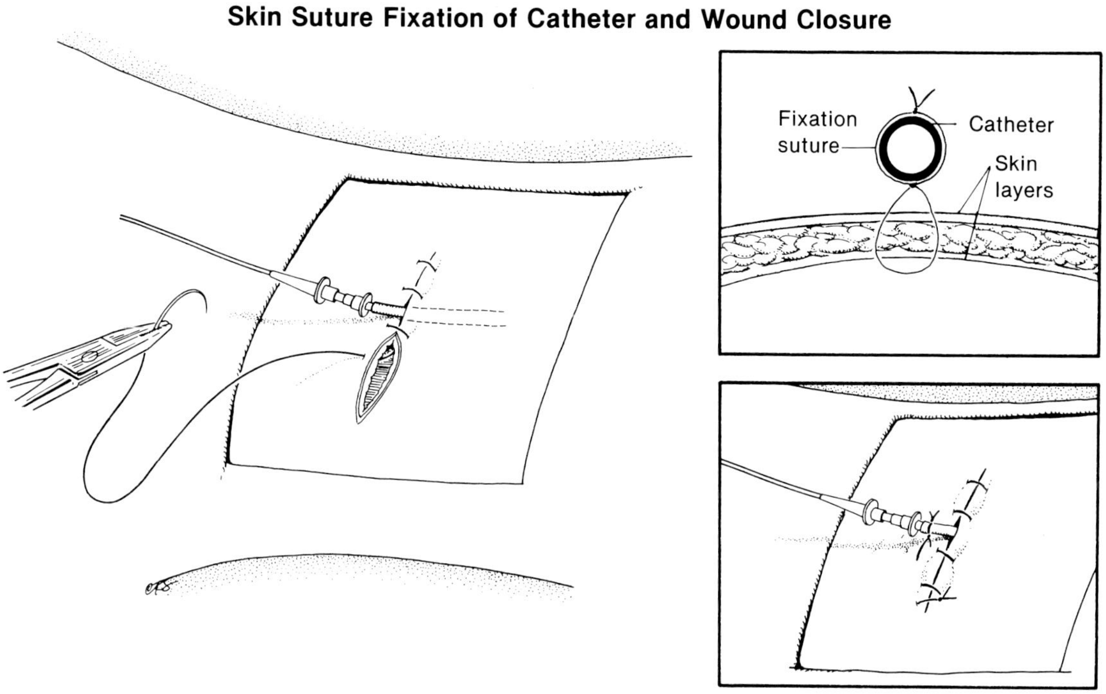

Figure 20–5 • Separate sutures are used for skin closure and fixation of the hub of the cutdown catheter.

Arterial Cutdown

An arterial cutdown is usually performed in the wrist with cannulation of the radial artery. Other cutdown sites include the dorsalis pedis, the posterior tibial, and occasionally the superficial temporal artery in the scalp. The brachial artery should not be used for arterial monitoring because of the high incidence of complications following prolonged cannulation of this vessel. Although the techniques are similar for other sites, some additional skill is required in the dissection. The technique for radial artery cutdown will be described and illustrated.

Indications for arterial cutdown consist of both a defined need for arterial access, and either a contraindication to the use of other available percutaneous sites (such as the femoral artery) or an inability to cannulate percutaneously an appropriate vessel (such as occasionally occurs in the neonate or pediatric age group). A careful Allen's test should be performed to demonstrate adequate collateral flow via the ulnar artery before proceeding with a radial cutdown.

The hand (or foot in the case of a dorsalis pedis or posterior tibial cutdown) should be immobilized using a splint and Kerlix roll (Fig. 20–7). A longitudinal incision is made over the palpated pulse approximately 1–2 cm proximal to the wrist. In cases in which the pulse is not easily palpable, incision is made lateral to the flexor carpi radialis tendon (Figs. 20–7A, 20–8A). Dissection is carried down sharply to the level of the superficial fascial layer. The fascia is divided sharply using Metzenbaum scissors to avoid injury to the artery. This particular technique differs from that used in the saphenous cutdown, where the fascia is separated using blunt clamp dissection. Once the artery has been identified, it is cannulated by a direct stick, usually using a 20 gauge intravenous catheter (or equivalent radial artery kit) (Fig. 20–8B). After the artery is pierced and good blood return observed, the catheter is gently advanced proximally in the artery. Proximal and distal ties are not used as in the venous cutdown. The wound is closed with a running 2-0 nylon suture, and the catheter is secured in a manner similar to venous cutdown (Fig. 20–8C).

IV. DISCUSSION

Decisions as to the site of venous cutdown and the type of catheter used will depend principally on the clinical indications. The distal saphenous vein (at the ankle) is most often the preferred site for acute trauma resuscita-

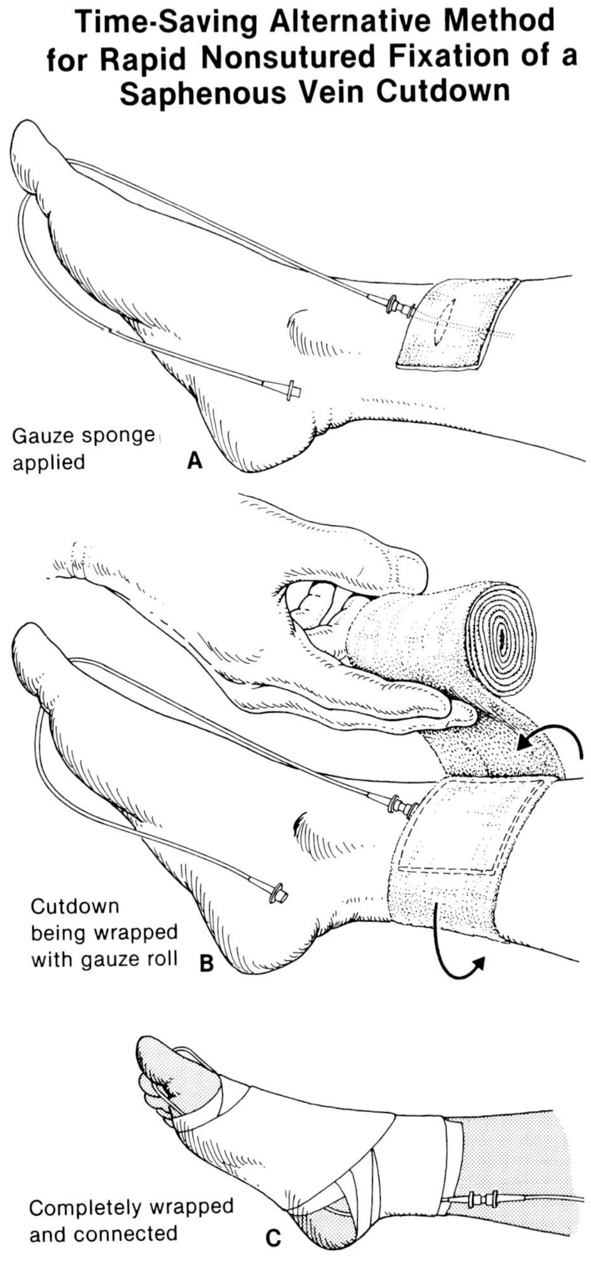

Figure 20–6 • Cutdown incision may be dressed with a gauze sponge and the tubing secured by the use of a gauze roll. The incision may be closed at a later time.

tion. Simultaneous bilateral cutdowns may be most easily placed under extreme resuscitation circumstances because that site generally produces minimal interference with other procedures (such as endotracheal intubation, tube thoracostomy, or diagnostic peritoneal lavage). The catheter size should be the largest available. Our preference has been to use a short segment of K-50 intravenous tubing. Ten gauge short intravenous catheters may also be used, if available.[3,4] Large-bore urology irrigation tubing connected to the intravenous solution will also allow for more rapid fluid infusions (Fig. 20–9). Catheters for monitoring central venous pressure (CVP) or pulmonary artery pressure, if placed by cutdown, are usually placed through forearm cutdown sites and should not be used for volume resuscitation.

The most common technical problems encountered are difficulty in locating the desired vein and difficulty performing the actual cannulation. In the case of

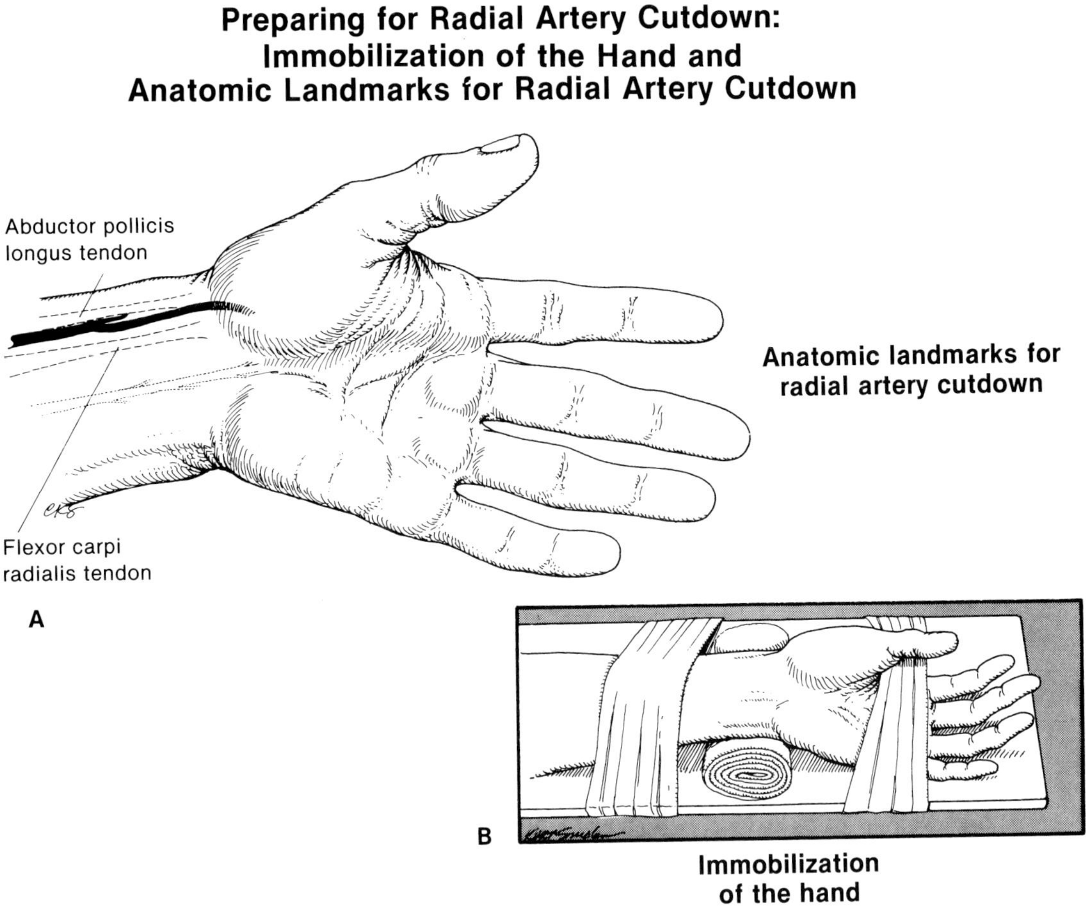

Figure 20–7 • Proper position of the hand and immobilization of the wrist is essential prior to beginning a radial arterial cutdown.

the saphenous cutdown, it should be remembered that the vein lies deep to the subcutaneous tissue, and veins encountered superficial to the fascial layer are generally not appropriate for cannulation. Most veins, particularly the distal saphenous vein, have a muscular coat and may be dilated using the hemostat to allow passage of the catheter if necessary, without fear of rupturing the vein. In cases where the distal saphenous vein is sclerosed from either intravenous drug injections or old phlebitis, another, more proximal site should be used. It is frequently necessary under these circumstances to use the saphenous vein in the proximal thigh.

There frequently is concern regarding the placement of venous lines distal to a potential injury site. If there is a strong suspicion of a proximal venous injury, then distal venous access should, in general, be avoided. Such injuries include penetrating trauma to the axillary or subclavian vessels in the case of an arm cutdown, and penetrating or crushing injuries to the lower extremity that might effect venous outflow through a distal saphenous cutdown. Pelvic fractures and penetrating abdominal trauma per se are not contraindications to the placement of a saphenous cutdown.

In the case of resuscitation from trauma, patients frequently have underlying fractures at sites that would otherwise be selected for venous cutdown. Careful examination should be performed to avoid, by the placement of a cutdown, converting a closed fracture to an open type of injury. Alternative sites should be selected if at possible.

The use of military antishock trousers (MAST) does not preclude the use of distal saphenous venous cutdowns (usually available and approachable), but the increase in venous resistance produced usually requires that fluid and blood infusion be performed using pressure bags.

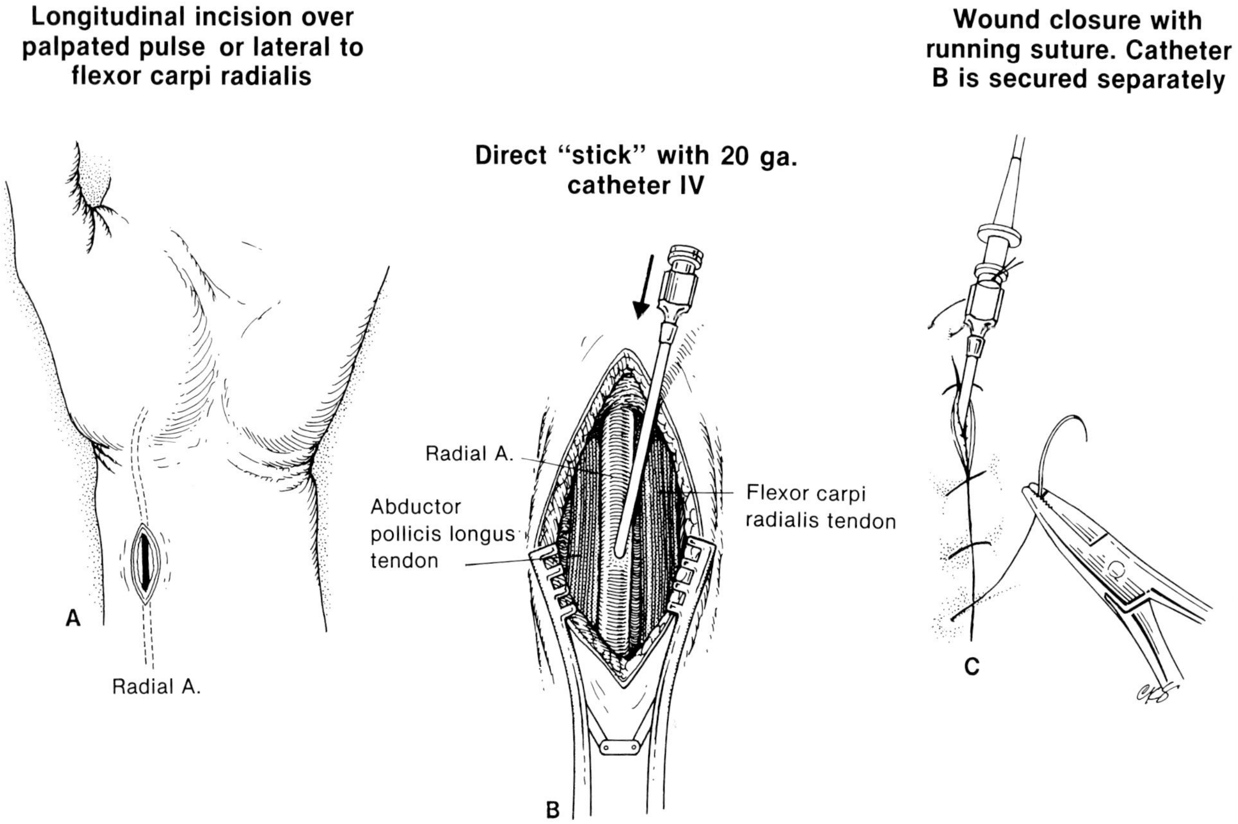

Figure 20–8 • Arterial cutdown differs from venous cutdown by the use of a longitudinal incision and the lack of proximal or distal ligatures.

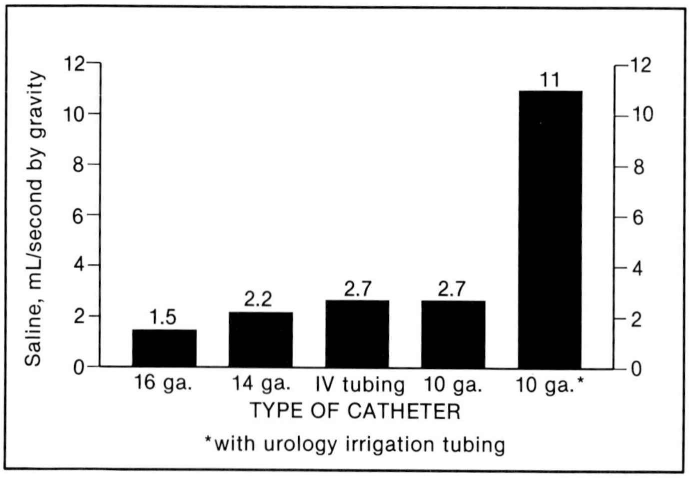

Figure 20–9 • Flow rates of normal saline under gravity flow obtained with various catheter types. (From Hansbrough JF, Cain TL, Millikan JS. Placement of 10 gauge catheter by cutdown for rapid fluid replacement. J Trauma 23:231–234, 1983; with permission.)

V. TECHNICAL ERRORS AND COMPLICATIONS

There are two major categories of early technical complications in the performance of cutdown cannulation (Table 20–1): (1) technical errors leading to difficult or aborted cannulations, and (2) injury to underlying structures such as the brachial artery or median nerve in the arm, or the greater saphenous nerve in the leg.

Most technical complications can be avoided by strict adherence to careful surgical technique and careful identification of landmarks and fascial planes. Careless dissection under "heat of battle" conditions, particularly in the forearm, has led to both nerve and arterial injuries.[5] These can be completely avoided by simply confining dissection to the subcutaneous tissue planes.

The late complications of venous or arterial cutdown are similar to those for percutaneously placed catheterization and include thrombosis, embolization, and infection. The rate of infection for cutdown venous and arterial catheterization is generally higher than that for percutaneous cannulation.[6,7] Lines placed under less than optimal conditions during resuscitation of hemodynamically unstable trauma patients are particularly prone to infection, as are lines placed in certain environments (the emergency department vs. the operating room). It has been our practice to remove all resuscitation lines for trauma within a 24-hour period of placement. Suppurative thrombophlebitis, sepsis and septic arthritis are all related infectious complications of venous cutdown.[8] Any patient with suspected infection should have the catheter removed immediately. Suppurative thrombophlebitis is diagnosed on clinical grounds and characterized by local cellulitis, thrombosis of the associated vein, and the aspiration or expression of pus from the vein. This is an indication for wide venectomy and parenteral antibiotics.[9]

Table 20–1 • Common Technical Errors in Cutdown Placement of Venous Catheter

- Incorrect placement of the incision
- Too small an incision made
- Initial incision not made completely through the dermis
- Small superficial veins other than the greater saphenous encountered with attempted cannulation
- Greater saphenous nerve injury or incorporation in ligature
- Venotomy made too proximally, with retraction under skin flap
- Imprecise venotomy: too small with difficulty cannulating, or vein transected with retraction
- Tubing cut incorrectly: too long, or not enough bevel

VI. REFERENCES

1. Talan DA, Simon RR, Hoffman JR. Cephalic vein cutdown at the wrist: comparison to the standard saphenous vein ankle cutdown. Ann Emerg Med 17:38–42, 1988.
2. Simon RR, Hoffman JR, Smith M. Modified new approaches for rapid intravenous access. Ann Emerg Med 16:44–49, 1987.
3. Dronen ST, Yee AS, Tomlanovich MC. Proximal saphenous vein cutdown. Ann Emerg Med 10:328–330, 1981.
4. Hansbrough JF, Cain TL, Millikan JS. Placement of 10 gauge catheter by cutdown for rapid fluid replacement. J. Trauma 23:231–234, 1983.
5. Finelli PF. Anterior interosseous nerve syndrome following cutdown catheterization. Ann Neurol 1:205–206, 1977.
6. Russell JA, Joel M, Hudson RJ, Mangano DT, et al. Prospective evaluation of radial and femoral artery catheterization sites in critically ill adults. Crit Care Med 11:936–939, 1983.
7. Band JD, Maki DG. Infections caused by arterial catheters used for hemodynamic monitoring. Am J Med 67:735–741, 1979.
8. Baker CC, Petersen SR, Sheldon GF. Septic phlebitis: A neglected disease. Am J Surg 138:97–103, 1979.
9. Zinner MJ, Zuidema GD, Lowery BD. Septic nonsuppurative thrombophlebitis. Arch Surg 111:122–125, 1976.

Chapter 21

Frederick G. Mihm, MD
Myer H. Rosenthal, MD

Pulmonary Artery Catheterization

OUTLINE

I. Introduction

Simplified techniques of pulmonary artery (PA) pressure monitoring were developed by 1953, but it was not until 1970 that a balloon-tipped PA catheter was introduced for clinical application.[1] In 1972, the determination of cardiac output by thermodilution was added to the pressure information provided by the PA catheter.[2] Still later the continuous measurement of mixed venous oxyhemoglobin saturation ($S_{\bar{v}}O_2$) using catheter fiberoptics (1975),[3] and measurements of right ventricular end diastolic volume (RVEDV) and right ventricular ejection fraction (RVEF) (1981) became available.[4] Pulmonary artery catheters with built-in electrodes or lumina for passing electrodes have been available for several years for dysrhythmia diagnosis and cardiac pacing.

The PA catheter in its various configurations (standard, fiberoptic, electrodes, etc) is an invasive medical device that has been associated with significant morbid and occasionally lethal events. Consequently the risk/benefit ratio of PA catheterization can be optimized when the physician has a clear indication for using this device, when he or she is well trained in venous access and PA catheterization techniques, and when he or she knows how to avoid the recognized complications, most of which are iatrogenic.

II. Indications

A. *General Considerations*

The PA catheter is a tool for obtaining information useful in the diagnosis, monitoring, and therapy of selected patients.[5] The direct information available includes vascular pressures (right atrium [RA], RV during placement, PA, and pulmonary artery occlusion pressure [PAOP]), cardiac output, blood oxygenation (RA/RV saturations during placement and mixed venous $S_{\bar{v}}O_2$, $P_{\bar{v}}O_2$), and measurements of right ventricular performance (RVEDV, RVEF) (Table 21–1).

Physicians considering PA catheterization desire the information it provides for several reasons:

1. It cannot be clinically obtained or even guessed reliably.[6-10]
2. Other devices (eg, the central venous pressure [CVP] catheter) provide either incomplete or misleading information.[11-17]
3. The information from the PA catheter makes a real difference. It helps confirm a diagnosis, directs therapy, or both.[6] Although many assume that outcome must be logically affected if the diagnoses made or therapies changed are clinically important, there is no proof that this is true.

Table 21–1 • PA Catheter Information

	Continuous	Intermittent
Vascular pressures	RA, PA	PAOP
Blood flow		CO
Blood oxygenation	$S_{\bar{v}}O_2$	$P_{\bar{v}}O_2$
RV performance		RVEF, RVEDV

While we await convincing outcome data, we must be satisfied with the justification of PA catheterization based on the likehood that its proper use confirms certain specific diagnoses (eg, tamponade), clinically significant events can be detected (eg, fluid overload, low cardiac output state), and potentially harmful therapies (eg, afterload reduction) can be titrated to optimal response.

From a diagnostic point of view, PA catheterization should be considered in patients who have hypotension (systolic or mean arterial pressure less than 90 or 60 mmHg, respectively) unresponsive to initial therapy; who have severe pulmonary edema (rales on examination, radiograph findings, and respiratory distress) of unknown cause;[8] or who are suspected to be in a low cardiac output state (Table 21–2). Clinicians must be particularly sensitive to the possibility of a low cardiac output in patients with renal insufficiency. Additionally, a number of specific disease states can be diagnosed or

Table 21–2 • Indications for PA Catheterization

Diagnosis	*Treatment*
Hypotension	Shock
Pulmonary edema	Coronary artery disease
Low cardiac output	Pulmonary edema
	Acute respiratory failure
	Renal insufficiency
	Fluid therapy
	Cardiac surgery
	Aortic surgery
	Pulmonary hypertension
	Dysrhythmias

at least suggested by information obtained from PA catheterization (Table 21–3).

From a monitoring or therapeutic perspective, Table 21–2 lists clinical situations encountered both inside and outside the operating room where PA catheterization should be considered. Clarification of each of these categories is necessary.

B. *Specific Indications*

1. SHOCK

Patients who have absolute (MAP < 60 mmHg, systolic < 90 mmHg) or relative hypotension and evidence of vital organ hypoperfusion with an associated metabolic acidosis are in shock; PA catheterization is usually indicated. This includes patients with cardiogenic or septic shock, patients with severe hypovolemic shock, and patients with shock of unknown cause. Patients with anaphylactic shock may not require PA catheterization if the diagnosis and treatment are made promptly.

2. CORONARY ARTERY DISEASE

Patients with acute myocardial infarction complicated by congestive heart failure or hypotension that does not respond readily to initial therapy are candidates for PA catheterization.

Patients with unstable angina or history of congestive heart failure who are to have major noncardiac surgery should have PA catheterization. In patients with stable, exercise-induced angina with no history of congestive heart failure, the indications are equivocal and depend in part on other associated diseases and the type of surgery planned. Patients who require noncardiac surgery with a recent history (less than 3 months) of a myocardial infarction have three times the risk of a perioperative reinfarction and should undergo PA catheterization for proper anesthetic management.[18] Nevertheless, the best anesthetic management can not guarantee that they will be protected from a myocardial reinfarction.

3. PULMONARY EDEMA

PA catheterization should be employed in patients who have cardiogenic pulmonary edema that does not respond to initial therapy, and those with moderately severe nonhydrostatic (permeability) pulmonary edema.

4. ACUTE RESPIRATORY FAILURE

Patients with nonneurologic causes of respiratory failure where hypoxemia is a prominent feature are good candidates for PA catheterization. Most important, fluid therapy must be very carefully managed in these patients in order to maintain cardiac output while minimizing pulmonary capillary hydrostatic pressures. In addition, titration of various respiratory therapies (tidal volume, PEEP) to maximize arterial oxygenation and minimize oxygen toxicity must also be monitored to avoid potential harmful effects on tissue oxygenation (decreased oxygen transport, maldistribution of blood flow). It may also be argued that PA catheterization is indicated in selected patients with respiratory insufficiency so that aggressive treatment may be used to prevent frank respiratory failure.

Table 21–3 • Specific Diagnostic Information from the PA Catheter

	RAP	PAOP	Other PA Catheter Findings
LV ischemia/infarction	—	↑	a,cv waves
Hypovolemia	↓—↑	↓	
RV infarction	↑	—	
Mitral regurgitation	—	↑	cv wave
Ventricular septal defect	↑	↑	O_2 saturation step-up
Pericardial tamponade	↑	↑	RAP ≈ RVEDP ≈ PADP ≈ PAOP
Pulmonary embolism	—	—	↑PAP
Cor pulmonale	↑	—	PAP, cv waves

5. Renal Insufficiency

With the awareness of the severe implications of acute renal failure in critically ill patients (mortality greater than 60%) and our general inability to reliably detect low cardiac output states, the aggressive use of PA catheterization has become commonplace in these individuals. Patients with progressive renal insufficiency despite conservative therapy should have PA catheterization unless the cause of renal deterioration is known to be untreatable. Finally, anesthesiologists should have a low threshold for PA catheterization in any patient undergoing surgery with stable renal insufficiency, especially those with creatinine clearances of less than 30 mL/min.

6. Fluid Therapy

There are many situations where confusion exists about the intravascular volume status of a critically ill patient. In the usual clinical setting, the patient is not in shock and is not hypotensive, and the focus of attention has usually been on oliguria that has been present for several hours. The oliguria did not respond to a volume challenge, but did respond to diuretics. Several hours later oliguria has recurred. When the physical examination of the patient is unrevealing, continued concomitant fluid and diuretic therapy seems contradictory, and diuretic therapy alone may be harmful and cause urine flow at the expense of renal insufficiency, PA catheterization is indicated.

7. Cardiac Surgery

It seems clear that not all patients who undergo cardiac surgery need PA catheterization, although the opposite has been argued.[19,20] Patients with coronary artery disease or valvular heart disease may benefit from PA catheterization if they have a history of chronic or ischemic-induced congestive heart failure, renal insufficiency, left main coronary disease,[21] or evidence at preoperative catheterization of left ventricular dysfunction or pulmonary hypertension (Table 21–4).[20] Patients with both mitral and aortic valvular disease are also at higher risk.[29]

8. Aortic Surgery

Patients who undergo aortic surgery may benefit from PA catheterization if they have a history of coronary artery disease (angina, previous myocardial infarction, or congestive heart failure) or renal insufficiency, as may those whose thoracic aorta is to be clamped without partial bypass.[23] The stress of aortic clamping to a full, beating heart is significant to patients at risk for ischemia, and PA catheterization provides both a meaningful monitor and a guide to therapy of any untoward events.[24–26] Indeed, a case can be made for all patients having aortic cross-clamping to receive PA catheterization, in that even 10% of patients without known cardiac disease may experience an untoward myocardial event with abdominal aortic cross-clamping.[23]

Table 21–4 • Indications for PA Catheterization in Cardiac Surgery

History–CHF, CRF, left main coronary artery disease
Catheterization–LVEDP > 20 mmHg resting, increase of 15 mmHg after injection of angiographic dye
Ejection fraction < 40%
Cardiac index < 2.0 l/min/m^2
Dyskinesis/akinesis ≥ 2 segments
Pulmonary hypertension with PA systolic > 50 mmHg
$S_{\bar{v}}O_2$ < 60%

CHF, Congestive heart failure; CRF, Chronic Renal Failure; LVEDP, Left Ventricular end-diastolic pressure.

9. Pulmonary Hypertension

Critically ill patients who are known or suspected to have pulmonary hypertension associated with systemic hypotension or respiratory failure should have PA catheterization. The underlying diseases associated with these situations include chronic obstructive pulmonary disease, pulmonary emboli, and primary pulmonary hypertension.

Patients with pulmonary hypertension are at high risk if they require general anesthesia and should have PA catheterization.[27]

10. Dysrhythmias

Patients with a bradydysrhythmia (complete heart block, sick sinus syndrome, etc) who also need a PA catheter can be ventricularly paced with the Pacing® or Paceport® PA catheter (Baxter-Healthcare Corporation, Irvine, Ca). The Pacing PA catheter may also be used for atrial pacing or atrial-ventricular pacing for patients dependent on atrial contraction for the maintenance of cardiac output.[28] The Pacing PA catheter can also provide overdrive atrial pacing of certain supraventricular tachydysrhythmias.

Finally, for the anesthesiologist, there may be still other patients who should have PA catheterization who do not belong in any of the above categories. These patients include elderly patients undergoing major surgery with expected large fluid losses; patients with pheochromocytoma;[29] patients with carcinoid syndrome, major trauma, and/or burns; patients with decompensated cirrhosis with bleeding and/or sepsis; and patients with severe peritonitis or pancreatitis.

Pulmonary artery catheterization has been shown to correctly detect venous air embolism in patients undergoing neurosurgical procedures in the sitting position.[30] However, because noninvasive monitors such as the precordial Doppler and end-tidal capnography are equally effective, PA catheterization for this reason alone has not been widely accepted.

Once a patient meets the initial criteria for PA catheterization, the indications for obtaining measurements of intermittent data must be addressed. There are obvious potential limitations to data that are only intermittently measured. The frequency with which intermittent data, especially cardiac output measurements, are acquired may have a dramatic impact on the usefulness of PA catheterization. In the case of cardiac output measurements, for example, these should be acquired at least every 3–4 hours in every patient. This practice is justified by the need to establish baseline cardiac function from which any acute deterioration can be properly assessed, and to detect any important early changes in cardiac output that may not be otherwise clinically detected by physical examination and vital signs. Changes in the indications for obtaining and using information from the PA catheter should be the basis for timely removal when the catheter is no longer needed.

III. How to Catheterize the Pulmonary Artery

A. *Equipment*

1. Introducer

Introducer sets (Fig. 21–1) are required for percutaneous PA catheter placement and include three main items: 7.5–8.5 French Teflon introducer (20 cm long) equipped with valves to prevent air entry into or blood loss from the introducer, a dilator, and a guide wire (0.035 inches by 30–50 cm). Introducers are also available with a side port that provides a "central" infusion line that is separate from the two vascular lumina on standard PA catheters. Introducer sets also have a plastic sheath that will keep sterile the entire length of the catheter that is outside the skin in case the catheter needs to be repositioned. An obturator or additional catheter is also available in some sets to replace the guide wire and dilator in a situation where the PA catheter will be placed at some later time (Fig. 21–1).

2. PA Catheters

Several configurations are available (Table 21–5), but all are thermodilution, balloon flotation catheters. Catheters may have various additional features depending on their application: an extra proximal infusion port for hyperalimentation (VIP®), five built-in pacing electrodes (three atrial, two ventricular) for atrial and/or ventricular pacing (Pacing) or a right ventricular (RV) lumen through which a single ventricular pacing electrode can be passed (Paceport), two fiberoptic bundles through which mixed venous oxygen saturation can be measured (oximetry), and an RV lumen and a fast response thermistor for determinations of RV ejection fraction or RV end-diastolic volume.

3. Connecting Tubing

The following are necessary:

One pressurized flush bag (normal saline with heparin, 2 units/mL) with dual lines to continuously flush (2 mL/hour) the proximal (RA) and distal (PA) lumina during pressure monitoring (Fig. 21–2).

One central line administration set (volutrol) for the sideport of the introducer.

One 500-mL bag of normal saline or 5% dextrose in water (D5W) with macrodrip set to attach to proximal lumen to fill 10-mL syringe for cardiac output measurements.

Additional line for any catheter with three lumina.

4. Transducers

Transducers should be flushed and zeroed. Although one transducer can be used for both PA and right atrial (RA) lumina where RA pressures are only needed intermittently (changed by turning a stopcock), it is preferable to have two transducers for these two pressures.

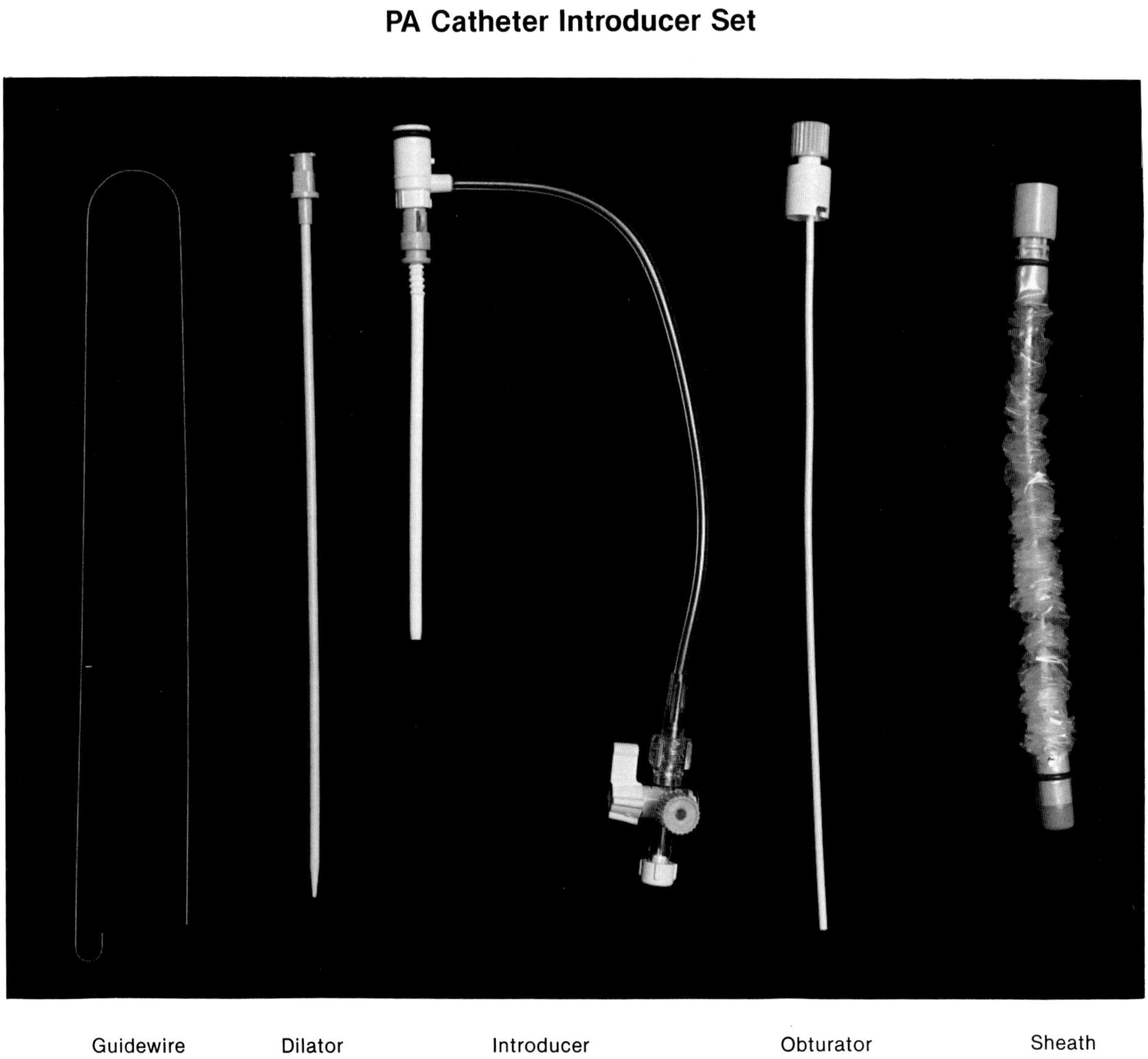

Figure 21–1 • Components of a standard introducer set are shown. Parts include a guide wire, dilator, introducer with sidearm, obturator, and plastic external catheter sheath. (Shown are parts of an Arrow Percutaneous Sheath Introducer kit, model AK-09802.)

Table 21–5 • Types of PA Catheters

	Size	Lumina	Lumen Sites
Standard	5F	2	Proximal/Distal
	7F	2	Proximal/Distal
VIP	7.5F	3	2 Proximal/Distal
Pacing	7.0F	2	Proximal/Distal
Paceport	7.5F	3	Proximal/RV/Distal
Oximeter	7.0F	2	Proximal/Distal
Oximeter VIP	8.0F	3	2 Proximal/Distal
Ejection fraction	7.5F	3	Proximal/RV/Distal

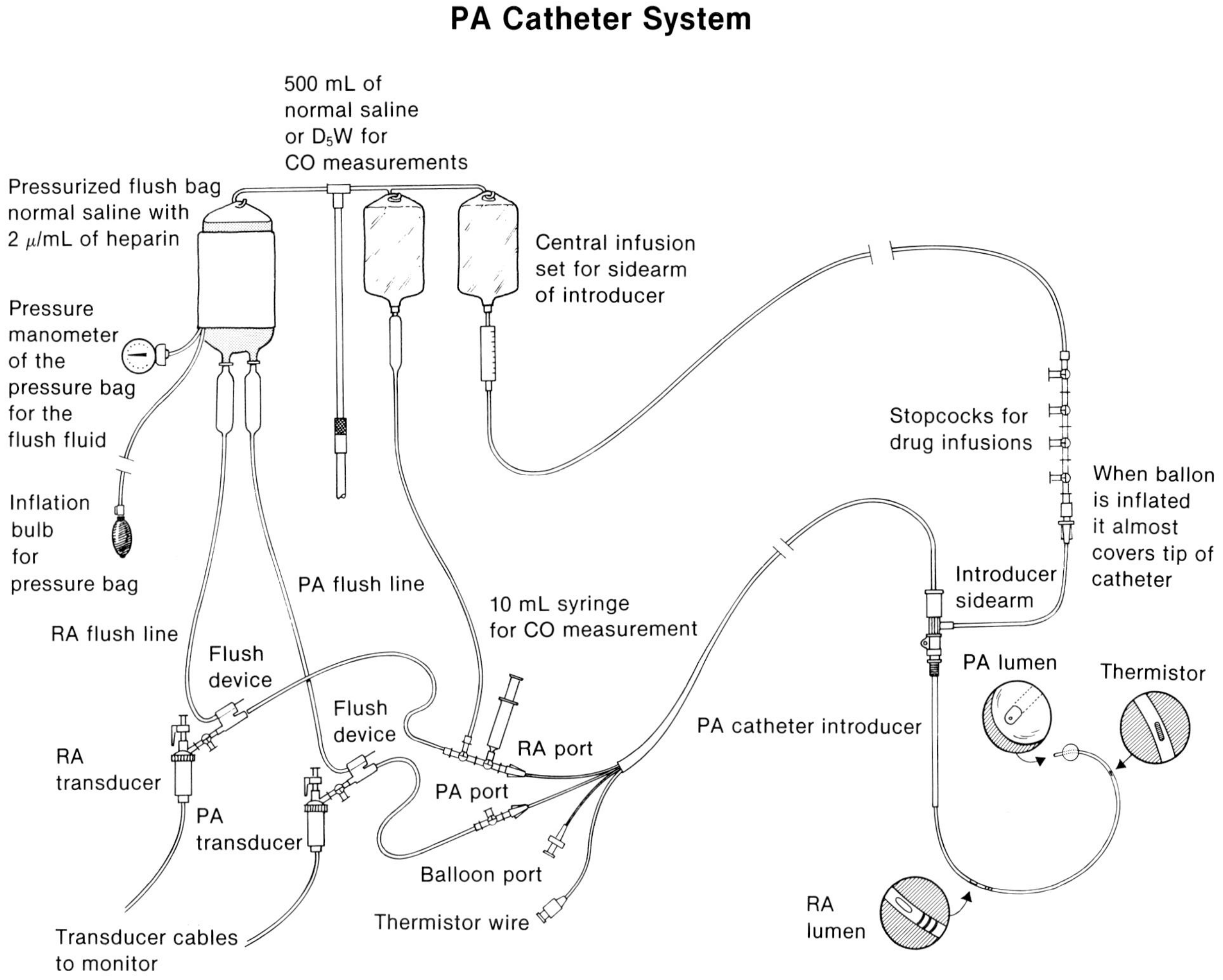

Figure 21–2 • The figure shows the various parts of the PA catheter system. RA = right atrium; PA = pulmonary artery; CO = cardiac output.

B. *Insertion*

1. Venous Access

The same considerations exist for PA catheterization as for central venous catheter placement discussed in Chapter 18, except that in place of the CVP catheter, the introducer and dilator are passed as one unit over the guide wire. The skin entry site must be enlarged with a No. 11 scalpel blade for the 8.5 French introducer (Fig. 21–3A). The physician should control the introducer/dilator and guide wire with one hand while twisting and advancing all three parts together with the other hand at the skin entry site (Fig. 21–3B). All the sites for CVP line placement can be used for placement of a PA catheter (internal and external jugular, subclavian, femoral and basilic veins).

Note: In placing the introducer through the external jugular vein, be careful how far the dilator extends past the end of the introducer. A short distance is desirable to guarantee that the dilator is not advanced too deeply into the normal curves of this vessel in the lower neck before the introducer enters the vessel (Fig. 21–4).

Once the PA catheter introducer is placed, the entire set (introducer, dilator, guide wire) can be left in situ. Alternatively, the guide wire and dilator can be removed and an obturator can be placed through the introducer while the PA catheter is removed from its packaging and examined. In either case, the introducer should be secured to the skin with a suture.

Note: Caution! Unrecognized dysrhythmias commonly occur at this point because the guide wire or the

(Text continued on p. 414)

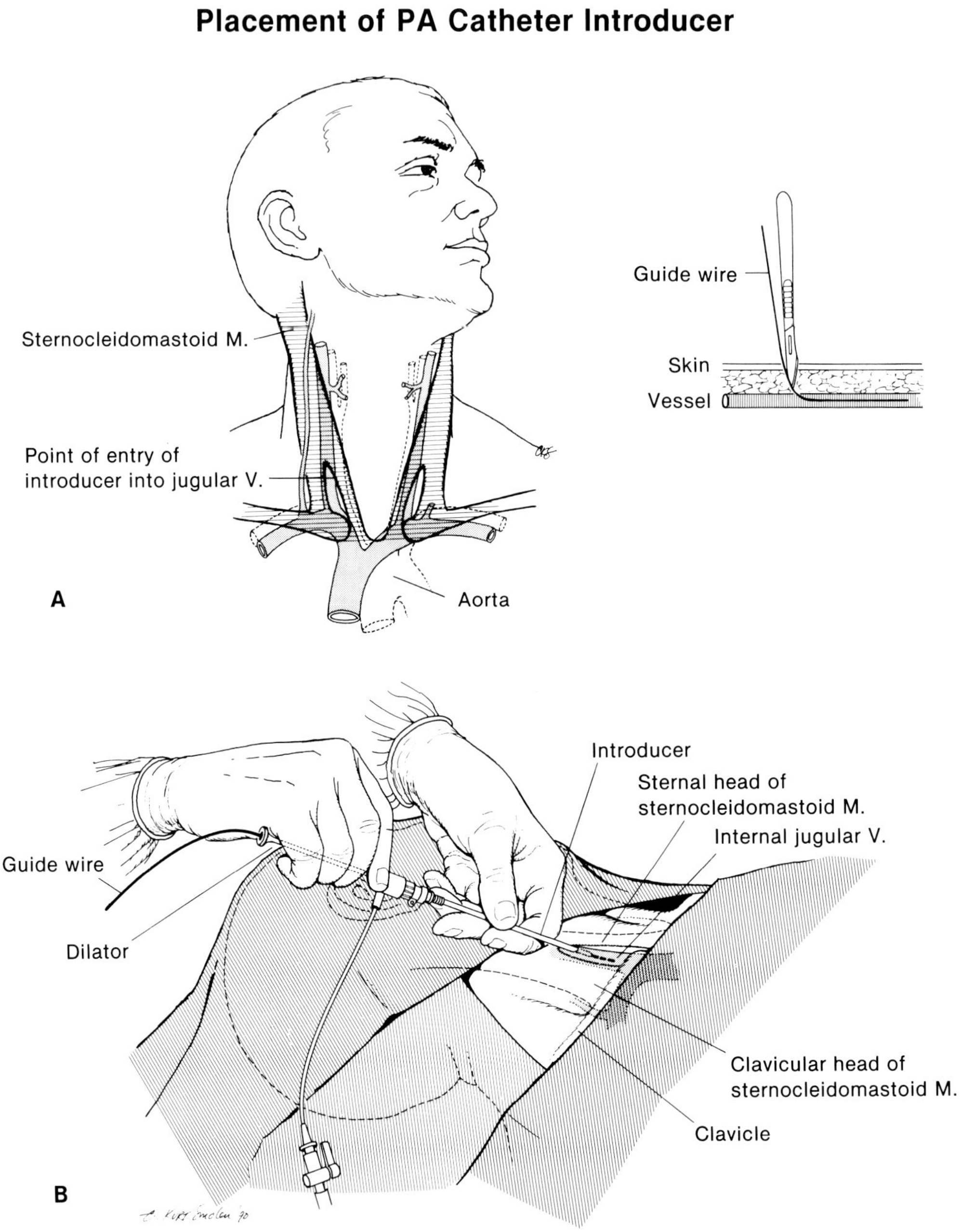

Figure 21–3 • (***A***) To place the introducer easily over the guide wire, the puncture site should be enlarged as shown with a #11 scalpel blade. (***B***) The introducer/dilator/guidewire should be advanced as one unit, using both hands as shown.

Introducer/Dilator Orientation

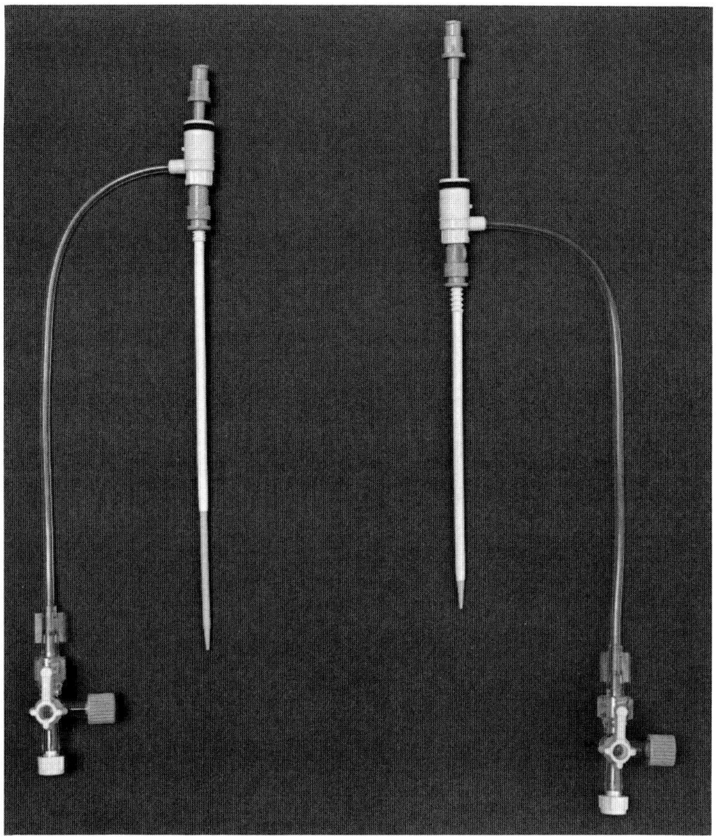

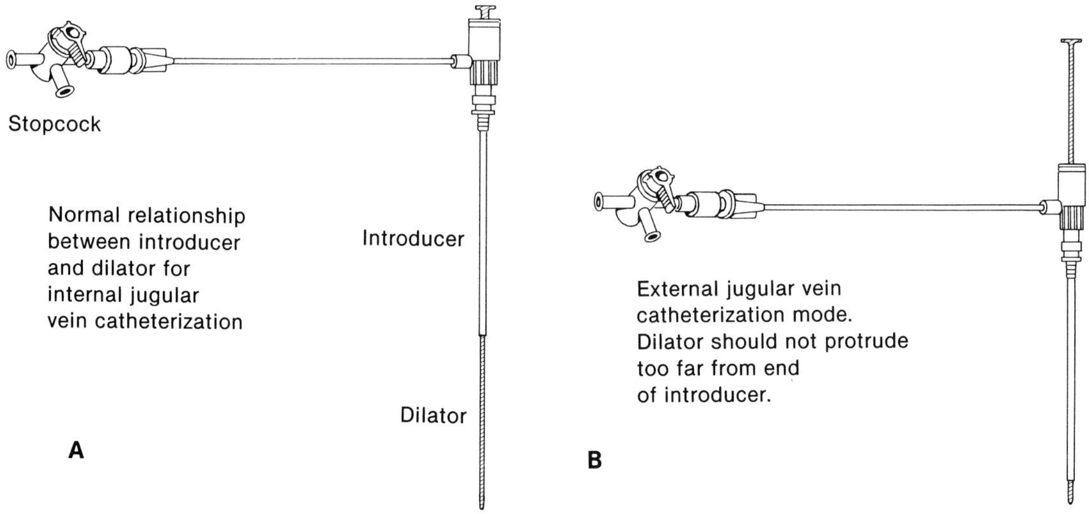

Figure 21–4 • (***A***) Orientation of the dilator and introducer for placement in internal jugular, femoral, and basilic veins is shown. (***B***) The introducer is moved closer to the tapered end of the dilator for placement in the external jugular vein. This orientation will help prevent the stiff end of the dilator from being advanced too deeply and perhaps perforating the vein; the stiff dilator should not be expected to negotiate the curved anatomy of the external jugular vein. A similar caution applies to the entry into the subclavian vein.

obturator is advanced too far and irritates (and sometimes perforates) the right ventricle.

2. System Check

After venous access has been accomplished, the following steps should be followed to check out the PA catheter and monitoring system.

- Calibrate the monitoring system, including the transducer, digital display, and paper printout or calibrated screen display (see Chapter 2).
- Note that it is always preferable to have a paper printout in addition to a screen display.
- Fix the height of the transducer so that it is at the level of the left atrium of the patient.
- Pass the external catheter sheath over the PA catheter, and tape the external catheter sheath to the PA catheter and the proximal PA catheter to the edge of the sterile field (Fig. 21–5).
- Inflate the PA catheter balloon (1.5 mL) and check for symmetry, extension of inflated balloon past the catheter tip, and complete passive deflation.

Note: *Do not* actively deflate the balloon in vitro or in vivo. This maneuver invariably overdeflates the balloon and invaginates a small part of the balloon into the balloon lumen. This is the most common cause of premature balloon rupture.

- Connect the thermistor cable to the cardiac output computer and check for a PA catheter fault signal.

Note: Most physicians do not take time to do this because manufacturing errors of the thermistor are rare.

- Attach the proximal and distal lumina to transducers and flush.
- Perform the shake–flick test (Fig. 21–6).[31] Coil the catheter in one hand and shake. If both lumina do not transmit high spiking waveforms on the oscilloscope screen (see Fig. 21–6A), then the system must be checked for air bubbles, disconnection, closed stopcocks, catheter kinks or knots, or monitor error. Next, with the hand that is holding the catheter, expose the end of the catheter by holding it at the 10-cm mark between thumb and index finger. With the other hand, flick the tip of the catheter and observe the oscilloscope screen (see Fig. 21–6B). The trace that shows a spike artifact clearly identifies the pressure transmitted from the distal lumen at the tip of the PA catheter. If no spike artifact is seen, check the system again for the same problems just mentioned above. After performing this test, flush the distal lumen again.

Maintaining Sterile Field for PA Catheterization

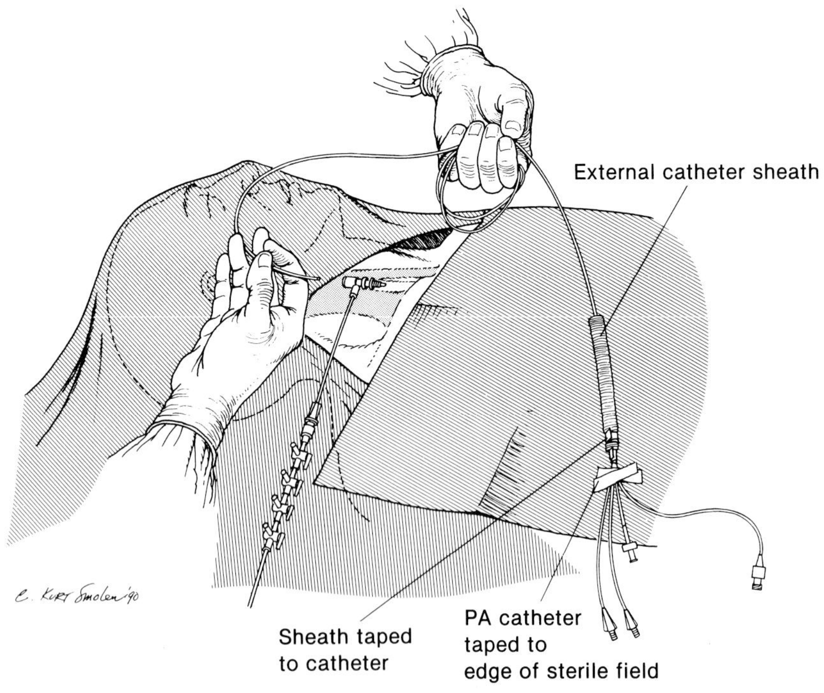

Figure 21–5 • The sterile field (triangle) for PA catheterization is shown. After the protective external catheter sheath has been passed over the catheter and positioned proximally, it can be secured with tape to the proximal end of the PA catheter. The PA catheter can also be secured by tape to one corner of the drapes to guarantee that the PA catheter is not inadvertently pulled off the sterile field.

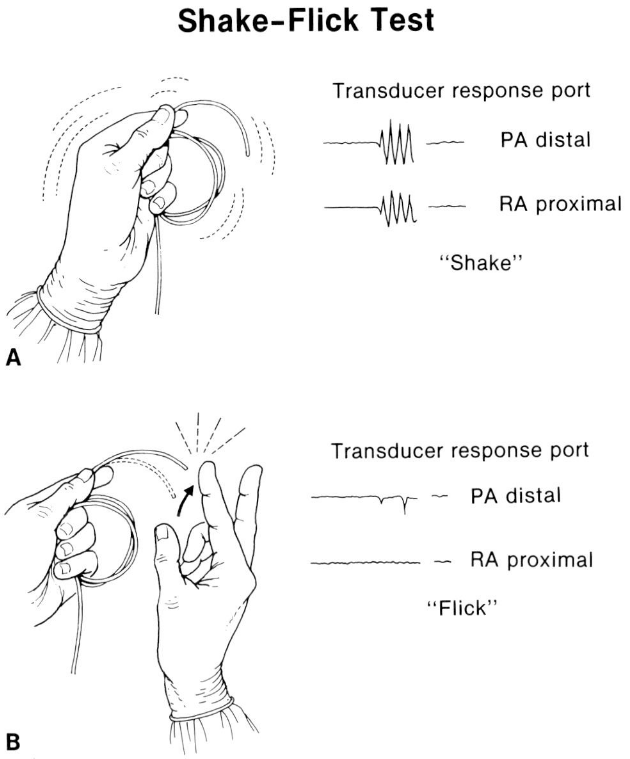

Figure 21-6 • The shake-flick test is demonstrated. (***A***) Shaking the catheter will produce deep spiking artifacts on the oscilloscope screen as shown from both the proximal (*RA*) and distal (*PA*) lumens. (***B***) When the catheter is held still and the exposed tip is flicked with a finger, a single deep-spike artifact should be seen on the oscilloscope screen, identifying the distal (*PA*) lumen and also providing a crude test for damping.

Note: This procedure not only identifies the distal lumen and insures its patency, but the size of the distal lumen spike can also be used as a semiquantitative test for damping if the force to flick the catheter and the screen calibration are kept relatively constant with each catheter placement.

3. PLACEMENT PROCEDURE

Remove the guide wire and dilator (or obturator) from the introducer sheath and cover the hub of the introducer with the thumb.

Pass the PA catheter through the introducer up to the 20-cm mark (two thin, circular marks) and stop.

Note: To avoid air embolism:

a. The maneuver described above should be performed in two phases as indicated.
b. The patient should be in a Trendelenburg position, if possible, unless the catheter is being placed via the femoral or basilic veins.

These two phases should be performed during mechanical inspiration if the patient is receiving ventilator support, or at the beginning of exhalation if the patient is spontaneously breathing. If the spontaneously breathing patient can cooperate (many will not or cannot), it is even safer to perform the maneuvers during episodes of breath-holding after inspiration.

The presence of valved introducers does not eliminate the risk of air embolism.[32]

Note: Before passing the catheter further, consider placing the patient back in a horizontal position, not only for patient comfort, but to allow accurate recording of right heart pressures during passage.

Inflate the balloon (1.0–1.5 mL) and begin to pass while observing the oscilloscope the screen.

Note: Inflate the balloon at the 20-cm mark, *before* the tip of the catheter enters the RV. Balloon inflation may not be possible at the 20-cm mark if the catheter is being passed from the basilic vein.

Note: The placement of a PA catheter can normally be accomplished by observing pressure tracings from the tip of the catheter and by knowing the characteristic features of the tracing as the catheter tip enters the various cardiovascular chambers (Fig. 21-7A–E).

Notice entry of the PA catheter into thorax by baseline variations caused by transmitted transpulmonary pressures.

Enter the right atrium (RA), and continue passing (see Fig. 21-7A–B).

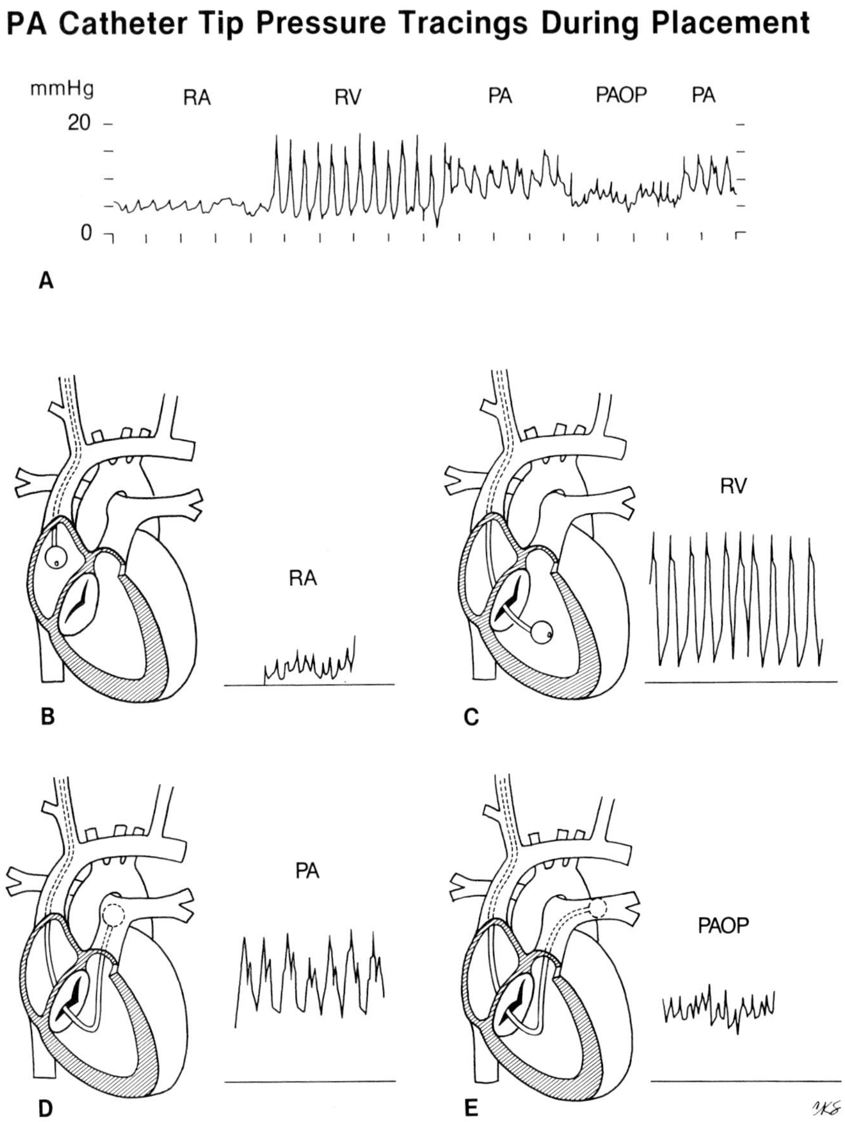

Figure 21–7 • Pressure tracings and chamber locations during PA catheterization are shown. (***A***) An entire PA catheterization is shown at the top of the figure. Specific chamber location and representative tracings are shown for the right atrium (*RA*) (***B***), right ventricle (*RV*) (***C***) pulmonary artery (*PA*) (***D***) and pulmonary artery occlusion pressure (*PAOP*) (***E***).

Note: The RA pressure trace is very similar in appearance to PAOP trace and frequently confuses physicians when the catheter enters the RV, coils up, then exits back into the RA.

Enter the RV and observe the relatively high amplitude (systolic) pressure waveforms, low RV diastolic pressures (usually 0–10 mmHg), the absence of a dicrotic notch, and similar angles of the upslope and downslope of the waveform (see Fig. 21–7A, C). Continue passing.

Note: The catheter tip should spend a minimum of time in the RV to decrease the incidence of dysrhythmias. Check catheter distance marks at entry into introducer and keep moving!

Enter the PA and observe the increase in diastolic pressure (consistent finding), presence of a dicrotic notch (not always transmitted well), and relatively sharp upslope compared to a more gradual downslope of the waveform (see Fig. 21–7A, D). Stop briefly to check the catheter distance again and then continue to pass slowly. Entry into the PA from the RV should require less than 20 cm of catheter advancement. If more catheter is needed, the catheter is probably coiling in the RV and should be repassed.

Obtain a PAOP and observe a decrease in the diastolic pressure (this is a consistent finding but the decrease may be small [1–2 mmHg]), damped pressure tracing (most of the time, but not always; ie, some patients transmit large — a and cv waves), and prompt return to PA pressure trace when the balloon is allowed to deflate passively (see Fig. 21–7A, E).

Note: As soon as the catheter is advanced to the point where the inflated balloon occludes a PA segment, a PAOP can be obtained. A PAOP tracing is defined as a tracing indicating a pressure measured at end-exhalation that is lower than the PAD measured at end-exhalation. The normal PAOP should not contain pathologic "a" or "cv" waves. The tracing should be reproducible with repeat balloon inflation. If there is still doubt, a blood gas sample can be obtained while the balloon is inflated (after discarding the first 3 mL). The sample obtained should reflect alveolar capillary gas pressures, which are generally highly oxygenated unless there are severe regional ventilation/perfusion abnormalities. Additionally, a fluid column higher than the measured pressure should run freely to indicate that there is no obstruction of the catheter tip or vascular obstruction beyond the tip.[33] These two latter maneuvers are rarely indicated.

Before securing the PA catheter, slowly inflate the balloon with a 3.0-mL syringe. If a PAOP tracing is obtained with 0.6 mL or less of inflation, withdraw the catheter 1–2 cm and recheck until 0.8–1.2 mL is required for vessel occlusion. If the PA catheter is placed through a tight-fitting valved introducer, there is no need to secure the PA catheter to the skin.

Note: This maneuver will remove excess or coiled lengths of catheter, and thereby help prevent spontaneous catheter wedging (balloon deflated).

Extend the external catheter sheath to cover the exposed external PA catheter and secure the end of the external sheath to the introducer. This will provide a degree of sterility so that the catheter can be repositioned, if necessary, after initial placement.[34]

IV. COMPLICATIONS

A. *General Considerations*

The many complications of PA catheterization include those associated with venous access and catheter placement, and complications observed after placement. Venous access complications are virtually identical to the complications with CVP venous access discussed in Chapter 18 and will not be discussed here. Complications during and after PA catheter placement are listed in Table 21–6. It is essential to understand that the vast majority of complications are iatrogenic and are avoidable. The incidence of serious complications has significantly decreased over the last 15 years, with only one catheter-related death reported in four recent prospective studies involving over 9,500 patients.[35–39]

Table 21–6 • PA Catheter Complications

Stress-induced myocardial ischemia	Trauma
Dysrhythmias	Thromboembolism
Coil/kink/knot	Infection
Failure to pass	Balloon rupture
Air embolism	Mesmerism
	Misinterpretation

B. *Specific Complications*

1. STRESS-INDUCED MYOCARDIAL ISCHEMIA

Any invasive procedure represents a stress, both physical and mental, to the patient. Patients with coronary artery disease are at particular risk of stress-induced myocardial ischemia during PA catheterization, especially if they are not receiving beta-blockade therapy.[40] Mental stress alone may cause symptomatically silent (heart rate less than 100 beats/minute, no chest pain) myocardial ischemia in over 70% of patients with coronary artery disease.[41,42] Anesthesiologists should also be aware that more than 15% of patients with coronary artery disease will arrive at the operating room with myocardial ischemia before invasive procedures have begun.[42]

Anesthesiologists who would use this information as a reason to place the PA catheter *after*[43] rather than *before* anesthetic induction and intubation are missing the potential value of the PA catheter in the periinduction/intubation assessment and treatment of the patient.[44] It is during this time that intraoperative ischemia and cardiac arrests are most likely to occur.[42,45]

Several clinical techniques have evolved to allow the safe placement of PA catheters in awake patients with coronary artery disease.[46,47] The following guidelines minimize the risk of stress-induced myocardial ischemia during PA catheterization.

- Develop good rapport and explain the procedure to the patient's satisfaction.

- Assess the patient adequately prior to beginning the procedure (heart rate, blood pressure, chest pain, leads II and V_5, anxiety).
- Continue beta-blockade therapy.
- Determine whether the patient can tolerate the Trendelenberg position (pulmonary edema or other lung disease) at all or for a limited time and choose the appropriate venous access site.
- Minimize pain by instilling 3–5 mL of local anesthetic along the venous access tract and place the local *prior to* prepping and draping. This provides adequate time for diffusion of the anesthetic.
- Administer oxygen by nasal prongs or mask.
- Be careful not to smother the patient with the drapes, which causes both physical (hypercapnia, hypoxemia, hyperthermia) and psychological (claustrophobia) stress.
- Maintain a constant awareness of the patient's physical and mental responses during the procedure and be ready to respond with verbal reassurance, supplemental local anesthesia, intravenous sedation, intravenous nitroglycerin for ischemia, etc. Indeed, many anesthesiologists routinely infuse low-dose nitroglycerin during the procedure, while continuously observing the arterial pressure and electrocardiogram (ECG).
- Keep your composure even if the procedure is not going well.

2. Dysrhythmias

Transient ventricular premature contractions are common during catheter placement and are usually caused by direct stimulation of the ventricle by the catheter. However, be aware that dysrhythmias may be a manifestation of myocardial ischemia. Other rhythm disturbances have occurred and include atrial premature beats,[48] ventricular tachycardia/fibrillation,[1,49] and bradycardia secondary to complete heart block. The latter event may occur in patients with preexisting left bundle branch block who develop transient injury to the right bundle branch system, resulting in complete heart block during PA catheter placement.[50] In patients without preexisting left bundle branch block, transient right bundle branch block is usually inconsequential.[51] Catheter-induced dysrhythmias have rarely resulted in death.[36] Direct irritation of the heart is more likely to occur during placement if the balloon is not inflated until the catheter tip has entered the RV and if knotting or coiling occurs.[48] After placement, the catheter tip may spontaneously fall back into the RV and cause dysrhythmias. Dysrhythmias are also more likely in patients with electrolyte disturbances (hypokalemia, hypocalcemia), hypotension, hypoxemia, and acidosis.[52] The following guidelines minimize the incidence and deleterious effects of dysrhythmias if they occur.

- Monitor the ECG continuously during catheter placement.
- Inflate the balloon as soon as the tip clears the introducer (20 cm).
- Pass the catheter without long pauses in the various chambers (RA, RV).
- When dysrhythmias occur, first stop passing the catheter, then withdraw the catheter out of the right side of the heart if they persist.
- Treat with xylocaine any premature ventricular beats that recur in each attempt to pass the catheter (50–100 mg intravenous boluses) to suppress ectopy during catheter placement.
- Cardioversion equipment should be readily available for immediate use if needed.

3. Coils, Kinks, and Knots

Coils, kinks, and knots may all occur during placement of a PA catheter. These events are complications because they may prevent proper catheter tip positioning and transmission of pressure tracings, and contribute to dysrhythmias or catheter trauma. Kinks or knots will necessitate catheter removal and may require a surgical procedure, particularly if intracardiac structures are snared. Invasive radiologic techniques may eliminate the need for surgery in many cases. If the catheter tip is positioned properly but coiling in the RV has occurred, slow withdrawal will usually effectively uncoil the catheter. This should be done even if a coiled catheter is not provoking any dysrhythmias, because if left alone coiling may cause the tip of the catheter to migrate further out into the lungs and cause spontaneous pulmonary artery occlusion.

The following guidelines minimize the risk of coils, kinks, and knots.

- Avoid inserting excessive lengths of catheter. Excessive lengths are determined by remembering the approximate distance to the RV from the various access sites: 35 cm from the right for internal jugular and subclavian veins, 45 cm from the left subclavian and internal jugular veins, 50 cm from the femoral veins, 60 cm from the right antecubital veins, and 70 cm from the left antecubital veins.
- Once in the RV, the catheter should pass into the PA within 15 cm, and obtain a PAOP within another 5–10 cm.

- Catheter withdrawal and reorientation and repositioning of the patient are preferable maneuvers, rather than excessive twisting of the catheter.
- Immersing or flushing a cold (sterile) solution through the catheter may increase its stiffness, improve chances for a successful pass, and minimize the need for excessive twisting of the catheter.

4. FAILURE TO PASS

In the initial report of balloon-floated PA catheters, failure to get into the PA and obtain a PAOP occurred 8% and 20% of the time, respectively.[1] The failure rate will decrease as an individual gains more experience, but there are other factors to consider. Pulmonary artery catheters may be difficult to pass in patients with severe pulmonary hypertension, enlarged RV chamber (Cor pulmonale, RV failure) or tricuspid regurgitation. When peripheral veins are the only access for PA catheter placement, venospasm can restrict catheter passage. Additionally, some very basic yet easily missed equipment system errors, calibration errors, and damping can turn a potential success into failure. Failure to pass from the RV to PA is the most common point of failure. The following maneuvers may be useful:

- Remove PA catheter and reorient the natural curve of the last 10 cm of the catheter posteriorly as it is passed.
- Have the patient hold a deep breath at inspiration.
- Change the patient's position; preferred position is left side down.
- Use fluoroscopy on rare occasions as needed.

5. AIR EMBOLISM

Although air embolism is a recognized complication of any central venous line placement, the risks are much higher with PA catheters because of the very large lumen (8.5 French) of the introducer.[53] Valved introducers greatly diminish this risk but do not eliminate it. Particular attention must be paid to this complication when placing PA catheters in spontaneously breathing patients who are in respiratory distress. Many of these people cannot or will not hold their breath after a deep inspiration, which would normally be the appropriate time to remove the guide wire and dilator (or obturator) from the introducer and pass the catheter. In order to avoid air embolism, this maneuver is best done in two steps, as previously suggested. For patients given controlled mechanical ventilation (CMV) or intermittent mandatory ventilation (IMV), these steps can be simply timed with the onset of a positive pressure breath. Access by femoral or antecubital vein will avoid air embolism as long as these sites are not elevated above heart level.

Air embolism can also occur by introduction through the catheter lumen, as well as especially after catheter balloon rupture. These volumes of air from the balloon are usually small and of no consequence, except in patients with right-to-left intracardiac shunts (small paradoxical emboli are always significant). Air embolism may also occur through the valved introducer at the time of PA catheter removal, or even through the subcutaneous tract after removal of the introducer.[32,54] Consider the following during PA catheter removal to minimize the risk of air embolism:

- Treat the valved end of the introducer as if it were an open 8.5 French lumen; ie, cover with your finger immediately and place a sterile obturator to fill the lumen.
- These large introducers should not be left in patients who are going to be transferred out of an intensively monitored environment (eg, the operating room, recovery room, or intensive care unit).
- When the introducer is removed, place antiseptic ointment over the skin entry site and rub the ointment over the area of the subcutaneous tract.
- If an air embolism occurs, administer 100% oxygen and place the patient in the left lateral head-down position. If a PA or CVP catheter is in place, attempt to aspirate air from RA and PA lumina.

6. TRAUMA

Pulmonary artery rupture is a rare but well-reported cause of death from PA catheters.[55] One recent study of 1400 patients has reported no incidents of PA rupture.[35] Although older patients with pulmonary hypertension and those undergoing cardiopulmonary bypass may be at greater risk, the usual causes are mistakes made during balloon inflation.[39] These mistakes include overinflation of the balloon, repeated and prolonged inflation times, and balloon inflation of an already wedged catheter. This latter error may result from misinterpretation of the pressure tracing in patients who transmit large "a" or "cv" waves to a wedged PA catheter. If these large waveforms are misinterpreted as PA pressure waveforms, balloon inflation may then be performed on an already-wedged catheter. The following precautions minimize the occurrence of PA rupture:

- During catheter placement, minimize the chance of spontaneous catheter wedging by assuring that at least 0.8–1.2 mL of balloon inflation are necessary to achieve a PAOP trace.
- After catheter placement, never begin balloon inflation unless a pulmonary artery pressure tracing is visible.

Note: Beware of large "a" or "cv" waves from an already wedged catheter.

- Inflate the balloon slowly, while observing the oscilloscope screen, *not* the syringe.

Note: *Stop* inflating if there is significant resistance in the syringe!

- Never use a predetermined inflation volume based on a previous measurement of PAOP. The correct volume to use is the minimum volume needed to obtain a PAOP at that time.

If PA rupture occurs, bleeding may occur in the lung parenchyma and not be detected until a chest radiograph is obtained. Frequently, however, PA rupture results in the dramatic onset of bleeding into the airway, which can be immediately life-threatening from rapidly developing hypoxemia with hypotension (hypovolemia plus hypoxic depression of myocardial function). The following suggestions may be life-saving:

- Deflate the PA catheter balloon.
- Administer 100% inspired oxygen.
- If the patient is intubated, apply 15–20 cm H_2O PEEP if tolerated.[39]
- Withdraw the PA catheter 1–2 cm and partially reinflate to divert blood flow away from the ruptured vessel.
- If the patient is intubated and bleeding out the airway, deflate the endotracheal tube cuff and advance the tube blindly into the right mainstem bronchus and inflate the cuff. A second small tracheal tube can be passed and used to ventilate the left lung. Alternatively, the head may be turned to right and the concavity of the endotracheal tube turned posteriorly; under these circumstances, the endotracheal tube has a good chance of entering the left mainstem bronchus. If the equipment is available, a double-lumen tube best separates the lungs.

Note: Because the vast majority of PA catheters flow to the right side, the rupture will have occurred on that side and a right endobronchial tube will mean that blood will continue to flow out of the tube. This maneuver will divert blood away from the left lung so that the patient can still be oxygenated. The left lung can be ventilated by placing a second endotracheal tube or by mask ventilation (with the right-sided endotracheal tube passing out the corner of the mouth under the mask). If blood stops coming out of the advanced endotracheal tube, ventilate the patient through this tube. It has either passed into the left bronchus with PA rupture on right, or it may have passed to the right (past the right upper lobe bronchus) and PA rupture has occurred in a left or in a right upper lobe vessel.

Note: Alternatively, a fiberoptic scope could be used to position the endotracheal tube in the nonbleeding side. A double-lumen endobronchial tube is the best alternative; however, both these maneuvers are time consuming and involve equipment not always immediately available.

- Tamponade the bleeding in the airway first with PEEP (see earlier) and then, with a balloon-tipped catheter placed into the bleeding bronchus by bronchoscopy, inflate the balloon to seal off the bronchus.[56]
- Perform emergency lung lobectomy, with or without the need for cardiopulmonary bypass.[57]

Cardiac perforation and valvular (tricuspid, pulmonic) incompetence may also occur as a result of direct catheter trauma. Perforation may result from advancing the guide wire too deeply or from the application of too much force during advancement of the catheter, and should be easily avoided. Perforation can also occur if the catheter tip falls back into the RV and the condition is not recognized. During difficult line placements, multiple catheter passes (both advancing and withdrawing) can damage the right heart valves or other intracardiac structures, but this trauma can be avoided by simply not using vigorous, forceful catheter manipulations.

Note: Never withdraw the PA catheter with the balloon inflated.

7. THROMBOEMBOLIC PHENOMENA

Thromboembolic phenomena such as mural thrombosis and aseptic valve vegetations[58] have been reported, although these complications are rare. In contrast, pulmonary emboli are considered common events when these catheters are used, but very few are clinically detectable, or of any known consequence.[59] As with any foreign body in the vascular system, the PA catheter serves as a focus for clot build-up. The amount of clot formed as a function of time reflects many factors, including the patient's illness, the presence of a coagulopathy or hypercoagulable state, catheter material, intimal damage, etc. The fact that clots form on PA catheters routinely, even in a few hours, frequently escapes notice or concern because these clots are "wiped" off (intravascularly) when the catheter is removed. It has been demonstrated that these clots range from 2 to 18 cm long and from 15 to 270 mg in mass on catheters in place only 1 to 3 hours.[60]

A frequent problem of clots forming on catheters is partial or complete occlusion of the lumina, which may dampen pressure tracings and prevent blood withdrawal for mixed venous sampling. Catheter clotting has also been occassionally associated with thrombocytopenia. Heparin impregnation of the catheter may decrease thromboembolic complications and is routinely performed by all PA catheter manufacturers.

Pulmonary infarction may result from migration of catheter clots or from direct occlusion of flow by the catheter (balloon inflated or deflated).[59] Fortunately, most pulmonary infarctions are asymptomatic, clinically unimportant radiographic findings. There is no convincing evidence that systemic heparinization is necessary for thromboembolic complications of the PA catheter. The most serious risk of pulmonary infarction is associated with prolonged balloon inflation, because a large vessel may be occluded. This complication will occur infrequently, as long as there is close observation for spontaneous catheter wedging and only short balloon inflation periods (less than 1 minute) are used.

Note: PA catheters with a locked balloon lumen valve are the most common cause of pulmonary infarction.

8. INFECTION

Infectious complications of PA catheters include minor site infections, thrombophlebitis, catheter sepsis, and endocarditis. Entry site infections can be minimized by daily dressing changes and appropriately timed catheter replacement at new sites. If cultures are positive from PA catheter tips, the catheter may have caused an infection or may be acting as a nidus of infection. In either case, the replacement catheter should be introduced from a new site. The risk of catheter-related septicemia increases significantly after 4 days;[61] this fact must be weighed against the need for continued PA monitoring, other accessible sites, the presence of a coagulopathy, etc. Pulmonary artery catheters should be suspect in patients with unresolving sepsis on appropriate antibiotics. In these situations, the catheter must be changed frequently.

9. BALLOON RUPTURE

Balloon rupture is almost always a complication of improper technique, although the fact remains that the latex rubber balloon does gradually lose elasticity with time. Improper techniques include reuse of catheters, overinflation of the balloon (manufacturers recommend 1.5 mL maximum volume for a 7 French TD-Edwards catheter), inflation of the balloon with a liquid instead of a gas (eg, air, carbon dioxide), and active rather than passive balloon deflation.

Note: There is no added confirmation that the balloon is completely deflated when active deflation is used instead of letting the balloon deflate passively. Return of a normal PA pressure trace is usually the only confirmation. If there is some question, obtain a chest radiograph. A hyperlucency around the tip of the PA catheter indicates that the balloon is still inflated. In this situation, attempt to actively deflate the balloon and replace the catheter.

10. MESMERISM

The "distraction" of PA monitoring is a real complication, particularly in the operating room, where the anesthesiologist works alone. Safe anesthesia delivery can be inversely related to the amount of invasive monitoring used if these monitors only serve to mesmerize the physician. The anesthesiologist must balance time spent debugging, calibrating, collecting, and calculating data from PA catheters with appropriate attention to other aspects of anesthetic management. Time distraction can occur in the intensive care unit as well as in the operating room.

Another aspect of mesmerism is a different type of distraction that occurs when the information from the PA catheter is valued above all other information about the patient. This is sometimes called the "just-tell-me-what-the-wedge-pressure-is syndrome"; it is an equally dangerous form of mesmerism.

11. MISINTERPRETATION

If all the previous risks have been avoided, and the catheter is in proper position, the last thing that can go wrong is that incorrect data are obtained or recorded.

Misinterpretation of the data results from equipment use errors, damping or ''fling'' phenomena, artifacts of transmitted airway and transpulmonary pressures, and the inability to interpret a PAOP tracing in the presence of ''a'' and ''cv'' waves.

a. Equipment Errors

Errors involving the pressure measuring equipment include inaccurate calibration of the monitoring system, particularly the transducer. Proper calibration of the transducer involves two points: zero reference to atmospheric pressure, and a second pressure (water or mercury column) applied to the transducer in the range of pressures to be measured. It must be remembered that the push-button calibration signal on many clinical monitors gives an electrical signal that ''simulates'' a given pressure on the transducer, so that the digital display can be two-point calibrated. The transducer must be calibrated first to zero by opening to atmosphere, then to a second pressure applied by a mercury column (eg, 50 mmHg). Because cm H_2O = 1.3 mmHg, a water column (eg, intravenous bottle) held 65 cm above and applied to a transducer = 50 mmHg. The transducer must be kept at right atrial level (~ 3–5 cm below the angle of Louis) for constant reference or else, despite correct calibration, erroneous data will be obtained. Fixing the transducer to the operating table or ICU bed is the best way to avoid this problem.

b. Damping and Fling

Damping sometimes refers to the effects of clot formation over the catheter tip, air bubbles, or apposition of the tip against the PA wall. Catheter *fling* may simply describe artifacts of catheter motion produced by cardiac contractions. Harmonic resonance more accurately describes the spiking artifacts produced when high frequency components of pressure wave signals match the resonating frequency of the fluid-filled monitoring system (includes catheter, extension tubing, in-line flush system, transducer) (Fig. 21–8).[62,63] The resonating frequency of a system can be altered significantly by changing the length of tubing or the material (eg, compliant vs. noncompliant tubing or transducer diaphragms). Because these changes are not always feasible, air bubbles are frequently introduced into the system to decrease fling. This method of ''uncontrolled'' damping is very crude and may cause overdamping. Adding air bubbles to the system will also decrease the natural frequency of the system, possibly enhancing ''ringing'' artifacts. Devices are available (eg, Accudynamic [Sorenson Corporation]) that have been shown to provide a controllable method of damping the monitoring system so that accurate pressure tracings can be obtained.[64] In addition, the ''square-wave test,'' performed with the Sorenson ''intraflo,'' is an example of an easily performed, objective test to determine if the system is under- or overdamped.[64]

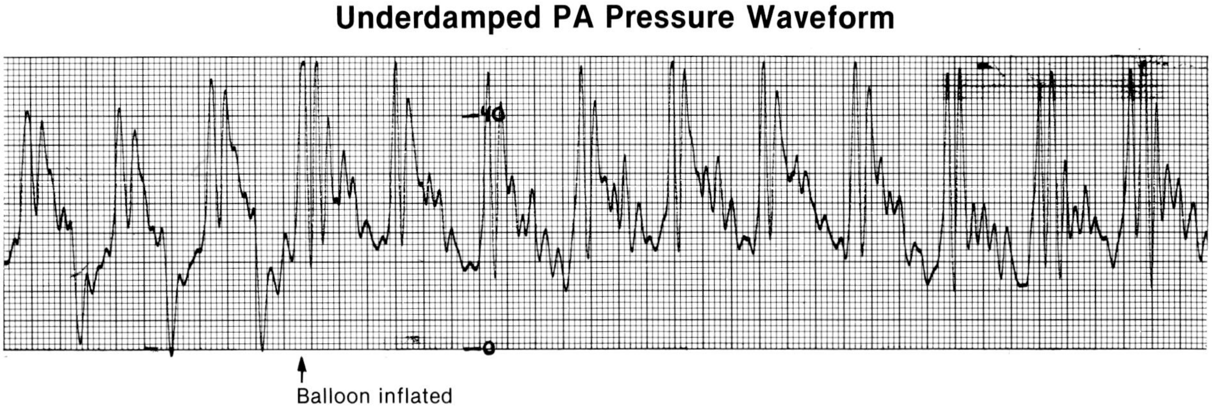

Figure 21–8 • PA pressure tracing demonstrating a classic underdamped system. Harmonic resonance causes the multiple spiking artifacts throughout the pressure tracing. Although no PAOP is obtained after balloon inflation, some of the spiking artifacts are removed, showing that the PAD is actually 15–17 mmHg, rather than 0 mmHg as seen in the early part of the tracing.

Table 21-7 • Respiratory-Induced Artifacts in PA Pressures

Respiratory Phase	Clinical Condition	Spontaneous Breathing	Mechanical Ventilation
Inspiration	Normal	Negative pressure	Positive pressure
Exhalation*	Normal	Negligible	Negligible
	Valsalva	Positive pressure	—
	Grunting	Positive pressure	—
	Purse-lip breathing	Positive pressure	—
	UAO	Positive pressure	—
	Bronchospasm	Positive pressure	Positive pressure
	CPAP/PEEP	Positive pressure	Positive pressure

*Normally there are negligible respiratory-induced PA pressure artifacts during exhalation because airway and pleural pressures approach zero during this phase of the respiratory cycle. However, pathologic conditions (Valsalva, grunting, purse-lip breathing, etc) must be recognized because they can produce significant positive pressure artifacts during exhalation that will result in falsely elevated PA pressures.

UAO, upper airway obstruction.

Overdamping produced by semiclosed stopcocks, clots, or air bubbles can usually be corrected by syringe aspiration. Although flushing the line is equally effective in removing bubbles, it should not be employed routinely to clear clots from the catheter lumen. Damping produced by catheter tip apposition to the vessel wall may require repositioning of the catheter.

c. *Transmitted Airway and Transpulmonary Pressures*

Transmitted airway and transpulmonary pressures are a serious cause of misinterpretation of the PA pressures. Pulmonary artery pressure measurements are absolute pressures by which we estimate actual transmural pressures. This estimation is valid as long as the pressure outside the PA vessel (which we do not measure) is close to atmosphere pressure. Negative pressure artifacts (subatmospheric pressure) may be transmitted to a PA catheter during the inspiratory phase of spontaneous breathing and may be extreme in patients with respiratory distress.[65] Positive pressure artifacts may appear during the inspiratory phase of positive pressure mechanical ventilation (Table 21–7). Positive pressure artifacts may also be transmitted during exhalation (spontaneous or mechanical ventilatory modes) if exhalation becomes an active process (eg, bronchospasm).[66] Any combination of the above artifacts can be seen in patients with PA catheters and may confuse the correct estimation of transmural vascular pressures. Because of the frequent use of muscle relaxants, intermittent mandatory ventilation, etc, the types of artifacts seen in a given patient may change minute by minute. In addition, the magnitude of pressure artifact transmission will depend on pulmonary/thorax compliance, position of the PA catheter, use of PEEP, patient effort, etc. Some of these factors will fluctuate over time in the same patient.

In order to obtain accurate PA pressure measurements during mechanical ventilation or spontaneous respirations, the following guidelines are suggested.

- Read pressures off a calibrated screen or preferably a paper printout. (Digital displays may be very inaccurate because they average over time.)[65]
- Establish the end-exhalation phases of either mechanical or spontaneous breaths, and read PAOP and PA pressures at these times only (Fig. 21–9).
- In patients with bronchospasm, pressure artifacts may exist in all parts of a respiratory cycle (mechanical or spontaneous ventilatory modes). The only way to obtain reliable PA pressure readings is to measure intrathoracic pressures (intrathoracic catheter[67] or esophageal balloon) and subtract this pressure from the observed PAOP or PA pressure. Alternatively, once the patient's bronchospasm is treated and has resolved, or if the patient is paralyzed, pressures during end-exhalation may again be measured.

These guidelines address the problem of intermittent pressure artifacts, but not the potential error induced by PEEP or CPAP. The amount of pressure transmitted will vary between patients, as well as in the same patient over time. Factors such as lung compliance, catheter position, mode of respiration, and level of PEEP, are important in determining how much of this airway

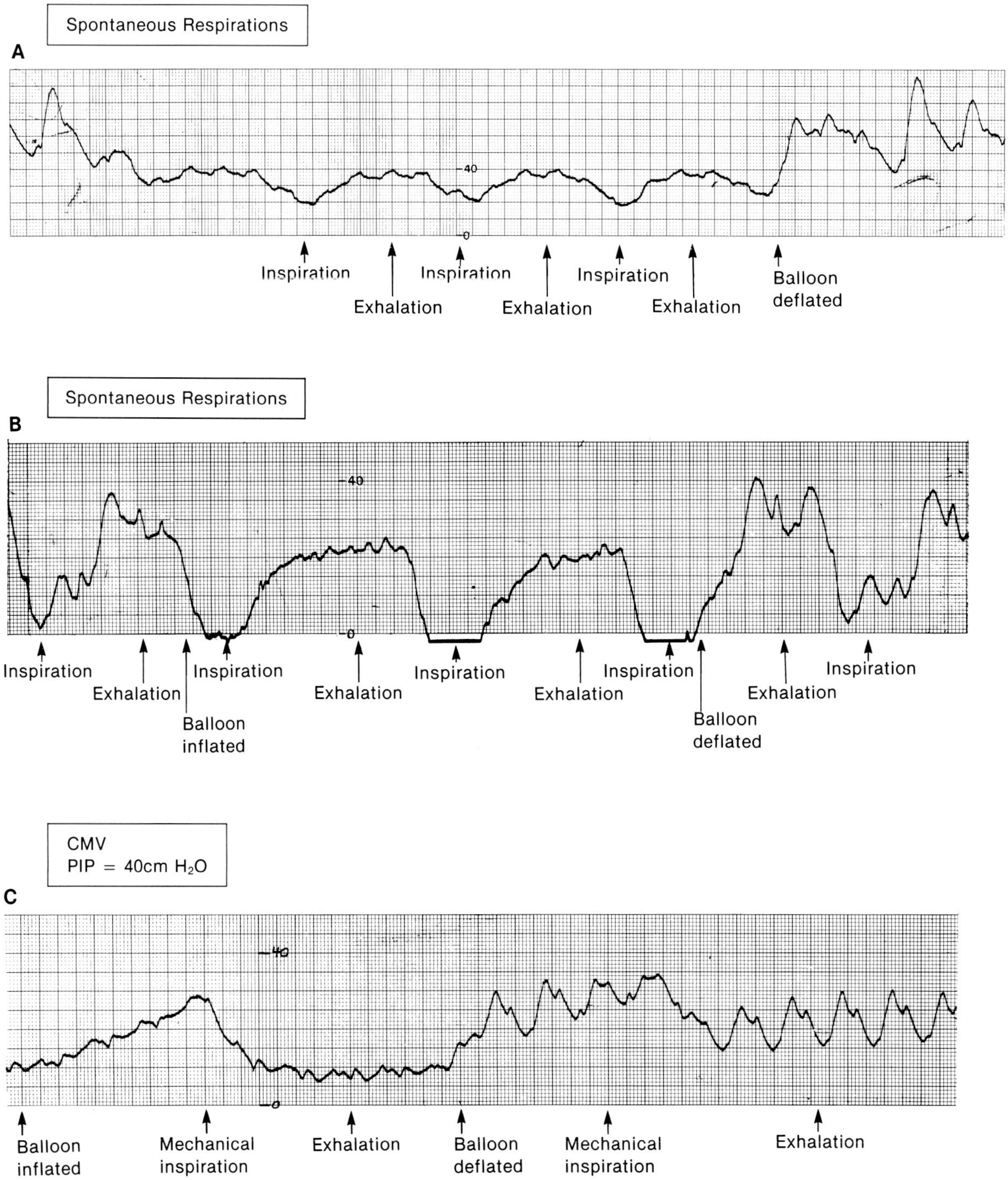

Figure 21–9 • Representative PA pressure tracings from patients in different respiratory modes are shown. (***A***) Spontaneous respirations: this patient has a PAOP of ~35 mmHg when measured at end-exhalation. His inspiratory efforts are generating about −15 mmHg intrapleural pressure, because during inspiration the PAOP tracing drops to 20 mmHg (35–15 = 20 mmHg). (***B***) Spontaneous respirations: this patient was in marked respiratory distress. While breathing with very stiff lungs, he generated tremendous negative pleural pressures. The PAOP tracing during inspiration was therefore as low as −40 mmHg (estimated). Reading during exhalation: PAD = 25 mmHg; PAOP = 20–22 mmHg. (***C***) Controlled mechanical ventilation (CMV): during CMV (peak inspiratory pressure [PIP] 40 cm H_2O), positive pressure artifacts are easy to identify during inspiration. Measured during exhalation, PAD is 15 mmHg; PAOP is 8 mmHg. During mechanical inspiration the PAOP artifactually increases to 28 mmHg (8 + 20 = 28 mmHg).

(continued)

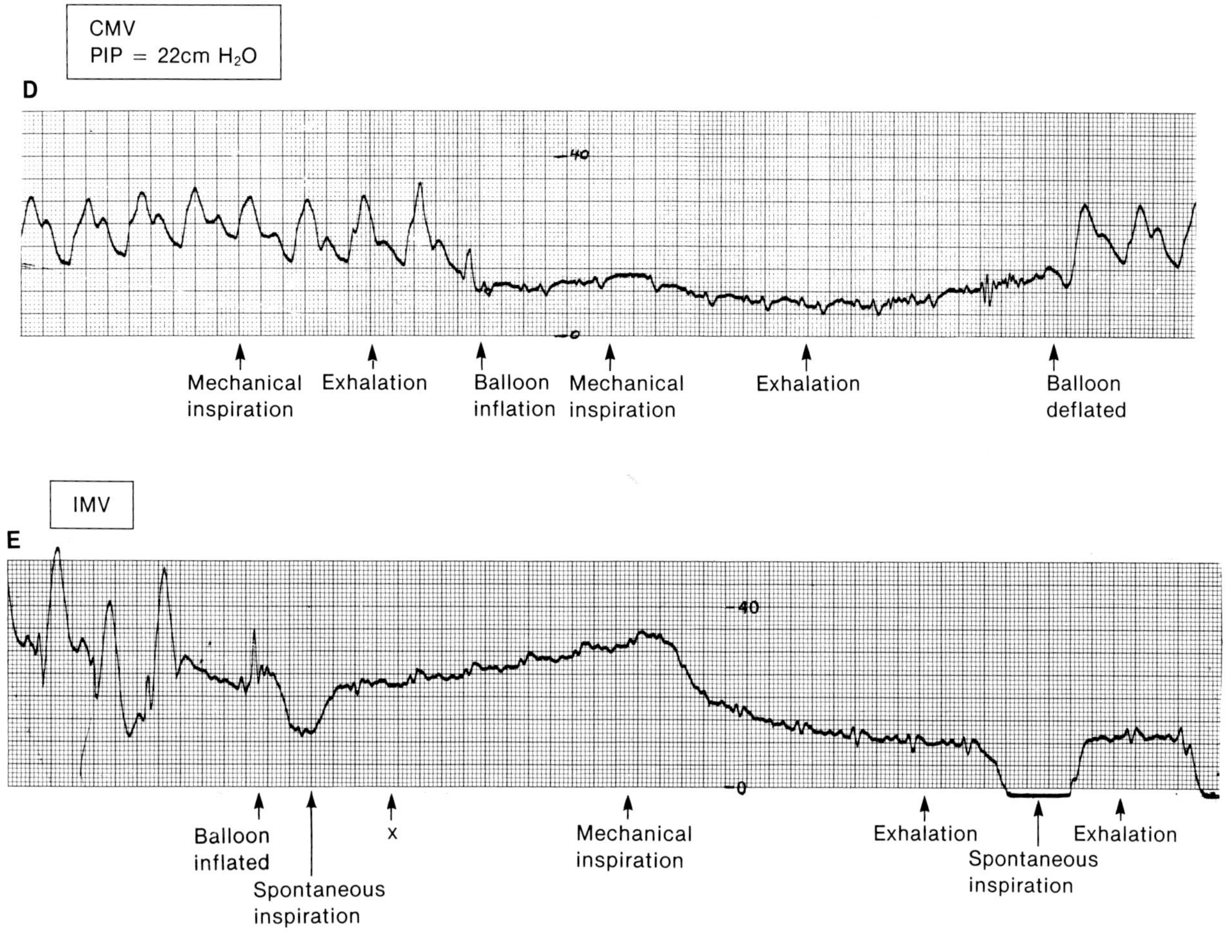

Figure 21–9 *(continued)*
(***D***) CMV: positive-pressure ventilation (peak inspiratory pressure, 22 cm H_2O) produces less marked inspiratory artifacts in this patient. Measured during exhalation, PAD = 15 mmHg, and PAOP = 7 mmHg. (***E***) Intermittent mandatory ventilation (IMV): PA pressure tracing during IMV can appear chaotic. On this tracing, after balloon inflation two periods of exhalation are identified, showing a PAOP = 10 mmHg. Exhalation after a mechanical inspiration or spontaneous inspiration should show the same value for PAOP. Notice that point x does not represent an exhalation point to read PAOP, because a mechanical inspiration immediately follows a spontaneous effort.

positive pressure will artifactually raise the PAOP. Stiff lungs and spontaneous respirations tend to "protect" against this artifact.[68] In addition, catheters positioned so that they face lung units under "zone 3" lung conditions (arterial > venous > alveolar pressure) will tend not to transmit PEEP pressure.[68–70] PEEP may convert lung zones from 3 to 2 and from 2 to 1. PEEP levels under 10 cm H_2O (7.7 mm Hg) are less likely to produce artifacts (Fig. 21–10).

The following guidelines for PA pressure monitoring pertain to patients on PEEP.

- In general, leave patients on PEEP, measure PAOP and PA pressures at end-exhalation, and ignore the level of PEEP being used. The rationale for this recommendation is that (a) most patients require less than 10 cm H_2O mmHg (7.7 mmHg) of PEEP; (b) patients who require PEEP usually have stiffer lungs, and airway pressure is less transmitted to the vasculature;[68] (c) PA catheters tend to "go with flow" and usually face zone 3 areas of the lung;[67] (d) the absolute transmural PAOP value, as a reflection of preload, is not nearly as important as changes in this variable for the evaluation of clinical events, and of various therapeutic interventions.
- If necessary, the PA catheter can be positioned so that the tip of the catheter lies below the level of the left atrium on a lateral chest film to further enhance the likelihood that it is facing a zone 3 lung area.

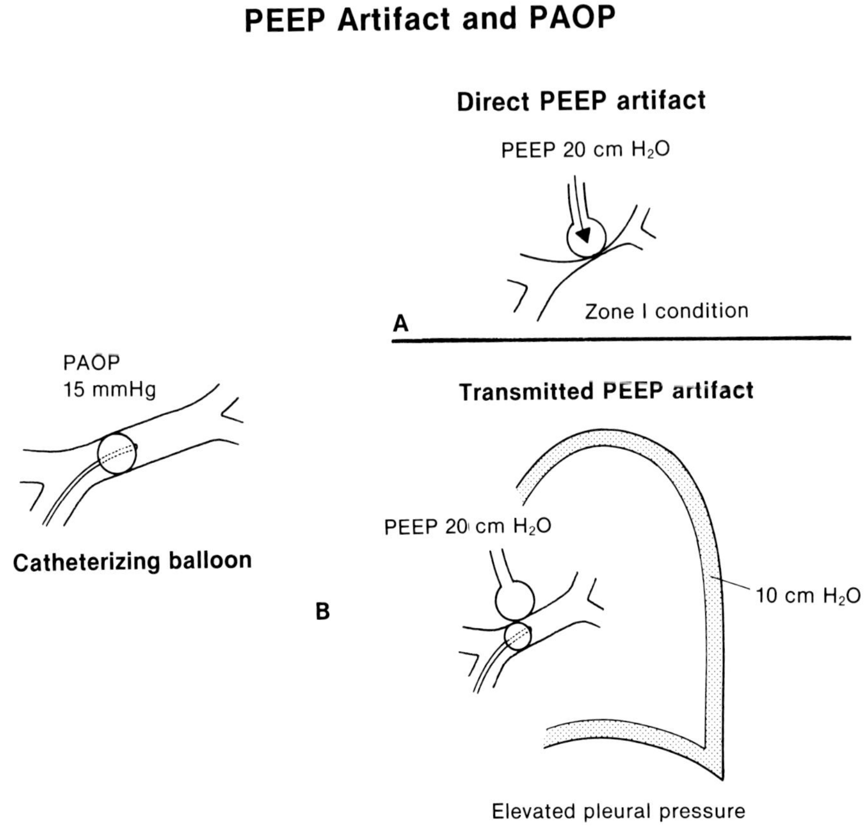

Figure 21–10 • Two possible mechanisms of PEEP artifact in the PAOP measurement are shown. In this example, the PAOP is 15 mmHg. (***A***) After balloon occlusion is accomplished, if the PA catheter tip faces a lung region under predominantly zone 1 conditions, then the PAOP will measure alveolar airway pressures. If the PAOP was 15 mmHg it would simply mean that alveolar pressures in that area of the lung were 20 mmHg (or ~20 cm H_2O) and that the PAOP was in this situation a measure of airway pressure rather than vascular pressure. (***B***) If the PA catheter tip after balloon occlusion faces primarily zone 3 lung units (the usual case), then alveolar pressures will not cause direct artifacts. However, PEEP may be transmitted through the lung and raise pleural pressures, as shown. In this case, a PAOP of 15 mmHg and a pleural pressure of 10 cm H_2O (or ~8 mmHg) means that the actual transmural PAOP is 7 mmHg (15–8 mmHg).

- When high levels of PEEP (> 15 cm H_2O) are used, accurate PAOP may be obtained by (a) measuring intrathoracic pressure with an intrathoracic catheter or esophageal balloon, or (b) while the PA catheter balloon is inflated, remove PEEP for less than 10 seconds, and record PAOP on and off PEEP (Fig. 21–11). This measurement need only be performed 1–2 times/day to document how much of the PEEP is transmitted to the PAOP. The second technique is quite simple compared to the first method, but is less desirable because loss of PEEP, even for a single breath, may result in a decrease in functional residual capacity. There is also concern that a sudden loss of PEEP may cause or exacerbate pulmonary edema. However, both of these statements must be balanced by the fact that intubated patients are routinely disconnected from PEEP during tracheal suctioning without any documented harm. Caution must be used in patients with severe hypoxemia, who may be very sensitive to PEEP removal.[71]

d. Pathologic "a" and "cv" Waves

Failure to identify and interpret transmitted left atrial "a" (atrial contraction) and "cv" (ventricular contraction) waves in a PAOP tracing may prevent accurate preload measurements and also lead to pulmonary infarction if spontaneous catheter wedging is not recognized (Fig. 21–12). Small a and c waves are commonly seen on balloon inflation. Pathologic (> 5 mmHg above baseline), large a waves occur with mitral stenosis (when sinus rhythm is present), junctional heart rhythms or complete heart block, atrial myxoma, and early acute heart failure associated with ischemia (Fig. 21–13).[72] In these situations, the last part of the a wave or the diastolic PAOP (the lowest part of the pressure trace measured at end-exhalation) will give the most reliable reflection of left ventricular filling pressures.[73]

Pathologic, or giant, cv waves occur with acute mitral regurgitation and may be seen on PAOP tracings of patients without an audible murmur.[74] The size of the cv wave does not always correlate with the magnitude of regurgitation.[75] Some patients with large cv waves do not have any mitral regurgitation and will be found to have mitral stenosis, congestive heart failure, or a ventricular septal defect.[76] In the presence of a large cv wave, simply measuring the *mean* PAOP at end-exhalation will give an artificially high estimate of left-ven-

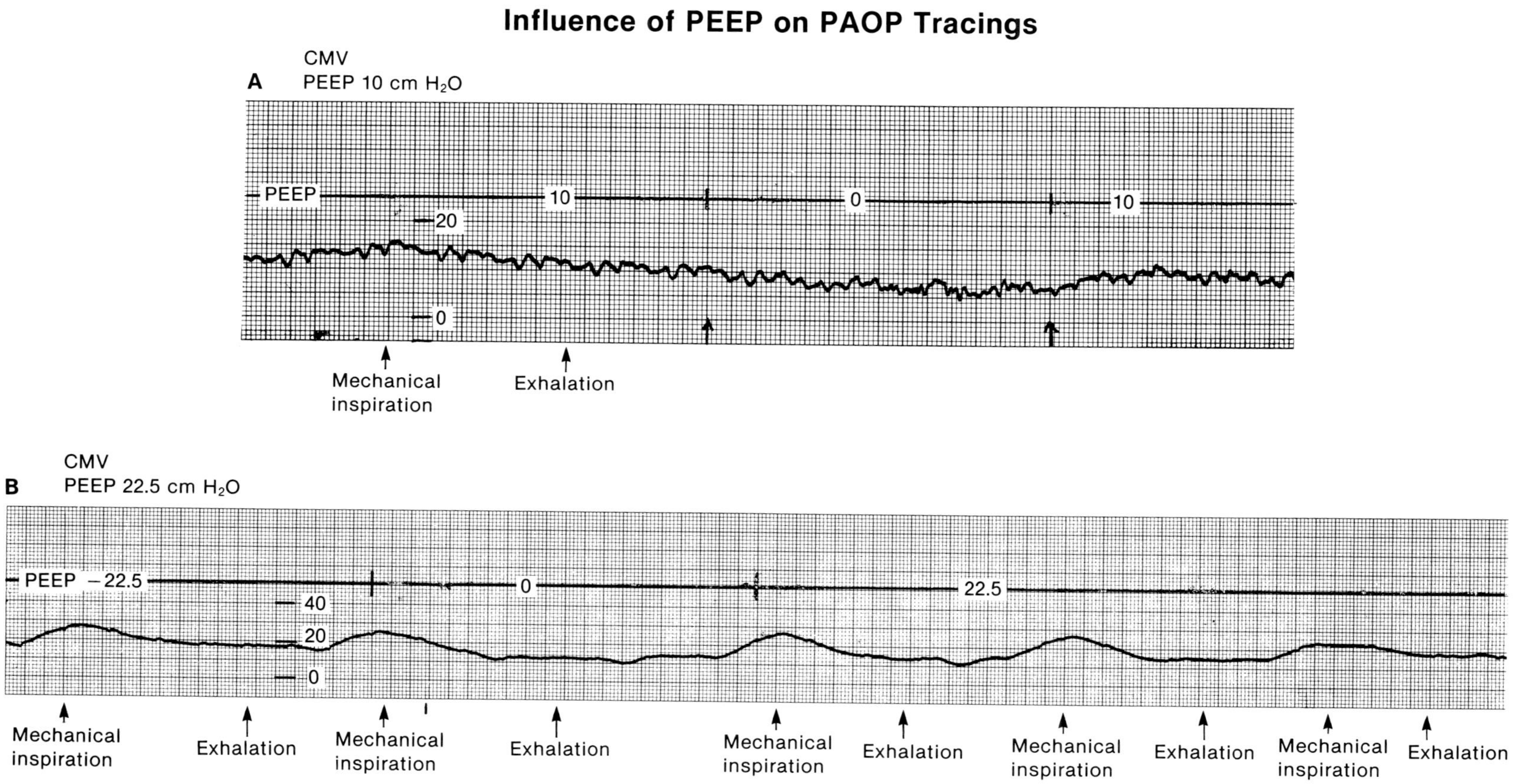

Figure 21–11 • PAOP tracings are shown in two cases where PEEP was withdrawn to determine the amount of PEEP-induced artifacts. (***A***) The PAOP falls quickly from 10 mmHg to 7 mmHg when 10 cm H_2O (7.7 mmHg) of PEEP is removed, and returns quickly to 10 mmHg when the PEEP is reapplied. Therefore, the PEEP-induced artifact in this patient is assumed to be ~3 mmHg. It is arguable as to whether the patient's hemodynamics are changing significantly during the few seconds required to do this maneuver. This maneuver is not necessary in most patients, because the PEEP-induced artifact is usually small (ie, <5 mmHg). (***B***) In this patient, who requires 22.5 cm H_2O (17.3 mmHg) PEEP, the PAOP value of 18 mmHg falls quickly to 12 mmHg off PEEP, then gradually returns over three respiratory cycles (exhalation at far right) to 18 mmHg after PEEP is reapplied. The PEEP-induced artifact in this patient appears to be about 6 mmHg. Even in this type of patient, the PAOP off PEEP does not generally need to be measured, as long as the clinician understands that some PEEP-induced artifact exists and integrates that knowledge with other information about the patient.

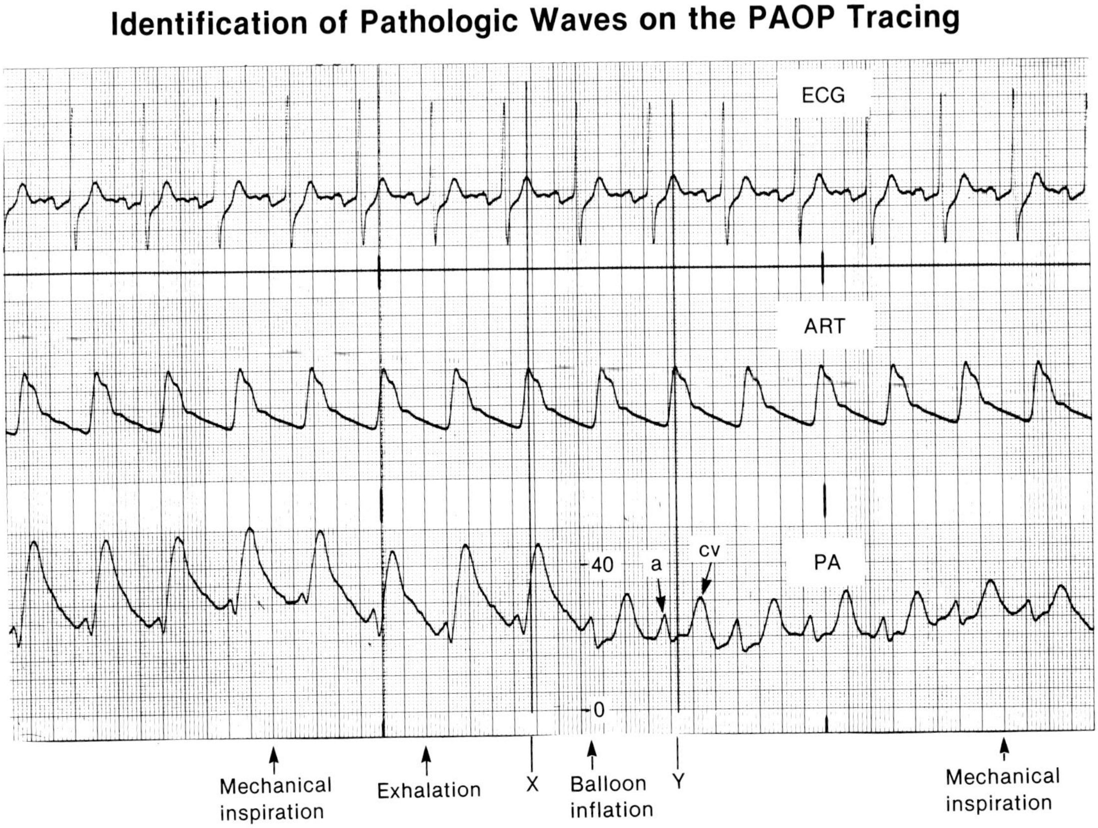

Figure 21–12 • The electrocardiogram (*ECG*), arterial (*ART*), and PA pressure tracings in a patient who has pathologic (>5 mmHg) a and cv waves visible on the PAOP tracing. Is the tracing after balloon inflation really a PAOP tracing? It is accepted as a PAOP tracing because after balloon inflation the lowest part of the tracing measured in exhalation (16 mmHg) is lower than the PAD measured in exhalation (19 mmHg), and the PA pressure returns promptly on balloon deflation (not shown).

To distinguish the a from the cv wave, the waves on the PA and PAOP tracing need to be compared with some other regular cardiac event (eg, electrocardiogram or systemic arterial pressure trace). Drawing lines through the peak of the T wave on the electrocardiogram or peak of the systemic arterial trace and then both through the PA pressure tracing (*line X*) and through the PAOP tracing (*line Y*) will identify the waves. The cv wave, relative to the PA pressure wave, occurs later in the cardiac cycle (ie, further to the right of the line), because both the PA and cv waves reflect systolic events of right and left ventricles respectively, and the cv wave has to be transmitted over a longer, more compliant path to be detected by the PA catheter (ie, LV–LA–pulmonary veins–pulmonary capillaries–pulmonary artery–PA catheter). (Conversely, the a wave always appears earlier than the PA pressure wave [ie, to the left of the line] because it reflects an event of diastole.) Note also that the geometric shapes of typical a and cv waves are isosceles triangles compared to the right-angle triangle shape of the PA pressure trace. In summary, this patient has a PAD of 19 mmHg, and a PAOP of 16 mmHg with a 25-mmHg a wave and a 30-mmHg cv wave.

tricular filling pressure. Because the large cv wave represents transmitted left ventricular systolic pressure, it should be ignored when trying to assess diastolic filling pressures. The remaining a wave (usually normal size) or the diastolic PAOP will best reflect left ventricular filling pressures (Fig. 21–14).

V. Discussion

A. *PA Pressures*

While we carefully avoid the potential complications of PA catheterization and also avoid pitfalls in interpreting

Onset of A Waves with LV Ischemia

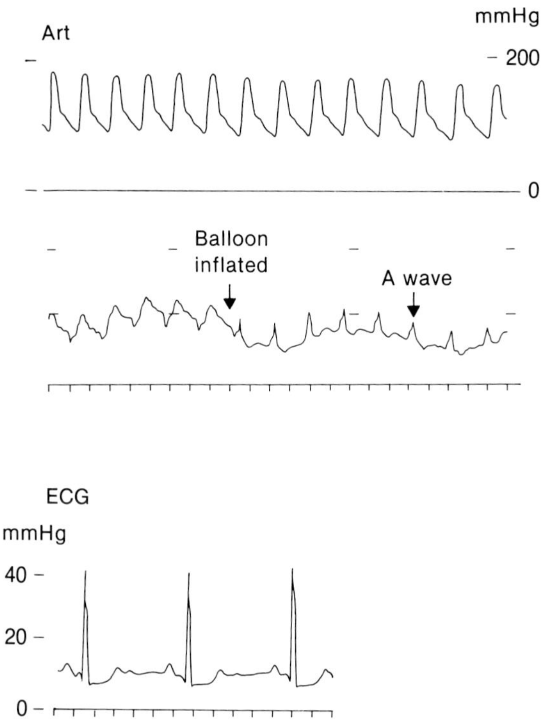

Figure 21–13 • PA pressure tracing of a patient who experienced angina just before anesthetic induction for coronary artery surgery. Associated with his symptoms were new ST segment depressions noted on his electrocardiogram and a new pathologic wave on his PAOP tracing. Lines drawn through the peak systemic arterial trace clearly demonstrate this wave to be an a wave because it occurs earlier than the PA pressure peak. PAD = 17 mmHg, PAOP = 15 mmHg with a 23-mmHg a wave. This a wave was not present when the PA catheter was initially placed, and disappeared (along with the chest pain and ST changes) a few minutes after starting a nitroglycerin infusion.

the PA pressure waveform, the limitations of what we have measured must be understood. As clinicians we would like to use the PAOP in two ways: (1) as an estimate of LV preload, and (2) as an estimate of pulmonary hydrostatic pressure. As discussed in Chapter 18, fluid infusion to augment or optimize preload in order to improve cardiac output must always be balanced against the danger of raising pulmonary hydrostatic pressures and thereby causing extravascular lung water (EVLW) accumulation (pulmonary edema) (Fig. 21–15).

1. PAD INSTEAD OF PAOP

In rare situations where the PAOP may be unobtainable, the PA diastolic pressure (PAD), measured carefully at end-exhalation, may be used as the next-best estimate of preload.[77] There are many clinicians, however, who never measure PAOP because they are concerned about interpretation problems as well as the risk of PA rupture. They also believe that the PAD tracks PAOP well enough for clinical decisions. Normally, the difference between the PAD and PAOP is less than 5 mmHg; however, this gradient may widen if pulmonary hypertension develops (eg, chronic obstructive pulmonary disease, pulmonary embolism). More important, pulmonary hypertension may be transiently caused by hypoxia, acidosis, drugs, etc, making the PAD–PAOP gradient change acutely. Therefore, changes in the PAD pressure may be misleading if they are always assumed to reflect changes in PAOP. When the PAOP is obtainable, the recommendation to measure the PAOP only once to determine the PAD–PAOP gradient, and then to follow the PAD exclusively is unsatisfactory because it ignores the dynamic relationship that may exist between these two pressures during the course of a patient's illness.[78]

2. PAOP AND PRELOAD

The PAOP measurement is at best a reasonable estimate of absolute or intracavitary LV filling pressure, assuming that conditions that may interfere with the relationship between the PAOP and LAP or the relationship between the LAP and LVEDP are not present (Fig. 21–16).[79] The conditions affecting the PAOP–LAP relationship all result in an overestimation of actual LV filling pressures. Such is not the case with the conditions affecting the LAP–LVEDP relationship. The LAP will overestimate LV filling pressures in patients with mitral stenosis as well as those with mitral regurgitation, particularly in the latter condition if the cv wave that is present is meaned for the PAOP value. In patients with longstanding mitral regurgitation, the cv wave may be attenuated and therefore not recognized because of a compliant left atrium, leading to a higher mean LAP/PAOP than the LVEDP. Conversely, aortic regurgitation may cause premature closure of the mitral valve, and therefore LAP will underestimate LV filling pressures.[77] In patients who undergo sudden worsening of LV compli-

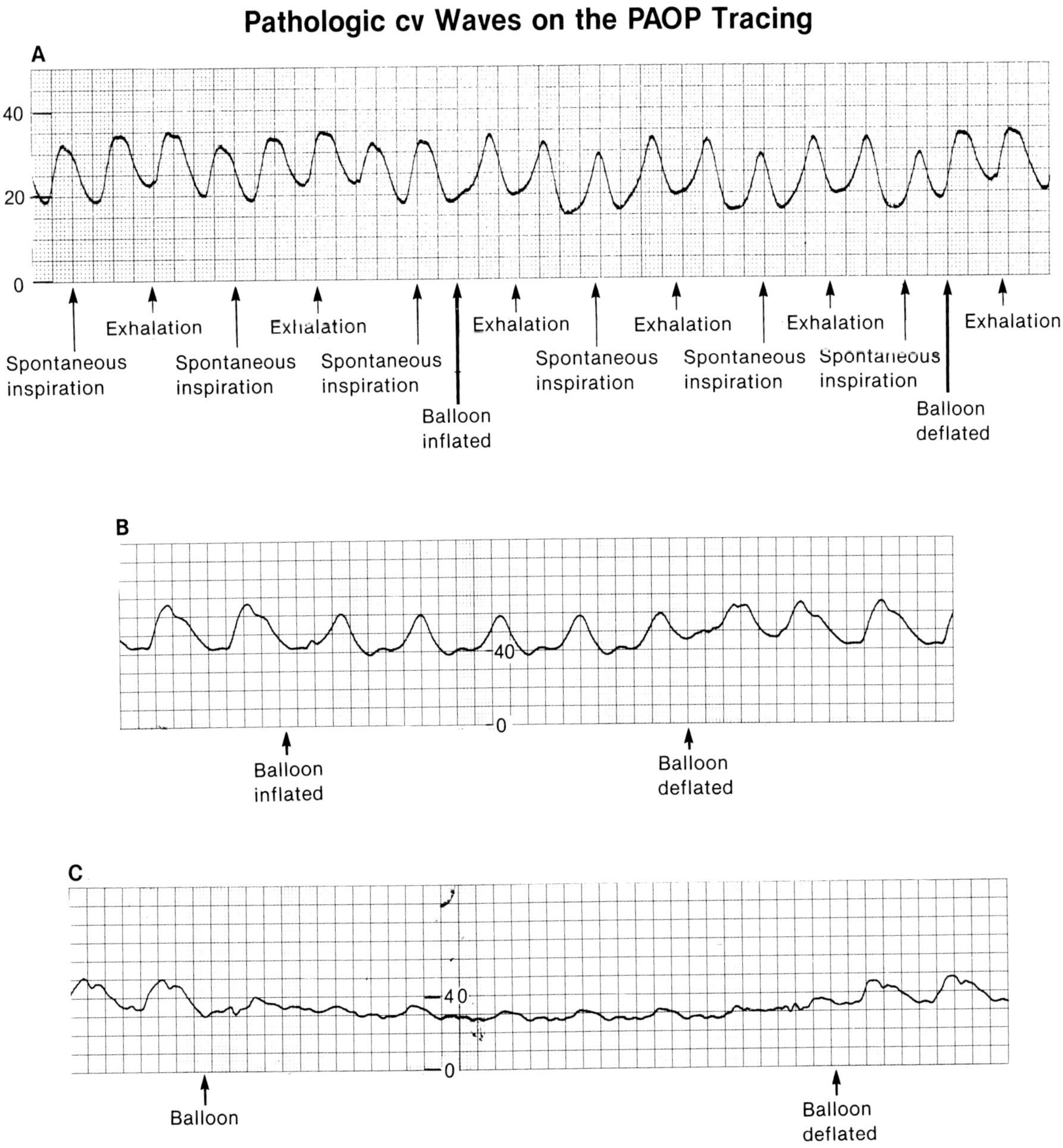

Figure 21–14 • PA pressure tracings of two patients with pathologic cv waves. (***A***) Note how, after balloon inflation, the waveform changes to an isosceles triangle shape. This is a PAOP trace because in exhalation the PAOP = 20 mmHg and the PAD = 23 mmHg. The cv wave peaks at 33 mmHg, making it almost as tall as the PA pressure peak. From this example, it is easy to see how PA catheters can become spontaneously wedged without recognition in patients with large cv waves. (***B***) A patient with significant PA hypertension associated with high filling pressures and a very large cv wave. PA = 67/42 mmHg, PAOP = 38 mmHg with a 60 mmHg (peak), 22 mmHg (pulse) cv wave. This patient was not in respiratory distress, but did have an audible murmur and rales heard more than halfway up his back. Note also that these are neglible respiratory artifacts on the PA and PAOP pressure tracing in this patient as in a few minutes after treatment with a nitroglycerin infusion. PAD = 35 mmHg, PAOP = 27 mmHg with minimal cv wave. (**C**) Same patient as in (*B*).

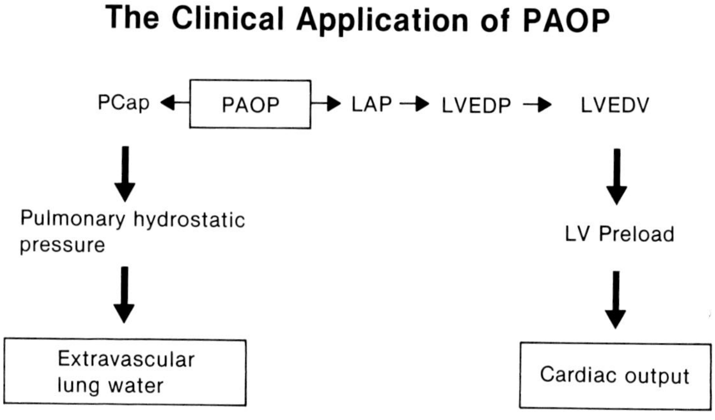

Figure 21–15 • The clinical application of PAOP. This is used as a guide to the level of left ventricular preload necessary to maintain an appropriate cardiac output, while also estimating pulmonary capillary hydrostatic pressure (*PCap*) and attempting to minimize the risk of pulmonary edema or elevation of extravascular lung water. LAP = left atrial pressure; LVEDP = left ventricular end-diastolic pressure; LVEDV = left ventricular end-diastolic volume.

ance (eg, ischemia) the mean LAP may underestimate LV filling pressures. The peak of the a wave has been suggested as a more accurate way of determining LV filling pressure in this situation.

Barring these mentioned conditions, the PAOP is a reasonably accurate estimate of intracavitary LV filling pressure. However, assuming that absolute measurements of LVEDP are close to transmural filling pressures of the left ventricle is not always correct. Similar to the problems of transmitted airway pressure affecting transmural PAOP pressure measurements, pericardial effusions or constriction and interventricular septal wall shifts may also result in net (transmural) LV distending pressures to be overestimated by absolute LVEDP measurements (Fig. 21–17). Assuming these conditions do not pertain to our patient and we have an absolute pressure that is a good estimate of transmural LVEDP, LV preload is still best thought of as a volume rather than a pressure (see Fig. 21–15).[33] As discussed in Chapter 18, the LV pressure–volume relationship normally is a curve, and this curve can be shifted chronically or very dynamically by the various conditions listed in Table 21–8 (Fig. 21–18). The dynamic conditions (ischemia, drugs) may affect the "stiffness" of the left ventricle over a period of minutes. For example, in a patient developing myocardial ischemia, it is understandable that the PAOP, accurately reflecting LVEDP, might increase, while LVEDV or preload remains unchanged. It should be equally understandable how, in that same patient, as myocardial ischemia resolves, the PAOP and LVEDP might decrease while LVEDV or preload remains unchanged. There are obviously many other possible per-

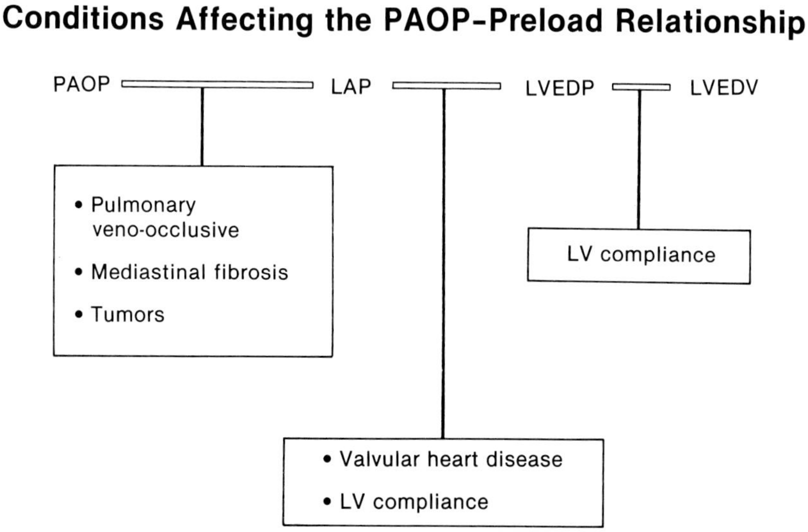

Figure 21–16 • The PAOP should track left ventricular end-diastolic volume (*LVEDV*). However, the various conditions shown intersecting this direct relationship will interfere with the relationship between PAOP and left atrial pressure (*LAP*), left-ventricular end-diastolic pressure (*LVEDP*) and, ultimately, LVEDV as a measure of left ventricular preload.

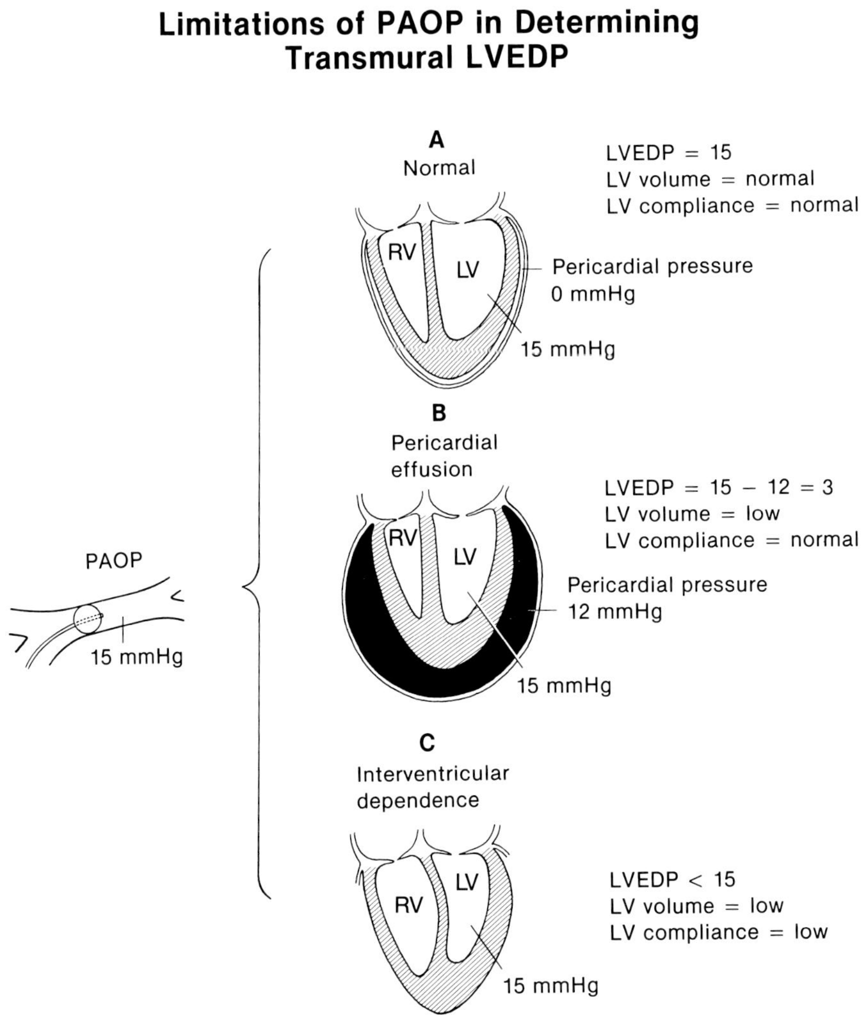

Figure 21–17 • Effects of pericardial effusions and RV distention on the relationship between absolute or intracavitary left ventricular filling pressure (LVEDP) and transmural LVEDP ($LVEDP_{tm}$) as reflected by PAOP. (***A***) In the normal situation where the PA catheter is functioning properly without artifacts or interfering diseases (eg, valvular disease, tumors, etc), the PAOP will closely reflect transmural LVEDP. In this example, the PAOP and LVEDP equal 15 mmHg. This absolute measure of LVEDP is the same as the actual distending pressure (also called transmural pressure) because the pericardial pressure is zero ($LVEDP_{tm} = 15 - 0 = 15$ mmHg). However, because the pericardial effusion (***B***) creates a pericardial pressure of 12 mmHg, actual transmural LVEDP = 3 mmHg (15 − 12 = 3 mmHg). In this case, left ventricular distending pressures are significantly overestimated by the PAOP of 15 mmHg. (***C***) Patients who develop cor pulmonale have right ventricular (RV) distention that can cause interventricular septal wall shift into the LV chamber. Although it is not as easily quantifiable, the net effect on transmural LVEDP is the same as seen with pericardial effusions: ie, although the PAOP reflects LVEDP of 15 mmHg, it overestimates LV preload.

Table 21-8 • Factors Affecting LV Compliance

Hypertrophy	Ischemia
Fibrosis	Drugs[†]
Infiltrative process*	Dilated cardiomyopathy

*Amyloidosis.

[†]Nitroglycerin, inotropic agents, beta-blockers.

mutations. The possibility that LV preload may change even though the PAOP, accurately measured and consistently reflecting LVEDP, remains unchanged is a possibility often overlooked in clinical practice. It is commonly believed that one measurement of cardiac output with its associated PAOP is adequate to guide future therapy, which is then aimed at maintaining the PAOP without the need to measure cardiac output again, because "we know what it is." Not only may we be unaware of changes in LV compliance, but changes in contractility or afterload and their effects on cardiac output may be unnoticed unless a measurement of cardiac output is made. The important message of this discussion is that clinically we cannot be assured of knowing the cardiac output on the basis of only the PAOP; hence, the importance of repeated measurements of cardiac output.

3. PAOP AND PCAP

With any decision to raise preload in the attempt to improve cardiac output comes the understanding that this maneuver will also raise capillary hydrostatic pressures throughout the body, but this is of particular concern in the lung. Because the pulmonary capillary pressure (Pcap) is the most important variable that

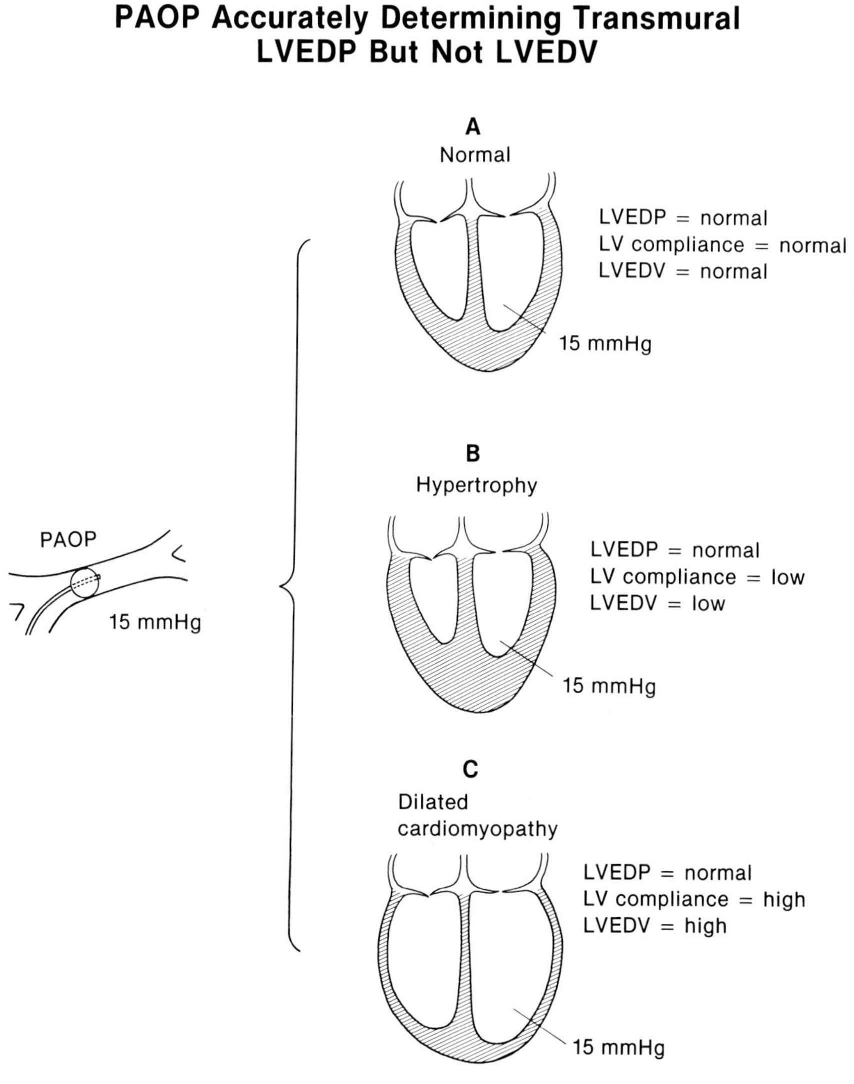

Figure 21-18 • Shown are possible relationships between LV distending (transmural) pressure, accurately measured by the PAOP, and LV end diastolic volume (LVEDV), which is considered a better reflection of preload. (***A***) Note that how the same PAOP of 15 mmHg, which accurately reflects transmural LVEDP in each of these examples, can be associated with a small LVEDV (low preload) in the patient with left ventricular hypertrophy (***B***) or a very large LVEDV (high preload) in the patient with a dilated cardiomyopathy (***C***), depending on pathologic changes in left ventricular compliance.

determines fluid flux in the lung, significant elevations of Pcap predictably cause accumulation of extravascular lung water (EVLW) and, eventually, sufficient water accumulation to be recognized clinically as pulmonary edema. In patients with acute respiratory failure, the potential harm of raising Pcap is magnified because of the well-recognized permeability injury these patients suffer.

The PAOP has traditionally been taken by clinicians as an estimate of Pcap and, in fact, the pulmonary *capillary* wedge pressure (PCWP), a term used in the past for PAOP, reflects this long-held assumption.

The measurement of Pcap is difficult to make, but estimates are possible by analyzing the pressure decay curve generated at the moment of PA balloon occlusion (Fig. 21–19).[80] Such estimates suggest that, in some patients, Pcap may be 5–10 mmHg higher than PAOP. Until these measurements are better understood and more broadly applied, it is prudent for clinicians to understand the possible significant underestimation of pulmonary hydrostatic pressures when assessing patients by the PAOP value.[81] This would appear particularly important in patients with a permeability injury of the lung and those with significant pulmonary hypertension as evidenced by a large difference between the PAD and PAOP.

B. *Mixed Venous Oxygen Saturation*

Although oxygen hemoglobin saturation in mixed venous blood ($S_{\bar{v}}O_2$) can be measured by sampling from the distal (PA) lumen,[82] the introduction of PA catheters equipped with fiberoptic bundles for light transmission has permitted accurate in vivo oximetry for continuous monitoring of $S_{\bar{v}}O_2$ (Fig. 21–20). This measurement has been proven accurate and reliable with negligible technical problems.[83,84] Some oximeter PA catheters perform better than others.[85] Oximeter PA catheters require little extra effort (other than calibration, which is simple and performed in 30 seconds) and still provide the same capability as the standard thermodilution PA catheters to measure cardiac output and PA pressures. It should be mentioned that PA oximeter catheters cost two to four times as much as standard 7.5 French thermodilution catheters, and whether they are cost effective overall depends on how the catheter is used.

1. Physiology

When oxygen demand increases above oxygen supply, monitoring of $S_{\bar{v}}O_2$ reflects the extent to which the

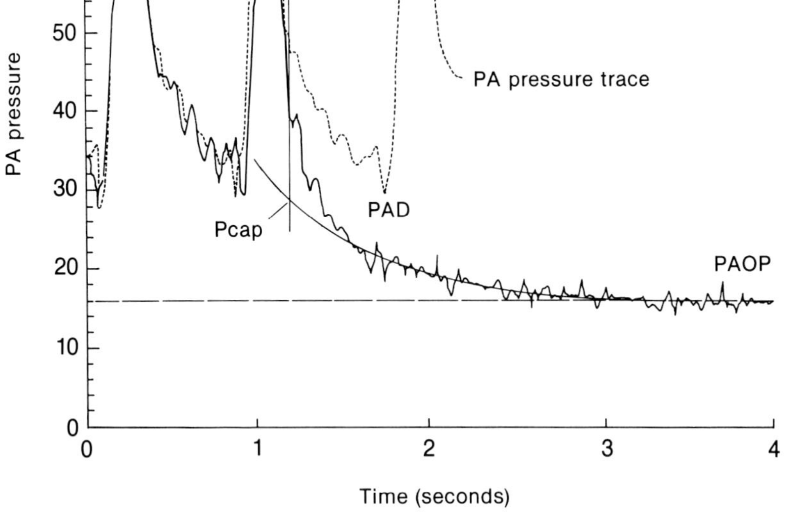

Figure 21–19 • A proposed method for estimating pulmonary capillary pressure (*Pcap*) is shown. The normal PA pressure is indicated by the dotted lines and superimposed on the pressure tracing during balloon occlusion (*solid line*). The point of intersection of two lines, one vertical at the moment of PA occlusion and the other on the exponential line fitted to the PAOP tracing, indicates the estimated Pcap value. The value of Pcap will always lie between the PAD and PAOP values.

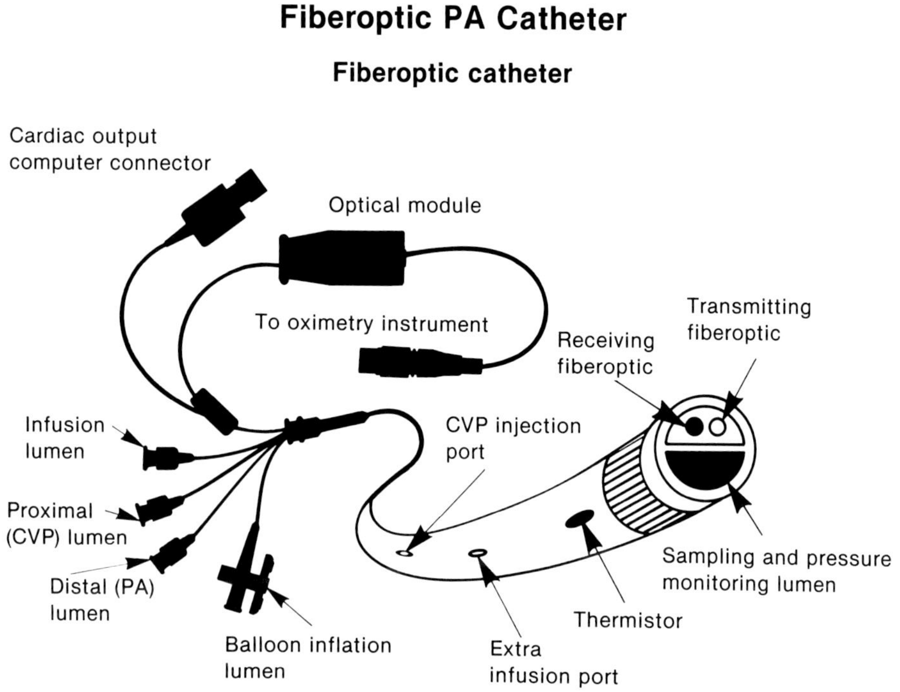

Figure 21–20 • The fiberoptic oximetry PA catheter is shown with its various features identified. The oximetry system uses one fiberoptic bundle to transmit three specific wavelengths of light sequentially and the other bundle to receive light reflected back in proportion to the amount of light absorbed by the hemoglobin in red blood cells (reflective spectrophotometry). (Shown is the Oximetrix Opticath, model P7110-EP8-H [Abbott Laboratories, Chicago, IL].)

body's various compensatory mechanisms are being used. These mechanisms include increasing cardiac output, increasing oxygen extraction, redistribution of blood flow, increased hemoglobin concentration (slow-responding mechanism), and increased arterial oxygen saturation (Fig. 21–21). Cardiac output can be tripled in normal adults (5–15 L/min) and has been documented to be more than 35 L/minute in athletes;[86] however, many critically ill patients have a limited cardiac reserve. Hemoglobin compensation is too slow for acute clinical events, but blood transfusion can be used to significantly increase oxygen supply. Arterial oxygen content can be increased only minimally with high inspired oxygen concentrations unless hyperbaric oxygen is used. In the critically ill patient with limited cardiac reserve, therefore, the major compensation for oxygen supply/demand imbalance will be increased extraction; ie, decreased $S_{\bar{v}}O_2$.[87]

In the clinical setting, there often is confusion between what is the optimal (sometimes thought to mean the highest) vs. the adequate cardiac output level in a given patient (Fig. 21–22). Physicians can increase cardiac output in many ways (fluids, drugs, pacing, vasodi-

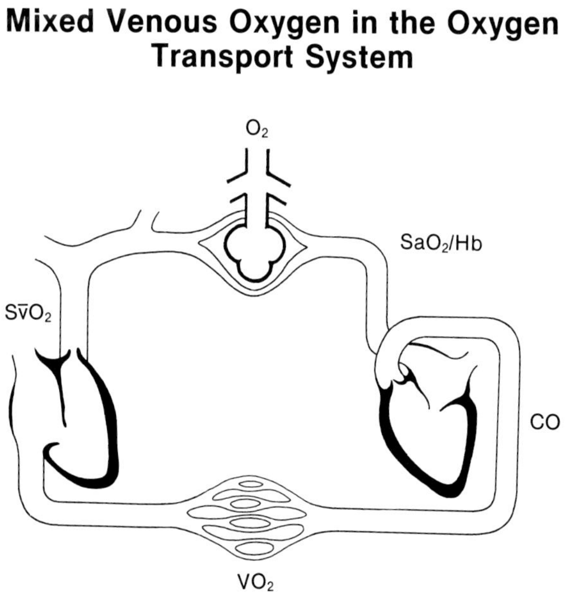

Figure 21–21 • Mixed venous oxygen hemoglobin saturation ($S_{\bar{v}}O_2$) normally reflects how well the body's needs for oxygen have been met. Healthy people can respond acutely to increased oxygen consumption ($\dot{V}O_2$) by increasing cardiac output (*CO*) and oxygen extraction. The latter will be reflected by a lowered $S_{\bar{v}}O_2$.

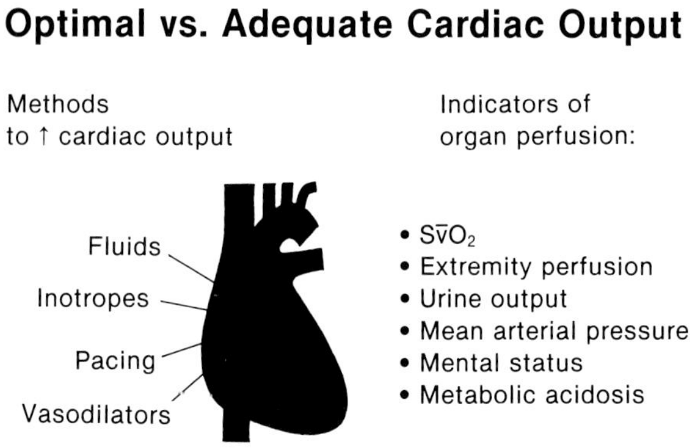

Figure 21–22 • Pictured on the left are the various techniques (fluids, drugs, pacing, vasodilators) used to increase cardiac output (CO), balanced against various indicators of organ perfusion on the right. Is it possible, in a given patient, that $S_{\bar{v}}O_2$ monitoring could resolve the dilemma about what cardiac output level is *adequate* rather than arbitrarily trying to achieve the *optimal* or highest cardiac output obtainable? More (ie, the highest cardiac output) is not always better, safe, or necessary.

lators), but this is frequently done at some cost in patients with coronary artery disease. How high a cardiac output is unnecessarily high? In our zealousness to restore vital organ perfusion, we may overshoot with inotropic therapy such that we achieve the highest cardiac output possible rather than stopping at the cardiac output that would have been adequate. Because one of the first responses to a slightly inadequate cardiac output is increased oxygen extraction from blood, which would be reflected by a low $S_{\bar{v}}O_2$, it is possible that this form of monitoring will help resolve this clinical dilemma.

2. Clinical Observations

$S_{\bar{v}}O_2$ levels below 30% have been associated with lactic acidosis and poorer prognosis in cardiogenic and traumatic shock.[88-91] Mixed venous oxygen has been shown to predict survival in patients with chronic obstructive pulmonary disease, primary pulmonary hypertension, and sepsis.[92,93] Further, $S_{\bar{v}}O_2$ has also been shown to be an ideal biologic variable to control rate-adjustable pacemaker systems.[94]

Results of several studies in acute care settings, primarily involving patients who have had cardiac surgery, have suggested that continuous monitoring is useful as an early warning indicator of low cardiac output or shock.[3,83,96-98]

a. *Examination of the Fick Equation*

The Fick equation:

$$\dot{V}O_2 = CO\,(C_aO_2 - C_{\bar{v}}O_2)$$

Solved for mixed venous oxygen:

$$S_{\bar{v}}O_2 \approx C_{\bar{v}}O_2 = C_aO_2 - \frac{\dot{V}O_2}{CO}$$

where $\dot{V}O_2$ = oxygen consumption, C_aO_2 = arterial oxygen content, $C_{\bar{v}}O_2$ = mixed venous oxygen content, and CO = cardiac output, reveals that $S_{\bar{v}}O_2$ may not always reflect cardiac output changes, but will reflect changes in other important variables such as arterial oxygenation, oxygen consumption, hemoglobin concentration, and distribution of blood flow. This type of monitoring has been criticized for its nonspecificity, but this is a problem only if other available information about the patient is ignored.[96] Monitoring $S_{\bar{v}}O_2$ may also be insensitive, when offsetting changes in arterial blood oxygen saturation (Sao2), hemoglobin, oxygen consumption, or cardiac output occur. Overly simplistic approaches to monitoring $S_{\bar{v}}O_2$ can be dangerous. Although a very low $S_{\bar{v}}O_2$ is not desirable, the reverse is not always true. Patients with cirrhosis or renal failure have peripheral shunts that result in high $S_{\bar{v}}O_2$ values. More disturbing are situations such as sepsis, pancreatitis, and burns, where high $S_{\bar{v}}O_2$ values (ie, $>$ 60%) may exist in the face of lactic acidosis.[9] A similar problem may occur in rare situations where oxygen uptake or use by the cell is blocked (eg, cyanide toxicity, carbon monoxide poisoning, methemoglobinemia).[99]

3. Indications for $S_{\bar{v}}O_2$ Monitoring

Clinicians are currently divided regarding the indications for $S_{\bar{v}}O_2$ monitoring, from one extreme of using the oximeter catheter every time PA catheterization is performed to the other extreme of never using this catheter. There are few data to support either position. A middle ground is to accept a list of indications, as suggested in Table 21–9.

In patients with severe respiratory failure associated with hypoxemia, the titration of PEEP therapy may be easily accomplished by following $S_{\bar{v}}O_2$.[100,101] With on-line $S_{\bar{v}}O_2$, the level of PEEP that best balances the improvement in arterial oxygenation with any untoward effect on cardiac output can be determined rapidly.[100] $S_{\bar{v}}O_2$ may also be valuable as an alternative to

Table 21–9 • Indications for $S_{\bar{v}}O_2$ Monitoring

Respiratory failure and severe hypoxemia
Dysrhythmias
Severe tricuspid regurgitation
Cardiogenic shock
Sepsis

the cardiac output measurement in patients with dysrhythmias or tricuspid regurgitation. Patients with certain dysrhythmias (frequent premature ventricular contractions, premature atrial contractions, atrial fibrillation, etc) have significant beat-to-beat variability in stroke volume, and triplicate determinations of cardiac output will reflect this variability. Poor reproducibility leaves doubts about what cardiac output determination to believe and makes any clinical deterioration or improvement difficult to appreciate. In patients with severe tricuspid regurgitation, the cardiac output may be erratic or unmeasurable by thermodilution (Fig. 21–23).

Patients in various phases of cardiogenic shock may undergo significant changes in cardiac output that are not appreciated because thermodilution measurements were not made at those times.[97,102] When cardiac output falls low enough to become clinically obvious (eg, falling blood pressure, urine output, etc), cardiac output measurements are made, but $S_{\bar{v}}O_2$ monitoring should lead to earlier diagnosis of this event. It has also been suggested that such monitoring is useful during weaning patients off intraaortic balloon counterpulsation as they recover from cardiogenic shock.[97]

Monitoring $S_{\bar{v}}O_2$ in patients at risk for sepsis has been proposed to detect the early evolution of this clinical problem. Once sepsis is established, a falling $S_{\bar{v}}O_2$ can provide immediate evidence for the development of the cardiogenic phase of septic shock.[93] In the hyperdynamic phase of sepsis, clinicians are frequently confused as to how much to augment cardiac output with fluids or inotropic agents. Some evidence supports using $S_{\bar{v}}O_2$ changes as a justification and endpoint to the augmentation of cardiac output in this clinical condition.[103] If $S_{\bar{v}}O_2$ remains stable as cardiac output (and thereby oxygen transport) is raised, then it suggests increased tissue extraction and further elevations of cardiac output are indicated. If $S_{\bar{v}}O_2$ increases with increasing cardiac output, then the therapy was not needed and can be withdrawn.

In addition to the list in Table 21–9, the oximeter PA catheter placed with the tip in the superior vena cava is considered useful when anatomic abnormalities and planned surgery preclude PA catheterization, eg, in patients with congenital heart disease.[104] $S_{\bar{v}}O_2$ monitoring has also been reported to be of specific value in the diagnosis of an unsuspected ventricular septal defect.[97] It is hoped that further clinical evaluations will clarify just

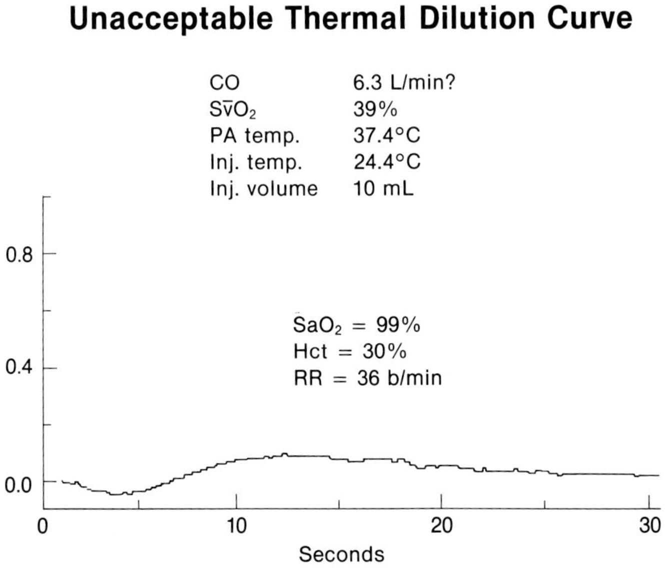

Figure 21–23 • Mixed venous oxygen saturation monitoring was a reasonable alternative to cardiac output measurements in this patient. An unacceptable thermodilution curve in a patient with severe tricuspid regurgitation is shown. This patient's cardiac output was not really 6.3 L/min. Repeated attempts at measuring thermodilution CO produced curves that looked severely attenuated, like the one shown. Calculated CO values were erratic and ranged from 1.2 to 7.5 L/min. Known about this patient was the following: oxygen consumption was probably near normal because her breathing was not labored, she was at bed rest, and she had a body temperature of 37.4°C. Arterial oxygenation was normal (SaO2 was 99% by pulse oximeter), and she had a near-normal hematocrit of 30%. With this information, the finding of a mixed venous oxygen saturation ($S_{\bar{v}}O_2$) of 39% was perfectly consistent with a low cardiac output state.

when and how this information ($S_{\bar{v}}O_2$) from a PA catheter is useful in improving patient care.

C. Right Ventricular Ejection Fraction

The use of ventricular washout curves to determine ventricular volumes has been known for over 30 years.[105] The measurement of right ventricular end diastolic volume (RVEDV) and cardiac output by thermodilution allow the derivation of right ventricular ejection fraction (RVEF). The accuracy and reproducibility of this technique are still a concern.[106,107]

There is no doubt that right ventricular function is particularly important in patients with acute pulmonary hypertension secondary to the adult respiratory distress syndrome, pulmonary embolism, or chronic obstructive lung disease.[108] Patients with right coronary artery disease are also at risk of developing severe right ventricular dysfunction.[109] Not surprisingly, the RVEDV measurement has been shown to be a better measure of right ventricular preload than pressure measurements.[110] Ventricular function assessment by cardiac output measurement can be misleading in some patients, who may show progressive increases in cardiac output in response to volume loading while ejection fraction decreases.[111] This finding suggests that the appropriate time to initiate inotropic support is when RVEF no longer increases to volume leading.[4] This may also be the point at which further RV volume loading causes RV distention and the well-known septal shift that can contribute to left ventricular dysfunction. Despite these interesting observations, the measurement of RVEDV/RVEF has not been widely accepted for clinical use. This position may change as the technique is further refined and its value is more extensively investigated.

VI. Summary

Pulmonary artery catheterization is an invasive, nontherapeutic procedure. After satisfactory indications for PA placement have been met, it should be approached with sufficient care to avoid the many known complications associated with its use. This procedure benefits patients only when physicians properly integrate the information that it provides, understanding its limitations, with the other known information about the patient, and then use sound clinical judgment to direct patient care.

VII. References

1. Swan HJC, Ganz W, Forester J, Marcus H, et al. Cardiac catheterization of the heart in man with use of a flow-direct balloon-tipped catheter. N Engl J Med 283:447–451, 1970.
2. Forrester JS, Ganz W, Diamond G, McHugh T, et al. Thermodilution cardiac output determination with a single flow-directed catheter. Am Heart J 83:306–311, 1972.
3. Krauss XH, Verdouw PD, Hugenholtz PG, Nanta J. On-line monitoring of mixed venous oxygen saturation after cardiac surgery. Thorax 30:636–643, 1975.
4. Jeevendra Martin JA, Snider MT, Farago LF, Burke JF. Thermodilution right ventricular volume: A novel and better predictor of volume replacement in acute thermal injury. J Trauma 21:619–626, 1981.
5. Matthay MA, Chatterjee K. Bedside catheterization of the pulmonary artery: Risks compared with benefits. Ann Intern Med 109:826–834, 1988.
6. Connors AF, McCaffee DR, Gray BA. Evaluation of right-heart catheterization in the critically ill patient without acute myocardial infarction. N Engl J Med 308:263–267, 1983.
7. Eisenberg PR, Jaffe AS, Schuster DP. Clinical evaluation compared to pulmonary artery catheterization in the hemodynamic assessment of the critically ill patient. Crit Care Med 12:549–553, 1984.
8. Fein AM, Goldberg SK, Walkenstein MD, Dershaw B, et al. Is pulmonary artery catheterization necessary for the diagnosis of pulmonary edema? Am Rev Resp Dis 129:1006–1009, 1984.
9. Forrester JS, Diamond G, Swan HJ. Correlative classification of clinical and hemodynamic function after acute myocardial infarction. Am J Cardiol 39:137–145, 1977.
10. Bayliss J, Nevell M, Ryan A, Thurston M, et al. Bedside haemodynamics monitoring: Experience in a general hospital. Br Med J (Clin Res) 287:187–190, 1983.
11. Civetta JM, Gabel JC, Laver MB. Disparate ventricular function in surgical patients. Surg Forum 22:136–139, 1971.
12. Toussaint GPM, Burgess JH, Hampson LG. Central venous pressure and pulmonary wedge pressure in critical surgical illness. Arch Surg 109:265–269, 1974.
13. Cohn JN, Tristani FE, Khatri I. Studies in clinical shock and hypotension via relationship between left and right ventricular function. J Clin Invest 48:2008–2018, 1969.
14. Bell H, Stubbs D, Pugh D. Reliability of central venous pressure as an indicator of left atrial pressure; a study in patients with mitral valve disease. Chest 59:169–173, 1971.
15. Lewis BM, Houssay HEJ, Haynes FW, Dexter L. The dynamics of both right and left ventricules at rest and during exercise in patients with heart failure. Circ Res 1:312–320, 1953.
16. Baek SM, Makabali GG, Bryan-Brown CW, Kusek JM, et al. Plasma expansion in surgical patients with high central venous pressure (CVP); the relationship of blood volume to hematocrit; CVP, pulmonary wedge pressure, and cardiorespiratory changes. Surgery 78:304–315, 1975.

17. Forrester JS, Diamond G, Chatterjee K, Swan HJ. Medical therapy of acute myocardial infarction by application of hemodynamic subsets. N Engl J Med 295:1356–1362, 1404–1413, 1976.
18. Rao TLK, Jacobs KH, El-Etr AA. Reinfarction following anesthesia in patients with myocardial infarction. Anesthesiology 59:499–505, 1983.
19. Lowenstein E, Teplick R. To (PA) catheterize or not to (PA) catheterize—that is the question. Anesthesiology 53:361–363, 1980.
20. Mangano DT. Monitoring pulmonary arterial pressure in coronary artery disease. Anesthesiology 53:364–370, 1980.
21. Moore CH, Lombardo TR, Allums JA, Gordon FT. Left main coronary artery stenosus: Hemodynamic monitoring to reduce mortality. Ann Thoracic Surg 26(5):445–451, 1978.
22. Sarin CL, Yalav E, Clement AJ, Braimbridge MV. The necessity for measurement of left atrial pressure after cardiac valve surgery. Thorax 25:185–189, 1970.
23. Attia RR, Murphy JD, Snider M, Lappas DG, et al. Myocardial ischemia due to infrarenalaortic cross-clamping during aortic surgery in patients with severe coronary artery disease. Circulation 53:961–965, 1976.
24. Braunwald E. Control of myocardial oxygen consumption. Am J Cardiol 27:416–432, 1971.
25. Ross J Jr, Braunwald E. The study of left ventricular function in man by increasing resistance to ventricular ejection with angiotension. Circulation 29:739, 1964.
26. Silverstein PR, Caldera DL, Cullen DJ, Davison JK, et al. Avoiding the hemodynamic consequences of aortic cross-clamping and unclamping. Anesthesiology 50:462–466, 1979.
27. Brooks JL, Kaplan JA. Cardiac diseases. In Katz J, Benumof J, Kadis LB (eds): Anesthesia and Uncommon Diseases. Philadelphia, WB Saunders, pp 287–289.
28. Zaidan JR, Freniere S. Use of a pacing pulmonary artery catheter during cardiac surgery. Ann Thoracic Surg 35:633–636, 1983.
29. Mihm FG. Pulmonary artery pressure monitoring in patients with pheochromocytoma. Anesth Analg 62:1129–1133, 1983.
30. Marshall WK, Bedford RF. Use of a pulmonary-artery catheter for detection and treatment of venous air embolism. Anesthesiology 52:131–134, 1980.
31. Mihm FG, Ashton JPA. Pulmonary artery catheters—the shake-flick test. Anesthesiology 59:262–263, 1983.
32. Bristow A, Batjer H, Chow V, Rosentein J. Air embolism via a pulmonary artery catheter introducer. Anesthesiology 673: 340–341, 1985.
33. Wiedemann HP, Matthay MA, Matthay RA. Cardiovascular-pulmonary monitoring in the intensive care unit. Part I. Chest 85:537–549, 1984.
34. Kopman EA, Sandza JG. Manipulation of the pulmonary artery catheter after placement: Maintenance of sterility. Anesthesiology 48:373–374, 1978.
35. Damen J, Bolton D. A prospective analysis of 1400 pulmonary artery catheterizations in patients undergoing cardiac surgery. Acta Anaesthesiol Scand 30:386–392, 1986.
36. Boyd KD, Thomas SJ, Gold J, Boyd AD. A prospective study of complications of pulmonary artery catheterizations in 500 consecutive patients. Chest 84:245–249, 1983.
37. Cohn JN, Franciosa JA, Francis GS, Archibald D, et al. Effect of short-term infusion of sodium nitroprusside on mortality rate in acute myocardial infarction complicated by left ventricular failure. N Engl J Med 306:1129–1135, 1982.
38. Pace NL. A critique of flow-directed pulmonary artery catheterization. Anesthesiology 47:455–456, 1977.
39. Shah KB, Rao TLK, Laughlin S, El-Etr AA. A review of pulmonary artery catheterization in 6,245 patients. Anesthesiology 61:271–275, 1984.
40. Lunn JK, Stanley TH, Webster LR, Bidwal AV. Arterial blood pressure and pulse-rate responses to pulmonary and radial arterial catheterization prior to cardiac and major vascular operations. Anesthesiology 51:265–269, 1979.
41. Rozanski A, Bairey CN, Krantz DS, Friedman J, et al. Mental stress and the induction of silent myocardial ischemia in patients with coronary artery disease. N Engl J Med 318:1005–1012, 1988.
42. Slogoff S, Keats AS. Does perioperative myocardial ischemia lead to postoperative myocardial infarction? Anesthesiology 62:107–114, 1985.
43. Dzelzkalus R, Stanley TH. Placement of the pulmonary arterial catheter before anesthesia for cardiac surgery: A stressful, painful, unnecessary crutch. J Clin Monit 1:197–200, 1985.
44. Streisand JB, Clark NJ, Pace NL. Placement of the pulmonary arterial catheter before anesthesia for cardiac surgery: Safe, intelligent, and appropriate use of invasive hemodynamic monitoring. J Clin Monit 1:193–196, 1985.
45. Keenan RL, Boyan CP. Cardiac arrest due to anesthesia: A study of incidence and causes. JAMA 253:2373–2377, 1985.
46. Quintin L, Whalley DG, Wynands JE, Morin JE. The effects of vascular catheterizations upon heart rate and blood pressure before aorto-coronary bypass surgery. Can Anaesth Soc J 28:244–247, 1981.
47. Waller JL, Zaidan JR, Kaplan JA, Bauman DI. Hemodynamic responses to preoperative vascular cannulation in patients with coronary artery disease. Anesthesiology 56:219–221, 1982.
48. Geha DG, Davis NJ, Lappas DG. Persistent atrial arrhythmias associated with placement of a Swan-Ganz catheter. Anesthesiology 39:651–653, 1973.
49. Cairns JA, Holden D. Ventricular fibrillation due to passage of a Swan-Ganz catheter. Am J Cardiol 35:589, 1975.
50. Thomson IR, Dalton BC, Lappas DG, Lowenstein E. Right bundle branch block and complete heart block caused by the Swan-Ganz catheter. Anesthesiology 51:359–362, 1979.
51. Luck JC, Engel TR. Transient right bundle branch block with (Swan-Ganz) catheterization. Am Heart J 92:263–264, 1976.
52. Wiedemann HP, Matthay MA, Matthay RA. Cardiovascular-pulmonary monitoring in the intensive care unit. Part 2. Chest 85:656–668, 1984.
53. Doblar DD, Hinkle JC, Fay ML, Condon BF. Air embolism associated with pulmonary artery catheter introducer kit. Anesthesiology 56:389–391, 1982.
54. Paskin DL, Hoffman WS, Tuddenham WJ. A new complication of subclavian vein catheterization. Ann Surg 179:266–268, 1974.
55. Pape LA, Haffajee CI, Markis JE, Ockene IS, et al. Fatal pulmonary hemorrhage: A complication of the flow-directed balloon-tipped catheter. Ann Intern Med 90:344–347, 1979.
56. Sprung CL. The Pulmonary Artery Catheter. Baltimore, University Park Press, 1983, 84–85.
57. Connor JP, Sandza JG, Shaw RC, Wolff GA, et al. Lobar pulmonary hemorrhage—an unusual complication of Swan-Ganz catheterization. Arch Surg 115:883–885, 1980.
58. Pace NL, Horton W. Indwelling pulmonary artery catheters: Their relationship to aseptic endocardial vegetations. JAMA 233:893–894, 1975.
59. Foote GA, Schabel SI, Hodges M. Pulmonary complications of the flow-directed balloon-tipped catheter. N Engl J Med 290:927–931, 1974.
60. Hoar PF, Wilson RM, Mangano DT, Hill D, et al. Heparin

bonding of pulmonary artery catheters to eliminate catheter thrombogenesis in man (abstract). Crit Care Med 9:144, 1981.
61. Maki DG, Cobb L, Garman JK, Shapiro JM, et al. An attachable silver-impregnated cuff for prevention of infection with central venous catheters: A prospective randomized multicenter trial. Am J Med 85:307–314, 1988.
62. Shinozaki T, Dean RS, Mazuzan JE. The dynamic responses of liquid-filled catheter systems of direct measurements of blood pressure. Anesthesiology 53:498–504, 1980.
63. Rothe CF, Kim KC. Measuring systolic arterial blood pressure: Possible errors from extension tubes or disposable transducer domes. Crit Care Med 8:683–689, 1980.
64. Gardner RM. Direct blood pressure measurement—dynamic response requirements. Anesthesiology 54:227–236, 1981.
65. Marin AG. Variables in pulmonary capillary wedge pressure: Variation with intrathoracic pressure, graphic and digital recorders. Crit Care Med 8:102–105, 1980.
66. Rice DL, Awe RJ, Gaasch WH, Alexander JK, et al. Wedge pressure measurement in obstructive pulmonary disease. Chest 66:628–632, 1974.
67. Downs JB. A technique for direct measurement of intrapleural pressure. Crit Care Med 4:207–210, 1976.
68. Berryhill RE, Benumof JL. PEEP-induced discrepancy between pulmonary artery wedge pressure and left atrial pressure: The effects of controlled vs. spontaneous ventilation and compliant vs. noncompliant lungs in the dog. Anesthesiology 51:303–308, 1979.
69. Roy R, Powers SR, Feustel PJ, Dutton RE: Pulmonary wedge catheterization during positive end-expiratory pressure ventilation in the dog. Anesthesiology 46:385–390, 1977.
70. Tooker J, Huseby J, Butler J. The effect of Swan-Ganz catheter height on the wedge pressure-left atrial pressure relationship in edema during positive-pressure ventilation. Am Rev Respir Dis 117:721–725, 1978.
71. DeCampo T, Civetta JM. The effect of short-term discontinuation of high-level PEEP in patients with acute respiratory failure. Crit Care Med 7:47–49, 1979.
72. Chambers DA, Kaplan JA. Tracing of left heart failure—not regurgitation. Anesthesiology 47:395, 1977.
73. Rahimtoola SH, Loeb HS, Ehsani A, Sinno MA, et al. Relationship of pulmonary artery to left ventricular diastolic pressures in acute myocardial infarction. Circulation 46:283–290, 1972.
74. Forrester JS, Diamond GA, Swan HJC. Bedside diagnosis of latent cardiac complications in acutely ill patients. JAMA 222:59–63, 1972.
75. Fuchs RM, Heuser RR, Yin FCP, Brinker JA. Limitations of pulmonary wedge V waves in diagnosing mitral regurgitation. Am J Cardiol 49:849–854, 1982.
76. Pichard AD, Kay R, Smith H, Rentrop P, et al. Large V waves in the pulmonary wedge pressure tracing in the absence of mitral regurgitation. Am J Cardiol 50:1044–1050, 1982.
77. Falicov RE, Resnekov L. Relationship of the pulmonary artery pressure to left ventricular end-diastolic and mean filling pressure in patients with and without left ventricular dysfunction. Circulation 42:65–73, 1970.
78. Bonner JT. Clinical use of the pulmonary artery (Swan-Ganz) catheter. Anesthesiology Rev 7:26–29, 1977.
79. Raper R, Sibbald WJ. Misled by the wedge: The Swan-Ganz catheter and left ventricular preload. Chest 89:427–437, 1986.
80. Collee GG, Lynch KE, Hill RD, Zapol WM. Bedside determination of pulmonary capillary pressure in patients with acute respiratory failure. Anesthesiology 66:614–620, 1987.
81. Siegel LC, Pearl RG, Shafer SL, Ream AK, et al. The longitudinal distribution of pulmonary vascular resistance during unilateral hypoxia. Anesthesiology 70:527–532. 1989.
82. Mihm F, Feeley TW, Rosenthal M, Raffin TA. The lack of effect of variable blood withdrawal rates on the measurement of mixed venous oxygen saturation. Chest 78:452–455, 1980.
83. Baele PL, McMichan JC, Marsh HM, Sill JC, et al. Continuous monitoring of mixed venous oxygen saturation in critically ill patients. Anesth Analg 61:513–517, 1982.
84. Stritter GM, Pearl RG, Mihm FG. Effect of heparinization of catheters on pulmonary artery oximetry. J Clin Monit 4:204–209, 1988.
85. Gettinger A, Detraglia MC, Glass DD. In vivo comparison of two mixed venous saturation catheters. Anesthesiology 66:373–375, 1987.
86. Ekblom B, Hermansen L. Cardiac output in athletes. J Appl Physiol 25:619–625, 1968.
87. Kandell G, Aberman A. Mixed venous oxygen saturation: Its role in the assessment of the critically ill patient. Arch Intern Med 143:1400–1402, 1983.
88. Kazarian KK, Sharma P, Caron N, Arias J, et al. Significance of mixed venous oxygen reserve in traumatic shock. Surg Forum 28:16–19, 1977.
89. Kasnitz P, Druger GL, Yorra F, Simmons DH. Mixed venous oxygen tension and hyperlatatemia: Survival in severe cardiopulmonary disease. JAMA 236:570–574, 1976.
90. Parr GVS, Blackstone EH, Kirklin JW. Cardiac performance and mortality early after intracardiac surgery in infants and young children. Circulation 51:867–874, 1975.
91. Kazarian KK, DelGuercio LRM. The use of mixed venous blood gas determinations in traumatic shock. Ann Emerg Med 9:179–182, 1980.
92. Kawakami Y, Kishi F, Yamamoto H, Miyamoto K. Relation of oxygen delivery, mixed venous oxygenation, and pulmonary hemodynamics to prognosis in chronic obstructive pulmonary disease. N Engl J Med 308:1045–1049, 1983.
93. Heiselman D, Jones J, Cannon L. Continuous monitoring of mixed versus oxygen saturation in septic shock. J Clin Monit 2:237–245, 1986.
94. Wirtzfield A, Goedel-Meinen L, Bock T, Heinze R, et al. Central venous oxygen saturation for the control of automatic rate-responsive pacing. Pace 5:829–835, 1982.
95. Waller JL, Kaplan JA, Bauman DI, Craver JM. Clinical evaluation of a new fiberoptic catheter oximeter during cardiac surgery. Anesth Analg 61:676–679, 1982.
96. Jamieson WRE, Turnbull KW, Larrieu AJ, Dodds WA, et al. Continuous monitoring of mixed venous oxygen saturation in cardiac surgery. Can J Surg 25:538–543, 1982.
97. Gore JM, Sloan K. Use of continuous monitoring of mixed venous saturation in the coronary care unit. Chest 86:757–761, 1984.
98. Birman H, Hag A, Hew E, Aberman A. Continuous monitoring of mixed venous oxygen saturation in hemodynamically unstable patients. Chest 86:753–756, 1984.
99. Norfleet EA, Watson CB. Continuous mixed venous oxygen saturation measurement: A significant advance in hemodynamic monitoring? J Clin Monit 1:245–258, 1985.
100. Fahey PJ, Harris K, Vanderwarf C. Clinical experience with continuous monitoring of mixed venous oxygen saturation in respiratory failure. Chest 86:748–752, 1984.
101. Divertie MB, McMichan JC. Continuous monitoring of mixed venous oxygen saturation. Chest 85:423–428, 1984.
102. Muir AL, Kirby BJ, King AJ, Miller HC. Mixed venous oxygen saturation in relation to cardiac output in myocardial infarction. Br Med J 4:276–278, 1970.

103. Wolf YG, Cotev S, Perel A, Manny J. Dependence of oxygen consumption on cardiac output in sepsis. Crit Care Med 15:198–203, 1987.
104. Fauss BG, Rah KH. Continuous mixed venous oxygen saturation monitoring for perioperative management of a boy undergoing a modified Fontan procedure. J Clin Monit 1:52–57, 1985.
105. Holt JP. Estimate of the residual volume of the ventricle of the dog's heart by two indicator dilution techniques. Circ Res 4:187, 1956.
106. Urban P, Scheidegger D, Gabathuler J, Rutishauser W. Thermodilution determination of right ventricular volume and ejection fraction: A comparison with biplane angiography. Crit Care Med 15:652–655, 1987.
107. Kay HR, Afshari M, Barash P, Webbler W, et al. Measurement of ejection fraction by thermal dilution techniques. J Surg Res 34:337–346, 1983.
108. Dhainant JF, Brunet F, Monsallier JF, Villemant D, et al. Bedside evaluation of right ventricular performance using a rapid computerized thermodilution method. Crit Care Med 15:148–152, 1987.
109. Hines R, Barash PG. Intraoperative right ventricular dysfunction detected with a right ventricular ejection fraction catheter. J Clin Monit 2:206–208, 1986.
110. Jardin F, Gueret P, Dubourg O, Farcot, JC, et al. Right ventricular volumes by thermodilution in the adult respiratory distress syndrome. Chest 88:34–39, 1985.
111. Mangano DT, Van Dyke DC, Ellis RJ. The effect of increasing preload on ventricular output and ejection in man. Circulation 62:535–541, 1980.

Chapter 22

•

Thomas G. Karagianes, MD

Electrocardiography

OUTLINE

I. Introduction

The electrocardiogram (ECG) is the record of the electrical activity of the heart and is typically displayed on a monitoring screen or on specialized graph paper. It is the most commonly monitored physiologic parameter in both the operating room (OR) and the intensive care unit (ICU). The American Society of Anesthesiologists mandates the continuous ECG monitoring of all patients receiving an anesthetic, and similar guidelines apply to ICU patients. Despite its ubiquitous usage, lack of understanding of certain aspects of ECG monitoring is not uncommon and diminishes its utility.

This chapter discusses the important factors involved in ECG monitoring: the characteristics of the various leads, the clinical setting, and the appropriate handling of the ECG signal. Methods for obtaining a good-quality ECG trace, potential sources of artifact, and safety concerns are addressed. The indications and procedural aspects of invasive ECG monitoring are also discussed. Emphasis throughout the chapter is on monitoring for dysrhythmias and myocardial ischemia, the primary functions of the ECG in the OR and ICU.

II. How to Monitor the Electrocardiogram (ECG)

A. *Essential Background Information on the Leads*

1. Bipolar Leads

Most ECG monitoring in the OR and ICU is performed with bipolar leads, using three electrodes (positive, negative, and reference). Bipolar leads measure the electrical potential between the positive and negative electrodes. Since the three limb leads (I, II, III) were introduced by Einthoven, numerous bipolar leads using electrodes placed on the chest or torso have been introduced for monitoring purposes. They are identified by the letter C (chest) appearing in the lead designation, usually as the first letter (eg, CB_5), but occasionally as the second (eg, MCL_1).

Bipolar recording is only possible with the lead selector switch in position I, II, or III. The polarity of the electrode and which is the reference electrode is dependent on the position of the monitor lead selector switch (Table 22–1). For example, position I will produce a negative right arm (RA) electrode and a positive left arm (LA) electrode. It is important to distinguish lead from lead selector position. The former denotes a specific electrode configuration, whereas the latter designates the polarity of the electrodes that may be placed anywhere. Because both the polarity and the location of the electrodes are selectable, the electrodes should be designated as positive, negative, or reference and by position in a bipolar arrangement. Referring to the electrode as RA, LA, or LL (left leg) is acceptable if the lead selector position is indicated, because this designates polarity. The electrode position must still be specified if it is in other than the standard position.

Placing the limb electrodes on the distal part of the extremities is neither practical nor necessary in the ICU or OR. Limb electrodes placed on the torso will produce an ECG essentially identical to one obtained from electrode placement on the distal extremities.[1,2] Thus, standard "limb" electrode position denotes the torso position, the details of which are offered in Fig. 22–1.

Table 22–1 • Standard Bipolar Limb Leads

Lead Selector	Negative Electrode	Positive Electrode	Reference Electrode
I	RA	LA	LL
II	RA	LL	LA
III	LA	LL	RA

2. Unipolar Leads

Unipolar leads record the electrical voltage from one electrode position and not the difference in potential between two electrodes. This requires a central terminal obtained by electronically connecting certain limb leads together through resistances of at least 5,000 ohms. Of the 12 standard ECG leads, all are unipolar except the three original limb leads. The position of the exploring electrode in the six precordial V leads is noted in Fig. 22–2.

Unipolar precordial recording requires five electrodes: three limb lead electrodes (RA, LA, LL), typically a reference electrode (RL), and the active chest (C) electrode. Unipolar leads are designated by the letter V (eg, V_5, aVL). The lead is named by the location of the

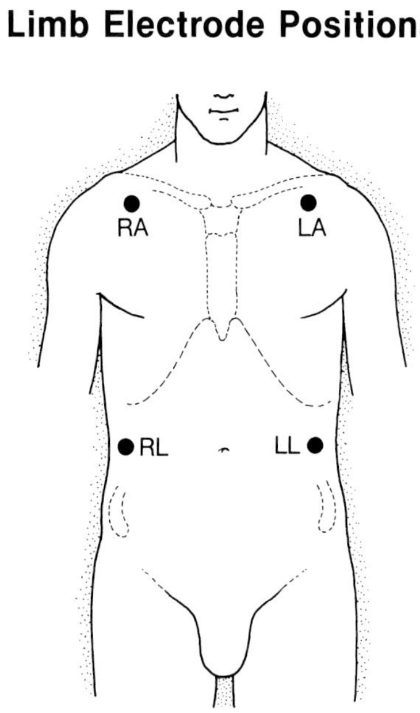

Figure 22–1 • Mason-Likar modification of limb electrode positions. RA and LA electrodes are placed 2 cm below the respective clavicle just medial to the deltoid muscle. LL electrode is placed halfway between the costal margin and the iliac crest in the anterior axillary line. The RL (reference) electrode may be placed in the corresponding position on the right, or in another position if more convenient.

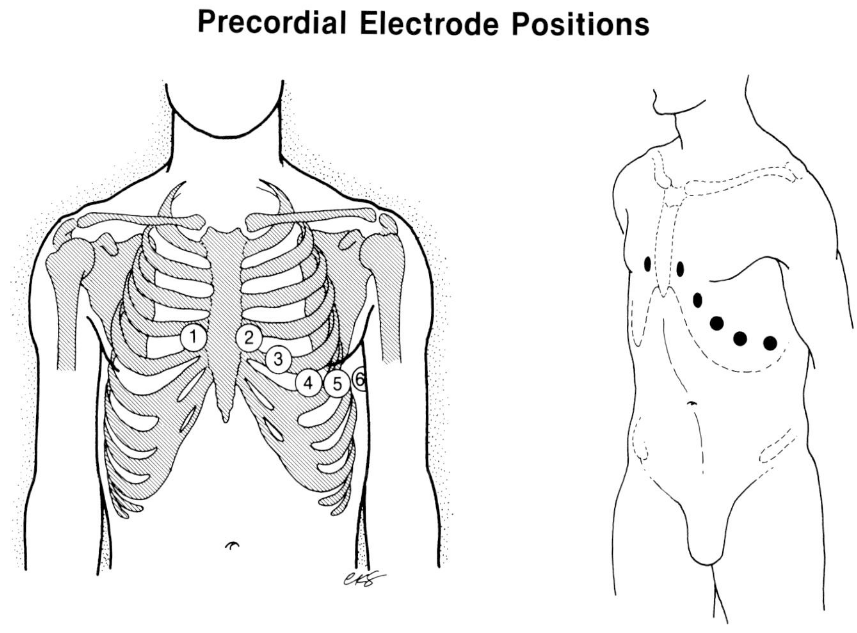

Figure 22–2 • Position of precordial electrodes. V_1 = fourth intercostal space at right margin of sternum; V_2 = fourth intercostal space at left margin of sternum; V_3 = midway between V_2 and V_4; V_4 = fifth intercostal space at left midclavicular line; V_5 = horizontal level of V_4 at left anterior axillary line; V_6 = same horizontal level as V_4 and V_5 at left midaxillary line.

C electrode (eg, V_5). The lead selector switch is placed in the V position.

Because augmented limb leads (eg, aVF) are rarely useful and the three standard limb leads and numerous bipolar chest leads can be obtained from the three-electrode format, a five-electrode format is primarily indicated for ischemia monitoring and certain unipolar invasive lead recordings. It may also be helpful in the evaluation of complex dysrhythmias, because more leads (seven) can be examined.

3. Reference Electrode

The reference electrode is handled differently depending on the type of monitor and whether a three- or five-electrode format is used. The important distinction is whether the reference electrode is either fixed or electronically rotated to the inactive electrode. Standard 12-lead ECG machines and the five-electrode format use the RL electrode as the reference electrode.

The situation with the three-electrode format is less standardized. Some older monitors use a fixed reference, limiting monitoring to one lead, a bipolar recording between the positive and negative electrodes. Newer monitors rotate the reference electrode, increasing the diagnostic potential of the electrode configuration, because three leads can potentially be monitored by switching the lead selector. In this situation, the monitoring cable usually does not have an RL electrode wire insertion site, using LL as the third insertion site instead. The importance of proper placement of the potentially active reference electrode is obvious. Some monitors provide the ability to obtain the three augmented limb leads (aVR, aVL, aVF) from the three-electrode format, but these leads offer little for monitoring purposes.

B. ECG Signal Handling

The manner of ECG signal handling by the monitor is commonly ignored, but can significantly alter the accuracy and usefulness of the ECG. Paper speed, voltage gain, and signal filtering will be addressed in reference to the intended use of the ECG and the American Heart Association (AHA) guidelines (Table 22–2).

1. Paper Speed

Without paper trace capability, the diagnostic usefulness of the ECG is severely limited. A paper trace should be available under most circumstances, because the "screen" ECG can be inadequate and unreliable.[3] Comparison of ECGs, interval timing, and ST segment and wave form analysis require a paper trace.

The reference paper speed for the 12-lead ECG is 25 mm/second. Using the same speed for monitoring facilitates comparison with previous ECGs, and ST segment changes are more easily detected. However, a continuous paper trace at this speed produces an unaccept-

Table 22-2 • ECG Signal Handling

ECG Parameter	Ischemia Monitoring	Dysrhythmia Monitoring
Paper speed	25 mm/sec	Capability of > 25 mm/sec
Gain	10 mm/mv	Capability of > 10 mm/mv
Frequency filters	≤ 0.05 Hz and ≥ 100 Hz	≤ 0.5 Hz and ≥ 50 Hz

able volume of output (90 m/hour). Recording at a slower speed (eg, 25 mm/minute) will provide a "crunched ECG" with a "periisoelectric band" comprising various periisoelectric ECG components, including the ST segment. If this band changes from baseline, then the paper speed can be increased to 25 mm/second to specifically evaluate for ST segment changes (Fig. 22–3).

An increasing number of monitors offer ST segment analysis, which substantially improves the ability to monitor continuously for ischemia and alleviates the problem of frequent examination of the paper trace.[4]

2. VOLTAGE GAIN

The AHA recommendation for gain is 10 mm/mV. Ischemia monitoring with the same gain allows quantitation of the ST segment change (eg, 2-mm ST depres-

Trend Monitoring for Myocardial Ischemia

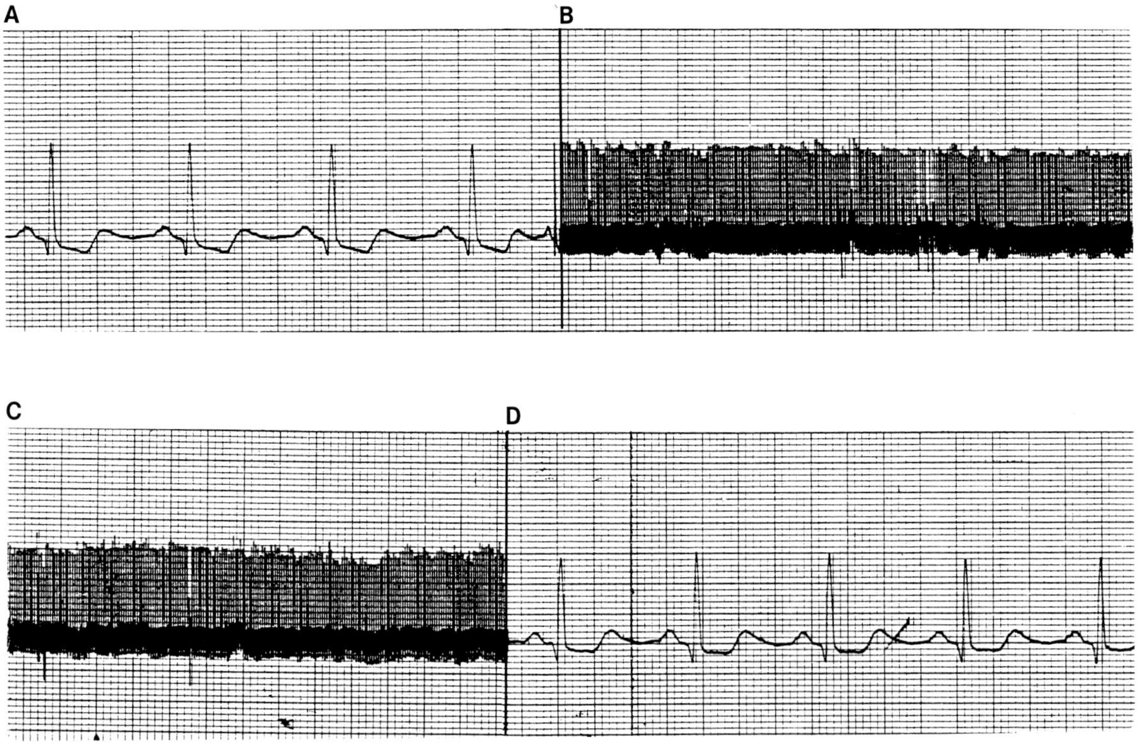

Figure 22–3 • (***A***) Electrocardiogram (ECG) recorded at 25 mm/sec demonstrating approximately 2-mm downsloping ST depression. (***B, C***) ECGs recorded at 25 mm/min. Note that the broad, dark periisoelectric band becomes smaller and less negative in progression from ***B*** to ***C*** after institution of intravenous nitroglycerin therapy. (***D***) 1-mm horizontal ST depression indicating that the change in the periisoelectric band was secondary to an ST segment change. The periisoelectric band is comprised of not only the ST segment, but also the p, Q, and T waves. Therefore, a change in this band can rarely be secondary to changes in these other components, which can be diagnosed by obtaining the ECG at 25 mm/sec.

sion) in relation to accepted diagnostic criteria. Different voltage standardization (eg, 0.5 or 2 × normal standard) is acceptable, but ST segment changes must be referenced to normal standardization. Dysrhythmia detection relies heavily on discerning atrial electrical activity; if this voltage is low, increasing the gain will enlarge the atrial waves and permit easier detection. Monitors permit the gain to be changed in either a graduated, stepwise fashion or a continuous fashion.

3. SIGNAL FILTERING

The stability of the ECG signal is dependent on frequency filtering, particularly of the low frequencies. Filtering improves signal stability but reduces diagnostic potential; therefore, a compromise must be achieved. Without low-frequency filtering, the ECG tends to drift off the paper or screen in response to low-frequency noise (eg, patient movement, breathing). High-frequency filtering reduces artifact from high-frequency noise (eg, shivering) and affects the faster components of the ECG, primarily the QRS complex. For a diagnostic quality ECG, the AHA guidelines for low-frequency (high pass) and high-frequency (low pass) filters are 0.05 Hz and 100 Hz, respectively. These guidelines should be followed when monitoring for ischemia. A low-frequency filter set too high will significantly alter the true ST segment; therefore, ischemia monitoring is poorly achieved with a highly filtered signal (Fig. 22–4).

Many monitors offer two frequency filter options, commonly designated as monitoring and diagnostic modes. Lack of standardization in the past has resulted in the use of a variety of frequency filters. For the monitoring mode, the high-pass filter is generally 0.5 Hz or 1 Hz, but is occasionally up to 4 Hz; the low-pass filter is typically either 30 Hz or 50 Hz. Newer monitors conform to the AHA guidelines for the monitoring mode of 0.5 Hz and 50 Hz, which will produce a stable

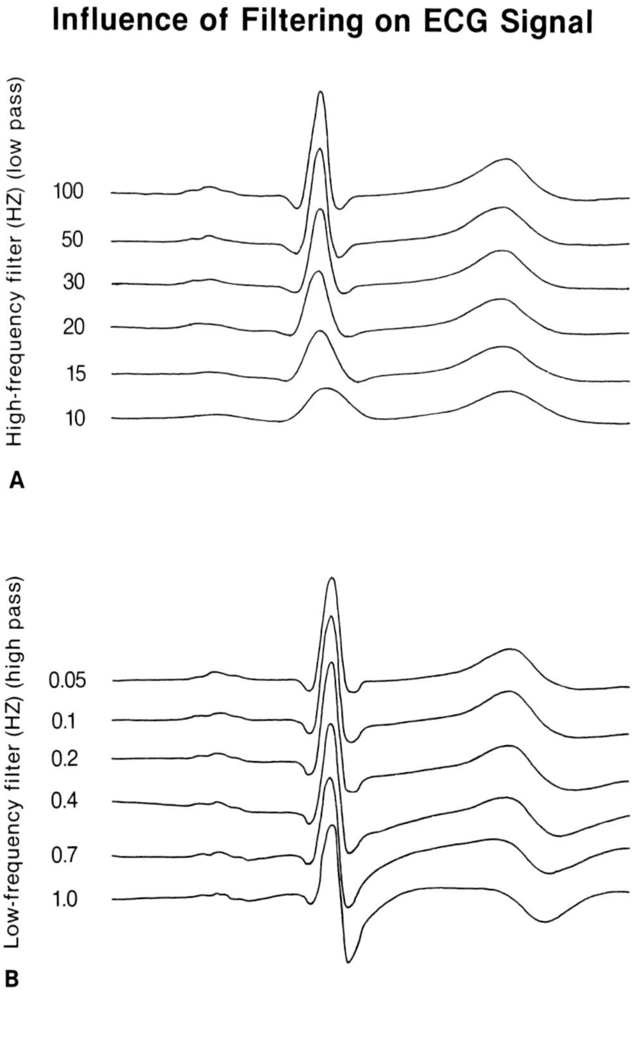

Figure 22–4 • The ECG is obtained at 200 mm/sec to clearly demonstrate the influence of filtering. High frequency filtering primarily effects the QRS complex, whereas low frequency filtering impacts on the ST segment and T wave. Note the marked impact on the ST segment and T wave by increasing the low frequency filtering, thereby inducing artifact and decreasing diagnostic potential.

signal but with diminished ischemia monitoring potential. The diagnostic mode frequency filters are also variable, but many newer monitors follow the AHA guidelines mentioned previously. Dysrhythmia monitoring is less dependent on frequency filtering, and diagnostic potential is usually not sacrificed with greater filtering (ie, monitoring mode). The diagnostic mode, however, may allow detection of unsuspected myocardial ischemia, and is the mode of choice for routine monitoring unless precluded by signal instability. The diagnostic mode should always be used for ischemia monitoring.

C. Detection of Myocardial Ischemia

Monitoring for myocardial ischemia is an important function of the ECG. All ischemia under general anesthesia is asymptomatic, and the majority of perioperative ischemic events are silent. Recent studies have documented the high incidence of silent ischemia in patients with coronary artery disease (CAD),[5-8] and it is reasonable to expect ICU patients with CAD to have an even greater incidence. Considering this high degree of silent ischemia, the ECG becomes an increasingly important monitor. Other modalities (eg, two-dimensional transesophageal echocardiogram) are more sensitive and specific for ischemia, but are not practical for continuous monitoring. The effectiveness of the ECG as an ischemia monitor is a function of (1) the degree and location of the ischemia, (2) the number and location of the ECG electrodes, and (3) how the ECG signal is handled (eg, frequency filtering).

Areas of ischemia may be missed if the chosen ECG lead does not examine that area; hence, the importance of selecting the appropriate lead to evaluate a potentially ischemic area (Table 22–3). In order of decreasing incidence, ischemia may involve the anterior, lateral, inferior, or posterior aspect of the left ventricle. Right ventricular ischemia is much less common and is frequently associated with inferior left ventricular ischemia.

Table 22–3 • Matching of Myocardial Area with Lead

Area	Lead
Anterior	$V_{2\text{-}6}$
Lateral	V_6, I, aVL
Infeior	II, III, aVF
Posterior	$V_{1\text{-}2}$, esophageal leads
Right ventricle	Right V leads (eg, V_4R)

Potentially ischemic areas can be identified in a number of ways. Coronary arteriography demonstrates stenotic arteries and thus indicates which myocardial areas may be in jeopardy. For example, a stenotic right coronary artery should focus monitoring on the inferior wall. Thallium testing, both exercise and dipyridimole, may also highlight ischemic areas and guide electrode placement. Review of previous ECGs during ischemia (eg, treadmill stress test) may demonstrate the ischemia-prone leads.

In research studies, ischemia diagnosis is enhanced by monitoring numerous leads, but this is not practical in the OR or ICU. The number of electrodes to be placed and leads to be monitored is a compromise between diagnostic potential and practicality. Furthermore, most ischemia will be evident in two or three appropriately chosen leads.

1. The V_5 and the Various C Leads

If "area focusing" studies are unavailable or not helpful, then which leads should be monitored? Based on treadmill stress test studies, approximately 90% of the ischemia evident on a 12-lead ECG is observed in lead V_5.[9] This is not surprising, because most ischemia involves the anterior or anterolateral regions of the left ventricle. The additional monitoring of lead II will augment V_5 by addressing stenotic right coronary artery-induced ischemia (inferior wall). Atrial dysrhythmia detection is also enhanced, because atrial activity is greater in lead II compared to V_5. Recently, the addition of lead V_4 to V_5 demonstrated improved sensitivity compared to the V_5 + 11 combination in the detection of intraoperative ischemia.[10] If this finding is reproduced, the addition of V_4 to V_5 should be considered.

Precordial V lead monitoring requires the five-electrode format; however, many monitors are limited to the three-electrode format. In this situation, a bipolar approximation of the V lead is used and will be termed the C lead.

AC lead requires the placement of only three electrodes. Most commonly, the positive electrode is placed in the V_5 position. However, if indicated, it may be placed in any "V" position. Numerous positions for the negative electrode have been used (Fig. 22–5). The second letter in the C lead is an abbreviation denoting the position of the negative electrode.

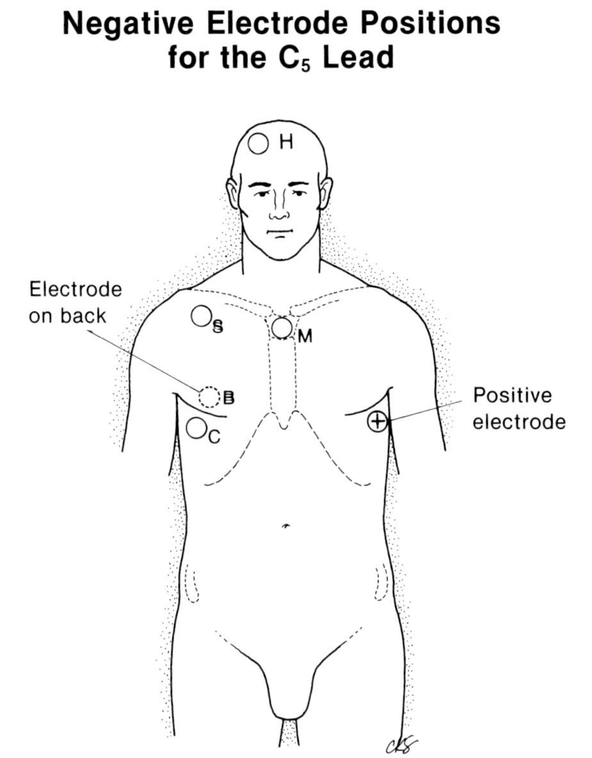

Figure 22–5 • Five positions for the negative electrode in a C_5 lead. CH_5 = head; CS_5 = subclavicular; CM_5 = manubrium; CB_5 = back, over midscapula; CC_5 = chest, anterior axillary line, right fifth intercostal space.

A common location for the negative electrode is beneath the right clavicle (subclavicular, CS_5). By placing the LL electrode in the standard position, greater versatility of this electrode configuration lead is obtained. Lead selector position I produces the CS_5 lead, and position II offers lead II with the advantages of enhanced inferior ischemia detection and greater dysrhythmia diagnosis potential (Fig. 22–6).

Two other C leads deserve mention. The CC_5 lead with the negative electrode placed in the right fifth intercostal space at the anterior axillary line has demonstrated good correlation with V_5 in stress test studies.[11] If the negative electrode is placed over the center of the right scapula on the back, then the CB_5 lead is obtained, which demonstrates good atrial activity, a potential benefit for dysrhythmia diagnosis.[12]

Which C_5 lead has the greatest diagnostic potential and whether it is an acceptable alternative to the V_5 lead in the ICU and OR has not been completely established. However, based on treadmill stress test studies[11] and a small number of patients studied in the OR,[12] C_5 leads appear to be a reasonable substitute for the V_5 lead. Nonetheless, high-risk patients should be monitored with the V_5 lead if possible (Fig. 22–7).

To summarize the major points involved in ischemia monitoring: Review available cardiac tests to ascertain ischemia-prone areas or leads that have previously demonstrated ischemia. Electrode placement and lead selection are guided by these data. If no guidance is provided by the tests, then lead V_5 and II should be monitored. If only the three-electrode format is available, a C_5 lead is selected. Lead CS_5 with the LL electrode in the standard position has the added capability of lead II monitoring by switching the lead selector from position I to II. Paper trace capability is necessary, particularly intermittent recording at 25 mm/second. Gain should conform to AHA guidelines, and signal frequency filtering must meet the AHA guidelines for a diagnostic quality ECG.

D. *Dysrhythmia Detection*

Detection of dysrhythmias is the most common function of the ECG in the OR and ICU. As with ischemia monitoring, the crucial question is which lead should be monitored. The lead most capable of demonstrating

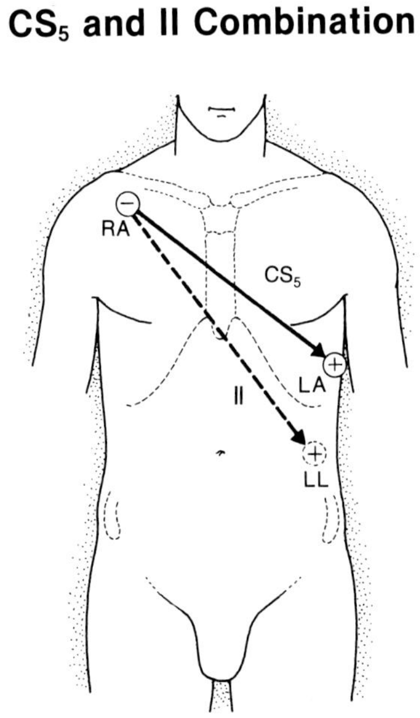

Figure 22–6 • Lead selector position I produces the CS_5 lead, and position II offers lead II. RA and LL electrodes are in standard position, and LA electrode is in the V_5 position.

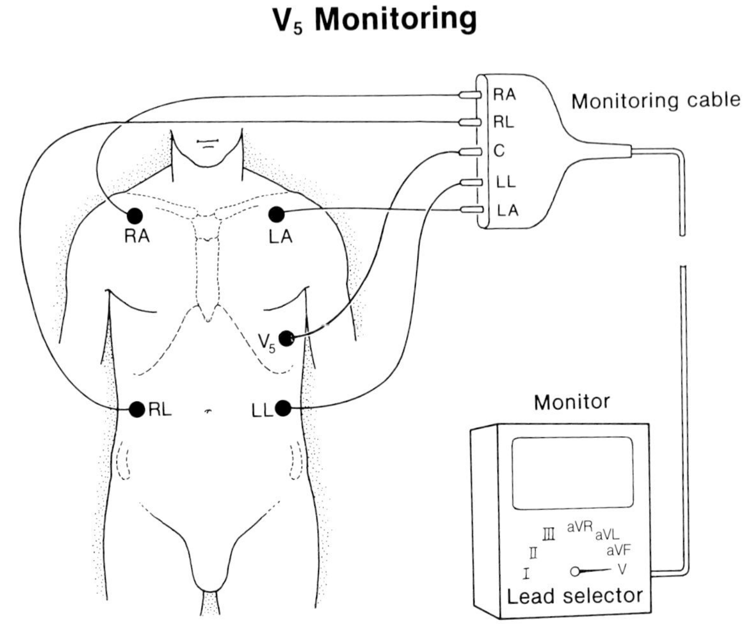

Figure 22–7 • Electrode placement and lead selector position for V_5 monitoring. Six other leads (I, II, III, aVR, aVL, aVF) may be monitored with this electrode configuration.

atrial activity is preferred, because detection of atrial activity is the single most important aspect in the diagnosis of dysrhythmias. As an example of the importance of atrial activity detection, consider the perplexing problem of a regular, wide complex tachycardia. Distinguishing ventricular tachycardia from supraventricular tachycardia with aberrancy is considerably easier if p waves are discernable and the degree of association and temporal relationship between the atrial and ventricular electrical activity can be established (Fig. 22–8).

1. LEAD II AND MCL_1 LEAD

Review of previous ECGs may indicate which lead offers the greatest atrial activity (at least in that rhythm). This is most commonly lead II or V_1, but may be different with an abnormal p-wave vector. Lead V_1 is also the single best lead in distinguishing ventricular ectopic beats from aberrantly conducted supraventricular beats. Most routine monitoring uses three electrodes placed on the torso, which produces bipolar leads, either the standard limb leads or the bipolar chest C leads. Of the numerous C leads, MCL_1 (''bipolar V_1'') (Fig. 22–9) has achieved the greatest popularity in the ICU. The assessment of more than one lead is often helpful in dysrhythmia diagnosis, particularly with complex dysrhythmias. The five-electrode format will produce six limb leads (three standard, three augmented) and one precordial lead (V_1); therefore, its use should be considered in patients with a history of complex dysrhythmias.

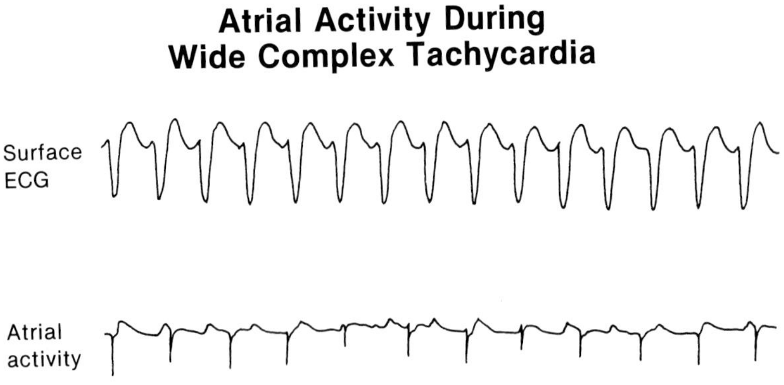

Figure 22–8 • Simultaneous recording of surface ECG demonstrating wide complex tachycardia and an invasive lead trace showing only atrial activity. Dissociation between the atria and ventricles (ventricular rate faster then atrial rate) indicates the rhythm is ventricular tachycardia and not supraventricular tachycardia with aberrancy.

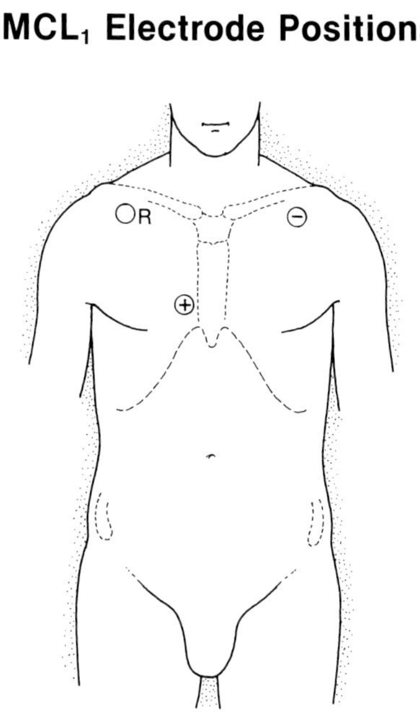

Figure 22–9 • The negative electrode is placed in the left subclavicular position and the positive electrode is in the V_1 position. The reference (*R*) electrode may be placed anywhere.

Signal handling restrictions for the ECG are less stringent when compared to those for ischemia monitoring. Filtering of frequencies below the usual range of 0.5 or 1 Hz will not appreciably affect the detection of atrial activity and may be necessary to produce a stable baseline. Despite this minor influence, the less-filtered diagnostic mode should be used (unless prohibited by a wandering baseline) to produce a truer ECG and increase the potential for detection of "incidental" ischemia.

The ability to increase the paper speed (> 25 mm/second) and thereby stretch the ECG signal out is useful, particularly with tachydysrhythmias. This can be helpful in finding atrial activity waves, which can be "buried" in a tachydysrhythmia recorded at slower speeds.

Quantitation of the voltage (eg, millimeters of ST depression) is not an issue with dysrhythmia detection. Therefore, if the atrial activity is low voltage and difficult to discern, the size of the atrial waves can be enhanced by increasing the gain.

In summation, greatest atrial activity is usually evident in lead II or V_1. Lead II can be monitored with the standard, three-electrode format, but V_1 cannot. Lead MCL$_1$ is therefore used as the bipolar approximation of V_1. For complex dysrhythmias, the five-electrode format with the precordial electrode in the V_1 position should be considered. A paper trace should be available and the ability to stretch the ECG out by increasing the paper speed is helpful. Signal frequency filtering should be the minimal necessary to provide a stable signal. The gain may be increased to enlarge the ECG in an attempt to discern the atrial activity. Analysis of more than one lead can be particularly helpful in the search for atrial activity and the assessment of that "FLB" (funny-looking beat).

E. *The Invasive Leads and the Atrial Electrogram (AEG)*

Invasive leads offer enhanced atrial electrical activity detection and are useful when atrial waves are not detected in the surface leads. Electrodes may contact the endocardial or epicardial surface of the heart or may be placed within the right atrium or esophagus. The ECG obtained from these leads has been termed the atrial electrogram (AEG).[13] Unlike surface lead nomenclature, the terms *unipolar* and *bipolar* refer to the number of electrodes in the recording device.

The relative size of the atrial (A) wave and QRS complex is variable in AEG traces; this can make separation and identification difficult. Certain bipolar leads, particularly those with closely spaced electrodes, may exhibit little if any ventricular activity, whereas unipolar leads tend to demonstrate discernable ventricular activity similar to a surface lead but with enhanced atrial activity (Fig. 22–10). The simultaneous recording of a surface lead will alleviate these potential problems, because the QRS complex can now be delineated by a timing comparison of the AEG trace with the surface lead trace (Fig. 22–11). Most newer monitors allow simultaneous recording of at least two leads, and most ECG machines allow simultaneous recording of three leads. If simultaneous recording is not available and atrial and ventricular rates are different, sequential recording and comparison of the invasive and surface leads will frequently allow identification of the QRS in the AEG trace. Alternatively, if simultaneous recording is unavailable and the QRS complex is not visualized with the bipolar AEG, one wire from an invasive electrode can be disconnected and attached to a newly applied surface electrode, thereby producing a unipolar AEG with a more apparent QRS complex.

Bipolar recording devices are generally preferred because they offer large A waves and can always be used

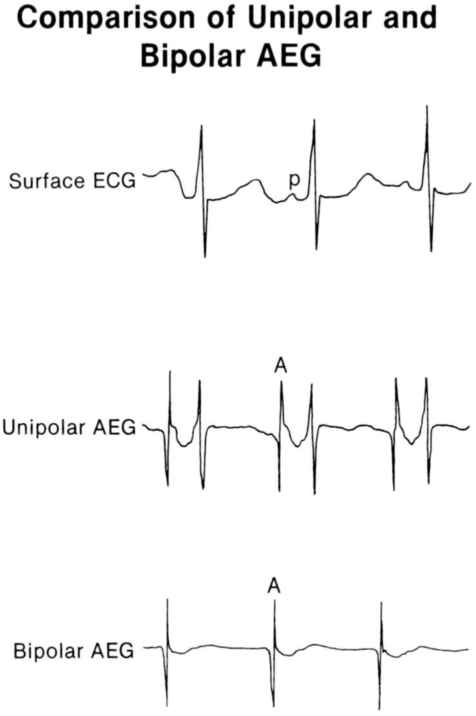

Figure 22–10 • Atrial (*A*) waves in an unipolar AEG have a variable size relationship to the QRS. A waves in a bipolar AEG tend to be larger than QRS, and frequently the QRS is poorly visible. Simultaneous recording of a surface lead is helpful in identification of the QRS complex in both types of AEG recordings. This will permit separation of A waves from the QRS.

in a unipolar fashion if indicated. The electrode wires to the invasive electrodes of the bipolar device may be switched on a trial and error basis to possibly aid dysrhythmia identification by offering different and potentially more recognizable complexes and waves (eg, upright atrial waves).

The electrode wire/electrode connections and surface electrode placement during AEG recording are primarily dependent on whether a three- or five-electrode format is used and whether the invasive device is unipolar or bipolar (Table 22–4).

A variety of methods exist for establishing the connection between the invasive electrode and the monitoring cable, depending on the type of electrode and the type of electrode wire. The most frequently used methods are noted in Fig. 22–12.

1. Esophageal Electrode

The proximity of the esophagus to the atria (particularly the left atrium) allows enhanced recording of atrial activity when electrodes are placed in it.[14,15] Detection of posterior ischemia is also improved by the proximity of this surface of the left ventricle to the esophagus,[16] although this is an infrequent use. Numerous types of esophageal electrodes have been used. Some involve placing either one or two electrically conducting metal electrodes in or

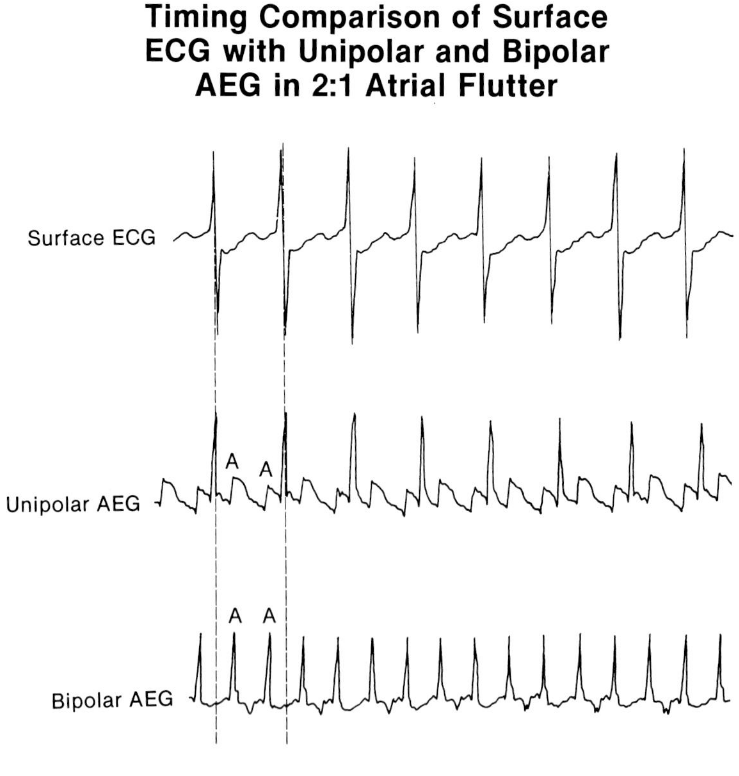

Figure 22–11 • 2:1 atrial flutter. Note the enhanced atrial activity waves present in the unipolar AEG, making rhythm diagnosis much easier compared to the surface ECG. Timing comparison of the surface ECG with the bipolar AEG is helpful in demonstrating two A waves for every one QRS complex.

Table 22-4 • Atrial Electrogram

Option	Recording Device	Electrode Site and Electrode Wire Attachments	Lead Selector	Simultaneous Leads	Comments
		3 Electrodes			
1	Unipolar	LA—standard RA—invasive LL—standard	I	II or III	Useful in IVECG since p wave changes resemble those of familiar option 3
2	Bipolar	RA—invasive LA—invasive LL—standard	I	II or III	May be difficult to visualize QRS from trace obtained only from invasive electrodes (lead selector I)
		5 Electrodes			
3	Unipolar	C—invasive 4 standard limb electrodes	V	Whichever shows QRS	Preferred option for 5 electrode unipolar recording and for IVECG
4	Bipolar	RA—invasive LA—invasive LL—standard RL—standard C—precordial	I	Whichever shows QRS	Same as option 2 except offers more simultaneous leads

around a tube such as a nasogastric tube.[17] Pill electrodes, which are swallowed,[18] and endocardial pacing leads have also been employed. An esophageal stethoscope with two electrodes, placed 7 and 20 cm from the distal end, is commercially available. The distal electrode in this lead is usually close to the posterior aspect of the left ventricle.

Electrodes are positioned to optimize the atrial wave size. Typically, a unipolar electrode is placed 30–40 cm from the teeth or nares. Optimal positioning of bipolar electrodes is more variable due to different electrode separation distances.

Esophageal leads are prone to low-frequency noise secondary to breathing and peristalsis. Increased filtering helps stabilize the signal. Monitors that permit a wide selection of low-frequency filters are optimal for this type of recording.

2. INTRACAVITARY ELECTRODE

Catheters are rarely placed in the heart or central veins solely for dysrhythmia detection, but central venous pressure (CVP) or pulmonary artery (PA) catheters can be used for this function by making them electrically conductive. This is accomplished by placing either electrolyte solution or a metal wire in the catheter lumen. Obtaining an AEG from the proximal port of the PA catheter requires signal processing methods that are not widely available.[19]

Both hypertonic saline (3% or greater) and sodium bicarbonate (8.4%) produce a better signal than normal (0.9%) saline.[20] A noisy or poor-quality trace frequently indicates the need to replenish the electrolyte solution. A metal hub connector is attached to the end of the catheter and is also filled with electrolyte solution. The electrical connection between the metal hub and the electrode wire is established with an insulated double alligator clip. A commercially available plastic hub connector with a metal insert alleviates the need for the alligator clips if a snap-on electrode wire is used (Fig. 22–12D). At the end of recording, the electrolyte solution should be flushed from the catheter to reduce electrical microshock hazard. Instead of electrolyte solution, a metal guide wire can be passed through the catheter until it barely protrudes from the end of the catheter, as evidenced by the marked increase in ECG voltage amplitude as the wire leaves the "insulation" of the catheter. The wire must be soft-tipped, preferably with a "J"

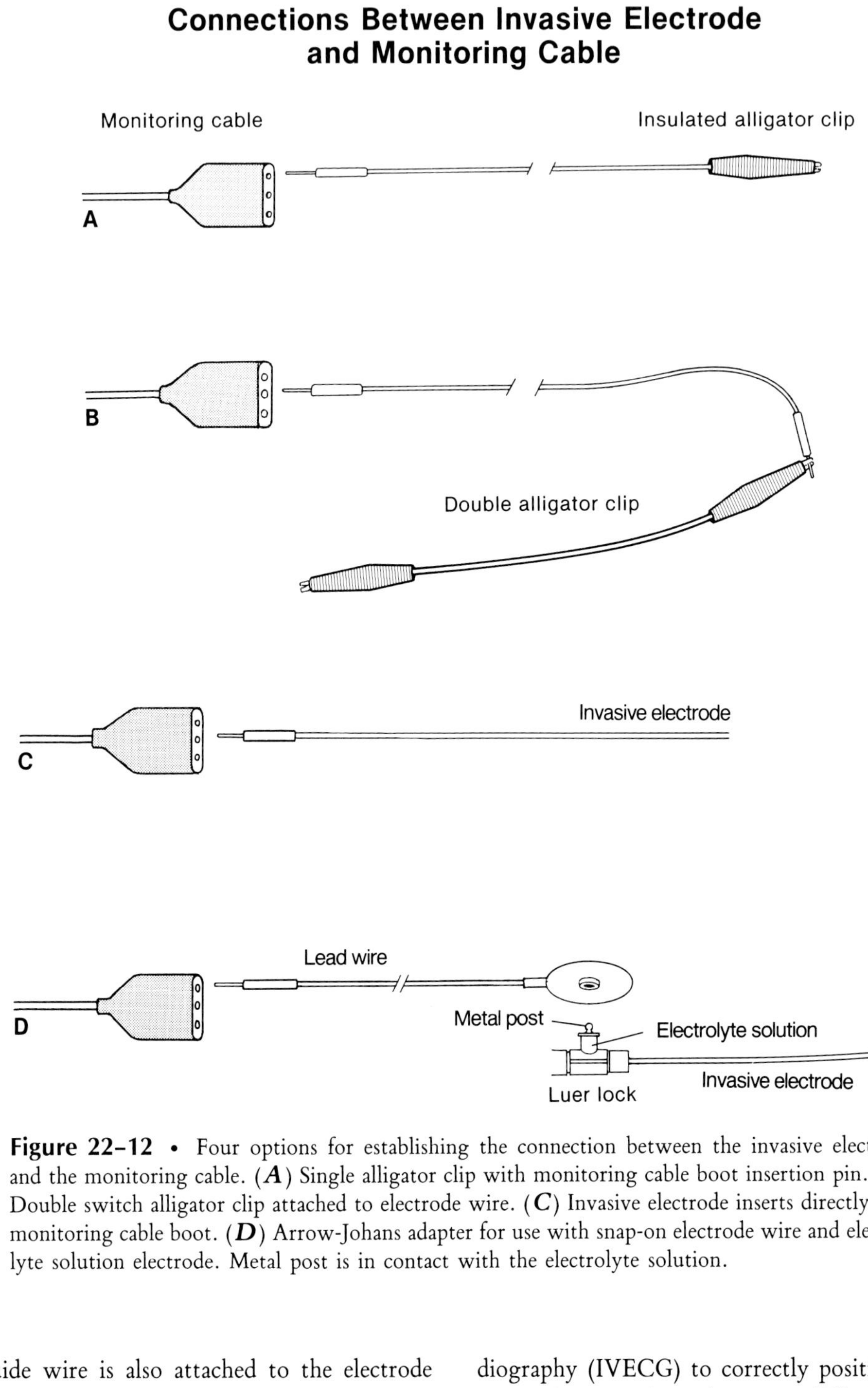

Figure 22–12 • Four options for establishing the connection between the invasive electrode and the monitoring cable. (***A***) Single alligator clip with monitoring cable boot insertion pin. (***B***) Double switch alligator clip attached to electrode wire. (***C***) Invasive electrode inserts directly into monitoring cable boot. (***D***) Arrow-Johans adapter for use with snap-on electrode wire and electrolyte solution electrode. Metal post is in contact with the electrolyte solution.

end. The guide wire is also attached to the electrode wire via an alligator clip. When not recording, the wire should be withdrawn into the catheter or, preferably, completely removed to diminish the risk of cardiac perforation, dysrhythmias, and electrical microshock.

3. Intravascular Electrocardiography

A variation of intracavitary ECG recording for dysrhythmia diagnosis is the use of intravascular electrocardiography (IVECG) to correctly position an air aspiration catheter in the right atrium.[21,22] The method is the same as for intracardiac recording, except that the ECG is recorded as the catheter traverses the central veins into the right atrium. The changes in the p wave guide placement by indicating catheter location (Fig. 22–13).

The most common recording method is to connect the invasive electrode to the C electrode wire with the four limb electrodes in standard position and the lead selector in the V position (Fig. 22–14). If only the three-

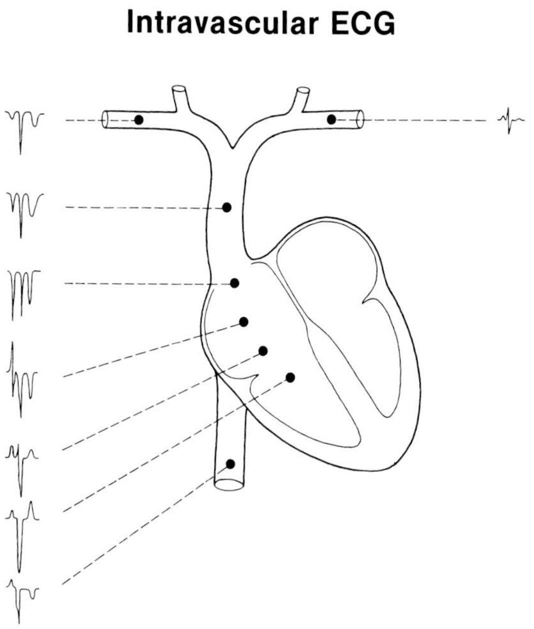

Figure 22–13 • ECG obtained from various sites in the central veins heart recorded via method described in Table 22–4, option 3. Biphasic p wave indicates mid–right atrial position.

electrode format is available, then the invasive electrode is attached to the LA electrode wire, the RA electrode is in the standard position, and the lead selector is placed in the I position. With this method, the p wave changes will more closely resemble those obtained with the five-electrode format (see Fig. 22–13). Actually, any electrode configuration with a positive invasive electrode should provide similar findings, although this has not been evaluated in the literature.

Which orifice of a multiorifice catheter acts as the "electrode" is unclear[19]; however, the proximal one is most likely.[23,24] If a guide wire is used as the electrode, the signal is received from the point of emergence from the catheter.[24]

4. ENDOCARDIAL ELECTRODE

Metallic electrodes in contact with the right atrial endocardium from either a pacing wire or specialized PA catheter can be used to record an AEG.[26] If the electrodes are not in contact with endocardium, then an intracavitary AEG is obtained.

5. EPICARDIAL ELECTRODE

At the time of cardiac surgery, pacing wires can be attached to the epicardial surface of the heart, typically the right atrium and right ventricle. The wires are brought out to the skin surface, where the external portion of the wires must be electrically insulated, usually by placing them in rubber surgical gloves. They are associated with rare complications and are removed usually by pulling them out when no longer needed. The atrial wires can be used to obtain an AEG by attaching them to the electrode wires with an insulated alligator clip.[13]

The wires may also be used for treatment of certain reentrant dysrhythmias via overdrive pacing. The previously discussed invasive electrodes also have this potential, but may not have the same efficacy as the epicardial wires.

III. TECHNICAL CONSIDERATIONS AND SAFETY CONCERNS

A. *Technical Considerations*

Although not technically complex by modern standards, technical problems do arise during ECG monitoring, particularly in the electrically unfavorable environments of the ICU and OR. The process of signal acquisition to signal display relies on a number of component elements. In order of decreasing frequency, problems may arise with the skin, electrodes, electrode wires, monitoring cable, and monitor. Connections between the components may also be the cause of a problem. The electrode–skin interface is the greatest cause of technical problems.

The proper application of electrodes is the single most important aspect in obtaining a good-quality trace. It will increase the amplitude of the signal as well as markedly decrease 60-Hz interference. The skin should be cleaned with alcohol and then dried. Abrading the skin with either cotton gauze or the abrading pad supplied with some electrodes is the next step. The electrode must make good contact with the skin and should not be placed over hairy areas or areas where bone contour will reduce skin contact. Large muscle mass areas should be avoided because of the possibility of electrical myopotential interference. If the electrode is in the surgical prep site, it should be covered with an occlusive dressing.

Sixty-hertz interference is the most common technical problem, with poor skin preparation being an important cause. Another source of interference is the electrode wire, which may act as an antenna. Twisting the electrode wires together will tend to diminish the an-

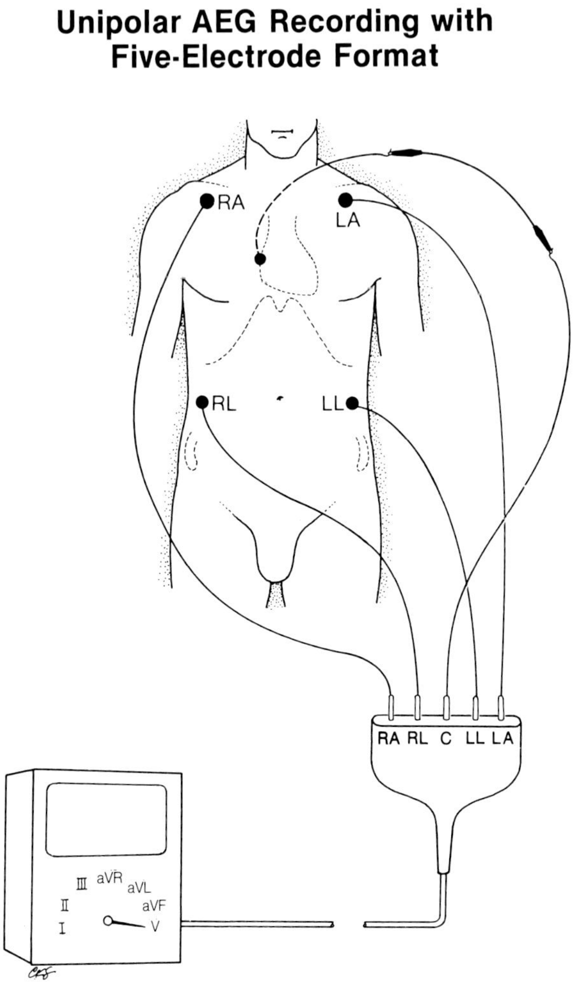

Figure 22–14 • Method for obtaining a unipolar AEG as listed in Table 22–4, option 3. It is the preferred option for five-electrode, unipolar recording and is primarily useful for IVECG positioning of an air-aspiration catheter.

tenna effect. Attention to keeping the wires and the monitoring cable away from electrical cords, motors, and electrically powered devices is important. Sequentially unplugging various devices may pinpoint the source of electrical interference. Many newer monitors are equipped with a 60-Hz notch filter to somewhat selectively diminish the 60-Hz interference.

A poor or absent signal may result from a problem anywhere from the monitor to the patient's skin. Breaks in the electrode wires or poor contact with the electrode, as well as poor electrode–skin contact, are common causes of this problem. A nonfunctional monitoring cable or a defective monitor are also possibilities.

An ECG signal simulator will help isolate the source of a technical problem (ie, no signal). After being attached to the monitoring cable, it provides a simulated ECG signal. The problem can therefore be separated into two areas: the monitor and cable or the more common source of the electrode wires, their attachment to the electrode, or the electrode–skin interface.

B. *Safety Concerns*

Electrical microshock to the heart producing ventricular fibrillation may arise when an invasive electrode is incorporated into an "electrical circuit." The ICU and OR are equiped with much electrical equipment, all of which has some degree of electrical current leakage and is capable of producing a microshock to the heart. Certain steps must be taken to minimize this risk when invasive electrodes are used (Table 22–5). All equipment not absolutely necessary should be unplugged (not just turned off) during the use of invasive electrodes. Electrode wires and connections (eg, alligator clips) should be well insulated and kept clear of electrical cords and metal surfaces. The patient must not be in contact with metal surfaces. The leakage current from the ECG monitor should conform to the AHA guideline of less than 10 μA.[27] Additionally, a battery-powered monitor may be used during recording.

Radio frequency from the electrosurgical unit (ESU) may produce burns if the current is grounded through an ECG electrode. The ESU current is normally captured via the large-surface-area dispersive elec-

Table 22–5 • Safety Checklist for Invasive Lead Recording

1. Connections (eg, electrode/electrode wire) are insulated.
2. Unnecessary electrical equipment around the patient is unplugged.
3. Ideally, monitor is battery powered.
4. Leakage current from monitor is $< 10\mu$A.
5. No metal contact with patient.
6. Remove guidewire or flush electrolyte solution from catheter when not recording.
7. Check ESU dispersive (grounding) pad for proper skin contact and function.
8. ESU protection filter between electrode wire and monitoring cable.
9. Limit or preferably eliminate electrosurgical unit usage.

ESU = electrosurgical unit

trode of the ESU, thereby distributing the current over a large area. This reduces the risk of burn to a negligible amount if the dispersive electrode is properly applied and functional. A nonfunctional dispersive electrode may result in the ECG electrodes fulfilling this function. Because the surface area of the electrodes is so much smaller, the current density is increased and the risk of burn is enhanced. Needle electrodes, because of their very small surface area, pose a particular problem in this regard. Small electrodes in general are prone to this problem and should probably not be used.[28,29]

Invasive electrodes pose a magnified risk because a burn in the tissue contacting the electrode (ie, heart or esophagus) may have serious consequences, although this complication has not been reported. Ideally, the ESU should not be used while invasive electrodes are in place. If this is not possible, extra care should be taken to insure the proper functioning of the ESU dispersive electrode. Additionally, an ESU protection filter capable of filtering frequencies greater than 20 kHz should be inserted between the electrode wire and monitoring cable.

IV. REFERENCES

1. Mason RE, Likar I, Biern RD, Ross RS, et al. Multiple lead exercise electrocardiography. Circulation 36:517–525, 1967.
2. Mason RE, Likar I. A new system of multiple-lead exercise electrocardiography. Am Heart J 1966:196–205, 1966.
3. Arbeit SR, Rubin IL, Gross H. Dangers in interpreting the electrocardiogram from the oscilloscope. JAMA 211:453–456, 1970.
4. Kotter GS, Kotrly KJ, Kalbfleisch JH, Vacins EJ, et al. Myocardial ischemia during cardiovascular surgery as detected by an St segment trend monitoring system. J Cardiothorac Anesth 1:190–199, 1987.
5. Schang SJ Jr, Pepine CJ. Transient asymptomatic S-T segment depression during daily activity. Am J Cardiol 39:396–402, 1977.
6. Cecchi AC, Dovellini EV, Marchi F, Pucci P, et al. Silent myocardial ischemia during ambulatory electrocardiographic monitoring in patients with effort angina. J Am Coll Cardiol 1:934–939, 1983.
7. Deanfield JE, Maseri A, Selwyn AP, Ribeiro P, et al. Myocardial ischemia during daily life in patients with stable angina: Its relation to symptoms and heart rate changes. Lancet ii:753–758, 1983.
8. Gottlieb SO, Gottlieb SH, Achuff SC, Baumgardner R, et al. Silent ischemia on Holter monitoring predicts mortality in high-risk post infarction patients. JAMA 259:1030–1035, 1988.
9. Blackburn H. The exercise electrocardiogram: technological, procedural, and conceptual development. In Blackburn H (ed): Measurement in Exercise Electrocardiography. Springfield, IL, Charles C Thomas, 220–258, 1969.
10. London MJ, Hollenberg M, Wong MG, Levenson L, et al. Intraoperative myocardial ischemia: Localization by continuous 12-lead electrocardiography. Anesthesiology 69:232–241, 1988.
11. Melicher VF Jr, Wolthius R, Keiser N, Stewart A, et al. A comparison of two bipolar exercise electrocardiographic leads to lead V_5. Chest 70:611–616, 1976.
12. Bazaral MG, Norfleet EA. Comparison of CB_5 and V_5 leads for intraoperative electrocardiographic monitoring. Anesth Analg 60:849–853, 1981.
13. Waldo AL, MacLean WAH, Cooper TB, Kouchoukos NT, et al. Use of temporarily placed epicardial atrial wire electrodes for the diagnosis and treatment of cardiac arrythmias following open-heart surgery. J Thorac Cardiovasc Surg 76:500–505, 1978.
14. Binkley PF, Bush CA, Kolibash AJ, Magorien RD, et al. The anatomic relationship of the esophageal lead to the left atrium. Pace 5:853–859, 1982.
15. Hammill SC, Pritchett ELC. Simplified esophageal electrocardiography using bipolar recording leads. Ann Intern Med 95:14–18, 1981.
16. Kates RA, Zaidan JR, Kaplan JA. Esophageal lead for intraoperative electrocardiographic monitoring. Anesth Analg 61:781–785, 1982.
17. Copeland GD, Tullis IF, Brody DA. Clinical evaluation of a new esophageal electrode with particular reference to the bipolar esophageal electrocardiogram. Am Heart J 53:862, 1959.
18. Arzbaecher R. A pill electrode for the study of cardiac arrhythmia. Medical Instrumentation 13:277, 1978.
19. Kint PP, Spaa W, Van Den Berg A, Muskens G, et al. Recording the right atrial electrogram through the fluid column of a pulmonary artery catheter. Crit Care Med 13:982–984, 1985.
20. Artru AA, Colley PS. The site of origin of the intravascular electrocardiogram recorded from multiorificed intravascular catheters. Anesthesiology 69:44–48, 1988.
21. Michenfelder JD, Terry HR Jr, Daw EF, Miller RH. Air embolism during neurosurgery: A new method of treatment. Anesth Analg 45:390–395, 1966.
22. Richards CC, Freeman A. Intra-atrial catheter placement under electrocardiographic guidance. Anesthesiology 25:388–391, 1964.
23. Johans TG. Multiorificed catheter placement with an intravascular electrocardiographic technique. Anesthesiology 64:411–413, 1986.
24. Warner DO, Cucchiara RF. Position of proximal orifice determines electrocardiogram recorded from multiorificed catheter. Anesthesiology 65:235–236, 1986.
25. Westheimer DN. Right atrial catheter placement: Use of a wire guide as the intravascular ECG lead. Anesthesiology 56:478–480, 1982.
26. Mantle JA, Massing GK, James TN, Russell RO Jr, et al. A multipurpose catheter for electrophysiologic and hemodynamic monitoring plus atrial pacing. Chest 72:285–290, 1977.
27. American Heart Association. AHA Editorial: electric safety standards for electrocardiographic apparatus. Circulation 61:669, 1980.
28. DeRosa JF, Gadsby PD. Radio-frequency heating under ECG electrodes. Medical Instrumentation 13:273, 1979.
29. Finlay B, Couchie D, Boyce L, Spencer E. Electrosurgery burns resulting from use of miniature ECG electrodes. Anesthesiology 41:263–269, 1974.

Chapter 23

Daniel M. Thys, MD
Zaharia Hillel, MD, PhD

Echocardiography

I. Introduction and Indications

Echocardiography is a powerful diagnostic tool that plays a major role in the noninvasive evaluation of patients with cardiovascular disease. In recent years, anesthesiologists have become very interested in the intraoperative application of this technology.[1] The development that triggered this interest was, undoubtedly, the introduction of transesophageal echo transducers. Early esophageal transducers, introduced in the mid-1970s, were primarily of the M-mode type, and therefore had limited applicability intraoperatively. Recent instruments incorporate not only M-mode, but also two-dimensional and Doppler examination techniques.

Modern instruments are commonly used for the intraoperative diagnosis of cardiovascular pathology as well as for the monitoring of global and regional myocardial function. Because of the transesophageal transducer's close proximity to the heart, the sound waves do not have to travel through bone, air, or fat, and the echo information obtained from the esophagus is usually of high technical quality. The advantages of the esophageal approach have lately also been recognized by cardiologists, who, as a result, now commonly subject some of their awake patients to esophageal examinations. Daniel et al have reported their experience with transesophageal echocardiography in 1300 patients, 92% of whom were conscious at the time of the examination and 42% of whom were outpatients.[2] The major reasons for specifically selecting the transesophageal, rather than the transthoracic, route are listed in Table 23–1.

Table 23–1 • Indications for Diagnostic Transesophageal Examinations

1. **Inability to perform an adequate transthoracic examination**
   Obesity
   COPD, emphysema
   Surgical dressings
2. **Specific view not available by transthoracic examination**
   Atrial appendages
   Descending thoracic aorta
   Coronary arteries
3. **Advantageous posterior transducer position**
   Atrial examination in the presence of a prosthetic atrioventricular valve.

COPD, chronic obstructive pulmonary disease

II. How To Do the Procedure

(See Color Figures at the Front of the Book)

A. *Principles of Echocardiography*

In echocardiography, harmless sound waves with a frequency beyond the audible range penetrate living tissues. The reflection of these waves provides information about cardiovascular structures and the blood flowing within these structures. Small transducers or probes transmit the electronic signals to the tissues, receive the reflected echoes, and pass the information on to very sophisticated processing electronics and computers. The computers generate images of the cardiac structures or measure blood flow characteristics. A simple schematic of an echo device is shown in Fig. 23–1. A more detailed discussion of technical aspects of echocardiography can be found in Thys et al.[3]

1. M-Mode Echocardiography

The most basic form of ultrasound imaging is *M-mode* echocardiography. In this mode, the density and position of all tissues in the path of a narrow ultrasound beam (ie, *along a single line*) are displayed as a scroll on a video screen. The scrolling produces an updated, continuously changing time plot of the studied tissue section, several seconds in duration (Fig. 23–2). Since this is a timed *motion display* (normal cardiac tissue is always in motion), it is called M-mode. Because only a very limited part of the heart is being observed at any one time and because the image requires considerable interpretation skills, M-mode is not currently used as a primary imaging technique. This mode is, however, useful for the precise timing of events within the cardiac cycle and is often used in combination with color flow Doppler for the timing of abnormal flows (see below). Quantitative measurements of size, distance, and velocity are also easily performed in the M-mode without the need for sophisticated analysis stations. Whenever a measurement includes a temporal component, the M-mode image is more advantageous than a two-dimensional (2-D) image because it is updated a thousand times each second. Thus, more subtle changes in motion or dimension can be appreciated.

2. Two-Dimensional Imaging

By rapid, repetitive scanning along *many different radii* within an area in the shape of a fan (sector) originating

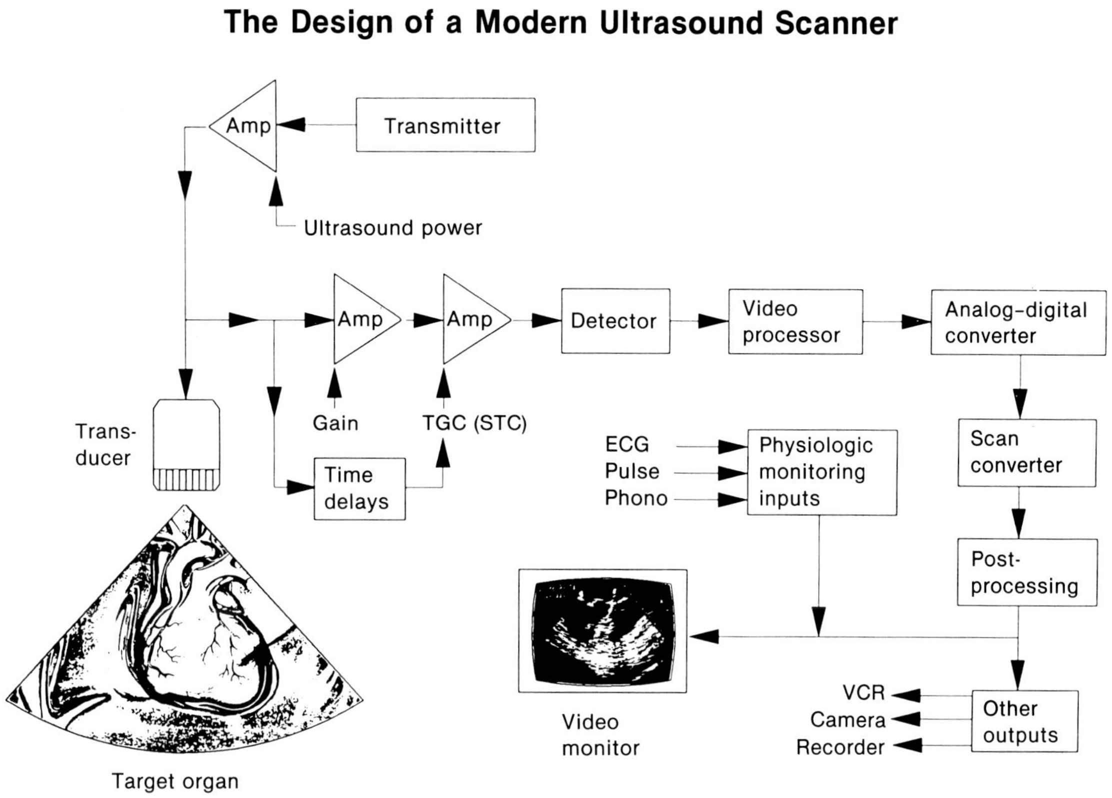

Figure 23–1 • Schematic representation of the design of a modern ultrasound scanner. The arrows indicate the directions for the flow of information or electronic power. AMP = electronic amplifier; TGC (*STC*) = time-to-gain (sensitivity–time) compensation; Pulse = pressure display channel; Phono = phonocardiogram record channel; VCR = video cassette recorder.

from the esophagus, echocardiography generates a 2-D image of a section of the heart. This image, which resembles an anatomic section and thus can be more easily interpreted, is called a *2-D scan* (see Color Fig. 1 and Fig. 23–10; these figures should be studied together). Information on structures and motion in the plane of a 2-D scan is updated 30 to 60 times per second. This produces a "live" (real-time) image of the heart. Scan-

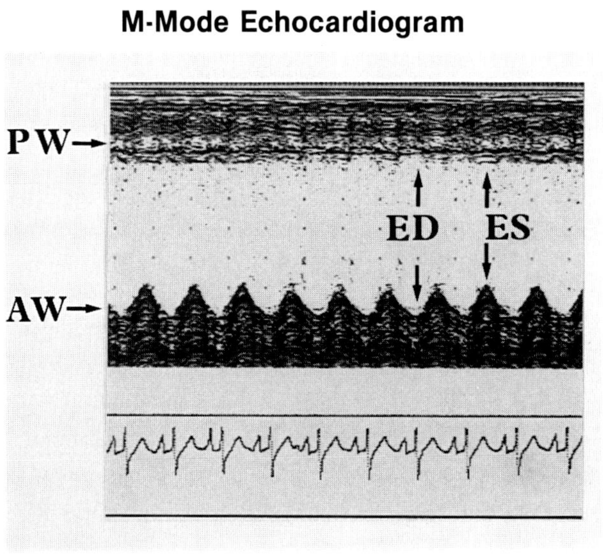

Figure 23–2 • M-mode echocardiogram of the left ventricle along the anterior–posterior diameter of its cross section with the corresponding ECG tracing below. Time is scanned along the horizontal axis, whereas tissue position and density are imaged along the vertical axis. Cyclic motion of the anterior ventricular wall (*AW*) is evident along with abnormal motion (akinesis) of the posterior ventricular wall (*PW*). ED = end-diastolic diameter; ES = end-systolic diameter.

ning 2-D echo devices scan the heart either by using a mechanically steered transducer or, as is common in many of the newer devices, an electronically steered ultrasound beam (phased-array transducer). Experimental probes with two transducers scanning in two orthogonal planes also exist.

3. Doppler Techniques

Information on blood flow dynamics can be obtained by applying Doppler frequency shift analysis to echoes reflected by the moving red blood cells.[1,5] Blood flow velocity, direction, and acceleration can be instantaneously determined. This information is different from that obtained in 2-D imaging and, hence, complements it.

The Doppler principle as applied in echocardiography states that the frequency of ultrasound reflected by a moving target (red blood cells) will be different from the frequency of the transmitted ultrasound. The magnitude and direction of the frequency shift is related to the velocity and direction of the moving target. The velocity of the target is calculated with the Doppler equation:

$$v = \frac{(cf_d)}{(2f_o \cos\theta)}$$

where v is the flow velocity, f_d the frequency shift, f_o the frequency of the emitted ultrasound, and Θ the angle between the ultrasound beam and the direction of blood flow. There are two basic Doppler measuring techniques: pulsed wave and continuous wave Doppler.

In *pulsed wave (PW) Doppler*, blood flow parameters can be determined at precise locations within the heart by emitting repetitive short bursts of ultrasound and analyzing the frequency shift of the reflected echoes after a specific time delay. The delay is proportional to the distance between the transducer and the location of the velocity measurements. The trade-off for the ability to measure flow *at precise locations* is that *ambiguous information* is obtained when flow velocity is very high. Pulsed wave Doppler measurements are performed with the same transducer as the one used for imaging.

The *continuous wave (CW) Doppler* technique uses continuous, rather than discrete, pulses of ultrasound waves. As a result, the region where flow dynamics are measured cannot be precisely localized. Blood flow velocity is, however, measured with great accuracy even at high flows.

Although many echo scanners have both PW and CW Doppler capabilities, most transesophageal probes, used for 2-D imaging, cannot perform CW measurements. Dedicated CW probes have two transducers, one of which continuously transmits ultrasound while the other continuously receives echoes. The display of Doppler color flow information is unique and is discussed in section F1 on pulsed wave Doppler analysis.

4. Color Flow Doppler

Advances in electronics and computer technology have allowed the development of *color flow Doppler (CFD)* ultrasound scanners capable of displaying blood flow within the heart in colors, in real time, while also showing 2-D images in black and white. In addition to showing the location, direction, and velocity of cardiac blood flow, the images produced by these devices allow one to estimate flow acceleration and to distinguish between laminar and turbulent blood flow. An example of a CFD image is shown in Color Fig. 2. Color flow Doppler echocardiography is based on the principle of multigated, pulsed wave Doppler.[6] According to this principle, blood flow is sampled at many locations, along many lines covering the entire imaging sector. At the same time, the sector is also scanned to generate a 2-D image.

Color flow Doppler imaging uses the three basic colors (red, blue, and green) used in standard color television. The color assignment is completely arbitrary. A picture element (pixel) on the video monitor screen corresponding to a location in the heart where the scanner has detected flow toward the transducer (the top of the image sector) is assigned the color red. Flow away from the direction of the top is assigned the color blue. In the most common color flow coding scheme, the faster the velocity (up to a limit), the more intense the color. Flow velocities that change by more than a preset value within a brief time interval (flow variance) have the color green added to either the red or the blue. Thus, they are mapped in brighter shades (hues) of red or blue. Both rapidly accelerating laminar flow (change in flow speed) and turbulent flow (change in flow direction) satisfy the criteria for rapid changes in velocity. To summarize, the brightness of the red or blue colors at any location and time is usually proportional to the corresponding flow velocity, while the hue is proportional to the temporal rate of change of the velocity. This color-coding map is depicted in Color Fig. 3.

Table 23–2 • Manufacturers of Echo Scanners with Transesophageal Capabilities

Acuson (Mountain View, CA)
Aloka/Corometrics (Wallingford, CT)
ATL (Bothell, WA)
Ausonics (Milwaukee, WI)
Diasonics (Milpitas, CA)
GE Medical Systems (Milwaukee, WI)
Hewlett-Packard (Andover, MA)
Hoffrel (South Norwalk, CT)
Siemens (Iselin, NJ)
Toshiba (Tustin, CA)
Vingmed/Interspec (Philadelphia, PA)

B. *Preparations*

1. EQUIPMENT

a. The Room and the Anesthesia Equipment

For intraoperative use, an operating room fully equipped for anesthesia is well suited. One necessary provision is that the room be sufficiently spacious to accommodate the rather bulky echo scanner without compromising patient care or safety.

For outpatient applications, a room with adequate privacy, an examination table, and a lighting system with dimming capabilities are necessary. Monitoring equipment must include a pulse oximeter, an electrocardiograph (ECG) monitor and a blood pressure cuff. An intravenous set-up should be available. Resuscitation drugs and a full resuscitation cart, including equipment for oxygen administration and airway management (suction, oral airway, face mask, air–mask–bag unit (AMBU), tongue depressor, laryngoscope, and endotracheal tube) must also be in the room.

b. The Ultrasound Equipment

Several ultrasound companies manufacture echo scanners that accommodate transesophageal transducers (Table 23–2). Although most of these devices share many common features, they do differ significantly in multiple important as well as trivial details. We herein attempt to provide generic technical descriptions and general set-up guidelines. For specific details on any particular device, the reader is referred to the particular manufacturer's technical manuals.

The Scanner. Most scanners are of medium refrigerator size and contain the following components (Fig. 23–3):

1. Scanner electronics (hidden from view)
2. Control pannel(s) (Fig. 23–4)
3. Transducer port(s) (connectors)
4. Viewing video monitor(s)
5. Video cassette recorder (optional, but invariably always there: VHS, Beta, or Super-VHS format)
6. Photography unit (optional, usually a Polaroid® unit)
7. Hard copy display (paper chart recorder, optional)

Ultrasound Scanner with Color Capability

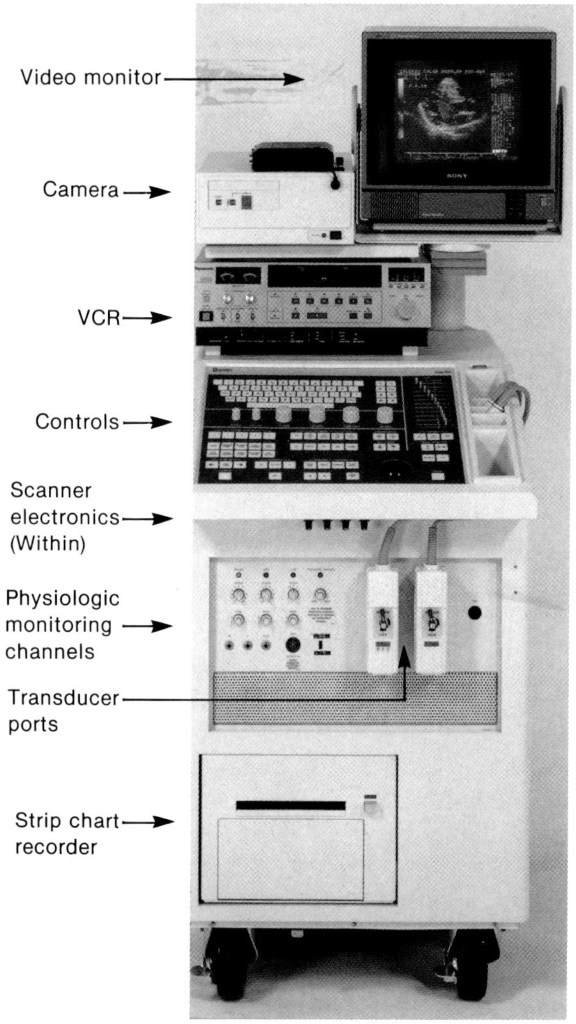

Figure 23–3 • An ultrasound scanner with Doppler color-flow capabilities and common accessories. Approximate size is 2.5 feet wide by 3.5 feet deep by 6 feet high.

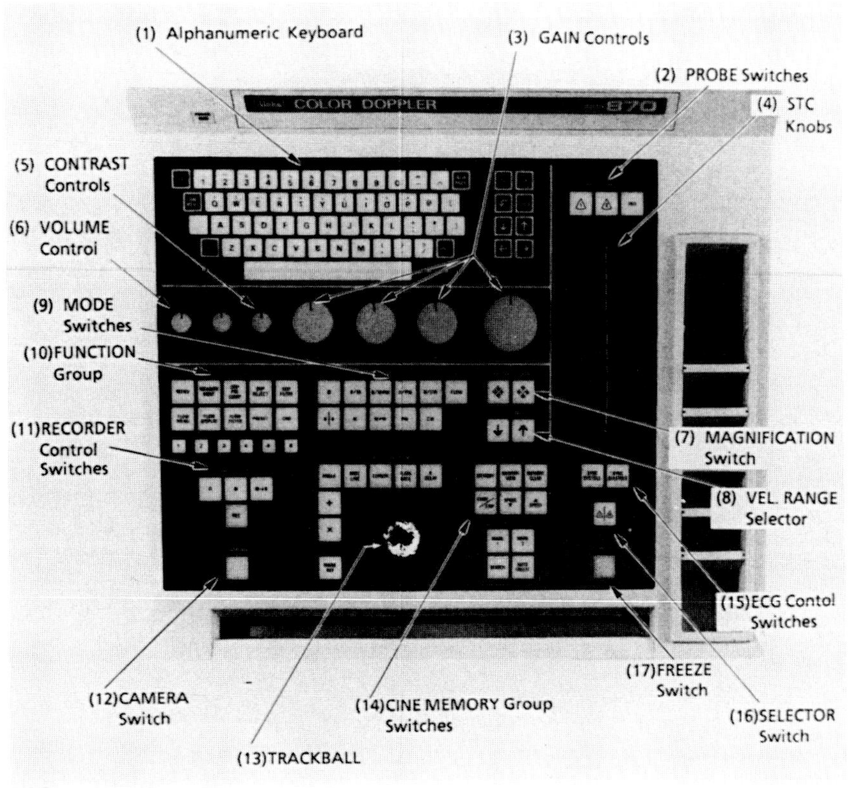

Figure 23–4 • The main control panel of a modern ultrasound scanner. The various controls are identified.

8. Speaker(s) for generating sound of the same frequency as the Doppler shift (happens to be in the audible range)
9. Additional monitoring channels: ECG, blood pressure (optional), sound (optional)

The Transducers. The transesophageal transducers for intraoperative use are based on the flexible gastroscope concept (Fig. 23–5). Most adult-size probes are approximately 100 cm long and 9 to 12 mm in diameter. The width at the transducer tip is often a couple of millimeters larger than the shaft diameter. The probes have either three or four types of motion. Two of these are linear motion (sliding) along the esophagus and rotation along the length of the shaft. In addition, all probes have 90° or more of up–down motion (flexion–extension, third degree of freedom), and most newer probes have less than 90° of left–right motion at the tip. Motion is controlled by knobs at the proximal end. Due to the distensibility of the esophagus and lack of rigidity of the surrounding anatomic structures, the orientation of the tip does not always correspond to the control settings. The probe tends to rotate along its length while the transducer tip is being oriented. For outpatient (''awake'') procedures, probes with shorter shaft length are desirable and available. Certain probes offer additional features, such as a fiberoptic channel for endoscopic visualization, a suction channel (gastroscopic vestiges), or a temperature gauge. On some probes, close-range resolution can be improved by adapting a fluid-filled balloon to the tip of the transducer. Recently, smaller esophageal transducers have been introduced for pediatric examinations. One such probe (Aloka, Wallingford, CT) has a transducer diameter of 0.6mm.

Basic Set-up (for all examinations):

1. Verify that the scanner/transducer complies with the maximum ultrasound energy limit allowed for transesophageal echocardiography (TEE) use.
2. Verify proper electrical grounding of the equipment and electrical isolation of both patient and equipment.
3. Check transducer tip surface for cracks or breaks (can cause electrical burns, current leakage, cardiac fibrillation). If the transducer is intact, it can be connected to the scanner.

Transesophageal Transducer
Head

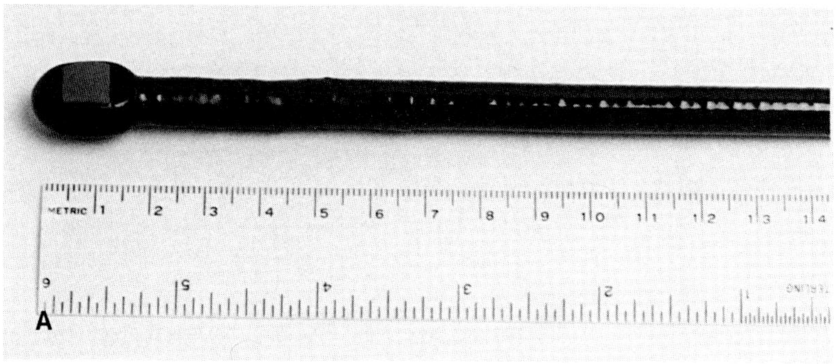

Entire transducer

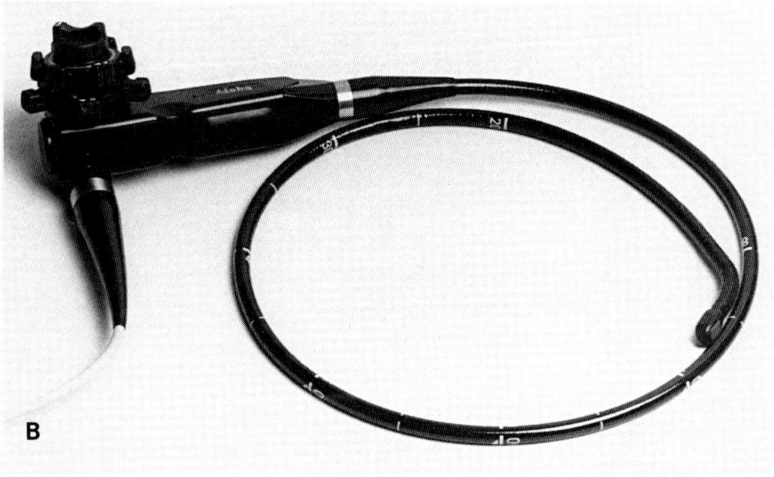

Figure 23-5 • (***A***) Transesophageal transducer head. (***B***) A modern transesophageal transducer (Aloka) with bidirectional motion of the tip. It interfaces with a Doppler color-flow scanner.

4. Set acoustic (ultrasound) transmit power control to zero (or lowest setting).
5. Connect scanner to a grounded electrical power source and turn power ON.
6. Dial a medium ultrasound power level (B-mode gain on some devices) and adjust the near to midfield TGC (or STC) controls to a middle-to-high range setting (see Fig. 23-4).
7. Check that the system is operational by verifying that gentle finger rubbing of the transducer surface produces a changing gray pattern on the video monitor.
8. Apply jelly (compatible with body mucosa) to the transducer head and observe white-out of the video screen.
9. Attach ECG cable and check operation of ECG monitoring channel.
10. Attach and check operation of optional monitoring channels.

2. Patient

Before attempting a transesophageal study, the following contraindications must be excluded:

1. Esophageal pathology: bleeding, varices (liver cirrhosis), diverticulae, strictures, severe swallowing problems, scleroderma, esophagitis, past surgery, and past irradiation to the mediastinum
2. Bleeding disorders or coagulation problems
3. Full stomach

At some institutions, antibiotic prophylaxis against endocarditis is used according to the American Heart Association guidelines for invasive procedures in high-risk patients.[7]

For ambulatory patients, cooperation and consent are mandatory.

a. *Place ECG Leads*

This is essential for the timing of observations within the cardiac cycle. In the anesthetized patient, two shoulder leads and a third placed on the forehead are often adequate. Because most echo scanners are programmed to monitor lead II, an adequate ECG signal will be obtained by attaching the left leg lead to the left shoulder, the left shoulder lead to the forehead, and the right shoulder lead to the right shoulder.

In addition to the physician performing the echo examination, a second person must be present to monitor the patient's vital signs and provide other assistance as necessary. This recommendation applies for studies in awake as well as anesthetized patients.

b. *Awake Study (Outpatient)*

Monitor vital signs (heart rate and rhythm, blood pressure, respiration, patient color) and establish intravenous access. Monitoring arterial oxygen saturation with a pulse oximeter is desirable but optional. A vagal response with bradycardia and hypotension, or *any* type of dysrhythmia, including asystole, can be potentially triggered during pharyngeal/laryngeal stimulation.

There are two ways of performing an ''awake'' transesophageal examination of the heart: with and without patient sedation. The choice between the two approaches seems to be based on philosophical or cultural differences, rather than on any scientific information. Some European groups (Germany and the Netherlands) do not use sedation, while others (France) and all groups in the United States prefer patient sedation.

Midazolam as a premedication or intravenously appears to produce excellent results.[8] Tranquilizing agents or small doses of short-acting narcotics can also facilitate a transesophageal examination in the conscious patient.

Topical anesthesia of the oropharynx can be accomplished with aerosol and viscous lidocaine or similar airway-compatible agents. Additional anesthesia can be obtained with a superior laryngeal block. Note that after pharyngeal anesthesia, normal swallowing is impaired for about an hour and that there is some risk of aspiration.

Drying of the pharynx can be accomplished with a 0.2-mg intravenous bolus of glycopyrrolate. This reduces secretions and the need for suctioning during the procedure. Make the patient aware of the anticholinergic effects of the medication.

c. *Study Under Anesthesia*

Minimal preparation is necessary because monitoring and intravenous access are already instituted. The endotracheal tube should be firmly secured because it could easily become dislodged or move during the procedure. Protect the eyes. Remove all esophageal instruments (temperatures probes, nasogastric tubes, esophageal stethoscopes) to avoid overdistention and a possible inadvertent advance into the stomach. Small instruments may be repositioned in the esophagus after placement of the TEE probe. We find that removal of the oral airway sometimes helps. Look for loose teeth or dental prostheses and observe standard precautions.

C. ***Probe Insertion***

1. THE CONSCIOUS PATIENT

After proper patient preparation (monitoring and sedation if desired), the patient is placed in the left lateral decubitus position. A bite guard may be slipped over the TEE probe (unnecessary if the patient is edentulous). The probe tip is flexed slightly and lubricated. With the head in a comfortable position, the patient is asked to open his or her mouth. Using gloved hands, the operator's left index finger should reach the posterior surface of the tongue. From there the finger will guide the probe shaft, which is advanced with the opposite hand down the oropharynx toward the esophageal opening. If resistance is encountered, the probe should be reoriented by rotation with the advancing hand or redirection with the left index finger in the mouth. The probe can also be reoriented at the distal steering controls, which should be left unlocked. Starting at about 15 cm from the teeth, the patient's swallowing should help esophageal entry. Proper topical anesthesia at this point minimizes gagging, while sedation minimizes apprehension and discomfort. Once the probe tip is beyond 20–25 cm from the teeth, gagging should subside, and the advance to a plane where the heart can be imaged should be easy and well tolerated.

2. PATIENT UNDER GENERAL ANESTHESIA

Insertion of the TEE probe is easier in the anesthetized than in the conscious patient because no response to the stimulation, such as gagging or coughing, occurs. The

Insertion of TEE Probe

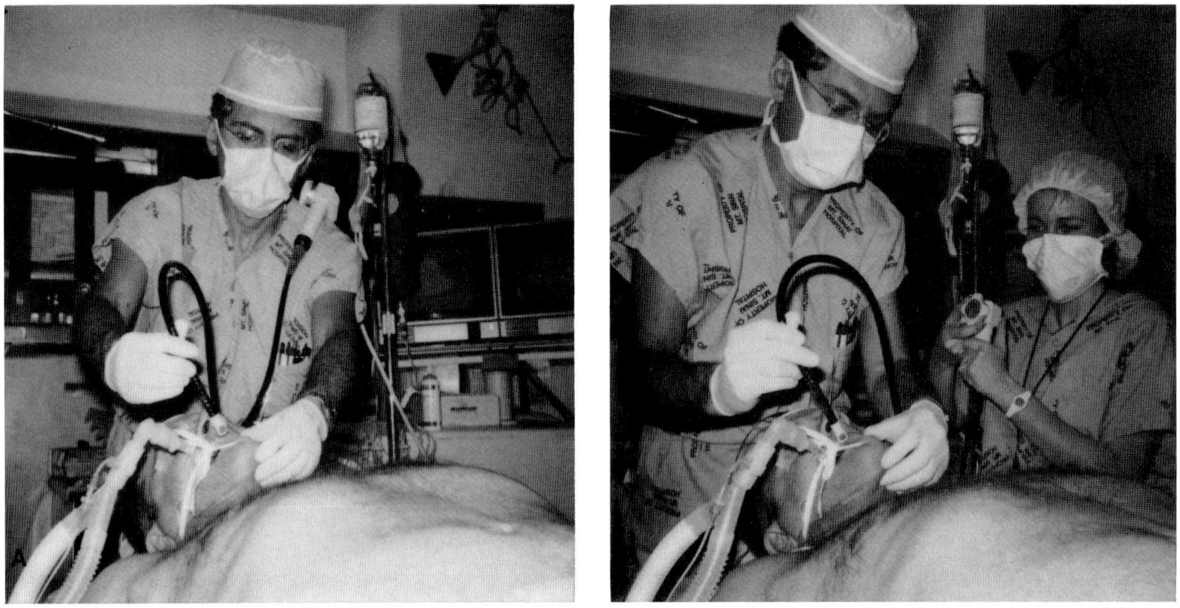

Figure 23–6 • Methods of inserting the transesophageal (TEE) probe in the anesthetized patient. (***A***) Single-handed with the distal end of the probe over the shoulder. (***B***) With the aid of an assistant.

patient is usually supine with the head in the midline, neutral position (no flexion or extension are normally necessary, but if the mandibular-oropharyngeal anatomy demands it, either slight flexion or extension at the neck may help). The control end of the probe can be positioned on the operating table next to the patient's head, held by an assistant, or placed on the operator's shoulder (Fig. 23–6). Most probes have locking left–right and up–down controls that must be placed in the neutral, unlocked position. With one hand the mandible is gently pulled upward (standard finger-spreading technique), while with the other hand the probe is inserted blindly into the mouth, in the posterior direction, with the transducer's face oriented anteriorly. At 16–18 cm from the incisors, the probe may pass into the esophagus, may become lodged in one of the *piriform sinuses,* or may coil in the pharynx. Although a minimal amount of resistance may be felt as the probe enters the esophagus (probably due to the close anterior proximity of the laryngeal structures), no attempt should be made to advance the probe against significant resistance. Resistance or inability to enter the esophagus may be circumvented by rotating the probe around its shaft during insertion, or by elevating the base of the tongue and the anterior pharyngeal wall. This anterior displacement of the mandible and tongue may be done by hand or with the aid of a laryngoscope. The laryngoscope can also be used for insertion under direct visualization of the esophageal opening. Deflation of the endotracheal tube cuff may be helpful in some cases. To avoid trauma to the pharynx, larynx, or esophagus, the procedure should be abandoned if undue difficulty is encountered with insertion.

The first images of cardiac structures will be obtained at about 30 cm. At this depth, the transducer should be rotated anteriorly until the great vessels become visible. If no identifiable image is seen and the screen is dark, check the acoustic power output control, the B-mode gain, and the TGC slide switches for the near field zone.

D. *The Two-Dimensional Examination*

1. Detailed Equipment Set-Up

The control panel of a modern ultrasound scanner is shown in Fig. 23–4, where the major controls are identified.

a. Ultrasound Transmission

Frequency/Probe Selection. Most scanners have a single TEE probe, which operates at a fixed frequency in the range of 3–5 MHz. Some of the newer devices may have more than one type of probe. The probe for adult patients may operate at one frequency, while a probe for pediatric use may operate at a higher setting. This is possible because lesser depths need to be scanned in pediatric subjects, thus allowing the use of a higher frequency and hence a higher resolution transducer. Most modern scanners automatically switch to the appropriate frequency when any compatible probe is attached.

Acoustic Power Level. Ultrasound power is transmitted into the examined tissue. For TEE studies it should probably not exceed 60–70 mW. The potential dangers related to the use of excess power are those of overheating and burning of the esophagus. To avoid these problems, some probes incorporate a thermometer near the transducer surface. It measures the local temperature, thus estimating tissue heating, and automatically interrupts ultrasound transmission if the temperature exceeds a predetermined value. Although no reports of heating or damage to the esophagus after TEE have been published, it is prudent to transmit as little power as necessary to image a particular structure. It is also prudent to set the power transmission control to its lowest setting between observations. For patients undergoing cardiac surgery, it is prudent to turn the power transmission control to its lowest setting during cardiopulmonary bypass because the esophagus may be less well perfused and thus less able to dissipate heat under those conditions.

Enhanced Image Resolution. Some of the new scanners can enhance the resolution in a region of interest by directing the scanner to spend more time interrogating that particular region than the remainder of the sector.

b. Ultrasound Reception

Depth Range. The maximum distance from the transducer surface at which tissues will be examined is set by adjusting the depth range. The available ranges vary from less than 5 cm to more than 20 cm and number from three to as many as seven ranges (depending on manufacturer). For a TEE examination, the deepest range necessary may be 15 cm. Transducers that operate at 5 MHz or higher have more limited depth ranges than those operating at 3.0 or 2.5 MHz. Indeed, at higher operating frequencies, signal penetration decreases while resolution increases.[9]

Gain. The brightness of the image is adjusted with the gain knob. It varies the degree to which the incoming echoes are amplified. With an increase in gain, all the returning echoes are amplified to the same degree. If an echo image is weak, one should first attempt to increase image brightness by adjusting the gain rather than by increasing the power output, which exposes the tissue to more heating risk. Too much gain, however, increases the background image noise (Fig. 23–7). In that situation, the power output should be increased or

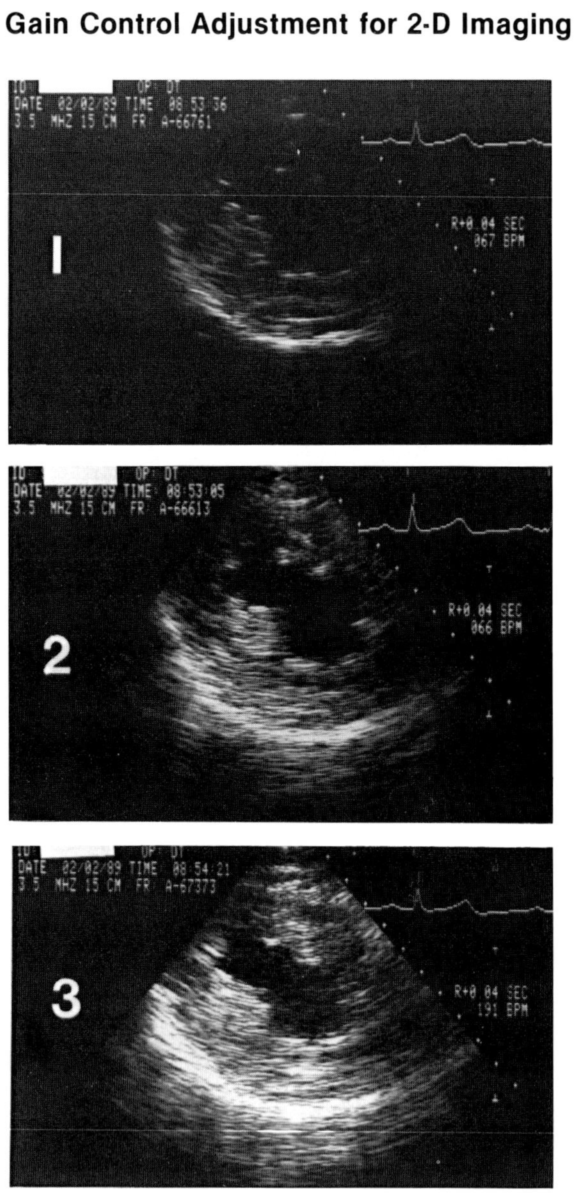

Figure 23–7 • Gain control adjustment for 2-D imaging. (***1***) Too little gain. (***2***) Adequate gain. (***3***) Excessive gain.

Time-to-Gain Adjustment

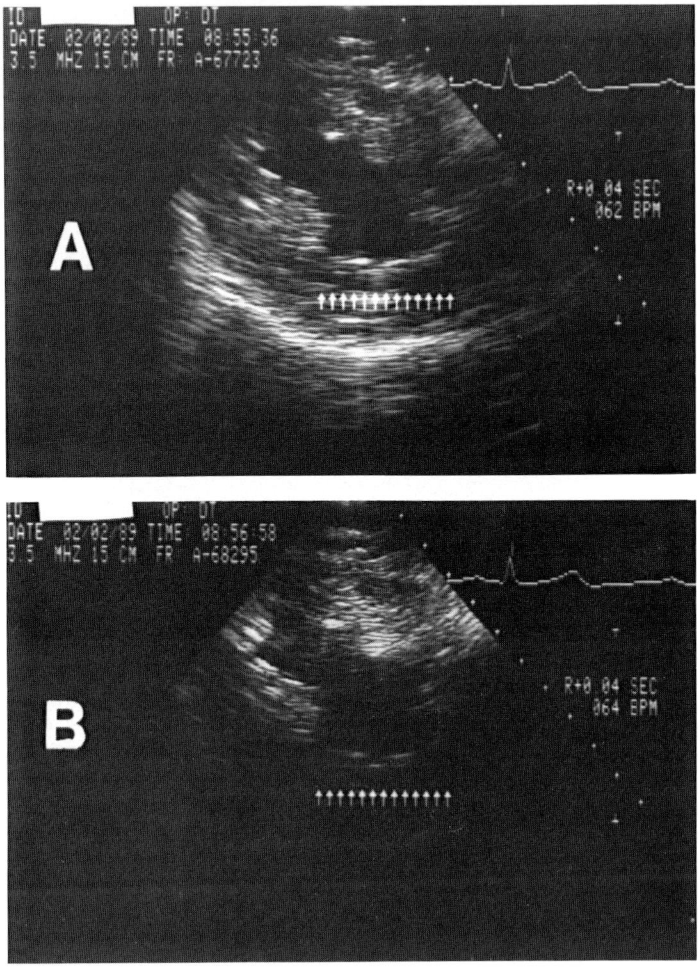

Figure 23–8 • The time-to-gain compensation in 2-D imaging. (***A***) Image obtained after optimal adjustment of TGC switches. (***B***) Inadequate adjustment of distal TGC. The anterior wall, indicated by the arrows, is inadequately visualized because TGC adjustment for that region was too low.

an adjustment in image processing parameters may be necessary (see below).

Time-gain compensation (TGC) or sensitivity-time compensation (STC). This is a selective amplification adjustment. The TGC control is usually composed of seven to eleven sliding switches that adjust the gain of signals from selected depths in the sector. This is an essential compensation for the unavoidable attenuation by scattering or absorption of transmitted and received signals. The farther the tissue location from the transducer or the denser the intervening tissue, the greater the attenuation and the greater the need for compensation. Thus, in general, the near-field tissues appear brighter and the far-field tissues darker. Scanners usually have a default setting, which is adequate. However, if *part of the image* is too bright or too noisy, the corresponding TGC switch (identified by trial and error) should be adjusted for less gain. Conversely, if any part of the image appears too dark, the corresponding TGC switch should be set for higher gain (see Fig. 23–8). When the entire image is too bright or too dark, a global gain adjustment should be made.

c. Image Generation (See Color Figures at the Front of the Book)

Image Formatting (orientation, polarity, and magnification). Some scanners allow selection of the image orientation on the video screen. The orientation is arbitrary, but the American Society of Echocardiography (ASE) has recommended that TEE images be displayed in the same manner as precordial echo images. According to this convention, the left heart in the short-axis or four-chamber views is imaged on the right side of the screen and the right heart on the left side of the screen (see Color Fig. 1, panel 6). A small symbol (diamond, circle, or square) near the sector's apex identifies the image orientation on the video screen relative to a mark on the transducer. It allows the examiner to maintain the same display orientation for different studies and indicates when the orientation has been changed.

The option to invert the image from left to right (see Color Fig. 2) or flip the image upside down may also be available. TEE echocardiographers usually display the apex of the sector at the top of the screen.

Most devices also offer a choice between bright echoes on a dark background (white-on-black image) or dark echoes on a bright background (black-on-white image). It is customary (perhaps for ease of viewing or increased perception) to image 2-D echoes as bright on a dark screen.

The magnification of the imaged tissue is set by the "depth" setting, because the imaging sector always fills the full screen and the maximum depth is always at the sector arc. Thus, in order to magnify the size of tissues in the near field, one can select a lower imaging depth. An alternative method and the only one that allows magnification of structures in the far field makes use of a digitally selected "region of interest," which is magnified as a postprocessing option (not available on all scanners).

Digital Gray Scale Processing. This image manipulation is performed after the image is generated in the device memory. It involves gray scale reassignments or the setting of cutoffs. Any echo intensity can be assigned a variety of arbitrary pixel brightnesses. The relations between image brightness and echo intensity can thus be changed to various curvilinear forms. High or low intensity signals can be completely eliminated from the brightness map. Examples of these manipulations are shown in Fig. 23–9.

2. Standard Anatomic Views

Although transesophageal echocardiography often provides images whose quality is unparalleled by the transthoracic method, the number of different views that can be obtained with this technique are fewer than with the transthoracic method.

Once the transducer tip reaches the level of the heart in the esophagus, a sequence of views, described in Table 23–3, can be obtained by advancing and orienting the probe from the base of the heart to the apex. There are three basic positions from which most views are obtained: the base of the heart, the left ventricular

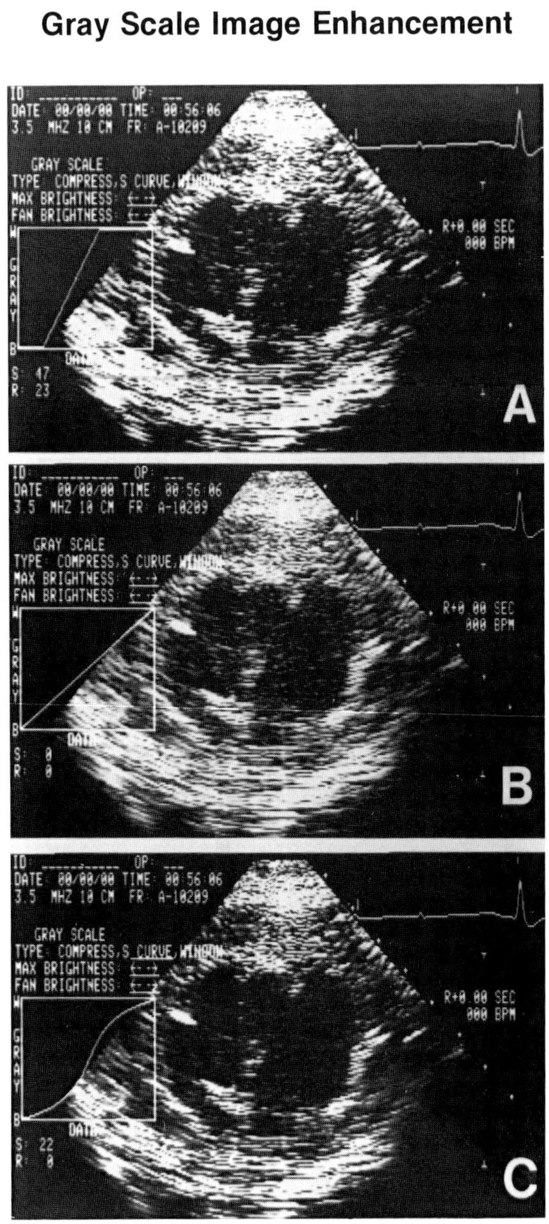

Figure 23–9 • Gray scale processing image enhancement. The same short-axis view of the left ventricle imaged in systole was subjected to three different types of gray scale postprocessing. A schematic of the signal strength to gray scale (pixel brightness) assignment is shown in the insert on the left of each panel. (***A***) The weakest echoes (the lowest 23rd percentile) have been eliminated, while intermediate strength echoes (from 60th percentile and up) have been enhanced by being assigned the highest pixel brightness. There is relatively little background noise inside the ventricular cavity, while the weaker endocardial echoes have been enhanced. (***B***) Image without gray scale postprocessing: echo signal strength and pixel brightness are linearly related. Note the high level of background noise in the cavity. (***C***) Similar manipulation as in panel ***A,*** except that a gradual suppression of weaker echoes and gradual enhancement of intermediate-strength echoes have been used. The cavity is nearly noise free, but the endocardial borders are not as well delineated as in panel ***A.***

Table 23-3 • Transesophageal Echocardiographic Views

Position	View	Depth	Details
Basal short-axis	Main pulmonary artery	~25 cm	
	Left atrial appendage		See also pulmonary veins
	Aortic root		See coronaries, pulmonic valve and pulmonary veins
	Aortic valve		Aortic leaflets, right and left atria, foramen ovale, tricuspid valve
Basal four-chamber	LV outflow tract	~30 cm	LV, LA aortic valve
	True four-chamber		LA, RA, LV, RV, mitral and tricuspid valves, septa
	Coronary sinus		
LV short-axis	Mitral valve	~35 cm	
	Mid papillary		RV is seen in short-axis
	Ventricular apex		
LV long-axis	Apical long axis	~40 cm	LV outflow tract
	Obtuse long axis		Lengthwise mirror image of parasternal long-axis view from the obtuse angle of the heart
Aortic cross-section	Descending thoracic aorta seen in the posterior thorax	≥30 cm	180° rotation of the probe along its length

level, and the apex of the heart (Fig. 23–10). At the base of the heart, several views that include the great vessels and the atria are obtained (see Fig. 23–10A, insets 1–4, and Color Fig. 1, panels 1–4). The aortic valve leaflets can often be easily visualized (see Fig. 23–10A, inset 4, and Color Fig. 1, panel 4). Aortic valve anatomy and function can be evaluated at this level. The valve leaflets should appear as thin lines when the valve is open as well as closed, and they should open almost fully to the aortic wall in systole and coapt fully in diastole. If the probe is retracted slightly, the take-off of the left main and right coronary arteries can be seen in good detail in most patients (see Color Fig. 1, inset 3, and Fig. 23–10A, inset 3). Although atherosclerotic plaques are probably difficult to demonstrate in this limited view, aneurysmal dilatation of the coronaries can be easily detected when present (Color Fig. 3). Blood flow in the great vessels and occasionally in the coronaries can be imaged using Doppler color flow at this level.

One to two cm farther down the esophagus and with slight extension of the probe tip, several different four-chamber views are obtained. In a four-chamber view (see Color Fig. 1, panels 5 and 6, and Fig. 23–10B, insets 5 and 6), a longitudinal section of each of the cardiac chambers is seen. The chambers can almost be seen in their entirety except for some atrial wall. Atrial and ventricular septal defects are easily visualized at this level and, using Doppler, flows across these defects can be imaged or estimated (Color Fig. 4). Both atrioventricular valves are also seen and their anatomy and function can be examined. Valve leaflet thickening, calcification (secondary to rheumatic or other heart disease), and prolapse can be detected. Valve opening and closing are also easily demonstrated in this view. Normal and abnormal flow across both atrioventricular valves can be imaged and estimated. The coronary sinus can also be visualized at this level (see Color Fig. 1, panel 7, and Fig. 23–10B, inset 7).

Advancing the probe farther in the esophagus to the level of the ventricles, several different short-axis views of the left ventricle (LV) can be obtained (in some patients the transducer has passed the gastric cardia and is in the stomach at this position). All short-axis views of a normally functioning LV share the full, circular image of the endocardium and a partial (occasionally complete) circular view of the epicardium. When the myocardial wall has a shape that deviates significantly from the circular doughnut shape, an oblique rather than a true cross-sectional plane should be suspected. This is undesirable if semiquantitative or quantitative measurements are to be performed on the image. The superior short-axis view at the mitral valve level shows valve anatomy and in diastole allows estimation of valve opening (or area by planimetry) (see Color Fig. 1, panel 8, and Fig. 23–10C, inset 8). Near the midventricular position both papillary muscles are imaged near the vertical diameter of the LV (see Color Fig. 1, panel 9, and Fig. 23–10B, inset 9). The midpapillary short-axis view im-

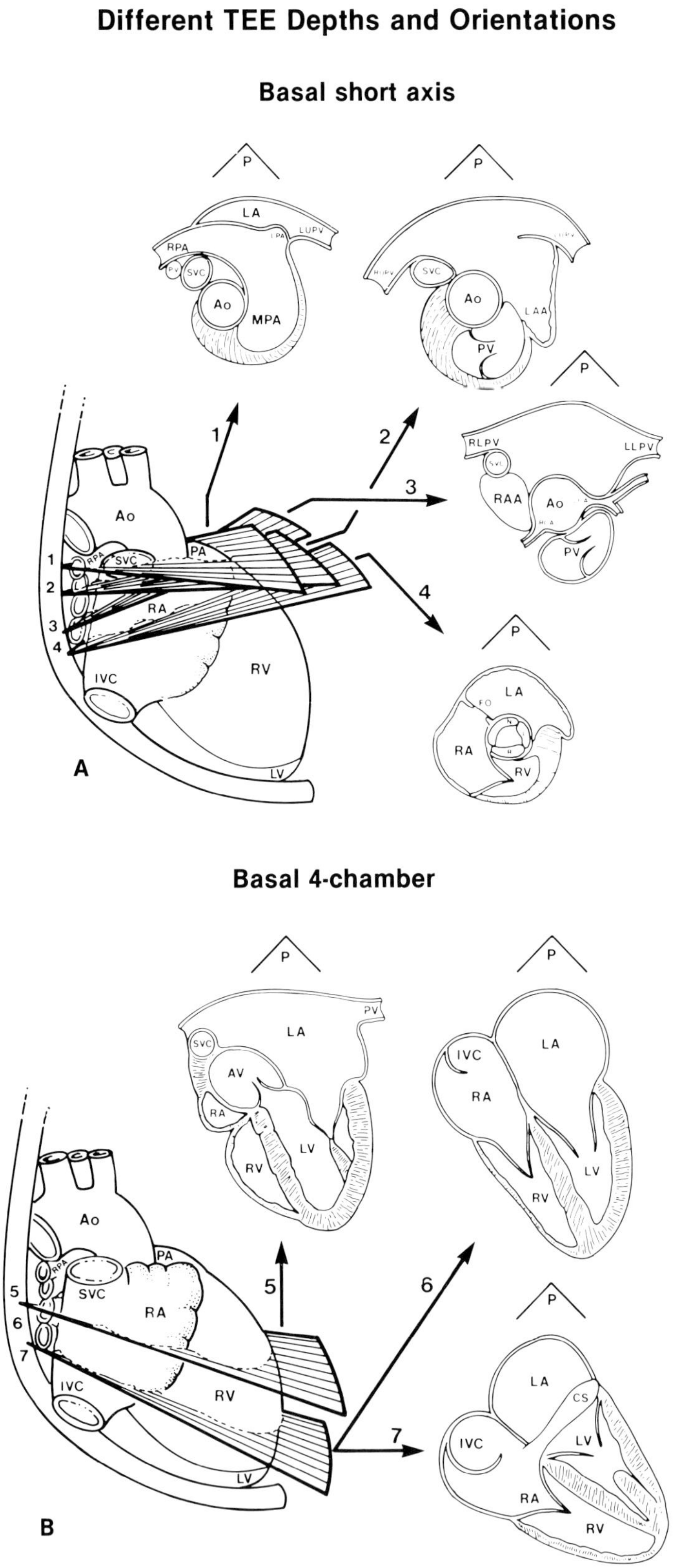

Figure 23–10 • Schematic representation of different transesophageal echocardiography (TEE) scan planes and the corresponding images. The *P* at the apex of the sector indicates that the transducer lies posteriorly to the imaged structure. (***A***) Basal short-axis views: (*1*) main pulmonary artery, (*2*) pulmonic valve, (*3*) aortic root and coronaries, (*4*) aortic valve. (***B***) Basal four-chamber views: (*5*) LV outflow tract, (*6*) classic four-chamber, (*7*) coronary sinus.

(continued)

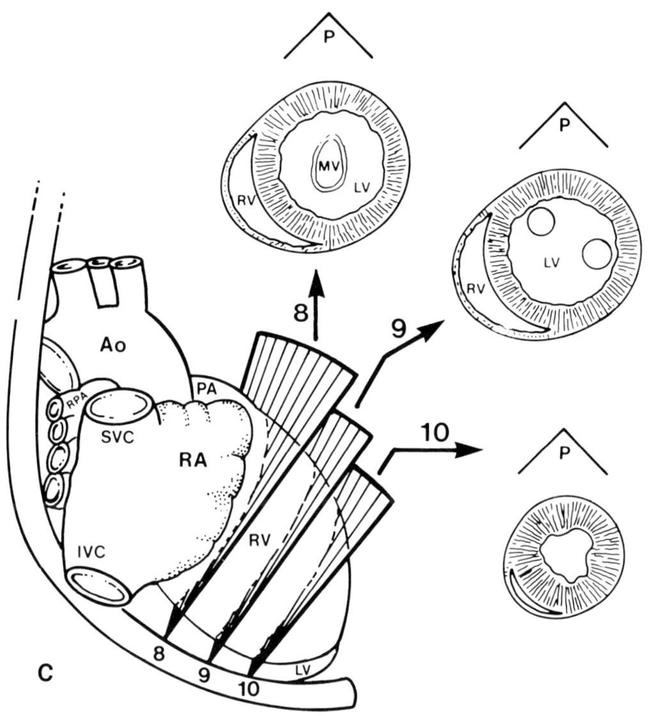

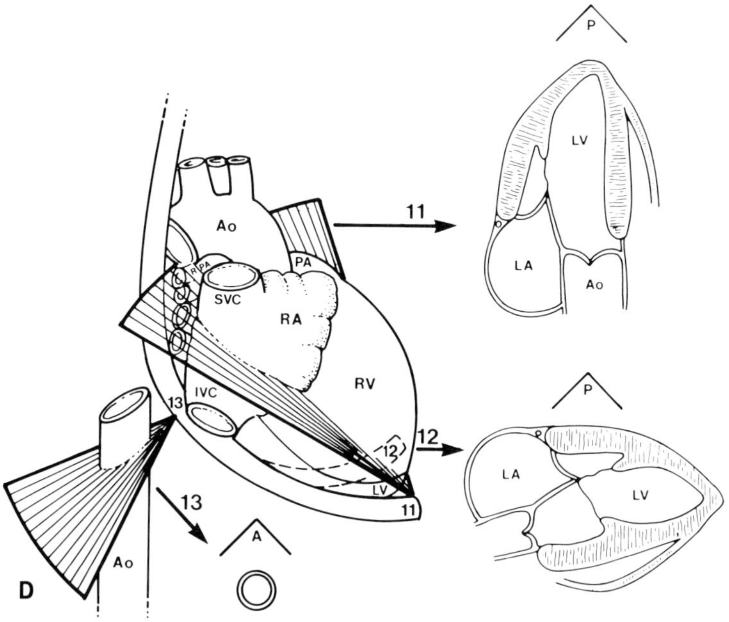

Figure 23–10 *(continued)*
(***C***) LV short-axis views: (*8*) mitral valve, (*9*) midpapillary muscle, (*10*) apical. (***D***) LV long-axis views: (*11*) apical, (*12*) obtuse angle. (*13*) Short-axis view of the descending thoracic aorta. A = anterior; Ao = aorta; AL = anterolateral papillary muscle; CS = coronary sinus; FO = fossa ovalis; IVC = inferior vena cava; LA = left atrium; LAA = left atrial appendage; LCA = left coronary artery; LPA = left pulmonary artery; LUPV = left upper pulmonary vein; LV = left ventricle; MPA = main pulmonary artery; PM = posteromedial papillary muscle; PV = pulmonic valve or pulmonary vein; RA = right atrium; RAA = right atrial appendage; RCA = right coronary artery; RLPV = right lower pulmonary vein; RPA = right pulmonary artery; RUPV = right upper pulmonary vein; RV = right ventricle; SVC = superior vena cava.

ages both papillary muscles in circular cross section and is the view most frequently used for qualitative or quantitative assessment of global or regional LV function. In this view the right ventricle (RV) is also seen in short-axis section but, in contrast to the LV, its shape is crescent-like or triangular. Following ASE recommendations for image orientation, the RV is to the left of the LV in this view. During RV overload or dysfunction, flattening or bulging of the interventricular septum into the LV cavity are easily noted in this view (Fig. 23–11).

When using the midpapillary muscle short-axis view to compare LV regional myocardial function or regional wall motion, it is important to maintain the transducer in the same relative position and orientation to the heart. This will be best accomplished by maintaining a view in which the exact shape of the papillary muscles and ventricular cavity are unchanged and by verifying that external markers, like the insertion points of the RV, are still in the same location.

By further advancing the probe with some flexion at the tip, one occasionally obtains an apical long-axis view of the left heart (see Color Fig. 1, panel 11, and Fig. 23–10D, inset 11). Flexion and leftward orientation at this depth images the left heart in long-axis section from its obtuse angle (see Color Fig. 1, panel 13, and Fig. 23–10D, inset 12). Sections of the descending thoracic aorta can be obtained in the vicinity of 30–35 cm in the esophagus by rotating the transducer posteriorly (see Color Fig. 1, panel 13, and Fig. 23–10D, inset 13). These images are helpful in patients with thoracic aortic dissections. Images from a patient with a descending aortic dissection are shown in Color Fig. 6.

E. *The M-Mode Examination*

1. Details of Set-Up

a. Single M-Mode Display

The M-mode line of imaging is set on a 2-D image. In devices with two video monitors, the 2-D and M-mode images are displayed on different screens. In single-screen devices, the screen can be shared by these two modes to allow side-by-side simultaneous viewing (B-/M-mode). This facilitates precise selection of the sampling direction while verifying that an adequate M-mode image is obtained. A simple control (joystick, trackball, or key) is used to move the sampling line along any radius within the 2-D sector. Time intervals are measured using the horizontal spacing between screen markers, while distances are obtained from the vertical marker ruler. The speed with which the image is swept can be adjusted, allowing enhanced time resolution.

M-mode image characteristics may be changed with the gain, contrast, or AGC controls. Some devices (Corometrics, Wallingford, CT; Diasonics, Milpitas, CA), allow selective magnification of any region within

Right Ventricular Hypertrophy

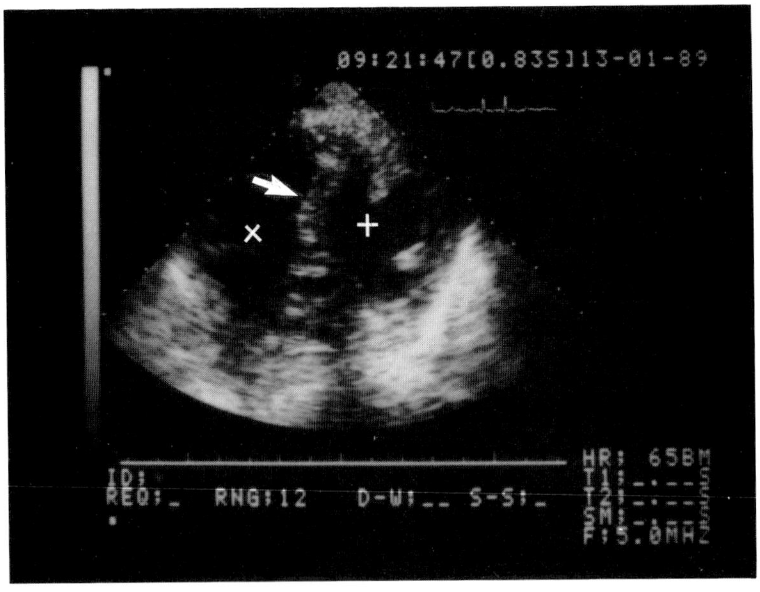

Figure 23–11 • Right ventricular hypertrophy leading to interventricular septal flattening demonstrated in a midpapillary short-axis view of the left ventricle (LV). The + symbol marks the LV cavity, the x symbol marks the RV cavity, and the arrow points to the septum.

the M-mode section while keeping the 2-D image unchanged in the dual-display mode. This magnifies the structures seen on M-mode, thus improving spatial resolution, while the exact part of the heart being examined can be seen in the 2-D image. On single-screen devices, after the initial M-mode setup, the 2-D part of the split-screen image may be replaced by full-screen M-mode.

b. Dual M-Mode Display

Some echo scanners can obtain M-mode information along two directions simultaneously. This feature makes relative timing of the motion of two valves or other complex time analyses easier. The location and the size of the regions of interest can be selected independently in a manner completely analogous to the single M-mode examination.

2. Standard M-Mode Parameters

Since the advent of 2-D imaging, M-mode has been used primarily for size or distance measurements. There are extensive tables providing normal values of anatomic parameters for the four cardiac chambers in both children and adults.[10] These measurements were performed using the leading-edge to leading-edge technique to eliminate the variability of line thickness secondary to gain adjustments.[11] Extrapolation of unidimensional cardiac parameters to multidimensional areas or cardiac volumes is fraught with errors secondary to geometric assumptions. Although largely replaced by 2-D indices, M-mode can be used to derive indices of LV performance such as circumferential shortening fraction (the unidimensional equivalent of ejection fraction [EF]), fractional shortening, rate of circumferential shortening, and ventricular wall velocity (see below). The rate parameters are obtained by dividing distances by time, which is easily measured on M-mode tracings.

F. Doppler Analysis

A standard Doppler examination begins with 2-D imaging of the anatomic region where flow is to be studied. When the Doppler section is switched on, a cursor line along which blood flow is sampled appears on the video screen and is manually directed to the region of interest. The Doppler signal is then imaged on a second screen, or on the same full or split half-screen as the 2-D image. For a moving object to produce a Doppler shift in ultrasound frequency, the relative orientation between the beam and the direction of flow (angle Θ) must be close to 0°. When Θ is less than 25°, the Doppler measured velocities are true velocities. For Θ greater than 25°, a correction must be applied (division by cosine Θ), because the velocity measured underestimates the true velocity.

To estimate angle Θ, the operator manually orients a second built-in cursor line in the estimated direction of flow. An internal computer then measures the angle between the ultrasound beam (first cursor line) and flow direction (Fig. 23–12). Mathematic conversion of measured velocity to true velocity is then performed as mentioned above. This compensation is not recommended for Θ greater than 60°, because a small error in Θ produces a large error in velocity.

Because heart tissue itself is in motion most of the time, it produces low-frequency Doppler signals (tissue moves much more slowly than red cells in normally flowing blood). Low-frequency filters in the range of 100 to 1000 Hz are available to cut off these unwanted signals, because they may be strong and interfere with the weaker flow signals. Improved signal cosmetics may also be achieved using the "reject" setting, which eliminates Doppler signals weaker than a selected strength.[5]

1. Pulsed Wave

In pulsed wave Doppler analysis, the precise location of flow sampling (the sampling volume) is selected with the aid of the 2-D image. The sampling volume is positioned along a directional cursor in the region of interest, using a trackball, joystick, or pushbuttons. The size of the sampling volume can also be selected by the operator. Its position can be further refined by maximizing the amplitude (greater mass of flow) or the pitch (higher velocity flow) of the Doppler audio signal. Because the signal is generated by many red cells within the sampling volume and each of these may have slightly different velocities, the flow signal actually represents an envelope of velocities. Modern echo devices display a power spectrum of this envelope. This is the spectrum of frequencies of the Doppler shift (velocities) plotted in increasing order on the vertical axis as a function of time on the horizontal axis (Fig. 23–13). Pixel brightness is proportional to the logarithm of the intensity of the echo at that velocity and point in time. Arbitrarily, flow toward the transducer is displayed above the zero frequency shift baseline (zero velocity line), while flow

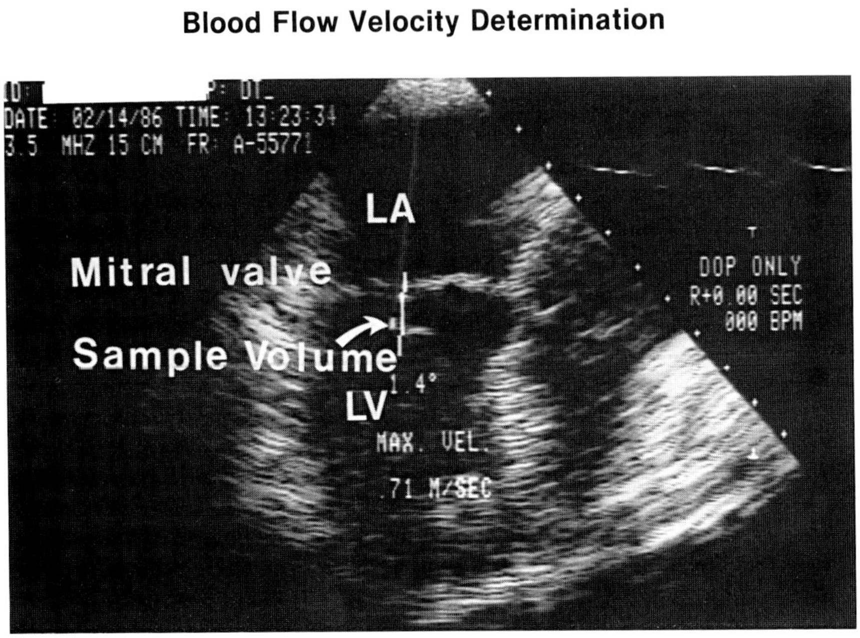

Figure 23–12 • Transmitral blood flow velocity determination by pulsed wave Doppler on a four-chamber view. LA = left atrium; LV = left ventricle. The angle between the Doppler beam and the assumed direction of blood flow is 1.4°. With the sample volume at this distance from the sector's apex, the maximum velocity that can be sampled at the location of the sample volume is 0.71 m/sec^{-1}.

away is displayed below this baseline. The power spectrum is characterized by the peak velocity (the maximum recorded frequency), the modal velocity (the dominant shift at any point in time, indicated by the brightest region in the spectral display), and several important time intervals, detailed below.

The basic Doppler flow parameters are computed as schematized in Fig. 23–21, using simple machine controls. They are the maximum or peak velocity, which is measured from baseline to the highest point in the frequency spectrum (the computer automatically calculates a peak velocity value). Flow time is the time from the beginning of the trace (detection of the first positive Doppler shift greater than a baseline selected above noise) until the end of the trace. Mean *temporal* velocity is computed as the area under the trace divided by the flow time. Time to peak is the time from start of the trace to the instant of maximum velocity. Flow acceleration is the ratio of maximum velocity and time to peak. Additional derived parameters include peak and mean pressure gradient, pressure halftime, and valve area. These parameters are based on a modification of Ber-

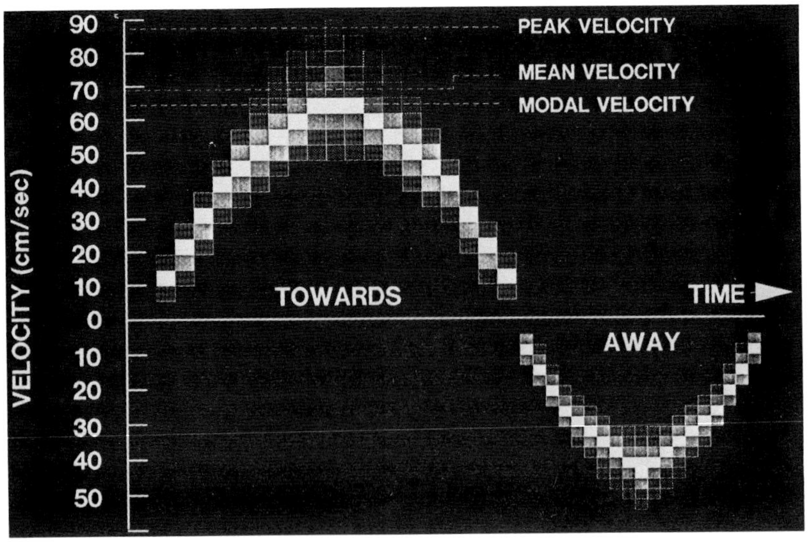

Figure 23–13 • Schematic representation of a Doppler power spectrum. Bidirectional flow is diagrammed. The brightness of the spectrum at any position is proportional to the number of red blood cells having the corresponding velocity at that time. Peak, modal, and mean velocities are indicated.

noulli's equation, which states that the pressure gradient (P) responsible for the flow is related to the maximum flow velocity (V_{max}) via the relation:

$$P = 4\ (V\ \max)^2$$

It is clear that the area of maximum velocity in a flow region must be determined to determine some of the derived parameters. Typical applications of Doppler analysis are mitral and aortic valve flow measurements (see below).

Normal Doppler-derived maximal flow velocities have been determined in children and adults for the mitral and tricuspid valves, the pulmonary artery, the aorta, and the LV.[12] In children, additional velocities have been determined in the superior vena cava (SVC), both atria, and both ventricular inflow tracts. Normally, the highest reported peak velocities occur in the descending aorta (1.7–1.8 m/sec^{-1}). Additional normal Doppler parameters include the LV ejection time ($\sim$300 m/sec), the aortic acceleration time ($\sim$100 m/sec), and the average aortic acceleration ($\sim$15 m/sec^{-2}).

In pulsed wave Doppler, ultrasound waves are emitted in a pulsatile manner at a finite pulse repetition frequency (PRF). Any velocity that produces a Doppler shift greater than PRF/2 (the Nyquist limit) is displayed in the opposite of the true direction, a condition called *aliasing*. With aliasing, flow toward the transducer is displayed below the baseline and vice versa. By selecting a high velocity range for the measurement, aliasing is eliminated in most situations. For a typical modern scanner, having high PRF capability (25 kHz) with a 2.5 MHz transducer operating in the highest velocity range, normal display aliasing occurs for velocities greater than $\sim$3 m/sec^{-1}. By shifting the baseline, spectra corresponding to velocities as high as 7 m/sec^{-1} can be displayed unambiguously. This is well above the normal flows mentioned earlier. Thus, signal aliasing presents a problem only with abnormally high flows, and even then it is easily identified.

2. CONTINUOUS WAVE

Continuous wave (CW) Doppler allows determination of velocities as high as 12 m/sec^{-1}. Such high velocities may be encountered in pediatric patients with congenital heart disease or in adults with severe valvular heart disease. Although at present CW Doppler is not available on TEE probes, it may become available in the near future. One common application of CW Doppler in the operating room is the determination of cardiac output by transesophageal measurement of descending aorta blood velocity and calculation of the stroke volume.[13] A modified esophageal stethoscope with two ultrasound transducers is used for this purpose. This method, however, still presents some practical problems.[14]

G. *Doppler Color Flow*

Color flow imaging is activated independently of black-and-white tissue imaging. A black-and-white 2-D image is obtained initially; the color flow imaging section is switched on subsequently. When flow imaging is active, some gray background from the cardiac chambers is automatically eliminated to produce a high-contrast, noise-free image and thus enhance color brightness. For color flow imaging, the acoustic power level selector should be adjusted to the minimum setting, which produces sharp image details and color flow.

1. IMAGE SIZE

Most echo scanners allow one to select several combinations of *flow sector size* and image sector size, each variable independently, and in several discrete steps in the range of 30° to 80°. This is an important feature, because in addition to image size, it affects the quality of the color flow display and the detection sensitivity at the high end of the velocity range. Choosing a smaller color sector (eg, 30° or 45°) allows the scanner to sample the area faster and hence more often. This updates the color flow information more frequently, leading to a higher *color frame rate* and a smoother flowing video display. A larger color sector slows down the rate of flow sampling, and very brief high velocity flows (eg, regurgitant valve jets) may be missed. Color sectors smaller than maximum (80° or 90°) can be selectively positioned anywhere within the full 2-D image sector.

2. GAIN

The flow image gain (controls sensitivity and color brightness) is adjusted to produce colors where appropriate, usually to a middle setting. In the absence of intracardiac communications, cardiac chamber walls should not display any color. Conversely, with a reasonable cardiac output, the diastolic flow across the mitral valve should be imaged in hues of blue, while the systolic flow through the LV outflow tract should be imaged in orange-red hues in a TEE four-chamber view (see Color

Fig. 2). The higher the gain setting, the larger the size and brightness of the colored areas displaying flow (see Color Fig. 3). Thus, when attempting to estimate abnormal flows such as valvular regurgitation or septal shunt flow, one should be aware that an inappropriate gain setting can lead to overestimation. Conversely, too low a gain setting will cause underestimation of normal flows or may cause the examiner to completely miss or overlook abnormal flow patterns. Excessive gain introduces color artifacts (noise). As these artifacts occur in the brighter part of the spectrum, they interfere with correct assessment of high velocity or turbulent flow. Flow gain should be adjusted to minimize this noise. As a final note, acoustic power interacts synergistically with gain in producing the color flow map, but should not be used to increase image or flow brightness except when imaging distant targets (unusual in TEE).

3. ALIASING

Red–blue color inversion occurs when the blood flow velocity exceeds the maximum velocity range (color Figs. 3 and 5). The upper limit of detectable velocity is determined by transducer frequency (not adjustable), the depth of the examination (adjustable), the size of the 2-D and color flow image sectors (adjustable), and the PRF (adjustable on some devices via the velocity range control). When color inversion occurs, the presence of aliasing can be verified by performing a standard PW Doppler examination in that region. A typical aliased power spectrum such as that shown in Color Fig. 7 should be obtained if the velocity limit is exceeded. If switching to the highest available velocity range at that depth and sector size does not remove the aliasing, shifting the color-coding baseline, just as for aliased PW Doppler, may help. In certain situations it may not be possible to remove color aliasing because very rapid flows, beyond the limits of the device, are present. This occurs with severely stenotic valves and some pediatric congenital shunts.

4. M-MODE COLOR FLOW DOPPLER

Blood flow can be imaged in an M-mode display in a very localized region of the heart along the line of the M-mode cursor. The advantage of this type of display is that, with the ECG signal as a clock, it is very easy to time any flow with precision in the cardiac cycle (see Color Fig. 5).

5. COLOR FLOW IMAGE ANALYSIS

When color flow was first introduced, there were expectations that it might be suitable to quantitate blood flow. An obvious quantitative application is the determination of the degree of mitral regurgitation. As a qualitative tool, Doppler color flow mapping was demonstrated to have sensitivity and specificity in the 90 percentile range for the intraoperative detection of mitral regurgitation (MR), using angiography as a gold standard.[15] It is probably the most sensitive method of detecting valvular regurgitation, because small, regurgitant jets can be demonstrated in many patients without any clinical or other evidence of valve disease.[16]

As with all echo modalities, however, color flow provides two-dimensional information obtained in a single plane at any given time. Because regurgitant valve jets are three-dimensional, their quantitation from color flow images is complex and not fully resolved. Initially, uniplanar indices such as regurgitant jet area, the ratio of jet area to LA area, and jet length were used.[17] Later, a multiplanar approach was taken, using either the maximum or the average jet area obtained from three orthogonal imaging planes.[18] Multiple time frames in the same imaging plane can also provide information on regurgitation, because larger jets persist longer and hence are seen in more frames. A regurgitant jet may be characterized by the regurgitant fraction or by its volume. Using benchtop mechanical models for mitral regurgitation (MR), it was demonstrated that jet volumes determined from single-plane color flow jet areas ($area^{3/2}$) overestimated true regurgitant volumes.[19] Jet area or volume did correlate well with the instantaneous flow rate. Another approach has been to calculate regurgitant jet momentum using velocity information extracted from the color flow map.

In spite of these difficulties, the clinical experience is promising. Intraoperative epicardial echocardiography performed in 68 patients undergoing cardiac surgery was found to be in complete agreement with angiography in grading MR on a 0 to 4+ scale in 72% of patients, and differed by one grade in 25%.[15]

H. *Physiologic Signals Display*

1. ELECTROCARDIOGRAPH (ECG)

Every ultrasound device permits display of the ECG on the video screen. Only a single lead, however, usually lead II, is available for monitoring. The size of the ECG trace and its position on the image screen are usually adjustable. This signal is of paramount importance for timing cardiac events and is available in all imaging as well as Doppler display modes. Color Fig. 5 shows an example of an atrial septal defect with abnormal flow into the right atrium. The ECG signal, superimposed upon the Doppler color flow M-mode, clearly demonstrates that the observed aliasing coincides with the atrial contraction.

a. ECG Synchronized Images

In advanced scanners, an ECG synchronization function permits observation of a 2-D image in real time at any fixed point within the cardiac cycle. This allows demonstration of the effect of a given manipulation on an echocardiographic observation at a particular point in the cardiac cycle. Examples are the effect of the Valsalva maneuver on the LV cavity size at end-diastole, or the effect of the finger-grip maneuver on the size of a mitral valve regurgitant jet imaged in the LA using color flow Doppler. Using a split-screen display, images at two fixed, selected points in the cardiac cycle can also be displayed continuously in real time.

2. Other Signal Displays

A phonocardiogram signal can also be displayed on the image screen. This may be of interest to cardiologists trying to time echo observations in relation to physiologic closing times of the valves or, in the case of a patient with a complex cardiac murmur pattern, to identify the physiologic or anatomic correlate of each component of the murmur.

Some echo devices have an additional unassigned display channel that could be used to monitor a hemodynamic parameter such as arterial pressure, for example, in either the 2-D or the M-mode. This may be useful in research applications or could in the future lead to a single monitoring screen that integrates the echo information with all the other hemodynamic information.

I. Non-Real-Time Image Manipulations

On nearly all the ultrasound devices, the operator has the ability to manually "freeze" or store a single image frame on the screen. This allows visualization and close scrutiny of any unusual transient anatomic or physiologic observation. It also allows one to perform quantitative measurements on line. Using this storage mode, however, it is somewhat difficult to capture a particular point in the cardiac cycle. For this reason, modes that acquire more than a single frame have been devised.

1. Image Storage

a. Cine Memory

One of the newest modes of information storage, present on the more modern devices, is the cine memory function. When activated, this mode captures in digital memory approximately one second's worth of very high fidelity image information. The information can then be played back, frame-by-frame, in several different ways. It can be replayed using a manually controlled trackball to step between frames. This allows the observer to spend any amount of time on any one frame. It can also be replayed continuously in repeating, endless-loop fashion, either at the same speed at which it was recorded or at a slower speed, allowing scrutiny of very brief transient observations.

b. Videotape

The video recorder is the most common long-term, mass-storage medium used in echocardiography. All devices come or can be equipped with a 1/2-inch VHS video cassette recorder (VCR), very similar to the VCR for home use. Higher-resolution "Super-VHS" or professional (3/4-in) VCRs are also available. Because the VCR is an analog type of storage medium, the quality of videotaped images is currently inferior to the real-time display or the digital cine memory replay. This makes for more difficult quantitative and sometimes qualitative image analysis.

c. Other Storage Media: Paper Chart, Photography, Digital Laser Disk

Photographic or digital paper chart recorders are available for most devices and are most useful for off-line, quantitative measurements of M-mode data scrolled in time (continuous time record). These devices can also provide prints of single frame 2-D images. Higher quality 2-D image prints and color flow Doppler images are obtained using either an instant Polaroid® type camera or a regular 35-mm camera with color film.

In addition to the standard photographic color record, very high fidelity color prints can be produced with color video printers (eg, Mitsubishi, Piscataway, NJ) from any digital or video source.

Digital image storage is possible on magnetic disk media. With the exception of the noninterchangeable hard disk, current floppy disks can store a very limited number of images because the amount of information in a single full video frame is on the order of 1 megabyte (10^6 bytes). Furthermore, current hardware and computer architecture do not allow rapid retrieval of image information. A new digital mass storage medium uses "write-once, read-many" digitally encoded laser disks. Using a mammoth-sized, 810-megabyte memory, it can store 24,000 frames or 800 different cine loops, each 30 frames long.

2. QUANTITATIVE IMAGE ANALYSIS

a. On-Line Analysis

All new echo devices and most of the older systems have built-in, computer-driven, quantitative image analysis packages. Analysis can be performed either on an individually stored frozen frame or on any frame played back from cine memory. For M-mode data, lengths, velocities, and time intervals can be measured. For 2-D or color flow images, lengths, areas, and angle relations can be measured, added, subtracted, divided, or substituted into formulas to obtain anatomic and physiologic parameters such as wall thickness, wall motion, cavity diameter, the area or volume of a cardiac chamber, and area or volume ejection fraction. For Doppler data, velocity, acceleration, and stroke volume/cardiac output (which needs 2-D information also) are measurable. All these measurements require some operator input in the form of pointing or line tracing on the video screen using a trackball or joystick. Doppler power spectra can be automatically traced once their beginning and end are identified. Unfortunately, automatic border tracing (endocardium or epicardium) of 2-D images is not yet available.

b. Off-Line Analysis

Off-line image analysis can be performed on video data. The data can be acquired from the scanner, in digital format, by a special data analysis station or from videotape playback on such a device. With direct digital retrieval, image quality is high but only limited amounts of information can be stored. The videotape stores tens of thousands of images, but of a lower quality. All the on-line analysis features are available on off-line stations. In addition, more sophisticated operations, such as wall motion or wall thickening analysis with digital readout and graphing as a function of image position, are possible (Fig. 23–14).

III. DISCUSSION OF THE PROCEDURE

A. *Global Ventricular Function*

1. SYSTOLIC FUNCTION

The classic determinants of systolic ventricular function are preload, afterload, and contractility. Although these were initially described as the determinants of systolic function in isolated muscle preparations, they since have been adopted in clinical medicine. A variety of hemodynamic variables has been used to estimate preload, afterload, and contractility in clinical practice; with these variables, global ventricular function is often evaluated. A large array of echocardiographic measures of preload, afterload, and contractility have also been described. The use of these echocardiographic measures, in combination with hemodynamic measurements, has enhanced our abilities to gauge the systolic function of the left ventricle.

a. Preload

Although in conventional hemodynamics preload is often estimated by measuring left ventricular filling pressures (pulmonary capillary wedge pressure or left ventricular end-diastolic pressure), in echocardiography it is determined by measuring left ventricular end-diastolic dimensions. In M-mode echocardiography a single ventricular diameter is often obtained, while in 2D echocardiography one or multiple tomographic cuts are recorded (see Color Fig. 1). The debate as to the number of cuts that are required to accurately represent ventricular volumes is ongoing and beyond the scope of this discussion.[20] In transesophageal echocardiography, one is often, for practical reasons, limited to a single, short-axis view at the level of the papillary muscles. Some evidence suggests that end-diastolic short-axis areas (EDA) measured at this level correlate reasonably well

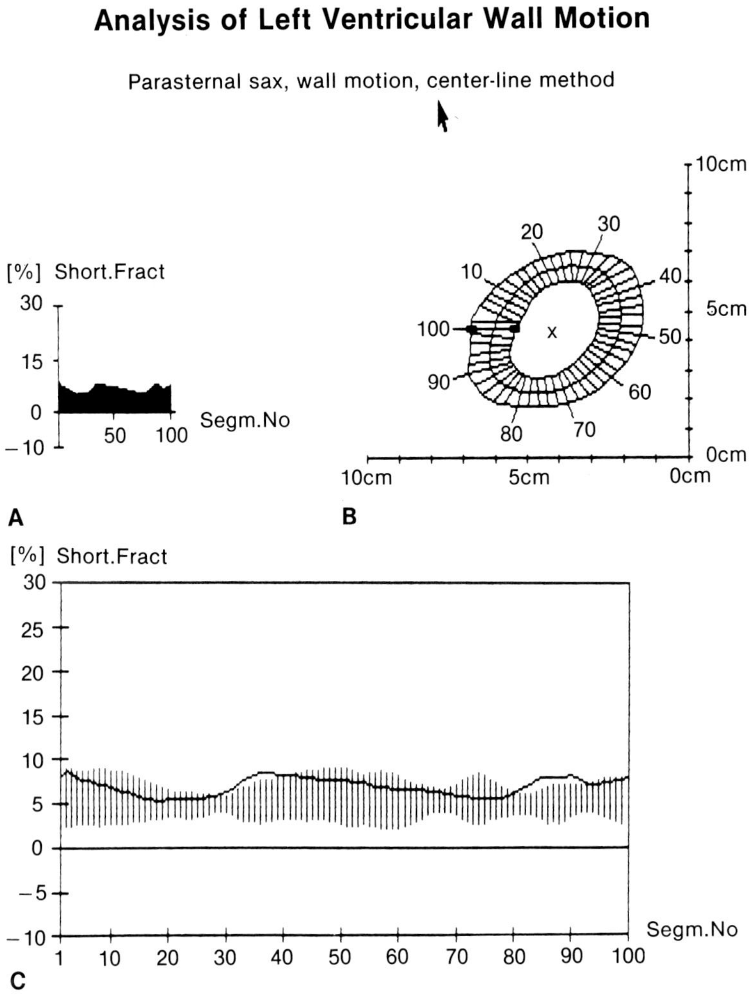

Figure 23–14 • Center-line analysis of left ventricular wall motion. (***B***) The inward motion of the endocardium during systole was measured by the device along 100 different lines. (***C***) The systolic motion (*solid line*) is compared with the standard deviation of the motion measured in normal subjects (*vertical lines*). (***A***) A compressed version of ***C***.

with end-diastolic volumes measured simultaneously using radionuclides.[21] In the operating room, a simple visual examination of the short-axis view at end-diastole will indicate whether the left ventricle is empty or full. If quantitative information is required, the endocardial outline must be electronically delineated and the end-diastolic area must be calculated (Fig. 23–15). It has been proposed that the end-diastolic area measured in this manner is a better index of preload than the pulmonary capillary wedge pressure (PCWP). We have compared PCWP and end-diastolic volumes (EDV), derived from short-axis areas at the level of the papillary muscles, as predictors of cardiac output in patients undergoing coronary artery surgery.[22] In our patients, strong correlations were observed between end-diastolic areas or end-diastolic volumes and cardiac index, although no significant correlation was found between pulmonary capillary wedge pressure and cardiac output. We thus concluded that end-diastolic dimensions obtained by 2-D echo provide a better index of left-ventricular preload than PCWP measured with conventional hemodynamic monitoring. In clinical practice, however, it is best to measure both the end-diastolic volume and the left ventricular filling pressure, because together they define the compliance of the left ventricle.

b. *Afterload*

Although afterload cannot be determined by echocardiography alone, the combination of ventricular dimensions with ventricular wall thickness and systolic arterial pressure yields end-systolic wall stress. Ventricular wall thickness is derived by calculating the difference between the epicardial and endocardial areas, while the ventricular dimension corresponds to the endocardial area.[23] The formula to calculate wall stress was derived by Sandler and Dodge from the basic Laplace equation:

$$Wallstress = \frac{(1.33 \times P \times LVEDD)}{4WT\ (1 + WT/LVEDD)}$$

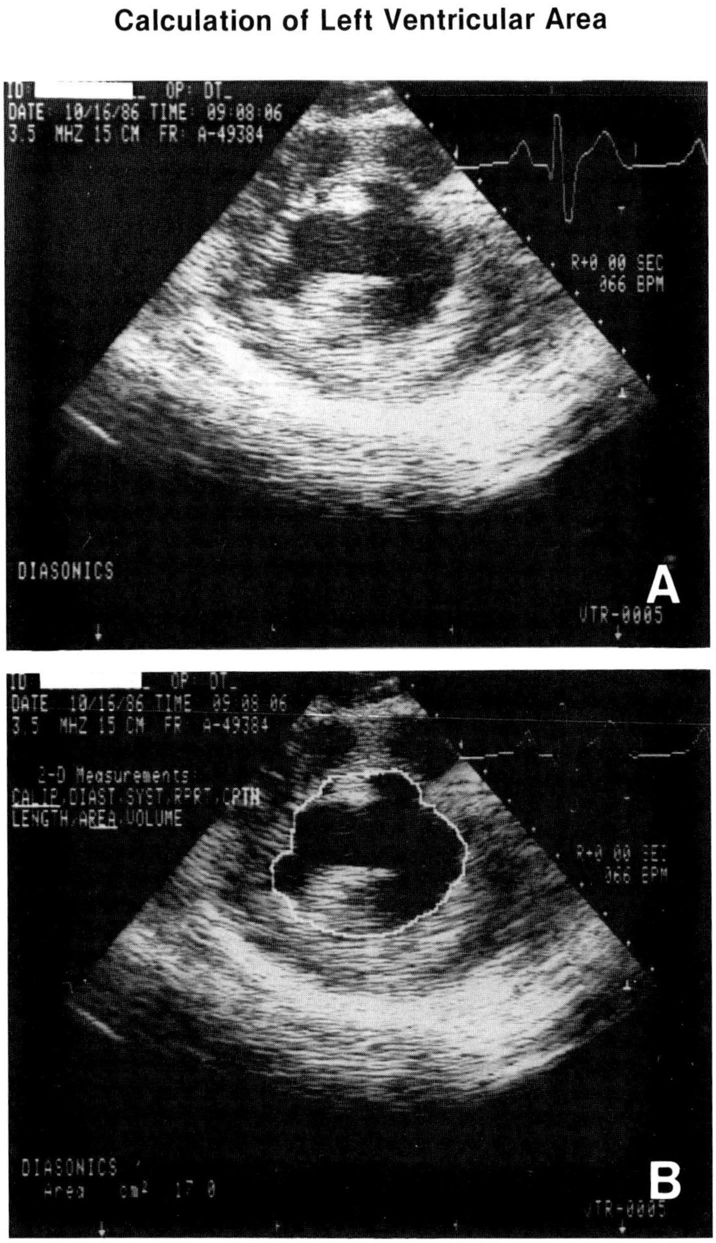

Figure 23–15 • (***A***) Midpapillary short-axis view of the left ventricle obtained at end-diastole (identified by the right edge of the ECG). (***B***) Same view after electronic delineation of the endocardium for the calculation of the ventricular area.

where *P* equals the systolic blood pressure, *WT* represents wall thickness, *LVEDD* represents the end-diastolic cavity dimension, and 1.33 converts mmHg to dynes / cm^{-2}.[24]

A simplified version of the wall stress equation states that:

$$Wallstress = \frac{(P \times LVEDD)}{WT}$$

where *P* equals systolic arterial pressure, *LVEDD* equals left ventricular end-diastolic dimension, and *WT* equals left ventricular wall thickness. Diastolic dimensions are selected because it is assumed that peak-systolic wall stress occurs during isovolumic ventricular contraction while the ventricle still possesses its diastolic anatomic configuration.

Elevations in wall stress have been observed in patients with left ventricular enlargement due to systemic hypertension, aortic stenosis, or aortic regurgitation.[25] Wall stress definitely provides a better index of afterload than systemic vascular resistance when forward stroke volume is not equal to the total ventricular ejection, as in mitral regurgitation or in the presence of a ventricular septal defect. Whether it also does so in patients without such lesions is unclear. In one animal study, it was observed that, during pharmacologic interventions, systemic vascular resistance and wall stress did not correlate well and occasionally varied in opposite directions.[26] In our cardiac surgical patients, we similarly found a poor correlation between systemic vascular resistance and end-systolic wall stress.[22] It remains to be determined whether systemic vascular resistance or wall stress will be most useful for the intraoperative evaluation of left ventricular function. The close association between wall stress and myocardial oxygen consumption, however, should provide a strong impetus for future investigations.

c. *Contractility*

Indices of contractility are traditionally divided into isovolumic and ejection phase indices. Echocardiography has been used to estimate contractility with either type of indices, although it is, by design, better suited for the evaluation of the ejection phase. In a different approach to the assessment of contractility, the use of newer indices, based on the study of the end-systolic pressure volume relation, has also been suggested.

Isovolumic Phase Indices. The isovolumic phase indices, such as dP/dt, are obtained during the isovolumic phase of systole, prior to the opening of the aortic valve. Because of technical and anatomic limitations, transesophageal echocardiography is not particularly well suited for the assessment of the isovolumic phase of the contraction (eg, cannot measure dP/dt). Some information on the isovolumic phase can, however, be gathered by measuring the length of the preejection period. The preejection period is the time between the onset of the QRS on ECG and the opening of the aortic valve on M-mode echocardiography (Fig. 23–16). The usefulness and limitations of the preejection period as well as the other systolic time intervals has extensively been reviewed elsewhere.[27,28]

Another measurement which is, to some extent, related to the isovolumic phase of the contraction is the maximal acceleration of blood flow in the aorta.[29] Maximal blood flow acceleration occurs in the early part of the left ventricular ejection and can be measured by Doppler echocardiography. In the ascending aorta, it is determined by the placement of a Doppler transducer in the suprasternal notch and by aiming the ultrasound beam at the aortic valve. A variety of studies have demonstrated that maximum blood flow acceleration, sampled in this manner, provides information of left ventricular contractility.[30–32] With transesophageal echocardiography, the ascending aorta cannot be adequately

M-Mode and the Projection Period

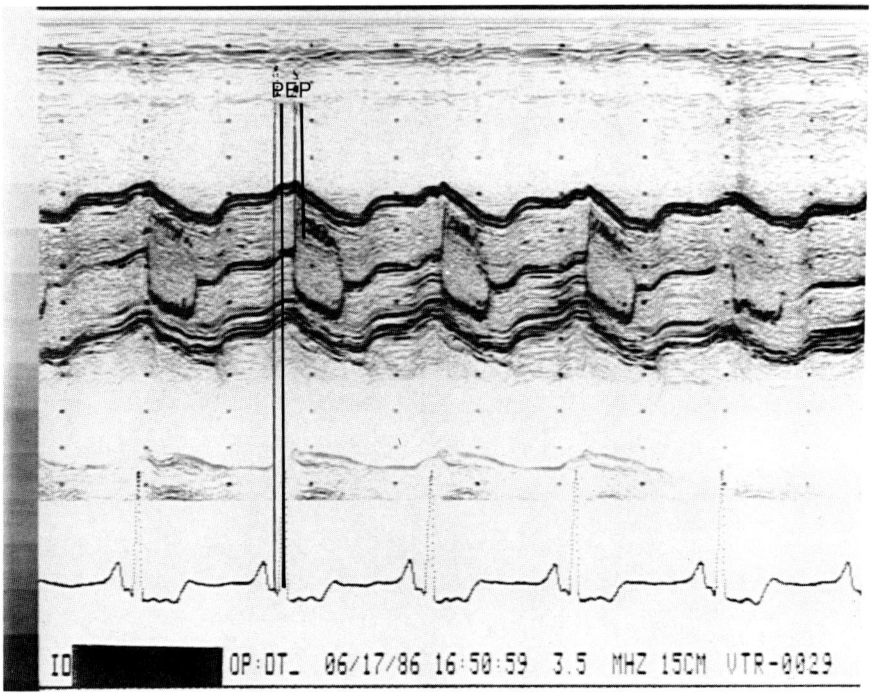

Figure 23–16 • M-mode across the aortic valve. The two continuous solid lines represent the walls of the aorta. With the opening of the aortic valve, a box-like structure appears. The time between the onset of the QRS on ECG and the opening of the aortic valve represents the preejection period (*PEP*).

visualized for Doppler flow measurements. Recently, however, an esophageal probe with a tip-mounted ultrasound crystal has become available for the sampling of blood flow velocity in the descending aorta[33] (Fig. 23–17A–B). Using this instrument, we noted a strong correlation between the maximum blood flow acceleration in the ascending and descending aorta.[34] We further observed that descending aortic blood flow acceleration, adjusted for afterload, contains information on left ventricular performance.

Ejection Phase Indices. Using echocardiography, contractility has been most frequently estimated with ejection phase indices. A wide array of ejection phase indices have been described, but all require that end-diastolic and end-systolic dimensions be measured. In M-mode echocardiography, these dimensions will often be simple linear, internal dimensions of the left ventricular cavity. The ratio of

$$\frac{(LVIDD - LVISD)}{LVIDD}$$

with *LVIDD* representing LV internal diastolic dimension and *LVISD* representing LV internal systolic dimension, will yield fractional shortening, a basic ejection phase index of contractility. Guidelines concerning the measurement of left ventricular internal dimensions have been published by the American Society of Echocardiography, and the interested reader is referred to their publication for specific recommendations.[35] Linear dimensions can also be converted to ventricular volumes. Although a variety of formulae have been proposed for these conversions, the most accurate results have been obtained with Teichholz's formula:[36]

$$V = \frac{(7 \times D^3)}{(2.4 + D)}$$

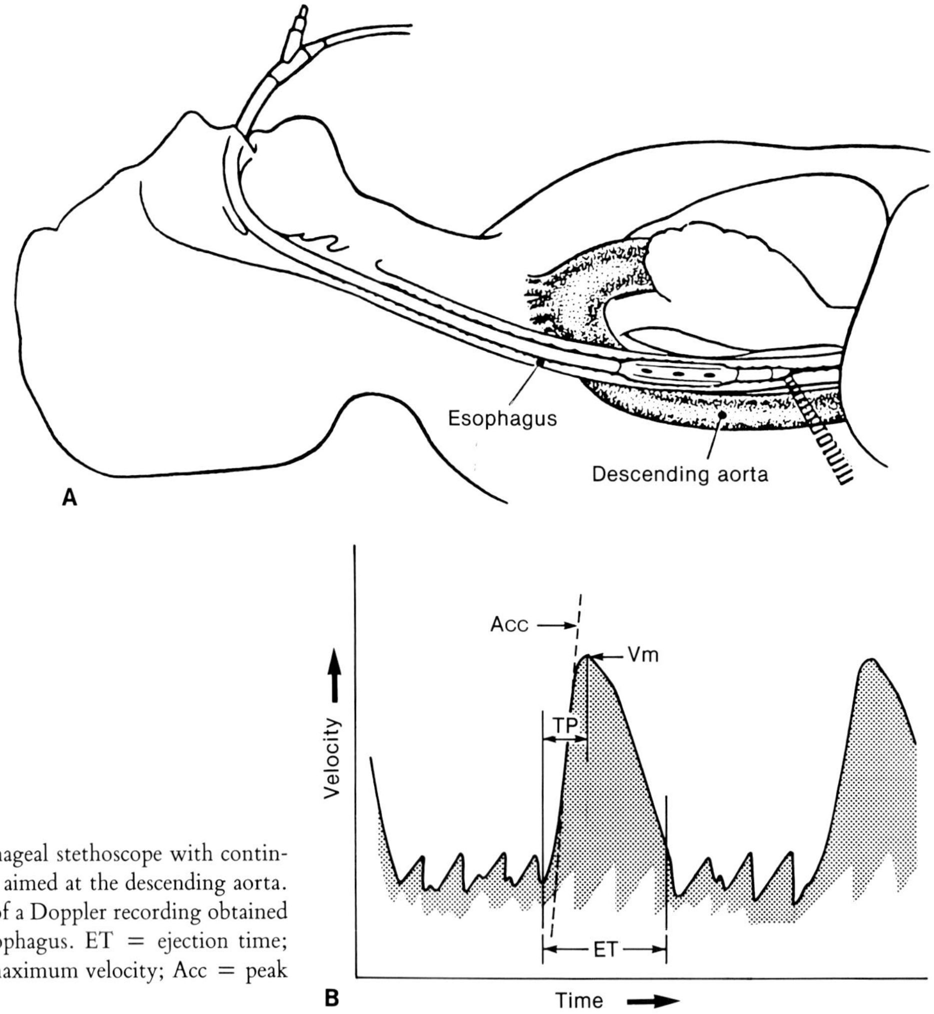

Figure 23–17 • (***A***) Esophageal stethoscope with continuous wave Doppler transducer aimed at the descending aorta. (***B***) Schematic representation of a Doppler recording obtained with the transducer in the esophagus. ET = ejection time; TP = time to peak; Vm = maximum velocity; Acc = peak acceleration.

where D represents a ventricular internal dimension. Even with this formula one must remember, however, that the measured linear dimension may not be representative of the whole ventricle and that the shape of the ventricle may be irregular due to regional wall motion abnormalities. Using the ventricular volumes, ejection fraction can then be calculated with the standard formula:

$$\frac{(LVEDV - LVESV)}{LVEDV}$$

where *LVEDV* is LV end-diastolic volume and *LVESV* is LV end-systolic volume.

In transesophageal echocardiography, one is often limited to a single, short-axis area dimension at the level of the papillary muscles. Once the end-diastolic and end-systolic endocardial areas have been delineated with the help of an electronic plotter, the contractility is estimated with the "fractional area shortening" (FAC) or "ejection fraction area" (EFA):

$$\frac{(LVEDA - LVESA)}{LVEDA}$$

where *LVEDA* represents end-diastolic area and *LVESA* is the end-systolic area. For all quantitative echocardiographic measurements, an average of at least four consecutive contractions is recommended, because considerable beat-to-beat variation is known to occur.

If transthoracic echocardiography is used, accurate ventricular volumes can be obtained by the combination of multiple tomographic cuts across the left ventricle. Whether such a multiplanar approach is necessary or desirable for the intraoperative determination of ventricular performance remains to be established.

End-Systolic Pressure Volume Relationship. Because both the isovolumic and ejection phase indices of contractility are significantly influenced by ventricular loading conditions, the use of load-independent indices has been explored. One such index is the left ventricular end-systolic pressure volume relationship (ESPVR).[37] For its measurement, multiple end-systolic pressures and volumes need to be measured during a rapid and preferably pronounced alteration in left ventricular preload (eg, vena cava occlusion). On a pressure volume diagram, the end-systolic pressure volume points will be positioned on a single line (Fig. 23–18). The slope of this line is relatively independent of loading conditions and proportional to contractility; the steeper the slope, the greater the contractility. The intraoperative determination of contractility by this technique has been hampered by difficulties in obtaining accurate ventricular volumes and pressures. Nonetheless, using single short-axis views and radial arterial pressures, we were able to confirm the linearity of the end-systolic pressure volume relationship and observed that, with the administration of known positive or negative inotropic agents, its slope changed in the predicted direction[38,39] (Fig. 23–19).

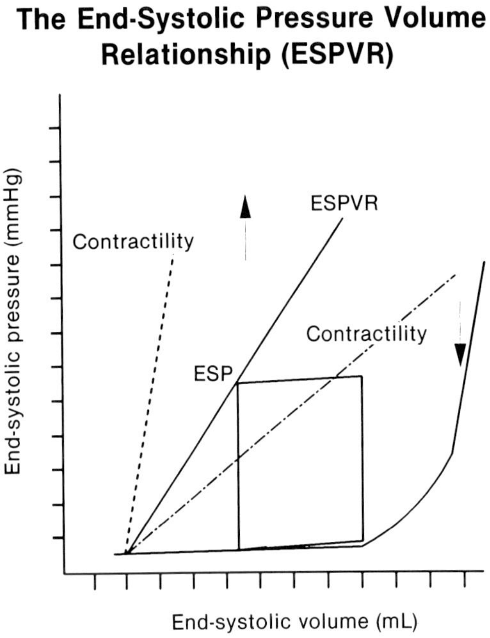

Figure 23–18 • Pressure–volume diagram with one loop representing a single cardiac cycle. ESP indicates the end-systolic point. If multiple ESPs were obtained by rapid preload alteration, they would be positioned on a single line, the end-systolic pressure volume relation (*ESPVR*). The slope of this line is proportional to contractility. It is steeper at higher contractility and flatter at lower contractility.

d. Intraoperative Applications

Differential Diagnosis. The use of intraoperative transesophageal echocardiography has been very beneficial in the differential diagnosis of hemodynamic disturbances. Under those circumstances, a rapid glance at the screen of the echoscanner often helps clarify the most complicated hemodynamic situations. In one report, for instance, Cahalan et al were able to establish that the etiology of a hypotensive episode was hypovolemia although the pulmonary capillary wedge pressure (PCWP) was normal.[40] In our experience, the information provided by 2-D echo has been particularly helpful

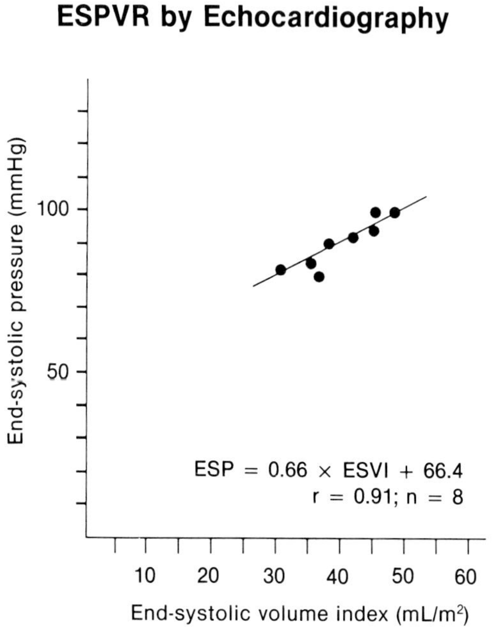

Figure 23–19 • End-systolic pressure volume relationship obtained by intraoperative echocardiography. The end-systolic volumes were calculated from single, short-axis views.

in the management of patients at the completion of cardiopulmonary bypass. At that time, the PCWP does not accurately reflect left ventricular preload, and fluid management or inotrope administration is better guided by 2-D echo information.[22] A fluid challenge may be indicated if a small LV cavity is noted in the presence of systemic hypotension and a low or normal PCWP. A large LV cavity with low ejection and systemic hypotension presents an indication for the administration of an inotrope.

Effect of Interventions. Intraoperative echocardiography has also been used to assess the effects of surgical and anesthetic interventions on global LV ventricular function. Ren et al evaluated the effects of myocardial revascularization or valve replacement on left ventricular function.[41] They noted that patients who underwent valve replacement for regurgitant lesions had a postoperative decrease in left ventricular function. Most patients undergoing myocardial revascularization had no change in LV ejection fraction, but those who suffered perioperative myocardial ischemia presented a significant reduction, from 52 ± 10% to 43 ± 12%. In patients undergoing aortic surgery, Roizen et al observed marked reductions in EFA during aortic cross-clamping, while only minimal changes in cardiac output were noted.[42] Reich et al have studied the effects of changes in the patient's position on left and right ventricular function. After placing patients in the Trendelenburg position, they observed significant changes in right ventricular function with little change in left ventricular function.[43] In other studies, the effects of various respiratory maneuvers, such as the application of PEEP, on ventricular function have been evaluated.[44,45]

Pharmacodynamics. It is not surprising that one of the first studies describing the use of echocardiography in anesthetized patients was a pharmacodynamic study.[46] Indeed, echocardiography appears ideally suited to obtain information on the cardiovascular effects of drugs without the use of invasive monitoring. In this early study, Barash et al studied the effects of halothane on ventricular function in healthy children. Data were obtained prior to the induction of anesthesia and at halothane concentrations ranging from 0.5% to 2.0%. At 2.0% halothane, they noted a 26% reduction in left ventricular ejection fraction. Since then, echocardiography has been used in numerous other studies to evaluate the cardiovascular effects of inhaled anesthetics.[47–49] The results of these studies have sometimes been conflicting.[20]

2. Diastolic Function

In the last 10 years it has been clearly recognized that, in some patients, the signs and symptoms of congestive heart failure are primarily due to diastolic dysfunction.[50–52] In these patients, various degrees of congestive heart failure are observed in the presence of normal or even increased left ventricular systolic function. The techniques most frequently used to assess diastolic function are radionuclide angiography and echocardiography.[53] Transesophageal echocardiography can also be used for the study of left ventricular diastolic function and is particularly well suited for this type of examination because of the close proximity of the esophageal transducer to the left atrium and mitral valve. In addition, with the transesophageal approach the ultrasound beam can easily be emitted in a plane that is nearly parallel to the blood flowing through the mitral valve. As a result of these favorable anatomic considerations, the velocity of mitral blood flow can be measured accurately by transesophageal Doppler echocardiography.

a. Technique and Interpretation

To assess diastolic function, the transesophageal transducer is positioned to obtain a four-chamber view of the heart. The examination begins by evaluating the size of each of the cardiac chambers and gauging the morphology and motion of the mitral valve. In the assessment of the mitral valve, particular attention should be paid to the integrity of the mitral valve apparatus (papillary muscles, chordae tendineae, etc) and to the systolic bulging or prolapse of the mitral valve leaflets into the left atrium. A more extensive assessment of valvular function also includes a Doppler color flow examination of the mitral and aortic valves. If such an examination reveals any suggestion of mitral or aortic regurgitation, the interpretation of the diastolic mitral flow velocity, as an indicator of diastolic ventricular function, must take these abnormal flows into account.

After valvular dysfunction has been excluded, the sample volume of the pulsed Doppler system is placed in the mitral inflow. The best location for the sample volume is in the center of the mitral flow, just slightly to the ventricular side of the mitral valve (see Fig. 23–17A). Flow velocity measured with the sample volume in this location will result in a typical flow velocity pattern (Fig. 23–20). After opening of the mitral valve, the early inflow into the left ventricle will be recognized as a large velocity peak (E peak). It is followed by a period of diastasis and a second, smaller velocity peak (A peak), representing the flow produced by the atrial contraction. Analysis of the diastolic inflow includes the analysis of the general velocity pattern (ratio of the E/A peak), measurement of peak E and A velocity, derivation of acceleration and deceleration for each peak, calculation of various time intervals, and integration of the total area, or parts of the area, under the velocity display (Fig. 23–21).

Velocity Patterns. Deviations from the normal diastolic velocity pattern have been described under various circumstances (Fig. 23–22). With tachycardia, fusion of the E and A peaks occurs while the A peak is absent during atrial fibrillation. In mitral regurgitation, the E peak is much larger than the A peak, and the E peak velocity exceeds values observed in normal people. The diastolic inflow of the patient with mitral stenosis is marked by high E peak velocity, prolonged deceleration from the peak velocity, and continuous flow throughout diastole. The most commonly observed abnormality is a reversal of the E/A ratio, indicating impaired left ventricular filling. Such abnormality has been noted with advanced age, ischemic heart disease, hypertrophic cardiomyopathy, secondary left ventricular hypertrophy, dilated cardiomyopathy, and in patients with right ventricular pressure overload.

E Peak Velocity. Recent animal and human studies have extensively investigated the determinants of E peak velocity. Variables that have been clearly recognized as determinants of E peak velocity include the left atrial V-wave pressure, the left ventricular relaxation rate, and the systemic arterial pressure. The E peak velocity varies directly with increasing left atrial pressure and inversely with increases in the rate of relaxation or

Velocity Across the Mitral Valve

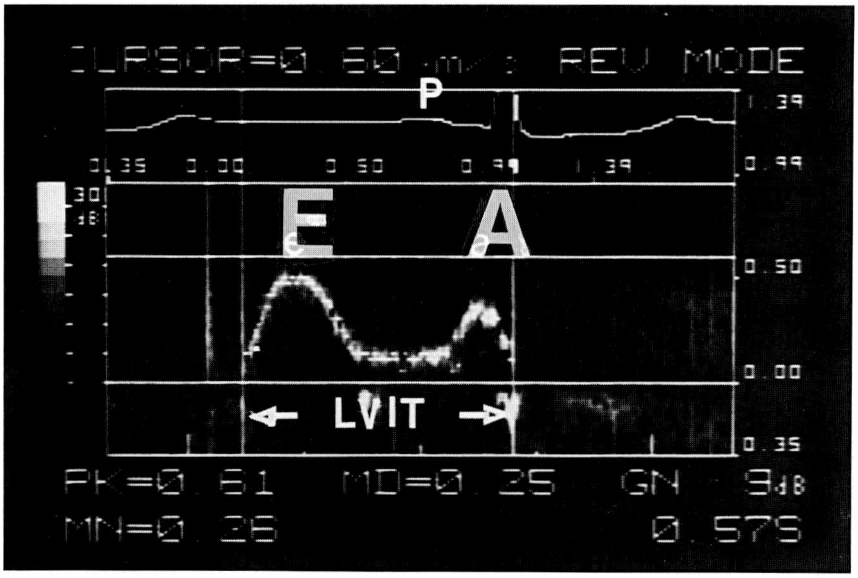

Figure 23–20 • Pulsed-wave Doppler recording obtained at the level of the mitral valve. The horizontal axis is the time axis, while the velocity spectrum is displayed on the vertical axis. The velocity measurements were made with a transesophageal transducer. The flow should thus be away from the transducer and below the baseline, but the image has been inverted electronically. E = early filling peak; A = atrial filling peak; P = p wave on the ECG; LVIT = left ventricular inflow time.

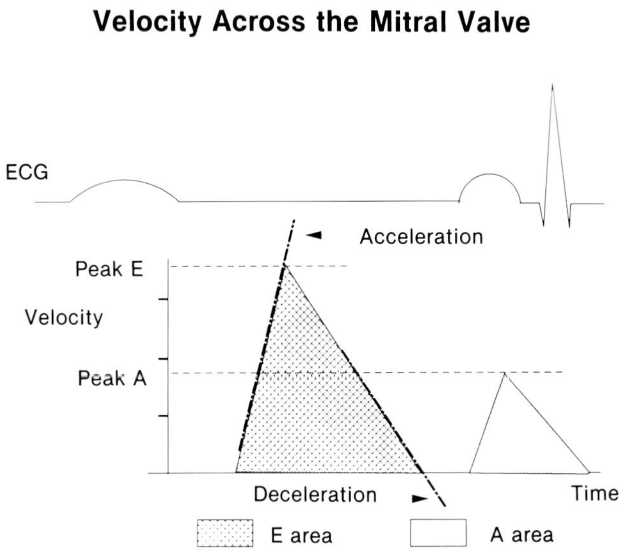

Figure 23–21 • Schematic representation of a Doppler velocity recording at the level of the mitral valve. The E peak corresponds to early ventricular filling, while the A peak represents the flow after atrial contraction.

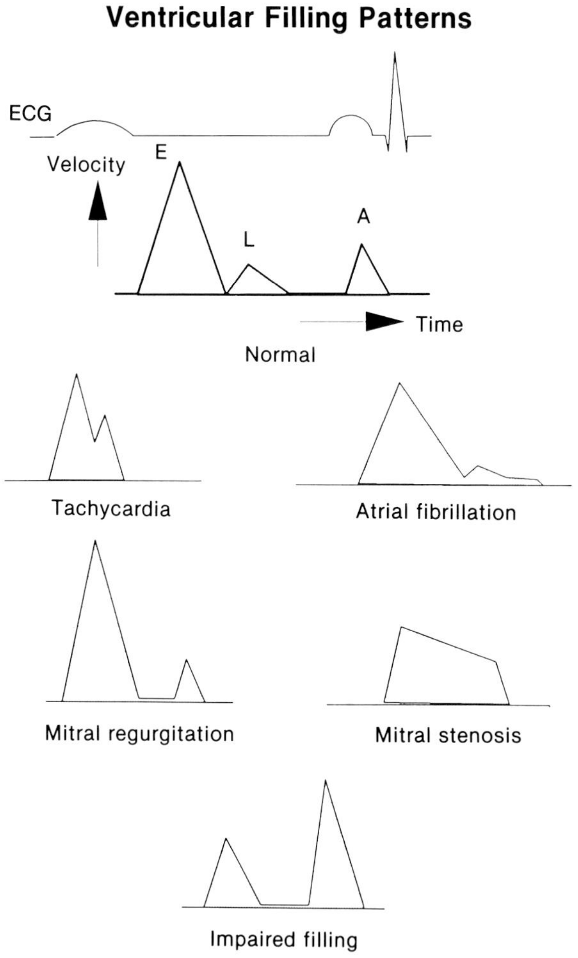

Figure 23–22 • Various ventricular filling patterns (see text).

systemic arterial pressure.[54] Other factors that have not been directly associated with the E peak velocity but are nonetheless important for the onset of diastolic flow encompass the ventricular suction effect and mitral ring recoil. The manner in which all these factors influence E peak velocity is complex and interrelated. Some studies suggest that changes in left atrial pressure have more pronounced effects than changes in left ventricular rate of relaxation. Interpretation of diastolic peak velocity will be further confounded by changes in heart rate.

Acceleration and Deceleration. Acceleration of flow in early diastole is the result of the pressure gradient between the left atrium and the left ventricle, while deceleration coincides with the reversal of the pressure gradient between these chambers.[55] Under normal circumstances, the average forward gradient associated with acceleration is significantly greater than the reverse gradient associated with deceleration. The determinants of E wave deceleration are similar to those of E peak velocity.

Area Integration. Integration of the *total* area under the flow velocity display has been used for the measurement of stroke volume. In the measurement of stroke volume, the flow velocity integral is multiplied with the cross-sectional area of the mitral valve. Various authors have proposed different models for the calculation of mitral valve cross-sectional area.[56,57] Using transesophageal echocardiography, Roewer et al have calculated stroke volume in 27 surgical patients. They obtained the stroke volume by multiplying the mitral flow velocity integral with the cross-sectional area of the mitral valve calculated from the mitral diameter measured at the mitral annulus during mid-diastole. A comparison of Doppler stroke volumes with those obtained by thermodilution yielded an excellent correlation, with a correlation coefficient of 0.951 and a standard error of the estimate of 0.34 L/min^{-1}.[58] However, LaMantia et al, who performed a similar study in 13 cardiac surgical patients, measuring the maximal mitral diameter, only found a modest correlation ($r = 0.68$) and a standard estimate of 0.92 L/min^{-1}.[59] When the results of various studies are compared, it is important to know which velocities (mean, mode, or peak) were selected for the calculation of the flow velocity integral, how the cross-sectional area of the mitral valve was calculated, and where the Doppler sampling volume was located. Because PW Doppler provides a spectral display of instantaneous velocities, different areas will be integrated if peak velocities, mean velocities, or the modes of the velocities are used (see Fig. 23–13). It is also important to know whether the measurement of the mitral orifice diameter was repeated at various cardiac outputs. It has indeed been well established that the size of the mitral orifice varies with varying flows. The importance of the sample volume location was demonstrated in a study by Dittmann et al.[60] They noted that stroke volume was underestimated when the sampling volume was placed at the mitral leaflet tips and overestimated at the mitral annulus.

Integration of *partial* areas under the flow velocity curve has been suggested for the assessment of ventricular diastolic function.[61] Some of the areas that have been studied include the areas for the first 33% of diastole, the first 50% of diastole, the area under the E peak (Ei), and the area under the A peak (Ai). Using the ratio of Ei to Ai, Pearson et al have observed an inverse linear relationship between age and early diastolic filling.[62] This observation suggests that with increasing age, the filling of the left ventricle becomes more dependent on atrial contraction. In children, Snider et al have found that the ratio of the area under the first 33% of diastole over the total area was larger in normal than in hypertensive children.[63] Conversely, the ratio of Ai over total area was larger in the hypertensives.

b. Intraoperative Applications

Diastolic function has been assessed intraoperatively by pulsed Doppler echocardiography in only a few studies. In cardiac surgical patients, we observed that some patients with normal mitral inflow patterns before cardiopulmonary bypass had signs of impaired ventricular filling after bypass.[64] More recently, Rinder et al have reported that diastolic filling was significantly impaired 2 hours after cardiopulmonary bypass. They noted a trend toward recovery by 4 hours, and a return to baseline by 18 hours.[65] Other potential intraoperative applications of the determination of diastolic mitral flow by pulsed Doppler echocardiography include the following:

Determination of Stroke Volume. The usefulness of mitral inflow measurement for the determination of cardiac output has been alluded to in the previous section. Further investigations will be required to define the optimal technique of mitral orifice measurement and to establish whether, in individual patients, changes in stroke volume can be accurately followed with this method.

Assessment of the Atrial Contribution to Stroke Volume. The contribution of the atrial contraction to ventricular filling is ideally studied by the measurement of mitral flow velocity. The area under the A peak will be directly proportional to the portion of the stroke volume contributed by the atrial contraction. In cardiac surgical patients, we have demonstrated that the decrease in cardiac output occurring as a result of the loss of the atrial contraction will be greater in patients with lower Ei/Ai ratio.[66] Others have used pulsed Doppler echocardiography to document increased cardiac output with atrioventricular vs. ventricular pacing, or to optimize atrioventricular delay intervals during atrioventricular sequential pacing.[67–69]

Detection of Ischemia. Because the rate of left ventricular relaxation is an important determinant of early ventricular filling, one would expect that impaired relaxation would result in impaired early ventricular filling. Ventricular relaxation is an energy-requiring process, and one of the early consequences of myocardial ischemia is an impairment in ventricular relaxation. When myocardial ischemia is produced by transient occlusion of a coronary artery, as during angioplasty, the observation of a rapid reduction in E peak velocity is suggestive of impaired relaxation. In one study, diastolic left ventricular dysfunction was the earliest change noted after coronary occlusion, and it often preceded the development of abnormal systolic function.[70] In another study, it was observed that acute ischemia not only altered early ventricular filling but also produced marked abnormalities in late ventricular filling.[71]

B. *Regional Ventricular Function*

Two-dimensional transesophageal echocardiography provides the anesthesiologist with the capability to assess regional myocardial performance intraoperatively. By nature, myocardial performance is regional and inadequate perfusion of the myocardium is, therefore, reflected in regional disturbances of myocardial performance such as regional wall thickening and regional wall motion abnormalities. Laboratory and clinical observation suggest that the assessment of these abnormalities is clinically useful, because they provide early and sensitive indications of ischemia. To clinically gauge regional performance, the motion of the endocardium and thickening of the ventricular wall are assessed in a number of ventricular segments.

On a short-axis view at the level of the papillary muscles, the cavity is usually divided into four segments corresponding to the coronary perfusion beds: the anterior, inferior, lateral, and septal segments. For a complete description of all myocardial wall segments, the reader is referred to the *Report of the American Society of Echocardiography, Committee on Nomenclature and Standards: Identification of Myocardial Segments.*[72] Having identified each of the segments, the systolic endocardial motion is graded as normal, hypokinetic (reduced motion), akinetic (lack of motion), dyskinetic (paradoxical motion), or hyperkinetic (increased motion) (Fig. 23–23). Wall thickening is similarly graded as normal, reduced thickening, absence of thickening, or wall thinning. Using transesophageal echocardiography and such an analysis, Smith et al detected that 24 of 50 high-risk patients developed intraoperative changes consistent with myocardial ischemia, while only six of these patients had ECG evidence of ischemia.[73] They concluded that transesophageal echocardiography was not only more sensitive than ECG in detecting myocardial ischemia, but was also able to diagnose an ischemic episode earlier and to predict the likelihood of progression to myocardial ischemia better. More recently, London et al have studied the natural history of segmental wall motion abnormalities (SWMA) detected intraoperatively.[74] They noted that new SWMA were common in their high-risk population and occurred more frequently than ECG changes. Deterioration of normal segments to akinesis or dyskinesis was less common than to hypokinesis, suggesting that changes in ventricular loading conditions may also have played a role in the genesis of the SWMA.

The influence of changes in loading conditions, specifically regional loading conditions, on regional myocardial performance is an unsettling problem that has not been adequately assessed because of experimental limitations. In a few experiments, however, the important effects of regional loading on regional performance have been documented. In a recent investigation, Goto et al used a highly instrumented, isolated heart model

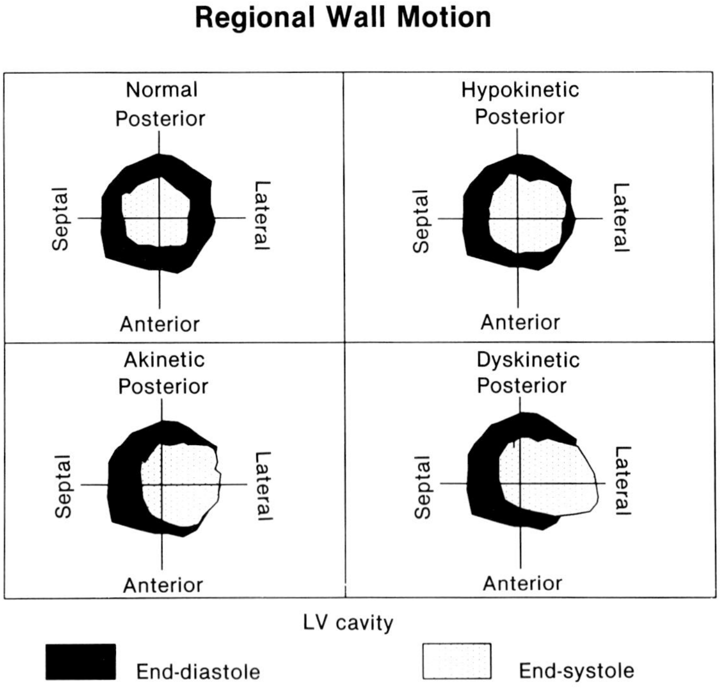

Figure 23–23 • Examples of end-diastolic and end-systolic outlines with normal regional wall motion and lateral hypokinesis, akinesis, and dyskinesis.

to explore whether the hyperkinesis in a nonischemic segment of a regionally ischemic ventricle was due to increased contractility or altered loading.[75] They observed that the essential mechanism for the hyperkinesis was a reduction in regional afterload due to intraventricular mechanical interaction between the ischemic and the nonischemic segments of the ventricle. Although the nonischemic segment showed pronounced hyperkinesis, its contractility was unchanged. Another example of intraventricular mechanical interaction is provided by the observation that nonischemic segments, immediately adjacent to ischemic segments, often display reduced motion due to tethering. Unfortunately, the effects of anesthetic agents on intraventricular mechanical interaction have not been systematically examined, and their contribution to the clinically observed SWMA is currently speculative.

C. *Valvular Function*

With intraoperative echocardiography (epicardial or transesophageal), the aortic and mitral valves can be clearly visualized and, with the use of color flow Doppler, the flow across these valves can be evaluated. It was natural, therefore, that echocardiography be evaluated for the intraoperative assessment of valvular function. The technique was expected to be of greatest benefit in the evaluation of valve repairs. Stewart et al reviewed 150 consecutive patients in whom intraoperative echocardiography had been used to determine the frequency with which the echo information influenced intraoperative decision-making.[76] They found that the echo information led to a change in surgical treatment in 15% of patients. In nine patients, valve replacement was avoided based on the echo information obtained prior to cardiopulmonary bypass. Echo information obtained after cardiopulmonary bypass led to further surgery in 13 patients: in six patients after repair for mitral regurgitation, in five with persistent aortic regurgitation after aortic valve repair, and in two patients with new regional wall motion abnormalities requiring additional coronary bypass grafting. The same group of investigators also compared transesophageal echocardiography with epicardial (from within the chest) echo for the intraoperative assessment of mitral valve repair.[77] They concluded that both techniques were comparable in assessing the severity of mitral regurgitation. The advantages of transesophageal echocardiography were that it did not interfere with surgery and allowed prolonged examinations, but epicardial echo allowed a more complete examination of the valve.

The intraoperative examination of valvular function requires considerable experience and clinical judgment. Anesthesiologists should approach this task with circumspection, because the potential for errors is great and the consequences of such errors could be dire (see "Complications").

D. *Other Considerations*

1. THORACIC AORTIC DISEASE

Because of its posterior location, the thoracic aorta is difficult to image by transthoracic echocardiography. With transesophageal echocardiography, however, most of the thoracic aorta, with the exception of the arch vessels, is easy to visualize. As a result, numerous investigators have explored the use of TEE in the diagnosis of thoracic aortic aneurysms and dissection. Erbel et al have recently reported on the diagnostic accuracy of transesophageal echocardiography for the diagnosis of acute aortic dissection in 164 patients.[78] They found that TEE had a 99% sensitivity and 98% specificity in diagnosing acute aortic dissection. Other investigators have reported similar results, and many experts now consider TEE the diagnostic modality of choice in thoracic aortic pathology.[79-84] Images of the ascending aorta are obtained by advancing the esophageal probe with the ultrasonic array facing anteriorly. To visualize the descending aorta, the transesophageal probe needs to be rotated 180°. In thoracic aneurysms, color flow Doppler will help differentiate the true from the false lumen, while in aortic dissection it may point to the site of an intima tear (see Color Fig. 6).

2. CONTRAST ECHOCARDIOGRAPHY

The ability of echocardiography to detect micron-sized bubbles within the circulation was first reported by Robissow and McKay.[85] They reported that microbubbles developed during decompression sickness could be directly imaged by ultrasound. Microbubbles are detectable because their air–liquid interface results in a large acoustic mismatch and near perfect reflection of ultrasound energy. In contrast echocardiography, the flow and distribution of microbubbles within the circulation are studied.

In clinical practice, contrast echocardiography is used to detect air embolism during cardiac and neurosurgical procedures. Oka et al have reported evidence of intracardiac air in 79% of patients after open cardiotomy vs. in 11% of patients without cardiotomy.[86] Topol et al reported similar findings, but found no association between the intracardiac air and postoperative focal neurologic deficit.[87]

Cucchiara et al have used transesophageal echocardiography in neurosurgical patients undergoing procedures in the sitting position. They reported being able to detect air embolism convincingly in nine of 15 neurosurgical patients using TEE, but only in seven patients using transthoracic Doppler.[88] In addition, they reported detection of paradoxical air embolism to the left heart in one patient without neurologic sequelae. In other applications of contrast echocardiography, contrast is injected into the circulation in an attempt to quantitate ventricular volumes or myocardial perfusion. In a dog model, the analysis of contrast washout curves has been used to obtain ejection fractions, which correlated well with angiographic ejection fractions ($r = 0.87$).[89] To quantitate myocardial blood flow, contrast has been injected in the aortic root or coronary arteries. Digital subtraction echocardiography is then applied to study the distribution of contrast within the myocardium. Time to peak contrast intensity and washout half-life have both been shown to be sensitive indicators of myocardial perfusion.[90,91]

3. Congenital Cardiac Disease

Echocardiography is now an intrinsic part of the diagnostic work-up of a child with congenital heart disease. Currently, many children are referred for corrective surgery on the basis of echo findings without undergoing cardiac catheterization. The use of intraoperative echocardiography has also seen a steady growth in pediatric cardiac surgery. In more than 100 cases, echo provided useful information about intracardiac shunt closure, relief of obstruction, redirection of blood flow, the quality of valve repair, and abnormalities that escaped detection on initial examination.[92,93] Greeley et al have reported on the use of echocardiography in 140 pediatric cardiac surgical patients.[94] They found that in 7% of these patients it significantly altered management. In 18 of their patients, additional repairs of residual defects were performed immediately, based on the intraoperative echo findings. With the recent introduction of pediatric transesophageal echo transducers, this aspect of intraoperative echocardiography should undergo rapid development in the near future.

IV. Complications

Although transesophageal echocardiography has been performed in many thousands of patients to date, it has so far been remarkably free of complications. Potential complications include damage to pharyngeal, laryngeal, esophageal, and gastric structures. Ruptures, tears, and hemorrhage are some of the possible complications. In two patients operated on in the sitting position, vocal cord paresis has been attributed to the use of transesophageal echocardiography.[87]

O'Shea et al have evaluated the safety of transesophageal echo in animals by excising the entire esophagus after continuous TEE use of variable duration.[95] They did not observe any significant mucosal or thermal injury.

An unusual but interesting complication was reported by Humphrey.[96] She described a patient in whom manipulations of the transesophageal transducer led to the undetected displacement of an esophageal stethoscope into the stomach. Only several weeks later was the errant stethoscope discovered and removed endoscopically.

Although the complications related to the mechanical aspects of transesophageal echocardiography fortunately have been very minimal, the complications related to incorrect interpretations have not yet been evaluated, but could be of much greater magnitude.

Anesthesiologists are often asked to make clinical judgments based on the interpretation of echo information. Although we approach this task with enthusiasm, it is worth remembering that most of us have not enjoyed formal training in echocardiography and are unable to dedicate our entire clinical practice to this field. In addition, some of the echo techniques are very new, not always fully understood, and not yet buttressed by large bodies of accumulated experience. The recent findings of Yoshida et al highlight the difficulties that one might encounter in the assessment of valvular function with color flow Doppler and suggest that the limits of normality may need to be redefined.[16] These investigators examined valvular function with transthoracic color flow Doppler in 211 apparently healthy volunteers. In their normal subjects, the prevalence rate of mitral regurgitation was 38% to 45%; of tricuspid regurgitation, 15% to 77%; and of pulmonary regurgitation, 28% to 88%. Regurgitant flow signals were never detected at the aortic valve. In an accompanying editorial, Sahn and Maciel discussed the clinical implications of these observations.[97] They also indicated that the esophageal echo window significantly increases the sensitivity of Doppler color flow for intracardiac flow events. If transesophageal echocardiography were used as a gold standard, the incidence of detectable valve regurgitation in healthy subjects would be substantially higher.

V. References

1. Hillel Z, Mikula S, Thys DM. The current state of intraoperative echocardiography in North America: Results of a survey. J Cardiothoracic Anesth 2:803–511, 1988.
2. Daniel WG, Mgge A, Schröder E, et al. Transesophageal echocardiography in clinical cardiology—indications, practicability, and risks. Circulation 78:II-227, 1988.
3. Thys DM, Hillel Z, Konstadt SN, Goldman M., et al. Intraoperative echocardiography. In Kaplan JA (ed). Cardiac Anesthesia. 2nd ed. Orlando, Grune & Stratton, 1987.
4. Hatle L, Angelsen B. Doppler Ultrasound in Cardiology. 2nd ed. Philadelphia, Lea & Febiger, 1984.
5. Kisslo J, Adams D, Mark DB. Basic Doppler Echocardiography. New York, Churchill Livingstone, 1986.
6. Kisslo J, Adams DB, Belkin RN. Doppler Color Flow Imaging. New York, Churchill Livingstone, 1988.
7. Keusch D, Hillel Z. Mitral valve prolapse: Anesthetic considerations. In Eisenkraft JB (ed). Progress in Anesthesiology. San Antonio, Texas, Dannemiller Memorial Education Foundation, 1987.
8. Seward JB, Khandheira BK, Oh JK, et al. Transesophageal echocardiography: Technique, anatomic correlations, implementation and clinical applications. Mayo Clin Proc 63:649, 1988.
9. Brown RE. Ultrasonography. St. Louis, WH Green, 1975.
10. Feigenbaum H. Echocardiography. 4th ed. Philadelphia, Lea & Febiger, 1986, 621–334 (Appendix A–D).
11. Feigenbaum H. Echocardiography. 4th ed. Philadelphia, Lea & Febiger, 1986.
12. Feigenbaum H. Echocardiography. 4th ed. Philadelphia, Lea & Febiger, 1986, 637–639 (Appendix F).
13. Mark JB, Steinbrook RA, Gugino LD, et al. Continuous noninvasive monitoring of cardiac output with esophageal Doppler ultrasound during cardiac surgery. Anesth Analg 65:1013–720, 1986.
14. Thys D, Hillel Z. Can the K-Factor be a source of inaccuracy in the determination of esophageal cardiac output? Anesthesiology 69: A239, 1988.
15. Czer LSC, Maurer G, Bolger AF, et al. Intraoperative evaluation of mitral regurgitation by Doppler color flow mapping. Circulation 76 (suppl III):III-98, 1987.
16. Yoshida K, Yoshikawa J, Shakudo M, et al. Color Doppler evaluation of valvular regurgitation in normal subjects. Circulation 78:840–847, 1988.
17. Miyatake K, Izumi S, Okamoto M, et al. Semi-quantitative grading of severity of mitral regurgitation by real-time two-dimensional Doppler flow imaging technique. J Am Coll Cardiol 7:82, 1986.
18. Helmcke F, Nanda NC, Hsiung MC, et al. Color Doppler assessment of mitral regurgitation with orthogonal planes. Circulation 75:175, 1987.
19. Davidoff R, Wilkins GT, Thomas JD, et al. Regurgitant volumes by color flow overestimate injected volumes in an in vitro flow model. J Am Coll Cardiol 9:110A, 1987.
20. Thys D, Hillel Z. Difference between M-mode and two dimensional echocardiography. Anesthesiology 68:645–646, 1988.
21. Clements FM, Harpole D, Quill T, et al. Simultaneous measurements of cardiac volumes, areas and ejection fractions by transesophageal echocardiography and first pass radionuclide angiography. Anesthesiology 69:A4, 1988.
22. Thys DM, Hillel Z, Goldman ME, et al. A comparison of hemodynamic indices by invasive monitoring and two-dimensional echocardiography. Anesthesiology 67:630–634, 1987.
23. Reichek N, Wilson J, St John Sutton M, et al. Noninvasive determination of left ventricular end-systolic stress: Validation of the method and initial application. Circulation 65:99, 1982.
24. Sandler H, Dodge HT. Left ventricular tension and stress in man. Circ Res 13:91, 1963.
25. Hartford M, Wilstand JCM, Wallentin I, et al. Left ventricular wall stress and systolic function in untreated primary hypertension. Hypertension 7:97, 1985.
26. Lang RL, Borow KM, Newman A, et al. Systemic vascular resistance: An unreliable index of afterload. Circulation 74:1114, 1986.
27. Weissler AM. Systolic time intervals. N Engl J Med 296:321, 1977.
28. Lewis RP, Rittgers SE, Forester WF, et al. A critical review of the systolic time intervals. Circulation 56:146, 1977.
29. Noble MIM, Trenchard D, Guz A. Left ventricular ejection in conscious dogs: 1. Measurement and significance of the maximum acceleration of blood from the left ventricle. Circ Res 19:139, 1966.
30. Bennett ED, Else W, Miller GAH, et al. Maximum acceleration of blood from the left ventricle in patients with ischaemic heart disease. Clin Sci 46:49, 1974.
31. Mehta N, Bennett DE. Impaired left ventricular function in acute myocardial infarction assessed by Doppler measurement of ascending aortic blood velocity and maximum acceleration. Am J Cardiol 57:1052, 1986.
32. Sabbah HN, Khaja F, Brymer JF, et al. Noninvasive evaluation of left ventricular performance based on peak aortic blood acceleration measured with a continuous-wave Doppler velocity meter. Circulation 74:323, 1986.
33. Freund PR. Transesophageal Doppler scanning versus thermodilution during general anesthesia. Am J Surg 153:490, 1987.
34. Thys DM, Hillel Z. Left ventricular performance indices by transesophageal Doppler. Anesthesiology 69:728, 1988.
35. Sahn DJ, DeMaria A, Kisslo J, et al. Recommendations regarding quantitation in M-mode echocardiography: Results of a survey of echocardiographic measurements. Circulation 58:1072, 1978.
36. Teichholz LE, Kreulen T, Herman MV, et al. Problems in echocardiographic volume determinations: Echocardiographicangiographic correlations in the presence and absence of asynergy. Am J Cardiol 37:7, 1976.
37. Suga H, Sagawa K. Instantaneous pressure-volume relationships and their ratio in the excised, supported canine left ventricle. Circ Res 35:117–106, 1974.
38. Hillel Z, Thys DM, Mindich BP, et al. A new method for the

intraoperative determination of contractility. Anesth Analg 65:S72, 1986.
39. Hillel Z, Thys DM, Mindich BP, et al. Intraoperative measurement of the effects of dopamine on left ventricular contractility. Anesthesiology 63:A25, 1985.
40. Cahalan M, Kremer P, Schiller N, et al. Intraoperative monitoring with two-dimensional transesophageal echocardiography. Anesthesiology 57:A153, 1982.
41. Ren JF, Panidis IP, Kotler MN, et al. Effect of coronary bypass surgery and valve replacement on left ventricular function: Assessment by intraoperative two-dimensional echocardiography. Am Heart J 109:281, 1985
42. Roizen M, Beaupre P, Alpert R, et al. Monitoring with two-dimensional transesophageal echocardiography. Comparison of myocardial function in patients undergoing supraceliac, suprarenal-infraceliac, or infrarenal aortic occlusion. J Vasc Surg 1:300, 1984.
43. Reich DL, Konstadt SN, Raissi S, et al. The Trendelenburg position and passive leg raising do not significantly improve cardiac performance. Crit Care Med 17:xxx, 1989.
44. Terai C, Venishi M, Sugimoto H, et al. Transesophageal echocardiographic dimensional analysis of four cardiac chambers during positive end-expiratory pressure. Anesthesiology 63:640, 1985.
45. Koolen J, Visser C, Wever E, et al. Transesophageal two-dimensional echocardiographic evaluation of biventricular dimension on function during positive end-expiratory pressure ventilation after coronary artery bypass grafting. Am J Cardiol 59:1047, 1987.
46. Barash P, Glanz S, Katz J, et al. Ventricular function in children during halothane anesthesia: An echocardiographic evaluation. Anesthesiology 49:79, 1978.
47. Rathod R, Jacobs H, Kramer N, et al. Echocardiographic assessment of ventricular performance following induction with two anesthetics. Anesthesiology 49:86, 1978.
48. Wolf WJ, Neal MB, Peterson MD. The hemodynamic and cardiovascular effects of isoflurane and halothane anesthesia in children. Anesthesiology 64:328, 1986.
49. Murray D, Vandewalker G, Matherne GP, et al. Pulsed Doppler and two-dimensional echocardiography: Comparison of halothane and isoflurane on cardiac functions in infants and small children. Anesthesiology 67:211, 1987.
50. Dodek A, Kassenbaum DG, Bristow JD. Pulmonary edema in coronary artery disease without cardiomegaly. N Engl J Med 25:1347, 1972.
51. Dougherty AM, Naccarelli GV, Gray EL, Hicks CH, et al. Congestive heart failure with normal systolic function. Am J Cardiol 54:778, 1984.
52. Topol EJ, Traill TA, Fortuin NJ. Hypertensive hypertrophic cardiomyopathy of the elderly. N Engl J Med 312:277, 1985.
53. Labovitz AJ, Pearson AC. Evaluation of left ventricular diastolic function: Clinical relevance and recent Doppler echocardiographic insights. Am Heart J 114:836, 1987.
54. Choong CY, Abascal V, Thomas JD, et al. Combined influence of ventricular loading and relaxation on the transmitral flow velocity profile in dogs measured by Doppler echocardiography. Circulation 78:672–683, 1988.
55. Courtois M, Kovacs SJ, Ludbrook PA. Transmitral pressure-flow velocity relation. Circulation 78:661–671, 1988.
56. Fisher DC, Sahn DJ, Allen HD, et al. The mitral valve orifice method for noninvasive two-dimensional echo Doppler determinations of cardiac output. Circulation 67:872–877, 1983.
57. Lewis JF, Kuo LC, Nelson JG, et al. Pulsed Doppler echocardiographic determination of stroke volume and cardiac output: Clinical validation of two new methods using the apical window. Circulation 70:425–431, 1984.
58. Roewer N, Bednarz F, Dziadka A, Schulte am Esch J. Intraoperative cardiac output determination from transmitral and pulmonary blood flow measurements using transesophageal pulsed Doppler. Anesthesiology 67:A639, 1987
59. LaMantia K, Harris S, Mortimore K, Davis E, et al. Transesophageal pulse-wave Doppler assessment of cardiac output. Anesthesiology 69:A1, 1988.
60. Dittman H, Voelker W, Karsch KR, et al. Influence of the sampling site and flow area on cardiac output measurements by Doppler echocardiography. J Am Coll Cardiol 10:818–823, 1987.
61. Kuo LC, Quinones MA, Rokey R, et al. Quantification of atrial contribution to left ventricular filling by pulsed Doppler echocardiography and the effect of age in the normal and diseased hearts. Am J Cardiol 59:1174–878, 1987.
62. Pearson AC, Labovitz AJ, Mrosek D, Williams GA, et al. Assessment of diastolic function in normal and hypertrophied hearts: Comparison of Doppler echocardiography and M-mode echocardiography. Am Heart J 113:1417–18, 1987.
63. Snider AR, Gidding SS, Rocchini AP, et al. Doppler evaluation of left ventricular diastolic filling in children with systemic hypertension. Am J Cardiol 56:921–626, 1985.
64. Thys DM, Hillel Z, Konstadt S, et al. The intraoperative evaluation of left ventricular filling by esophageal Doppler echocardiography. Proceedings of the 8th Annual Meeting of the Society of Cardiovascular Anesthesiologists, Montreal, Canada, 1986, 80.
65. Rinder CS, Wheeler LR, Alpern WD. Pulsed Doppler assessment of diastolic function before and after cardiopulmonary bypass. Anesthesiology 69:A2, 1988.
66. Konstadt S, Reich D, Thys D, et al. Predicting the hemodynamic response to ventricular pacing with pulsed Doppler echocardiography. Scientific Abstracts. Society of Cardiovascular Anesthesia, 1989.
67. Stewart WJ, Dicola VC, Harthorne W, et al. Doppler ultrasound measurement of cardiac output in patients with physiologic pacemakers. Am J Cardiol 54:308, 1984.
68. Haskell RJ, French WJ. Optimum Av interval in dual chamber pacemakers. PACE 9:670, 1986.
69. Pearson AC, Janosik DL, Redd RM, et al. Prediction of hemodynamic benefit of physiologic pacing from baseline Doppler-echocardiographic parameters. PACE 10:127A, 1987.
70. Labovitz AJ, Lewen MK, Kern M, et al. Evaluation of left ventricular systolic and diastolic dysfunction during transient myocardial ischemia produced by angioplasty. J Am Coll Cardiol 10:748–455, 1987.
71. Bowman LK, Cleman MW, Cabin HS, et al. Dynamics of early and late left ventricular filling determined by Doppler two-dimensional echocardiography during percutaneous transluminal coronary angioplasty. Am J Cardiol 61:541–545, 1988.
72. Henry WL, DeMaria A, Feigenbaum H, et al. Report of the American Society of Echocardiography Committee on Nomenclature and Standards: Identification of Myocardial Wall Segments. Raleigh, NC, American Society of Echocardiography, 1982.
73. Smith J, Cahalan M, Benefiel D, et al. Intraoperative detection of myocardial ischemia in high risk patients: Electrocardiography versus two-dimensional transesophageal echocardiography. Circulation 72:1015, 1985.
74. London MJ, Tubau JF, Wong MG, et al. The natural history''

of segmental wall motion abnormalities detected by intraoperative transesophageal echocardiography: A clinically blinded, prospective approach. Anesthesiology 69:A7, 1988.
75. Goto Y, Igarashi Y, Yamada O, et al. Hyperkinesis without the Frank-Starling mechanism in a non-ischemic region of acutely ischemic excised canine heart. Circulation 77:468, 1988.
76. Stewart WJ, Currie PJ, Lytle BW, et al. The role of intraoperative echocardiography during cardiac valvular surgery. J Am Coll Cardiol 11:217A, 1988.
77. Currie PJ, Stewart WJ, Salcedo EE, et al. Comparison of intraoperative transesophageal and epicardial color flow Doppler in mitral valve repair. J Am Coll Cardiol 11:20A, 1988.
78. Erbel R, Rennollet H, Engberding R, et al. Detection of aortic dissection by transesophageal echocardiography. A multi-center cooperative study. Circulation 78:II-297, 1988.
79. Mohr-Kahaly S, Erbel R, Steller D, et al. Aortic dissection detected by transesophageal echocardiography. Int J Card Imaging 2:31, 1987.
80. Borner N, Erbel R, Braun B, et al. Diagnosis of aortic dissection by transesophageal echocardiography. Am J Cardiol 54:1157, 1984.
81. Mohr-Kahaly S, Rennollet H, Wittlich N, et al. Follow-up of aortic dissection by transesophageal color Doppler echocardiography. Circulation 76:IV-3s7, 1987.
82. Gussenhoven EJ, Taams MA, De Jong N, et al. Transesophageal echo in the diagnosis of thoracic aortic pathology. Circulation 78:II-298, 1988.
83. Chan KL. Aortic disease in suspected aortic dissection—a transesophageal echo study. Circulation 78:II-298, 1988.
84. Freeman WK, Khanderia BK, Oh JK, et al. Thoracic aortic pathology by transesophageal echocardiography. Circulation 78:II-298, 1988.
85. Robissow GJ, McKay RS. Ultrasonic imaging of in vivo bubbles in decompression sickness. Ultrasonics 9:225, 1971.
86. Oka Y, Boriwaki K, Hong Y, et al. Detection of air emboli in the left heart by M-mode transesophageal echocardiography following cardiopulmonary bypass. Anesthesiology 63:109, 1985.
87. Topol EH, Humphrey LS, Bashan M, et al. Value of intraoperative left ventricular microbubbles detected by transesophageal two-dimensional echocardiography in predicting neurologic outcome after cardiac operations. Am J Cardiol 56:773, 1985.
88. Cucchiara RF, Nugent M, Seward JB, et al. Air embolism in upright neurosurgical patients: Detection and localization by two-dimensional transesophageal echocardiograhy. Anesthesiology 60:353, 1984.
89. Rovai D, Nissen S, Elion J, et al. Contrast echo washout curves from the left ventricle: Application of basic principles of indicator-dilution theory and calculation of ejection fraction. J Am Coll Cardiol 10:125, 1987.
90. Rovai D, Lombardi M, Ferdeghini E, et al. Color-coded functional imaging of myocardial perfusion by contrast echocardiography. Circulation 76:IV-504, 1987.
91. Zotz R, Kann B, Brennecke R. Evaluation of PTCA by videointensitometric analysis of contrast echocardiograms. Circulation 76:IV-505, 1987.
92. Maurer G, Czer L, Bolger A, et al. Intraoperative color Doppler flow mapping for repair of congenital hearth disease. Circulation 74:II-37, 1986.
93. Hagler DJ, Seward JB, Tajik J, et al. Intraoperative two-dimensional color flow imaging. Circulation 74:II-36, 1986.
94. Greeley WJ, Ungerleider RM, Stanley T, et al. Intraoperative echocardiography and color flow imaging during pediatric cardiovascular anesthesia and surgery. Anesthesiology 69:A778, 1988.
95. O'Shea J, D'Ambra M, Magro C, et al. Transesophageal echocardiography: Is it safe to the esophagus? An in vivo study. Circulation 78:II-1656, 1988.
96. Humphrey LS. Esophageal stethoscope loss complicating transesophageal echocardiography J Cardiothoracic Anesth 2:356, 1988.
97. Sahn DJ, Maciel BC. Physiological valvular regurgitation: Doppler echocardiography and the potential for iatrogenic heart disease. Circulation 78:1075-1077, 1988.

Chapter 24

Edward A. Meathe, MS

Determination of Cardiac Output

OUTLINE

I. INTRODUCTION

The monitoring of heart rate and vascular pressure provides information for assessing the performance of the cardiovascular system. If a more comprehensive assessment is required, cardiac output is also monitored. The classic means of measuring cardiac output is the *indicator dilution method.* Clinically, this method involves the injection into the vascular system of a known amount of a suitable indicator, the passage of that indicator through a mixing chamber, and its subsequent detection and quantification at a downstream site. The injection site is usually a central venous location, often the right atrium. The mixing chamber is the right ventricle. Detection of the diluted indicator is done either in the pulmonary artery or at a systemic arterial site. Two indicator substances, indocyanine green dye (dye dilution) and cold fluid (thermodilution), are in common use, with thermodilution as the dominant technique. Recently, the use of ultrasonic Doppler techniques to continuously measure blood velocity has become available to the clinician. Doppler systems rely on sophisticated electronic processing of ultrasonic signals to measure vessel diameter and the velocity profile across that vessel. Integration of this profile over a cardiac cycle provides an indication of stroke volume. As the cost of using these new continuous techniques declines, the single–time-point assessment of cardiac output using an indicator dilution technique may be replaced by the continuous measurement of blood flow.

II. HOW TO DO THE PROCEDURES

A. *Green Dye*

The earlier of the two indicator dilution techniques mentioned, the *green dye method* usually involves the injection of 2 mL of indocyanine green dye into the central venous circulation. After mixing in the ventricles, it is detected and quantified at an arterial site. Detection is accomplished by continuously withdrawing blood from the artery through a densitometer, which measures the change in the optical density of the blood at a wavelength specific to the dye. The preparation for this procedure is as follows:

1. Mix the green dye powder with its diluent to achieve a concentration of 2.5 mg/mL.
2. Draw the dye to be used for the output determination into a 2-mL glass syringe; use 2 mL for an adult patient and 1 mL for a child.
3. Draw 10 mL of saline flush solution into a 12-mL syringe. Connect this syringe to one port of a three-way stopcock. Connect the syringe containing the dye to the other port of the stopcock. Adjust the rotor of the stopcock so that all ports are occluded. Shield the syringes from ambient light until ready for use. The dye solution should be used within 10 hours of preparation.
4. Configure the densitometer according to the manufacturer's instructions, indicating the amount of dye to be injected. Connect a syringe pump so that arterial blood can be withdrawn through the densitometer's cuvette. Place a 60-mL syringe in the syringe pump. Connect a stopcock, a 4-foot pressure tube, and a final stopcock to the syringe (in that order). Coat the barrel of the syringe, and fill the pressure tubing with heparinized saline (1–3 units/mL). Place a sterile cap on the distal port of the pressure tubing until ready to connect to the intraarterial line.
5. Connect the male port of the stopcock attached to the dye syringe to the central venous pressure (CVP) catheter port. The distal port of this catheter should be located in the proximity of the right atrium.
6. Connect the distal end of the tubing attached to the syringe pump to the intraarterial line. Fill the tubing with arterial blood.
7. Begin the continuous withdrawal of arterial blood through the densitometer at a rate of approximately 40 mL/min for adults or 25 mL/min for children. When blood is flowing through the cuvette, adjust the densitometer's output to zero. This is usually accomplished by depressing a switch.
8. Adjust the rotor of the stopcock attached to the syringe of dye so that the dye may be injected into the CVP catheter. Rapidly inject the dye. *Immediately* after the dye has been injected, adjust the stopcock to open the syringe of flush solution to the patient, and rapidly flush the dye into the circulation.
9. Observe the output of the densitometer. A concentration curve characteristic of indicator dilution should be inscribed: A rapid rise in concentration should be followed by an exponential decay not returning completely to the original baseline, and by a second shallow rise indicative of recirculation. When the digital display of the densitometer indicates that a cardiac output has been calculated, stop the syringe pump and infuse the blood just withdrawn. Record the cardiac output.
10. Following the same procedure, a second output determination should be made. The two values should be averaged to arrive at the final value of cardiac output.

B. *Thermodilution*

The most common technique used to determine cardiac output is *thermodilution.* This technique is based on the temperature change resulting from the dilution of a liquid at one temperature (the indicator) by a liquid at a higher temperature (the blood). To accomplish this, a Swan-Ganz catheter is inserted into the central circulation so that the proximal port is in the right atrium, and the catheter thermistor is in the pulmonary artery (Fig. 24–1). A known volume of solution, at a known temperature, is injected into the right atrium via the right atrial (RA) port. The indicator solution mixes with the blood in the right ventricle before being ejected into the pulmonary artery, where the resulting fall in blood temperature is measured by the thermistor, which is integrated into the wall of the catheter.

The injectate solution may be 5% dextrose in water or normal saline. The temperature of the injectate may be either held at room temperature or cooled to approximately 0° C. A typical cold injectate system is shown in Fig. 24–2. A bag of sterile injectate solution is connected to a length of delivery tubing. A section of this tubing is coiled and should be placed in an insulated container of crushed ice and water. The remaining length of tubing terminates at a one-way check valve. A 10-mL syringe is attached to the valve, along with a flow-through housing (used to monitor the temperature of the injectate) and a three-way stopcock. The stopcock is inserted into the proximal port of the Swan-Ganz catheter. The third port of the three-way stopcock is used to monitor the central venous pressure (right atrial pressure). After the tubing is assembled, it should be completely filled with injectate solution, taking care to eliminate all air bubbles. A temperature probe is inserted into the flow-through housing and then connected to

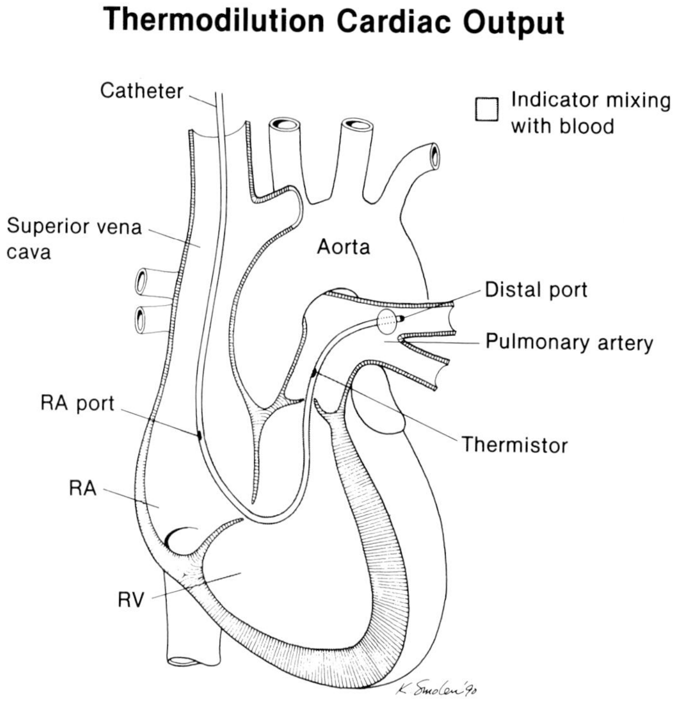

Figure 24–1 • To perform thermodilution cardiac output measurements, a Swan-Ganz catheter is first advanced into the central circulation. When properly positioned, the distal port is in one of the branches of the pulmonary artery and the catheter thermistor is located in or near the main pulmonary artery. The proximal port (*RA port*) is located in the right atrium. The indicator is injected through the RA port. After injection, the indicator moves from the right atrium into the right ventricle, where it is mixed with the patient's blood (*shaded area*). It then flows into the pulmonary artery, where the decrease in temperature is monitored by the thermistor.

the cardiac output computer. The thermistor located in the catheter is also connected to the computer. If room-temperature injectate is to be used, the delivery system is simplified by the removal of the cooling coil and the elimination of the need for an ice bucket. The following procedure may then be used when making a cardiac output determination:

1. Enter the appropriate computation constant into the cardiac output computer. Follow the manufacturer's recommendations when selecting this constant.
2. Verify that the distal port of the Swan-Ganz catheter is located in the pulmonary artery. A pulmonary artery pressure waveform from the transducer/monitor system connected to the distal port will validate the location.
3. Verify that the proximal port is located in or near the right atrium. A pressure that has a central venous contour, rising with a mechanical breath or falling with a spontaneous breath, and a value appropriate for this location are sufficient.
4. Verify the integrity of the catheter thermistor and its connections to the computer by monitoring the patient's blood temperature using the computer system. If an inappropriate value, or no value, is displayed, the thermistor and its connections must be checked.
5. If the proximal port is being used to infuse any drug, aspirate the solution from the catheter. This will avoid the potential of a bolus infusion of the drug during the cardiac output determination.
6. Turn off, if possible, any high-flow-rate infusions. This eliminates their effect as an additional indicator in the output determination. If a side-port introducer was used to insert the Swan-Ganz catheter, occlude the port during this procedure.
7. Adjust the three-way stopcock attached to the proximal port of the Swan-Ganz catheter so that the injectate system is in communication with the right atrium.
8. Without activating the computer, aspirate approximately 10 mL of injectate solution into the syringe connected to the injectate delivery system. Rapidly inject the solution into the patient. This will purge the warm fluid from the catheter and thus insure greater uniformity of the subsequent determinations. This does not need to be done when room-temperature injectate is used.
9. Aspirate the desired volume of injectate into the syringe, press the start button on the computer, and immediately and smoothly inject the contents of the syringe into the patient. The entire volume should be delivered at a rate equal to or greater than 10 mL in 4 seconds.
10. When the acquisition of the thermodilution curve and the calculation of the cardiac output are complete, the computer will display the cardiac output value. The contour of the thermodilution curve should be reviewed to determine its acceptability.

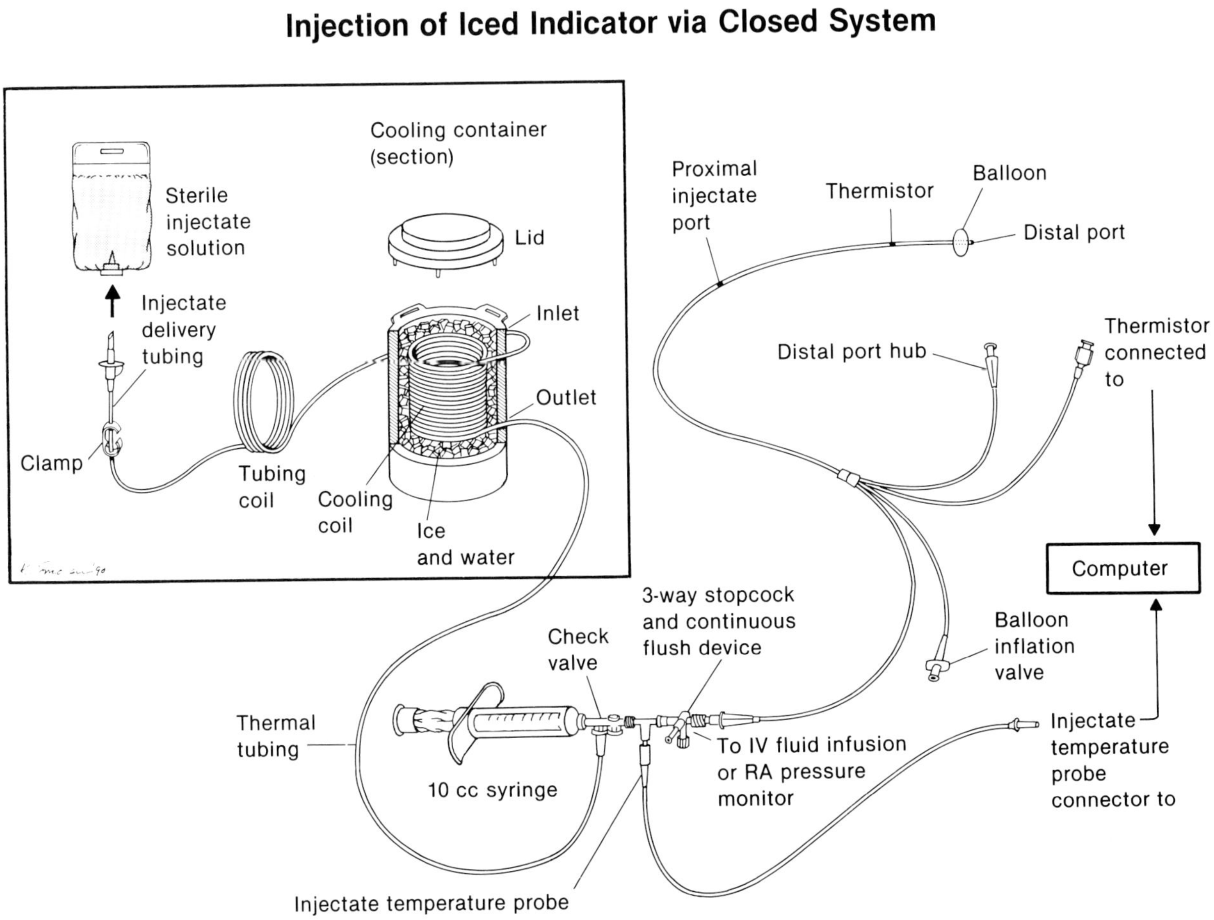

Figure 24–2 • This diagram represents a closed injectate delivery system for the administration of a cold indicator. The sterile indicator solution is contained in the bag shown on the left. A continuous length of tubing transports the indicator to the patient. A length of this tubing is coiled in a mixture of ice and water stored in an insulated container. This cools the injectate to between 0° and 4° C. When it is time to determine cardiac output, 10 mL of indicator is drawn into the syringe and injected into the patient through the proximal port of the catheter. A check valve at the syringe blocks indicator from passing back into the delivery system during injection. Injectate temperature is measured using a temperature probe inserted into the flow-through housing distal to the syringe.

If additional determinations of cardiac output are desired, they should follow as soon as possible after the previous determination. When the sequence of determinations is complete, all system connections and infusions should be returned to their original predetermination settings.

III. Discussion of the Procedures

A. *Green Dye*

A typical green dye indicator dilution curve is shown in Fig. 24–3. It is characterized by a rapid upswing in the concentration curve, followed by an exponential decrease in concentration until recirculation occurs. The curve then begins to rise again, but only slightly. The computer determines the cardiac output using the following formula:

$$CO = \frac{I \times 60}{C \times T}$$

where CO = cardiac output (L/min); I = amount of indicator injected (mg); 60 = seconds in one minute; C = average concentration of indicator occurring at the sampling site as a result of the initial injection (ignoring the recirculation); and T = time (sec).

Thus, the output computer must not only monitor the concentration of dye in the arterial blood being

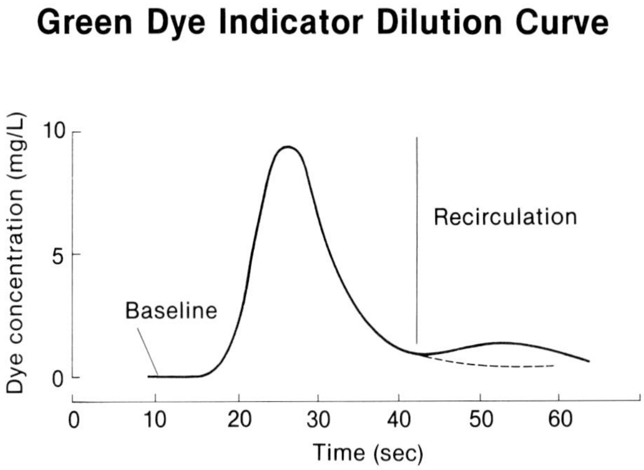

Figure 24–3 • This figure represents a normal green dye indicator dilution curve. Arterial blood is drawn through a cuvette, which measures the concentration of dye in the blood. The concentration rises rapidly to a peak and then begins an exponential decline to the baseline value. However, recirculation of the dye prevents the curve from returning to baseline. The cardiac output is determined by calculating the area under the curve produced by the initial dye injection (recirculation must be ignored).

drawn through its cuvette; it must also integrate the area under the curve up to a point on the downslope where recirculation begins. It must then extrapolate the remainder of the curve, determine the area under this section, and add it to the area determined up to the point where recirculation began. Any situation that distorts the shape of the concentration curve may compromise the accuracy of the determination. A right-to-left shunt at the level of either the atria or the ventricle would produce a curve with two peaks. A left-to-right shunt would prolong the downslope of the curve and produce an inaccurate cardiac output value. An incompetent cardiac valve would produce a similar effect. It is imperative, then, that the contour of the curve be assessed after each output determination. If it deviates from the typical curve, the result of that determination should be suspect, and the source of the error identified.

B. *Thermodilution*

As with the dye dilution technique of cardiac output determination, the thermodilution technique produces a characteristic indicator dilution curve (Fig. 24–4). It begins with a rapid decrease in temperature, usually manifested as a rising curve, followed by an exponential decay to the predetermination (baseline) temperature. A recirculation curve is not seen with thermodilution because the blood is quickly warmed back to body temperature as it passes through the circulation. The computer determines the cardiac output using the following formula:

$$CO = \frac{1.08 \times C_T \times 60 \times V_I \times (T_B - T_I)}{\int_0^{\infty} \Delta T_B(t)dt}$$

$$CC = 1.08 \times C_T \times 60 \times V_I$$

where CO = cardiac output (L/min); C_T = correction for injectate temperature rise; V_I = volume of the injectate (mL); T_B = initial blood temperature (°C); T_I = initial injectate temperature (°C); 60 = seconds in one minute; and 1.08 = ratio of (density × specific heat of the injectate) to (density × specific heat of blood). A computation constant (CC) is supplied for the Swan-Ganz catheter, which consists of the product of several terms in the above equation:

The thermodilution cardiac output computer provides a mechanism for the entry of the computation constant, acquisition of the initial blood temperature from the catheter thermistor, and acquisition of the injectate temperature from the probe located in the flow-through housing of the delivery system. It also integrates the area

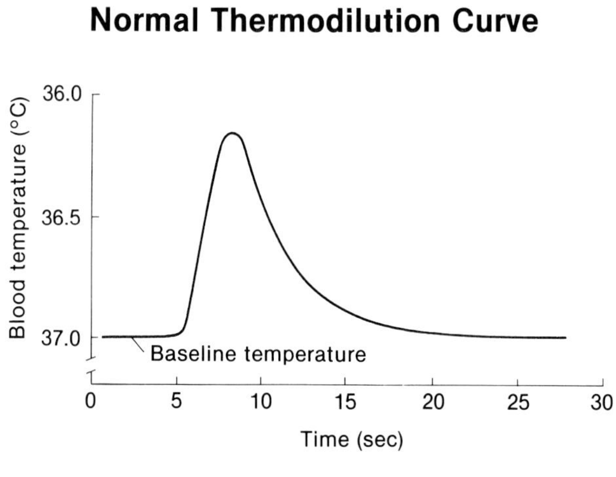

Figure 24–4 • Indicator dilution using a thermal indicator typically produces a curve with the above contour. It is characterized by a rapid fall in blood temperature (shown here with a positive slope), followed by an exponential decay returning to the baseline temperature. Patients with a high cardiac output generate small curves, whereas low cardiac outputs produce large curves. Some situations produce aberrations in the curve which may be indicative of an inaccurate output determination. These situations and their remedies are listed in Table 24–1.

under the thermodilution curve. Although recirculation is not a problem with thermodilution, variations in pulmonary artery blood temperature other than those caused by the injectate are often present. These variations may be caused by ventilation moving cooler air into the lungs and cooling the blood, or by the infusion of other fluids not at body temperature.[1] These extraneous variations in blood temperature make it difficult for the computer to determine when to stop the integration of blood temperature change and calculate the cardiac output. To eliminate this potential difficulty, the computer terminates its integration of the curve at some percentage of the peak height, usually at 30%. It then extrapolates the area from that point, adding it to the initial area.

The accuracy of the determination will be compromised if any of the variables in the cardiac output equation are in error. The computation constant may be compromised by:

1. The inappropriate selection of computation constant for the catheter being used (for example, selecting the computation constant for a 7 French catheter when a 5 French is used).
2. An altered injectate volume, or the delivery of an imprecise volume.
3. Adding extension tubing between the injection syringe and the proximal injection port, thus increasing the amount of heat gained by the indicator as it enters the body. This is only significant when using a cold injectate solution.

The most significant term in the cardiac output equation is the integral of the blood temperature change (the area under the thermodilution curve). Any situation that distorts the contour of this curve may lead to an erroneous output determination. Potential problems, possible causes, and their remedies are listed in Table 24–1.

Although thermodilution produces a value measured in liters per minute, it is in fact making the determination over a 10- to 20-second interval. Thus, the value displayed by the computer is representative of flow during this short sampling interval. The thermodilution technique may be accurate for this time interval, but it may not represent flow over a longer period of time. Performing multiple measurements and averaging the results will help determine a meaningful value of cardiac output. Under normal circumstances, it is recommended that three sequential measurements be made and averaged. Even in the hemodynamically stable patient, variations of 5% to 15% between measurements could be expected.

Variability may also be due to physiologic factors, such as changes in pulmonary artery temperature, variation in heart rate, cardiac arrhythmias, valvular insufficiencies, intracardiac shunts, and other causes of hemodynamic instability.[2] Errors produced by the user involve incorrect catheter positioning, warming of the injectate, or uneven injection rates.

Ventilation can have a significant influence on the variability of the cardiac output, and hence on the value determined over a short period of time with the thermodilution technique. The effect is dependent on the type of ventilation. During a spontaneous breath, the decrease in pleural pressure increases venous return, and thus augments cardiac output. During a mechanical breath, however, pleural pressure increases, and cardiac output falls. Injection of the indicator at the same point in the respiratory cycle may be done, but the data will be skewed, reducing data scatter but also overall accuracy.[3] Studies show that there is no satisfactory moment for indicator injection under changing conditions[4]. The mean of a large series of measurements shows good correlation with other methods. Under these circumstances it is best to increase the number of determinations, use cold injectate to create a larger change in blood temperature, and accept a 15% to 20% data scatter as reasonable in such instances.

The clinician may choose between room-temperature and a cold (iced) injectate. The use of room-temperature injectate is more convenient, avoiding the use and cost of ice, water, and the associated container. However, iced injectate provides a larger temperature change for a given cardiac output and injectate volume. This may be significant in cases where there are fluctuations in the baseline temperature or other manifestations of hemodynamic instability. Iced injectate should be used in cases where a low injectate volume is employed ($<$ 10 mL) or when cardiac output is expected to be high ($>$ 8 L/min). In many clinical situations, room-temperature injectate yields satisfactory results.[5,6] However, if scattered cardiac output readings occur, or clinical indications show significant hemodynamic instability, one should use the largest volume of iced injectate possible (up to 10 mL) and average five determinations, made at random points in the ventilatory cycle.

It is possible to obtain reproducible results without obtaining accurate results. If a consistent error—long injection time or uneven injection, for example—is made with each determination, the results may exhibit

Table 24–1 • Problems Indicated by Thermodilution Curves

Problem	Possible Causes	Remedies
1. Random or cyclic variations in the patient's baseline blood temperature. These variations affect the results most under conditions of high flow, small injectate volumes, and room temperature injectate.	• Mechanical ventilation • Other variations in regional venous return (coughing, shivering, or other abnormal respirations)	For all causes: • Increase injectate volume to 10 mL (if permissible for patient). • Use iced instead of room temperature injectate. • Synchronize injections to a phase of respiration (eg, end-expiration).
2. Patient's baseline blood temperature shows significant drift.	• Administration of IV fluids • Rewarming patient from a hypothermic condition	For all causes: • Increase injectate volume to 10 mL (if permissible for patient). • Use iced instead of room-temperature injectate. • Attempt to stabilize the patient's temperature.
3. Downslope of curve deviates significantly from an exponential.	• Catheter thermistor is positioned against the wall of the pulmonary artery or catheter tip is advanced too far into the pulmonary artery.	• Pull catheter back until full or near-full balloon inflation produces a wedge tracing.
	• Cardiac shunt	• If present, the accuracy of the cardiac output values will be questionable, depending on the severity of the shunt.
	• Kinked catheter injection lumen or injection not smooth	• Release any exterior kinks. Internal kinks may be verified by radiograph. Inject smoothly and rapidly.
4. Thermodilution curve does not return to the original baseline.	• Shift in blood temperature baseline during injection. May be due to administration of IV fluids or other changes in blood temperature.	• Try to stabilize the patient's temperature. Turn off any IV infusions (if possible) during the determination.
	• Cardiac shunt	• If a shunt is present, the accuracy of the determination may be in question, depending on the severity of the shunt.
5. A thermodilution curve is not seen for more than 15 sec following the start of the injection.	• Low stroke volume or low flow rate	• The cardiac output measurement will not be affected.
	• Delayed injection: 10 mL in more than 4 sec	• Inject smoothly and rapidly. Check to make sure that the catheter is not kinked, thus making it more difficult to inject.
6. Change in blood temperature too small to be used by the cardiac output computer.	• Using room temperature injectate with a hypothermic patient (ie, blood temperature $<34°$ C)	• Use only iced injectate with hypothermic patients.

(continued)

Table 24-1 • Problems Indicated by Thermodilution Curves (Continued)

Problem	Possible Causes	Remedies
	• The injectate temperature is greater than 25° C, possibly due to a warm room.	• Use iced instead of room-temperature injectate.
7. A thermodilution curve was not detected within 30 sec after beginning the injection.	• Catheter tip is either advanced too far into the pulmonary artery, or the thermistor is positioned against the wall of the artery.	• Pull the catheter back until a full or near-full balloon inflation produces a wedge tracing.
8. The amplitude of the thermodilution curve is greater than the computer can accommodate.	• The injectate volume is too large for the patient (eg, in pediatric patients).	• Reduce the injectate volume. If still too much signal, switch to room temperature injectate.
	• The incorrect injection port was used (ie, the distal lumen was used instead of the proximal lumen, or a bolus of cold solution was infused through a distal lumen during the determination).	• Inject through the proximal lumen. Do not bolus solutions through the distal lumen during a determination.

little variation but still be in error. Strict adherence to good procedure and an awareness of the potential sources of error will alleviate this problem.

IV. Complications

A. *Green Dye*

Two anaphylactic deaths have been reported following Cardio-Green (indocyanine green) dye administration during cardiac catheterization.[7] One of these was in a patient with a history of sensitivity to penicillin and sulfa drugs. Cardio-Green dye contains sodium iodide and should be used with caution in patients who have a history of allergy to iodides. Some commercially available Water for Injection may be incompatible with Cardio-Green dye; therefore, the dye should be dissolved in the aqueous solvent provided with the product. The total dose of dye injected should be kept below 2 mg/kg.

B. *Thermodilution*

Complications associated with the determination of cardiac output using the thermodilution technique are few. The most frequent complications occur with the insertion and manipulation of the Swan-Ganz catheter. However, the slowing of sinus rhythm during the injection of iced indicator solution has been reported.[8] It is important to monitor the patient's electrocardiogram during the cardiac output determination, from injection of the indicator to display of the result. If bradycardia follows the injection of the cold indicator, the indicator should be changed to room temperature if possible. Since the determination of cardiac output by this means requires direct access to the vascular system, the sterility of the injectate delivery system should be insured and maintained. Most manufacturers provide closed injectate systems for the delivery of both iced and room-temperature indicators. These should be used whenever possible.

V. References

1. Wetzel RC, Latson TW. Major errors in thermodilution cardiac output measurement during rapid volume infusion. Anesthesiology 62:684–687, 1985.
2. Weil MH: Measurement of cardiac output. Crit Care Med 5:117–119, 1977.
3. Snyder JV, Powner DJ. Effects of mechanical ventilation on the measurement of cardiac output by thermodilution. Crit Care Med 10:677–682, 1982.
4. Jansen JRC, Schreuder JJ, Bogaard JM, et al. Thermodilution

technique for measurement of cardiac output during artificial ventilation. J Appl Physiol 51:584–591, 1981.
5. Vennix CV, Nelson DH, Pierpont GL. Thermodilution cardiac output in critically ill patients: Comparison of room-temperature and iced injectate. Heart Lung 13:574–578, 1984.
6. Nelson LD, Anderson HB. Patient selection for iced versus room temperature injectate for thermodilution cardiac output determinations. Crit Care Med 13:182–184, 1985.
7. Package insert for Cardio-Green dye. Becton Dickinson Microbiology Systems, 1988.
8. Harris AP, Miller CF, Beattie C, et al. The slowing of sinus rhythm during thermodilution cardiac output determination and the effect of altering injectate temperature. Anesthesiology 63:540–541, 1985.

Chapter 25

Stephen M. Hahn, MD
Nora Goldschlager, MD

Treatment of Cardiac Dysrhythmias

OUTLINE

I. Introduction

Changes in cardiovascular function during general anesthesia may be hazardous, especially in the patient with organic heart disease or significant preoperative dysrhythmias. Myocardial ischemia may result, leading to hemodynamic dysfunction or to atrial or complex ventricular rhythms including ventricular tachycardia and ventricular fibrillation. Certain operative procedures increase vagal tone, leading to sinus bradycardia or atrioventricular (AV) block. Prompt recognition of these dysrhythmias followed by appropriate therapy is critical to avoid the occurrence of sustained or life-threatening cardiovascular dysfunction. In this chapter, we will describe the procedures necessary to treat these dysrhythmias. Recognition and management of specific dysrhythmias will also be discussed.

II. Electrical Techniques to Terminate Dysrhythmias

A. *Electrical Cardioversion*

Synchronized direct-current (DC) cardioversion is the emergent or elective application of an electrical shock delivered by a defibrillator/cardioverter to the myocardium in order to change an abnormal cardiac rhythm to a normal one (Fig. 25–1). By delivering a shock of sufficient strength, a critical mass of myocardial tissue is depolarized simultaneously, allowing the emergence of the dominant normal rhythm.

Defibrillator/cardioverters have a control mechanism that allows synchronization of the electrical shock with the R wave of the QRS complex as recorded by a surface electrocardiogram (ECG) (Fig. 25–2). Synchronization allows the cardioverter to avoid delivery of the shock during the vulnerable period of myocardial tissue (usually at or near the peak of the T wave), thus reducing the chance of inducing ventricular fibrillation. Synchronization is what distinguishes electrical countershock (cardioversion) from defibrillation, in which the shock can be delivered at any time during the P-QRST complex. Newer defibrillator/cardioverters are being developed to calculate transthoracic impedance when the paddles (electrodes) are placed on the patient's chest. Assessment of impedance allows for automatic energy level adjustment, thus potentially maximizing the efficacy of termination of the abnormal rhythm.[1] Direct-current (DC) cardioversion may be used to convert any tachycardia (with the exception of ventricular fibrillation) to sinus rhythm. Elective DC cardioversion is performed in patients whose tachydysrhythmia is hemodynamically relatively well tolerated, whatever its mechanism. In many instances, antidysrhythmic medications are attempted prior to elective DC cardioversion. Rapid rate or mechanism of tachycardia are not per se indications to perform immediate cardioversion.

Emergent DC cardioversion should be performed in any patient with a tachydysrhythmia (other than sinus tachycardia or digitalis-toxic rhythm) that results in hemodynamic compromise, congestive heart failure, or angina, and that does not respond promptly to medical management.

1. Technique

Synchronized DC cardioversion should always be performed with the patient sedated unless there is loss of consciousness associated with the tachydysrhythmia. If possible, an anesthetist or anesthesiologist should be in attendance when endotracheal intubation is required. The choice of sedative-hypnotic agents should be individualized. For elective procedures, the patient should fast for at least 6 hours. A critical care unit is the proper location for all *elective* cardioversions because blood pressure and ECG monitoring equipment is required, along with the equipment necessary for cardiopulmonary resuscitation. After cardioversion, whether or not it is successful in restoring normal cardiac rhythm, the patient should remain under close observation until he or she is awake and cardiac rhythm is stable. Antidysrhythmic agents may be administered prior to cardioversion and continued if sinus rhythm is restored. The choice of antidysrhythmic agent and duration of therapy will depend on the precardioversion rhythm and the specific clinical setting in which it occurs. When performing DC cardioversion, these procedural guidelines should be observed:

1. Perform a 12-lead ECG to evaluate the P wave, QRS morphology, and rate(s) of the abnormal rhythm. Attach the patient to the monitor of the defibrillator/cardioverter directly (see Fig. 25–1), or attach the cardioverter to the ECG output of the bedside monitor. This depends on the particular equipment available. The QRS complex

Defibrillator/Cardioverter

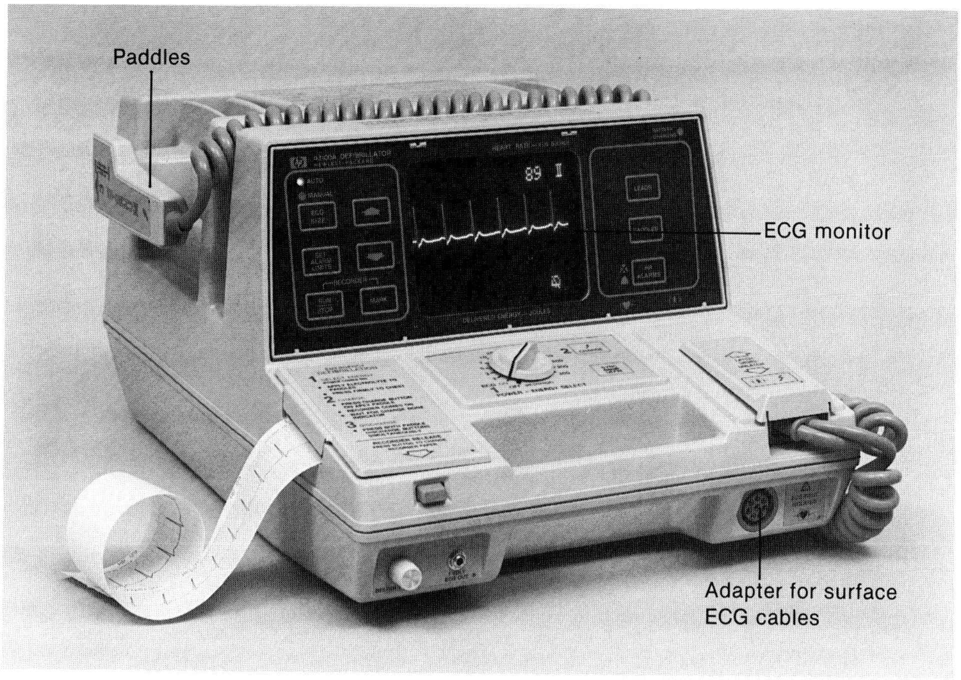

Figure 25–1 • Defibrillator/cardioverter. Surface ECG cables from the patient may be attached directly to the defibrillator/cardioverter or to a standard bedside monitor.

Control Panel of Defibrillator/Cardioverter

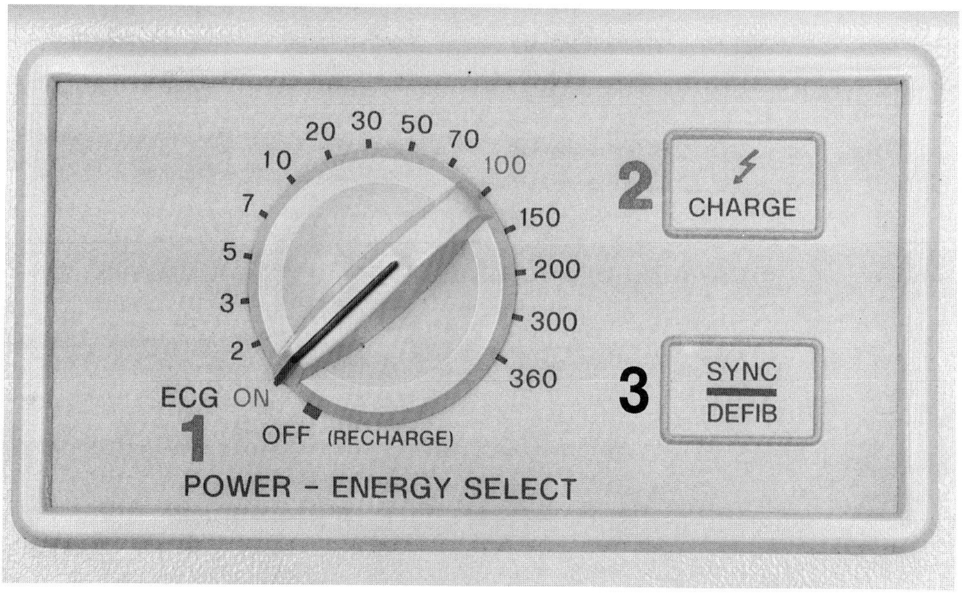

Figure 25–2 • Closeup of the control mechanisms for the defibrillator/cardioverter. After the QRS complex has been displayed on the monitor, activate the synchronized circuit (*SYNC*) for cardioversion or the defibrillation circuit (*DEFIB*) for defibrillation (*3*). When ready to deliver electrical energy, select the energy level required (*1*) and charge the capacitor (*2*). See text for details.

DC Cardioversion Treatment of Paroxysmal AV Nodal Reentrant Tachycardia

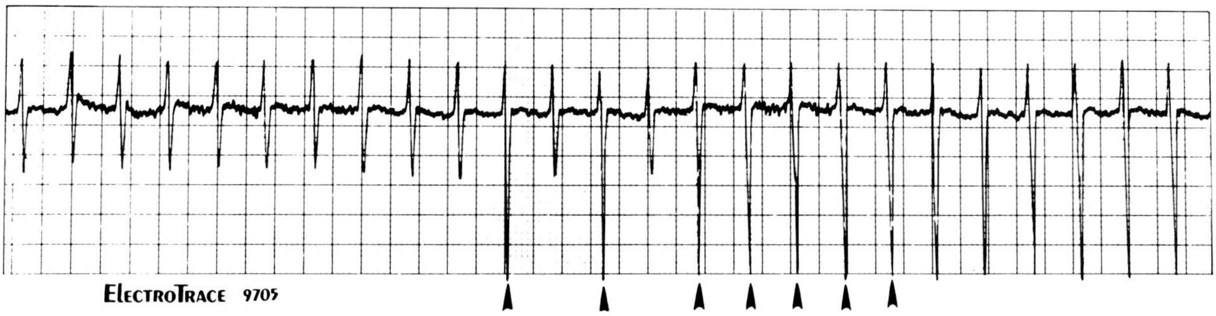

Figure 25-3 • Bedside monitor tracing recorded in a patient with paroxysmal AV nodal reentrant tachycardia at the time of DC cardioversion. The first arrow indicates activation of the synchronization button of the cardioverter/defibrillator. Note the superimposition of the synchronization signals (*arrows*) onto the patient's QRS complexes, elongating them. The precise point of superimposition reflects the time during the QRS complex that the cardioverting shock will be applied, and must be assessed and validated by the physician.

displayed on the monitor should be upright, using the surface ECG lead having the tallest R wave (usually a precordial lead).

2. Activate the synchronized circuit of the defibrillator/converter (see Fig. 25–2). The ECG monitor should show the cardioverter signal superimposed on the patient's QRS complex (Fig. 25–3); its position indicates the precise time of delivery of the cardioverting shock. If the time of shock delivery is not considered optimal, the surface ECG lead being monitored should be changed.
3. Apply a conductive medium such as electrode paste, saline-soaked gauze pads, or preformed disposable electrode pads to the chest wall.[2-4] Alcohol pads should be avoided.
4. Select the electric energy required, and charge the capacitor (see Fig. 25–2). The minimal amount of current necessary to convert the rhythm should always be used; this will depend on the rhythm itself, the clinical setting including medications and plasma electrolytes, and possibly the patient's body habitus.[5-7] The energy delivered to the myocardium during the shock will be approximately 80% to 90% of the selected (stored) energy, because of energy losses in the equipment and across the chest wall.
5. Place the paddles on the chest wall. Incorrect paddle placement is the most common cause of cardioversion failure.[8] One of three positions is most often employed. In the standard method, one paddle is placed to the left of the left nipple in the anterior axillary line, and the second paddle is placed to the right of the upper sternum at the second intercostal space and below the clavicle (Fig. 25–4). This is the most commonly used position and is achieved most rapidly. In the second (anteroposterior) method, one paddle is placed anteriorly over the high right parasternal area, and the second paddle is placed posteriorly in the left infrascapular area (Fig. 25–5). In the third (apex-posterior) method, one paddle is placed anteriorly to the left of the palpated cardiac apical impulse. The second paddle is placed posteriorly in the right infrascapular area. There is no documented advantage of one configuration over the other in terms of cardioverting energy required or overall success rate.[7]
6. Check the cardiac rhythm on the monitor. The cardioverting shock should be precisely synchronized to the R

Standard Paddle Placement

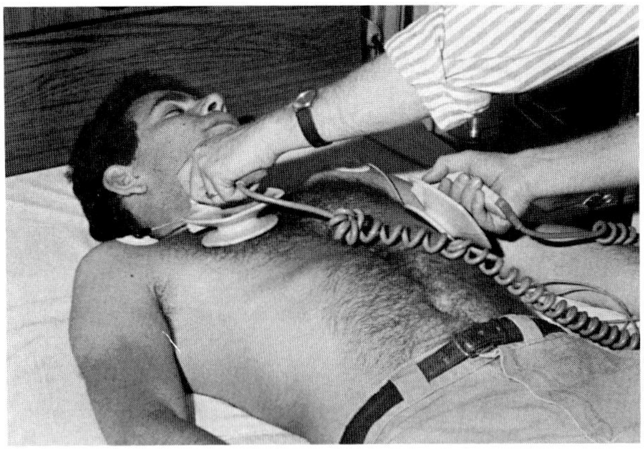

Figure 25–4 • The standard paddle placement for defibrillation/cardioversion. One paddle is placed to the left of the left nipple in the anterior axillary line; the second paddle is placed to the right of the upper sternum at the second intercostal space and below the clavicle.

Anterior and Posterior Paddle Placement

Anterior view

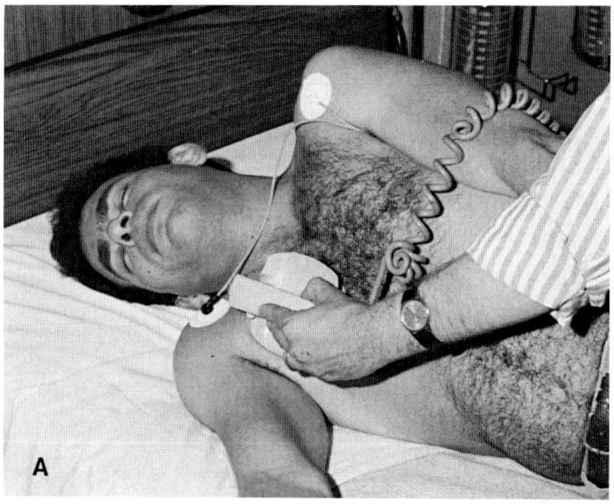

Posterior view

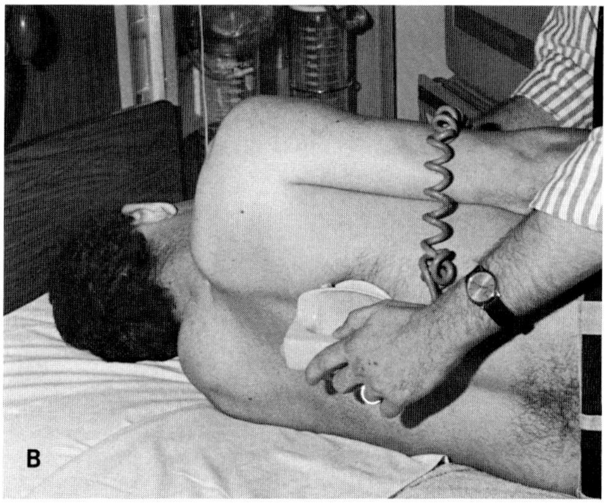

Figure 25–5 • (***A***) Anterior view of paddle placement using the anteroposterior method of defibrillation/cardioversion. The anterior paddle is placed over the high right parasternal area. (***B***) Posterior view of paddle placement using the anteroposterior method of defibrillation/cardioversion. The posterior paddle is placed in the left infrascapular area.

wave of the ECG (the earliest and tallest portion of the QRS complex in patients with bundle branch block) to avoid inappropriately timed shock delivery and possible ventricular fibrillation.

7. Clear the area, making certain that no personnel are directly or indirectly in contact with the patient.
8. Apply firm pressure to each paddle to achieve good contact with the chest wall.
9. Deliver the shock by pressing the discharge buttons on the paddles simultaneously until skeletal muscle contraction is seen, indicating delivery of the shock (Fig. 25–6).
10. Reassess the cardiac rhythm and treat accordingly. If the initial cardioversion is unsuccessful, the procedure may be repeated using higher levels of energy.

Patients with implanted cardiac pacing systems deserve special mention. Pacing leads provide a low-impedance pathway down which current may flow and produce an electric burn. Care should be taken not to place the cardioverter's paddles close to the pacing lead(s). If a temporary pacing system is in place, the external pulse generator should be turned off and, whenever possible, temporarily disconnected from the electrode catheter. In patients with permanent pacemakers, the cardioverting paddles should be placed along an imaginary line perpendicular to the implanted electrodes to avoid damage to the lead electrodes and to prevent myocardial burns. The paddles should not be placed within 3–5 inches of the implanted pacemaker generator. After cardioversion, the pacing and sensing functions of the implanted generator, including telemetric and programming capability should be completely assessed by qualified personnel. Pulse generators (as well implanted cardioverter/defibrillators) are protected against conventional electroshock delivery by means of diodes and other protective circuitry that provide resistance to power surges.[9]

The Defibrillator/Cardioverter Paddles

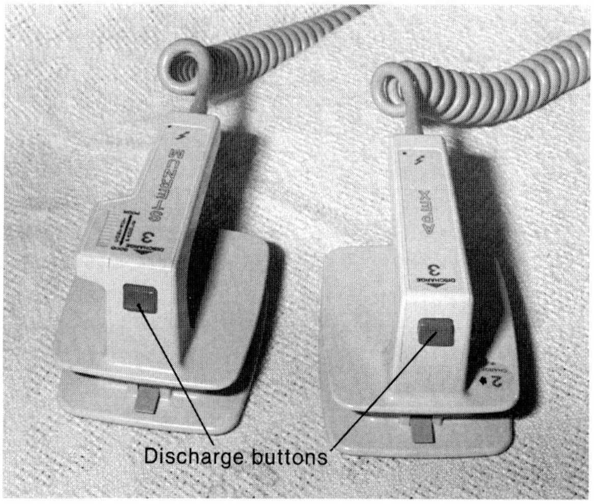

Figure 25–6 • Closeup of the defibrillator/cardioverter paddles. The shock is delivered by pressing the discharge buttons simultaneously until skeletal muscle contraction is seen.

2. Complications of Direct Current Cardioversion

The major complications of DC cardioversion are postconversion dysrhythmias, systemic embolization, myocardial trauma, postconversion hypotension, and chest wall burns. Postconversion dysrhythmias include bradycardia, bradycardia-dependent tachycardias, and other tachydysrhythmias. These are often short-lived and require no specific therapy. Ventricular fibrillation occurs in up to 5% of patients after DC cardioversion and is almost always due to improper synchronization of the cardioverting shock on the QRS complex of the ECG.[10] Clinically recognized embolism occurs in 1% to 2% of all patients undergoing cardioversion and is usually related to the presence of a large left atrium or ventricle.[11-13] Patients at high risk for embolism (such as those with cardiomyopathy, mitral valve disease, and thrombus demonstrated by echocardiography) should be anticoagulated before the procedure. Routine anticoagulation in all patients, however, is not generally recommended.

Myocardial trauma of clinical significance is not common after cardioversion, although transient ST-segment elevation and small rises in creatine kinase do occur.[14-16] The MB fraction of plasma creatine kinase is often normal and should not confound the diagnosis of acute myocardial infarction, even if multiple shocks have been administered. Occasionally, a patient may develop postconversion hypotension, often associated with low cardiac output and pulmonary edema. The etiology of this syndrome is not known but may be related to intense autonomic discharge; management is supportive, and the outcome favorable.[12]

The risk of significant injury from cardioversion to the equipment operator or other medical and paramedical staff is small. However, any person who is in contact with the patient may receive an electric shock. All staff must be electrically isolated from the patient and his or her bed during delivery of the shock.

Direct-current cardioversion may cause malignant dysrhythmias if performed in patients whose rhythms represent digitalis toxicity; the procedure is therefore contraindicated in these patients. The usual rhythms encountered are ectopic (automatic) atrial tachycardia with 2:1 atrioventricular (AV) block, and bidirectional tachycardia (Table 25–1 and Fig. 25–7). A digoxin level in the "toxic" range is not necessarily a contraindication to cardioversion, unless the rhythm itself is, or is suspected to be, the result of digitalis toxicity. It is not necessary to discontinue digitalis therapy before cardioversion unless there is clinical or electrocardiographic evidence of digitalis toxicity.

Patients with evidence of both sinus node dysfunction and paroxysmal supraventricular tachycardias (bradycardia–tachycardia syndrome) should undergo cardioversion with caution, since postconversion asystole or marked bradycardia may occur.[17] Bradycardia–tachycardia syndrome should be suspected in any patient with atrial flutter or fibrillation whose ventricular rate is slow in the absence of AV nodal blocking agents. Temporary transvenous pacing should be employed if DC cardioversion is deemed necessary in this clinical circumstance.

B. *Defibrillation*

Defibrillation is the asynchronous mode of electric shock used to terminate ventricular fibrillation. The procedure involves delivery of a current of sufficient strength to depolarize and render refractory a critical mass of fibrillating myocardium. The magnitude of the defibrillating current necessary to terminate the rhythm will depend on the resistance of the subject and the mass of the fibrillating myorcardium. Defibrillation is an emergency procedure and is the only effective therapy for ventricular fibrillation.

Controversy exists regarding the initial energy level selected for defibrillation. Recent studies suggest that excessively high current may produce myocardial damage and actually hinder resuscitation.[18,19] Therefore, we recommend that 200 J be used initially, with increases up to 300–360 J, if additional attempts are made.

1. Technique

Defibrillation should be instituted at the earliest possible time after ventricular fibrillation has been identified. If the patient is not being electrocardiographically monitored, abrupt cardiovascular collapse with absence of blood pressure and pulse should be assumed to be due to ventricular fibrillation. The technique of defibrillation is described below:

1. Initiate basic life support measures.
2. Evaluate the cardiac rhythm if the patient is attached to a monitor. If "quick look" paddles are available, apply conductive medium to the paddles and place the paddles on the patient's chest. The patient's rhythm will be transmitted through the paddles and appear on the monitor of the defibrillator/cardioverter. Continuous electrocardio-

Table 25–1 • Etiology of Tachydysrhythmias

Tachydysrhythmias generally due to digitalis toxicity

- Atrial fibrillation with high degree or complete AV block:
  - QRS rate regular
  - QRS rate showing group beating (type I or II exit block)
- Automatic (nonparoxysmal) junctional tachycardia
- Ectopic (automatic) atrial tachycardia with AV block
- Bidirectional tachycardia

Tachydysrhythmias generally not due to digitalis toxicity

- Atrial fibrillation (with controlled or rapid, irregular ventricular response)
- Atrial flutter
- Multifocal atrial tachycardia
- AV nodal reentrant tachycardia
- Accelerated junctional or ventricular rhythm

Regular Wide-Complex Bidirectional Tachycardia

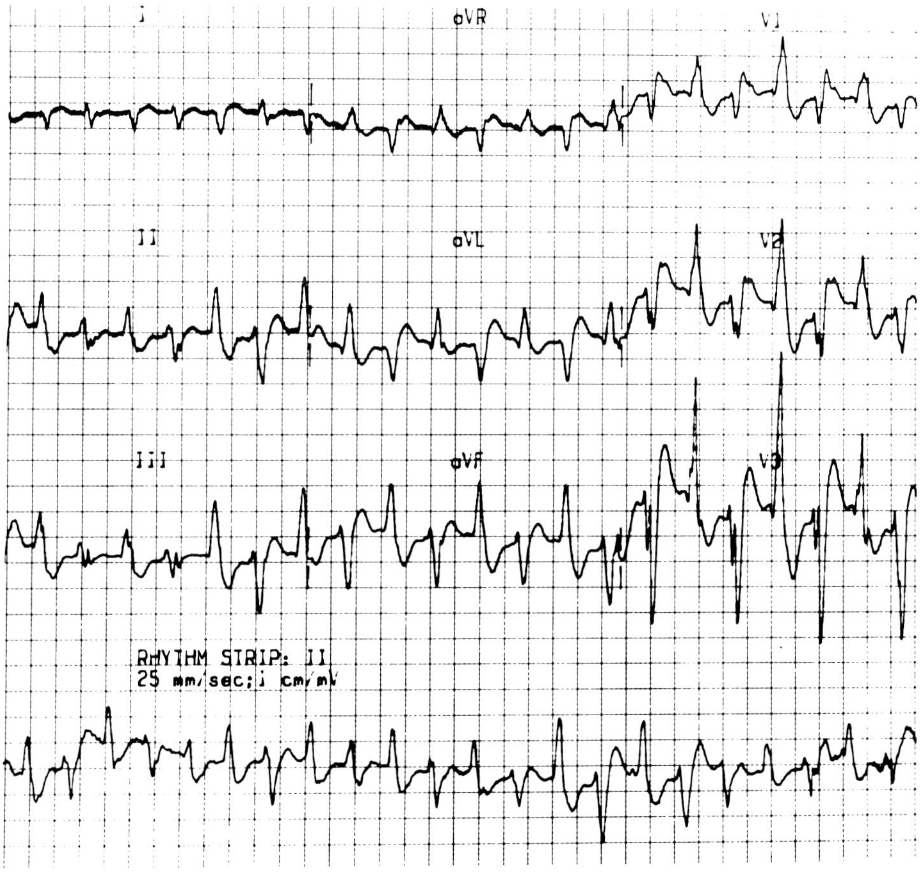

Figure 25–7 • Electrocardiogram (V4–V6; not shown) with Lead II rhythm strip illustrating a regular wide-complex bidirectional tachycardia in a patient whose serum digoxin level is 4.6 ng/mL. Atrial activity is not clearly seen. The QRS complex morphology alternates in polarity in each lead. This potentially life-threatening arrhythmia may require the administration of digoxin-specific antibodies.

graphic monitoring (using standard surface electrodes) should be instituted as soon as it is feasible.

3. If ventricular fibrillation is present, proceed with defibrillation.
4. Apply conductive material to the paddles or to the patient's chest.
5. Turn on the defibrillator; be sure that the equipment is functioning in the "defibrillating" (and not "synchronized") mode (see Fig. 25–2). If the synchronous mode is used for defibrillation, the defibrillating shock might fail to be delivered, since the device might not detect QRS deflections of large enough amplitude to trigger it.
6. Select the energy level desired, and charge the capacitor (see Fig. 25–2).
7. Place the paddles properly on the chest, applying firm pressure. The standard, anteroposterior, or apex-posterior method (as previously described) may be used.
8. Recheck the cardiac rhythm on the monitor.
9. Clear the area and check that no personnel are directly or indirectly in contact with the patient.
10. Deliver the electric energy by pressing both paddle discharge buttons simultaneously (see Fig. 25–6); wait for evidence of delivery of the defibrillating shock (skeletal muscle contraction).
11. Reassess the cardiac rhythm and check for pulses; measure blood pressure.
12. If ventricular fibrillation is still present, repeat the procedure immediately using higher energy levels. Additional steps for refractory ventricular fibrillation are described later in this chapter.

An alternative method to external paddle defibrillation involves the use of large self-adhesive pads that can both monitor the ECG and defibrillate the patient (Fig. 25–8). These pads are placed on the patient's chest wall and then attached to a defibrillator/cardioverter which can be charged at the time of recognition of ventricular fibrillation.[20,21] These large adhesive pads are particularly advantageous because they can be placed in advance in patients at high risk for a malignant ventricular dysrhythmia. They can remain in place throughout the high-risk period. The speed of defibrillation may thus be increased and the hazards to the operator reduced.

The ability to successfully defibrillate a patient decreases in the presence of cardiovascular collapse with associated acidosis, hypoxia, local ionic imbalance (especially hyperkalemia), and continued myocardial ischemia. The duration of ventricular fibrillation is also important. If ventricular fibrillation has been present for less than 2 minutes, attempts at defibrillation will be successful about two thirds of the time;[22] if it has been present for more than 2 minutes, the chances for successful defibrillation decrease to approximately 50%.[22]

Disposable ECG Monitoring/Defibrillation Pads

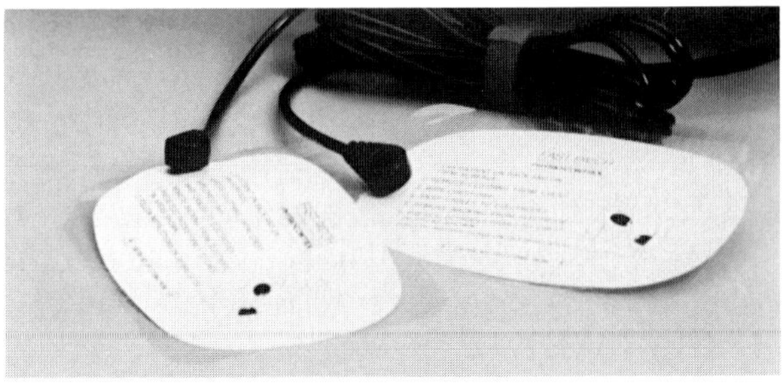

Figure 25–8 • Disposable self-adhesive defibrillation pads for electrocardiographic (ECG) monitoring and defibrillation.

2. COMPLICATIONS OF DEFIBRILLATION

Defibrillation in patients with pacemakers requires special caution. Pacemaker generators are designed so that the sensing and pacing circuitry is protected from excessive electric energy, but the protective mechanisms may fail on occasion, resulting in pulse generator malfunction.[23–27] Guidelines for defibrillation of patients with pacemakers are similar to those previously described for patients undergoing cardioversion. The integrity of all programmable parameters of the pacing system should be evaluated as soon as the patient is stabilized. Pulse generators that have the capability of transmitting stored information by telemetry should be interrogated to evaluate previously programmed parameters. Failure of pulse generator function (including capability to be interrogated and programmed) to return to normal within a reasonable period of time mandates generator replacement.

C. *Temporary Cardiac Pacing*

Temporary cardiac pacing is the delivery of an electric stimulus to the heart using a temporary pacing system that causes electric depolarization and subsequent mechanical contraction. The technique was first introduced in 1952 using external transcutaneous pacing electrodes.[28] Indications for temporary cardiac pacing have expanded over the years to include the termination and prevention of both atrial and ventricular tachydysrhythmias, prevention of significant bradyarrhythmias in patients at high risk (especially those with anterior wall myocardial infarction), and evaluation of coronary reserve and cardiac function.

Temporary cardiac pacing can be achieved by using one of several systems: transcutaneous, transthoracic, transesophageal, or transvenous. The external pulse generator and the pacing electrodes are essential parts of each of these systems. External pulse generators for all techniques except transcutaneous pacing have several features that allow for proper regulation of pacing function (Fig. 25-9). The output control dial regulates the magnitude of the pacing stimulus, measured in milliamperes (mA). The lowest output at which capture of myocardial tissue occurs, the *pacing threshold*, is determined by turning the output clockwise from its lowest output setting. A second control dial on the pulse generator allows the desired rate of impulse delivery to be set. Another control dial on the pulse generator allows selection of the demand or fixed-rate (asynchronous) mode of pacing. This control is usually called the *sensitivity dial*, and reflects the amplitude in millivolts (mV) of the electric signal that will be sensed by and inhibit the

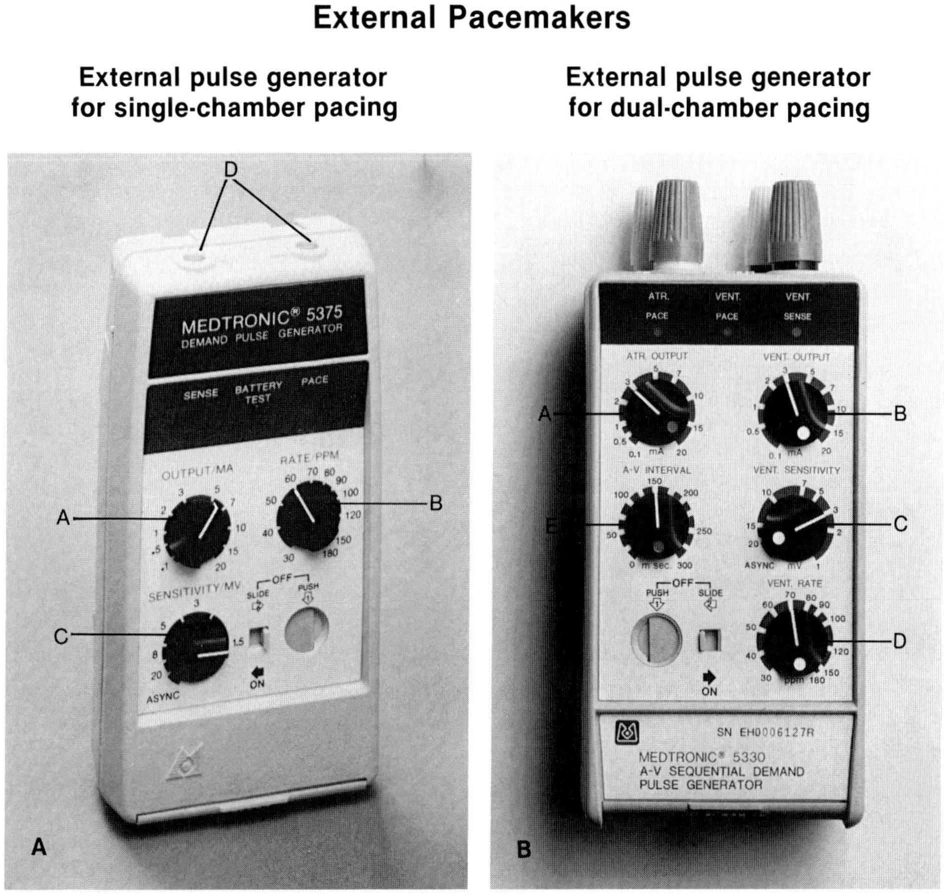

Figure 25-9 • External pacemakers. (***A***) External pulse generator for single chamber pacing. The output control dial (*A*) regulates the magnitude of the pacing stimulus. The rate control dial (*B*) allows the operator to set the desired pacing rate in pulses per minute. The sensitivity dial (*C*) allows selection of the demand or fixed-rate asynchronous (*ASYNC*) mode of pacing. When the demand mode of pacing is chosen, the sensitivity dial (*C*) can be manipulated to reflect the amplitude of electrical signal in millivolts (mV), which will be sensed by the pulse generator, inhibiting it. The distal and proximal electrodes to the pacing catheters are attached to the negative and positive poles (*D*) of the pulse generator, respectively. (***B***) External pulse generator for dual chamber pacing (atrial and ventricular). The atrial output control dial (*A*), ventricular output control dial (*B*), ventricular sensitivity dial (*C*), and ventricular rate dial (*D*) have functions similar to those of the single chamber pulse generator. The AV interval dial (*E*) regulates the delay between atrial and ventricular pacing pulses.

pacemaker generator. In the fixed-rate (asynchronous) mode, the pulse generator transmits electric impulses at regular intervals, determined by the rate selected. If spontaneous cardiac electric activity is present, competition between paced and spontaneous depolarizations may cause ventricular (or atrial) dysrhythmias, which can be life threatening. This pacing mode can be used when no spontaneous cardiac activity is present; however, the demand mode is always preferred.

When using the demand mode, a pacing rate is selected. If the intrinsic heart rate is higher than the selected rate, the pulse generator output is inhibited. If the intrinsic heart rate is lower than the selected pacing rate, or if a spontaneous QRS complex (or P wave) does not occur within the period of time determined by the selected pacing rate, the pulse generator transmits an output pulse. In the demand mode, the pulse generator is inhibited by spontaneous atrial or ventricular (or both) electric activity, depending on the location of the electrode(s) within the heart.

Indicator lights on the pulse generator illuminate when a pacing pulse is generated and when a spontaneous QRS (or P) complex is sensed. Single and dual chamber pulse generators are available for ventricular (or atrial) (see Fig. 25–9A) and atrioventricular sequential pacing (see Fig. 25–9B).

The electrode systems created for temporary cardiac pacing vary with the pacing technique employed and are described below. Most modern electrodes are bipolar; however, unipolar systems do exist.

1. Transcutaneous Pacing

Transcutaneous or *external* cardiac pacing provides a means of electrically pacing the heart in clinical situations not amenable to transvenous pacing. It also provides a means of pacing prior to the institution of other forms of pacing. Transcutaneous pacing operates by passing current to the myocardium using electrodes placed on the skin surface (Fig. 25–10). In its early development, transcutaneous pacing was associated with unacceptable side effects, including painful stimulation of the cutaneous nerves and underlying skeletal muscle, in the great majority of patients. Recent improvements in design allow the device to be reasonably well tolerated by most patients; however, mild sedation is usually required.[29–31] The external pacing system uses two large surface low-impedance electrodes placed on the anterior and posterior chest wall (see Fig. 25–10). The long pulse duration of 20–40 milliseconds and the available current output of several hundred milliamperes are necessary to

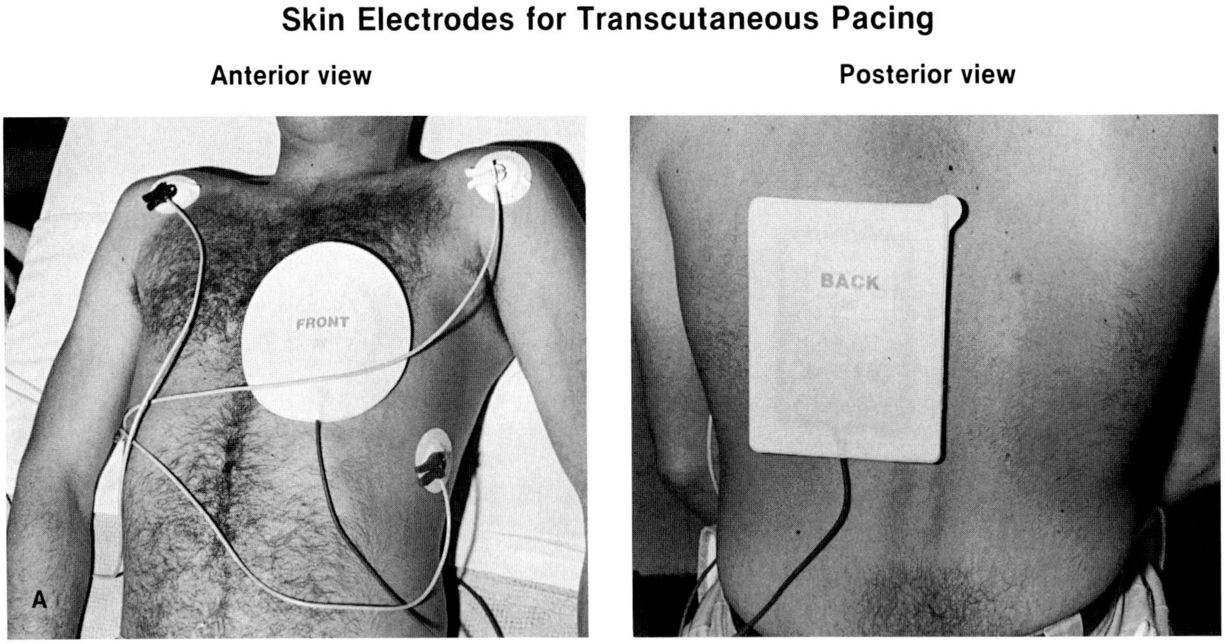

Figure 25–10 • Self-adhesive skin electrodes for transcutaneous pacing. Their large size is dictated by the fact that the electrical energy they deliver must penetrate the chest wall and thoracic structures to reach the myocardium in order to stimulate it. (***A***) Anterior view of the self-adhesive skin electrode which is placed over the apex of the heart in the V2–V3 position. (***B***) Posterior view of the self-adhesive skin electrode, which is placed to the left of the spine just below the scapula at the midheart level.

overcome the impedance offered by the chest wall and intrathoracic structures. The transcutaneous pacemaker paces the ventricle and inhibits pacer stimulus output when it senses ventricular electric activity, thus functioning in a VVI (demand) mode.

a. Technique

Transcutaneous pacing is performed in the intensive care unit, operating room, cardiac catheterization suite, or emergency room. Equipment and drugs necessary for cardiac resuscitation should be readily available. Transcutaneous pacing is instituted as follows:

1. Attach the patient to the pacer monitor via the surface electrodes (Fig. 25–11A). The posterior electrode is placed to the left of the spine just below the scapula at the mid-heart level. The anterior electrode is placed over the apex of the heart in the V2–V3 position. Patients with cardiomegaly may require repositioning of the electrodes if ventricular capture cannot be achieved.

Transcutaneous Pacemaker System

Overview

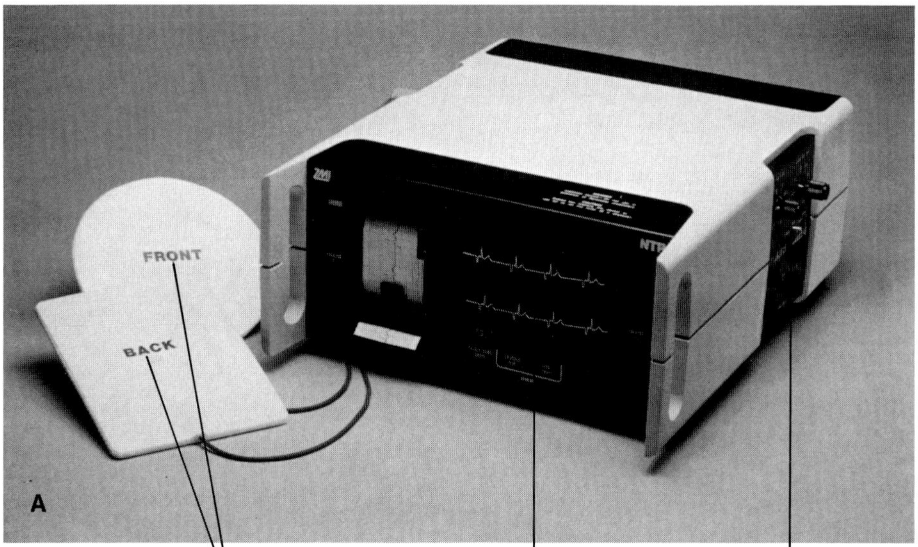

Self-adhesive skin electrodes (see Fig. 25–10)

Surface ECG monitor

Control panel (see Fig. 25–11B)

Control panel

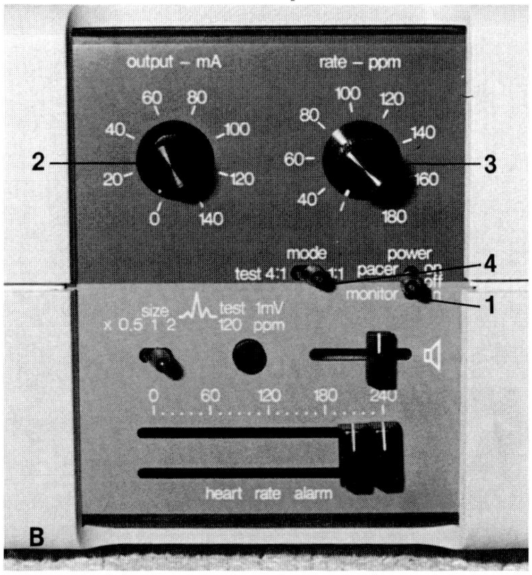

Figure 25–11 • (***A***) Overview of the transcutaneous pacemaker system. The patient is attached to the ECG monitor via the self-adhesive skin electrodes which are placed as shown in Fig. 25–10. (***B***) Control panel for the transcutaneous pacemaker system. After establishing the surface ECG rhythm on the monitor, flip the power switch to the "monitor on" position (*1*). Set the output control to zero mA (*2*). Turn the rate control to an appropriate level (*3*). When ready to pace, flip the power switch to the "pacer on" position (*4*). Turn the output control (*2*) until capture is achieved.

2. Turn the power switch of the pulse generator to the monitor-on position to monitor the cardiac rhythm (Fig. 25–11B).
3. Set the output control to zero mA.
4. Turn the rate control to a level deemed appropriate for the patient.
5. Turn the power switch to the pacer-on position, which allows for both ECG monitoring and pacing.
6. Turn the output control until capture is achieved.

   The pacing pulses are 40 msec in duration and should not be confused with QRS complexes (Fig. 25–12). If capture is occurring, the pacer output pulse will be followed by a QRS complex, best seen on the pacemaker generator's oscilloscope and strip chart recording. However, significant distortion of the QRS complex will be present on the bedside rhythm monitor (or electrocardiographic machine recording) (see Fig. 25–12B). Capture should always be verified by palpating the pulse. Skeletal muscle twitching occurs at a stimulus output of 30 mA, but capture does not usually occur until 35 to 80 mA. In an emergency setting, the output should be quickly turned to the maximum level. After capture has been documented, decrease

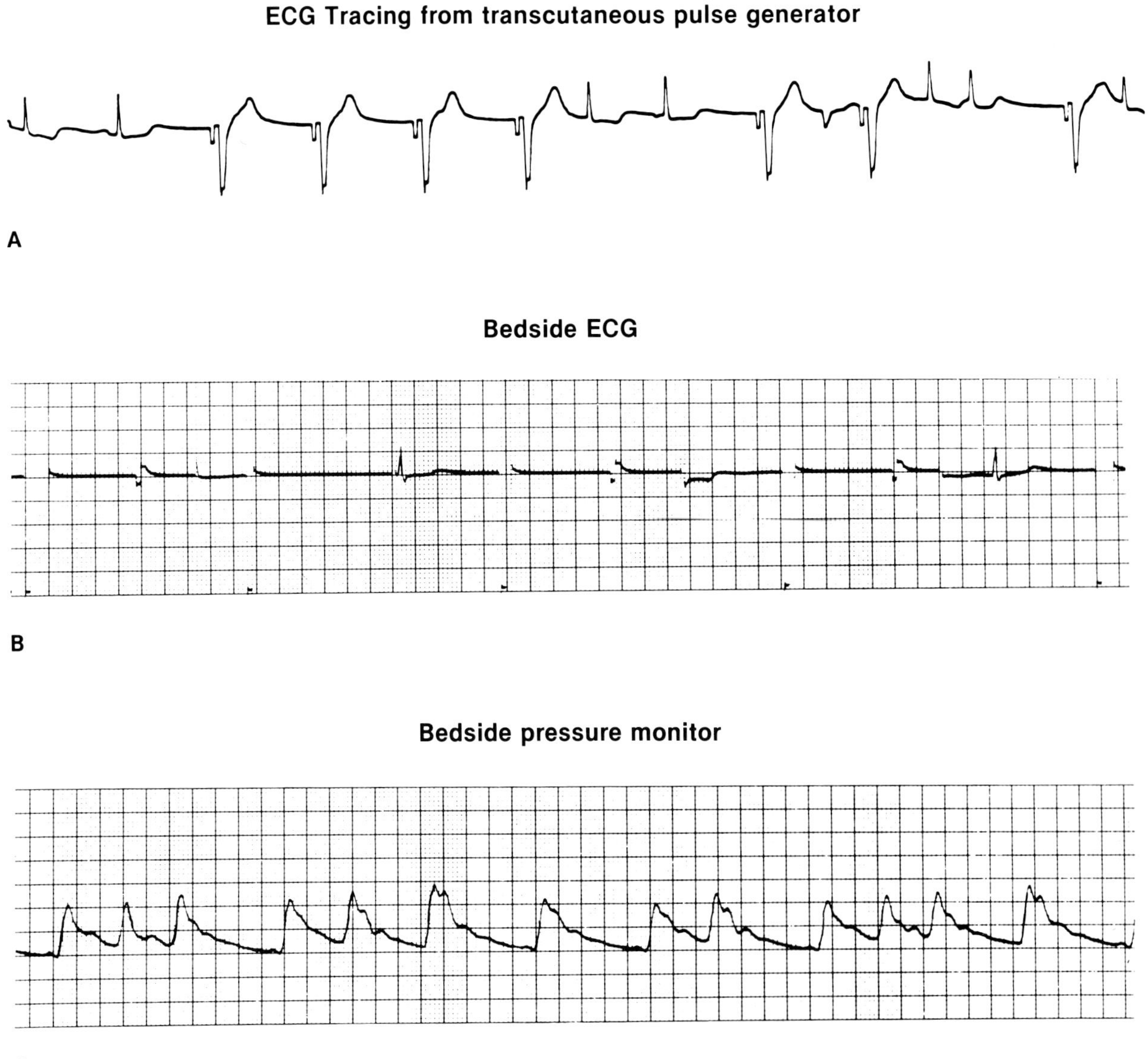

Figure 25–12 • ECG tracings recorded from the strip chart recorder of the transcutaneous pulse generator (***A***), and from the bedside ECG (***B***) and intravascular pressure monitor (***C***), simultaneously recorded. The pacing output pulses and ensuing QRS complexes (the third to sixth, ninth, tenth, and thirteenth QRS complexes) are easily seen in strip ***A***. However, in the bedside recording, the pacing output pulses associated with ventricular capture saturate the channel completely, totally obscuring the paced QRST complexes. All clearly visible QRS complexes are spontaneous.

the output to approximately 10% above capture threshold for patient comfort.
7. Check the patient's arterial pulse for evidence of peripheral perfusion.

Pacing function may be maintained in a demand or fixed-rate (asynchronous) mode. The radiographic appearance of the transcutaneous electrodes is unique and should not be confused with intrapulmonary processes (Fig. 25–13).

The advantages of transcutaneous pacing include ease of use, the lack of invasive procedures, and prophylactic use in high-risk patients. Its disadvantages include local discomfort, obscuring of the bedside-monitored rhythm by large stimulus artifacts, and concealing of monitored arterial pulse waves by skeletal muscle contractions.

b. Complications

Complications of transcutaneous pacing are uncommon and include local irritation from cutaneous nerve stimulation, local skeletal muscle contraction, failure to sense or capture, and, rarely, precipitation of ventricular tachycardia or ventricular fibrillation.[29]

Falk and associates have found that external cardiac pacing is effective in most patients studied, although this success rate is not achieved in all reported series.[32] The majority of pacing failures occur in patients during the advanced stages of cardiopulmonary arrest. The opportunity for successful transcutaneous pacing in patients with cardiac arrest of greater than 15 minutes' duration is about 33% to 45%.[29,33] It is unclear from the literature if transvenous pacing would produce better results in this setting. The hemodynamic effect of transcutaneous pacing appears to be similar to that achieved with transvenous pacing. It is reasonable to suggest that the hemodynamic and clinical effects of temporary pacing, whatever the technique, depend more on the condition of the myocardium and the circulation than on the location of the electrodes.

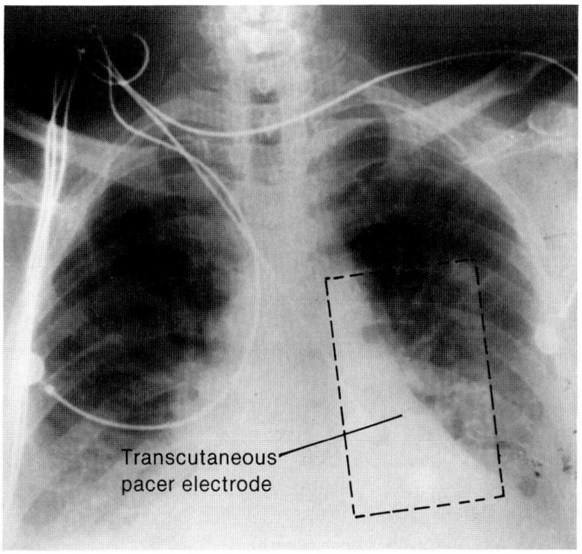

Figure 25–13 • Portable anteroposterior chest radiograph illustrating the appearance of the large surface electrode applied to the posterior thorax (*dotted line*). The anterior electrode overlies the cardiac shadow and is not seen.

2. TRANSTHORACIC PACING

Transthoracic pacing is a technique of percutaneous placement of cardiac pacing wires into the ventricular cavity or onto the ventricular wall through a transthoracic needle (Fig. 25–14). The reliability of this technique is poor, and it is a highly invasive and potentially morbid procedure. Transthoracic pacing is performed only in an emergency setting, usually during a cardiac arrest in which transvenous pacing cannot be accomplished rapidly or in which transcutaneous pacing is not available or successful. The reported incidence of successful capture with transthoracic pacing varies from 5% to 90%, although typically it is 20% to 40%.[34] Often, however, electric capture is not followed by mechanical systole.

Transthoracic pacing should be reserved for situations of utmost gravity in which no other pacing system is feasible. External pacing should always be employed first because it is probably as efficacious (if not more) and is associated with significantly less morbidity. Transthoracic pacing should never be used in awake or stable patients.

a. Technique

Transthoracic pacing can be performed in approximately 35–40 seconds. While the intracardiac needle is being placed, cardiopulmonary resuscitative procedures should be halted to decrease the chance of myocardial or lung damage.

1. Prepare the subxiphoid area in a sterile fashion, if time permits.
2. While CPR is transiently stopped, insert the transthoracic needle and trochar (see Fig. 25–14) in the left xiphocostal space and direct it toward the left shoulder or sternal notch at an angle of 30° to 45° to the skin (Fig. 25–15).

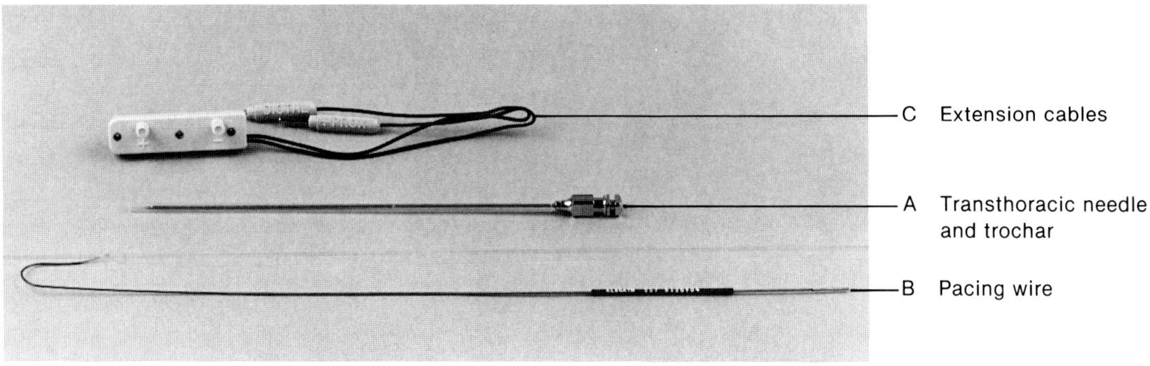

Figure 25–14 • The transthoracic pacemaker system. Components include transthoracic needle and trochar (*A*), J-shaped pacing wire (*B*), and extension cables (*C*).

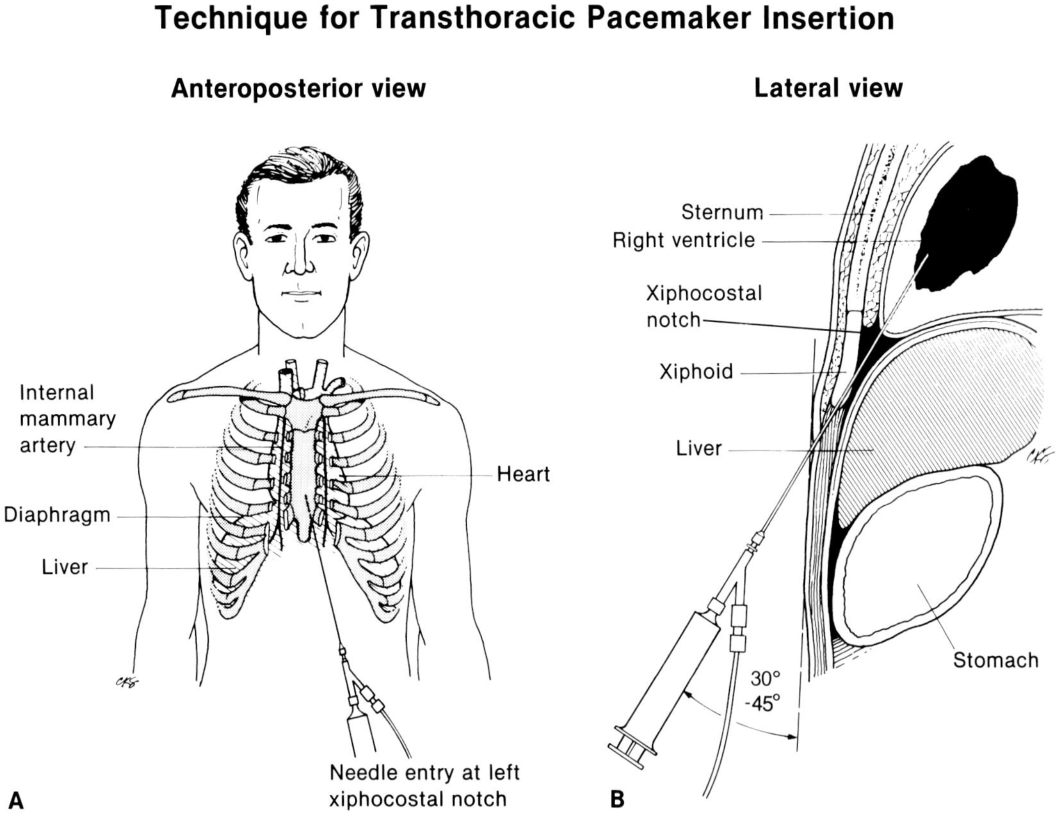

Figure 25–15 • Technique for transthoracic pacemaker insertion. Prepare the subxiphoid area in a sterile fashion (***A***). Insert the transthoracic needle and trochar into the left xiphocostal space and direct it toward the left shoulder or sternal notch (***A***) at an angle of 30° to 45° (***B***). Advance the needle 4 inches and remove the trochar. Aspirate through the needle. If no blood is obtained, reinsert the needle. Once blood is aspirated, advance the J-shaped pacing wire through the needle into the cardiac cavity. Withdraw the needle and attach the pacing wire to the pulse generator via the positive terminal on the extension cables. The cables are then connected to the pulse generator (see Fig. 25–9).

Exceeding a 45° angle to the skin could result in pneumothorax or laceration of intraabdominal structures.

3. Advance the needle approximately three fourths of its length, or 4 inches, and remove the trochar.
4. Aspirate through the needle. Aspirated free-flowing blood confirms the presence of the needle within the ventricle. If no blood is aspirated, withdraw the needle and reinsert. Resume CPR when it is confirmed that the needle is in the heart.
5. Advance a J-shaped pacing wire through the needle (see Fig. 25–14). Thread the wire into the cardiac cavity, and withdraw the needle. Only the pacing wire should exit from the chest.
6. Attach the pacing wire to the pulse generator via the extension cables.
7. Turn on the pulse generator and select the sensitivity. The clinical situation often allows the sensitivity control to be turned to the asynchronous position to insure fixed-rate pacing.
8. Set the rate to an appropriate level.
9. Turn the output control dial to its maximum or until capture occurs. Then lower the output to about 10% above the capture threshold. Make sure that atrial pacing is not occurring (Fig. 25–16).
10. Check the patient's arterial pulses to assess mechanical cardiac function.

If pacing is unsuccessful, the pacing wire should be manipulated to change its position, and all lead connections should be rechecked. If the patient has been stabilized, verify the position of the wire, and perform an anteroposterior and cross-table lateral chest radiograph to exclude a pneumothorax. Obtain a 12-lead ECG to confirm capture, and document the morphology of the paced complexes. If the pacing wire is in the right ventricular cavity (as it should be), there should be an upright paced QRS complex in leads I, aVL, and V6, and a negative QRS complex in lead V1, reflecting the left bundle branch block pattern caused by right ventricular depolarization preceding left ventricular depolarization. A decision should then be made about the need for a transvenous pacing system.

b. Complications

The major complications of transthoracic pacing include myocardial or coronary artery laceration, pericardial tamponade, pneumothorax, and hepatic or gastric damage.[34,35]

3. TRANSESOPHAGEAL PACING

Temporary *transesophageal* pacing was introduced in 1957.[36] This technique of cardiac pacing is relatively noninvasive and safe. It is generally quite effective for atrial pacing because of the proximity of the electrode to the left atrium, but provides inconsistent ventricular pacing. Because of this limitation, transesophageal pacing has been used only for atrial pacing of limited dura-

Transthoracic Pacing

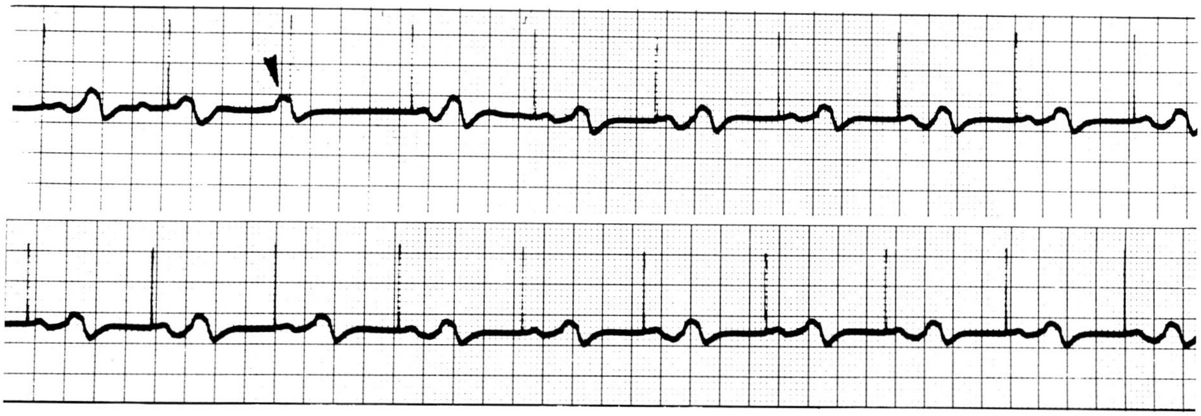

Figure 25–16 • Transthoracic pacing illustrating atrial, rather than ventricular, pacing. Standard lead insertion procedures had been followed. The fact that atrial pacing is occurring suggests that a large right atrium occupied the retrosternal area normally occupied by the right ventricle. It is conceivable that the paced complexes are in fact ventricular and that the paced QRS complex is extremely broad (0.48 sec) due to acidosis and hyperkalemia. However, the third QRS complex in the top strip (*arrow*), not preceded by a pacing stimulus, reveals the true QRS morphology.

tion (less than 1 hour). It should not be used in patients who require temporary pacing for hemodynamic support.

The indications for atrial pacing include the termination of reentrant supraventricular tachydysrhythmias using atrial overdrive pacing,[37] the diagnosis of cardiac rhythm by documenting atrioventricular dissociation, the assessment of conduction system abnormalities by demonstrating atrioventricular block at rapid paced rates, and the diagnosis of myocardial ischemia by demonstrating ischemic ST-T abnormalities at rapid paced rates.

a. *Technique*

1. The *pill electrode* is a bipolar electrode enclosed in a gelatin capsule with thin wire leads attached (Fig. 25–17). Have the patient swallow the pill electrode with a few sips of water.
2. When the electrode is approximately 40 cm from the teeth (and well beyond the left atrium), connect the wires to a preamplifier by way of an extender cable (Fig. 25–18). The right arm and left arm output cables from the preamplifier are then connected to the right and left arm input cables to the ECG machine. The right arm output from the preamplifier is also connected to the patient's right arm. The right and left leg cables from the ECG machine are connected to the patient in the usual fashion (see Fig. 25–18B).
3. Monitor lead I, and slowly withdraw the electrode a few centimeters at a time. Optimal position, near the left atrium, is obtained when the maximal voltage in the atrial electrogram (the P wave) is seen. The atrial deflection in this position should be 2 to 3 times the height of the ventricular deflection (which corresponds to the QRS complex).
4. When proper position is insured, tape the electrode wires to the patient's chin. Remove the wires from the ECG machine and connect them to the pulse generator to begin pacing.
5. Set the appropriate rate, pulse duration, and current levels on the pulse generator. Turn the power switch to the "on" position. Finally, move the pacer switch to the "on" position when pacing is desired. Radiographic confirmation of electrode placement is not necessary.

The Pill Electrode

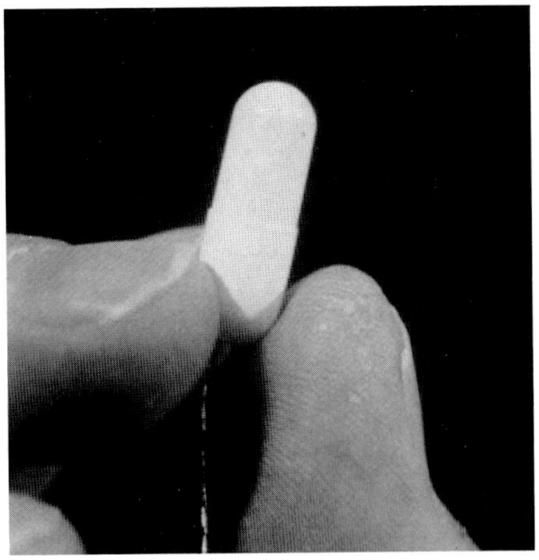

Figure 25–17 • The pill electrode. This bipolar electrode with thin wire leads attached is encased in a gelatin capsule.

b. *Complications*

Complications of transesophageal pacing include gastrointestinal discomfort, dysrhythmias (nonsustained atrial fibrillation and ventricular tachycardia), phrenic nerve stimulation, and brachial plexus stimulation. In addition, the transesophageal pacing catheter is fairly easy to dislodge, leading to failure to capture.

4. Transvenous Pacing

The *transvenous* method of temporary cardiac pacing is the most widely employed. Transvenous pacing catheters may be placed in the right atrium, the right ventricle, or both chambers. Although most transvenous pacing is ventricular, the ability to place catheters in both atrium and ventricle permits dual chamber pacing (AV sequential pacing), which may have beneficial hemodynamic effects in certain clinical settings.[38–41]

The pacing catheters used for transvenous ventricular pacing include balloon flotation, semiflotation, traditional (stiff), and combined Swan-Ganz ventricular pacing catheters (Fig. 25–19). The buoyancy of flotation and semiflotation catheters allows cardiac flow to direct them into the right ventricle, an advantage in emergency situations. The balloon-flotation catheter is 100 cm in length, with markers at 10-cm intervals beginning from the catheter tip. The two electrodes (tip and ring) at the end of the catheter are separated by a latex balloon. At the proximal end of the catheter are two pins for insertion into the negative and positive poles of the pacemaker generator, and a stopcock used for inflation of the balloon. Traditional or stiff electrode catheters cannot be floated into the ventricle and must be positioned using fluoroscopic guidance. Transvenous atrial pacing is usually accomplished using a J-shaped catheter,

Transesophageal Pacing

The system

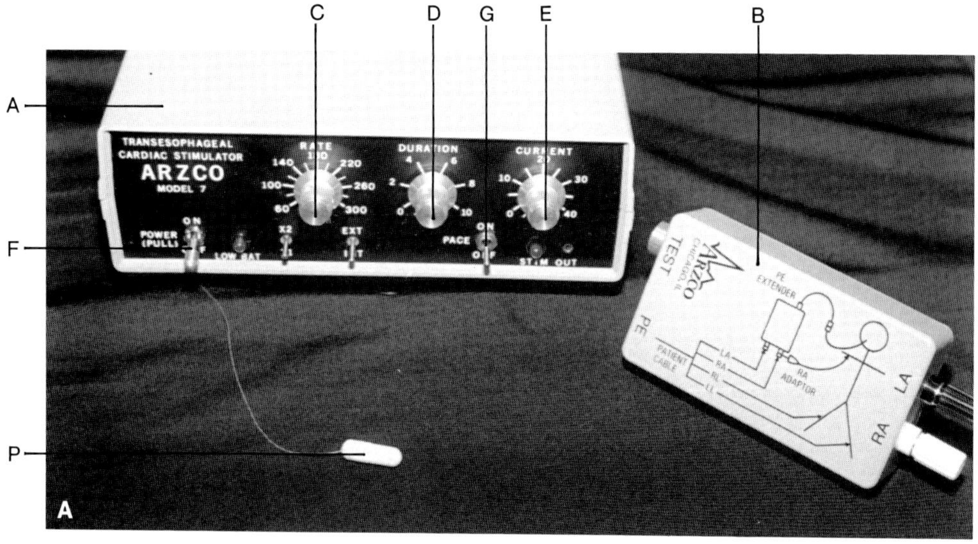

Schema for Esophageal Electrode Recording

Lead and cable connection

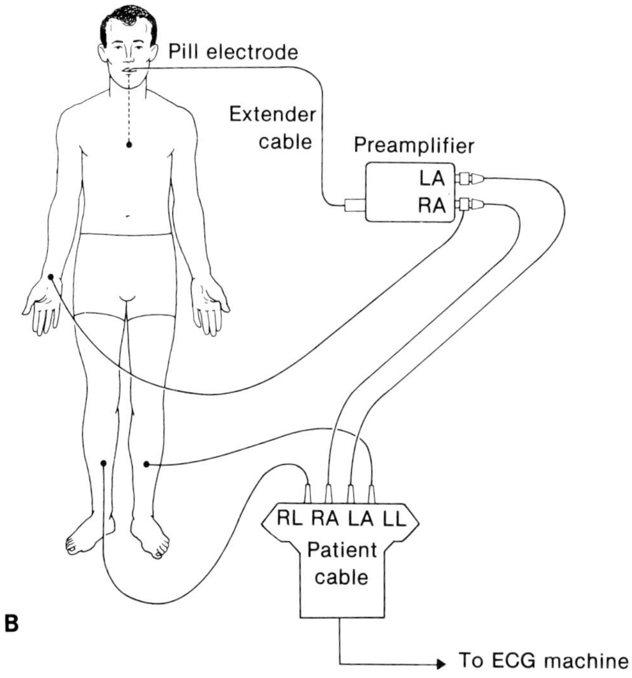

Figure 25–18 • Transesophageal pacing. (***A***) The pulse generator (*A*) and preamplifier (*B*) for transesophageal pacing. After the pill electrode (P) is swallowed, proper placement is ensured. When pacing is desired, the electrode is connected to the pulse generator. The rate (*C*), duration of impulse (*D*), and current levels (*E*) are set with the appropriate dials. The power switch (*F*) and pacer switch (*G*) are moved to the "on" positions when pacing is desired. (***B***) Proper lead and cable connections with the pill electrode and preamplifier. The pill electrode is connected to the preamplifier via an extender cable after it is swallowed. The right and left arm output cables from the preamplifier are then connected to the right and left arm input cables to the ECG machine. The right arm output from the preamplifier is also connected to the patient's right arm. The right and left leg cables from the ECG machine are connected to the patient in the usual fashion. Lead I of the ECG machine is monitored for placement.

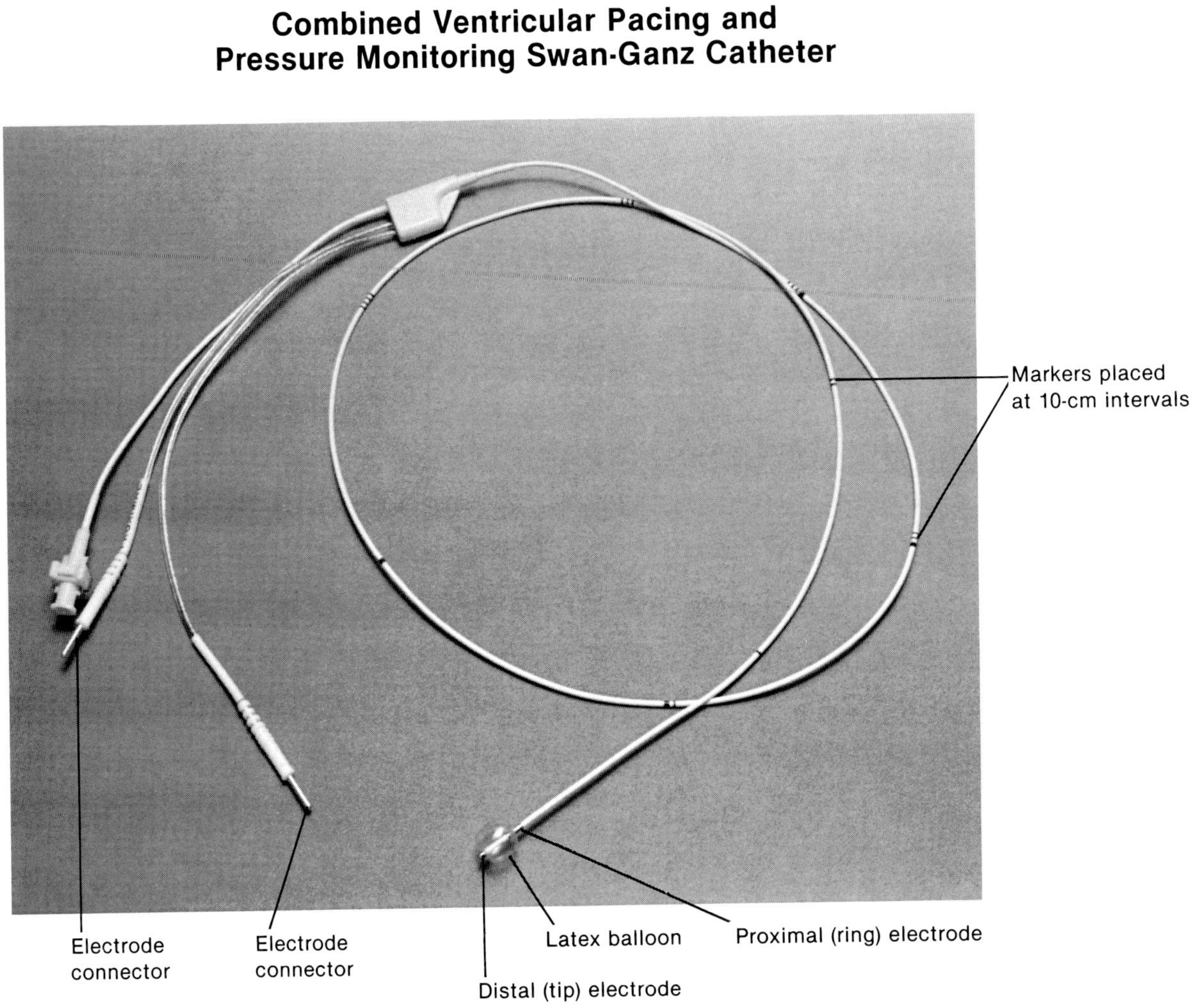

Figure 25–19 • Combined Swan-Ganz ventricular pacing catheter. The two electrodes (tip and ring) are located at the end of the catheter and separated by a latex balloon. The balloon allows for flotation of the catheter into the ventricle as described in the text. At the other end of the catheter are connectors (pins) for insertion into the pacemaker generator. (Reproduced with permission of Baxter Healthcare Corportion, Santa Ana, CA.)

which allows placement from the subclavian vein into the right atrial appendage.[42] The traditional pacing catheter may also be used for atrial pacing.

Dual chamber (AV sequential) pacing can be accomplished by placing separate atrial and ventricular pacing catheters. The disadvantage of this system is that it may require two separate attempts at venous access. Recently, however, a double-lumen sheath has been developed to allow placement of the two pacing catheters from the same venous site. Alternatively, multipolar pacing catheters with several electrodes attached to the catheter allow two or more ring electrodes to remain positioned within the right atrial cavity, while the tip electrode is placed into the right ventricular cavity.

a. Technique

Temporary pacing catheters may be inserted under direct visualization using fluoroscopy, or by using the unipolar electrogram recorded from the distal (tip) electrode to guide passage into the heart. Fluoroscopy is mandatory when a stiff pacing catheter is used and in the femoral vein approach; it is strongly advised when most atrial pacing leads are to be placed.

Obtaining central venous access is the first step in placing a transvenous pacemaker. The sites available include the left subclavian vein, the left or right internal jugular vein, the femoral vein, and the antecubital vein. Each site has its own advantages and disadvantages. The left subclavian vein is probably the best approach in emergent situations because the anatomy is fairly constant from patient to patient, the pacing catheter is more easily passed through the tricuspid valve, and better electrode stability is achieved. However, the risk of pneumothorax is increased, and puncture of the subclavian artery is a possibility. The internal jugular vein is the preferred site in nonemergent situations because it is easily accessed and allows easy passage of the electrode catheter through the tricuspid valve; in addition, there is a lower incidence of pneumothorax in comparison to the subclavian approach. The left internal jugular vein is less desirable than the right internal jugular vein because of its usually more tortuous course. The femoral vein is often used in elective situations in which the cardiac catheterization laboratory can be used because this vein is easily accessed. Antecubital veins are generally used only in patients with bleeding disorders or in those receiving anticoagulant therapy; access is by cutdown rather than by percutaneous approach because the ability to control bleeding is better. Sterile technique should always be used during placement of the transvenous electrode catheter.

The technique of positioning balloon-flotation or semiflotation pacing catheters with the aid of the unipolar electrogram is described below.

1. Attach the limb leads of a surface ECG recorder to the patient.
2. Advance the electrode catheter through the cannula until the catheter tip reaches the superior vena cava (approximately 10–20 cm from the insertion site when using the internal jugular venous approach).
3. At this point, an intracardiac unipolar electrogram is monitored to verify the position of the catheter (Fig. 25-20). Connect the wire from the distal (tip) electrode to the V lead of the ECG machine with a double alligator clip or specially constructed connector, and record the V lead of the ECG. A simultaneous recording of a surface ECG lead and the intracardiac electrogram should be made whenever possible, using a multichannel recording device.
4. With the balloon inflated, advance the pacing catheter slowly into the right atrium across the tricuspid valve and into the right ventricular apex. Deflate the balloon after placement in the right ventricular apex. The recorded intracavitary unipolar electrogram identifies the position of the tip electrode as the procedure is performed (see Fig. 25-20). When the catheter tip is in the superior vena cava, only the ventricular electric signal is recorded, due

Passage of a Transvenous Electrode Catheter

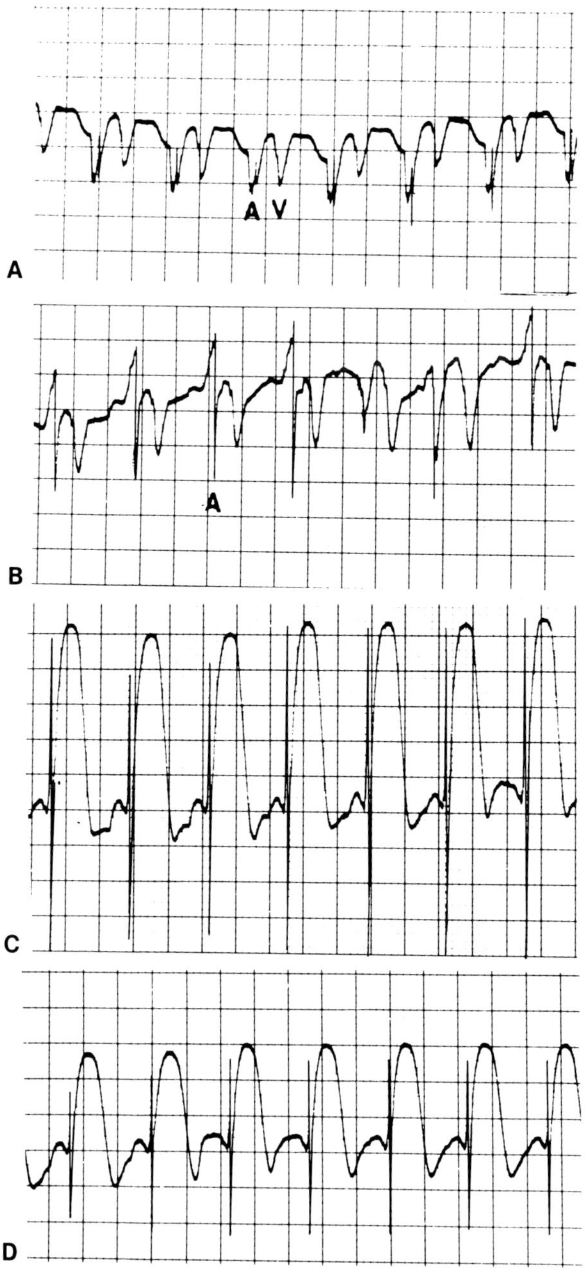

Figure 25-20 • Noncontinuous recordings of a tip (distal) unipolar electrogram during passage of a temporary transvenous electrode catheter into the apex of the right ventricle. (***A***) The catheter is within the body of the right atrium. The atrial (*A*) signal exceeds the amplitude of the ventricular (*V*) signal. (***B***) Level of the tricuspid valve. The atrial signal has better definition. (***C***) Endocardial surface of the right ventricle. Atrial electrical activity is no longer recorded. The ventricular signal has an RS configuration. The ST segment is elevated to 2.5 mV. (***D***) Same tracing as (***C***), but recorded at half-standard (0.5 cm = 1 mV) to visualize the entire signal morphology.

to its large magnitude (5–10 mV). As the catheter approaches the right atrium from the superior vena cava, the atrial electric signal increases in size in comparison to the ventricular signal. The atrial signal is usually of brief duration and triphasic. As the catheter tip approaches the tricuspid valve, the two signals are of approximately the same magnitude. Once the electrode catheter crosses the tricuspid valve and enters the right ventricle, the ventricular signal becomes larger. Half or quarter standard may be required on the ECG machine to record the entire signal. Close to the right ventricular apex, there should be little if any atrial signal, since atrial signal magnitude is in the range of only 1–4 mV (see Fig. 25–20). The ventricular signal should be of an rS or RS configuration. When the catheter is in good apposition with the endocardium of the right ventricle, the ST segment of the unipolar electrogram will demonstrate elevation, called the *current of injury.* In this position, ventricular capture should be expected, and sensing function should be normal. Incorrect pacing catheter position is suggested by the presence of the atrial signal on the unipolar electrogram and by absence of the current of injury. If simple manipulation of the catheter fails to correct the problem, fluoroscopy is required. When repositioning the pacing catheter, it is best to withdraw the lead into the right atrium and recross the tricuspid valve.

5. Determine the unipolar and bipolar pacing thresholds. To determine the bipolar pacing threshold, attach the tip (distal) electrode of the pacing catheter to the negative pole of the pulse generator and the ring (proximal) electrode to the positive pole of the pulse generator (see Fig. 25–9). Set the pacing rate to exceed the patient's spontaneous rate, and set the mode of function to demand (sensitivity control in the full clockwise position). Increase the output until capture is established. Ventricular pacing should be achieved at current outputs of about 1 mA whenever possible. The final output setting should be 1.5 to 2 times the capture threshold. To determine the unipolar pacing threshold, attach the tip or ring electrode to the negative pole of the pulse generator, and a surface electrode (such as an ECG-monitoring electrode) to the positive pole, and proceed as outlined above. Care must be taken to isolate the unused wire of the electrode catheter from surrounding objects.
6. Check both a ring and tip unipolar electrogram by attaching the terminal from the respective electrodes to the V lead of the ECG machine and recording the V lead. The ring unipolar electrogram should demonstrate an rS configuration with normal-appearing or inverted T waves. The ST segment is usually not elevated. The tip electrogram may have a higher signal amplitude than the ring electrogram. The ventricular signal has an rS or RS configuration, and ST-segment elevation is present. Determine the amplitude of the ventricular signal. Test the sensing threshold by turning the sensitivity control dial counterclockwise toward the asynchronous position. When sensing is lost, pacer output stimuli will occur at the previously selected rate. The point at which this occurs is a relative measure of ventricular signal amplitude. The final sensitivity setting should be well below this threshold.
7. Check the bipolar electrogram by attaching the terminals from the ring and tip electrodes to the left and right arm leads of the ECG machine, respectively, and by recording lead I. The leg leads of the ECG machine should remain on the patient. Since the bipolar signal (and not the unipolar electrogram) is what is sensed by the external pulse generator, it is very important to measure the amplitude of this signal. Test the sensing threshold as outlined above.
8. Check all connections for tightness. Encase the pulse generator in a rubber glove. This will prevent stray current from the environment from reaching the pacing catheter and the heart.
9. Confirm the electrode catheter placement using electrocardiographic and radiographic criteria. If the pacing catheter is properly placed at the apex of the right ventricle, a paced 12-lead ECG should show a superiorly directed mean frontal plane axis and a left bundle branch block pattern (Fig. 25–21). Occasionally (in 5%–10% of patients), a right bundle branch block pattern is recorded in the right precordial leads even if the catheter is placed properly.[43] On an AP chest radiograph, the tip electrode should be located to the left of the spine and directed inferiorly. On the cross-table lateral chest radiograph, the catheter should be directed anteriorly and inferiorly.
10. Obtain a 12-lead paced ECG and AP and cross-table lateral chest radiographs, daily to confirm continued proper placement (see Fig. 25–21B–C). Lead dislodgement will usually require repositioning to insure stability of pacing and sensing function. The chest radiograph should also be evaluated for pneumothorax, lead migration, and lead fracture; the latter is extremely unusual (see Fig. 25–21C).

There are alternatives to insertion of balloon-flotation catheters with the aid of the unipolar electrograms. One such method involves identification of the pacer output pulse and associated ventricular capture on the surface 12-lead ECG to determine the location of the intracardiac catheter. This technique is described below.

1. Attach the pins of the catheter electrodes to the pacemaker generator before insertion of the catheter.
2. Set the rate on the pulse generator to exceed the patient's intrinsic rate. Set the current output to its maximum, and

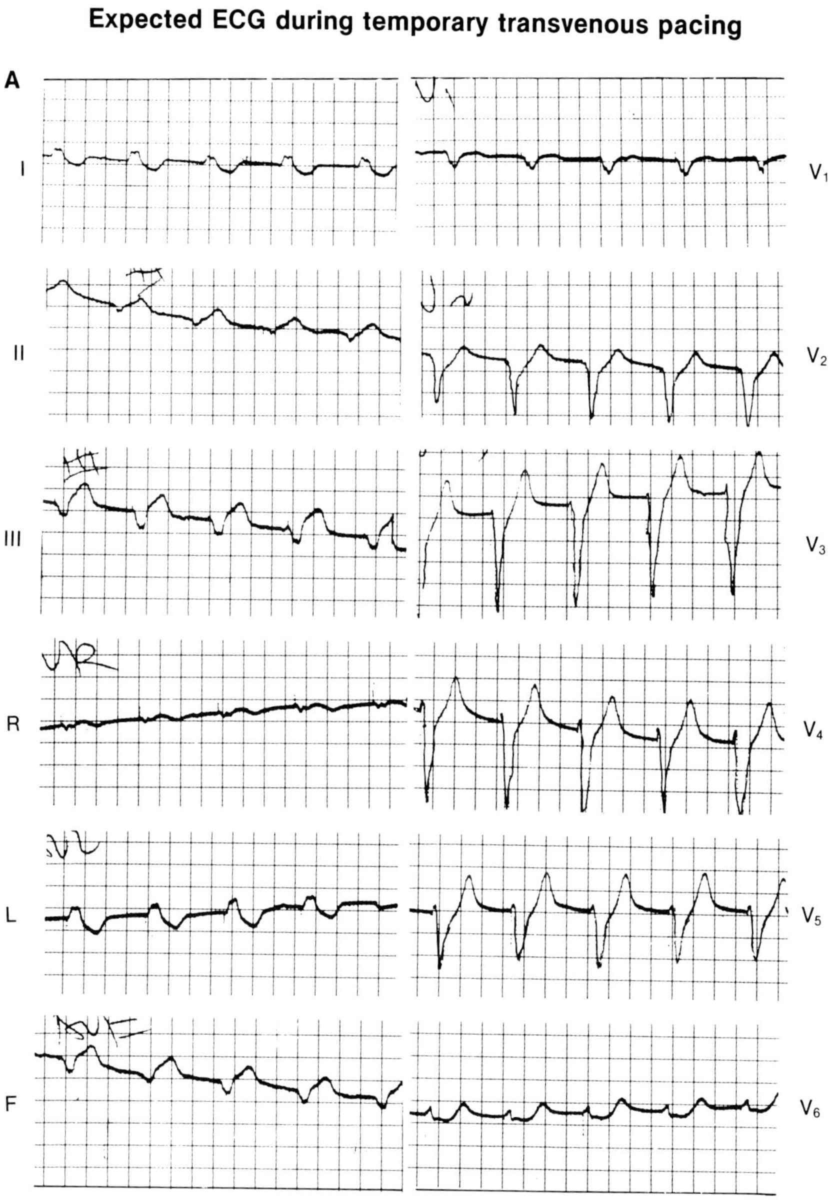

Figure 25–21 • (*A*) Paced 12-lead ECG obtained immediately after temporary transvenous pacing was established. All QRS complexes are paced. The mean frontal plane QRS axis is directed superiorly, yielding negative complexes in leads II, III, and aVF, and upright complexes in leads aVR and aVL. A left bundle-branch block pattern indicates right ventricular depolarization occurring before left ventricular depolarization, the expected situation when pacing from the right ventricle.

(continued)

ECG during temporary transvenous pacing with tip of pacing catheter in right ventricular outflow tract

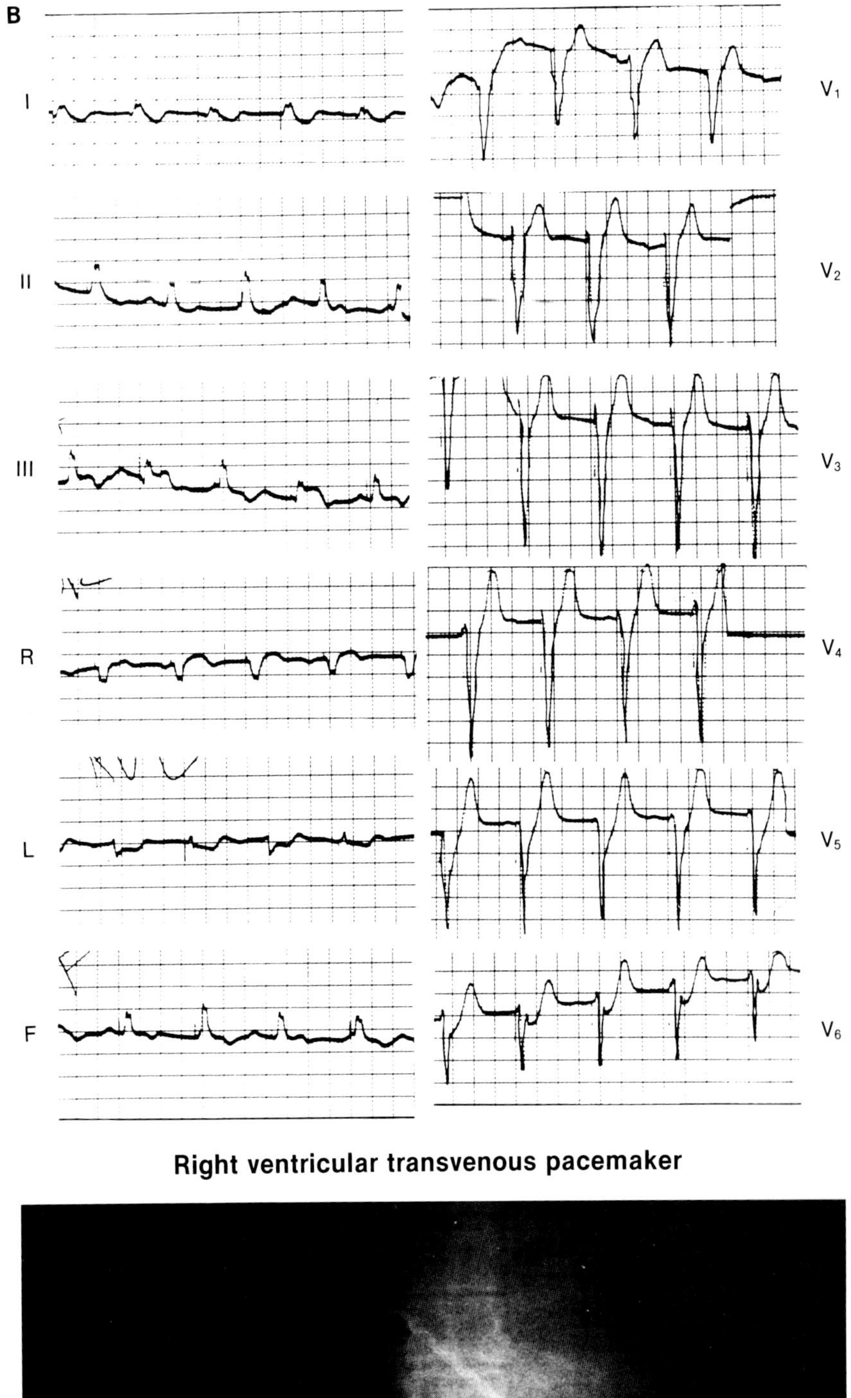

Right ventricular transvenous pacemaker

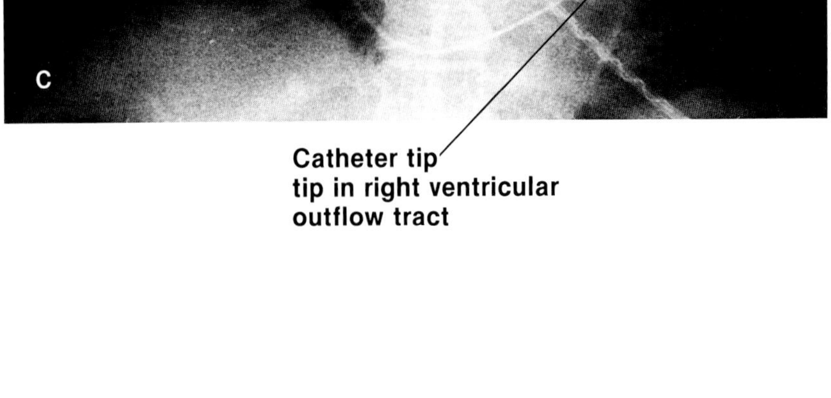

Figure 25–21 *(continued)*
(***B***) Paced 12-lead ECG, and AP chest radiograph obtained in the same patient 2 days later. All QRS complexes are paced. A left bundle-branch block pattern is still present, indicating right ventricular pacing. However, the mean frontal plane axis is now directed inferiorly, yielding upright complexes in leads II, III, and aVF. (***C***) The chest radiograph shows the tip of the pacing catheter directed superiorly, in the right ventricular outflow tract. Repositioning of the pacing lead was required.

turn the sensitivity control toward its full clockwise position to pace in a demand mode.

3. While passing the balloon catheter into the heart, the surface ECG is recorded. When contact with the endocardium is established, the ECG will show a pacing stimulus followed by a captured QRS complex. Confirm catheter placement as described above.
4. Obtain a daily paced 12-lead ECG and chest radiograph. This method of electrode catheter placement should be used only in emergent situations since optimal positioning is not insured.

b. Complications

Pacemaker-related complications and malfunction, including sensing and pacing failure, lead migration, and myocardial penetration or perforation, can be minimized in several ways. Inexperienced operators should not insert catheters without close supervision. The 12-lead ECG should always be evaluated for paced QRS morphology and axis as well as for sensing and pacing functions. Pulse generator batteries should be checked frequently. Recording the unipolar and bipolar electrograms in patients who are not pacemaker-dependent is also helpful. Transvenous pacing catheters should be replaced in a new site every 3 to 4 days to decrease the risk of infection and thromboembolism.

The reported complication rate for transvenous cardiac pacing is significant, varying from 4% to 20%.[44–46] The risk increases if the pacing system is placed in an emergency setting. Pneumothorax, infection, venous thrombosis, pulmonary embolism, air embolism, dysrhythmias, serious bleeding, myocardial penetration or perforation, pericardial tamponade, and arterial trauma are the major complications reported. Pneumothorax, arterial trauma, air embolism, and serious bleeding are the direct result of obtaining central venous access (see Chapter 20). Proper technique, including placing the patient in the Trendelenberg position during catheter insertion to decrease or eliminate the amount of air entering the thoracic structures, will help prevent these complications. Rigorous line care after catheter insertion will help prevent infection. Venous thrombosis is a major complication of pacing catheters placed in the femoral vein and varies in incidence from 25% to 35%.[47,48] Venous thrombosis may be associated with a significant incidence of pulmonary embolism.[48] Avoiding the femoral approach, except for catheters kept in place for just a few hours, will reduce this complication. Ventricular dysrhythmias are the most common dysrhythmic complication of transvenous pacing. As with any intracardiac catheter, its placement against the right ventricular inflow or outflow tracts is usually the cause of these dysrhythmias. Repositioning of the catheter is required, and antidysrhythmic drug therapy should be avoided. Nonsustained ventricular dysrhythmias are also seen commonly during initial passage of the catheter into the heart.

Myocardial penetration or perforation is a serious complication of transvenous pacing with a reported incidence of 2% to 30%.[49] Fortunately, pericardial tamponade is quite uncommon. The diagnosis of myocardial perforation should be suspected if the patient complains of chest pain or if a pericardial friction rub is heard after the insertion of the pacing lead. Other findings that should raise the level of suspicion of penetration include failure to sense or capture and a change in the configuration of the paced QRS complex. If myocardial penetration or perforation is suspected, tip (distal) and ring (proximal) unipolar electrograms must be obtained. The tip unipolar electrogram morphology will differ from its configuration at initial insertion, manifesting as Rs or pure R wave configuration. It may resemble a surface ECG recording of lead V4, V5, or V6, depending on the direction of the perforating lead. The ST segment is not elevated, and the T wave resembles a normal precordial T wave. The proximal unipolar electrogram may also be altered, depending on the precise location of the ring electrode. A chest radiograph will not routinely detect penetration or perforation. If the diagnosis is still in doubt after evaluating the unipolar electrogram, a two-dimensional echocardiogram should be obtained to confirm the location of the tip of the pacing catheter.[50] Once the diagnosis of perforation or penetration is confirmed, the catheter must be repositioned if pacing malfunction is present or if the patient is experiencing chest pain. Pulling back on the catheter slightly usually does not suffice because the lead tends to migrate back through the tract originally created. The catheter should therefore be pulled back into the right atrium and reinserted into the ventricle. Fluoroscopy is recommended. If there is evidence of significant pericardial effusion or tamponade, urgent pericardiocentesis is indicated (see Chapter 27).

The incidence of pacing system malfunction, which includes failure to sense (undersensing), oversensing, and failure to capture, ranges from 14% to about 37%.[44–46] Failure to sense the patient's native depolarizations (undersensing) can result in the delivery of a pacing stimulus inappropriately early (Figs. 25–22 and 25–23). Repetitive

Failure to Sense in a Temporary Transvenous Pacing System

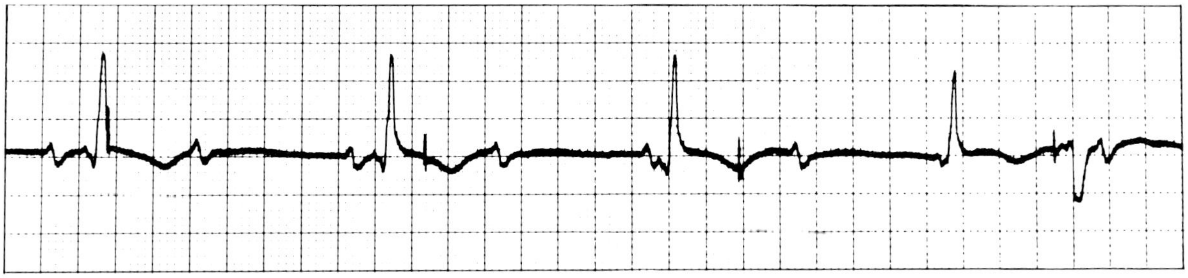

Figure 25–22 • Lead II rhythm strip illustrating failure to sense in a patient with an acute inferior wall myocardial infarction and a temporary transvenous pacing system placed for complete AV block. The pacing stimuli are being delivered at a rate of 35/min to display their occurrence throughout the QRST complex. The fourth pacing stimulus falls outside the refractory period of the ventricles and captures appropriately. The delivery of a pacing output pulse on the QRST complex can, under some clinical circumstances, cause repetitive ventricular beating, including ventricular fibrillation. The pacing artifacts have been retouched for clarity.

ventricular beating, ventricular tachycardia, or ventricular fibrillation can result.

Undersensing is usually caused by poor positioning of the temporary pacing catheter or by a poor intracardiac signal. Less commonly, it can be caused by generator malfunction or lead fracture. If failure to sense is diagnosed, a 12-lead ECG and an AP and cross-table lateral chest radiograph should be obtained to assess catheter position and look for lead fracture. Poor intracardiac signal quality is common and results from myocardial ischemia, acid–base disorders, ventricular dilatation, electrolyte abnormalities, and the use of certain drugs, particularly class I antiarrhythmic agents. Unless potentially life-threatening dysrhythmias result from failure to sense, careful observation may be all that is indicated. If intervention is required, several management options are open. First, the sensitivity

Pacer-Induced Ventricular Tachycardia

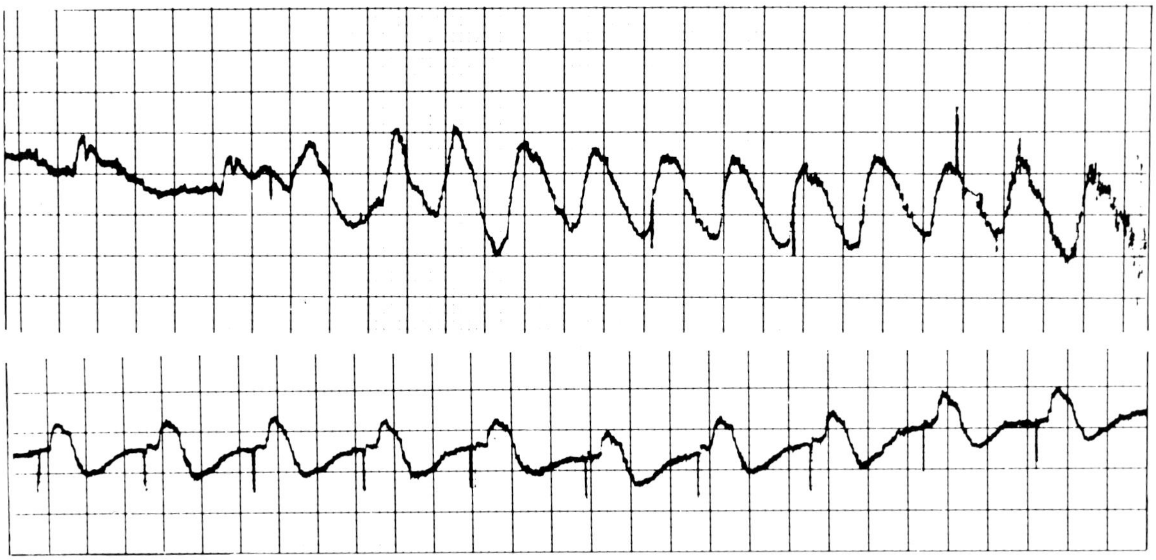

Figure 25–23 • MCL_1 rhythm strip showing pacemaker-induced ventricular tachycardia in a patient with an acute anterior wall myocardial infarction. Failure to sense the patient's spontaneous QRS complexes results in the delivery of a pacing stimulus at the beginning of the downstroke of the T wave (*top*). Pacing pulses are emitted during the ventricular tachycardia, indicating that not all tachycardia complexes are sensed. The monomorphic ventricular tachycardia that resulted was converted to sinus by increasing the rate of the pacemaker generator, capturing the ventricle (*bottom*) and gradually slowing the paced rate (*not shown*).

control of the pulse generator can be set to the full demand position. This maneuver allows the generator to sense signals of small magnitude (around 1 mV) (see Fig. 25–9). If catheter malposition is suspected, repositioning of the catheter is indicated. If lead fracture is diagnosed, the catheter must be replaced. Finally, if poor intracardiac signal is the problem, the electrode catheter can be unipolarized to augment the intracardiac signal (Fig. 25–24). This is done by connecting the negative terminal of the pulse generator to the intracardiac electrode that has the greatest signal magnitude, and the positive terminal of the pulse generator to a surface electrode (a standard bedside-monitoring electrode is fine for this purpose). The end of the unused catheter electrode is encased in a rubber stopper or glove to prevent accidental conduction of current directly into the heart. When the pacing system is thus unipolarized, both the bipolar and the tip and ring unipolar signals must be recorded daily to assess changes in intracardiac signal magnitude so that optimal sensitivity settings may be selected.

Oversensing, or sensing of unwanted signals, may be dangerous if it results in pauses in paced rhythm due to inhibition of generator output. Oversensing may be the result of sensing of atrial electric activity (if the lead electrodes are situated near the tricuspid valve), sensing of T waves, or sensing of electric signals from the environment. Management consists of turning the sensitivity control toward the asynchronous position until the unwanted signals are no longer sensed, removing the offending external environmental signals, or repositioning the catheter.

Failure to capture is one of the most common pacing system malfunctions. Failure to capture may be intermittent or complete and may, if the patient is 100% paced, be manifested by type I or type II exit block (Fig. 25–25). Failure to capture is frequently a preterminal occurrence, where it is a harbinger of electromechanical dissociation.[21] Failure to capture results from lead malposition, increased myocardial stimulation threshold, loose connections, myocardial penetration or perforation, and lead fracture

Technique for Unipolarization of a Transvenous Pacemaker System

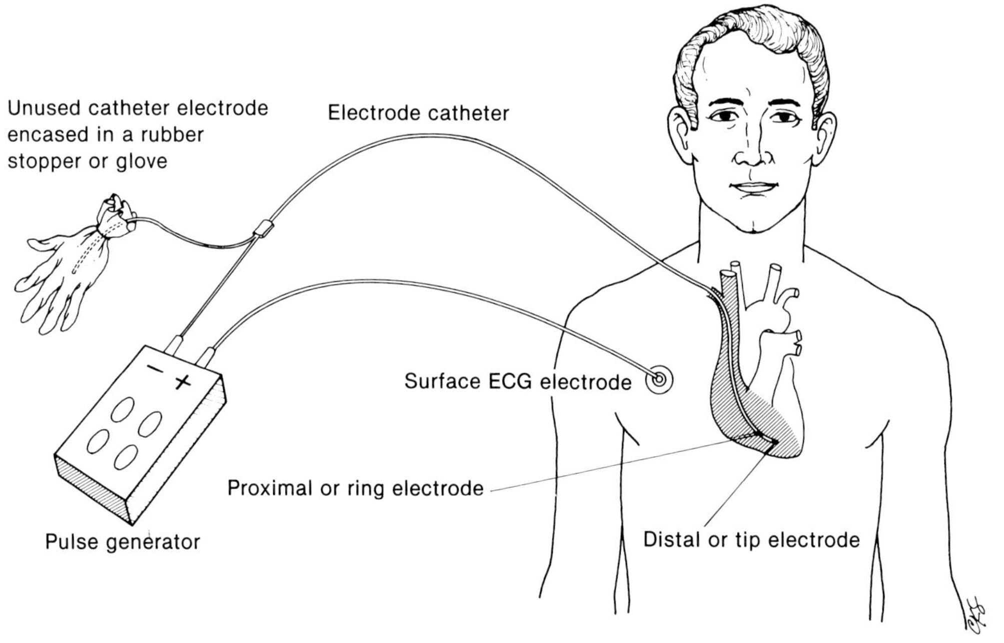

Figure 25–24 • Technique for unipolarization of a transvenous pacemaker system. The negative terminal of the pulse generator is connected to the intracardiac electrode, and the positive terminal is connected to a surface electrode. The unused catheter electrode is encased in a rubber stopper or glove to prevent accidental conduction of current directly into the heart. When the pacing system is unipolarized, bipolar and unipolar (both tip and ring) signals must be evaluated daily to assess changes in intracardiac signal magnitude, so that optimal sensitivity changes may be selected.

Temporary Pacing with Intermittent Failure to Capture

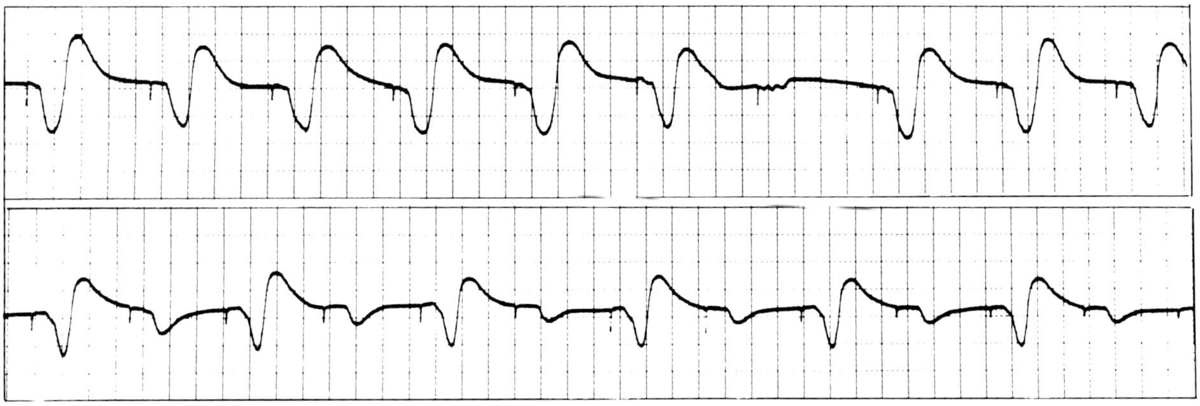

Figure 25–25 • MCL_1 recording from a terminally ill patient with a temporary pacing system in place. Intermittent failure to capture is present: the seventh pacing stimulus (*top*) and every alternate pacing stimulus (*bottom*) are unassociated with QRS complexes. The paced QRS complexes follow the pacer output pulse by 0.12 seconds, indicating first-degree exit block from the pacing electrodes to the surrounding myocardium. This phenomenon is also known as *pacemaker latency*. The undulations in the baseline following the episodes of noncapture might represent local muscle depolarization insufficient to produce a true QRS complex on the surface ECG. Most QRS complexes were unassociated with a pulse (electromechanical dissociation); the patient expired shortly after this recording was made.

or pulse generator malfunction. Increased myocardial stimulation threshold is often caused by hyperkalemia, myocardial necrosis, acidosis, shock, or a high concentration of type I antidysrhythmic agents (especially flecainide).[52] Management options include increasing the output current until consistent capture occurs; correcting any hemodynamic, drug, or electrolyte abnormalities if present; and evaluating for lead malposition, lead fracture, loose connections, and myocardial perforation. In emergency settings, low-dose intravenous corticosteroids (40 mg of methylprednisolone) or low-dose isoproterenol may be used to restore temporary pacing function.

D. *Carotid Sinus Massage*

Carotid sinus massage (CSM) is a simple bedside maneuver that may be useful in diagnosing and treating cardiac rhythm disturbances. It is widely used in the termination of paroxysmal reentrant supraventricular tachycardias and to diagnose sinoatrial and atrioventricular nodal disease. The mechanism of some tachycardias may also be revealed with CSM by decreasing conduction at the AV node and allowing the atrial rhythm to be seen. Other clinical uses of CSM include the diagnosis of carotid sinus hypersensitivity syndrome, the evaluation of pacing function of a permanent cardiac pacemaker by slowing the patient's spontaneous rate, and the diagnosis of latent digitalis toxicity.[53]

1. TECHNIQUE

The patient should be supine and a blood pressure cuff placed. Continuous ECG monitoring is mandatory; however, in most instances, a critical care unit is not necessary. Atropine should be available at the bedside, and a defibrillator should be nearby. The following steps should be employed:

1. Obtain a blood pressure and ECG strip.
2. Extend the patient's neck, and turn the head to the contralateral side (Fig. 25–26).
3. Auscultate both carotid arteries for the presence of bruits. The presence of bruits is a contraindication to CSM.
4. Massage the right carotid sinus first, since it is more effective in slowing ventricular rate than left carotid massage. In addition, if a cerebral embolic event were to occur as a result of CSM, it would be less damaging in the nondominant hemisphere.
5. Locate the carotid artery pulsation with gentle palpation. Press the index and middle fingers against the carotid pulsation at the angle of the jaw (see Fig. 25–26). Gentle pressure should be applied first, since some patients (especially elderly patients) may have hypersensitive carotid sinuses, making

Carotid Sinus Massage

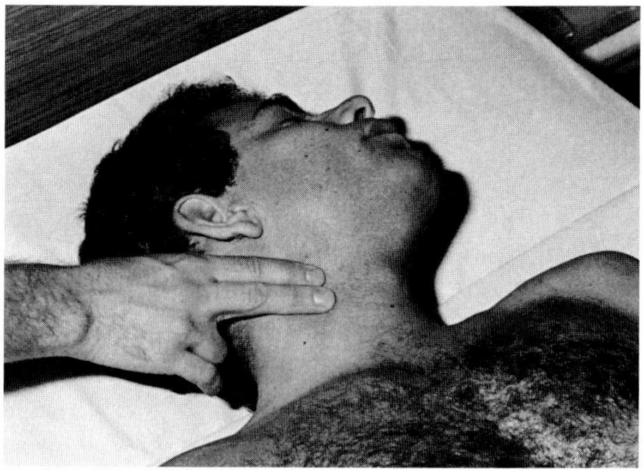

Figure 25–26 • Carotid sinus massage. Position of the patient's head and neck and the operator's fingers for the performance of carotid sinus massage. The carotid artery is palpated and the area is then massaged for up to 5 seconds.

prolonged sinus arrest or AV nodal block possible. Apply firm pressure if no diagnostic or therapeutic benefit is initially obtained and if no adverse event occurs.

6. Perform the massage in an up-and-down motion for 5 to 10 seconds.
7. Evaluate the cardiac rhythm strip and blood pressure during the CSM.
8. If the desired diagnostic or therapeutic effect is not obtained, CSM may be repeated on the same side in a different location. It is also possible to perform CSM on the contralateral side.
9. Obtain a repeat blood pressure and 12-lead ECG at the end of the procedure or if complications occur.

2. COMPLICATIONS

Complications of CSM are uncommon. Mechanical obstruction of the carotid artery and cerebral vascular events have been reported.[54-56] Because of this, CSM should not be performed in patients with carotid bruits, known cerebrovascular disease, or a history of a cerebrovascular accident or transient ischemic attack.

Carotid sinus massage may induce nonsustained ventricular tachycardia and, rarely, has been reported to cause sustained ventricular tachycardia or ventricular fibrillation.[57-63] Asystole has been reported only once with CSM.[53] Prolonged sinus arrest may result but is easily treated with a precordial thump or a cough.

E. *Precordial Thump*

The *precordial thump* was first described in 1920 by Schott, who reported that a blow to the chest restored the pulse in a patient who had suffered a Stokes-Adams attack.[64] Since that time, there have been reports of its success in ventricular asystole, ventricular tachycardia, and ventricular fibrillation.[65-68] Other workers, however, have reported only marginal clinical benefit, and a significant incidence of adverse effects including the induction of ventricular fibrillation.[69] Based on these limited data, the American Heart Association, in its *Guidelines for Advanced Cardiac Life Support*, recommends the use of a single precordial thump for witnessed cardiac arrests when a defibrillator is not available, and for patients with monitored ventricular tachycardia when a palpable pulse is present.[70]

The mechanism by which the precordial thump is effective is not fully known. It may achieve conversion of abnormal rhythms by causing electromechanical transduction, in which a low-energy current that traverses the chest wall to the myocardium is produced as the result of the mechanical blow. This electric impulse then depolarizes a reentrant pathway in the myocardium, interrupting the abnormal rhythm. Because relatively small amounts of electric energy are created by the mechanical blow to the chest, only those rhythms that are terminated by low levels of energy are likely to respond to the precordial thump. Another possible mechanism of action is the induction of a premature ventricular systole that interrupts a reentrant pathway or creates electric activity during ventricular asystole.

1. TECHNIQUE

The precordial thump is performed as follows:

1. Identify the rhythm on the monitor.
2. Raise a fist 8–12 inches above the sternum, and deliver the fleshy part of the hypothenar eminence to the lower sternum with moderate pressure. Never deliver enough pressure to break ribs (Fig. 25–27).
3. Evaluate the monitor quickly for a change in rhythm.

2. COMPLICATIONS

The precordial thump does have the potential to make a cardiac rhythm less stable. In one uncontrolled study in the prehospital setting, 12 of 27 patients with ventricular tachycardia (VT) were thumped into more malignant rhythms, which included asystole, ventricular fibrillation

Precordial Thump

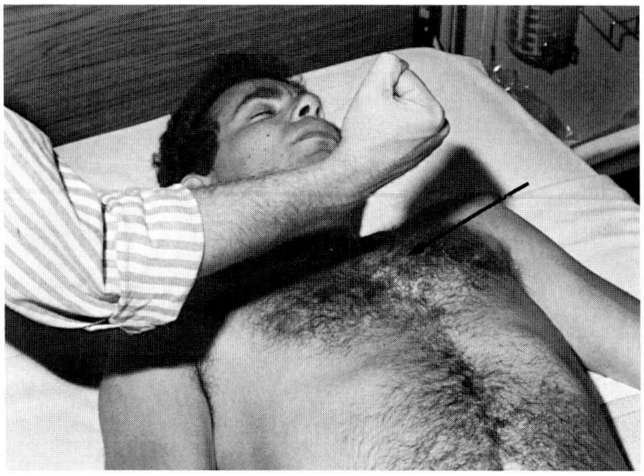

Figure 25–27 • Precordial thump. Position of the fist relative to the chest wall for the performance of the precordial thump. The fist should fall on the lower sternum.

(VF), and electromechanical dissociation.[69] The authors postulated that hypoxia and acidosis in the field may have contributed to the complications seen in their study.

III. CARDIAC DYSRHYTHMIAS: RECOGNITION AND MANAGEMENT

A. *Atrial Tachydysrhythmias*

Tachydysrhythmias may arise from any portion of the heart and are classified as either supraventricular or ventricular. *Supraventricular tachydysrhythmias* arise from the sinus node, atrium, coronary sinus, AV node, or His bundle. *Ventricular tachydysrhythmias* arise from the Purkinje system or ventricular muscle. The detrimental consequences of tachydysrhythmias include rapid rate and loss of AV synchrony, leading to impaired ventricular filling and hemodynamic compromise (hypotension and pulmonary edema) or ischemic cardiac pain.

1. SINUS TACHYCARDIA

Sinus tachycardia is defined as an increase in the rate of discharge of the sinus node to greater than 100/minute. The P waves are normal and are followed by QRS complexes. If the rate is extremely rapid, the P waves may be buried in the preceding T waves, confounding interpretation of the rhythm. Carotid sinus massage should be attempted to transiently slow the rate, allowing the identification of the P waves. The rate is rarely above 150/minute unless the plasma catecholamine levels are extremely high, as in acute myocardial infarction, pulmonary edema, cocaine intoxication, or pheochromocytoma.[71]

Sinus tachycardia is a physiologic response to stress. Such stresses include exertion, pain, fever, anxiety, hypovolemia, myocardial infarction, and congestive heart failure. Treatment of sinus tachycardia is directed at finding and treating the underlying condition. Intravenous or oral beta-blocking agents should be used with caution and only in situations in which the tachycardia is detrimental to hemodynamic stability (myocardial infarction or ischemia). Propranolol, metoprolol, or esmolol may be used.

2. PAROXYSMAL SUPRAVENTRICULAR TACHYCARDIA

Paroxysmal supraventricular tachycardia (PSVT) is a reentry tachydysrhythmia involving the AV node alone (intra-AV nodal reentry) or the AV node and an extra-AV nodal bypass tract (for example, a Kent bundle in the Wolff-Parkinson-White [WPW] syndrome) (Fig. 25–28). The patient with PSVT generally has at least two pathways within the AV node: one is a slow-conducting pathway and the other is a fast-conducting pathway having a long refractory period. During normal sinus rhythm, the fast-conducting pathway typically conducts the electric impulse to the ventricle. If an impulse, usually a premature impulse, is blocked in the fast pathway due to its long refractory period but conducts down the slow pathway, it can reexcite the previously blocked fast pathway in a retrograde fashion, provided that sufficient time has elapsed for the fast pathway to recover. The reentry impulse may fail to propagate further or may find the slow pathway repolarized and able to conduct in an antegrade fashion, setting up a reentry tachycardia.

The typical ECG in PSVT reveals a regular, narrow QRS complex tachycardia (see Fig. 25–28). The P waves occurring before, after, or during the QRS complex are inverted in leads II, III, and AVF due to retrograde atrial depolarization. Often PSVT is initiated by a premature atrial depolarization with a prolonged PR interval. If bundle branch block or antegrade conduction via an extra-AV nodal bypass tract is present, the QRS complex will be wide, making PSVT difficult to distinguish from ventricular tachycardia (VT). If VT or a bypass tract cannot be excluded, therapy for VT must be instituted because the treatment for PSVT (AV nodal

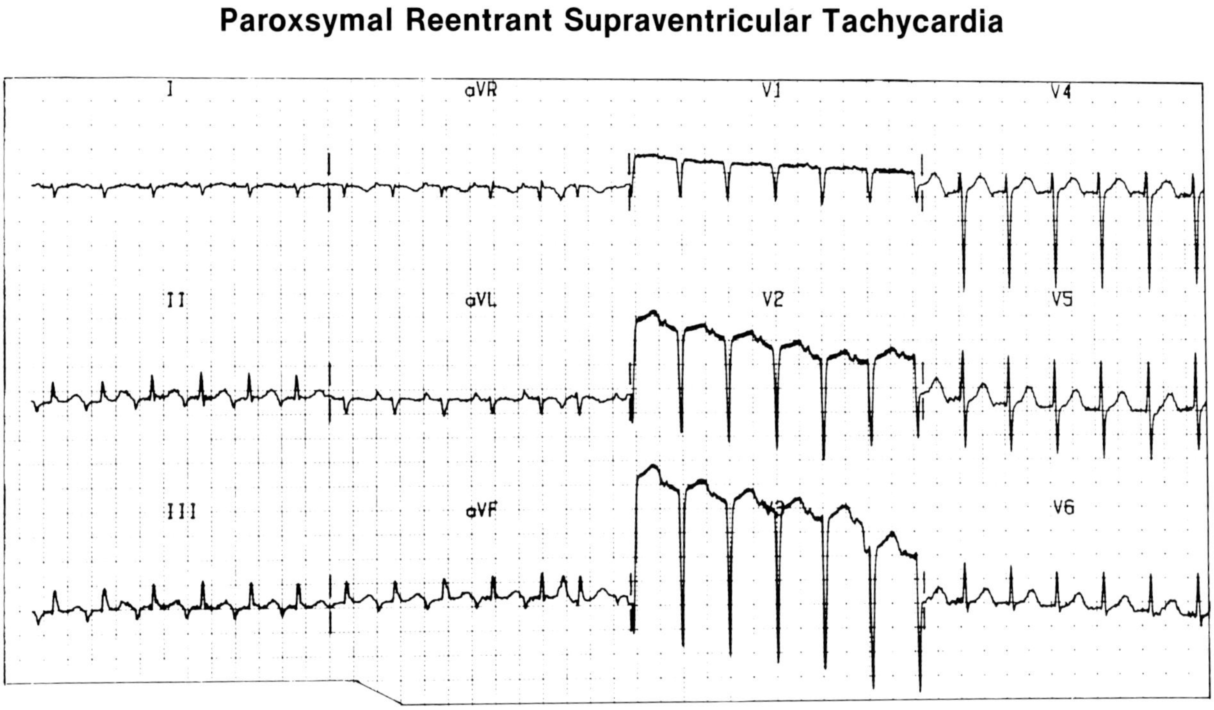

Figure 25–28 • Paroxysmal reentrant supraventricular tachycardia illustrating a rapid, regular narrow QRS complex tachycardia with inverted P waves in the inferior leads, indicating retrograde atrial depolarization. The RP interval exceeds the PR interval. This patient has a concealed left-sided AV bypass tract. During this tachycardia the blood pressure was normal and the patient had no symptoms. The rhythm terminated to normal sinus rhythm after 7.5 mg of intravenous adenosine.

blocking agents) might have adverse hemodynamic consequences if the rhythm is ventricular in origin.

The major goal of treatment is PSVT is to slow the ventricular rate and terminate the rhythm. Slowing the ventricular rate can be accomplished by delaying impulse conduction within the reentry pathway, in either a retrograde or antegrade direction. Always attempt CSM first unless there is a contraindication. Valsalva maneuvers may also terminate the rhythm. However, neither maneuver should be expected to be effective if hemodynamic instability or high catecholamine levels exist. The drug of choice is intravenous adenosine; intravenous verapamil may also be used (Fig. 25–29). Intravenous esmolol is also useful because of its short half-life. Occasionally, intravenous procainamide will also convert the rhythm. Synchronized DC cardioversion is effective if pharmacologic agents or CSM fail. Usually 15–50 J of energy is sufficient. If higher energy levels are needed, as when the tachydysrhythmia is associated with congestive heart failure, 100 and 200 J may be used. Atrial overdrive pacing is required if other methods of therapy fail, and should be performed in the cardiac catheterization laboratory by experienced personnel. Emergency cardioversion, rather than pharmacologic treatment, is mandatory if myocardial ischemia, pulmonary edema, or hemodynamic compromise is present.

3. ATRIAL FLUTTER

Atrial flutter is a supraventricular rhythm characterized by sawtooth flutter waves (Fig. 25–30). It is an unstable rhythm that often converts to atrial fibrillation or normal sinus rhythm spontaneously, depending on the underlying clinical situation. The clinical consequences of atrial flutter depend on the underlying cardiac status and the ventricular rate. The loss of atrial contribution to cardiac output may lead to a decrease in cardiac output, hypotension, ischemic chest pain, syncope, or pulmonary edema. Atrial flutter is encountered in patients with structural cardiac disease, pulmonary disease, myocardial infarction, and pericardial disease. It is also a transient complication of pneumonia, thyrotoxicosis, and cardiac surgery.

The atrial rate in flutter is usually 280–320/minute. Ventricular rates vary due to different AV conduction ratios (see Fig. 25–30). If the ventricular rate is rapid, flutter waves may not be easily identified. With CSM or other

Treatment of Paroxysmal Reentrant Tachycardia with Verapamil

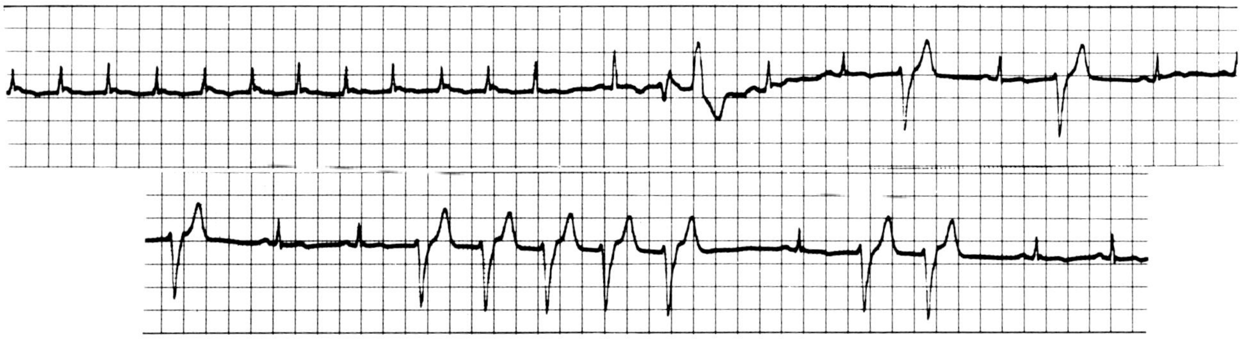

Figure 25–29 • Reentrant supraventricular tachycardia converted to normal sinus rhythm after 5.0 mg intravenous verapamil. Ventricular extrasystoles are commonly observed after conversion of this rhythm using pharmacologic agents, for reasons that are not clear.

vagal maneuvers, AV conduction may delay enough to allow the flutter waves to be identified. The QRS complexes are narrow, unless bundle branch block or an AV nodal bypass tract are present.

The selection of electric or pharmacologic treatment for atrial flutter depends on the clinical circumstances. Atrial flutter, as a complication of an acute illness such as pneumonia, requires only rate control and treatment of the illness. However, rate control can be difficult to achieve in flutter. In the setting of underlying cardiac disease, DC cardioversion is usually required and is generally preferred. Pharmacologic conversion of atrial flutter may be difficult but can be attempted in the asymptomatic patient prior to electric conversion, and in patients who fail electric conversion. In patients with hypotension, pulmonary edema, or angina, DC cardioversion is mandatory .

Synchronized DC cardioversion is performed using low-level energy (20 J). Energy levels may be increased to 50 or 100 J. For control of ventricular rate, digoxin is the agent of first choice, but this agent alone may not slow the ventricular rate. Increasing the total dose beyond what is recommended in efforts to achieve rate control may lead to digitalis toxicity. Pharmacologic agents that may be administered in addition to, or substituted for, digoxin include verapamil, esmolol, propranolol, or diltiazem (Table 25–2). Pharmacologic conversion is attempted with a type IA antidysrhythmic agent (quinidine or procainamide) but only after adequate rate control or a full digitalizing dose is achieved. Otherwise, administration of a

Atrial Flutter

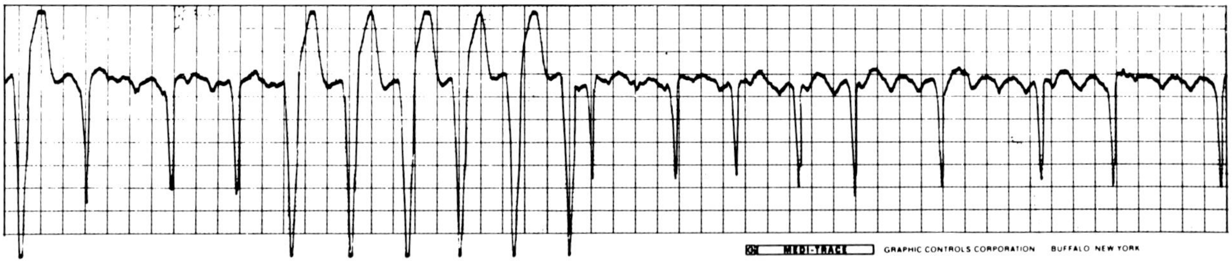

Figure 25–30 • Lead III illustrating atrial flutter with varying AV conduction, from 2:1 to 4:1. The classic sawtooth pattern of the flutter waves is best appreciated in the inferior leads. In this example, the wide QRS complex rhythm is due to rate-dependent intraventricular aberration and not to ventricular tachycardia. It is often extremely difficult to distinguish intraventricular aberration from ventricular tachycardia in the presence of supraventricular tachydysrhythmias.

Table 25-2 · Commonly Used Dosages for Pharmacologic Treatment of Cardiac Dysrhythmias

Drug	Dosage
Propranolol	1 mg IV every 5 min to a total of 3 mg
Metoprolol	5 mg IV every 5 min to a total of 15 mg; 50 mg PO every 8 hr
Esmolol	500 μg/kg IV load over 1 min followed by a continuous infusion of 50–300 μg/kg/min. After 5–30 min, if the rhythm or rate is not controlled, the IV load is repeated and the infusion is increased to 100 μg/kg/min. The infusion may subsequently be increased after 5–30 min intervals to 150, 200, 250, and 300 μg/kg/min; each increase in the infusion is preceded by the 500 μg/kg IV load.
Verapamil	2.5–10 mg IV over 2–3 min; a repeat dose may be given after 20–30 min; 80 mg PO every 8 hr
Digoxin	0.25–0.50 mg IV or PO initially, followed by 0.25 mg PO or IV every 4–6 hr until the rate is controlled or a total of 1.25–1.50 mg is administered over 24 hr
Diltiazem	0.25 mg/kg IV load, followed by 0.001–0.002 mg/kg IV/min; 30–120 mg PO every 6 hr
Quinidine	200–600 mg PO every 6 hr after an oral load of 600 mg (12 mg/kg)
Procainamide	100 mg every 5 min IV load up to a total of 1 g or until hypotension occurs, QRS complex widens by 50%, or the dysrhythmia is terminated; continuous IV infusion of 1–6 μg/min; oral load of 500–1000 mg (14 mg/kg) followed by 350–1000 mg every 3–6 hr
Lidocaine	1 mg/kg IV loading dose which may be repeated 5 min after the first dose; continuous IV infusion of 1–4 mg/min
Isoproterenol	1–6 μg/min IV continuous infusion
Magnesium sulfate	2–5 g IV over 30–60 min; 100–300 mg continuous infusion
Epinephrine	0.5–1.0 mg IV over 30–60 sec; may be repeated every 5–10 min during cardiac arrest
Bretylium	5 mg/kg IV load; continuous infusion of 1–2 mg/min
Atropine	0.5–1.0 mg IV bolus every 5 min up to a total dose of 2.0 mg
Amiodarone	800–1600 mg/day PO for 1–3 weeks; load followed by a maintenance dose of 400–600 mg/day

type I agent may result in a more rapid ventricular rate due to the development of 1:1 conduction of the flutter impulses. When sinus rhythm has been restored, antidysrhythmic therapy is continued. Atrial overdrive pacing is successful in terminating atrial flutter in 30% to 80% of all patients, and in 70% to 80% of selected patients.[72] It should be considered after other forms of treatment have failed or emergently if DC cardioversion is unsuccessful.

4. ATRIAL FIBRILLATION

Atrial fibrillation is characterized by disorganized atrial electric activity that results in the absence of effective atrial contraction. The ECG does not show discrete P waves, but displays small irregular undulations in the baseline. Variable AV conduction leads to the classic irregularly irregular ventricular rhythm. The ventricular rate is usually between 100 and 180/minute. Patients who present with atrial fibrillation and a ventricular rate of less than 100/min may have underlying sinoatrial or AV nodal disease. The QRS complex is usually normal; a wide QRS complex is the result of a bundle branch block, or conduction via an extra-AV nodal bypass tract. Intermittent wide QRS complexes following long–short RR intervals are generally due to aberrant intraventricular conduction and are called *Ashman's phenomenon.* However, long–short RR sequences also favor the occurrence of ventricular extrasystoles, so the differential diagnosis may be difficult, and one must rely on morphologic criteria. Recognition of digitalis toxicity in the setting of atrial fibrillation consists of identifying high-grade or complete AV block and an ectopic pacemaker that stimulates the ventricular rhythm. Because ectopic pacemakers discharge at regular intervals, the ventricular response will be regular (Fig. 25–31). Type I (Wenckebach) or type II exit block may occur from the ectopic focus to ventricular myocardium leading to the expected changes in the RR intervals.[73] Ventricular premature complexes, junctional tachycardia,

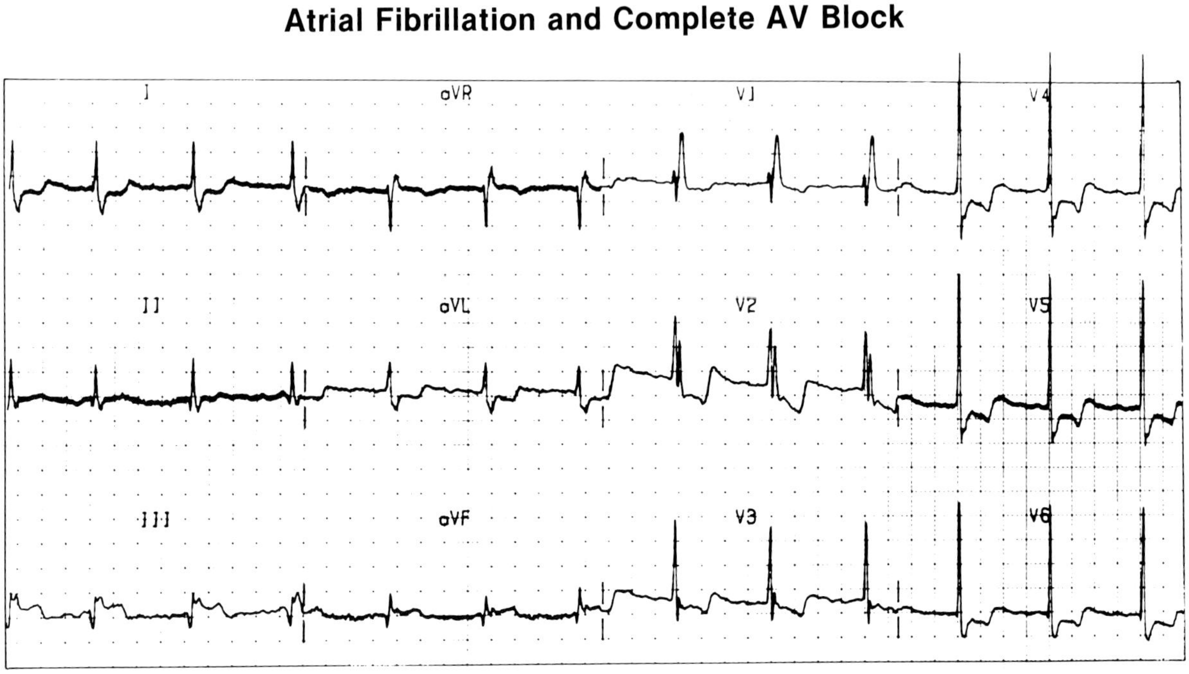

Figure 25–31 • Twelve-lead ECG recorded in a patient whose serum digoxin level was 3.0 ng/dL. The atrial rhythm is fibrillation but the ventricular rate is regular. A regular QRS rhythm in the presence of atrial fibrillation implies the existence of complete AV block (usually at the level of the AV node) with the QRS rhythm originating in a subnodal focus which discharges at regular intervals. Inferior wall myocardial infarction and right bundle-branch block pattern are also present in this tracing.

VT, or VF in the setting of atrial fibrillation may also signify digitalis toxicity.

The treatment of atrial fibrillation depends on the specific clinical circumstance. Emergent synchronized DC cardioversion should be performed in patients with hemodynamic compromise, pulmonary edema, or myocardial ischemia who do not respond to simple medical management. The majority of patients will demonstrate no untoward effects from atrial fibrillation once ventricular rate is controlled. Treatment should begin by slowing the ventricular rate; conversion to sinus rhythm can then be considered. Conversion to sinus rhythm results in improved cardiac performance, especially in patients with noncompliant ventricles or mitral stenosis.

Digoxin is given to slow the ventricular response in atrial fibrillation (see Table 25–2). Alternative drugs for rate control that may be added to or substituted for digoxin include verapamil, esmolol, propranolol, or diltiazem. Digoxin and direct-acting AV nodal blocking agents are contraindicated in patients with atrial fibrillation and a wide QRS complex rhythm when the presence of VT or extra-AV nodal bypass tracts cannot be excluded. Conversion to sinus rhythm is accomplished with synchronized DC cardioversion or using a type I antidysrhythmic agent. Pharmacologic conversion may be less desirable than electric conversion in certain patients because of a significant incidence of drug failure and prodysrhythmic complications. If electric conversion is desired, oral quinidine or oral or intravenous procainamide should be administered before and after the procedure to help maintain sinus rhythm. Energy levels should start at 100 J and increase by 100 J with each subsequent attempt. It is usually not necessary to increase energy levels beyond 200 J, but exceptions do occur. Patients suspected of having underlying AV nodal disease (those presenting with normal or slow ventricular rates in the absence of medication) should either not be electrically cardioverted at all, or should have a temporary transvenous ventricular pacing system in place during the procedure for rate support. Similarly, patients whose rhythm is suspected of being due to digitalis toxicity should not be electrically cardioverted, as malignant postconversion ventricular arrhythmias can occur.[74]

Most patients with atrial fibrillation should be anticoagulated for 2 to 3 weeks before and several weeks after pharmacologic or electric cardioversion. Again, this decision should be individualized. Unless otherwise contraindicated, patients with mitral stenosis, dilated cardiomyopathy, large left atria, atrial fibrillation of long duration, or a history of thromboembolic phenomena should be anticoagulated.

5. ECTOPIC (AUTOMATIC) ATRIAL TACHYCARDIA

Any cardiac tissue capable of undergoing diastolic depolarization to reach threshold and discharge is called *automatic tissue.* In some circumstances, abnormal impulse formation occurs in this tissue, leading to enhancement of the intrinsic firing rate and ectopic (or automatic) tachycardias. Digitalis toxicity, severe congestive heart failure, severe chronic obstructive pulmonary disease, alcohol ingestion, and acute myocardial infarction are all clinical settings in which automatic atrial tachycardias can occur.

The atrial rate in automatic atrial tachycardias is between 150 and 200/minute. The AV conduction ratio is usually 1:1, but higher ratios reflecting type I or type II AV block can occur. The presence of AV block should suggest that the rhythm is digitalis-toxic. The ectopic P waves have a normal axis, a short duration, and peaked morphology. If P waves are not seen, CSM may slow the rate enough to allow them to be identified. There should be no change in atrial rate with CSM, and the tachycardia will not terminate with such a maneuver.

Therapy depends on the specific etiology identified. Digitalis should always be discontinued if it is a part of the patient's medical regimen. Other therapy for digitalis toxicity may be necessary. Usually, DC cardioversion is not successful; it is dangerous if digitalis toxicity is present.[74] Antiarrhythmic agents are generally not useful. In specific instances, electrophysiologic study may be warranted. Treatment is supportive.

6. MULTIFOCAL ATRIAL TACHYCARDIA

Multifocal atrial tachycardia (MAT) is an automatic rhythm characterized by P waves of varying morphologies, varying PR intervals, and an irregular ventricular rhythm (Fig. 25–32). Usually, AV conduction is 1:1, although AV block can occur. Patients with chronic obstructive pulmonary disease or severe metabolic derangements often exhibit MAT. It rarely causes significant hemodynamic compromise. Care must be taken to avoid misdiagnosing this rhythm as atrial fibrillation.

Therapy is primarily directed to the underlying condition. Electrolyte replacement, especially of magnesium and potassium, and aggressive therapy to maximize respiratory function should be undertaken. Verapamil has been used to control the ventricular rate in MAT, but its effect is transient and variable. Usually, MAT is unresponsive to other antiarrhythmic agents and to DC cardioversion.

7. ACCELERATED JUNCTIONAL RHYTHM AND JUNCTIONAL TACHYCARDIA

Accelerated junctional rhythm is the result of enhanced automaticity of the AV junction and is *not* caused by AV block (Fig. 25–33). The rate of this rhythm is usually 60–120/minute. Atrioventricular dissociation is present because the ventricles are depolarized by the junctional focus and the atria are depolarized by their independent mechanism, which is usually the sinus node. No specific therapy is indicated unless digitalis toxicity is suspected, in which case digitalis should be discontinued and a serum digoxin level obtained.

Junctional tachycardia is encountered in the setting of severe congestive heart failure, recent open heart surgery, hypokalemia, inferior wall myocardial infarction, or digitalis toxicity. The rate of this rhythm is 120 to 200/minute. The ECG reveals QRS complexes of supraventricular origin. Retrograde conduction to the atria or AV dissociation may be present. Withholding digitalis and treating any underlying disease are the mainstays of therapy.

8. PREEXCITATION SYNDROMES

Preexcitation syndromes are characterized by premature activation of the ventricles by an atrial impulse that is partly or wholly conducted down an anomalous pathway rather than through the AV node. This results in the absence of the conduction delay normally seen at the AV node. Wolff-Parkinson-White (WPW) syndrome is the classic example of ventricular preexcitation.

The ECG will show various abnormalities depending upon the specific accessory pathway present. In WPW conduction, the impulse is conducted to the ventricles down the bundle of Kent. The ECG will reveal a shortened PR (less than 0.12 sec), a widened QRS (greater than 0.12 sec), and a slow-rising slur (delta wave) on the initial portion of the QRS complex. Other preexcitation syndromes will reveal a normal PR interval with a wide QRS complex having a delta wave (Mahaim connection), or a short PR interval with a normal QRS complex.

Many dysrhythmias occur in patients with preexcitation syndromes. The most common are paroxysmal AV nodal reentry tachycardias (PSVT). If antegrade conduc-

Multifocal Atrial Tachycardia

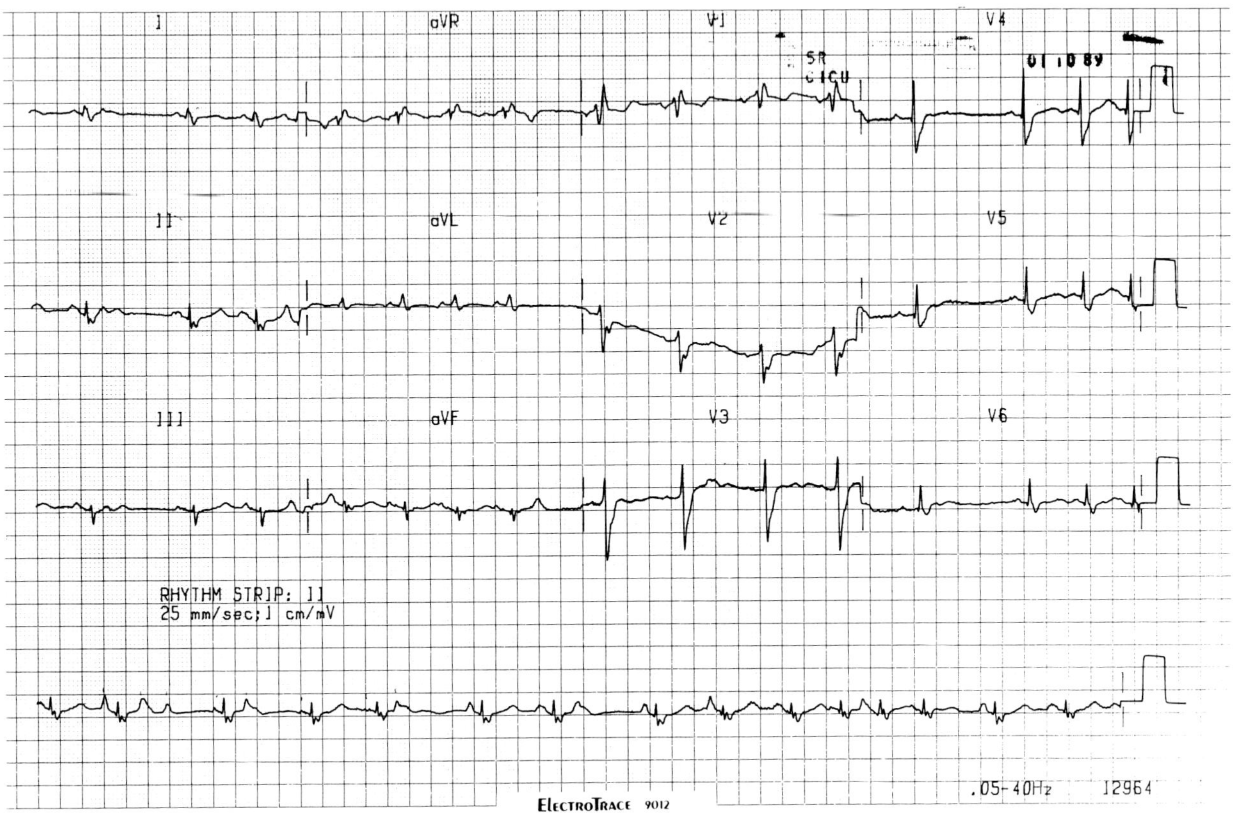

Figure 25–32 • Multifocal atrial tachycardia. Lead II (rhythm strip) reveals the varying morphology of the P waves and the varying PR intervals. Many atrial impulses are not conducted to the ventricles, illustrating that AV block can occur. The patient had no symptoms.

tion within the reentry circuit occurs down the accessory pathway, a wide QRS complex tachycardia may result, depending on the type of pathway. Atrial flutter and atrial fibrillation may both occur; conduction of these rapid atrial impulses down the accessory pathway results in a poorly tolerated rapid tachycardia, often with wide QRS complexes and fusion beats. Atrial fibrillation, PSVT, and atrial flutter may all be difficult to distinguish from ventricular tachycardia in this setting. In atrial flutter or fibrillation, AV nodal blocking agents and digitalis are contraindicated. Instead, DC cardioversion should be considered.

B. *Ventricular Tachydysrhythmias*

The important ventricular tachydysrhythmias include ventricular premature complexes, monomorphic ventricular tachycardia, polymorphic ventricular tachycardia, bidirectional ventricular tachycardia, and ventricular fibrillation.

1. Ventricular Premature Complexes

Ventricular premature complexes (VPCs) are the most common dysrhythmias in adults. The ECG will reveal a wide QRS complex (usually greater than 0.12 sec) that is not preceded by a premature P wave. The T wave is commonly in the opposite direction to the QRS complex. Often, but not always, a full compensatory pause (the interval between the normal QRS complexes preceding and following the VPC is twice the normal PP interval) occurs after the VPC. Occasionally, fusion beats will be identified. By general definition, three consecutive VPCs constitute ventricular tachycardia.

There is little evidence that suppression of VPCs will alter the risk of developing more malignant ventricular dysrhythmias.[75] When frequent VPCs are encoun-

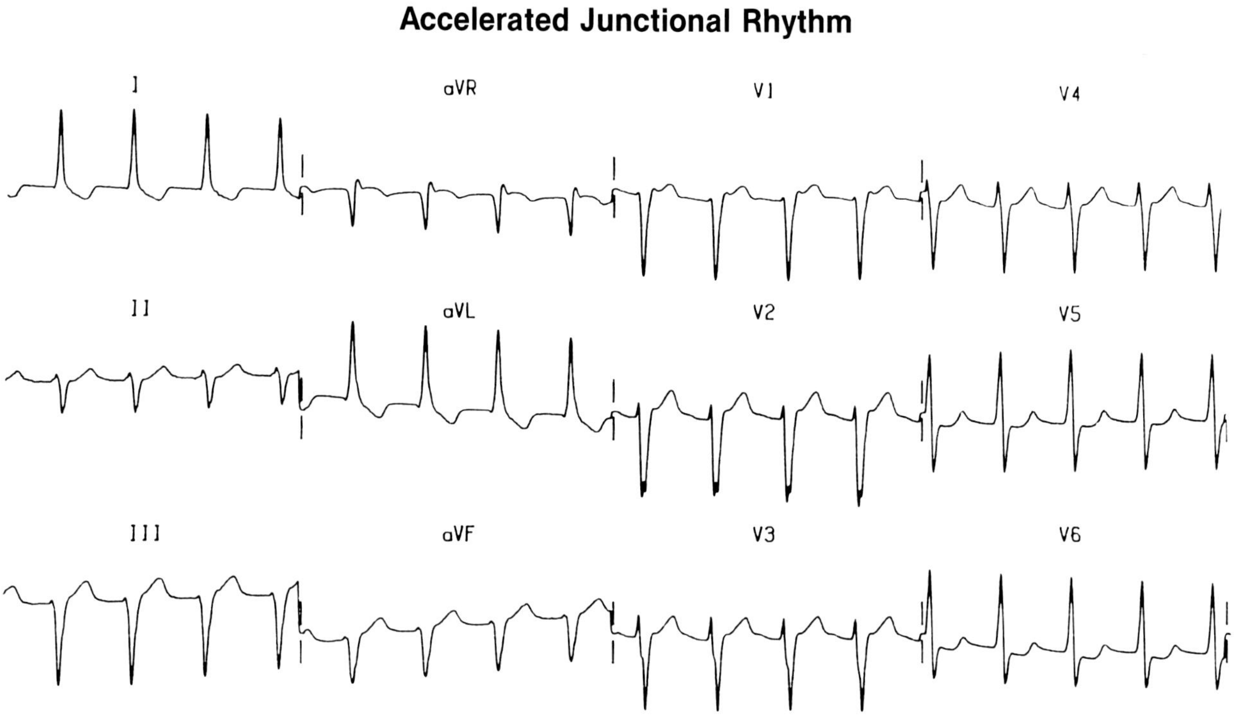

Figure 25–33 • Accelerated junctional rhythm in a patient with dilated cardiomyopathy who is receiving digitalis. The QRS rhythm is regular and a mild intraventricular conduction delay is present. The mean frontal plane QRS axis is superiorly directed. P waves are not clearly seen but appear to deform the terminal portions of the QRS complexes. The rhythm resolved spontaneously.

tered, especially in a hospital setting, one must assess the patient for adequate oxygenation and fluid and electrolyte balance. Isolated VPCs of uniform morphology require no therapy unless they occur frequently (more than 5/min) in the setting of an acute myocardial infarction. Symptomatic or "malignant" VPCs (multiform extrasystoles, doublets, and triplets) occurring in the setting of an acute myocardial infarction generally require suppression. Intravenous lidocaine or procainamide is commonly used. Intravenous atropine is effective when the sinus rate is slow and the VPCs are felt to be bradycardia dependent.

2. MONOMORPHIC VENTRICULAR TACHYCARDIA

Monomorphic ventricular tachycardia (VT) is a wide complex rhythm of ventricular origin with a uniform morphology (Fig. 25–34). It may or may not be sustained ($>$30 sec or associated with immediate hemodynamic collapse). The etiologies of monomorphic VT include ischemic heart disease, cardiomyopathies, electrolyte disturbances, and prodysrhythmic effect of some antidysrhythmic drugs. A search for hypoxia and electrolyte disturbances is mandatory in all patients who present with VT.

The rate of monomorphic VT is usually between 100 and 220/minute. The rhythm may be irregular or regular. During slower ventricular tachycardias, P waves can be identified, indicating that AV dissociation may be present. Retrograde ventriculoatrial (VA) conduction may also be present; VA association is not diagnostic of VT. There is usually a superior frontal plane QRS axis, and the QRS complexes across the precordium can be similar in morphology (concordance). The QRS complexes are wide (usually greater than 0.12 sec), although fusion beats may be present if AV dissociation with capture is present.

It may be difficult to distinguish VT from supraventricular tachycardia with aberrant intraventricular conduction.[76] A 12-lead ECG should always be performed to make this determination. Table 25–3 describes some of the differentiating features. If a 12-lead ECG is not revealing and there is insufficient time to perform more sophisticated electrophysiological studies, the dysrhythmia should be treated as if it were VT.

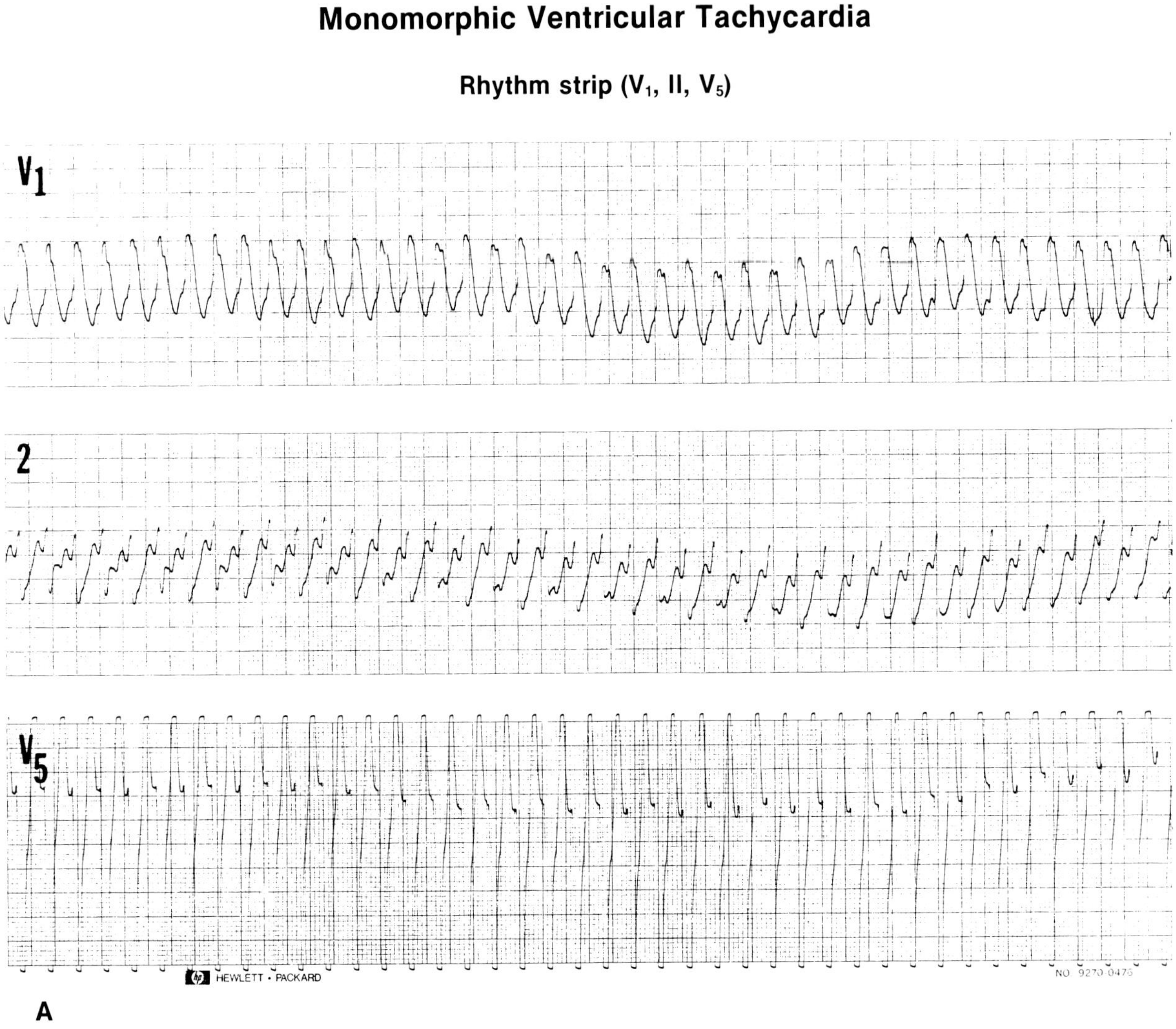

Figure 25-34 • Monomorphic ventricular tachycardia demonstrating a superiorly directed frontal plane QRS axis and concordance of QRS morphology in the precordium. The QRS complexes are wide (>0.12 sec) but no fusion beats are present.

(continued)

Table 25-3 • Differential Diagnosis of Wide QRS Complexes

Aberrant Supraventricular with Intraventricular Conduction Delay	Ventricular
Preceded by a premature P wave	No preceding premature P wave
rSR′ in V1	R, RR′, or QR in V1
Rs with wide S in V6	QR or rS in V6
Fixed coupling absent	Fixed coupling present
QRS duration usually <0.14 sec	QRS duration usually >0.14 sec
QRS complexes resemble a defined bundle branch block pattern	Superior frontal plane axis
Discordance of QRS complex morphology in the precordial leads	Concordance of QRS complexes in the precordial leads
	AV dissociation
	Fusion complexes
	RBBB pattern, QRS duration >0.14 sec
	LBBB pattern, QRS duration >0.16 sec
	LBBB pattern, right axis deviation

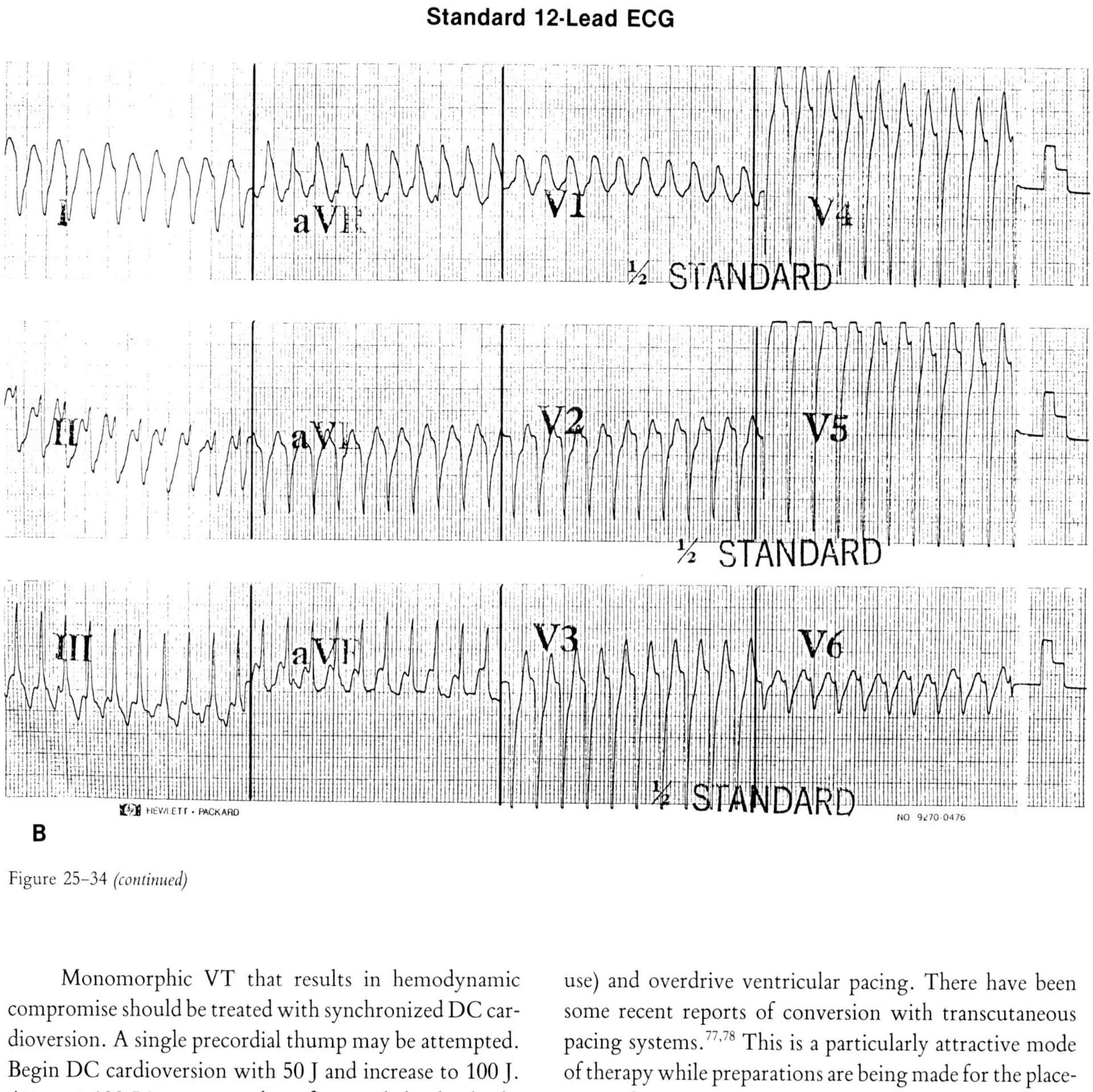

Figure 25–34 *(continued)*

Monomorphic VT that results in hemodynamic compromise should be treated with synchronized DC cardioversion. A single precordial thump may be attempted. Begin DC cardioversion with 50 J and increase to 100 J. Attempt 100-J increments thereafter until the dysrhythmia is terminated or until maximal energy level is reached (360 J). After successful electric cardioversion, intravenous lidocaine should be administered. If successful electric cardioversion has not occurred, intravenous lidocaine, procainamide, and bretylium may be used in succession, each followed by attempts at DC cardioversion.

Monomorphic VT that is well tolerated or causes only mild hypotension can be treated initially with drugs. Lidocaine is the drug of first choice. Intravenous procainamide is then administered if lidocaine is ineffective (see Table 25–2). Synchronized DC cardioversion should be employed in VT that is refractory to drug therapy. Other potentially useful therapies in refractory VT are oral amiodarone (the intravenous form is not available for general use) and overdrive ventricular pacing. There have been some recent reports of conversion with transcutaneous pacing systems.[77,78] This is a particularly attractive mode of therapy while preparations are being made for the placement of a transvenous pacemaker.

3. POLYMORPHIC VENTRICULAR TACHYCARDIA

Polymorphic VT is a wide QRS complex tachycardia of ventricular origin with a continuously varying QRS morphology (Fig. 25–35). If the rhythm appears to undulate around an isoelectric baseline and the QT interval is prolonged, it is called *torsade de pointes*. Polymorphic VT is usually nonsustained and has an irregular rate. Among the causes of polymorphic VT, including torsade de pointes, are acute myocardial ischemia and infarction, antidysrhythmic drugs (especially type I agents), hypokalemia, hypomagnesemia, and congenital QT-interval prolonga-

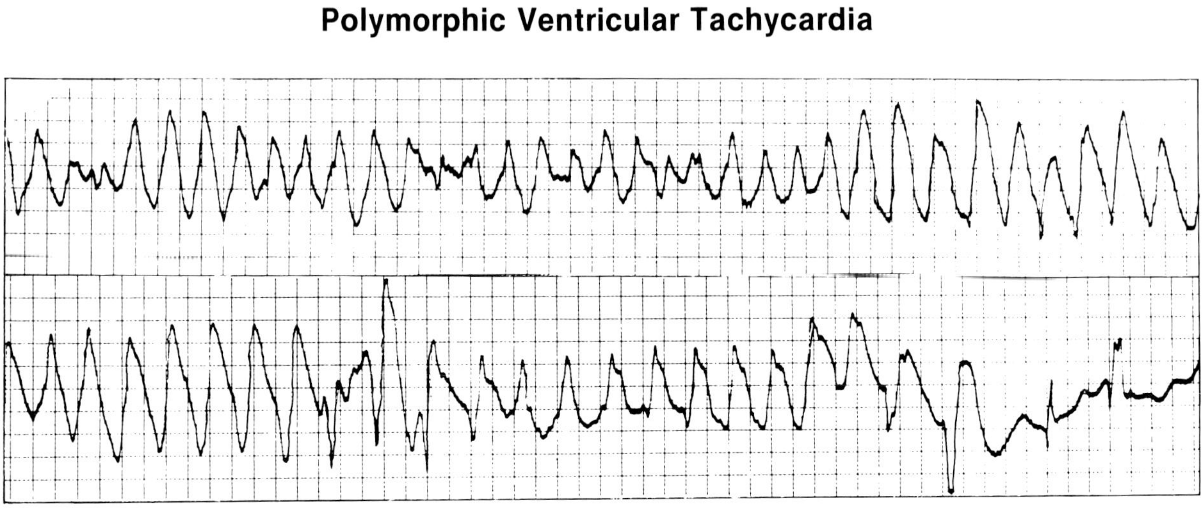

Figure 25–35 • Continuously recorded lead MCL_1 tracing in a patient with long QT interval and episodes of nonsustained polymorphic ventricular tachycardia. In this example, the *torsade de pointes* was due to hypokalemia and hypomagnesemia; the patient was taking no medications. With potassium replacement and intravenous magnesium therapy, the rhythm was eventually abolished. Patients receiving type I antiarrhythmic agents who present with this rhythm are demonstrating the prodysrhythmic effects of these drugs. Whereas the QT interval is always long in *torsade de pointes,* a long QT interval does not predict the rhythm.

tion. This rhythm has a tendency to degenerate to VF, making early intervention mandatory.

Overdrive transvenous pacing is the therapy of choice in polymorphic VT; atrial pacing is preferred to ventricular. A pacing rate exceeding the underlying sinus rate is usually required. All drugs that might have caused the rhythm should be discontinued. While preparations are being made for placement of the temporary pacing system, some therapy may be required. Isoproterenol may be useful, especially if the VT is bradycardia-dependent (see Table 25–2). Intravenous magnesium sulfate is often extremely effective. Some patients with hypokalemia will respond to the administration of intravenous potassium but only after magnesium has been replaced. Lidocaine has been used successfully in isolated cases but the effect is not consistent. Finally, if the rhythm has caused hemodynamic compromise, angina, or pulmonary edema, and has not responded to initial medical management, synchronized DC cardioversion can be attempted, but only if the rhythm is relatively sustained. If termination has been accomplished by pharmacologic or electric means, a transvenous pacing system should be inserted and overdrive suppression instituted to prevent further dysrhythmias.

4. Accelerated Ventricular Rhythm

Accelerated ventricular rhythm is a benign rhythm often seen in the setting of myocardial ischemia but not necessarily caused by it. The intrinsic firing rate of the ventricles is enhanced above its normal 30–40/min. The rhythm emerges as an escape rhythm when the sinus rate slows, and it disappears as the sinus rate increases. Its onset and offset are characterized by the presence of fusion complexes. No treatment is indicated because it is rarely rapid and causes no hemodynamic compromise.

5. Ventricular Fibrillation

Ventricular fibrillation (VF) is a lethal ventricular rhythm characterized by a lack of distinct P waves, QRS complexes, or T waves. Either a sine wave or an irregular undulation of the isoelectric baseline is inscribed on the surface ECG. Many of the cardiac arrests reported each year in the United States are attributable to VF, which is fatal within 3 to 5 minutes if untreated.[70] Ventricular fibrillation occurs in the same clinical circumstances as VT.

Basic CPR should be instituted. Immediate defibrillation, using either standard paddles or disposable external defibrillator pads, is the treatment of choice. Defibrillation should begin with 200 J, and repeated with 300 J. If the second shock does not defibrillate the patient, a third shock at maximal energy (360 J) should be administered. This is followed by intravenous epinephrine (see Table 25–2) and a repeat defibrillation attempt at 360 J. If treatment continues to be unsuccessful, intravenous lidocaine is given followed by defibrillation at 360 J. Bretylium is then administered and defibrillation at 360 J repeated. Further resuscitation efforts should follow the American Heart Association's guidelines for VF.[70]

C. *Bradydysrhythmias*

Bradydysrhythmias include sinus bradycardia, sinoatrial exit block, sinus pauses, and AV block.

1. SINUS BRADYCARDIA

Sinus bradycardia is a slowing of the sinus node firing rate below 60/min. The P waves are normal and followed by QRS complexes with constant PR intervals. Sinus bradycardia results from the vagotonia associated with an inferior myocardial infarction, right ventricular infarction, increased intracranial pressure, visceral distension, endotracheal suction, endotracheal intubation, or vagal maneuvers. It may also result from the administration of AV nodal blocking agents.

Usually no therapy is required. If hemodynamic compromise with symptoms of cerebral hypoperfusion occurs, intravenous atropine may be given. If atropine has no effect, temporary cardiac pacing, either transcutaneous or transvenous, should be instituted. Isoproterenol can increase the sinus rate and enhance AV conduction, but it is contraindicated in critically ill patients because it causes peripheral vasodilatation, is prodysrhythmic, and increases myocardial oxygen demand.

2. SINOATRIAL EXIT BLOCK

Sinoatrial exit block can take the form of first-, second-, or third-degree block. First-degree sinus exit block cannot be identified on the 12-lead ECG and is not clinically relevant. Third-degree sinoatrial exit block is indistinguishable from sinus arrest (described below). Second-degree sinoatrial exit block may be either type I or type II. Type II is characterized by the absence of sinus activity at intervals that are a multiple of the underlying PP interval. Type I is characterized by group beating with the PP intervals progressively shortening prior to the pause in P wave rate (the sinus impulse has failed to be conducted to the atrium). The PP interval that brackets the nonconducted sinus impulse is less than twice the preceding PP interval.

Sinoatrial exit block does not usually cause symptoms unless prolonged pauses occur. The exit block is caused or contributed to by enhanced vagal tone or drugs (especially digoxin or type Ia antidysrhythmic agents). Rarely, it is associated with an acute myocardial infarction. Treatment, when necessary, is the same as outlined for sinus bradycardia.

3. SINUS ARREST

Sinus arrest or *sinus pause* is the loss of spontaneous sinus activity in the absence of atrial depolarization from a subsidiary pacemaker (Fig. 25–36). Sinus arrest is usually caused by intrinsic sinus node dysfunction. Other etiologies include enhanced vagal tone and hyperkalemia.

Sinus Arrest with Junctional Escape

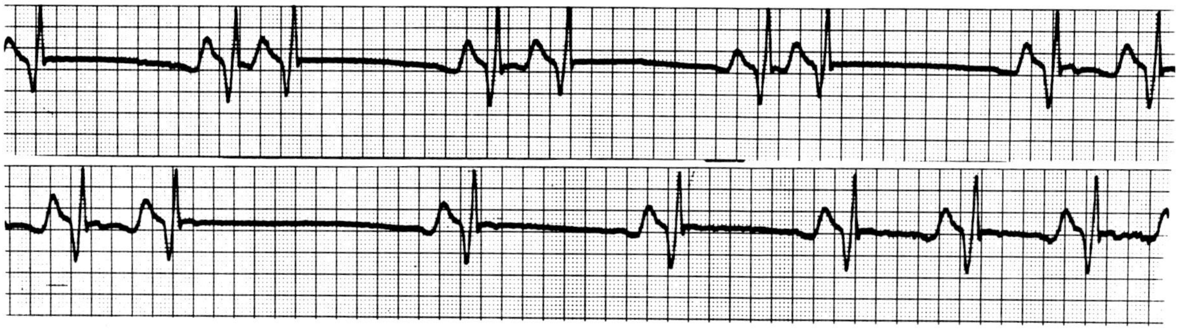

Figure 25–36 • Continuously recorded lead MCL_1 rhythm strip in a patient admitted for evaluation of syncopal episodes. The atrial rhythm is sinus, but the rate is extremely slow and variable. Several pauses in rhythm are terminated by junctional escape complexes. The junctional escape complexes themselves occur only after prolonged pauses, suggesting disease within the AV node and His bundle. In addition, intraventricular conduction is abnormal, showing a right bundle-branch block pattern. This patient was taking no medication and his electrolytes were normal. Permanent dual chamber pacing eliminated the syncopal spells.

This rhythm can be exacerbated by digitalis therapy, especially if vagal tone is high.[79] If the sinus arrest is of short duration, no therapy is indicated. If the pauses are prolonged or associated with hemodynamic compromise, intravenous atropine should be administered and temporary cardiac pacing considered.

4. Atrioventricular Block

Atrioventricular (AV) block is the delay or interruption of impulse conduction from the atria to the ventricles. It is also classified as first-, second-, or third-degree block. The actual anatomic location of the block may be at the AV node, His bundle, or in the bundle branches. The prognosis of AV block depends on the anatomic location of the lesion and the underlying cardiac disease.

First-degree AV block is defined electrocardiographically as a PR interval exceeding 0.20 to 0.21 seconds. The block most commonly occurs at the level of the AV node, although it may also occur at infranodal areas. When it occurs at the AV node, the QRS complex is narrow and normal-appearing.

Second-degree AV block results in intermittent failure of impulse conduction from the atria to the ventricles. Type I (Wenckebach) second-degree AV block usually occurs at the level of the AV node and causes little in the way of hemodynamic compromise unless the sinus rate is slow and the AV conduction ratio is low (3:2, 2:1). It is the result of increased vagal tone, drug effect, or myocardial ischemia or infarction (especially involving the inferior wall). Type I second-degree AV block is characterized by progressive prolongation of the PR intervals, followed by a nonconducted P wave. The atrial rate and rhythm are regular. The ventricular rate is lower than the atrial rate. The RR interval that brackets the nonconducted P wave is less than twice the prior RR interval.

Type II second-degree AV block is characterized by constant PR intervals prior to the nonconducted P wave. This form of AV block usually occurs at the level of the His bundle or, more commonly, at the bundle branches. Its more distal location carries a poor prognosis for the development of symptomatic AV block.

Third-degree (complete) AV block is the complete absence of impulse conduction between the atria and ventricles. The block may occur at the AV node or at infranodal levels. When it is located at the AV node, a junctional escape rhythm is often established having regular narrow QRS complexes with a rate of 40–60/minute. Complete AV block at the AV node is caused by increased vagal tone, drugs, or myocardial ischemia or infarction. It may be transient. The prognosis varies with the clinical situation and with any underlying heart disease, and is usually benign. When third-degree AV block occurs at the level of the His bundle or bundle branches, a ventricular escape rhythm should ensue, having wide QRS complexes with a rate of less than 40/min. Complete AV block occurring at this more distal site is caused by intrinsic conduction system disease and by acute myocardial infarction. The atrial rate is normal and the atrial rhythm regular. There is no relationship between the atrial and ventricular rhythms.

Intravenous atropine followed by ventricular or atrioventricular pacing is indicated in all instances of AV block associated with hemodynamic compromise, pulmonary edema, ventricular dysrhythmias, or angina. If the site of block is subjunctional, however, atropine may have no effect.

IV. References

1. Kerber RE, Martins JB, Kienzel MG, Constantin L, et al. Energy, current, and success in defibrillation and cardioversion: Clinical studies using an automated impedance-based method of energy adjustment. Circulation 77:1038–1046, 1988.
2. Ewy GA, Taren D. Impedance to transthoracic direct current, discharge: a model for testing interface material. Med Instrumentation 22:47, 1978.
3. Ewy GA, Taren D. Comparison of paddle electrode pastes used for defibrillation. Heart Lung 6:847–850, 1977.
4. Aylward PE, Kieso R, Hite P, Charbonnier F, et al. Defibrillator electrode-chest wall coupling agents: Influence on transthoracic impedance and shock success. J Am Coll Cardiol 6:682-686, 1985.
5. Kerber RE, Sarnat W. Factors influencing the success of ventricular defibrillation in man. Circulation 60:226–230, 1979.
6. Kerber RE, Grayzel J, Hoyt R, Marcus M, et al. Transthoracic resistance in human defibrillation: Influence of body weight, chest size, serial shocks, paddle size and paddle contact pressure. Circulation 63:676–682, 1981.
7. Kerber RE, Jensen SR, Grayzel J, Kennedy J, et al. Elective cardioversion: Influence of paddle-electrode location and size of success rates and energy requirements. N Engl J Med 305:658–662, 1981.
8. DeSilva RA, Margolis B, Lown B. Determinants of success during inhospital defibrillation. Peter Bent Brigham Hospital, Harvard University School of Public Health, Boston, MA.
9. Levine PA, Barold S, Fletcher RD, Talbot P. Adverse acute and chronic effects of electric defibrillation and cardioversion on implanted unipolar cardiac pacing systems. J Am Coll Cardiol 1:1413–22, 1983.
10. Goldschlager N. Cardiovascular disorders. In Luce JM, Pierson DJ (eds). Critical Care Medicine. Philadelphia, WB Saunders, 1988, 15–133.
11. Selzer A, Kelly JJ Jr, Johnson RB, Kerth WJ. Immediate and long-term results of electric conversion of arrhythmias. Prog Cardiovasc Dis 9:90–104, 1966.
12. Resnekov L, McDonald L. Complications in 220 patients with

cardiac dysrhythmias treated by phased direct current shock, and indications for electroconversion. Br Heart J 29:926–936, 1967.
13. Mancini J, Goldberger AL. Cardioversion of atrial fibrillation: Consideration of embolization, anticoagulation, prophylactic pacemaker, and long-term success. Am Heart J 104: 617–1621, 1982.
14. Ehsanin A, Ewy GA, Sobel BE. Effects of electric countershock on serum creatine phosphokinase (CPK) isoenzyme activity. Am J Cardiol 37:12–18, 1976.
15. Chun PKC, Davia JE, Donohue DJ. ST-segment elevation with elective DC cardioversion. Circulation 63:220–224, 1981.
16. Ovsyshcher IA, Ilia R, Wanderman KL. Conduction disturbance and ST elevation following cardioversion. Isr J Med Sci 20:736–738, 1984.
17. Ferrer MI. The Sick Sinus Syndrome. Mount Kisco, NY, Futura Publishing, Inc, 59–62.
18. Weaver WD, Cobb LA, Copas MK, Hallstrom AP. Ventricular defibrillation: A comparative trial using 175-J and 320-J shocks. N Engl J Med 307:1101–1106, 1982.
19. Kerber RE. Energy requirements for defibrillation. Circulation 74(Suppl IV):1-119, 1986.
20. Kerber RE, Margins J, Kennedy J, et al. Self-adhesive pre-applied electrode pads for defibrillation and cardioversion. J Am Coll Cardiol 3:815–820, 1984.
21. Kerber RE. External defibrillation: New technologies. Ann Emerg Med 13:794–797, 1984.
22. Dalzell GW, Cunningham SR, Wilson CM, Allen JD, et al. Ventricular defibrillation: The Belfast experience. Br Heart J 58:441–446, 1987.
23. Giedwoyn JO. Pacemaker failure following external defibrillation. Circulation 44:293, 1971.
24. Aylward P, Blood R, Tonkin A. Complications of defibrillation with permanent pacemaker in situ. PACE 2:462–464, 1979.
25. Palac RT, Hwang MH, Klodnycky ML, Loeb HS. Delayed pulse generator malfunction after D.C. countershock. PACE 4:163–167, 1981.
26. Das G, Eaton J. Pacemakers malfunction following transthoracic countershock. PACE 4:487–490, 1981.
27. Gould L, Patel S, Chokshi AB. Pacemaker failure following external defibrillation. PACE 4:575–577, 1981.
28. Zoll PM. Resuscitation of the heart in ventricular standstill by external electric stimulation. N Engl J Med 247:768, 1952.
29. Zoll PM, Zoll RH, Falk RH, Clinton JE, et al. External noninvasive temporary cardiac pacing: Clinical trials. Circulation 71:937–944, 1985.
30. Hedges JR, Syverud SA, Dalsey WC, Feero S, et al. Prehospital trial of emergency transcutaneous cardiac pacing. Circulation 76:1337–1343, 1987.
31. Rosenthal E, Thomas N, Quinn E, Chamberlain D, et al. Transcutaneous pacing for cardiac emergencies. PACE 11:2160–2167, 1988.
32. Falk RH, Zoll PM, Zoll RH. Safety and efficacy of noninvasive cardiac pacing: A preliminary report. N Engl J Med 309:1166–1168, 1983.
33. Noe R, Cockrell W, Moses HW, Dove TT, et al. Transcutaneous pacemaker use in a large hospital. PACE 9:101-104, 1986.
34. Wharton JM, Goldschlager N. Indications for temporary cardiac pacing. In Saksena S, Goldschlager N (eds). electric Therapy for Cardiac Arrhythmias. Philadelphia, WB Saunders (in press).
35. Brown CG, Gurley HT, Hutchins GM, MacKenzie EJ, et al. Injuries associated with percutaneous placement of transthoracic pacemakers. Ann Emerg Med 14:223–53, 1985.
36. Shafiroff BGP, Linder J. Effects of external electric pacemaker stimuli on the human heart. J Thoracic Surg 33:544–550, 1957.
37. Gallagher JJ, Smith WM, Kerr CR, Kasell J, et al. Esophageal pacing: A diagnostic and therapeutic tool. Circulation 65:336–341, 1982.
38. Chamberlain DA, Leinbach RC, Vassaux CE, Kastor JA. Sequential atrioventricular pacing in heart block complicating acute myocardial infarction. N Engl J Med 282:577–582, 1970.
39. Hartzler GO, Maloney JD, Curtis JJ, Barnhorst DA. Hemodynamic benefits of atrioventricular sequential pacing after cardiac surgery. Am J Cardiol 40:232–236, 1977.
40. Reiter MJ, Hindman MC. Hemodynamic effects of acute atrioventricular sequential pacing in patients with left ventriucular dysfunction. Am J Cardiol 49:687–692, 1982.
41. Topol EJ, Goldschlager N, Ports TA, et al. Hemodynamic benefit of atrial pacing in right ventricular myocardial infarction. Ann Int Med 96:594–597, 1982.
42. Littleford PO, Pepine CJ. A new temporary atrial pacing catheter inserted percutaneously into the subclavian vein without fluoroscopy: A preliminary report. PACE 4:458–464, 1981.
43. Barold SS, Falkoff MD, Ong LS, Heinle RA. Normal and abnormal patterns of ventricular depolarization during cardiac pacing. In Barold SS (ed). Modern Cardiac Pacing. Mount Kisco, Futura Publishing, Inc, 1985, 545–569.
44. Austin JL, Preis LK, Crampton RS, Beller GA, et al. Analysis of pacemaker malfunction and complications of temporary pacing in the coronary care unit. Am J Cardiol 49:301, 1982.
45. Krueger S, Rakes S, Wilkerson J, Stuber RR, et al. Temporary pacemaking by general internists. Arch Intern Med 143:1531, 1983.
46. Hynes JK, Holmes DR Jr, Harrison CE. Five-year experience with temporary pacemaker therapy in the coronary care unit. Mayo Clin Proc 58:122–126, 1983.
47. Pandian NG, Kosowsky BD, Gurewich V. Transfemoral temporary pacing and deep vein thrombosis. Am Heart J 100:847–851, 1980.
48. Nolewajka AJ, Goddard MD, Brown TC. Temporary transvenous pacing and femoral vein thrombosis. Circulation 62:646, 1980.
49. Morelli RL, Goldschlager N. Temporary transvenous pacing: Resolving postinsertion problems. J Crit Illness 2:73–80, 1987.
50. Switzer DF, Nanda NC. Doppler-echocardiographic assessment of cardiac pacemakers. Cardiol Clin 3:631–655, 1985.
51. Morelli RL, Goldschlager N. The technique of inserting a transvenous pacing catheter. J Crit Illness 2:63–73, 1987.
52. Dohrmann ML, Goldschlager NF. Myocardial stimulation threshold in patients with cardiac pacemakers: Effects of physiologic variables, pharmacologic agents, and lead electrodes. Cardiol Clin 3:527–537, 1985.
53. Lown B, Levine SA. The carotid sinus: Clinical value of its stimulation. Circulation 23:766, 1961.
54. Askey JM. Hemiplegia following carotid sinus stimulation. Am Heart J 31:131–137, 1946.
55. Zeman FD, Siegal S. Monoplegia following carotid sinus pressure in the aged. Am J Med Sci 213:603, 1947.
56. Brannon ES. Hemiplegia following carotid sinus stimulation: Case report. Am Heart J 36:299–300, 1948.
57. Meredith HC, Becwith JR. Development of ventricular tachycardia following carotid sinus stimulation in paroxysmal supraventricular tachycardia. Am Heart J 39:694–695, 1950.
58. Mathews CA. Ventricular tachycardia induced by carotid sinus stimulation. J Maine Med Assoc 60:135–137, 1969.
59. Greenwood RJ, Dupler DA. Death following carotid sinus pressure. JAMA 181:605–609, 1962.
60. Porus RI, Marcus FI. Ventricular fibrillation during carotid sinus stimulation. N Eng J Med 268:1338–1342, 1963.
61. Alexander S, Ping WC. Fatal ventricular fibrillation during carotid sinus stimulation. Am J Cardiol 18:289–291, 1966.

62. Hilal M, Massumi R. Fatal ventricular fibrillation after carotid sinus stimulation. N Engl J Med 275:157–185, 1966.
63. Cohen MV. Ventricular fibrillation precipitated by carotid sinus pressure: Case report and review of the literature. Am Heart J 84:681–686, 1972.
64. Schott E. Uber ventrikelstillstand (Adams-Stokes'sche Anfalle) nebst bemerkungen uber andersartige arhythmien passagerer. Natur Deutsches Arch Klin Med 131:211–229, 1920.
65. Scherf D, Bornemann C. Thumping of the precordium in ventricular standstill. Am J Cardiol 5:30–40, 1960.
66. Harwood-Nash D. Thumping of the precordium in ventricular fibrillation. S Afr Med J 36:28–281, 1962.
67. Pennington JE, Taylor J, Lown B. Chest thump for reverting ventricular tachycardia. N Engl J Med 283(22):1192, 1970.
68. Morgera T, Baldi N, Chersevani D, Medugno G, et al. Chest thump and ventricular tachycardia. PACE 2:69, 1979.
69. Miller J, Tresch D, Horwitz L, Thompson BM, et al. The precordial thump. Ann Emerg Med 13:791, 1984.
70. American Heart Association. Textbook of Advanced Cardiac Life Support. Dallas, American Heart Association, 1987.
71. Benditt DG, Benson W Jr, Dunnigan A, Gornick CC, et al. Atrial flutter, atrial fibrillation, and other primary atrial tachycardias. Med Clin N Am 68:895, 1984.
72. Greenberg ML, Kelly TA, Lerman BB, DiMarco JP. Atrial pacing for conversion of atrial flutter. Am J Cardiol 58:95–99, 1986.
73. Kastor JA, Yurchak PM. Recognition of digitalis intoxication in the presence of atrial fibrillation. Ann Intern Med 67:1045, 1967.
74. Lown B. electric reversion of cardiac arrhythmias. Br Heart J 29:469, 1967.
75. German LD, Ideker RE. Ventricular tachycardia: mechanisms, diagnosis, and management. Med Clin N Am 68:919, 1984.
76. Akhtar M, Shenasa M, Jazayeri M, Careves J, et al. Wide QRS complex tachycardia: Reappraisal of a common clinical problem. Ann Int Med 109:905–912, 1988.
77. Luck JC, Grubb BP, Artman SE, Steckbeck RT. Termination of sustained ventricular tachycardia by external noninvasive pacing. Am J Cardiol 61:574–577, 1988.
78. Estes NA III, Deering TF, Manolis AS, Salem D, et al. External cardiac programmed stimulation for noninvasive termination of sustained supraventricular and ventricular tachycardia. Am J Cardiol 63:177–183, 1989.
79. Schmidt PJ, Ezri MD, Denes P. Cardiac arrhythmias: Update 1987. Dis-a-Month 33:365–432, 1987.

Chapter 26

Robert C. Mackersie, MD

The Pneumatic Antishock Garment

OUTLINE

I. INTRODUCTION

The pneumatic antishock garment is a three-compartment, inflatable, rubberized or polyvinyl trouser suit developed as an aid in treating hypovolemic hypotension. The device has been referred to by a variety of other names including MAST (military antishock trousers), external counterpressure device, G-suit, antishock trousers, and shock pants. External counterpressure was originally used in 1903 by Crile to alleviate hypotension during surgery.[1] The device was reintroduced in 1956 by Gardner, and later applied in the resuscitation of hemorrhagic shock victims during the Vietnam War.[2,3] The favorable wartime experience with MAST garments led to their subsequent use, beginning in 1973, for the prehospital treatment of civilian trauma.[4] Since that time, numerous reports have described the salutary effects of MAST suits in the prehospital setting and have led to their current widespread use. In addition to the treatment of hypovolemic shock, MAST suits are now being applied to the prehospital treatment of cardiac arrest.

A. *Physiologic Effects of MAST Application*

A variety of physiologic alterations associated with the use of external counterpressure have been reported.[5-20] The proposed mechanisms by which the MAST suit exerts its hemodynamic effects include (1) return of blood from peripheral venous capacitance pools to the central circulation; (2) increasing systemic vascular resistance; (3) tamponade of bleeding vessels; (4) splinting of fractures and the secondary reduction of associated blood loss; and (5) autotransfusion (Fig. 26–1).

The relative importance of these effects depends on the specific injury. Reports on the clinical use of the MAST suit found that its application produced increases in systolic blood pressure.[4,19,21] These pressure increases are attributed mainly to an increase in systemic vascular resistance (SVR).[11,22] Bivins and associates determined that less than 5% of total blood volume was displaced with the inflation of the MAST suit, and concluded that this effect was less important than the increases in SVR.[5] In an independent study using radioisotope scans, Hanke

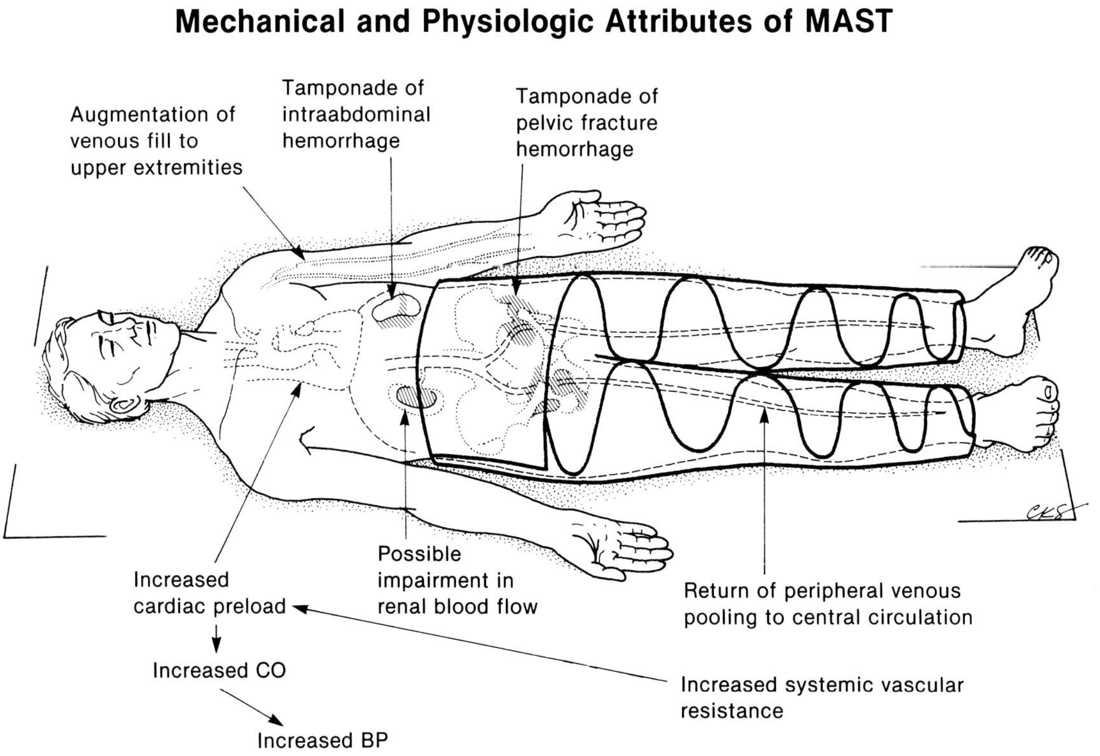

Figure 26–1 • Mechanical and physiologic effects of external counterpressure from military antishock trousers (MAST). CO = cardiac output; BP = blood pressure.

and coworkers similarly determined that blood volume displacement alone was unlikely to produce the observed hemodynamic associated with MAST inflation.[6]

The ability of the MAST suit to tamponade bleeding vessels has been demonstrated both for intraabdominal hemorrhage and for pelvic fractures.[23-25] Ex vivo studies have further demonstrated the ability of external counterpressure to transmit increased surrounding pressure to a bleeding vessel and thus reduce the rate of leakage.[7] Although controlled randomized human studies examining the efficacy of MAST for hemorrhage control are not available, animal studies and clinical reports using historic controls suggest that external counterpressure is consistently associated with reductions in blood loss.

In addition to its hemodynamic effects, the MAST suit may have additional effects on pulmonary, metabolic, and renal function (Figs. 26–1 and 26–2). The effects of MAST trousers on pulmonary function are unclear. Although increased peak inspiratory pressure and decreases in pulmonary function tests have been observed; apparently, MAST suit inflation does not appear to affect pulmonary function in normal individuals.[18-20] Clinical experience suggests that certain patients with diminished ventilatory capacity (eg, quadriplegics and patients with head injuries or severe chest contusions) may suffer some degree of respiratory embarrassment with MAST inflation.[14] Patients without these types of injuries generally have sufficient reserves to overcome the increase ventilatory work imposed by MAST suit inflation.

MAST suit inflation has been found to produce both increases and decreases in renal blood flow.[12,17] It has been demonstrated in both dogs and humans, however, that the increases in blood pressure associated with MAST usage are not secondary to MAST-induced increases in plasma renin activity.[15,16]

By causing significant increases in central venous pressure, MAST trousers have the potential for producing elevated intracranial pressure (ICP), and their use in patients with significant head injury has been questioned. Palafox and colleagues and Cram and associates both found increases in ICP with MAST inflation but not at clinically significant levels.[9,10] In a study of head-injured patients with ICP less than 20, Gardner and colleagues also found no significant ill effects of MAST suit inflation.[13] Given the increase in mortality associated with hypotension in head-injured patients, it would ap-

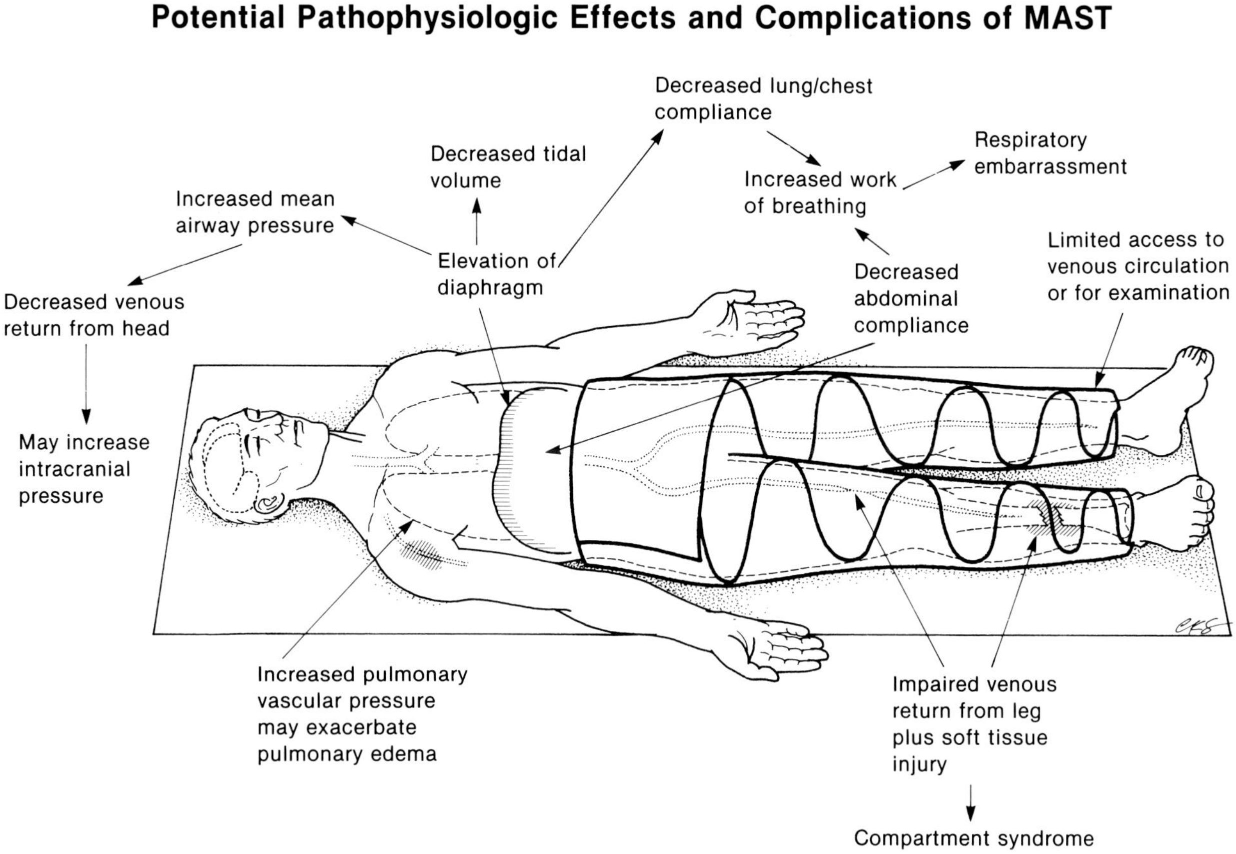

Figure 26–2 • Potential pathophysiologic effects and complications of external counterpressure from MAST. In most patients the respiratory and intracranial pressure effects are clinically minor (see text for full explanation).

pear that the potentially adverse effect of increased ICP is more than outweighed by the benefits of maintaining cerebral perfusion pressure through the use of external counterpressure.[26]

II. INDICATIONS AND CONTRAINDICATIONS

The indications for MAST application have been expanded in recent years to include both trauma and nontrauma patients (Table 26–1). In the prehospital setting, the MAST suit may be applied for the treatment of serious hypovolemic hypotension (eg, systolic blood pressure less than 90 mmHg) and the stabilization of pelvic and long-bone fractures. Nonhypovolemic hypotension, such as occurs with cardiac tamponade and high cervical spine injuries, may also respond to the increase in preload provided by external counterpressure.

On arrival at the hospital, hypotensive patients with nontraumatic intraabdominal hemorrhage, such as those with ruptured abdominal aortic aneurysms or ectopic pregnancy, may benefit from MAST application. The use of MAST garments under these circumstances is not a substitute for surgical hemostasis or good volume resuscitation. The MAST suit can effect improvement in blood pressure, however, and may reduce the degree of ongoing hemorrhage during resuscitation and preparation for operative intervention. In some instances, definitive care will involve transfer to another facility with the MAST suit in place.

There is accumulating evidence that the MAST suit may be effective in the treatment of nonhypovolemic cardiac arrest as well as hypovolemic shock. Most studies examining MAST effects on cardiopulmonary resuscitation have demonstrated improvements in blood pressure and atrial pressures, and some studies show improvements in cerebral blood flow.[27,28] In a randomized study, Mahoney and Mirick showed improved survival with the use of MAST garments in patients with prehospital arrest and either ventricular fibrillation or pulseless idioventricular rhythm.[29]

Table 26-1 • Indications for MAST Application

Prehospital (in transport to definitive care facility)
- Hypovolemic hypotension (BP <90–100 mmHg)
- Hypotension associated with spinal cord injury
- Hypotension secondary to cardiac tamponade (?)
- Stabilization of recognized pelvic/femoral fractures associated with hypovolemia

Emergency department (prior to definitive care)
- Refractory hypotension secondary to pelvic fractures
- Cardiac arrest (particularly ventricular fibrillation and pulseless idioventricular rhythms)
- Refractory hypotension secondary to ruptured ectopic pregnancy
- Refractory hypotension secondary to ruptured aortic aneurysm

Extended in-hospital application (part of definitive care)
- Control of hemorrhage associated with pelvic fractures
- Control of nonoperative intraabdominal or retroperitoneal hemorrhage (?)

The prolonged application of the MAST suit following resuscitation has been used mainly for the control of pelvic fracture hemorrhage and, on rare occasion, the control of nonoperative intraabdominal or retroperitoneal hemorrhage. Reports have attested to its effectiveness in definitive hemorrhage control under these circumstances.[23-25] Decisions regarding extended MAST application, however, are often complex and should be made in conjunction with careful surgical evaluation and by persons experienced in the use of MAST garments.

Injured patients with contraindications to MAST application are few, since the majority of potential MAST candidates are young and otherwise healthy. The only absolute contraindications to the use of the MAST suit are cardiogenic shock and congestive heart failure with pulmonary edema. In both cases, the increased afterload and preload produced by MAST inflation may increase the cardiac workload and exacerbate cardiac failure.

A number of relative contraindications to MAST application exist; in these, the benefit of increasing blood pressure must be weighed against specific adverse effects (Table 26-2). Advanced pregnancy should be regarded as a relative contraindication, although little information is available concerning the fetal effects of MAST. By increasing central arterial and venous pressures, MAST inflation may exacerbate hemorrhage above the diaphragm and should be used with caution in patients with these injuries, particularly in cases where the bleeding cannot be controlled by direct pressure. Foreign bodies impaled in the abdomen (knives, fenceposts, steel railing, etc) should always be left undisturbed prior to laparotomy, making MAST application difficult or in some cases impossible. Diaphragmatic rupture, flail chest, or high cervical cord injuries may impair ventilatory capacity. In these cases, MAST inflation may further compromise ventilation, leading to acute respiratory failure and the need for intubation and mechanical ventilation. Patients with neurologic and thoracic injuries who require MAST inflation should be monitored carefully for ventilatory failure.

The use of MAST for tension pneumothorax and cardiac tamponade is controversial. In most injuries, myocardial function is not impaired, and MAST-induced increases in afterload will not exacerbate cardiac failure. A major physiologic derangement with both of these injuries is diminished end-diastolic filling volume. Since MAST acts to increase central venous pressure, end-diastolic filling volume and cardiac output and arterial pressure all should increase. Davis and associates demonstrated precisely these changes in a canine model of cardiac tamponade.[8] Similar hemodynamic changes may be produced by MAST inflation for tension pneu-

Table 26-2 • Contraindications and Relative Contraindications to MAST Application

- Cardiogenic shock (not full arrest)
- Pulmonary edema and congestive heart failure
- Advanced pregnancy
- Major supradiaphragmatic hemorrhage
- Abdominal impalement
- Injuries leading to ventilatory compromise:
  - Ruptured diaphragm with visceral displacement
  - Flail chest or pulmonary contusion
  - High cervical cord injuries
- Tension pneumothorax

mothorax, but the already high intrathoracic pressures created by a tension pneumothorax may be worsened by MAST inflation leading to ventilatory failure. The immediate treatment for hypotension secondary to tension pneumothorax remains needle decompression of the involved hemithorax, *not* MAST suit application.

III. How to Use the MAST Suit

The standard MAST garment consists of three compartments: abdominal, right leg, and left leg. The compartments, which can be inflated and deflated independently, are connected to a foot pump for inflation, and to a manometer to measure suit pressure (Fig. 26–3). In the prehospital setting, the MAST suit is placed on a spine board before the patient is transferred and positioned. The patient is then placed on top of the MAST suit and the suit fastened. Placing the MAST suit on a patient already supine on a board requires a slightly different technique. The MAST trouser is initially unfolded and opened so that the Velcro fasteners may be secured appropriately on the outside of the patient. It is important to make sure the suit is not placed in an inside-out position. The patient's legs are then elevated, and the suit is positioned under the legs and up as high as the buttocks (Fig. 26–4A). Traction is applied for lower extremity fractures. The abdominal portion of the MAST suit is then placed into position by lifting the patient's hips (Fig. 26–4B). All three compartments are then closed and fastened using the Velcro strips attached to the MAST suit flaps (Fig. 26-4C–D). A poorly applied garment will not provide effective counterpressure and may become dislodged during transport. For this reason, it is important to obtain a snug fit by carefully opposing the Velcro flaps (see Fig. 26–4D). In a normal-sized adult, the MAST trouser will extend to approximately a hand's width above the umbilicus. In particularly small adults or in children, a pediatric-sized MAST suit should be used if available.

In normotensive patients who are at risk for major abdominal, retroperitoneal, or extremity hemorrhage, the MAST suit is positioned in the manner described and left in place and uninflated during prehospital trans-

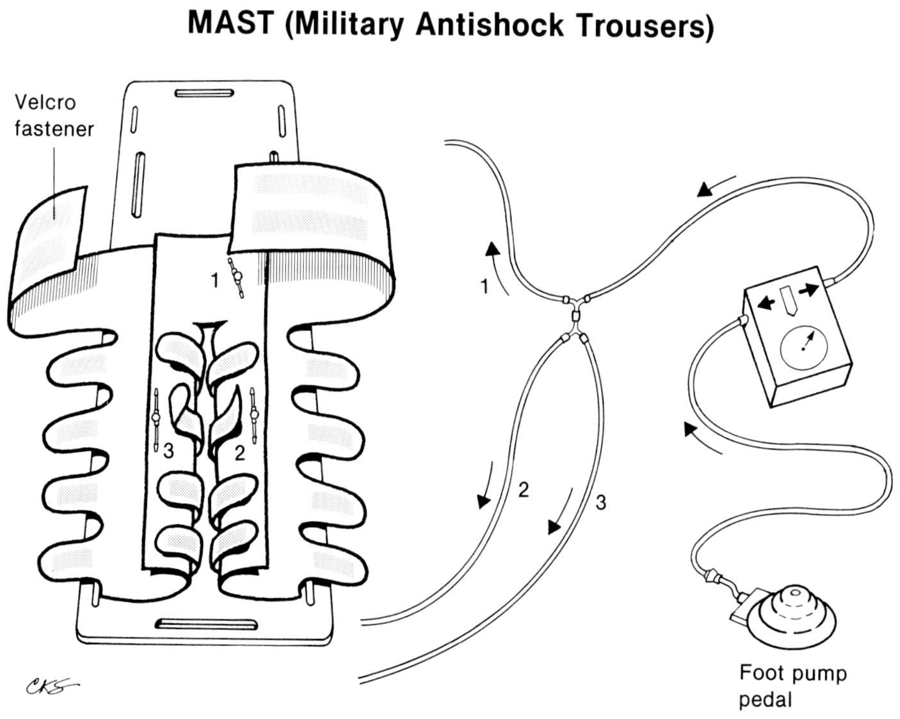

Figure 26–3 • Military antishock trousers (MAST). (1) abdominal compartment; (2) left leg compartment; (3) right leg compartment. Each compartment can be inflated and deflated separately by appropriate setting of the stop valves. Velcro fasteners hold the MAST suit around the patient.

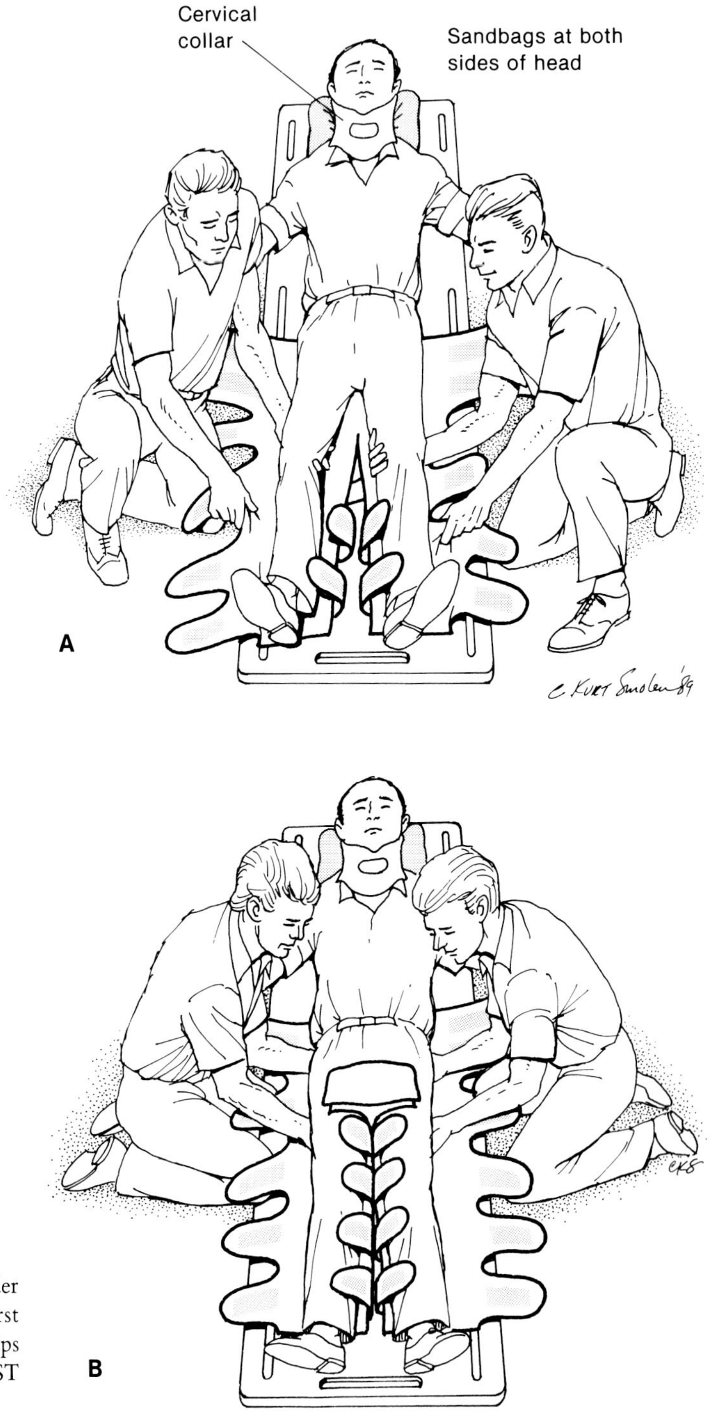

Figure 26–4 • How to place the MAST suit under and around a supine patient. (***A***) MAST suit is first positioned under legs and buttocks. (***B***) Lifting hips allows positioning of abdominal portion of the MAST suit.

port. In hypotensive patients, all three compartments of the MAST suit are inflated simultaneously using either a foot pump and connecting tubing or by "blowing up" the suit manually (Fig. 26–5). In selected patients, only the leg portions of the MAST suit may be inflated and the need for abdominal compartment reevaluated. The abdominal compartment of the MAST suit should never be inflated independently of the leg compartments because a tourniquet effect may occur, causing increased venous pooling in the legs and diminished central blood volume. All valves should be open during inflation and closed following inflation. If a manometer is available, MAST suits should be initially inflated to a pressure between 60 and 80 mmHg.[6] Pressures up to 100 mmHg

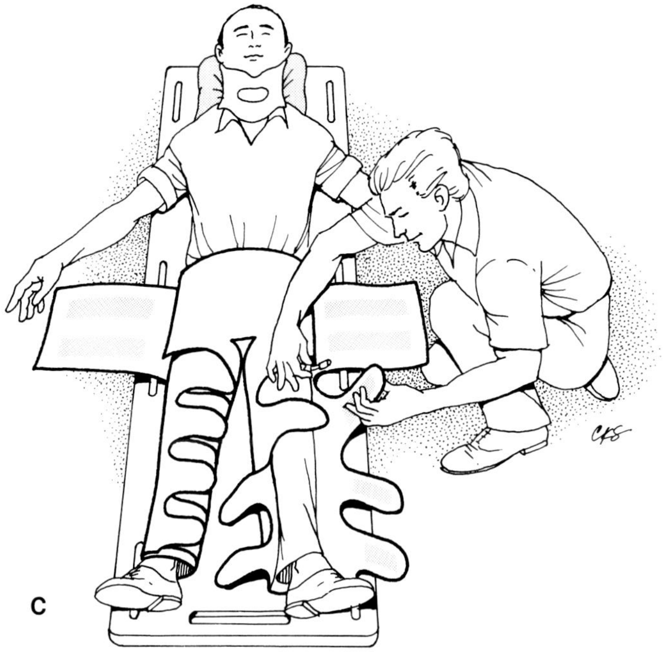

C

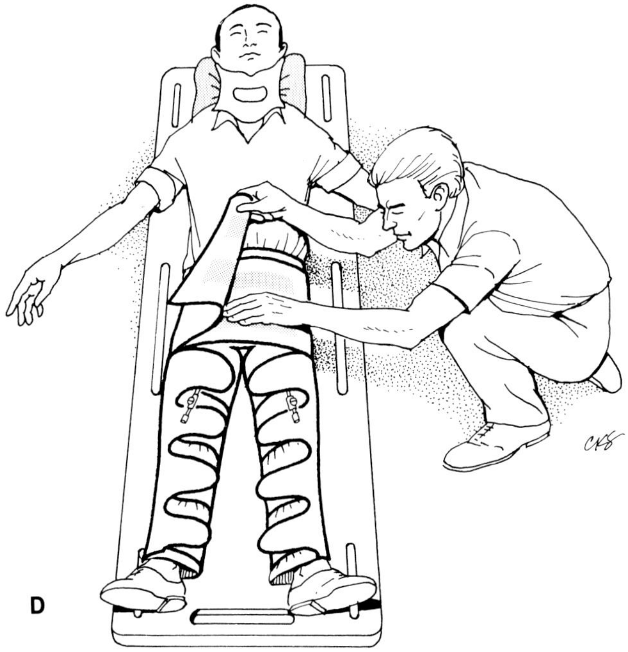

D

Figure 26–4 *(continued)*
(*C*) Leg compartments are secured by Velcro fasteners. (*D*) Abdominal compartment is securely fastened.

may be used if necessary to obtain a greater than blood pressure effect. In the cases where a manometer is not available, inflation is continued until the Velcro fasteners just begin to slip.

All patients should be closely monitored during MAST inflation. Pulse, blood pressure, and respiratory rate are useful measures of the hemodynamic effects of MAST inflation and provide signs of early ventilatory compromise (Fig. 26–6).

Deflation of the MAST suit is performed in a careful, stepwise manner. Patients who have had the suit applied for hypotension or control of hemorrhage should have a systolic pressure of approximately 100 mmHg before deflation is contemplated. Large-bore intravenous

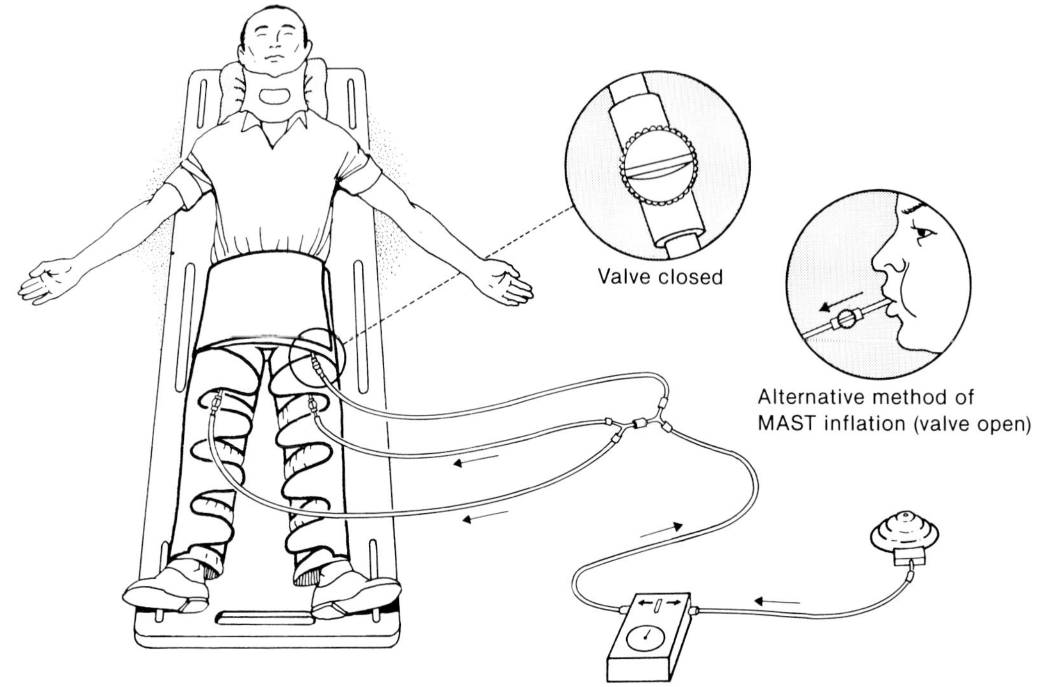

Figure 26–5 • When the valves to the three compartments are open and the foot pump is compressed repetitively, the compartments are inflated. The pressure is retained by turning the valves to a closed position. Deflation of the compartments occurs when the valve is disconnected from the tubing (rapid loss). In preparation for inflation, all three compartments are connected to pump using rubber tubing. MAST may also be inflated manually (per os; see text).

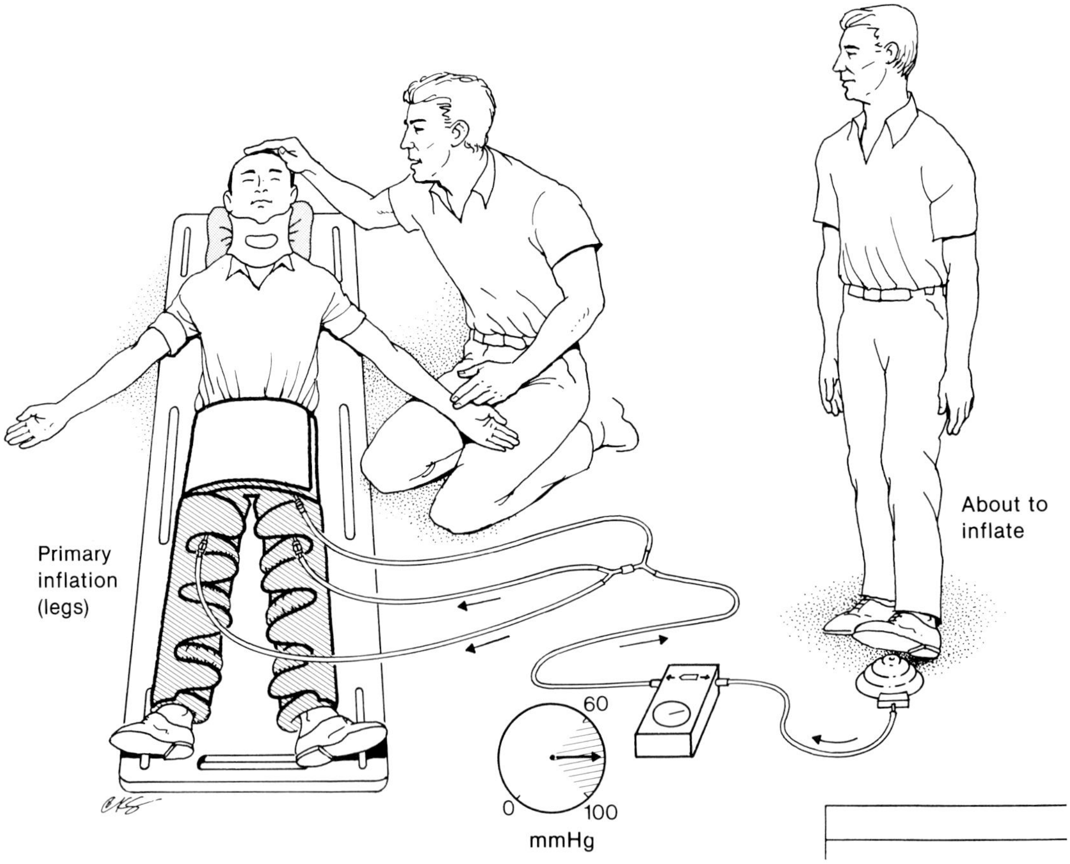

Figure 26–6 • Legs are inflated first to a measured pressure of 60–100 mmHg. Patient's vital signs are closely monitored.

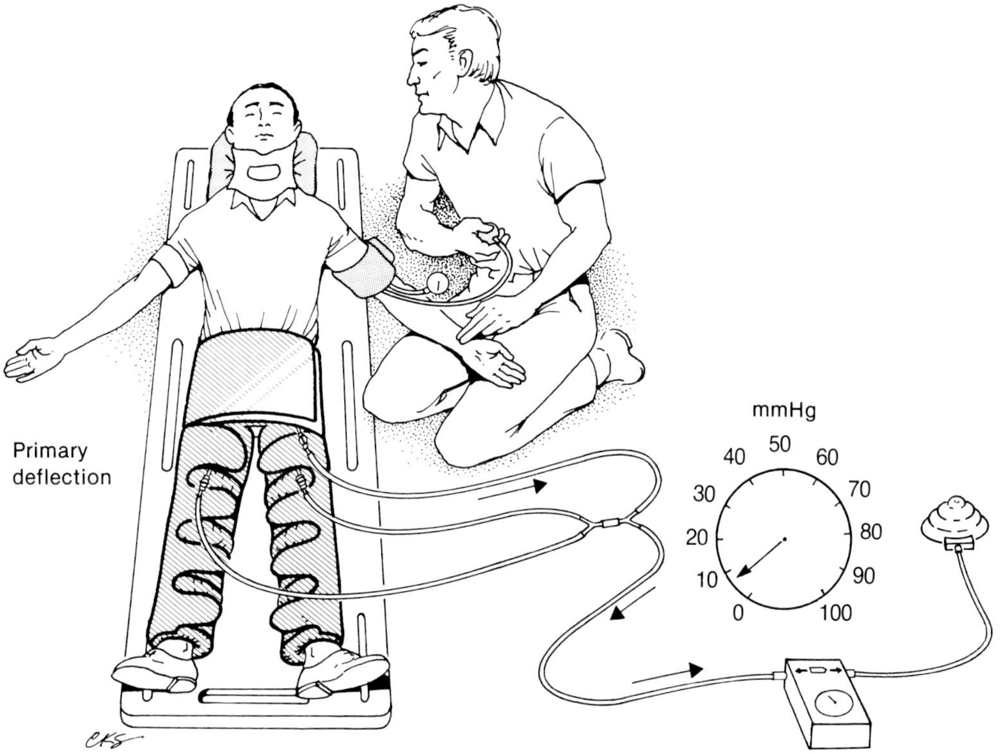

Figure 26–7 • MAST deflation begins with the abdominal compartment. The patient is carefully monitored for recurrent hypotension.

access should always be obtained prior to deflation. The abdominal portion of the MAST suit is deflated first with frequent monitoring of blood pressure and the administration of additional crystalloid or blood products as needed (Fig. 26–7). Recurrent hypotension under these circumstances is an indication for complete reinflation of the abdominal compartment. If the abdominal compartment is successfully deflated without recurrent hypotension, then the MAST suit is deflated one leg at a time with similar monitoring of vital signs. The MAST suit may be removed if ongoing hemorrhage has been controlled and further need is no longer anticipated.

IV. COMPLICATIONS

As the use of external counterpressure has increased, so has the recognition of a variety of associated problems and complications (Table 26–3). Ventilatory embarrassment may occur as a result of increased pressure and reduced compliance of the abdominal compartment, particularly with injuries that act directly to reduce ventilatory capacity (as previously discussed).

The potential for adverse MAST effects on ICP following severe head injury exists, but has not been well defined. In patients on positive pressure ventilation, MAST trousers may act to increase ICP by increasing central venous pressure and mean intrathoracic pressure, thereby decreasing venous return from the head. Although these effects have not been significant in laboratory studies or in patients with normal ICP, the tendency for MAST application to exacerbate an already elevated ICP is unknown.[13]

Table 26–3 • Problems and Complications Associated with MAST Application

- Increased work of breathing and ventilatory embarrassment
- Bullae and skin necrosis (prolonged application)
- Compartment syndrome (prolonged application)
- Relative over inflation (elderly patients)
- Limited access to patient for examination and procedures
- Increased metabolic acidosis
- Exacerbation of hemorrhage above the diaphragm (?)
- Exacerbation of increased intracranial pressure following head injury (?)
- Precipitous hypotension secondary to incorrect deflation

Prolonged application of the MAST suit (longer than 2 hours) has been associated with metabolic acidosis, skin necrosis, and compartment syndrome. Metabolic acidosis may occur with MAST deflation and is presumably secondary to reperfusion of vascular beds in the lower abdomen or extremities with washout of accumulated lactic acids. Acidosis may also reflect inadequate resuscitation. A worsening arterial base deficit should prompt a reassessment of possible ongoing hemorrhage and volume status.[30]

Bullae and skin necrosis have been reported with prolonged application of MAST garments, and there have been several reports of lower-extremity compartment syndrome and muscle necrosis both with and without associated fractures.[23,31-33] Virtually all cases of compartment syndrome reported in association with MAST usage have occurred with periods of MAST inflation exceeding 2 hours, or the use of high MAST pressures. Patients with tibia/fibula fractures or lower-extremity crush injuries are at particularly high risk. If extended MAST application is needed to control bleeding (eg, from pelvic fractures), lesser pressures (below 50 mmHg) should be used, and the suit should be deflated and reinflated periodically.

Proper application and inflation of the MAST suit may limit patient access for examination and procedures. Although examination is difficult with the MAST suit in place, important therapeutic and diagnostic procedures (eg, cutdowns, lavage) should be performed as needed. Despite increased resistance to venous flow, lower extremity cutdowns may be placed, and adequate infusion rates obtained using pressure bags.

Sudden deflation of the MAST suit may precipitate severe hypotension in patients who have adequate systolic blood pressure but remain profoundly hypovolemic. Rapid MAST reinflation and continued fluid resuscitation will usually restore the blood pressure. Deflation of the MAST suit should always be gradual, with frequent blood pressure monitoring.

V. Discussion

The primary indication for the use of external counterpressure remains the treatment of hypovolemic shock. The MAST suit will never be a substitute for restoration of circulating blood volume, and its application generally should not take priority over the placement of large-bore intravenous lines and fluid/blood administration. External counterpressure may occasionally be used as a means of definitive control of hemorrhage (eg, pelvic fracture bleeding), but should be applied only in very specific instances within which operative management is either unsafe or ineffective.

The number and variety of reported complications have increased with the widespread use of external counterpressure. Most of the associated complications are related to either excessive inflation pressures or prolonged use. As with any drug or operative procedure, the relative risks and benefits for MAST applications must be carefully assessed for each patient. Indiscriminate use will increase morbidity.

The accumulated experience with external counterpressure is enormous, with an estimated 2 million uses since 1973.[34] Despite many anecdotal reports and uncontrolled studies in the literature, it has become clear that external counterpressure dependably improves blood pressure, increases cardiac output, and decreases hemorrhage from certain types of injuries. Despite these apparent beneficial effects on blood pressure, the overall effect on patient survival of the prehospital application of MAST garments remains controversial. Reports attesting to improved survival have used historic controls[3,4] or have been completely uncontrolled studies.[21] Several comparative studies on the prehospital use of MAST using similar patient groups have failed to show any improvement in survival rates associated with the use of the garment.[35-37] All of these studies, however, were carried out in short transit time systems and involved predominantly penetrating trauma.

The lack of observed effect on survival with MAST application, despite hemodynamic improvement raises additional questions: (1) Are the adverse effects of MAST important enough to offset the observed hemodynamic improvements in terms of overall patient survival? (2) Is early hemodynamic improvement without restoration of circulating blood volume an unimportant determinant in patient survival? Further clinical and laboratory investigations will be needed to address these questions and to define the proper role of external counterpressure in the treatment of hypovolemic shock.

VI. References

1. Crile GW. The resuscitation of the apparently dead and a demonstration of the pneumatic blood pressure. Trans South Surg Gyn Assoc 16:361–370, 1904.

2. Gardner WJ, Dohn DR. The antigravity suit (G-suit) in surgery. JAMA 162:274–276, 1956.
3. Cutler BS, Daggett WM. Application of the G-suit: To the control of hemorrhage in massive trauma. Ann Surg 173:511–514, 1971.
4. Kaplan BC, Civetta JM, Nagel EL, et al. The military antishock trouser in civilian prehospital emergency care. J Trauma 13:843–848, 1973.
5. Bivins HG, Knopp R, Tiernan C, Dos Santos PAL, et al. Blood volume displacement with inflation of antishock trousers. Ann Emerg Med 11:409–412, 1982.
6. Hanke BK, Bivins HG, Knopp R, Dos Santos PAL. Antishock trousers: A comparison of inflation techniques and inflation pressures. Ann Emerg Med 14:636–640, 1985.
7. Eddy DM, Wangesteen SL, Ludewig RM. The kinetics of fluid loss from leaks in arteries tested by an experimental ex vivo preparation and external counterpressure. Surgery 64:451–458, 1968.
8. Davis JW, McKone TK, Cram AE. Hemodynamic effects of military anti-shock trousers (MAST) in experimental cardiac tamponade. Ann Emerg Med 10:185–185, 1981.
9. Cram AE, Davis JW Kealey GP, Kassell NF. Effects of pneumatic antishock trousers on canine intracranial pressure. Ann Emerg Med 10:28–31, 1981.
10. Palafox BA, Johnson MN, McEwen DK, Gazzaniga AB. ICP changes following application of the MAST suit. J Trauma 21:55–59, 1981.
11. Lee HR, Blank WF, Massion WH, Downs P, et al. Venous return in hemorrhagic shock after application of military antishock trousers. Am J Emerg Med 1:7–11, 1983.
12. Holcroft JW, Link DP, Lantz MT, Green JF, et al. Venous return and the pneumatic antishock garment in hypovolemic baboons. J Trauma 24:928–937, 1984.
13. Gardner SR, Maull KI, Swensson EE, Ward JD. The effects of the pneumatic antishock garment of ICP in man: A prospective study of 12 patients with severe head injury. J Trauma 24:896–900, 1984.
14. Gilbert RD. Depression of respiratory function by pneumatic antishock trousers in traumatic quadriplegia. Ann Emerg Med 12:378–381, 1983.
15. McCabe JB, Johantgen SR, Ventriglia WJ, et al. Effect of antishock trouser inflation on plasma renin activity during hemorrhagic shock. Ann Emerg Med 13:17–21, 1984.
16. McGivern D, Hardcastle A, Miller JG, et al. Modification of the normal postural changes in plasma renin activity by the application of positive pressure to the legs. Clin Endocrinol 11:105–109, 1979.
17. Shenasky JH, Gillenwater JY. The effects of external abdominal counterpressure on renal function. Surg Forum 21:528–530, 1970.
18. Burchard KW, Slotman GJ, Jed E, Singh AK, et al. Positive pressure respirations and pneumatic antishock garment application: Hemodynamic response. J Trauma 25:83–89, 1985.
19. Espinosa MH, Updegrove JH. Clinical experience with the G-suit. Arch Surg 101:36–39, 1970.
20. Abraham E, Gong H, Tashkin DP, Baraff LJ, et al. Effect of pneumatic trousers on pulmonary function. Crit Care Med 18:754–757, 1982.
21. Civetta JM, Nussenfeld SR, Rowe TR, Hirschman JC, et al. Prehospital use of the military anti-shock trouser (MAST). JACEP 5:581–587, 1976.
22. Gaffney FA, Thal ER, Taylor WF. Hemodynamic effects of medical anti-shock trousers (MAST garment). J Trauma 21:931–937, 1981.
23. Burdick JF, Warshaw AL, Abbot WM. External counterpressure to control postoperative intra-abdominal hemorrhage. Am J Surg 129:369–373, 1975.
24. Brooks DH, Grenvik A. G-suit control of massive retroperitoneal hemorrhage due to pelvic fracture. Crit Care Med 1:257–260, 1973.
25. Batalden DJ, Wickstrom PH, Ruiz E, et al. Value of the G-suit in patients with severe pelvic fracture. Arch Surg 109:326–328, 1974.
26. Eisenberg H, Cayard C, Papanicolau A, Weiner R, et al. The effects of three potentially preventable complications on outcome after severe closed head injury. In: Ishii S, Nagai H, Brock M (eds). Intracranial Pressure V. New York, Springer-Verlag, 1983, 549–553.
27. Neimann JT, Criley JM, Rosborough JP, et al. Predictive indices of successful cardiac resuscitation after prolonged arrest and experimental cardiopulmonary resuscitation. Ann Emerg Med 14:521–528, 1985.
28. Warren ET, Pass HI, Crawford FA. External cardiopulmonary resuscitation augmented by the military antishock trousers. Am Surg 49:651–654, 1983.
29. Mahoney BD, Mirick MJ. Efficacy of pneumatic trousers in refractory prehospital cardiopulmonary arrest. Ann Emerg Med 12:8–12. 1983.
30. Davis JW, Shackford SR, Mackersie RC, Hoyt DB. Base deficit as a guide to volume resuscitation. J Trauma 28:1464–1467, 1988.
31. Bass RR, Allison EJ, Reines HD, Yeager JC, et al. Thigh compartment syndrome without lower extremity trauma following application of pneumatic antishock trousers. Ann Emerg Med 12:382–384, 1983.
32. Johnson BE. Anterior tibial compartment syndrome following use of MAST suit. Ann Emerg Med 10:209–210, 1981.
33. Godbout B, Burchard KW, Slotman GJ, Gann DS. Crush syndrome with death following pneumatic antishock garment application. J Trauma 24:1052–1056. 1984.
34. McSwain NE. Pneumatic anti-shock garment: State of the art 1988. Ann Emerg Med 17:506–525, 1988.
35. Mackersie RC, Christensen JM, Lewis FR. The prehospital use of external counterpressure: Does MAST make a difference? J Trauma 24:882–887, 1984.
36. Mattox KL, Bickell WH, Pepe PE, et al. Prospective randomized evaluation of antishock MAST in post-hypotension. J Trauma 26:779–786, 1986.
37. Bickell WH, Pepe PE, Bailey ML, Wyatt CH, Mattox KL. Randomized trial of pneumatic antishock garments in the prehospital management of penetrating abdominal injuries. Ann Emerg Med 16:653–658, 1987.

Chapter 27

•

John W. Danforth, MD

Pericardiocentesis

OUTLINE

I. INTRODUCTION

The term *pericardiocentesis,* a contraction of the expression *pericardial paracentesis,* refers to the process of aspirating fluid from the pericardial space. The evacuation of pericardial fluid can be accomplished either surgically or percutaneously, for both diagnostic and therapeutic purposes, and under both elective and emergent circumstances. Romero is credited with performing the first recorded pericardiotomy in 1815.[1] Twenty-five years later, Shuh introduced a percutaneous method for draining pericardial fluid.[2] This technique was later refined by Singleton[3] and Blalock[4] in the 1930s and 1940s for the treatment of cardiac tamponade sustained as a result of penetrating cardiac trauma.

This chapter focuses on the percutaneous technique. Although the advent of new technology has substantially enhanced the safety of this approach, the morbidity associated with percutaneous pericardiocentesis remains significant, and thus there is considerable controversy regarding the relative merits of this approach vs. the surgical alternative.

II. INDICATIONS

A. *Percutaneous vs. Surgical Approach: General Overview*

Although the percutaneous approach was introduced more than 100 years ago, skepticism has persisted concerning the clinical value of this technique.[5,6] In 1980, for example, Becker wrote that " . . . the entire procedure should be abandoned in favor of the safer and more reliable approach of surgical intervention."[7] As a result of this skepticism, considerable controversy has evolved regarding the indications for the percutaneous approach.[5,6] In retrospect, it would appear that this skepticism has been perpetuated by the facts that (1) both the surgical and percutaneous techniques can be used to accomplish the same objective, and (2) the relative merits of the two approaches remain unresolved. This latter uncertainty stems in large part from the fact that the relevant technology and clinical indications for pericardiocentesis have continued to change with sufficient rapidity that there exists insufficient data from which to draw reliable conclusions.

It is clear that the morbidity associated with the performance of percutaneous pericardiocentesis was substantial during the 1940s and 1950s. However, the recent advent of a variety of techniques and monitoring systems, including the electrocardiographic method for monitoring the depth of needle penetration,[8] the Seldinger technique,[9] and high-resolution fluoroscopy and echocardiography,[10] have all contributed to reducing the incidence of complications sustained during the course of this procedure.

Despite these developments, the morbidity associated with this procedure remains significant. A recent survey by Guberman, for example, demonstrated that percutaneous pericardiocentesis was associated with a 7% major complication rate (eg, RV laceration in 3 of 46 patients).[11] In retrospect, it is entirely conceivable that the growing tendency to perform pericardiocentesis among increasingly debilitated individuals has contributed to the perceived morbidity of this procedure. It appears that the clinical condition of patients who present to medical attention with pericardial disease has been steadily deteriorating over the past 50 years. In this regard, it is well recognized that patients with infectious pericarditis currently tend to be older and less immunocompetent than their clinical counterparts of the 1940s.[12] It is presumed that this circumstance reflects the advent of recently developed chemotherapeutic regimens, transplant immunosuppressive therapies, radiation therapy, and the onset of the AIDS epidemic.[11,13] Regardless of the circumstances, the prognosis of patients who currently require pericardiocentesis tends to be poor. According to a survey by Markiewicz and associates, 67% of their patients who underwent pericardiocentesis between 1976 and 1982 died within 1 day to 1 year following completion of a successful procedure.[14] Also, it is likely the poor prognoses of the individuals who require pericardial drainage have adversely influenced the perception of many physicians concerning the morbidity of the procedure itself.

With the exception of cardiac tamponade, an indication for which the percutaneous approach is generally well accepted, it is likely that considerable uncertainty will persist concerning the relative merits of the surgical vs. percutaneous approach. Hence, it is reasonable to assume that the decision to proceed with either approach should be based on the relative risk–benefit profile of the particular procedure for the individual patient. For example, the presence of a large pericardial effusion tends to reduce the risk associated with percutaneous aspiration and thus favors this approach, whereas the presence of loculations or a history of previous bypass surgery tends to enhance the risk of percutaneous aspiration and favors the surgical alternative.[6,15,16] Of note is the fact that bypass surgery tends to provoke the development of pericardial adhesions that approximate the wall of the right ventricle to the pericardium, limiting the amount of fluid that can accumulate within the anterior free space. In this regard, both Wong and Engleman have reported a 50% failure rate for percutaneous pericardiocentesis performed among patients who had undergone prior bypass surgery.[6,16]

B. *General Indications (Diagnosis and Treatment)*

In general, percutaneous drainage of the pericardium can provide valuable information concerning the etiology of occult pericardial fluid collections and can permit pericardial decompression. For these reasons, pericardiocentesis is generally indicated among patients with either pericardial effusions of unsuspected etiology (for diagnosis) or evidence of hemodynamic compromise secondary to pericardial fluid accumulation (for treatment).

Before reviewing the specific indications for pericardiocentesis, it must be recognized that the clinical manifestations of many of these conditions tend to be subtle.[17] For example, in an autopsy survey of 189 patients with documented metastatic involvement of the pericardium, Thurber and coworkers reported that only 8.5% of the patients were found to have pericardial metastases ante mortem.[18] However, pericardial metastases accounted for the immediate cause of death in 36% of the 55 symptomatic patients in this series, and this condition contributed significantly to patient demise in an additional 49%.[18] Among 35 patients with tuberculosis, Rooney and associates reported that 7 individuals died from unsuspected pericardial involvement.[19] And Markiewicz and colleagues further observed that tamponade was not suspected among several patients in their review until a chest radiograph disclosed the presence of an enlarged cardiac silhouette and clear lung fields—despite the fact that many patients presented with typical signs and symptoms of this condition.[14] In short, the clinical manifestations of pericardial disease and tamponade tend to be subtle, and a high index of suspicion is frequently required to make the appropriate diagnosis.

C. *Specific Indications*

1. CARDIAC TAMPONADE

Cardiac tamponade constitutes the most frequent indication for percutaneous pericardiocentesis, and there exists little question concerning the value of this procedure in this circumstance. Among selected individuals, this procedure can be life saving. The difficulty in this circumstance does not concern utility of the procedure, but rather, identifying the indication. The diagnosis of cardiac tamponade can frequently prove elusive, for a variety of reasons. For example, we now recognize that many patients with tamponade physiology do not manifest signs and symptoms considered to be characteristic of this disorder. In a study of 56 medical patients with tamponade, for example, Guberman and associates observed that the majority tended to be normotensive and did not necessarily have a quiet precordium.[11] The central venous pressure (CVP) can be normal among volume-depleted individuals with tamponade physiology.[23] A pulsus paradoxus frequently does not develop among individuals who develop tamponade physiology with underlying atrial septal defects, aortic regurgitation, severe aortic stenosis, and uremia with severe left ventricular dysfunction.[11] Finally, pericardial effusions can become very large without embarrassing the cardiovascular system.[20-22]

In addition to these difficulties, the pulsus paradoxus and an elevated central venous pressure (CVP) constitute relatively nonspecific physical findings for tamponade. For example, the presence of a pulsus paradoxus has been associated with a number of unrelated conditions including (1) acute and chronic obstructive airway disease, (2) shock, (3) pulmonary emboli, (4) constrictive pericarditis, (5) right ventricular infarction, (6) restrictive cardiomyopathy, and (7) tense ascites.[11] Similarly, Krikorian reported that only 62% of 123 patients with pericardial effusions and elevated CVP who underwent pericardiocentesis were initially determined to have tamponade physiology (see Table 27–1).[5]

It should be recognized that the echocardiogram can be a misleading indication of tamponade on rare occasions. For example, both the echo-free space created by tense ascites and pericardial fat have been erroneously interpreted to represent pericardial fluid.[24,25] For these reasons, it is often helpful to install a Swan-Ganz catheter among patients with presumed cardiac tamponade to confirm the diagnosis before proceeding with pericardial decompression.

2. EFFUSIVE-CONSTRICTIVE PERICARDITIS

Effusive-constrictive pericarditis was first described by Burchell in 1954 and refers to a condition characterized by combined pericardial constriction and cardiac tamponade physiology.[26] Effusive-constrictive pericarditis has been reported in conjunction with tuberculosis, uremia, radiation, trauma, neoplasms, viral pericarditis, and pyogenic pericarditis.[27] Although the pathophysiology reflects the coexistence of both constriction and tamponade, the clinical features resemble tamponade.[27] The evacuation of pericardial fluid provides only partial relief, and definitive therapy ultimately requires a pericardiectomy.[27]

As in the case of cardiac tamponade, the diagnosis of this entity frequently proves elusive. The constricting layer of pericardium can be deceptively thin.[28] Performing a right heart catheterization before attempting pericardial decompression is frequently helpful in making the diagnosis.[5] Classically, the left and right ventricular

Table 27–1 • Distribution of Initial Diagnoses Among 123 Patients with Elevated CVP and Pericardial Effusions who Underwent Pericardiocentesis at Stanford

62%	Tamponade
17%	Constriciton
16%	Congestive heart failure
5%	Superior vena cava syndrome

(Data from Krikorian JG, Hancock EW. Pericardiocentesis. Am J Med 65:808–814, 1978; with permission.)

Y descents cannot be detected prior to decompression of the pericardium and become increasingly apparent during the process of removing fluid from the pericardial space.[26]

3. Pyogenic Pericarditis

In general, surgical drainage is recommended for patients with suspected pyogenic involvement of the pericardium. Among critically ill patients with relatively large pyogenic effusions, however, percutaneous pericardiocentesis has been advocated.[13] Although their findings are controversial, Bouwels and associates contend that surgical drainage among debilitated individuals carries a considerable morbidity, whereas percutaneous drainage among patients with large effusions tends to be well tolerated.[13] Despite this observation, percutaneous drainage will not prove sufficient among patients with pericardial adhesions and loculated effusions and thus should not be considered definitive therapy among the large majority of patients with pyogenic pericarditis.

4. Tuberculosis

Although uncommon, tuberculous pericarditis must be considered in the differential diagnosis of any pericardial effusion of undetermined etiology. Among patients with suspected tuberculous pericarditis, a pericardial biopsy, performed in conjunction with the pericardiocentesis, frequently enhances the diagnostic yield of the procedure relative to culture of the pericardial fluid alone (85% vs. 40%).[19] Biopsy provides immediate results, whereas pericardial cultures frequently require 4 to 6 weeks to yield positive results.

5. Malignancy

Among patients with metastatic involvement of the pericardium, percutaneous pericardiocentesis is frequently indicated to confirm the diagnosis and to decompress the pericardium.[6,29,30] Typically, the diagnostic yield of this procedure is particularly high for metastatic lung and breast tumors involving the pericardium.[5] However, false negative cytologies have been reported among patients with lymphomatous involvement of the pericardium.[5] For further discussion of the diagnostic potential of percutaneous pericardiocentesis among patients with malignant involvement of the pericardium, I recommend the review by Yazdi and associates.[31]

6. Uremic Pericarditis

The role of percutaneous pericardiocentesis among patients with pericardial fluid accumulation secondary to uremic pericarditis remains unclear.[32–37] It is conceivable that several varieties of uremic pericarditis exist and that the response to therapy depends on the type of uremic pericarditis submitted to treatment. Among patients with uremic pericarditis who have not been dialyzed, routine dialysis is sufficient to resolve the effusion in approximately 90% of individuals.[35,36] Among patients who develop uremic pericarditis while the condition is being managed on dialysis, the dialysis alone is generally ineffective, with a response rate of less than 40%.[37] Currently, therapeutic pericardiocentesis is recommended for patients with uremic pericarditis who fail to respond to intensive dialysis or require steroid therapy.[38,39]

III. How to Do Percutaneous Pericardiocentesis

A. *Preoperative Evaluation*

In 1951, Kotte and McGuire reported that 18 of 21 physicians had observed at least one fatality related to pericardiocentesis.[40] In 1965, Kilpatric and Chapman reported similar findings.[41] Although these experiences antedate the advent of cardiac catheterization laboratories, high-resolution fluoroscopic equipment, sensitive on-line hemodynamic monitors, soft-tip catheters, and so forth, they do point out the potential morbidity of this procedure when performed blind and underscore the need to take advantage of all the relevant technology that has evolved to enhance the safety of this procedure.

Provided that the patient's condition is sufficiently stable to permit a thorough evaluation, I recommend a two-dimensional echocardiogram and a right heart catheterization before proceeding with percutaneous pericardiocentesis. Few would argue with the utility of a preoperative echocardiogram, which provides helpful information concerning the amount of fluid that has accumulated within the pericardial space, the presence or absence of adhesions, and the optimal entry point.[42,44,45] However, the need to perform a right heart catheterization remains less well accepted. Although performing a right heart catheterization is somewhat controversial for all percutaneous pericardiocentesis candidates, I recommend it whenever feasible because it provides useful information concerning the diagnosis of cardiac tamponade, the diagnosis of effusive-constrictive pericarditis, and the hemodynamic response to pericardial decompression.[5]

In addition, the procedure should be performed within the cardiac catheterization laboratory or another suitable procedure room, and preferably within a hospital with thoracic surgery capability (see Table 27–2).[6] According to Krikorian, "The procedure should be performed by experienced persons, in a setting in which maximum diagnostic and physiologic information can be obtained and where alternative surgical therapy is promptly available."[5] It is frequently helpful to review the case with the surgical service in the event that their services are required.[46]

B. *Relevant Anatomy*

The anterior aspect of the pericardium is attached to the manubrium and xiphoid by means of the superior and inferior pericardiosternal ligaments.[55] Inferiorly, the pericardium is attached to the left hemidiaphragm and the central diaphragmatic tendon. The posterior aspect of the pericardium is attached directly to the esophagus and indirectly to the spinal column by the pericardiovertebral ligament.[55]

Among supine patients, pericardial fluid generally accumulates anterior to the right ventricle[55] and not posterior to the left ventricle, as has been suggested in several echocardiography textbooks.[56-59] This conclusion derives from a study by Gale and associates that used computed axial tomography (CAT scans) to determine the normal distribution of pericardial fluid among supine patients with pericarditis (Fig. 27–1).[55] The result seems entirely reasonable given the fact that the density of the heart exceeds the density of pericardial fluid. Although echocardiography seems to indicate that pericardial fluid normally collects posterior to the left ventricle, this is probably due to the effect of the lateral decubitus position (the optimal patient position for echocardiographic evaluation) on the distribution of pericardial fluid. In the lateral decubitus position, the heart is suspended by the base, allowing pericardial fluid to accumulate beneath the left ventricle. Furthermore, among patients studied in the lateral decubitus position, the fluid that accumulates anterior to the right ventricle frequently cannot be visualized by echocardiography, largely because of the reflection of the incident sound beam by bone.

Several anatomic considerations favor the subxiphoid approach (described below) for percutaneous pericardiocentesis including the fact that (1) the surface of the pericardium is roughly perpendicular to the tract of a needle introduced via this approach (Fig. 27–2),[46] and (2) the pericardial fluid tends to accumulate anterior to the right ventricle within a region of the mediastinum that is readily accessible using this approach. Occasionally, it is helpful to elevate the torso of the patient 15° in reverse Trendelenberg position at the outset of the procedure to enhance drainage of the pericardial fluid into the inferior-anterior aspect of the pericardium, the region most accessible by the subxiphoid approach.[60]

Table 27–2 • Advantages of Performing Percutaneous Pericardioscentesis in the Cardiac Catheterization Laboratory

- Fluoroscopic availability for identification of the atrioventricular groove and location of the right coronary artery
- Fluoroscopic availability to permit confirmation of the needle tip location within the pericardial space by means of contrast injection
- Presence of sensitive hemodynamic monitors and polygraphs to document changes in the intracardiac and intrapericardial pressure patterns
- Presence of arrhythmia monitors
- Presence of a trained crew that can respond appropriately in the event of a complication

Computed Axial Tomogram of a Patient with a Pericardial Effusion

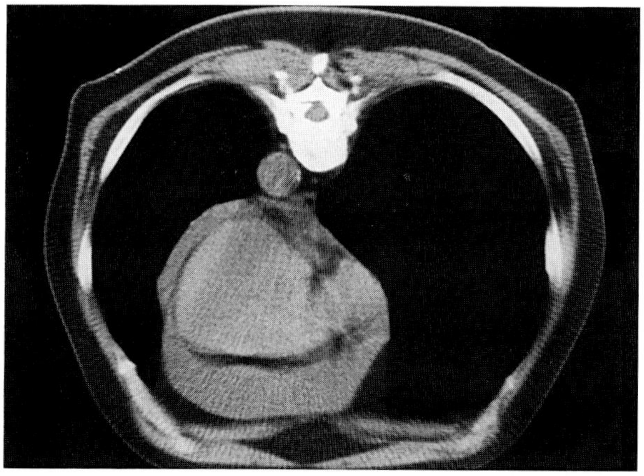

Figure 27–1 • Computed axial tomogram of the thorax of a supine patient with a pericardial effusion. Note that the majority of the effusion is located anterior to the right ventricle. (Courtesy of Dr Gale.)

Relevant Pericardial Anatomy

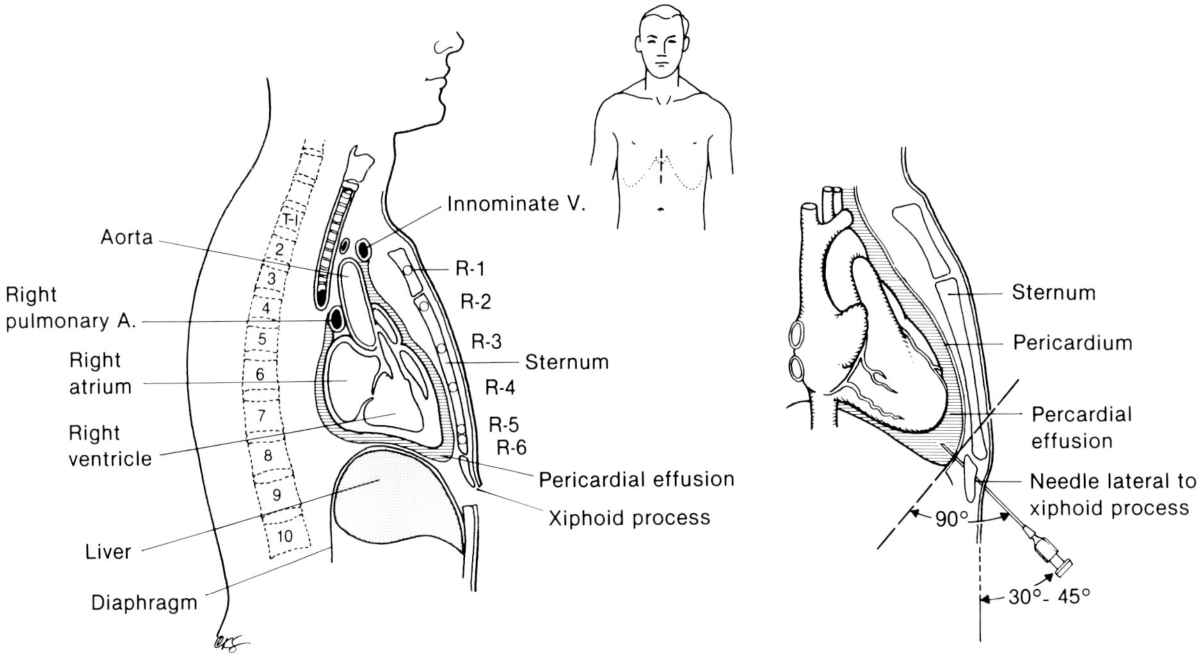

Figure 27–2 • Sagittal view of the thorax indicating the orientation of the pericardial needle, introduced via the subxiphoid approach, relative to the surface of the pericardium. Note that the needle enters the skin to the left of the xiphoid (see Fig. 27–3), and that the needle enters the pericardial space at right angles to the pericardium when inserted using this approach.

C. *The Percutaneous Procedure*

Under optimal circumstances, this procedure should be performed in either the cardiac catheterization laboratory or a suitable procedure room. Although fluoroscopy is generally available in this setting, I recommend the concomitant use of the electrocardiographic technique to assess the depth of needle penetration. In anticipation of the need to use the electrocardiogram, it is frequently most convenient to apply the four ECG limb leads before applying the surgical drapes to the patient. Once the patient is properly prepped, draped, and locally anesthetized, the operator should make a stab wound approximately 1 inch below the left xiphocostal angle and left costal margin in the region depicted in Fig. 27–3 and blunt-dissect the adjacent subcutaneous tissue. This will be used to accommodate the pericardial needle. The 1-inch margin enables the operator to direct the needle immediately below the ribcage with minimal difficulty (Fig. 27–4A–B). Once the superficial direction is complete, the operator should connect a suitable short-bevel 9- to 15-cm needle[61] to a 10-mL syringe. In turn, this assembly should be attached to the V1 lead of the electrocardiogram with a double-ended sterile alligator clip

Optimal Entry Point for Pericardiocentesis Needle

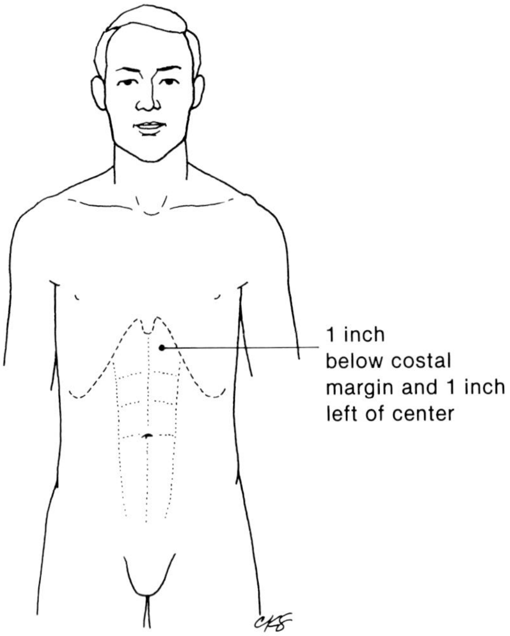

Figure 27–3 • Anterior view of the xiphoid indicating the optimal entry point for the pericardiocentesis needle. Note that the optimal entry point is approximately 1 inch below the costal margin and 1 inch to the left of the midline.

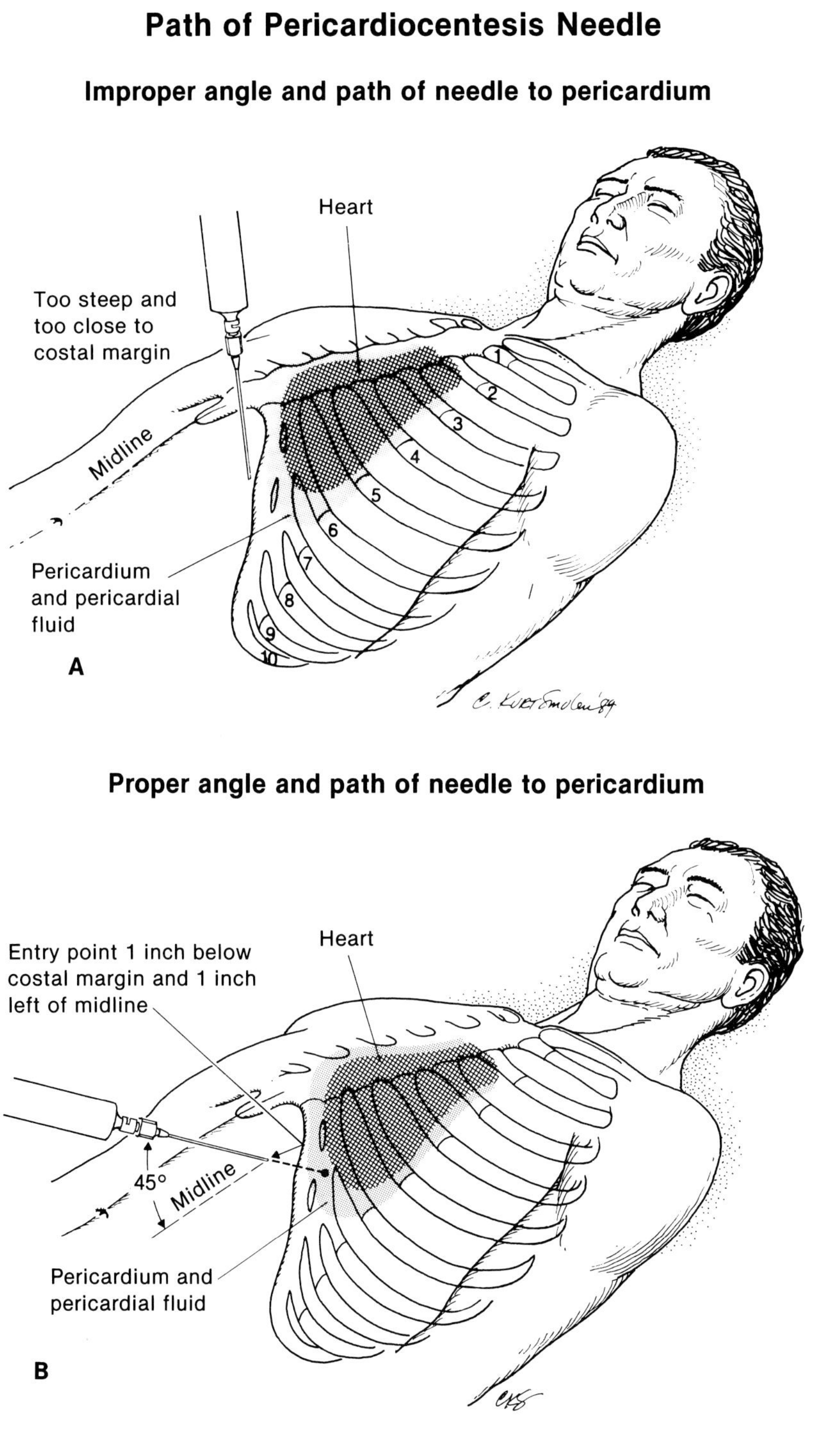

Figure 27–4 • Path of pericardiocentesis needle. (***A***) Sagittal view of the subcostal margin in the region of the pericardial needle entry point indicating the difficulty that can transpire when the needle is introduced less than 1 inch below the left costal margin. (***B***) Sagittal view of the subcostal margin in the region of the pericardial needle entry point, indicating that the introduction of the needle well below the left costal margin permits further insertion of the needle at the appropriate angle to the skin.

as illustrated in Fig. 27–5.[9] (Cook, Inc., of Bloomington, IN, makes an 18 gauge, thin-wall 9-cm needle suitable for this purpose that will accommodate a 0.038-inch guide wire.) The needle should be advanced slowly in the posterior and superior direction, into the stab wound, with the superior axis of the needle directed toward the left shoulder and the posterior axis at a 45° angle to the skin (Fig. 27–6).[60] Gentle suction should be applied to the syringe during this process.

The configuration of the electrocardiographic complex or the appearance of fluid within the syringe should be used to provide some feedback concerning the depth of needle penetration. In general, the pericardium is particularly sensitive and most patients will experience

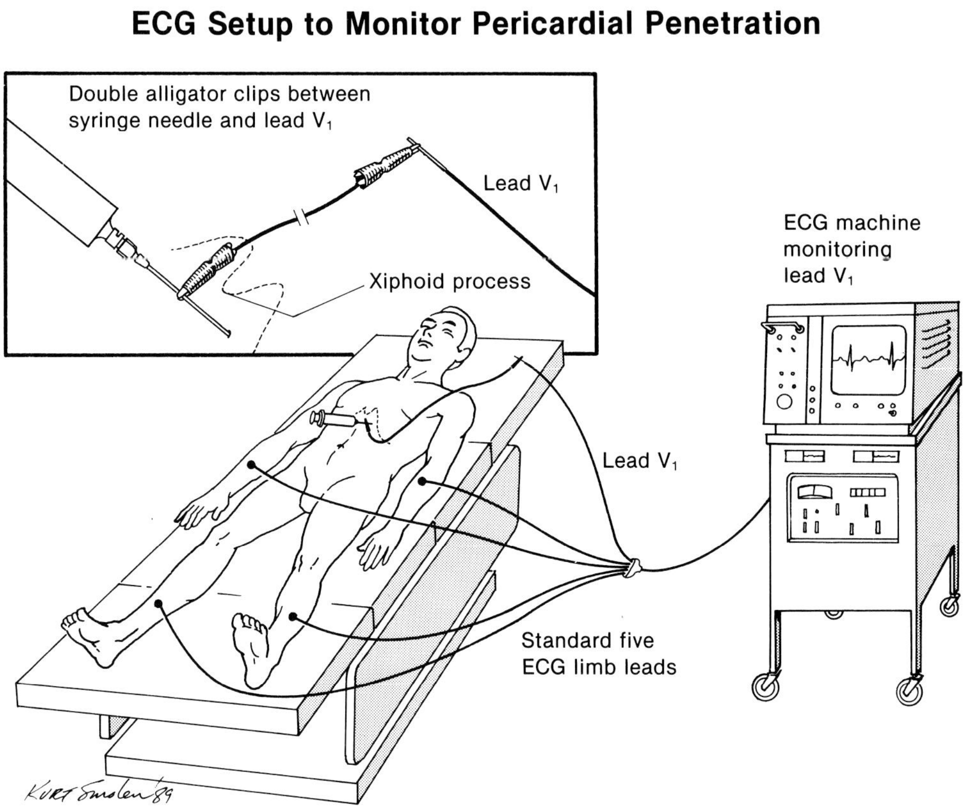

Figure 27–5 • Electrocardiographic setup required to monitor the depth of penetration of the pericardial needle consists of an electrocardiogram, standard limb leads, a V_1 precordial lead, sterile double-ended alligator clips, and a pericardiocentesis needle. The electrocardiogram should be preset to monitor the V_1 lead as the needle is introduced into the pericardium.

some discomfort as the needle penetrates the tissue layer.[46] Nonetheless, it is frequently helpful to monitor the ECG and evaluate the characteristics of the fluid withdrawn to assess the location of the tip of the needle, particularly among patients with relatively small pericardial effusions.

Typically, penetration of the myocardium provokes an electrocardiographic current of injury. Although the ECG approach is helpful, it does have some drawbacks. For example, this approach does not protect against laceration of the right coronary artery (RCA), which lies within the AV groove along the epicardial surface. Occasionally, this approach does not protect against penetration of the right ventricle because this structure is relatively thin. On rare occasions, this approach can fail among individuals in whom the epicardium has been replaced largely by neoplasm.[62]

Analysis of the fluid withdrawn into the syringe also can be used to assess the depth of needle penetration. For example, the fluid can be inspected for the presence of clot formation. In general, pericardial fluid will not clot, whereas blood withdrawn from the right ventricle will thrombose. Although this rule applies in most circumstances, fluid withdrawn from patients with hemopericardium will also frequently clot, so the operator must consider the patient's underlying condition when relying upon this general principle. Determination of the pH, PCO_2, and PO_2 can also be used to distinguish pericardial fluid from central venous blood contained within the right ventricle. Balakrishnan has reported that the PO_2 is lower and that the PCO_2 is higher in the pericardial fluid relative to the central venous blood.[64] Kindig has further reported that the pH of pericardial fluid is generally lower than the corresponding pH of the central venous blood.[65] A pH of less than 7.1 generally suggests an inflammatory state (eg, systemic lupus erythematosus or bacterial pericarditis).

Among patients who undergo the procedure in the cardiac catheterization laboratory, several other techniques in addition to monitoring the ECG and analyzing the characteristics of the aspirated fluid can be used to provide information concerning the depth of needle pen-

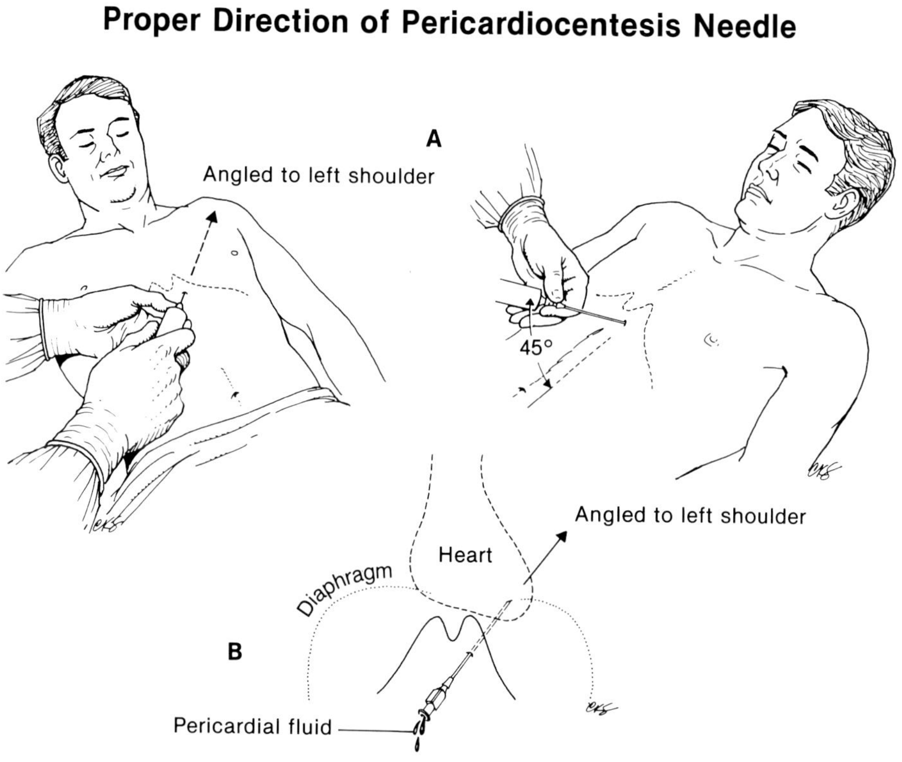

Figure 27–6 • Anterior and side views of the chest indicating the preferred axes of insertion for the pericardial needle. (***A***) The axis in the frontal plane should be directed toward the left shoulder. (***B***) The axis in the sagittal plane should be directed superiorly and posteriorly at an angle of 45° to the skin surface.

etration. For example, radiographic contrast medium can be injected into the pericardiocentesis needle under fluoroscope control.[60,66] Provided that the tip of the needle is located within the pericardium, the contrast injected simply accumulates within the pericardial space. In the event that the needle tip has penetrated the right ventricle, the injected contrast mixes with the blood coursing through the right ventricle, briefly delineates the contour of the right ventricular cavity, and subsequently passes out of the field of view with the circulation. If echocardiography is used to direct the procedure, saline can be injected into the needle to produce a cloud of echoes within the cavity penetrated by the tip of the needle.[67] Finally, the configuration of the pressure generated within the space penetrated by the needle can also be used to assess the intracavitary position of the tip. In this regard, Zattoni has observed that the pressure within the pericardial space increases during diastole, whereas the pressure generated within the right ventricle clearly decreases during this time frame.[63]

Once the operator is convinced that the tip of the needle is within the pericardial space, the syringe should be removed and a 0.038-inch flexible J wire should be advanced within the pericardial space (Fig. 27–7A). A suitable catheter should then be installed over the guide wire (eg, by means of the Seldinger technique) to permit aspiration of the pericardial contents without exposing the patient to the risk of withdrawing the fluid with the use of the sharp needle (see Fig. 27–7B–D).[9,68] The selection of the most appropriate catheter to be installed at this juncture should be based on the anticipated period of time that pericardial drainage will require. If procedure is performed strictly for diagnostic purposes, I recommend the use of a 4 or 5 French linear endhole multipurpose catheter. Insertion of this type of catheter frequently does not require the use of a dilator. If the procedure is performed to evacuate fluid, a multifenestrated 6 to 8 French pigtail catheter is recommended (Fig. 27–8).[45,69] This catheter can be left in place for several days and permits chronic percutaneous access to the pericardial space. Indications for chronic pericardial drainage include large pericardial effusions, life-threatening effusions, recurrent effusions, and acute/traumatic effusions.[13,45] The pigtail configuration offers several advantages over the linear endhole configuration. First, the curvilinear design of the catheter renders it relatively

Inserting Sheath for Pericardiocentesis Catheter

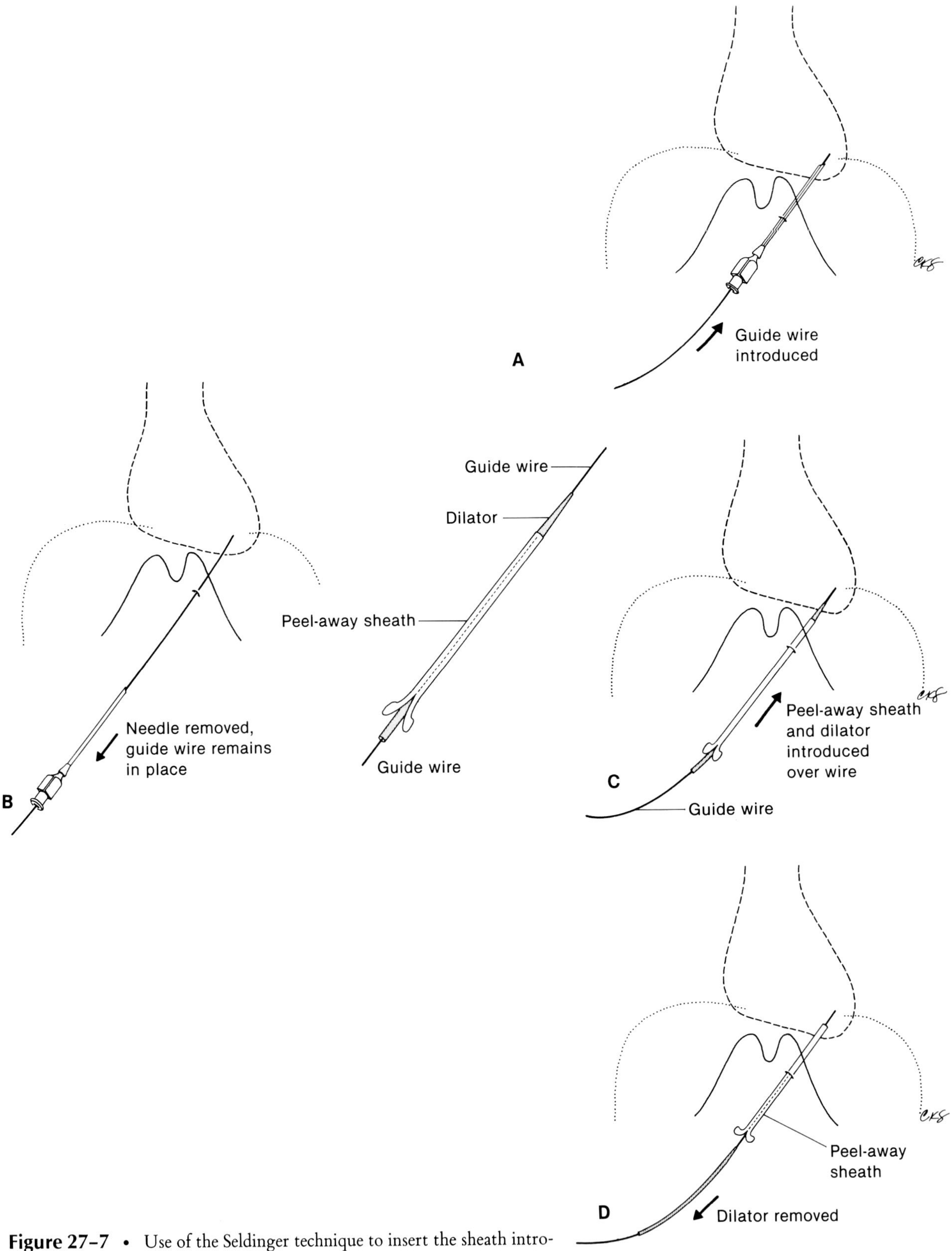

Figure 27–7 • Use of the Seldinger technique to insert the sheath introducer for the pericardiocentesis catheter. (***A***) The Seldinger technique involves the insertion of a guide wire. This approach circumvents the risk of aspirating the pericardial contents with a sharp needle. (***B***) The needle is removed. (***C***) The dilator and pacemaker peel-away sheath are introduced over the guide wire. (***D***) The dilator is removed.

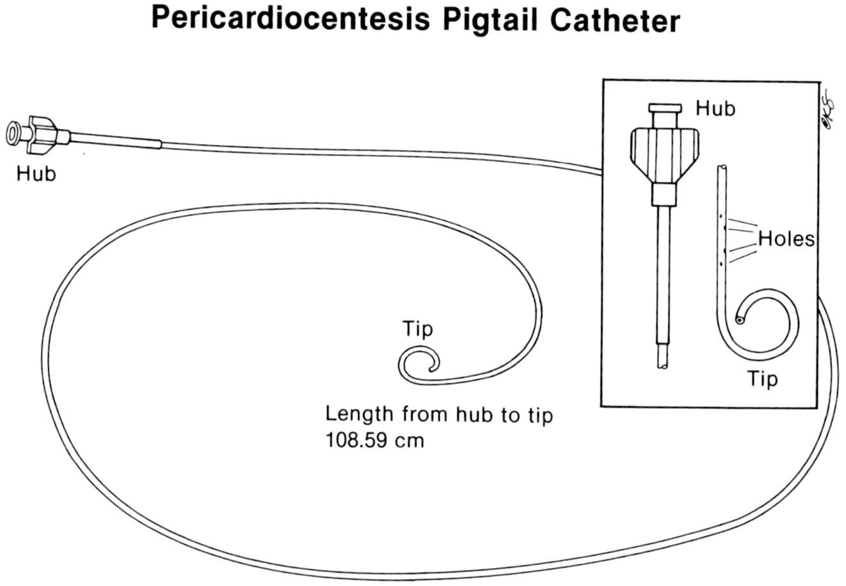

Figure 27–8 • The pericardiocentesis pigtail catheter has a curved nontraumatic end.

atraumatic. Moreover, the pigtail catheter tends to remain patent for longer periods of time than its linear endhole counterpart because it is multifenestrated along the medial and radial aspects of the pigtail curve. Most pigtail catheters tend to assume an orientation parallel to the surface of the pericardium, consequent with the process of removing pericardial fluid. The medial and radial distribution of catheter fenestrations tends to limit the incidence of obstruction created by direct apposition of the pericardial tissue planes onto the surface of the catheter.

Although it is feasible to simply introduce a pigtail catheter over a guide wire, following dilatation of the guide wire track with a standard dilator (see Fig. 27–7B–C), I have found that the uncurled pig-tail catheter tends to buckle when advanced in this manner. In addition, the nontapered distal aspect of the pigtail catheter tends to hang up on the various tissue planes during the process of advancing the catheter. For these reasons, I recommend the use of pacemaker peel-away sheath to accommodate a pigtail catheter in this circumstance (see Figs. 27–7C–D and 29–9).[70] This approach provides a channel for the catheter into the pericardial space that can be removed following introduction of the catheter. Once the catheter has been installed, the initial fluid withdrawn should be sent for cell count, culture (TB, fungal, and bacterial), and cytology. The latter sample should be sent in a heparinized container.

In addition to these general recommendations, it is often helpful to tailor the procedure to meet the needs of the particular patient. Among patients with hemodynamic instability secondary to tamponade physiology, the procedure must be performed emergently. For immunocompromised patients, meticulous antiseptic preparation of the anticipated incision site is recommended. Among patients with suspected chylous effusions, it is often helpful to use a large-bore needle or catheter to drain the relatively viscous fluid.[47,48] For patients with presumed tuberculous pericarditis, a pericardial biopsy in conjunction with the pericardiocentesis frequently enhances the diagnostic yield of the procedure, as previously indicated. Among debilitated patients with purulent pericardial effusions who are considered candidates for percutaneous pericardial drainage, a percutaneous drain should be installed during the course of the procedure. For patients with pyogenic pericarditis secondary to *Haemophilus influenzae,* Bennett has recommended the use of intrapericardial streptokinase infusions (via the pericardial drain) to expedite the evacuation process.[49] The pericardial fluid that accumulates in this circumstance tends to be particularly thick, and the infusion of streptokinase can effectively reduce the viscosity of this pericardial fluid. Bennett notes that streptokinase has been previously infused within intrapleural drains for similar purposes without provoking systemic bleeding complications.[50] Among patients with suspected effusive-constrictive pericarditis, it is frequently helpful to install a Swan-Ganz catheter at the outset and record the impact of the pericardiocentesis on the RA (right atrial), PCW (pulmonary capillary wedge), and RVEDP (right

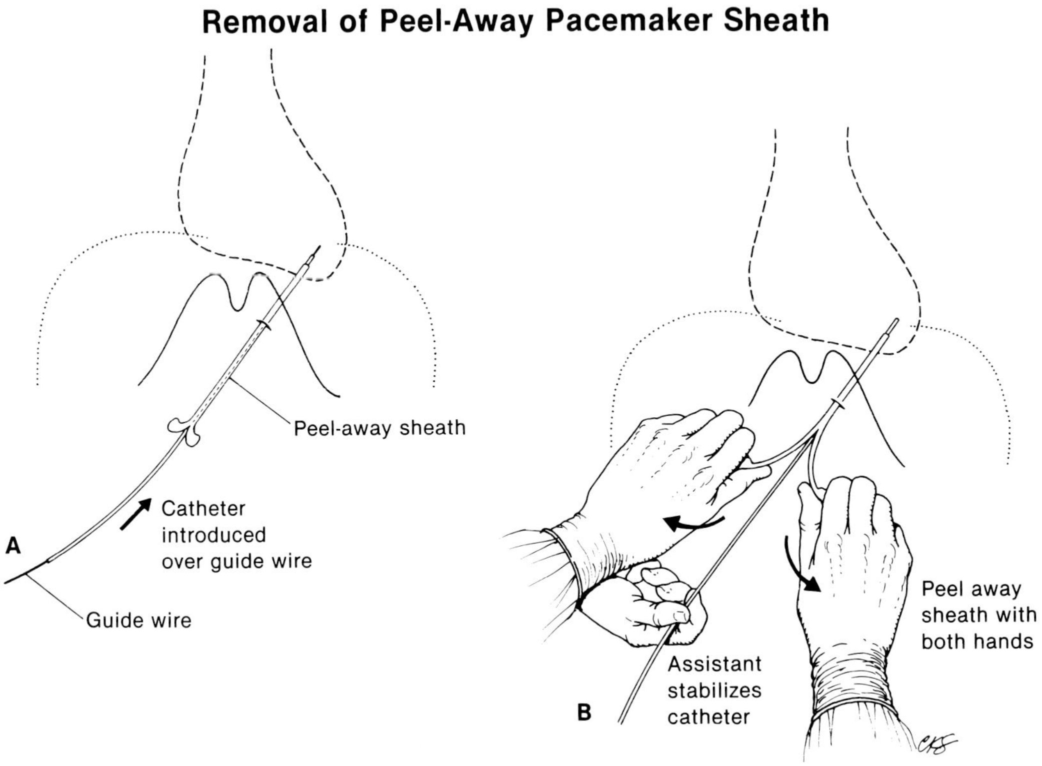

Figure 27–9 • Removal of the peel-away pacemaker sheath. Although conventional sheaths can be used in lieu of the peel-away variety, this approach permits the operator to discard the sheath (***B***) following insertion of the catheter into the pericardial space (***A***).

ventricular end-diastolic) pressure waveforms (Fig. 27–10). Typically, the aspiration of pericardial fluid from these patients results in the appearance of a sharp Y descent in these pressure waveforms. I recommend an American-Edwards (Irvine, CA) 7.5F Pace-Port Swan-Ganz catheter. This catheter contains a separate channel that terminates within the right ventricle and was designed to accommodate a pacing wire. However, this lumen can be attached to a pressure transducer, permitting the operator to monitor the RA, RVEDP, and PCW simultaneously. To evaluate the contour of the RA and PCW pressure curves, it is frequently helpful to use the 20 mmHg scale on the hemodynamic monitor.

Considerable preparation should precede a percutaneous pericardiocentesis among patients with presumed malignant pericardial effusions. The decision to perform this procedure should involve the cardiologist, the oncologist, and the thoracic surgeon.[14] Among individuals with suspected malignant pericardial effusions and no evidence of tamponade, it is generally preferable to perform the pericardiocentesis in the morning to preclude the need to store overnight the unprepared cells recovered during the course of the procedure. Among patients with a confirmed diagnosis who require therapeutic palliation, a decision should be made a priori concerning the need to perform tetracycline pericardial sclerosis. The performance of percutaneous tetracycline sclerosis has been found to be safe and effective.[52–54] In a series by Davis and associates, no late sequelae (eg, constriction) were detected among patients who had received this form of sclerosis.[54] The articles by Shepherd[53] and Smith[71] supply further details concerning this technique. The success of this procedure is directly related to the degree of fluid evacuation achieved.[52] Clearly, inadequate fluid evacuation will result in the suboptimal approximation of pericardial tissues and a suboptimal result.[52]

D. Postprocedure Maintenance of Pericardial Drainage Catheters

Left unattended, these catheters tend to become obstructed, and several suggestions on preventing this oc-

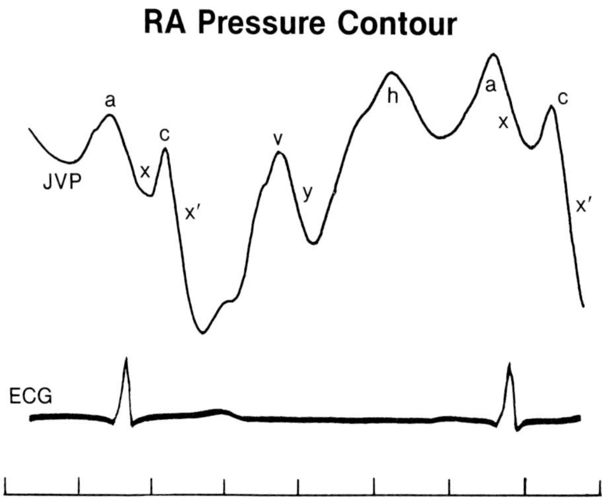

Figure 27–10 • Normal appearance of the right atrial (*CVP*) pressure contour indicating the appearance of the Y descent. The amplitude of the Y descent is frequently diminished among patients with tamponade and enhanced among patients with constriction.

currence have evolved. Lock has recommended that the operator cut several additional and relatively large-bore side holes into the distal shaft of the fenestrated pigtail catheter at the outset of the procedure.[69] Kopecky has recommended the practice of draining the pericardial space intermittently and infusing the drainage catheter with heparin when not in use.[45] In support of this approach, he cited a substantially reduced incidence of catheter obstruction with intermittent vs. continuous catheter drainage (2/9 vs. 1/33 obstructions). With respect to the latter recommendation, Patel has described an elegant system that permits continuous flush of the pericardial drain (Intraflo, Sorenson Research).[72]

IV. COMPLICATIONS

The incidence of complications related to percutaneous pericardiocentesis has clearly decreased over the past 20 years, due mainly to the advent of newer technologies that have dramatically contributed to the safety of this procedure.[40,41] Despite this progress, however, it should be remembered that when this procedure is performed blind, it is associated with a high and, by today's standards, unacceptable morbidity and mortality.[40,41] For this reason, every effort should be made to perform the procedure under optimal circumstances as described above.[5]

Despite the availability of fluoroscopy, echocardiography, and other such techniques, the incidence of complications related to percutaneous pericardiocentesis remains significant. The most common complications include perforation of the right ventricle, laceration of the right coronary artery, pneumothorarax, and infection of or trauma to the abdominal organs.[7,71] The right ventricular free wall tends to be a relatively thin structure, so perforation always remains an imminent possibility. This complication is generally well tolerated with the exception of patients managed on anticoagulants. Among this patient population, the risk of developing secondary hemopericardium remains significant. If perforation is suspected, the operator should let go of the needle whenever possible during evaluation of the depth of needle penetration. Efforts to stabilize the motion of a needle that has penetrated the right ventricular free wall can result in further laceration of this structure (the right ventricular tear can widen as the ventricle moves about an immobilized needle). As indicated previously, patients with small pericardial effusions or a history of previous bypass surgery are at increased risk for perforation of the right ventricle during this procedure.[6,15,16]

Although infrequent, laceration of the right coronary artery (RCA) remains the single most morbid complication related to this procedure. The right coronary artery lies within the right atrioventricular groove on the epicardial surface of the heart (Fig. 27–11). Thus it is particularly susceptible to penetration during the course of a percutaneous pericardiocentesis, performed via the subxiphosternal approach described earlier. The epicardial distribution of this vessel and its branches can allow perforation to occur without the development of an electrocardiographic current of injury. For these reasons, the use of fluoroscopy is strongly encouraged during percutaneous pericardiocentesis to identify the location of the AV groove and reduce the risk of inadvertent RCA penetration.

In conclusion, it must be recognized that the advent of new technology is largely responsible for the fact that percutaneous pericardiocentesis can be performed with an acceptable morbidity and mortality. Every effort should be made to take advantage of the added safety these technologies afford. Despite the data that have accrued to date concerning the morbidity of blind pericardiocentesis, some physicians still perform this procedure at the bedside. It is likely that the complications sustained as a result of this practice will continue to fuel the debate that currently persists concerning the relative merits of the percutaneous vs. surgical approach for

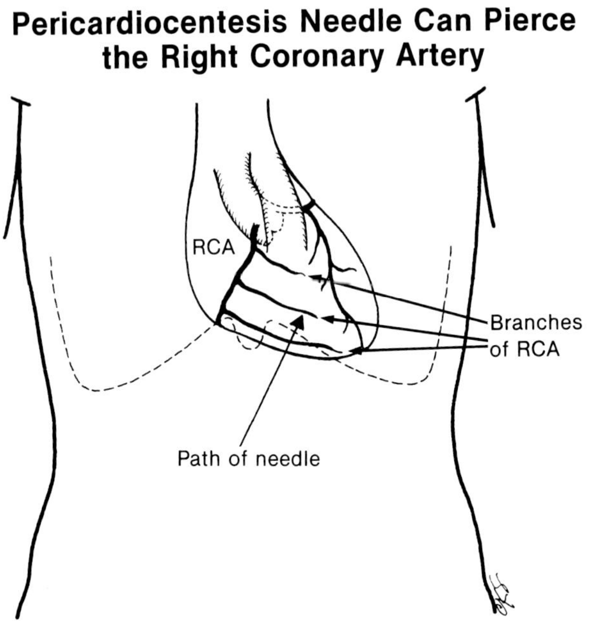

Figure 27–11 • Location of the right coronary (*RCA*) artery within the atrioventricular (*AV*) groove. Note that the acute marginal branches of the RCA course across the surface of the right ventricle and hence remain susceptible to laceration during the course of a percutaneous pericardiocentesis, despite the use of fluoroscopy and efforts to direct the needle away from the AV groove.

draining pericardial fluid. Properly performed among appropriate patient populations, percutaneous pericardiocentesis is a effective method for decompressing the pericardium and can be accomplished with relatively low morbidity and mortality.

V. References

1. Husson HM, Merat FV. Extrait d'un memoire de M. le docteur F. Romero, medecin de Catalogne, sur l'hydrothorax et l'hydropericarde; et du raport qui en a ete fait par MM Husson et Merat. Bull Fac Med Paris Soc Suc 4:373, 1815.
2. Shuh F. Erfahrungen uber die Paracentese der Brust und des Herzbeutels. Med Jahrb Osterr Staates Wien (neuste Folge 24) 33:388, 1841.
3. Singleton AO. Wounds of the heart and a discussion of the causes of death. Am J Surg 20:515, 1933.
4. Blalock A, Ravitch MM. A consideration of the nonoperative treatment of cardiac tamponade resulting from wounds of the heart. Surgery 14:157, 1943.
5. Krikorian JG, Hancock EW. Pericardioscentesis. Am J Med 65:808–814, 1978.
6. Wong B, Murphy J, Chang CJ, Hassenhein K, et al. The risk of pericardioscentesis. Am J Cardiol 44:1110–1114, 1979.
7. Becker RM. Management of pericardial effusion. Am J Cardiol 45:188, 1980.
8. Bishop LH Jr, Estes EH Jr, McIntosh HD. Electrocardiogram as safeguard in pericardioscentesis. JAMA 162:264–265, 1956.
9. Stewart JR, Gott VL. The use of a Seldinger wire technique for pericardioscentesis following cardiac surgery. Ann Thorac Surg 35:467–468, 1983.
10. Ekberg O, Nilsson PE, Aspelin P. Ultrasound guided percutaneous drainage of pericardial fluid with an indwelling catheter. Fortschr Rontgenstr 145:413–416, 1986.
11. Guberman BA, Fowler NO, Engel PJ, Gueron M, et al. Cardiac tamponade in medical patients. Circulation 3:633–639, 1981.
12. Klacsmann PG, Bulkley BH, Hutchins GM. The changed spectrum of purulent pericarditis: An 86 year autopsy experience in 200 patients. Am J Med 63:666–673, 1977.
13. Bouwels L, Jansen E, Janssen J, Cheriex E. Successful longterm catheter drainage in an immunocompromised patient with purulent pericarditis. Am J Med 83:581–583, 1987.
14. Markiewicz W, Borovick R, Ecker S. Cardiac tamponade in medical patients: Treatment and prognosis in echocardiographic era. Am Heart J 111:1138–1142, 1984.
15. Murphy JW, Wong B, Hassanein K. Identification of echocardiographic findings predicting the success of pericardioscentesis (abstr). Presented at the International Cardiovascular Congress II: Non-invasive Diagnosis. Phoenix, Arizona, February, 1979.
16. Engleman RM, Spencer FC, Reed GE, Tice DA. Cardiac tamponade following cardiac surgery. Circulation 41(Suppl II):165–171, 1969.
17. Press OW, Livingston R. Management of malignant pericardial effusion and tamponade. JAMA 257:1088–1092, 1987.
18. Thurber DL, Edwards JE, Achor RWP. Secondary malignant tumors of the pericardium. Circulation 26:228–241, 1962.
19. Rooney JJ, Crocco JA, Lyons HA. Tuberculous pericarditis. Ann Int Med 72:73–78, 1970.
20. Hancock EW. Cardiac tamponade. Med Clin North Am 63:223–237, 1979.
21. Evans JM, Walter CW, Hellems HK. Alterations in the circulation during cardiac tamponade due to pericardial effusion: An experimental study employing cardiac catheterization. Am Heart J 39:181–187, 1950.
22. Schepers GWH. Tuberculous pericarditis. Am J Cardiol. 9:248–276, 1962.
23. Antman E, Cargill V, Grossman W. Low-pressure cardiac tamponade. Ann Int Med 91:403–406, 1979.
24. D'Cruz IA. Echocardiographic simulation of pericardial effusion by ascites. Chest 85:93–95, 1984.
25. Rifkin RD, Isner JM, Carter BL, Bankoff MS. Combined posteroanterior subepicardial fat simulating the echocardiographic diagnosis of pericardial effusion. JACC 3:1333–1339, 1984.
26. Burchell HB. Problems in the recognition and treatment of pericarditis. Lancet 74:465–470, 1954.
27. Rasaretnam R, Chanmugam D. Subacute effusive constrictive epicarditis. Br Heart J 40:44–48, 1980.
28. Cooper DKC, Sturridge MF. Constrictive epicarditis following Coxsackie virus infection. Thorax 31:472–474, 1976.
29. Smith FE, Lane M, Hudgins PT. Conservative management of malignant pericardial effusion. Cancer 33:47–57, 1974.
30. Biran S, Brulnian G, Klein E, Hochman H. The management of pericardial effusion in cancer patients. Chest 71:182–186, 1977.
31. Yazdi HM, Hajdu SI, Melamed MR. Cytopathology of pericardial effusions. Acta Cytologica 24:401–412, 1980.
32. Jahn H, Kieny R. Management of pericardial heart disease in

uremia: Tap, drain, fenestration or pericardiectomy? Contr Nephrol (Basel) 33:197–209, 1982.
33. Fox HE, Yee JM, Weaver JC, Dugan DJ, et al. Pericardial drainage operations in the management of uremic pericarditis. J Thorac Cardiovasc Surg 73:504–510, 1977.
34. Morin JE, Hollomby D, Gonda A, Long R, et al. Management of uremic pericarditis: A report of 11 patients with cardiac tamponade and a review of the literature. Ann Thorac Surg 22:588–592, 1976.
35. Buselmeier TJ, Davin TD, Simmons RL, Najarian JS, et al. Treatment of intractable uremic pericardial effusion. JAMA 240:1358–1359, 1978.
36. Leehey DJ, Daugirdas JT, Ing TS. Early drainage of pericardial effusion in patients with dialysis pericarditis. Arch Int Med 143:1673–1675, 1983.
37. Daugirdas JT, Leehey DJ, Popli S, McCray GM, et al. Subxiphoid pericardiostomy for hemodialysis-associated pericardial effusion.
38. Quigg RJ, Idelson BA, Yoburn DC, Hymes JL, et al. Local steroids in dialysis-associated pericardial effusion. Arch Int Med 145:2249–2250, 1985.
39. Buselmeier TJ, Davin TD, Simmons RL, Hull AR. Trans Am Soc Artif Intern Organs 23:719–722, 1977.
40. Kotte JH, McGuire J. Pericardial paracentesis. Mod Concepts Cardiovasc Dis 20:102–103, 1951.
41. Kilpatric ZM, Chapman CB. On pericardioscentesis. Am J Cardiol 16:722–728, 1965.
42. Frsiedman MJ, Sahn DJ, Haber K. Two-dimensional echocardiography and B-mode ultrasonography for the diagnosis of loculated pericardial effusions. Circulation 60:1644–1649, 1979.
43. Weisse AB. Loculated pericardial effusion in acute pericarditis: Diagnosis by combined echocardiographic and radioisotopic techniques. Chest 76:113–115, 1979.
44. Kessler KM, Bilsker MS, Manasa M, Laignhold M, et al. Pericardial web: Extensive pericardial adhesions associated with idiopathic pericarditis. Am Heart J 111:602–603, 1986.
45. Kopecky SL, Callahan JA, Tajik AJ, Seward JB. Percutaneous pericardial catheter drainage: Report of 42 consecutive cases. Am J Cardiol 58:633–635, 1986.
46. Treasure T, Cotter L. Practical procedures: How to aspirate the pericardium. Br J Hosp Med 24:488–489, 1980.
47. Wilmshurst PT, Burnie JP, Turner PR. Chylopericardium, chylothorax, and hypobetalipoproteinaemia. Br Med J 293:483–484, 1986.
48. Torrington KG, Youkey JR. Simultaneous idiopathic chylopericardium and chylothorax. S Med J 74:357–359, 1981.
49. Bennet EV. Purulent pericarditis (letter). J Thorac Cardiovasc Surg 87:640–642, 1984.
50. Berglin E, Ekroth R, Teger-Nilsson AC, William-Olsson G. Intrapleural instillation of streptokinase. Effects on systemic fibrinolysis. Thorac Cardiovasc Surg 29:124–126, 1981.
51. Ortbals DW, Avioli LV. Tuberculous pericarditis. Arch Int Med 139:231–234, 1979.
52. Treatment of malignant pleural and pericardial effusions. Medical Letter 23:59–60, 1981.
53. Shepherd FA, Ginsberg JS, Evans WK, Scott JG, et al. Tetracycline sclerosis in the management of malignant pericardial effusion. J Clin Oncol 3:1678–1682, 1985.
54. Davis S, Rambotti P, Grigani F. Intrapericardial tetracycline sclerosis in the treatment of malignant pericardial effusion: An analysis of thirty-three cases. J Clin Oncol 2:631–636, 1984.
55. Gale ME, Kiwak MG, Gale DR. Pericardial fluid distribution: CT analysis. Radiology 162: 171–174, 1987.
56. Feigenbaum H. Echocardiography. Philadelphia, Lea & Febiger 1976, 419–437.
57. Weyman A. Cross-sectional echocardiography. Philadelphia, Lea & Febiger, 1982, 482–485.
58. Moss A. Gamsu G, Genant H. Computed Tomography of the Body. Philadelphia, WB Saunders, 1983, 414–421.
59. Naidich D, Zerhouni E, Siegelman S. Computed Tomography of the Thorax. New York, Raven, 1984, 275–278.
60. Singham KT. Percutaneous cannulation of large pericardial effusions. Cathet Cardiovasc Diagn 5:209–212, 1979.
61. MacAlpin RN. Percutaneous catheter pericardioscentesis. Eur Heart J 1:287–291, 1980.
62. Sobol SM, Thomas HM, Evans RW. Myocardial laceration not demonstrated by continuous electrocardiographic monitoring occurring during pericardioscentesis. N Engl J Med 292:1222–1223, 1975.
63. Zattoni J, Siani C, Perria B. Electromanometric confirmation of needle position in haemopericardium with severe tamponade. Br J Anaesth 53:1223–1225, 1981.
64. Balakrishnan S, Hartman CW, Grinnan GL, Bartel AG, et al. Pericardial fluid gas analysis in hemorrhagic pericardial tamponade. Ann Thorac Surg 27:55–58, 1979.
65. Kindig JR, Goodman MR. Clinical utility of pericardial fluid pH determination. Am J Med 75:1077–1079, 1983.
66. Hayward R, Treasure T, Swanton H, Emanuel R. Drainage of Neoplastic pericardial effusions. Lancet 1:1018–1019, 1983.
67. Chandraratna PAN, First J, Langevin E, O'Dell R. Echocardiographic contrast studies during pericardioscentesis. Ann Int Med 87:199–200, 1977.
68. Seldinger SI. Catheter replacement of the needle in percutaneous arteriography: A new technique. Acta Radiol 39:368–79, 1953.
69. Lock JE, Bass JL, Kulik TJ, Fuhrman BP. Chronic percutaneous pericardial drainage modified pigtail catheters in children. Am J Cardiol 53:1179–1182, 1984.
70. Jansen EW, Vincent JG, Fast JH, Tavilla G. Treatment of pericardial effusion. J Thorac Cardiovasc Surg 91:794–797, 1986.
71. Smith F, Luse M, Hudgins P. Conservative management of malignant pericardial effusion. Cancer 33:47–57, 1974.
72. Patel AK, Kosolcharoen PK, Nallasivan M, Kronke GM, et al. Catheter drainage of the pericardium: Practical method to maintain long-term patency. Chest 92:1018–1021, 1987.

Chapter 28

•

John W. Danforth, MD
Brigid Doyle Ide, MS, RN

Intraaortic Balloon Counterpulsation

OUTLINE

I. Introduction

The *intraaortic balloon counterpulsation pump* (IABCP) was originally developed to provide a means for mechanically minimizing and perhaps preventing the development of myocardial ischemia among individuals with critical coronary artery disease and hemodynamic instability. The pump was designed to simultaneously increase myocardial oxygen supply and decrease myocardial oxygen demand. The term *counterpulsation* refers to the process of decreasing the systolic blood pressure while increasing the diastolic blood pressure and is the principal mechanism of action of this device.[1] Despite the advent of considerable new technology, intraaortic balloon counterpulsation (IABC) remains the only available intervention capable of accomplishing these objectives simultaneously.[2]

A. History

The clinical potential of counterpulsation was first investigated by Clauss and coworkers in 1961.[1] These investigators accomplished counterpulsation by sequentially aspirating and injecting blood through the femoral artery during systole and distole. The first intraaortic counterpulsation balloon pump was designed, assembled, and subsequently tested by Moulopoulos and Topaz, while they were both working at the Cleveland Clinic.[3] At the time, Moulopoulos was a visiting cardiologist from Athens and Topaz was a graduate student at Purdue University. The device was first used clinically during the course of a resuscitation attempt involving a patient of Dr. Mason Sones.[4] Thereafter, the device was used only sporadically. No patient subjected to the insertion of this particular device survived.[4] In 1966, The Artificial Heart Program of the National Heart Institute began funding further development of a similar device. This effort culminated in the first successful clinical application of IABC in 1968.[5] Thereafter, interest in counterpulsation increased exponentially. In 1970, Mundth proposed the idea of using IABC to stabilize shock patients during surgery.[6] In 1973, Buckley reported the successful use of IABC among patients who could not be weaned from cardiopulmonary bypass, now the most common indication for counterpulsation.[7,8]

The past two decades have witnessed considerable improvement in the design of both the counterpulsation pump and balloon catheter, improvements that have contributed substantially to enhancing the risk–benefit profile of this intervention. A number of features have been added to the original counterpulsation pump, including failsafe electrocardiographic (ECG) trigger systems and automatic readjustment systems that compensate for changes in heart rate. Despite the fact that the current state-of-the-art pumps have become substantially more sophisticated, they are designed to be more user friendly than the first-generation models (Fig. 28–1).

A number of design modifications of the balloon catheter have been introduced over the past 20 years to facilitate the process of catheter introduction. Among these improvements are a dual lumen system that accommodates a guide wire (and thus permits the percutaneous introduction of the catheter), the use of reversible bonding on the surface of the balloon component (to permit the manufacture and distribution of these catheters in the prefolded configuration), and the development of lower profile catheters (Fig. 28–2).[10,11]. As a note of interest, some of the earlier balloons contained two segments. The distal segment was intended to partially obstruct the distal aorta, enhancing cerebral and coronary blood flow.[9] Although an intriguing concept, this design was subsequently abandoned in favor of a single-chamber system.

B. Mechanism of Action

As indicated previously, the IABCP simultaneously enhances myocardial oxygen supply and diminishes myocardial oxygen demand.[12-14] Both phenomena transpire in response to the sequential inflation and deflation of the balloon component of the catheter during the course of the cardiac cycle (Figs. 28–3 and 28–4). Abrupt deflation of the balloon during systole leads to a reduction in the systolic blood pressure,[17] systemic vascular resistance,[18,19] and left ventricular volume.[20-22] These responses, in turn, lead to a reduction in left ventricular wall stress and myocardial oxygen demand.[15] The principal determinants of myocardial oxygen demand include heart rate, systolic blood pressure, left ventricular contractility, and left ventricular volume.[15] Balloon pump-mediated reduction in myocardial oxygen demand has been observed in the open-chested dog[22-25] and in the awake pig with artificially induced coronary artery disease,[26] as well as among patients with hypotension or refractory angina.[27]

Datascope Intraaortic Balloon Pumps

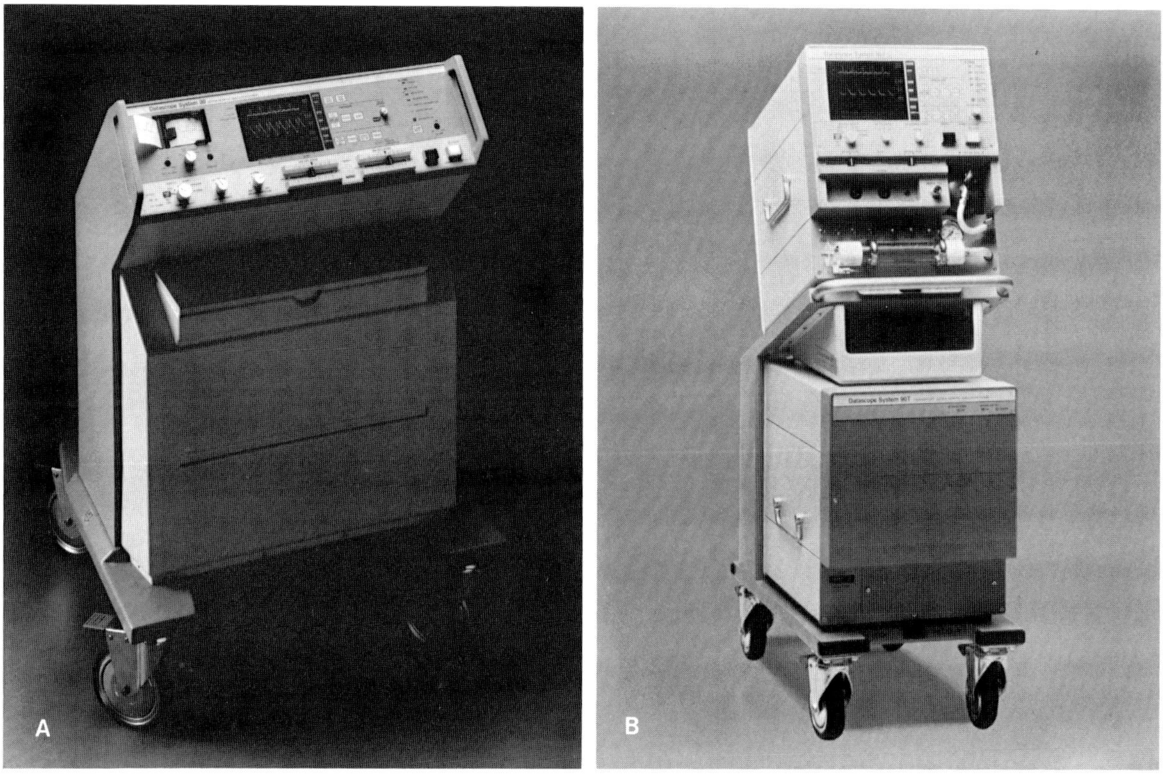

Figure 28–1 • (***A***) New Datascope System 90 intraaortic counterpulsation balloon pump (IACBP) that features simple, automatic operation. (***B***) New Datascope 90T transport intraaortic balloon pump.

Abrupt inflation of the counterpulsation balloon during diastole leads to a substantial increase in the systemic diastolic blood pressure.[28] It was originally assumed that this augmentation in diastolic blood pressure would invariably lead to enhanced coronary blood flow, myocardial perfusion, and hence improved myocardial oxygen supply. The principal determinants of myocardial oxygen supply were known to include the diastolic filling time, the coronary perfusion gradient (eg, the difference between the systemic diastolic pressure and the left ventricular end-diastolic pressure), and the integrity of the coronary vascular system.[16] Indeed, a number of investigators reported that counterpulsation augmented both regional coronary[14,29–36] and myocardial collateral[32,37–39] blood flow during the course of both clinical and animal laboratory studies. However, others did not observe similar results.[27,40] In a study by Leinbach and associates, for example, no increase in coronary blood flow was observed among individuals with severe coronary artery diseases following the institution of IABC.[27]

In retrospect, it is entirely conceivable that the disparity in coronary blood flow response to counterpulsation relates to the impact of the autoregulatory system on coronary artery blood flow.[41] Among normotensive individuals, the autoregulatory system governs coronary blood flow. This system functions to maintain adequate coronary blood flow over a wide range of alterations in both filling times and coronary perfusion gradients.[40] Myocardial oxygen demand constitutes the single most important factor affecting the autoregulatory system.[16] Among normotensive laboratory animals with an intact autoregulatory system, investigators have determined that the institution of IABC results in a reduction in coronary blood flow.[41] Presumably, this reduction in blood flow reflects the reduction in myocardial oxygen demand that frequently transpires following the institution of counterpulsation and the corresponding response of the autoregulatory system to this supply–demand imbalance.[29,40]

In the setting of cardiogenic shock, autoregulation has little impact on coronary blood flow because myocardial oxygen demand invariably exceeds oxygen supply.[42] Hence, myocardial blood flow becomes critically dependent on the coronary perfusion pressure gradient

Second Generation Datascope Catheter

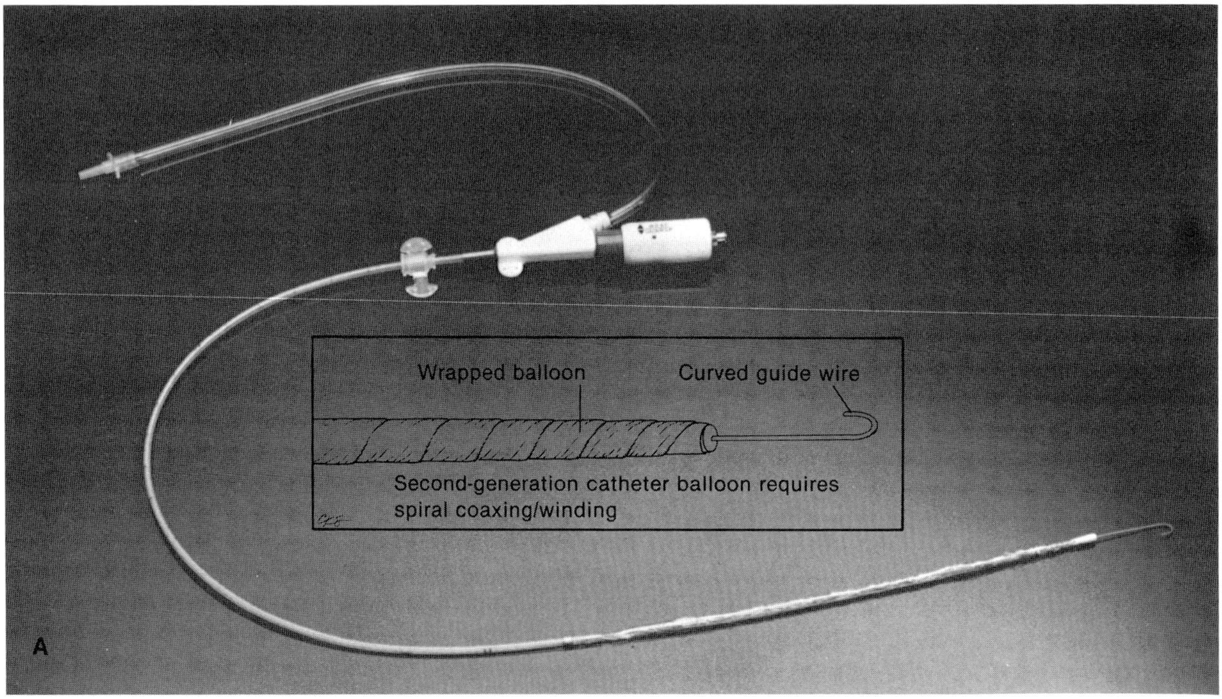

Rotary Device for Balloon

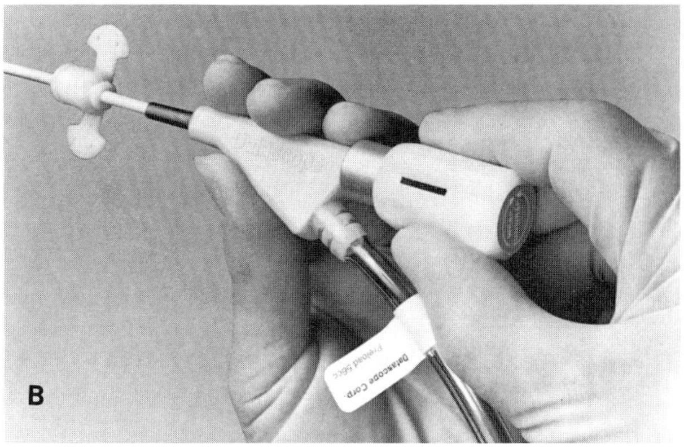

Figure 28–2 • (***A***) Second generation Datascope intraaortic balloon catheter with rotatable stylet. Preparation of this catheter requires coaxial rotation of the balloon around the stylet. (***B***) Closeup view of the rotational device that is continuous with the stylet in the balloon of the catheter shown in ***A***.

(continued)

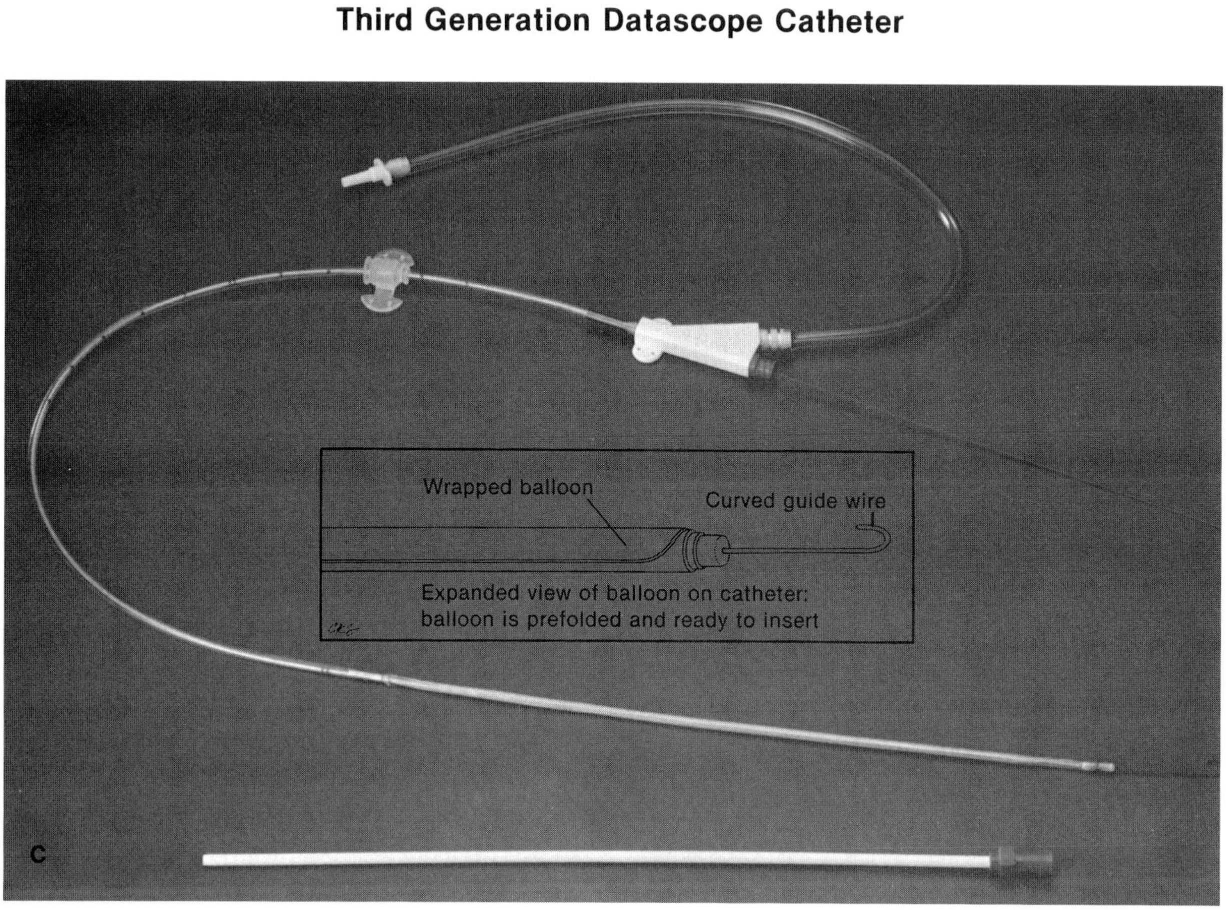

Figure 28–2 *(continued)*
(*C*) Third generation Datascope catheter and sheath. The balloon component of this catheter does not require preparation. It is folded longitudinally, and reversible bonding is used to maintain the low cross-sectional profile.

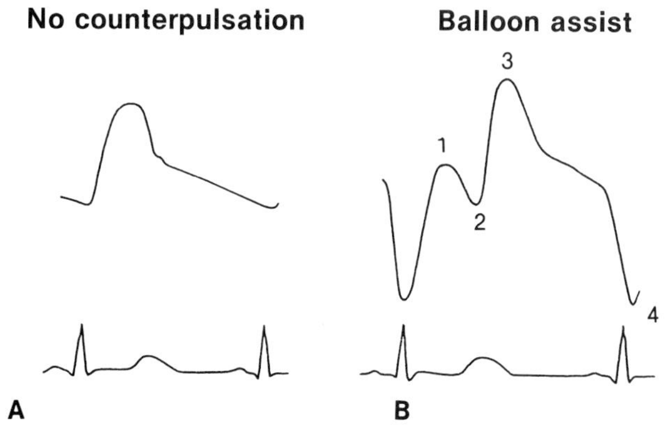

Figure 28–3 • Arterial pulse pressure waveform without counterpulsation (***A***) and with counterpulsation (***B***). 1 = assisted systole; 2 = point at which diastolic notch would appear; 3 = diastolic augmentation; 4 = assisted aortic end-idiostolic pressure. (Satler LF, Rackley CE. Assessment of adequate circulatory assist during intra-aortic balloon counterpulsation. Cardiovasc Clin 16: 141–149; with permission.)

(eg, the systemic diastolic pressure minus the left ventricular end-diastolic pressure).[40,43] In this circumstance, the institution of IABC has been shown to enhance coronary artery blood flow, and hence myocardial oxygen supply.[36] The increase in coronary blood flow that transpires following the institution of IABC among hypotensive patients and laboratory animals probably reflects the favorable impact of counterpulsation on both the systemic diastolic blood pressure and the left ventricular end-diastolic pressure, the two components of the coronary perfusion gradient.[12,28]

In the previously mentioned study by Leinbach and associates, in which no increase in coronary blood flow was found following the institution of IABC, the patients were normotensive.[27] Conversely, in the studies by Mueller[36] and others,[40] in which IABC was noted to provoke a significant increase in coronary blood flow, the patients were hypotensive.[36]

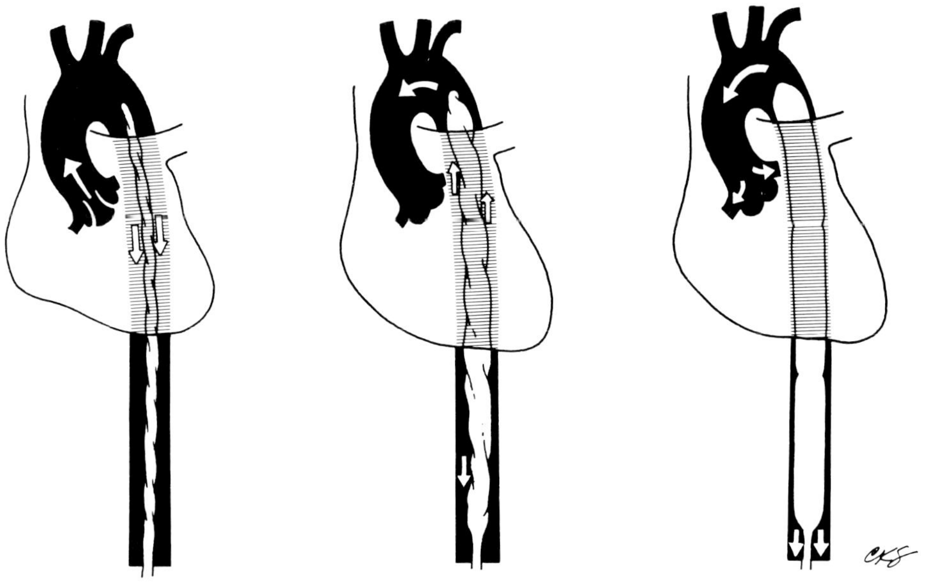

Figure 28–4 • Corresponding flow diagram indicating direction of blood flow with and without balloon inflation.

Under appropriate circumstances, IABC has been shown to do the following:

- Decrease left ventricular preload,[12,28] afterload,[17] and volume[20–22]
- Augment coronary blood flow[14,29–36] and collateral blood flow[32,37–39]
- Decrease myocardial lactate production[22]
- Improve ECG production[22]
- Improve ECG evidence of ischemia[20,44,45]
- Improve left ventricular contractile function[12,20,28,40]
- Reduce the frequency and intensity of anginal symptoms[44,45,47]
- Decrease the frequency of ventricular ectopy[48]
- Decrease the mortality among selected individuals requiring bypass surgery.[22,49–52]

For reasons that remain unclear, the beneficial effects of IABC tend to persist for 48 to 72 hours, and thereafter begin to taper among the majority of individuals.[18,53]

II. Indications

A. *General Considerations*

Considerable controversy persists concerning many of the indications for IABC. Although in theory counterpulsation offers several advantages over conservative therapy, the risks associated with this approach remain considerable and are frequently prohibitive. For example, counterpulsation is most effective among individuals with well-preserved left ventricular function. Hence it is reasonable to presume that counterpulsation pumps should prove beneficial when installed prophylactically in normotensive high-risk bypass surgery patients. Although this approach was originally recommended for such patients, advances in the delivery of general anesthetics, the delivery of cardioplegia, and the performance of bypass surgery have progressed to the extent that its risks outweigh its benefits among the majority of individuals.[9,28,49–53,54,55] Bolooki has reported that the incidence of preoperative prophylatic balloon pump insertion decreased from 12% in 1976 to 5% in 1983, and it is likely that this trend will continue.[28] Vijayanagar[54] and others[55] similarly have reported very favorable survival statistics among a series of patients with left main coronary artery disease who underwent bypass surgery with infrequent use of counterpulsation prophylaxis.

The advent of improved monitoring systems for use in the cardiac catheterization laboratory and of nonionic contrast agents has further decreased the need to stabilize patients with balloon pump counterpulsation prior to coronary arteriography and angioplasty. Despite the changes that have evolved and will inevitably continue to evolve concerning the indications for IABC, it is likely that two fundamental considerations will persist. First, each operator should weigh the relative risks and benefits of this intervention against the corresponding risks and benefits of the alternative therapeutic options before making the decision to proceed with counterpulsation. As technology improves, it is likely that the indications for counterpulsation will continue to diminish. Second, each operator should make every effort to reserve counterpulsation for patients who have a potentially reversible underlying disease process and at least moderately preserved left ventricular function. With respect to the latter consideration, it should be recognized that the beneficial impact of counterpulsation is largely contingent on the function of the left ventricle. The prognosis for the majority of candidates for counterpulsation is ultimately dependent on the reversibility of the underlying disease process. The IABC procedure is most effective among patients with moderate and reversible left ventricular dysfunction.[53] Conversely, it is not particularly effective among individuals with severe or irreversible ventricular dysfunction.[53] Okada and coworkers determined that counterpulsation offered no benefit among mongrel dogs with experimentally induced infarctions involving more than 50% of the muscle mass of the left ventricular free wall.[56] This is in large part explained by the fact that an intraaortic balloon pump by itself is incapable of generating forward blood flow.[57-59] Not surprisingly, the left ventricular stroke work index (LVSWI) has been reported to be the most important factor predicting survival among individuals requiring counterpulsation assistance.[53] Among individuals with an LVSWI >22 g $\cdot$m/m^2 and a pulmonary capillary wedge pressure (PCWP) <22 mmHg, survival generally exceeds 90%.

B. *Intraoperative and Postoperative Left Ventricular Failure*

The recent improvements in technology, cardioplegia, anesthetic delivery, and surgical techniques have decreased the morbidity and mortality of bypass surgery to the extent that the relative merits of counterpulsation have become difficult to predict.[8,9,54,60] As a result, many authorities have recommended that counterpulsation be reserved for those individuals who require this support intraoperatively, and that the use of preoperative prophylactic counterpulsation should be severely limited.[9,54,60]

Currently, 4% of bypass surgery patients require intraoperative IABC assistance, and inability to wean a patient from cardiopulmonary bypass currently constitutes the single most common indication for IABC.[8,53] In comparison to catecholamine therapy, which is the alternative to IABC in this circumstance, IABC augments cardiac function without aggravating myocardial oxygen demand.[9] Bolooki has proposed the following criteria for the emergent use of counterpulsation intraoperatively:

Definitive Criteria

1. Difficulty in weaning patient from cardiopulmonary bypass after 30 to 45 minutes (or three attempts) at low flow rates above 500 mL/min
2. Hypotension (<60 mmHg mean) and low cardiac index (<1.8 L/min/m^2) with high PCWP (>25 mmHg) despite pressor agents and afterload reduction
3. Continued postoperative use (if IABC was initiated before surgery).

Relative Indications

1. Requirement for large doses of pressor agents
2. Malignant dysrhythmia with evidence of intraoperative infarction not well controlled with drug therapy.[53]

Occasionally, IABC is required for patients who were successfully weaned from cardiopulmonary bypass and admitted to the intensive care unit, but who then required temporary left ventricular support.[9] Typically, it is the development of postoperative hypotension that presages the need to install an IABCP in this circumstance. Clearly, every effort should be made to rule out other common etiologies for hemodynamic compromise (eg, hypovolemia, tamponade, anemia, hypoventilation) including the insertion of a Swan-Ganz catheter and the like, before proceeding with counterpulsation in this patient population.

C. *Coronary Angioplasty Prophylaxis*

In contrast to the circumstance described above, prophylactic counterpulsation remains strongly recommended for selected individuals with either unstable angina or hemodynamic instability who are candidates for percutaneous transluminal coronary angioplasty.[61-63] Szatmary and coworkers have reported particularly favorable results following the use of combined counterpulsation and angioplasty among a population of patients with unstable angina.[64]

D. *Unstable Angina Refractory to Conventional Medical Therapy*

The large majority of patients with unstable angina will respond to conventional medical therapy. In this situation, the decision to install an IABCP should be reserved for those patients who have failed these measures. In general, approximately 2% of patients with unstable angina will require counterpulsation.[28] The majority of individuals with refractory angina (85% to 90%) will respond to this intervention.[65] Unlike antianginal therapy, counterpulsation does not compromise left ventricular function or provoke diastolic hypotension. For these reasons, counterpulsation constitutes a rational therapeutic option for patients with unstable angina and either critically depressed left ventricular function or hemodynamic instability.

E. *Postinfarction Left Ventricular Dysfunction and Shock*

Although one of the most common indications for counterpulsation, the effectiveness of IABC in this circumstance has been discouraging, particularly among those individuals who are not considered candidates for bypass surgery (Table 28–1). Cardiogenic shock constitutes the most common cause of death among hospitalized patients admitted with an acute myocardial infarction (MI).[66-68] The development of postinfarction cardiogenic shock generally reflects the loss of more than 40% of the left ventricular muscle mass.[69,70] According to Bolooki, approximately 3.8% of patients who present with an acute MI will require IABC.[28]

F. *Potential Impact on Infarct Size*

Despite these data, it is entirely conceivable that counterpulsation could be used to limit infarct size in humans. Roberts and colleagues have demonstrated that counterpulsation favorably influences infarct size among laboratory animals, if started within 3 hours following the onset of an experimentally induced infarction.[74] Other laboratory investigators have reported similar results.[45,75] Some encouraging clinical data exist as well. For example, Gutovitz and associates reported that CPK-MB blood levels remain elevated for a protracted period of time among individuals in shock, suggesting that myocardial necrosis continues to evolve among these individuals.[76] Leinbach and coworkers reported evidence of infarct size reduction among five patients who underwent counterpulsation within 6 hours following the onset of symptoms.[77] However, other studies in which counterpulsation was begun later in the course of the infarction have failed to reveal any benefit from the standpoint of infarct size reduction.[78-80]

In the case of acute MI, it is likely that counterpulsation functions to delay, rather than to prevent, the onset of necrosis. If this is the case, it suggests that IABC must be instituted before the onset of substantial myocardial necrosis and combined with bypass surgery, if it is to be used effectively to contain myocardial infarct size. Bolooki has reported that early intervention with IABC reduces infarct size among patients who present with an acute MI and undergo prompt surgical revascularization.[81] Similarly, DeWood and associates have reported that IABC and bypass surgery within 16 hours following the onset of chest pain resulted in a 34% (71.4% vs. 47.3%) reduction in long-term mortality among patients presenting in cardiogenic shock.[82] Of interest, the 5 patients who sustained a reduction in infarct size in the study by Leinbach and associates were ultimately determined to have sustained spontaneous coro-

Table 28–1 • In-hospital Mortality with Counterpulsation

Author	Year	Post-MI Shock (%)	Intraoperative Use (%)
Jackson[71]	1977	22	33
Watanabe[49]	1978		68
Forssell[72]	1979	33	
Tobias[2]	1979	19	26
Kafrouni[73]	1984	25	60
Goldberger[8]	1986	20	57.6

nary recannalization.[77] Among six other patients in this study who demonstrated persistent coronary occlusion, IABC did not influence infarct size.

G. *Rupture of the Left Ventricular Free Wall, Interventricular Septum, or Papillary Muscle*

Counterpulsation has been shown to be a life-saving procedure among patients who sustain infarct-related complications (eg, hypotension, dysrhythmias) resulting from rupture of the left ventricular free wall, the interventricular septum, and the papillary muscles.[9,83] In an autopsy study involving 1001 patients, approximately 4.7% of infarct victims sustained myocardial rupture.[84] Moreover, complications related to myocardial rupture account for approximately 10% of all in-patient deaths among patients admitted with an acute MI.[85] As a result, rupture constitutes the third most important etiology for postinfarction mortality.[86] Rupture generally develops during the course of the first 4 days postinfarction. It occurs more commonly among patients with a history of hypertension, and women tend to be at greater risk for this complication than men.[83] The most common clinical indications of rupture include the development of persistent chest pain, bradycardia, and hypotension.[83]

Although myocardial rupture carries a grave prognosis, counterpulsation has been used successfully to stabilize patients prior to surgical correction of this condition.

Rupture of the papillary muscle results in severe mitral regurgitation and pulmonary edema. In this circumstance, counterpulsation decreases left ventricular afterload and thus reduces the severity of the regurgitation. Rupture of the interventricular septum results in a left-to-right shunt with acute volume overload of the right ventricle, together with diminished left ventricular forward flow. In this circumstance, IABC has been shown to reduce left ventricular afterload, improve forward flow into the aorta, and diminish the severity of the shunt.[9,19] Goldberger and associates reported 80% survival among five patients who sustained rupture of the interventricular septum with the use of counterpulsation and timely surgical intervention.[8] Rupture of the free wall results in the accumulation of blood in the pericardial space and tamponade physiology. Although counterpulsation has been found to be useful in this circumstance as well, patient survival following the development of this disorder is critically dependent on early recognition of the condition and emergent decompression of the pericardial space.

H. *Refractory Ventricular Arrhythmias*

Among selected patients, counterpulsation has been shown to be effective in suppressing the development of presumed ischemically-mediated dysrhythmias.[53] Such dysrhythmias frequently prove refractory to conventional antiarrhythmic therapy. Hanson has reported improvement or resolution in the frequency of ventricular ectopy among 19 of 22 patients with the use of IABC.[48]

I. *Myocardial Contusion*

The literature contains several case reports that describe the use of counterpulsation in the treatment of patients who develop partially reversible left ventricular dysfunction and hemodynamic compromise following blunt cardiac injury.[87-89] Although the mechanism is currently unclear, Orlando and coworkers have proposed that counterpulsation might enhance left ventricular endocardial perfusion and improve right ventricular performance in this circumstance.[87] Transient right ventricular dysfunction is a well-recognized complication of blunt trauma to the chest. There is considerable speculation that redistribution of myocardial blood flow with secondary endocardial hypoperfusion commonly develops following myocardial contusion.[87]

J. *Septic Shock*

The role of counterpulsation in the treatment of septic shock remains particularly controversial.[90] Few would argue that the insertion of an IABC in septic patients carries a substantial risk. Nonetheless, some data suggest that counterpulsation could be beneficial for selected individuals with septic shock and congestive heart failure (CHF). The mortality among individuals with both CHF and septic shock approaches 100%, whereas the mortality for septic shock alone ranges between 50% and 80%.[90-92] For these reasons, IABC has been recommended for the treatment of individuals with septic shock and a low output state.[90,93]

K. Miscellaneous

Additional indications for counterpulsation include drug overdoses with profound myocardial depression, severe anaphylaxis, and aortic stenosis.[94,95] In the case of aortic stenosis and hemodynamic compromise, counterpulsation should only be considered among patients who are candidates for surgical repair. Because of the outflow tract obstruction created by the stenotic valve, IABC among these individuals enhances perfusion without affecting afterload.[95]

L. Contraindications

The primary contraindications for IABC include moderate to severe aortic valvular insufficiency and aortic dissection.

III. The Intraaortic Balloon Counterpulsation Procedure

A. Patient Selection

Because of the morbidity associated with the insertion of an IABCP, the physician must make every reasonable effort to gain as much information as possible concerning the reversibility of the patient's condition and the patient's potential for subsequent bypass surgery before committing to the procedure. Among patients in shock, IABC by itself does not confer a reduction in mortality.[8,79,82,96] Conversely, emergent counterpulsation and timely bypass surgery have resulted in a very favorable impact on mortality among these individuals (Table 28–2).[73,81,97,98]

For these reasons, we recommend performing both a right and a left heart catheterization among patients under consideration for counterpulsation to confirm the individual's cardiac function and to assess his or her potential for revascularization before proceeding with the insertion of an intraaortic counterpulsation catheter.

Because it is advisable to use fluoroscopy during insertion of the counterpulsation balloon catheter and it is frequently necessary to assess the coronary anatomy of a patient under consideration for counterpulsation, we have become accustomed to performing both procedures sequentially, through the same arteriotomy, in the cardiac catheterization laboratory. Among particularly unstable patients, the latter objective can frequently be accomplished by simply injecting a single dose of nonionic contrast media within the left main coronary artery and recording the run-off in the right anterior oblique (RAO) 30° projection at the start of the procedure. If the patient's distal anatomy appears amenable to engraftment, further views can be obtained once the balloon pump has been installed and the patient has been stabilized.

In addition to coronary arteriography, it is frequently advantageous to obtain a distal aortogram among patients under consideration for counterpulsation.[99–102] The incidence of complications sustained during insertion of a counterpulsation balloon catheter is directly related to the severity of the atheromatous disease contained within the peripheral vasculature.[103,104] In a survey of 794 patients who underwent IABC at Massachusetts General Hospital, Perler observed that virtually all the complications attributed to counterpulsation were sustained among individuals with severe peripheral

Table 28–2 • Survival with and without Bypass Surgery for Patients who Undergo IABC in the Setting of Cardiogenic Shock

Author	Year	Without Bypass Surgery (Medical) (%)	With Bypass Surgery (Surgical) (%)
Resnekov[97]	1977	12.5	88
DeWood[82]	1980	28.6**	52.7**
Kafrouni[73]	1984	25	52
Alcan[98]	1984	26	83

**Refers to long-term mortality.

vascular disease.[102] Furthermore, peripheral vascular disease occurs commonly among patients who are candidates for counterpulsation,[105] and it is frequently clinically silent. In the angiographic study of Bahn and associates, 44% of the candidates for IABC were found to have evidence of either tortuous vessels, lumenal stenoses, or projecting atheroma.[105] Peripheral vascular disease was not suspected at the time of the procedure among three fourths of the patients who sustained complications in the study by Perler.[102]

B. *Preoperative Evaluation*

All pertinent laboratory values should be reviewed before any patient is transferred to the procedure room or cardiac catheterization laboratory to undergo insertion of an intraaortic balloon catheter. The arteriotomy created during this procedure must be sufficient to accommodate an 11 French sheath (measuring approximately 4 mm in diameter), so failure to recognize the presence of an underlying condition (eg, coagulopathy) could have grave clinical consequences.

C. *Percutaneous vs. Surgical Approach*

The femoral approach (using the Seldinger technique) to the percutaneous insertion of a prewrapped 10.5 French intraaortic balloon catheter within the aorta will be described below. Although IABC has been clinically available since the late 1960s, percutaneous insertion of the counterpulsation balloon catheter was not feasible before the advent of the current generation of over-the-wire systems in 1982. Previously, it was necessary to surgically install the catheter. The surgical approach required exposing the femoral artery and engrafting a conduit onto the vessel to accommodate the catheter (Fig. 28–5). According to Goldberger and associates the suc-

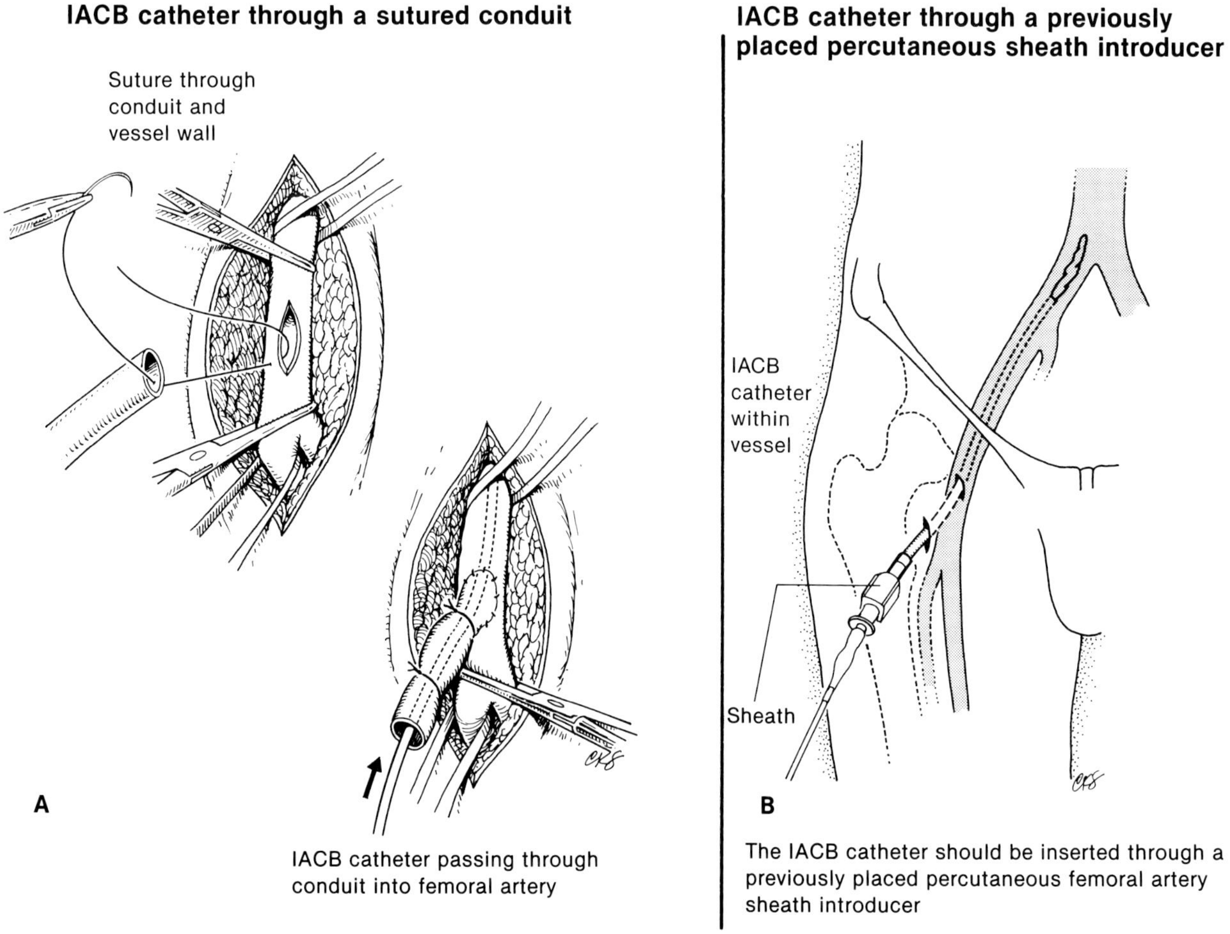

Figure 28–5 • (*A*) Surgical technique vs. percutaneous technique (*B*) for the insertion of a IACB catheter. Note that the surgical technique requires the construction of a conduit.

cess rate of the percutaneous and surgical methods is approximately the same (eg, 98% for the percutaneous approach vs. 97.3% for the surgical approach).[8] Despite this similarity, it is not presently clear which method carries the greater morbidity, and there is considerable discrepancy in the literature on this point. Some authors have reported an increased incidence of complications following the percutaneous approach.[8,35,106,107] Others have reported an increased incidence of complications following the surgical approach.[108,109] Finally, several reports indicate a similar incidence of complications following both approaches.[110,111] However, it appears that the percutaneous approach is less likely to lead to an infection[109] and that the surgical approach is preferable for patients with severe peripheral vascular disease, femoral grafts, or high femoral bifurcations.[100]

D. Technique for Catheter Insertion

The procedure should be performed either in a procedure room, cardiac catheterization laboratory or radiology suite where fluoroscopy is available.[104] Although it is possible to advance an intraaortic counterpulsation balloon catheter retrograde within the aorta without the aid of fluoroscopy under emergent circumstances, the morbidity of the procedure is sufficient to warrant the use of fluoroscopy in the majority of cases.

Before preparing and draping the patient, both femoral regions should be reexamined to assess clinically the relative patency of both vessels. Frequently, the firm procedure table provides better support for this aspect of the physical examination than a hospital mattress and permits a more careful evaluation. Once the examination is completed, the inguinal area least suspected of vascular obstruction should be prepped and draped in accordance with usual cardiac catheterization techniques. During this aspect of the procedure, it is frequently helpful to review the contents of the catheterization kit to determine that it contains all of the critical components and to prepare the counterpulsation balloon catheter for introduction according to the instructions provided with the device. We prefer to use the prewrapped 10.5 French 40-mL Dacor balloon catheter. This device does not require preparation (eg, evacuation, wrapping), and the surface of the wrapped balloon is considerably more lubricated than conventional balloon catheters that must be introduced with the balloon component wrapped in a spiral configuration (see Fig. 28–2).

Following the administration of local anesthesia (using approximately 6–10 mL of 1% lidocaine without epinephrine), an incision should be made in the skin, directly superficial to the pulse of the femoral artery and preferably several centimeters (ie, 1–3 cm) below the inguinal ligament. The incision should be of sufficient length (ie, 0.5 cm) to accommodate the femoral sheath. Access below the inguinal ligament reduces the risk of entering the superficial femoral artery (Fig. 28–6). According to Todd and coworkers, the smaller superficial femoral vessel is more prone to develop thrombosis and require thrombectomy when cannulated than is the common femoral vessel.[112]

Every effort should be made to enter the femoral artery in the center of the vessel. Misalignment of the needle enhances the risk of lacerating the vessel during the course of the procedure.[113] To locate the center of the femoral artery, it is frequently helpful to place the first and second fingers of one hand firmly on either side of the pulse, and aim between them with an 18 gauge intravenous catheter as illustrated in Fig. 28–7. The needle should be advanced swiftly through the vessel, with moderate cephalad angulation. Note that the axis of the needle in the frontal plane parallels the axis of the leg. The common femoral artery bifurcates at the level of the umbilicus and assumes a cephalocaudal course at the level of the inguinal ligament (see Fig. 28–6). Note that the bevel of the needle should be angled cephalad as well, for reasons illustrated in Fig. 28–8.

Following insertion of the needle, the stylet should be removed. If the vessel has been penetrated properly, removal of the stylet should not result in backbleeding. At this juncture, the needle should be slowly withdrawn until vigorous pulsatile backbleeding is observed (see Fig. 28–8A). It is frequently helpful to place the third finger of the hand controlling the needle on the skin of the patient and use the thumb and forefinger to withdraw the needle with a gentle twisting motion. Figure 28–9 shows this withdrawal motion but after the guide wire has been inserted. This approach provides some stability during the process of removing the needle, minimizes the need to use excessive force, and finally, permits the completion of this aspect of the procedure with one hand.

Once sufficient backbleeding occurs, a 0.038-inch (0.097-cm), full-length (140-cm) J wire should be advanced within the needle, cephalad to the level of the diaphragm, under fluoroscopic control according to the standard Seldinger technique (see Fig. 28–8B). The wire should not be forced against resistance under any circumstance. In the event that the backbleeding obtained is not brisk, it is sometimes helpful to readjust the angle of the needle so that it is more coaxial with the vessel.

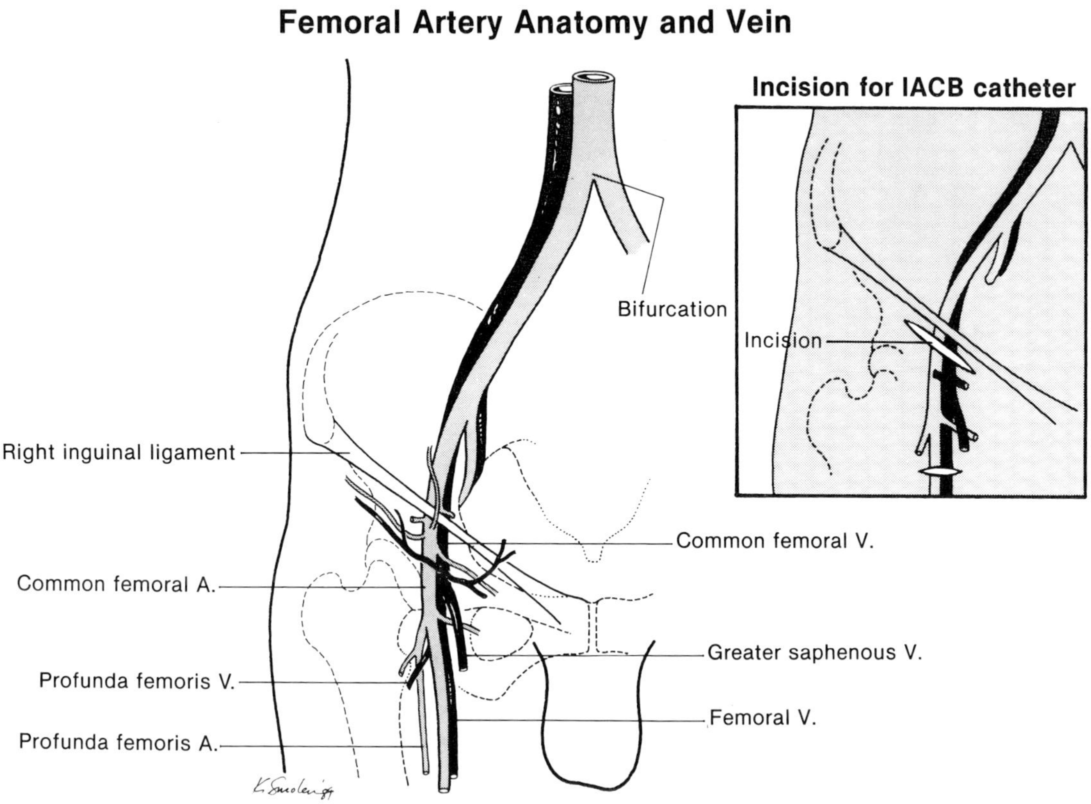

Figure 28–6 • Anterior view of the arterial circulation to the leg at the level of the inguinal ligament. Note the location of the superficial femoral branch. The inset shows the locations of the incision for intraaortic bottom insertion by the femoral route.

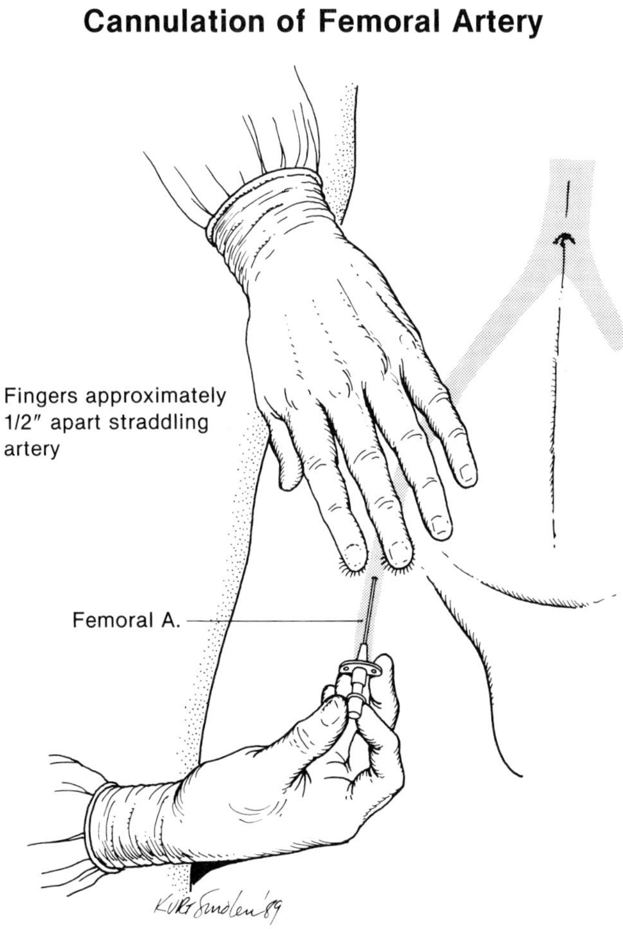

Figure 28–7 • It is frequently helpful to straddle the pulse with two fingers when attempting to locate the femoral artery. The axis of the needle is parallel to the long axis of the leg.

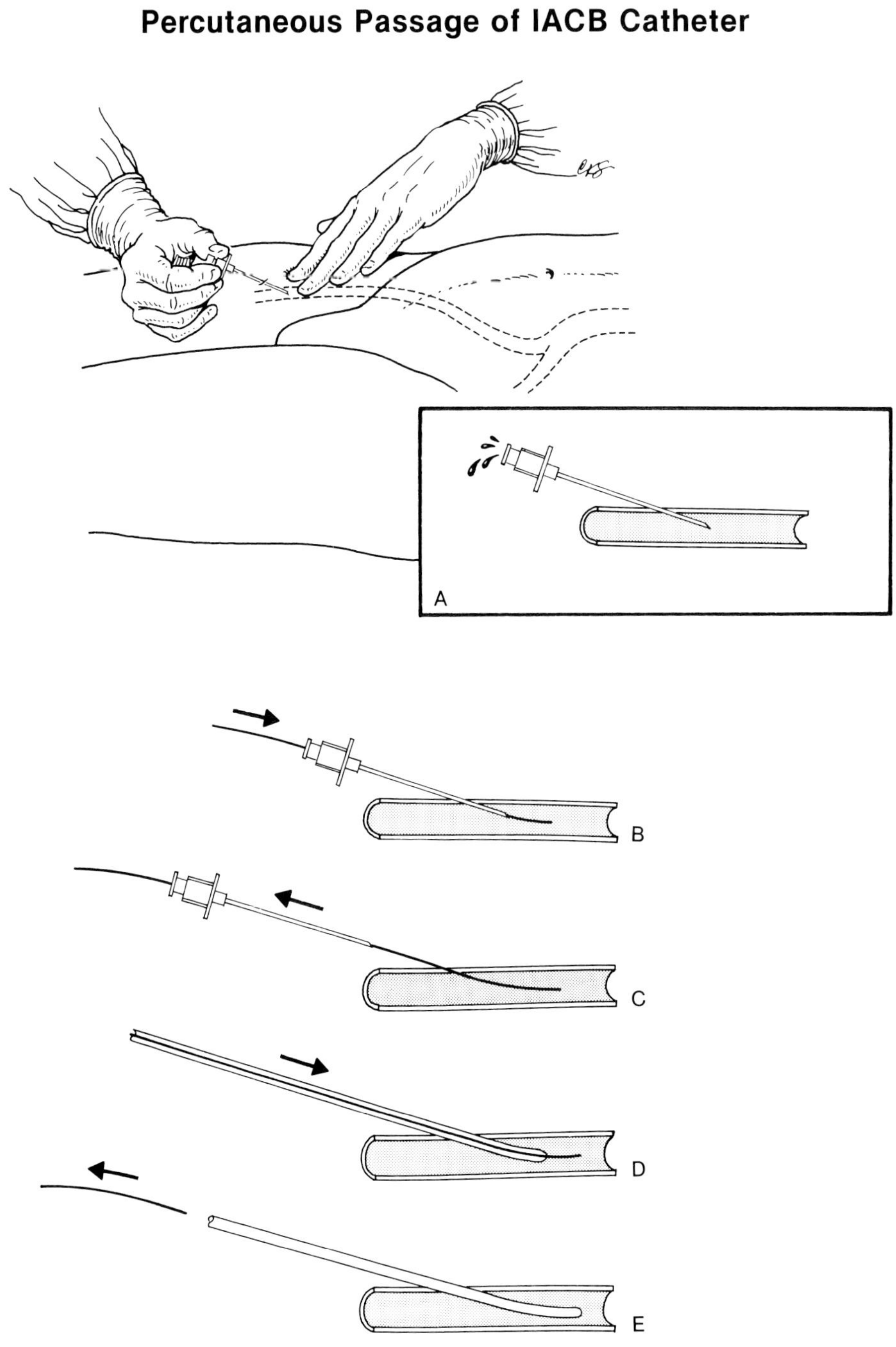

Figure 28–8 • Seldinger technique. (***A***) Insertion of the needle into the artery. The bevel of the needle should be angled cephalad. (***B***) Insertion of guide wire into needle. (***C***) Removal of needle over guide wire. (***D***) Insertion of femoral sheath over guide wire. (***E***) Removal of guide wire.

Following removal of the needle over the guide wire (see Fig. 28–8C), dilate the arteriotomy created so it will accommodate the 11 French sheath (see Fig. 28–8D). A 7 French catheter is available for pediatric use. The dilatation is generally accomplished by using two dilators of progressively larger size (an 8 French and a 10 French) in sequence. Hemostasis is best achieved during the dilator exchange process by applying firm pressure above and below the incision site (Fig. 28–10). Note that pressure should be applied sufficiently cepha-

Removal of Needle Over Guide Wire

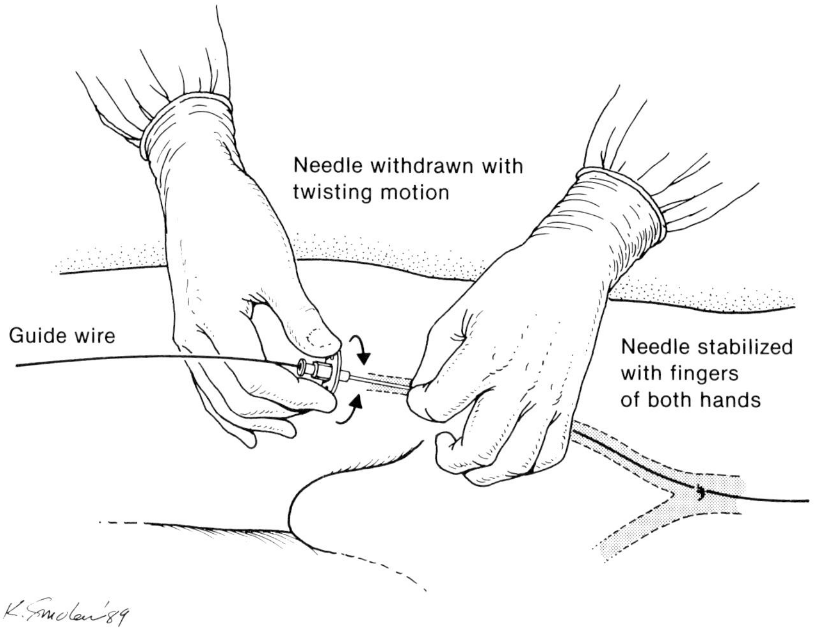

Figure 28–9 • Technique for removing the Seldinger needle. Note that two hands are used to stabilize the needle and that withdrawal of the needle is accomplished with a twisting motion.

Digital Pressure on Femoral Artery

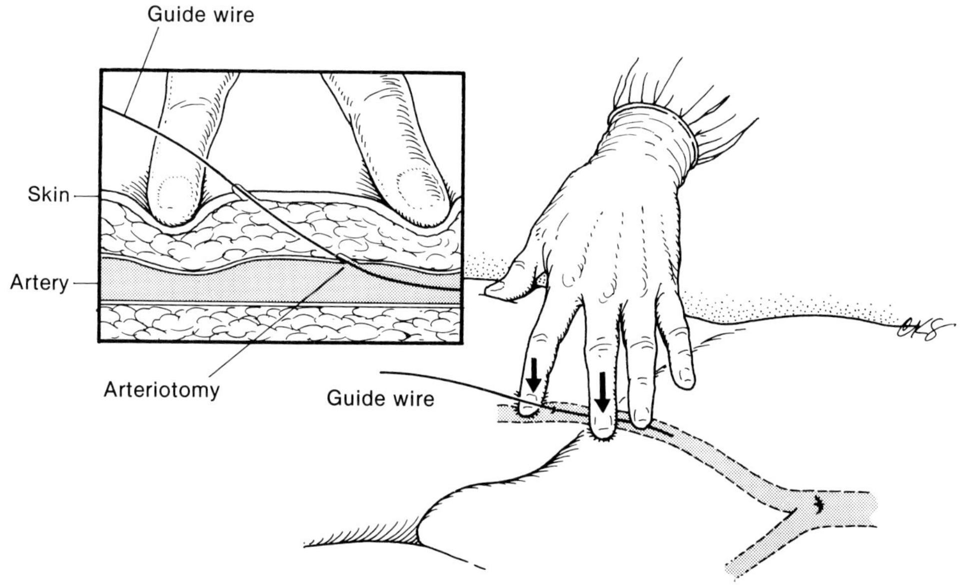

Figure 29–10 • To achieve adequate hemostasis following removal of the Seldinger needle, apply pressure to the femoral artery both above and below the incision site. Because the level of the arteriotomy is frequently cephalad to the level of the skin incision, it is often necessary to apply pressure with the fingers spread relatively wide apart, so that the pressure applied encompasses both the incision site and the arteriotomy.

lad during this aspect of the procedure to encompass the arteriotomy site. Not infrequently, a hematoma will develop following removal of the first dilator, because an unobstructed 8 French arteriotomy has been created, and the operator has applied pressure at the level of the skin incision and hence caudal to the level of the arteriotomy itself. Frequently, the 11 French dilator and sheath can be introduced at one time (see Fig. 28–8D). Among patients with tortuous vessels, a longer sheath can be used (eg, 45 cm) to expedite the process of introducing the balloon catheter and to minimize the potential for intraarterial trauma.[114]

Although standard practice involves removing both the guide wire and dilator at this juncture (see Fig. 28–8E), using the thumb of one hand to cover the end of the sheath to obtain hemostasis, it is preferable to remove only the dilator, leaving the guide wire within the aorta, and to use a hemostat to prevent backbleeding (Figs. 28–11 and 28–12). Rubber tubing is inserted over the ends of the hemostat to minimize the potential for traumatizing the sheath during this aspect of the procedure. This approach eliminates the need to reengage the aorta with a guide wire, provides superior hemostasis, permits the operator to use both hands to advance the counterpulsation balloon catheter over the extracorporeal aspect of the guide wire, and minimizes the risk of blood loss during insertion of the catheter with in the lumen of the intraarterial sheath. With regard to the latter advantage, the conventional approach requires the operator to remove his or her thumb *before* the catheter tip can be installed within the lumen of the sheath. Since the sheath contains a relatively large bore and communicates directly with the aorta, considerable blood loss can occur during this process, regardless of the proficiency of the operator. (It should be further recognized that the backbleeding often obscures the orifice of the sheath.) Conversely, the use of a hemostat permits the operator to introduce the tip of the counterpulsation balloon catheter within the lumen of the sheath before backbleeding occurs. Once the hemostat is removed, the catheter itself functions to impede blood loss. One of the authors has used this approach on many occasions and has never observed the development of significant trauma to the sheath as a result of this approach.

Once introduced over the guide wire and into the sheath, the catheter should be advanced under fluoroscopic control to within 4 cm of the origin of the left subclavian artery.[65] Introduction of the catheter beyond this point has been reported to provoke dissection of the aorta. The current consensus is that trauma generated by the repeated impaction of the tip of the linear catheter against the curvilinear lumenal surface of the aortic arch

Removal of Dilator from Femoral Artery Sheath

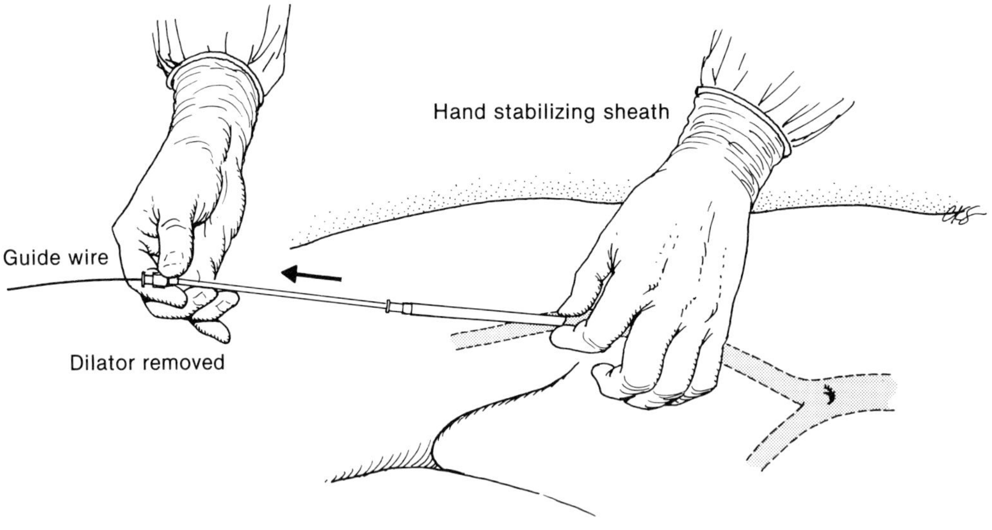

Figure 28–11 • Removal of the dilator following insertion of the 11.5 F femoral sheath. Depending on the technique preferred by the operator, the guide wire may or may not be removed at this juncture (see Figs. 28–12 and 28–13).

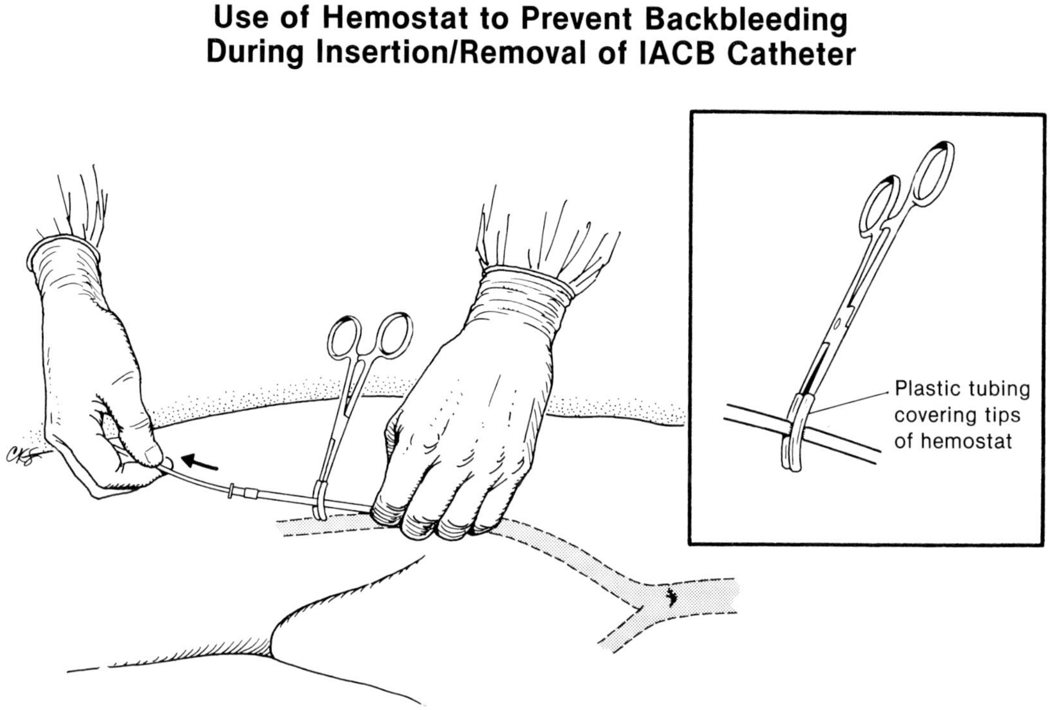

Figure 28–12 • Instead of using one's thumb to cover the hub of the sheath and provide hemostasis, backbleeding can be prevented by clamping the sheath with a hemostat. The tips of the hemostat must be covered if this approach is to be used. Segments of IV tubing are particularly suitable for this purpose.

during the course of each balloon inflation underscores the development of dissection under this circumstance.[115]

If the procedure must be performed without the aid of fluoroscopy, one can estimate the length of catheter to be inserted by simply placing the prepared catheter on the draped patient so that the proximal tip lies adjacent to the angle of Louis, with the distal end adjacent to the femoral sheath, and marking the sheath accordingly.[108] Once installed in this manner, the position of the catheter subsequently can be confirmed by means of a chest radiograph (see below).

Once the catheter has been advanced to the desired level within the aorta, the sheath should be partially withdrawn. Thereafter, the movable plastic cap, encompassing the catheter shaft, should be advanced along the length of the catheter and secured to the distal aspect of the sheath to create a hemostatic interface between the catheter and the sheath.

Following introduction of the catheter, the patient should be started on heparin, administered by continuous intravenous infusion in sufficient quantity to achieve full anticoagulation. Subramanian has also recommended the use of prophylactic low-molecular-weight dextran, and Bregman has recommended the administration of prophylactic cimetidine to patients who require counterpulsation.[10,108]

E. *Adjustment of The Balloon Inflation–Deflation Cycle*

The inflation–deflation cycle of the balloon should be adjusted so that the balloon inflates at the beginning of diastole and deflates before the onset of systole. Most balloon pumps are designed to be triggered by the electrochardiographic R-wave signal. However, the timing of the inflation can be adjusted with reference to either the ECG or the arterial pulse pressure waveform. We believe that, in general, the use of the arterial pulse pressure waveform is preferable for adjustment of the pump function. It has been our practice to install a radial arterial catheter to monitor pulse pressure among patients requiring counterpulsation. Although the balloon catheter itself contains a lumen that can be used for this purpose, it has been our experience that thrombus formation frequently accumulates within this channel among the majority of patients with prolonged use.

When adjusting the pump function with the use of the pulse pressure profile, the inflation trigger should be adjusted to coincide with the dicrotic notch, which reflects closure of the aortic valve and the beginning of diastole (Fig. 28–13). Earlier inflation increases the left ventricular afterload, potentially provokes early closure of the aortic valve, aggravates aortic regurgitation, and compromises diastolic augmentation (Fig. 28–14).[57] Later inflation invariably offsets the duration of balloon inflation and thus compromises the function of the pump (Fig. 28–15).

The deflation signal should be adjusted, following adjustment of the inflation signal, to maximize the diastolic augmentation (reflected by the amplitude of the diastolic pressure recording) and to minimize the left ventricular afterload (reflected by the nadir of the diastolic trough created by the counterpulsation) (see Fig. 28–13). For most practical purposes, both of these objectives can be accomplished by adjusting the deflation signal cursor to maximize the depth of the diastolic trough.[57] The contour of the trough is a function of both the patient's underlying pulse pressure and the impact of counterpulsation. *Early deflation* limits the balloon inflation time, compromises the function of the pump, and adversely affects the degree of afterload achieved. This circumstance, in turn, results in the generation of a suboptimal diastolic trough (Fig. 28–16). Conversely, *delayed deflation* compromises the time interval between the completion of balloon deflation and the onset of systole, and thus limits the time available for afterload reduction (Fig. 28–17). This results in the generation of a suboptimal trough as well. For these reasons, optimal adjustment of balloon deflation can frequently be achieved, for all practical purposes, by adjusting the deflation cursor with the aim of maximizing the trough generated with counterpulsation. Further suggestions concerning the proper adjustment of the pump can be found under "Troubleshooting Counterpulsation Pump Malfunction."

F. Postinsertion Management of the Catheter and Pump Adjustment

Once the balloon catheter has been installed, the pump adjusted, and satisfactory counterpulsation achieved, the sheath should be sutured in place with the use of the eyelets contained in the hemostatic cap. No sutures should be secured to the catheter shaft itself, because readjustment of the catheter position is occasionally required following inspection of the postoperative chest radiograph. The introduction site should then be cleansed and a suitable dressing applied. A chest radiograph should be obtained to confirm the position of the balloon. Note that the location of the distal aspect of the catheter will change depending on the position of the patient.[116]

Although the proper function of an IABCP does not permit appreciable flexion at the level of the hip, most patients with satisfactory cerebral perfusion find it more comfortable to lie with their torso slightly elevated (<30°) following insertion. Because the catheter is tethered to the patient's leg, this position forces the catheter to advance several centimeters cephalad within the aorta. For this reason, Biddle and coworkers have advocated that the chest radiograph should be obtained with the patient in this position to screen for this possibility.[116] Finally, the patient's hemodynamic profile (ie, PCWP, CO, and PVR) should be reassessed following the institution of counterpulsation. In the event that the patient is found to have a relatively low filling pressure following counterpulsation, fluids should be administered to achieve a PCWP of 15–20 mmHg.[49]

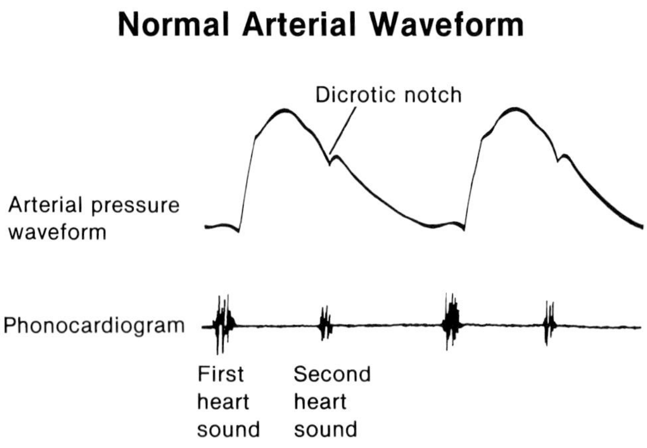

Figure 28–13 • The normal carotid arterial pulse with dicrotic notch.

Timing Errors in Early Inflation

Inflation of IACB prior to aortic valve closure

Waveform characteristics:
- Inflation of IACB prior to dicrotic notch.
- Diastolic augmentation encroaches onto systole (may be unable to distinguish)

Physiologic effects:
- Potential premature closure of aortic valve
- Potential increase in LVEDV and LVEDP or PCWP
- Increased left ventricular wall stress or afterload
- Aortic regurgitation
- Increased MVO_2 demand

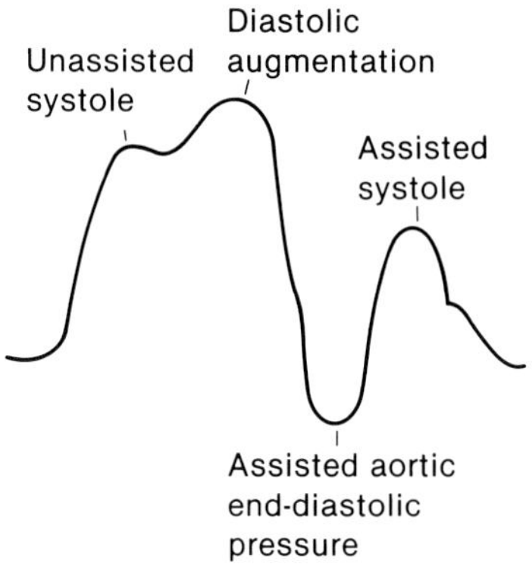

Figure 28–14 • Waveform characteristic of early inflation causing compromised diastolic augmentation. (Satler LF, Rackley CE. Assessment of adequate circulatory assist during intra-aortic balloon counterpulsation. Cardiovasc Clin 16: 141–149; with permission.)

Timing Errors in Late Inflation

Inflation of IACB markedly after closure of the aortic valve

Waveform characteristics:
- Inflation of the IACB after the dicrotic notch
- Absence of sharp V
- Suboptimal diastolic augmentation

Physiologic effects:
- Suboptimal coronary artery perfusion

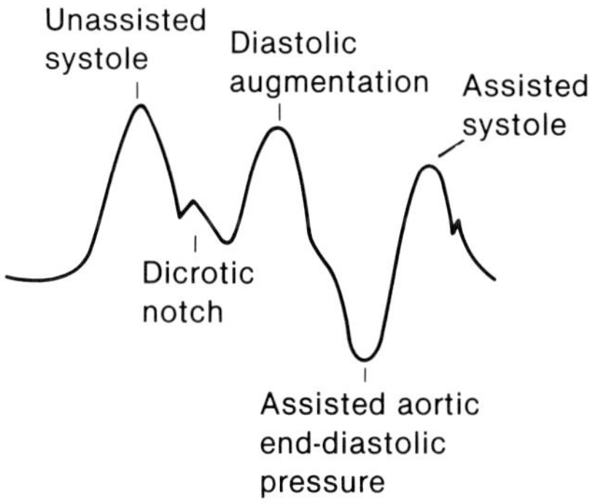

Figure 28–15 • Waveform characteristic of late balloon inflation and hence suboptimal diastolic augmentation. (Satler LF, Rackley CE. Assessment of adequate circulatory assist during intraaortic balloon counterpulsation. Cardiovasc Clin 16: 141–149; with permission.)

Timing Errors in Early Deflation

Premature deflation of the IACB during the diastolic phase

Waveform characteristics:
- Deflation of IACB is seen as a sharp drop following diastolic augmentation
- Suboptimal diastolic augmentation
- Assisted aortic end diastolic pressure may be equal to or greater than the unassisted aortic end diastolic pressure
- Assisted systolic pressure may rise

Physiologic effects:
- Suboptimal coronary perfusion
- Potential for retrograde coronary and carotid blood flow
- Angina may occur as a result of retrograde coronary blood flow
- Suboptimal afterload reduction
- Increased MVO_2 demand

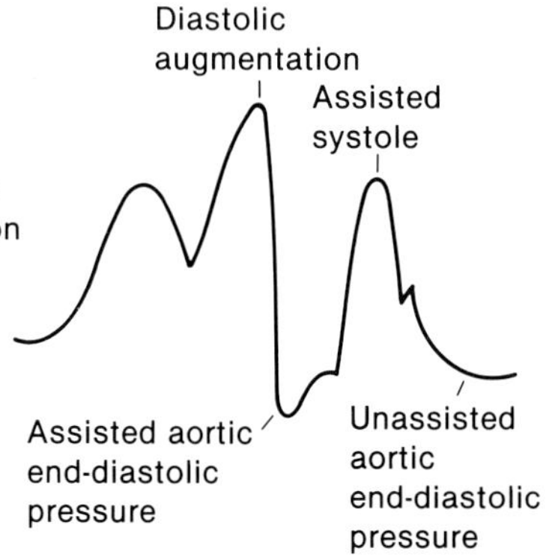

Figure 28–16 • Early deflation is characterized by wide U-shaped segments. (Modified from Satler LF, Rackley CE. Assessment of adequate circulatory assist during intraaortic balloon counterpulsation. Cardiovasc Clin 16: 141–149.)

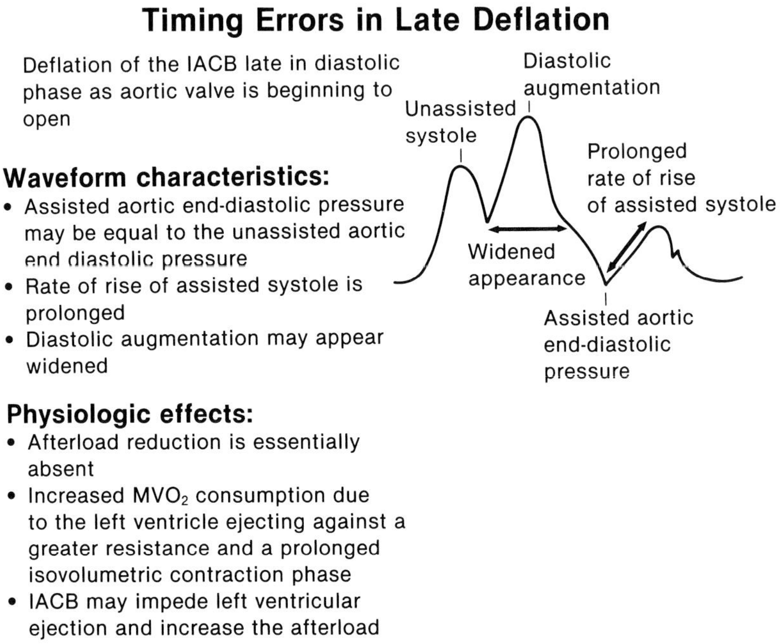

Figure 28–17 • Late deflation commonly results in a compromised trough (*arrow*) and hence suboptimal after-load reduction. (Modified from Satler LF, Rackley CE. Assessment of adequate circulatory assist during intraaortic balloon counterpulsation. Cardiovasc Clin 16: 141–149.)

During the course of the subsequent counterpulsation, the perfusion to the ipsilateral lower extremity should be reassessed, and the timing of the balloon inflation–deflation cycle readjusted, at least once during each nursing shift. In general, assessment of the perfusion to the lower extremity can be accomplished most readily by daily Doppler evaluation.[65,101] It is necessary to routinely readjust the inflation–deflation cycle of the pump because changes in heart rate have a profound impact on the function of conventional counterpulsation pumps. Conventional balloon pumps are triggered by the ECG, and the timing of the onset of both systole and diastole (eg, the dicrotic notch) varies with the onset of ventricular depolarization (eg, the QRS complex) depending on the heart rate. Furthermore, the duration of diastole, and hence the optimal duration for balloon inflation, is affected by changes in heart rate.

In addition to routine pump readjustment, the patient's hemoglobin, hematocrit, and platelet count should be reassessed on a daily basis throughout the duration of counterpulsation. Counterpulsation frequently provokes hemolysis and thrombocytopenia.[55,102,105] Bolooki estimates that patients generally require transfusion with one unit (250 mL) of packed red cells for every 48 hours of counterpulsation.[53]

G. *Troubleshooting Counterpulsation Pump Malfunction*

General troubleshooting guidelines can be applied to most machines regardless of their manufacturer (Datascope, Kontron, Aries, or Mansfield). Functional problems with balloon pumps fall into three interrelated categories: operator-related, patient-related, and pump-related.

1. Operator-Related Problems

The clinical potential of the pump is critically dependent on proper adjustment and is ultimately dependent on the level of knowledge of the practitioner caring for the patient. Because the majority of patients who require counterpulsation become dependent on the pump for survival, the practitioner must be able to determine the origin of problems when they arise and to promptly rectify these troublesome situations as necessary. The training required to independently operate a balloon pump generally derives from formal in-service classes and hands-on experience. Proficiency requires regular use of the equipment. If counterpulsation pumps are used infrequently within an institution, then resource personnel must be identified who can assist in both the delivery of care and the troubleshooting process.

2. Patient-Related Problems

The therapeutic potential of the IABCP is particularly dependent on the physiologic status of the patient. The following is a list of several common clinical conditions that have been found to compromise the function of counterpulsation balloon pumps, together with a list of corresponding troubleshooting strategies and caveats.

a. Low-Amplitude QRS Complex

Find the lead with the tallest R wave. If standard lead placement fails to provide an adequate R-wave trigger, try an anterior-posterior lead placement (positive lead on the chest and negative lead on the back at the midscapula level).

b. Tachycardia

Identify and treat the cause of the tachycardia. Use helium for the shuttle gas to the balloon because the dispersion time for helium is shorter than for CO_2. Reduce the support to a 1:2 beat/augmentation ratio. This allows adequate and complete pressure-vacuum sequencing. Decrease the exchange volume per beat in the balloon.

c. Atrial Fibrillation

Correct the rhythm and control rate. Use automatic timing mode if available. This mode employs an algorithm of the mechanical and electrical events that allows the machine to preset, track, and adjust the timing for various heart rates. Consider a 1:2 timing ratio if the rate cannot be controlled.

d. Premature Atrial or Ventricular Depolarizations

Treat the arrhythmia. The machine should sense the premature depolarization and recycle to augment the ectopic beat. If this sequence does not occur, choose a monitoring lead that minimizes the difference in amplitude between the normal and premature depolarizations. Select the automatic timing mode.

e. Pacemakers

Review the pacemaker logic built into the machine sensing circuitry. Decide if the trigger stimulus should be the pacer spike or the patient's intrinsic QRS complex. The decision to use the pacer spike for the trigger is most appropriate for patients who are virtually 100% pacemaker dependent.

f. Cardiac Arrest

The arterial pressure generated during CPR is frequently adequate to trigger the balloon pump, provided that the arterial pulse pressure trigger option is selected. On some machines, the internal rate mode can be selected to provide completely machine-driven intermittent balloon inflation. Although this approach diminishes the risk associated with a dormant balloon, it does not provide any hemodynamic benefit.

g. Hypotension: Inadequate Augmentation

Reassess the status of the patient and the timing of the balloon inflation–deflation cycle. Make sure that the balloon is not partially contained within the sheath. Many balloon catheters have markers along the shaft that can be used to determine the coaxial relationship of the catheter relative to the sheath.

Check the pneumatic tubing for kinks that might impede the rate of gas exchange. Remove any condensation that might have accumulated within the pneumatic tubing apparatus.

Refill the balloon with the shuttle gas. Many models require the balloon to be refilled every 2 hours. Depending on the model, this can be accomplished either manually or automatically. Check the integrity of the automatic component.

Check the gas reservoir in the tank.

Confirm that the balloon catheter is not contained within a false lumen of the aorta. This can be accomplished by injecting contrast medium into the lumen of the balloon catheter and inspecting the contrast run-off fluoroscopically.

3. PUMP-RELATED PROBLEMS

Many of the following problems can be avoided by compliance with a routine schedule for maintenance. Reference to the operator's manual will generally provide appropriate instruction in the event that an alarm is triggered. Because of the critical condition of most patients who require counterpulsation, a back-up unit must be available in the event that a malfunction develops in the primary unit resulting in compromised pump function. The following are machine-oriented problems that can occur regardless of manufacturer.

a. Excessive Condensation

Excess condensation may occur in the catheter's extension or external system components. Dispel the moisture by disconnecting the patient from the pneumatic part of the IABCP at the point most proximal to the patient. Allow the machine to pump for 20–30 seconds. Water will be expelled. Reconnect, refill the balloon, and resume pumping.

b. *Pneumatic Drive Vacuum Loss*

Slow gas leaks can trigger the machine alarms. The operator can override these alarms if the leak is not sufficient to adversely effect the function of the pump. Discrete external leaks may be mended temporarily with bone wax, eliminating the need to exchange the catheter.

Evaluate the patient's heart rate.

Tachycardias will diminish the responsiveness of the pneumatic system. If the tachycardia cannot be controlled, reduce the pump frequency to 1:2 as described above.

If a mechanical malfunction is identified, telephone the service department of the company that manufactures the pump machine, and transfer the patient to the standby IABCP.

c. *Balloon Leak or Rupture*

Plaque abrasion, traumatic insertion, or a manufacturing defect can cause the balloon to leak or rupture. Blood may appear in the balloon catheter. Place the machine on standby. Replace the balloon as necessary.

d. *Patient Disconnected from the IABCP*

Reattach the IABCP, refill the balloon, and resume pumping.

e. *Battery Depletion*

Operate on AC power only until the battery is recharged (time varies with models). It is necessary to switch machines if the patient must be transported to another facility or location within the hospital.

H. *Weaning from Counterpulsation*

Every effort should be made to delay the process of withdrawing counterpulsation support until the patient no longer requires the administration of inotropic agents.[65] Amsterdam has recommended that patients meet the following minimal performance criteria before counterpulsation is electively withdrawn:

1. Systolic blood pressure >90 mmHg
2. Cardiac index >2.0 L/min
3. Left ventricular filling pressure <20 mmHg
4. Heart rate <100 DPM[40]

The time required to successfully wean an individual from counterpulsation is clearly dependent on the patient's underlying pathophysiology. In general, however, the time required to wean an individual from counterpulsation support is approximately equal to 25% of the time that the patient has required counterpulsation.[53]

Weaning can be accomplished in two ways. The classical approach involves tapering the number of balloon inflations relative to the patient's heart rate. Advocates for this approach recommend that the anticipated time required to wean an individual should be divided into three equal intervals and that the counterpulsation ratio should be tapered from 1:1 to 1:2 to 1:3 at the beginning of each interval.[53,73] Because 1:3 counterpulsation affords little or no circulatory support, it can be used to predict the patient's hemodynamic response following removal of the balloon catheter.[53]

Alternately, weaning can be accomplished by maintaining the counterpulsation ratio and decreasing the volume to which the balloon inflates during diastole.[53] Bolooki recommends that the balloon volume should be decreased in increments of 25% (eg, 75%, 50%, 25%) in equivalent time intervals.[53] The heparin infusion should be discontinued approximately 1 hour before removal of the balloon catheter.

I. *Balloon Catheter Removal*

The sheath that accommodates the counterpulsation catheter does not contain a check valve, so both the sheath and catheter should be removed simultaneously. Although removing the sheath and catheter is relatively straightforward, a few considerations warrant discussion. First, the skin surrounding the incision site frequently becomes tender, particularly following protracted counterpulsation. Therefore, the administration of local anesthesia is generally recommended at the outset. Second, the operator should permit some backbleeding through the arteriotomy immediately after removing the catheter and sheath to evacuate any potential clot formation.[117] During the course of counterpulsation, thrombus accumulates on the intravascular surface of the catheter despite the administration of anticoagulation. Removal of the catheter can dislodge this thrombotic material within the vascular system in the region of the arteriotomy and provoke the development of thromboemboli. Because patients frequently sustain thromboembolic complications during this aspect of the procedure, some authorities have recommended the routine insertion of a Fogarty embolectomy catheter, following the removal of the catheter and prior to the application of hemostatic compression.[102]

Given the size of the arteriotomy, the presence of relative thrombocytopenia and the recent administration of anticoagulation, it is frequently necessary to maintain digital compression for 45 to 60 minutes following removal of the catheter and sheath to achieve satisfactory hemostasis. As indicated earlier, digital compression should be performed at this juncture according to the technique illustrated in Fig. 28–13. The force applied during this process should be adjusted to maintain hemostasis and yet permit perfusion to the ipsilateral lower extremity.[112]

IV. COMPLICATIONS

In general, the incidence of clinically evident complications related to IABC ranges from 5% to 15% (Table 28–3).[53] However, the incidence of actual complications, determined on the basis of necropsy studies, is substantially higher.[104,108] According to Isner and associates, 36% of patients evaluated post mortem were found to have sustained one or more complications attributed to balloon pump counterpulsation.[104] However, only 25% of these complications were identified ante mortem.

A number of possibilities have been proposed to explain this disparity, among them the fact that the baseline clinical state of most patients requiring counterpulsation tends to be catastrophic, a circumstance that frequently masks signs and symptoms related to the development of complications.[104,108] A considerable delay can transpire between the onset of dissection following the insertion of an IABCP and the development of the clinical manifestations of this complication.[108] In addition, several investigators have observed that IABCPs can function normally despite the presence of a significant dissection of the aorta.[102,104] Finally, others have observed that many of the reports concerning the incidence of complications sustained as a result of counterpulsation do not include the adverse consequences sustained among individuals in whom the catheter could not be advanced.[108]

Table 28–3 • Incidence of Vascular Repair for Catheter-Related Complications[113] (%)

0.6	Diagnostic cardiac catheterization
0.9	Percutaneous transluminal angioplasty
5.2	Transfemoral balloon valvuloplasty
11.5	Intraaortic balloon counterpulsation

(Data from Skillman JJ, Kim D, Baim DS. Vascular complications of percutaneous femoral cardiac interventions. Arch Surg 123:1207–1212, 1988; with permission.)

As a result, the actual incidence of complications related to counterpulsation remains unknown. However, there is sufficient clinical evidence to draw the following conclusions.

A. *Risk Factors*

The incidence of complications attributed to counterpulsation is directly related to the presence and severity of peripheral vascular disease.[103] Women are at additional risk,[103] as are patients who are obese[113] or have diabetes.[100,118] The size of the counterpulsation catheter installed.[113] The duration of counterpulsation by itself does not constitute a risk factor for arteriovascular complications.[109,119] However, Freed and associates have reported that patients who require protracted counterpulsation are prone to the development of fevers and bacteremia.[120]

B. *Aortic Dissection*

As discussed earlier, dissection generally transpires during the process of inserting the catheter and sheath. Occasionally, malposition of the catheter tip can provoke dissection of the aortic arch. Aortic dissection occurs more commonly than previously suspected and is generally fatal.[53,104,116,121]

C. *Ipsilateral Lower-Extremity Ischemia*

The incidence of ipsilateral lower-extremity ischemia can approach 30%.[53] However, the incidence of amputation and major functional loss secondary to the insertion of an intraaortic counterpulsation balloon catheter is less than 1%.[28,100] Pedal pulses commonly disappear following insertion of a counterpulsation balloon catheter and reappear after removal of the device.[53] The absence of pedal pulses following the removal of the catheter often indicates the presence of lower-extremity thromboemboli.[102] On rare occasions, the creation of a transpubic femoral–femoral crossover graft is indicated for patients who are critically dependent upon counterpulsation and who develop ipsilateral ischemia with compromised access to the contralateral femoral system.[65,122]

D. Hemolysis

Hemolysis occurs commonly during the course of counterpulsation. Bolooki has recommended that patients should receive approximately 1 unit of packed red cells for every 48 hours of counterpulsation.[53]

E. Miscellaneous

Several additional complications have been attributed to counterpulsation, including bacteremia,[123] splenic infarction,[124] foot drop,[73] and spinal cord paralysis.[125–127]

Because of the high incidence of complications associated with the performance of IABC, we recommend that the insertion and removal of counterpulsation catheters and the adjustment of the pump function be undertaken only by the most experienced operators. This recommendation is supported by Goldman and colleagues, who reported a 14.4% complication rate among the first 90 patients to undergo counterpulsation at their institution, followed by a 6% complication rate for the subsequent 100 patients.[109]

V. References

1. Clauss RH, Birtwell WC, Albertal G, et al. Assisted circulation: The arterial counterpulsator. J Thorac Cardiovasc Surg 41:447–458, 1961.
2. Tobias MA, Challen PD, Franklin CB, Phillips G, et al. Intraaortic balloon counterpulsation; Clinical experience. Anaesthesia 34:844–854, 1979.
3. Moulopoulos SD, Topaz S, Kolff WJ. Diastolic balloon pumping (with carbon dioxide) in the aorta: A mechanical assistance to the failing circulation. Am Heart J 63:669, 1962.
4. Igo SR, Hibbs CW, Trono R, Fuqua JM, et al. Intraaortic balloon pumping: Experience with 325 patients. Artif Organs 3:249–256, 1978.
5. Kantrowitz A, Tjonneland S, Freed PS, Phillips SJ, et al. Initial clinical experience with intra-aortic balloon pumping. J Am Med Assoc 203:113, 1968.
6. Mundth Ed, Yurchak PM, Buckley MJ, Leinbach RC, et al. Circulatory assistance in emergency direct coronary artery surgery for shock complicating acute myocardial infarction. N Eng J Med 283:1382, 1970.
7. Buckley MJ, Craver JM, Gold HK, Mundth ED, et al. Intraaortic balloon pump assist for cardiogenic shock after cardiopulmonary bypass. Circulation 47–48(Suppl 3):90, 1973.
8. Goldberger M, Tabak SW, Shah PK. Clinical experience with intra-aortic balloon counterpulsation in 112 consecutive patients. Am Heart J 111:497–502, 1986.
9. Swanton RH. Who requires balloon pumping? Intensive Care Med 10:271–273, 1984.
10. Subramanian VA, Goldstein J, Sos TA, McCabe JC, et al. Preliminary clinical experience with percutaneous intra-aortic balloon pumping. Circulation 62:(Suppl 1):123–129, 1980.
11. Leinbach RC, Goldstein J, Gold HK, Moses JW, et al. Percutaneous wire-guided balloon pumping. Am J Cardiol 49:1707, 1982.
12. Weber KT, Janicki JS. Intraaortic balloon counterpulsation. Am Thorac Surg 17:602, 1974.
13. Soroff HS, Giron F, Ruiz U, Birtwell WC, et al. Physiologic support of heart action. N Engl J Med 280:68, 1969.
14. Sponitz HM, Covell JW, Ross J, Braunwald E. Left ventricular mechanics and oxygen consumption during arterial counterpulsation. Am J Physiol 217:1352, 1969.
15. Sonnenblick EH, Skelton CL. Oxygen consumption of the heart: Physiological principals and clinical implications. Mod Conc Cardiovasc Dis 40:9, 1971.
16. Gorlin R. Coronary Artery Disease. Philadelphia, WB Saunders, 1976, 71.
17. Aroesty JM, Weintraub RM, Paulin S, O'Grady GP. Medically refractory unstable angina pectoris. II. Hemodynamic and angiographic effects of intraaortic balloon counterpulsation. Am J Cardiol 43:883–888, 1979.
18. Ehrich DA, Biddle TA, Kronenberg MW, Yu PN. The hemodynamic response to intraaortic balloon counterpulsation in patients with cardiogenic shock complicating acute myocardial infarction. Am Heart J 93:274–279, 1977.
19. Weiss AT, Engel S, Gotsman CJ, Shefer A, et al. Regional and global left ventricular function during intraaortic balloon counterpulsation in patients with acute myocardial infarction shock. Am Heart J 108:249–254, 1984.
20. Steele P, Jenkins M, Battock D, Pappas G, et al. Isosorbide dinitrate and intraaortic balloon pumping in preinfarction angina: Effects on central circulatory dynamics. Chest 69:712–717, 1976.
21. Nichols AB, Pohost GM, Gold HK, Leinbach RC, et al. Assessment of left ventricular function on-and-off intra-aortic balloon pump support by gated cardiac blood pool scanning (abstr). Circulation 55(Suppl 3):132, 1977.
22. Feola M, Weiner L, Walinsky P, Kasparian H, et al. Improved survival after coronary bypass surgery in patients with poor left ventricular function: Role of intraaortic balloon counterpulsation. Am J Cardiol 39:1021–1026, 1977.
23. Lefemine AA, Low HBC, Cohen ML, Lunzer S, et al. Assisted circulation. III. The effect of synchronized arterial counterpulsation on myocardial oxygen consumption and coronary flow. Am Heart J 64:789, 1962.
24. Braunwald E, Covell JW, Moroko PR, Ross J. Effects of drugs and of counterpulsation on myocardial oxygen consumption: Observations on the ischemic heart. Circulation 40(Suppl 4):220, 1969.
25. Sugg WL, Martin LF, Webb WR, Ecker RR. Influence of counterpulsation on aortic right and left coronary blood flow following ligation of the left circumflex coronary artery. Thorac Cardiovasc Surg 59:345, 1970.
26. Laas J, Campbell CD, Takanashi Y, Pick RL, et al. Failure of

intraaortic balloon pumping to reduce experiment myocardial infarct size in swine. J Thorac Cardiovasc Surg 80:85–93, 1980.
27. Leinbach RC, Buckley MJ, Austen WG, Petschek HE, et al. Effects of intra-aortic balloon pumping on coronary flow and metabolism in man. Circulation 43(Suppl 1):77, 1971.
28. Bolooki H. Clinical Application of Intra-Aortic Balloon Pump. 2nd ed. Mount Kisco, NY, Futura Publishing, Inc, 1984.
29. Fuchs RM, Brin KP, Brinker JA, Guzman PA, et al. Augmentation of regional coronary blood flow by intra-aortic balloon counterpulsation in patients with unstable angina. Circulation 68:117–123, 1983.
30. Hirsch LJ, Lluch S, Katz LN. Counterpulsation effects of coronary blood flow and cardiac oxygen utilization. Circ Res 19:1031, 1984.
31. Feola M, Haiderer O, Kennedy JH. Intraaortic balloon pumping (IABP) at different levels of experimental acute left ventricular failure. Chest 59:68, 1971.
32. Watson JT, Willerson JT, Fixler DE, Sugg WL. Temporal change in collateral coronary blood flow in ischemic myocardium during intraaortic balloon pumping. Circulation 5(Suppl 2):–, 1974.
33. Willerson JT, Watson JT, Platt MR. Effect of hypertonic mannitol and intraaortic balloon counterpulsation on regional myocardial blood flow and ventricular performance in dogs during myocardial ischemia. Am J Cardiol 37:514, 1976.
34. Saini VK, Hood WB Jr, Hechtman HB, Berger RL. Nutrient myocardial blood flow in experimental myocardial ischemia. Circulation 52:1086, 1975.
35. Gill CC, Wechsler AS, Newman GE, Oldham HN. Augmentation an redistribution of myocardial blood flow during acute ischemia by intraaortic balloon pumping. Ann Thorac Surg 16:444, 1973.
36. Mueller H, Ayres SM, Conklin EJ, Gianelli S, et al. The effects of intra-aortic counterpulsation on cardiac performance and metabolism in shock associated with acute myocardial infarction. J Clin Invest 50:1885, 1971.
37. Swank M, Singh HM, Flemma RJ, Mullen DC, et al. Effect of intraaortic balloon pumping on nutrient coronary flow in normal and ischemic myocardium. J Thorac Cardiovasc Surg 76:538–544, 1978.
38. Jacobey JA, Taylor WJ, Smith GT, Gorlin R, et al. A new therapeutic approach to acute coronary occlusion. II. Opening dormant coronary collateral channels by counterpulsation. Am J Cardiol 11:218, 1963.
39. Reneman RS, Jageneau AHM, Schaper WKA, Brouwer FAS, et al. Influence of counterpulsation on collateral circulation after acute occlusion of the left anterior descending coronary artery in dogs. Cardiovasc Res 45:–, 1972.
40. Amsterdam EA, Awan NA, Lee G, Low R, et al. Intra-aortic balloon counterpulsation:rationale, application and results. Cardiovasc Clin 16:79–96.
41. Williams DO, Korr KS, Gewirtz H, Most AS. The effect of intraaortic balloon counterpulsation on regional myocardial blood flow and oxygen consumption in the presence of coronary artery stenosis in patients with unstable angina. Circulation 66:593, 1982.
42. Mueller H, Ayres SM, Grace WT. Principal defects which account for shock following acute myocardial infarction in man: Implications for treatment. Critical Care Medicine 1:27–38, 1973.
43. Powel WJ Jr, Daggett WM, Magro AE, Bianco JA, et al. Effects of intraaortic balloon counterpulsation on cardiac performance, oxygen consumption, and coronary blood flow in dogs. Circ Res 26:753–764, 1970.
44. Weintraub RM, Voukydis PC, Aroesty JM, Cohen SI, et al. Treatment of preinfarction angina with intraaortic balloon counterpulsation and surgery. Am J Surg 34:809, 1974.
45. Maroko PR, Bernstein EF, Libby Y P, DeLaria GA, et al. Effects of intraaortic balloon counterpulsation on the severity of myocardial ischemia injury following acute coronary occlusion. Circulation 45:1150, 1972.
46. Iskandrian AS, Colby J, Hakki A-H, Boston B, et al. Effect of intraaortic balloon pumping on left ventricular function: Evaluation by radionuclide ventriculography. Clin Cardiol 7:211–216, 1984.
47. Gold HK, Leinbach RC, Sanders CA, Buckley MJ, et al. Intraaortic balloon pumping for control of recurrent myocardial ischemia. Circulation 47:1197–1203, 1973.
48. Hanson EC, Levine FH, Kay HR, Leinbach RC, et al. Control of post-infarction ventricular irritability with the intraaortic balloon pump. Circulation 62(Suppl 1):130, 1980.
49. Watanabe H, Johnson WD, Shore RT, Kayser KL. Use of Intraaortic balloon pumping (IABP) in clinical cardiac surgery and management of patients with IABP. Japan J Surg 8:282–290, 1978.
50. Gunstensen J, Goldman BS, Scully HE, Huckell VF, et al. Evolving indications for preoperative intraaortic balloon pump assistance. Ann Thorac Surg 22:535–545, 1976.
51. Kaplan JA, Craver JM, Jones EL, Sumpter R. The role of the intraaortic balloon pump in cardiac anesthesia and surgery. Am Heart J 98:580–586, 1979.
52. Brandt B, Wright CB, Doty DB, Rossi NP, et al. Surgical treatment of left main coronary artery disease: Operative risk. Surgery 87:436–440, 1980.
53. Bolooki H. Current status of circulatory support with an intra-aortic balloon pump. Cardiol Clin 3:123–133, 1985.
54. Vijayanagar R, Bognolo DA, Eckstein PF, Toole JC, et al. The role of intra-aortic balloon pump in the management of patients with main left coronary artery disease. Cathet Cardiovasc Diagn 7:397–401, 1981.
55. Jones EL, Craver JM, King SB, Kaplan JA, et al. Analysis of factors in the survival of patients with left main coronary artery disease. J Thorac Cardiovasc Surg
56. Okada M, Shiozawa T, Iizuka M, Okuno K, et al. The effect of intraaortic balloon pumping (IABP) on cardiogenic shock due to acute myocardial infarction. Kobe J Med Sci 30:35–41, 1984.
57. Satler LF, Rackley CE. Assessment of adequate circulatory assist during intra-aortic balloon counterpulsation. Cardiovasc Clin 16:141–149.
58. Reeves TJ, Blinks JR, Cox JR Jr, Danilowicz PA, et al. Mechanically assisted circulation: The status of the NHLBI program and recommendations for the future. Artif Organs 1:39–58, 1977.
59. Lee FA. Treatment of the hemodynamically unstable patient. Cardiol Clin 6:63–79, 1988.
60. Rajai HR, Hartman CW, Innes BJ, Bartel AG, et al. Prophylactic use of intra-aortic balloon pump in aortocoronary bypass for patients with left main coronary artery disease. Ann Surg 187:118–121, 1978.
61. Alcan KE, Stertzer SH, Wallsh E. DePasquale NP, et al. The role of intra-aortic balloon counterpulsation in patients undergoing percutaneous transluminal coronary angioplasty. Am Heart J 105:527–530, 1983.
62. Szatmary LJ, Marco J, Fajadet J, Caster L. The combined use of diastolic counterpulsation and coronary dilatation in unstable angina due to multivessel disease under unstable hemodynamic conditions. Int J Cardiol 19:59–66, 1988.
63. Murphy DA, Craver JM, Jones EL, et al. Surgical revasculariz-

ation following unsuccessful percutaneous transluminal coronary angioplasty. J Thorac Cardiovasc Surg 84:342, 1982.
64. Szatmary LJ, Marco J. Haemodynamic and antiischemic protective effects of intra-aortic balloon counterpulsation in high risk coronary heart patients undergoing percutaneous transluminal coronary angioplasty. Cor Vasa 29:181–191, 1987.
65. Jorge E. Pierce WS. Mechanical support or replacement of the heart. Cardiovasc Clin 17:361–379, 1987.
66. Scheidt S, Ascheim R, Killip T. Shock after acute myocardial infarction: A clinical and hemodynamic profile. Am J Cardiol 26:556, 1970.
67. Killip T, Kimball JT. Treatment of myocardial infarction in a coronary care unit: A two year experience with 250 patients. Am J Cardiol 20:457, 1967.
68. Gunnar RM, Loeb HS, Rahimtoola SH. Hemodynamic studies in shock with myocardial infarction. In Gunnar RM, Loeb HS, Rahimtoola SH (eds). Shock in Myocardial Infarction. Orlando, FL, Grune & Stratton, 1974, 113.
69. Page DL, Caufield JB, Kastor JA, DeSanctis R, et al. Myocardial changes associated with cardiogenic shock. N Engl J Med 285:133, 1971.
70. Harnarayan C, Bennett MA, Pentecost BL, Brewer DB. Quantitative study of infarcted myocardium in cardiogenic shock. Br Heart J 32:728, 1970.
71. Jackson G, Cullum P, Pastellopoulos A, MacArthur A, et al. Intraaortic balloon assistance in cardiogenic shock after myocardial infarction or cardiac surgery. Br Heart J 39:598–604, 1977.
72. Forssell G, Nordlander R, Nyquist O, Schenck-Gustavsson K. Intraaortic balloon pumping in the treatment of cardiogenic shock complicating acute myocardial infarction. Acta Med Scand 206:189-192, 1979.
73. Kafrouni G. Intraaortic balloon counterpulsation. Am J Surg 147:731–734, 1984.
74. Roberts AJ, Alonso DR, Combes JR, et al. Role of delayed intraaortic balloon pumping in treatment of experimental myocardial infarction. Am J Cardiol 41:1202–1208, 1978.
75. Sugg WL, Webb WR, Ecker RR. Reduction of extent of myocardial infarction by counterpulsation. Ann Thorac Surg 7:311, 1969.
76. Gutovitz AL, Sobel BE, Roberts R. Progressive nature of myocardial injury in selected patients with cardiogenic shock. Am J Cardiol 41:469, 1978.
77. Leinbach RC, Gold HK, Harper RW, et al. Early intraaortic balloon pumping for anterior myocardial infarction without shock. Circulation 58:204, 1978.
78. Flaherty JT, Weiss JL, Becker LC, et al. Failure of intraaortic balloon pumping and intravenous nitroglycerin to reduce scintigraphic indices of infarct size (abstr). Circulation (Suppl 3):120, 1983.
79. O'Rourke MF, Norris RM, Campbell TJ, et al. Randomized controlled trial of intraaortic balloon counterpulsation in early myocardial infarction with acute heart failure. Am J Cardiol 47:815, 1981.
80. Flaherty JT, Becker LC, Weiss JL, Brinker JA, et al. Results of a randomized prospective trial of intraaortic balloon counterpulsation and intravenous nitroglycerin in patients with acute myocardial infarction. J Am Coll Cardiol 6:434–446, 1985.
81. Bolooki H. Myocardial revascularization after acute infarction. Am J Cardiol 36:395, 1975.
82. DeWood MA, Notske RN, Hensley GR, Shields JP, et al. Intraaortic balloon counterpulsation with and without reperfusion for myocardial infarction shock. Circulation 61:1105–1112, 1980.
83. Pifarre R, Sullivan HJ, Grieco J, Montoya A, et al. Management of left ventricular rupture complicating myocardial infarction. J Thorac Cardiovasc Surg 86:441–443, 1983.
84. London RE, London SB. Rupture of the heart. A critical analysis of 47 consecutive autopsy cases. Circulation 31:202, 1965.
85. Rassmussen S, Leth A, Kjoller E, Pedersen A. Cardiac rupture in acute myocardial infarction. Acta Med Scand 205:11, 1979.
86. Hochreiter C, Goldstein J, Borer JS, Tyberg T, et al. Myocardial free-wall rupture after acute myocardial infarction: Survival aided by percutaneous intraaortic balloon counterpulsation. Circulation 65:1279–1282, 1982.
87. Orlando R III, Drezner AD. Intraaortic balloon counterpulsation in blunt cardiac injury. J Trauma 23:424–427, 1983.
88. Snow N, Lucas AE, Richardson JD. Intraaortic balloon counterpulsation for cardiogenic shock from cardiac contusion. J Trauma 22:426–429, 1982.
89. Demas C, Flancbaum L, Scott G, Trooskin SZ. The intraaortic balloon pump as an adjunctive therapy for severe myocardial contusion. Am J Emerg Med 5:499–502, 1987.
90. Mercer D, Doris P, Salerno TA. Intra-aortic balloon counterpulsation in septic shock. Can J Surg 24:643–645, 1981.
91. Wilson RF, Sarver EJ, Rizzo J. Hemodynamic changes, treatment and prognosis in clinical shock. Arch Surg 102:21–4, 1971.
92. Wilson RE, Ali M, Anand V, McCarthy B, et al. Effects of vasoactive agents in clinical septic shock. In Forscher BK, Lillehei RC, Stubbs SS (eds). Shock in Low and High-Flow States. Proceedings of a Symposium at Brook Lodge, Augusta, Michigan, June 1–3, 1971. Excerpta Medica (Amsterdam) 269, 1972.
93. Foster ED, Subramanian VS, Vito L, Hechtman HB, et al. Response to intra-aortic balloon pumping. Am J Surgery 129:464–71, 1975.
94. Raper RF, Fisher M. Profound reversible myocardial depression after anaphylaxis. Lancet 1:386–388, 1988.
95. Folland ED, Kemper AJ, Khuri SF, Josa M, et al. Intraaortic balloon counterpulsation as a temporary support measure in decompensated critical aortic stenosis. J Am Coll Cardiol 5:711–6, 1985.
96. Limet R, Demoulin JC, Fourny J. Five years experience with intraaortic balloon pumping: The changing indications and the emergence of prognostic indices. Acta Cardiol 35:121–130, 1980.
97. Resnekov L. Circulatory support and early cardiac surgery in the management of cardiogenic shock complicating myocardial infarction. Ann Clin Res 9:134, 1977.
98. Alcan KE, Stertzer SH, Wallsh E, Bruno MS. DePasquale NP. Current status of intra-aortic balloon counterpulsation in critical care cardiology. Crit Care Med 12:489–495, 1984.
99. Vignola PA, Swaye PS, Gosselin AJ. Percutaneous intraaortic balloon pumping: New problems and dilemmas. Cathet Cardiovasc Diagn 9:117–118, 1983.
100. Martin RS, Moncure AC, Buckley MJ, Austen WG, et al. Complications of percutaneous intra-aortic balloon insertion. J Thorac Cardiovasc Surg 85:186–190, 1983.
101. Sutorius DJ, Majeski JA, Miller SF. Vascular complications as a result of intra-aortic balloon pumping. Am Surg 45:512–516, 1979.
102. Perler BA, McCabe CJ, Abbott WM, Buckley MJ. Vascular complications of intraaortic balloon counterpulsation. Arch Surg 118:957–962, 1983.
103. Gottlieb SO, Brinker JA, Borkon M, Kallman CH, et al. Identification of patients at high risk for complications of intraaortic balloon counterpulsation: A multivariate risk factor analysis. Am J Cardiol 53:1135–1139, 1984.

104. Isner JM, Cohen SR, Virmani R, Lawrinson W, et al. Complications of the intra-aortic balloon counterpulsation device: Clinical and morphologic observations in 45 necropsy patients. Am J Cardiol 45:260–267, 1980.
105. Bahn CH, Vitikaineu KJ, Anderson CL, et al. Vascular evaluation for balloon pumping. Ann Thorac Surg 27:474–477, 1979.
106. Goldberg MJ, Rubenfire M, Kantrowitz A, et al. Intraaortic balloon pump insertion: A randomized study comparing percutaneous and surgical techniques. J Am Coll Card 9:515, 1987.
107. Kantrowitz A, Wasfie T, Freed PS, Rubenfire M, et al. Intraaortic balloon pumping 1967 through 1982: Analysis of complications in 733 patients. Am J Cardiol 57:976–983, 1986.
108. Bregman D, Cohen SR. Mechanical techniques of circulation support: A percutaneous intra-aortic balloon device. Artif Organs 7:38–48, 1983.
109. Goldman BS, Hill TJ, Rosenthal GA, Scully HE, et al. Complications associated with use of the intraaortic balloon pump. Can J Surg 25:153–156, 1982.
110. Alcan KE, Stertzer SH, Wallsh E, et al. Comparison of wire-guided percutaneous insertion and surgical insertion of intraaortic balloon pumps in 151 patients. Am J Med 75:24, 1983.
111. Hauser AM, Gordon S, Gangadharan V, Ramos RG, et al. Percutaneous intraaortic balloon counterpulsation: Clinical effectiveness and hazards. Chest 82:422–425, 1982.
112. Todd GJ, Bregman D, Voorhees AB, Reemtsma K. Vascular complications associated with percutaneous intra-aortic balloon pumping. Arch Surg 118:963–964, 1983.
113. Skillman JJ, Kim D, Baim DS. Vascular complications of percutaneous femoral cardiac interventions. Arch Surg 123:1207–1212, 1988.
114. Nichols AB, Weiss MB, Bregman D, Casarella WJ. Percutaneous intra-aortic balloon insertion in patients with aorto-iliac disease. Cathet Cardiovasc Diagn 7:443–9, 1982.
115. O'Rourke MF, Shepherd KM. Protection of the aortic arch and subclavian artery during intraaortic balloon pumping. J Thorac Cardiovasc Surg 65:543, 1973.
116. Biddle TL, Stewart S, Stuard ID. Dissection of the aorta complicating intraaortic balloon counterpulsation. Am Heart J 92:781–784, 1976.
117. Rodigas PC, Finnegan JO. Technique for removal of percutaneously placed intraaortic balloons. Ann Thorac Surg 40:80–81, 1985.
118. Alderman JD, Gabliani GI, McCabe CH, Brewer CC, et al. Incidence and management of limb ischemia with percutaneous wire-guided intraaortic balloon catheters. J Am Coll Cardiol 9:524–30, 1987.
119. Shahian DM, Neptune WB, Ellis FH Jr, et al. Intraaortic balloon pump morbidity:A comparative analysis of risk factors between percutaneous and surgical techniques. Ann Thorac Surg 36:444, 1983.
120. Freed PS, Wasfie T, Zado B, Kantrowitz A. Intraaortic balloon pumping for prolonged circulatory support. Am J Cardiol 61:554–557, 1988.
121. Beckman CB, Geha AS, Hammond GL, et al. Results and complications of intra-aortic balloon counterpulsation. Ann Thorac Surg 24:550, 1977.
122. Alpert J, Parsonnet V, Goldenkranz RJ, et al. Limb ischemia during intraaortic balloon pumping:indication for femoro-femoral crossover graft. J Thorac Cardiovasc Surg 79:729–734, 1980.
123. Grantham RN, Munnell ER, Kanaly PJ. Femoral artery infection complicating intraaortic balloon pumping. Am J Surg 146:811–814, 1983.
124. Busch HM, Cogbill TH, Gundersen AE. Splenic infarction: Complication of intra-aortic balloon counterpulsation. Am Heart J 109:383–385, 1985.
125. Macoviak J, Stephenson LW, Edmunds LH, Harken A, et al. The intraaortic balloon pump: An analysis of five years' experience. Ann Thorac Surg 29:451–457, 1980.
126. Seifert PE. Late paraplegia resulting from intraaortic balloon pump. Ann Thorac Surg 41:700–702, 1986.
127. Rose DM, Jacobowitz IJ, Acinapura AJ, Cunningham JN. Paraplegia following percutaneous insertion of an intra-aortic balloon. J Thorac Cardiovasc Surg 87:788–797, 1984.

Section IV

•

Central Nervous System Procedures

Chapter 29

Theodore J. Sanford, Jr, MD

Electroencephalography

OUTLINE

I. INTRODUCTION

The monitoring of certain cardiovascular, pulmonary, and renal functions during anesthesia and surgery has become routine. In fact, even the use of invasive modalities to measure cardiac output, mixed venous oxygen saturation, and arterial blood pressure is now common. It is now widely accepted that the noninvasive measurements of arterial oxygen saturation, end-tidal carbon dioxide, and continuous arterial blood pressure are not only accurate but also correlate well with the clinical condition of the patient. Observed changes in these monitors provide information for patient assessment that alert the clinician and allow appropriate intervention.

The electroencephalogram (EEG) is a record of the cerebral electrical activity and is used to monitor neurologic activity near the brain surface. It was suggested long ago that monitoring the intraoperative EEG could assess anesthetic depth and also indicate and prevent potential cerebral impairment. However, only in the last 10 years have technical and clinical improvements made EEG monitoring in the operating room feasible. Although attempts to correlate depth of anesthesia and other physiologic situations with changes in the EEG are not new, the on-line computerized processing of the EEG has the potential to result in the real-time, clinically useful application of electroencephalography to the practice of anesthesiology.

This chapter focuses on recent technical changes in processing of EEG information, indications for EEG monitoring, how to apply and set up the EEG in the operating room, and finally, the changes (both normal and abnormal) that occur during general anesthesia and specific types of surgery.

A. *Historical Aspects of Electroencephalographic (EEG) Monitoring*

Although EEG monitoring is one of the oldest electronic monitors used in medicine, continuous intraoperative EEG monitoring with the standard 16-lead machine has not been feasible for several reasons. Older equipment required a technician to run the machine; the size and complexity of equipment precluded simple operating room logistics; and the volume and complexity of the record precluded easy and simple review (Table 29–1). These factors created major problems with real-time interpretation.[1] For example, an EEG record running at the commonly used speed of 60 mm/second would produce a data record 216 meters long each hour! One can easily see that to compare a current EEG tracing to a record made 20 minutes earlier would require the review of many tens of feet of paper. Thus, there was a need for computerized recording and presentation of the EEG in a fashion that would allow the clinician to easily interpret changes in frequency, amplitude, and symmetry. The evolution of the processed EEG has made it possible to interpret the changes and trends in the EEG that are difficult to discern visually from a raw EEG recording.

Table 29–1 • Problems with Standard 16-Lead EEG

1. Size and complexity of equipment
2. Need for a technician to operate machine
3. Volume and complexity of the record
4. Need for person trained to read raw EEG
5. Problem of real-time interpretation

B. *Techniques of Computerized EEG Analysis*

A lot of confusion surrounding present-day computerized EEG analysis arises from the numerous display formats and the computer-aided techniques for analyzing the raw EEG. These include display formats and methods that generate a single derived value (univariant descriptor) that is plotted as a linear function on a polygraph, and methods that convert the raw EEG by power spectral analysis into a three-dimensional display. The bottom line of computer analysis of the EEG is the conversion of the EEG from the time domain into a frequency (most desirable) and an amplitude (less desirable) domain. There are three main conversion techniques: period analysis, power spectral analysis, and aperiodic analysis.

1. PERIOD ANALYSIS

Period analysis is the simplest of the methods of computer EEG analysis. It counts the frequency of occurrence of an event such as the number of times the fundamental EEG wave crosses the zero-axis in a certain time period. This value is then averaged over time, and results are used to generate a single derived value that can be plotted as a linear function of time on a polygraph. Examples of instruments that use period analysis include the Cerebral Function Monitor and the Klein Analyzer.

a. *Cerebral Function Monitor*

An early attempt at manipulation of the raw EEG into a single value was a commercial device known as the *Cerebral Function Monitor (CFM).*[2] This monitor uses a single bipolar lead rather than a montage of leads; however, there is also a second lead system to monitor for artifact. Unlike other processed EEG devices that convert the raw EEG signal from the time to frequency domain, the CFM remains in the time–amplitude domain.

A single value was derived from the raw EEG by an algorithm that multiplied amplitude and frequency and was plotted on semilogarithmic paper. The results were presented as a band whose thickness of the band indicated the amount of variability of the signal (Fig. 29–1). However, the algorithm used was unable to differentiate between large slow waves and small fast waves if the product was the same. This trace supposedly varied from the baseline with the onset of anesthesia and with changes induced by vascular events such as carotid artery clamping.

The CFM was found to be more sensitive to major changes in the EEG than visual interpretation of the raw EEG.[3] The derived product (amplitude × frequency) of this monitor was thought by some to be an adequate representation of global cerebral function and was recommended for use especially in cardiac surgery and following the resuscitation of patients after cardiac arrest (see Fig. 29–1).[4] However, this technique filtered out both high- and low-frequency EEG waves, occasionally hid frequency changes, and needed very slow paper speeds for recording a readable display. Thus information was lost, acute changes were difficult to detect in real time, and it was recommended that techniques that analyzed frequency and amplitude separately be used. In addition, correlation with a standard EEG was difficult. It remains to be seen if the updated version of the CFM, which has separate outputs for amplitude and frequency data, will prove to be more useful.

b. *Klein Analyzer*

The *Klein analyzer* is also a period analyzer that uses the zero-crossing method to obtain the amplitude (AO) and the average zero-axis crossing frequency (FO) of the fundamental waveform.[4] There is further processing of the signal, generating two additional amplitudes (A1, A2) and frequencies (F1, F2). The process results in a single value for the fundamental wave, which is thought to correlate with changes in the EEG induced by drugs or surgical events. Like the CFM, the derived values are plotted in a linear fashion against time on a polygraph (Fig. 29–2). The simplicity of this approach to EEG analysis makes the Klein analyzer attractive and awaits further development.

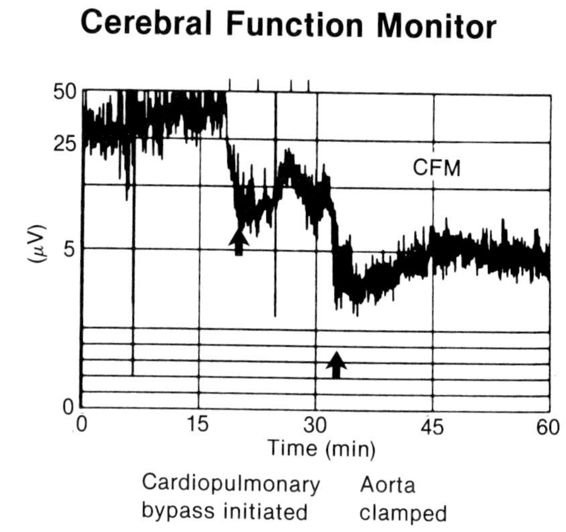

Figure 29–1 • An example of the display from a cerebral function monitor (CFM). The thickness of the band indicates the variability of the signal. The lower edge of the band represents the lowest peak-to-peak amplitude, while the upper edge of the band indicates the highest peak-to-peak amplitude. This display demonstrates the changes in the CFM over 1 hour of cardiac surgery. The patient was placed on cardiopulmonary bypass at about 18 minutes (*left arrow*), and then had the aorta clamped at 32 minutes (*right arrow*); each event resulted in a decrease in activity. Note that the CFM trace is not smooth, but contains numerous electrocautery spikes. (Adapted from Glaria AP, Murray A. Comparison of ECG monitoring techniques: An evaluation during cardiac surgery. Electroencephalogr Clin Neurophysiol 61:323–330, 1985.)

2. POWER SPECTRAL ANALYSIS

The most commonly used technique for processed EEG analysis is *power spectral analysis* (Fig. 29–3). The raw EEG signal is manipulated by a technique known as *fast Fourier transform,* which takes an epoch of time and mathematically separates the data and reduces complex waveforms to equivalent sine waves, providing frequency and amplitude information. Further manipulation of the data results in a power spectrum (amplitude^2)

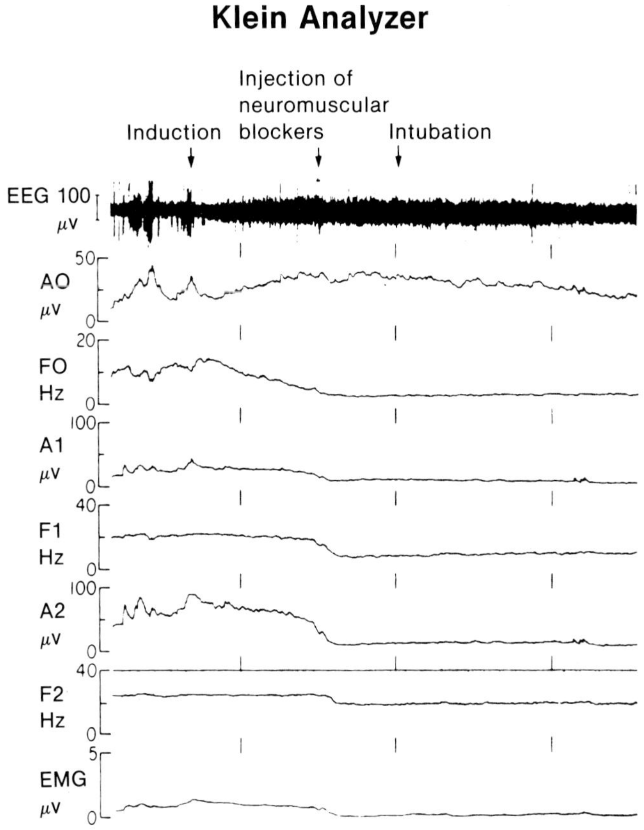

Figure 29–2 • The output from the Klein analyzer recorded during a fentanyl induction. The increase in the amplitude (*A0*) is characteristic of fentanyl analogue inductions as the EEG shifts to lower frequencies (*F0*). Note the sudden decrease in the other variables (*A1, F1, A2, F2, A0*) after muscle relaxants were given. The variables (*A0, A1, A2, F0, F1, F2*) are defined in the text. EMG = electromyograph (used to rule out muscle artifact). (Smith NT, Dec-Silver H, Sanford TJ, Westover CJ, et al. EEGs during high-dose fentanyl-, sufentanil, or morphine-oxygen anesthesia. Anesth Analg 63:386–383, 1984).

that can be plotted as a power vs. frequency histogram. If the time epochs are small, changes in the EEG can be followed continuously and almost in real time.

Power spectral analysis has many advantages and is incorporated in many contemporary computerized EEG instruments. Its advantages are that it retains most of the information from the raw EEG and detects small changes in frequency and amplitude. By retaining and displaying frequency data along the whole spectrum of the EEG, changes in one frequency cannot be counterbalanced or cancelled out by changes in another frequency, as occurs in an averaging technique. Power spectral analysis can also be computer enhanced to display four separate channels of EEG simultaneously and may allow for the monitoring of regional changes. Additionally, it is agreed that changes in spectral analysis are well correlated to clinical conditions. However, further attempts at enhancing the display by using various techniques of smoothing and averaging are believed to alter the accuracy and resolution of the frequency spectrum.

a. Displays of the Power Spectrum

Following fast Fourier transform calculations, it is necessary to present an otherwise massive amount of data in a simple, useful format for rapid interpretation by the clinician. Numerous displays have been designed from the resultant power spectrum. Two of these are the *compressed spectral array (CSA)* and a Grey scale display known as *density modulated spectral array (DSA)* (Fig. 29–4). These displays are linear plots of the derived power spectrum [(amplitude)^2 vs. (frequency)] against a third variable, time. The plots are presented in a manner that simulates a three-dimensional plot (see Fig. 29–4). These displays are updated at specified time intervals that present new data as an overlay of the previous time period. Disadvantages of the CSA include the loss of data hidden behind the updated display and confusion about time and amplitude of the hidden data (Fig. 29–5). On the other hand, the DSA can be read from afar, and may allow for earlier detection of frequency shifts. The DSA format is incorporated in the display of

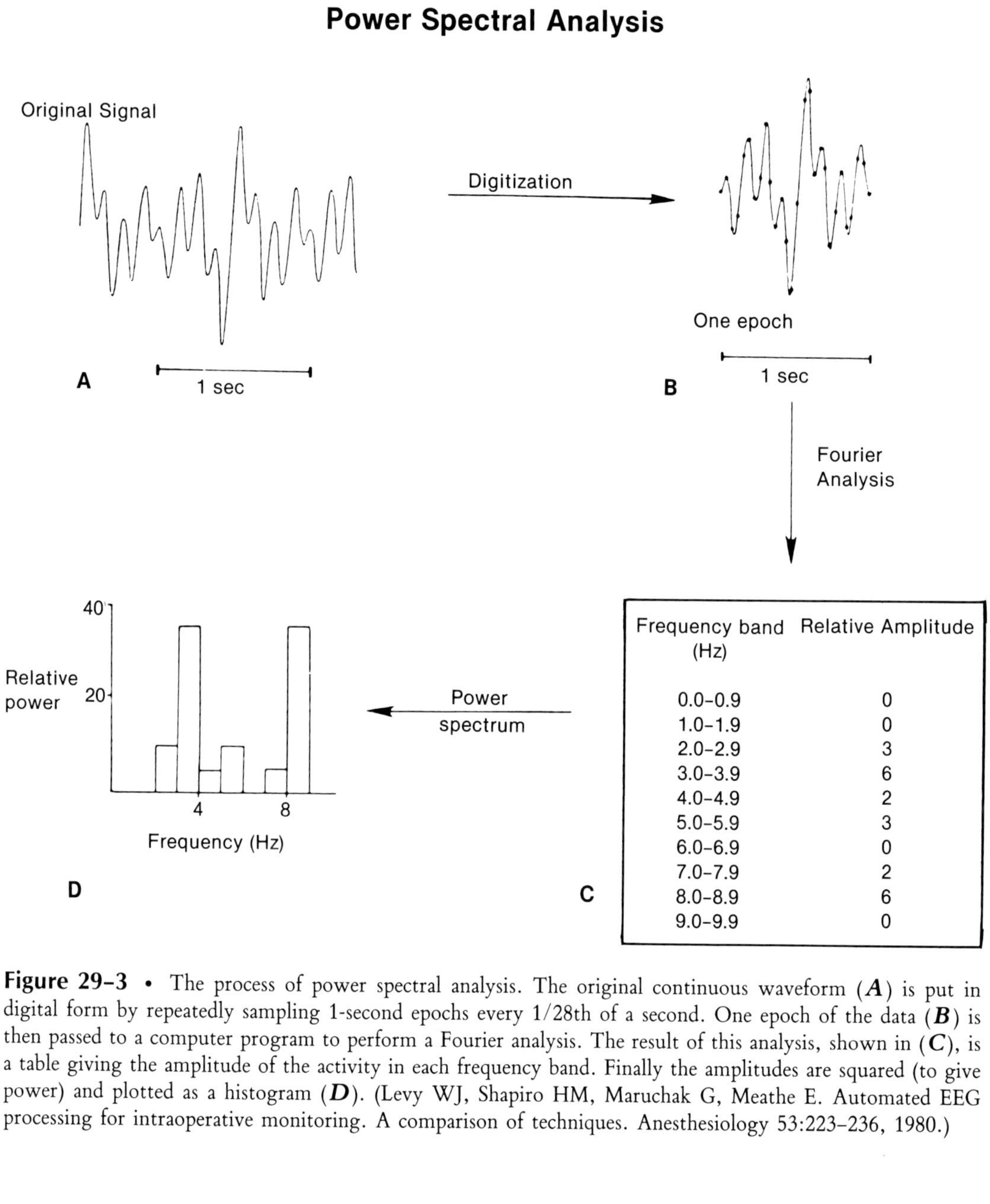

Frequency band (Hz)	Relative Amplitude
0.0–0.9	0
1.0–1.9	0
2.0–2.9	3
3.0–3.9	6
4.0–4.9	2
5.0–5.9	3
6.0–6.9	0
7.0–7.9	2
8.0–8.9	6
9.0–9.9	0

Figure 29–3 • The process of power spectral analysis. The original continuous waveform (***A***) is put in digital form by repeatedly sampling 1-second epochs every 1/28th of a second. One epoch of the data (***B***) is then passed to a computer program to perform a Fourier analysis. The result of this analysis, shown in (***C***), is a table giving the amplitude of the activity in each frequency band. Finally the amplitudes are squared (to give power) and plotted as a histogram (***D***). (Levy WJ, Shapiro HM, Maruchak G, Meathe E. Automated EEG processing for intraoperative monitoring. A comparison of techniques. Anesthesiology 53:223–236, 1980.)

the Neurotrac analyzer (Interspec, Conshohocken, PA). In addition, the DSA has been colorized and incorporated in the Cerebro Trac 2500 (SRD Ltd, Moshav Shorashim, Israel). The generation of these displays by computer processing of the EEG are reviewed in detail by Levy and associates.[1]

3. APERIODIC ANALYSIS

Some authors believe that the random or stochastic nature of the EEG and the finite time periods of each epoch render aperiodic analysis more useful than power spectral analysis. The technique of *aperiodic analysis* was described by Demetrescu in 1975 and was eventually incorporated into the Lifescan monitor (Diatek, San Diego, CA).[6] Instead of averaging a large number of waveforms over a given epoch, each waveform is mapped in relationship to its frequency, amplitude, and time of occurrence (Fig. 29–6). To accomplish this, the EEG signal is divided into three components: 1–8 Hz, 9–30 Hz, and a composite signal, having the potential to contain spikes, that is read as an artifact. Each component mea-

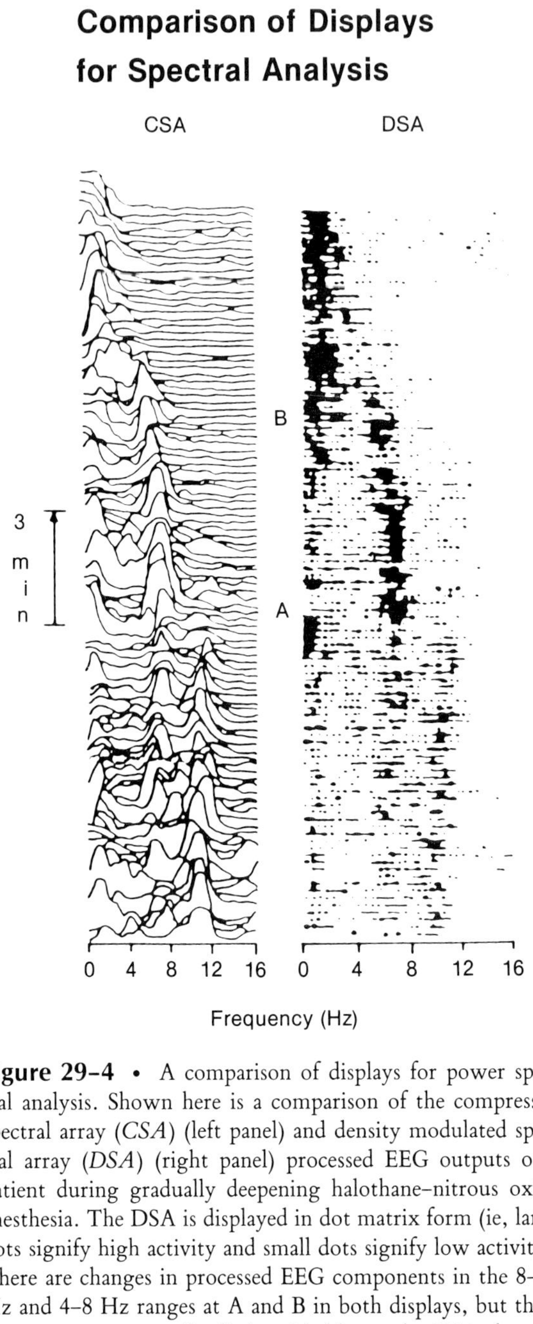

Figure 29-4 • A comparison of displays for power spectral analysis. Shown here is a comparison of the compressed spectral array (*CSA*) (left panel) and density modulated spectral array (*DSA*) (right panel) processed EEG outputs of a patient during gradually deepening halothane-nitrous oxide anesthesia. The DSA is displayed in dot matrix form (ie, large dots signify high activity and small dots signify low activity). There are changes in processed EEG components in the 8–12 Hz and 4–8 Hz ranges at A and B in both displays, but these changes are more easily distinguishable on the DSA than on the CSA. (Levy WJ, Shapiro HM, Maruchak G, Meathe E. Automated EEG processing for intraoperation monitoring. A comparison of techniques. Anesthesiology 53:223–236, 1980.)

sures the period of each wave in accordance with conventional EEG practice. Slow and fast waves are detected differently. Detection of fast waves requires only consecutive peaks and valleys (Fig. 29–7), whereas detection of slow waves requires the presence of zero-crossings between the highest peaks and lowest valleys (Fig. 29–8).[7]

The computer detects waves peaks, valleys, zero-crossings, and length of time between valleys. A *wave* is defined by detecting a valley, a peak, and then another valley. The *period* of the wave is the time between valleys. *Frequency* is defined as the reciprocal of the period. The data are stored in memory as the frequency (Hz), amplitude (fV), and the time of occurrence of each wave. The processed EEG is then displayed on a color screen that can be programmed to display both right and left cerebral hemispheres using a time scale from 5 to 30 minutes/screen. Frequency is displayed on the x-axis from values of 0.5 to 30 Hz. The power of each wave is calculated on the basis of the amplitude^2 and is displayed as a vertical "telephone pole" proportional to the amplitude. The position of each telephone pole is plotted on the screen at a point along the x-axis corresponding to the frequency of the wave and on the y-axis determined by the time of occurrence. This display is continuously updated and is presented as a real-time EEG analysis as a progression of telephone poles. These telephone poles are also color coded to represent the various frequencies (eg, delta, theta). In addition, the current version of this system of analysis is able to continually display the spectral edge frequency (see later). The Lifescan monitor, like other processed EEG monitors currently in use, has the advantage of being relatively easy to use, because it requires a simple five-lead montage and minimal set-up time and maintenance. There is a significant amount of recent literature describing the use of the Lifescan monitor and the effects of various anesthetics and other changes induced by surgery or other clinical conditions (see the later section on interpretation).

C. *Univariant Descriptors of the Raw EEG*

For the processed EEG to be a useful monitor, no matter what technique of computerized analysis or display is used, the reader of the EEG must be familiar with the patterns that correlate with various clinical conditions. To further enhance the ability of the clinician to interpret the intraoperative EEG, there has been an effort to develop numerically derived parameters or univariant descriptors that quantify various aspects of the raw EEG and to correlate these data with clinical data. Examples of these descriptors include spectral edge frequency, median power frequency, and peak power frequency (Fig. 29–9).

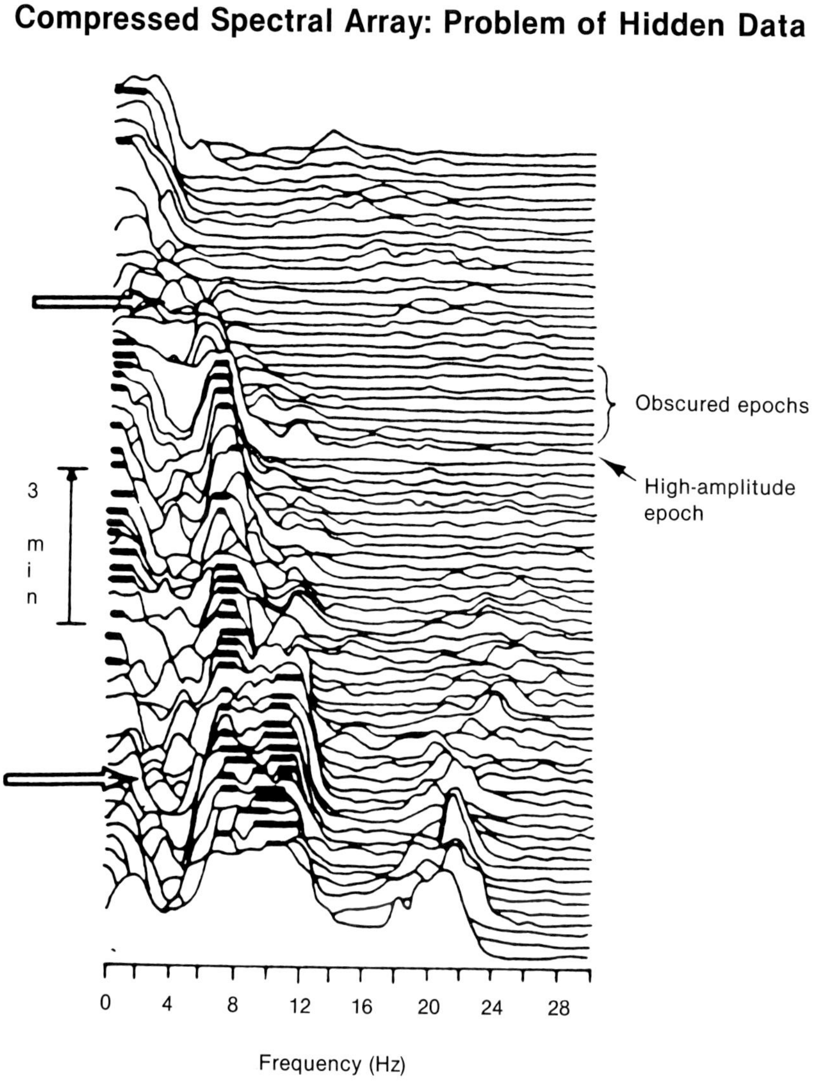

Figure 29-5 • An example of problems with the linear display of the CSA. (1) Loss of data. An epoch of high-amplitude activity is shown obscuring part of the data in subsequent epochs for almost 3 minutes. Many changes in the 0–7 Hz range of the EEG during this time would not be detectable. In an effort to prevent an even greater loss of data when very high amplitude activity occurs, "hills" may be truncated, as indicated by the heavy horizontal lines. Unfortunately, this only changes the amount of the data lost; it does not prevent some of the loss. (2) Confusion of time and amplitude. Because time and amplitude of the EEG spectrum are displayed on the same axis, an identifiable baseline is needed to estimate the amplitude. The low-amplitude, high-frequency segment of the epoch often serves as such a baseline. However, in areas such as those identified by the hollow arrows, it may be difficult or impossible to identify baseline and estimate EEG activity. (Levy WJ, Shapiro HM, Maruchak G, Meathe E. Automated EEG processing for intraoperative monitoring. A comparison of techniques. Anesthesiology 53:223–236, 1980.)

1. SPECTRAL EDGE FREQUENCY

Spectral edge frequency (SEF), as defined by Rampil, is the upper-frequency limit of the statistical distribution of the frequency spectrum (ie, the +2 standard deviation point).[8] As originally described, it was measured downward from the 97th percentile. However, the most commonly used SEF is the so-called *SEF-95,* meaning that 95% of the EEG power lies at frequencies below the SEF-95. To put it more simply, the SEF is the highest frequency at which a significant amount of energy is present in the EEG (see Fig. 29-9). The SEF is an optional parameter on most current EEG-processing machines. It is usually displayed as an overlay on the processed EEG or as a number that is the frequency of the calculated SEF.

Rampil and associates studied the usefulness of the SEF in a group of patients undergoing carotid endarterectomies.[9] They defined a significant change in cerebral well-being as a change of 50% or more in the SEF-95. This study demonstrated that significant changes in the EEG, indicative of cerebral ischemia, were for the most part detected intraoperatively with the SEF-95 and that these changes were predictive of gross neurologic outcome. Rampil and associates also showed that the SEF was useful in providing a rapid, simple, and sensitive indication of anesthetic depth. However, SEF should never be the sole parameter used to detect cerebral ischemia.[10] Instead, the SEF should be viewed in conjunction with other changes in the processed EEG, such as loss of symmetry or the presence of an artifact when monitoring for the presence or absence of ischemia. The SEF has also been used to set up a computer controller for delivery of anesthesia.[11]

Operational Principle of Lifescan™

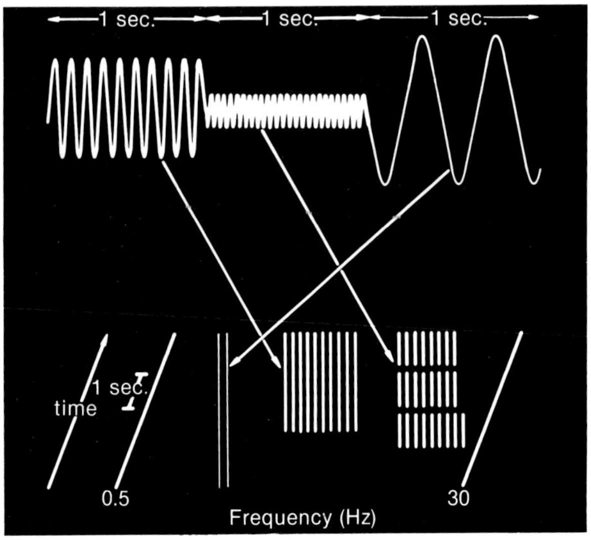

Figure 29-6 • The operational principle of the Lifescan EEG analyzer. The algorithm used searches for the local extremes of the raw EEG waveform. For each peak and valley detected (top) the amplitude and time of occurrence are measured. The amplitude of each wave after processing is assigned to a "telephone pole," which is then correlated with its frequency of occurrence (bottom). To detect the simultaneous occurrence of low frequency (delta or theta waves), a fast- *and* a slow-wave detection process are performed (see Figs. 29-7 and 29-8). Colors are assigned to the various "telephone poles" depending on the frequency of the wave. Note that not all of the waves can be represented on the screen, since the screen would become too crowded. (For more details of the aperiodic analysis algorithm see Gregory TK, Pettus DC. An electroencephalographic processing algorithm specifically intended for analysis of cerebral electrical activity. J Clin Monit 2:190–197, 1986.)

2. Median and Peak Power Frequencies

The *median power frequency (MPF)* is defined as that frequency that lies at the midpoint of the EEG power distribution (ie, 50% of the total power of the EEG power is at frequencies less than the MPF, and 50% of the total power of the EEG lies above the MPF) (see Fig. 29-9). The MPF has been used clinically to help develop a closed-loop feedback control for anesthesia.[12] When compared with other descriptors such as SEF, total power, and frequency band ratios, the MPF has been found to be a very useful indicator of the depth of anesthesia.[13] The MPF is a more sensitive descriptor of anesthetic depth than other descriptors. However, one of the drawbacks of using the MPF or even the SEF to serve as controlling parameters for anesthesia delivery is that not all anesthetics have the same effect on the EEG and the univariant descriptors. The MPF may be useless unless the effects of these individual anesthetics, as well as combinations of these anesthetics, are known.

The *peak power frequency (PPF)* is the frequency with the greatest power in the spectrum (ie, the mode of the spectrum) (see Fig. 29-9). Its disadvantage, like the MPF, is that it excludes the very low-frequency or delta wave band end of the power spectrum. Thus, use of the PPF to monitor high-dose fentanyl anesthesia, which results in a marked shift into the low-frequency delta band, would result in misinterpretation of the EEG.

3. Other Univariant Descriptors of the Raw EEG

In addition to the processed forms of the EEG, there have been other attempts to use the data from the raw EEG. One such suggestion is the grouping of data from each epoch of the aperiodic analysis into descriptors such as the following: number of waves, percent of power, total power, mean power per wave, cumulative percent power for each of 30 one-Hz intervals, the total number of waves, total power, and mean power per wave for all frequencies combined.[14] This grouping is an effort to differentiate the effects of various drugs and clinical events on specific portions of the EEG. For example, the effects of opiates such as fentanyl and alfentanil produced different, easily recognizable changes in the processed EEG when compared with thiopental.[14] Efforts to break up the EEG as described are also an effort to judge the depth of anesthesia and the need for more or less anesthetic.[15] The most recent univariant descriptor of the EEG is the *burst suppression ratio,* which is suggested as a way to quantify the burst suppression phenomenon and may even be used to describe the EEG signature of various anesthetics.[16] The usefulness of any of these univariant descriptors of the EEG still needs to be documented.

D. *Which Processed EEG Should I Buy?*

There are many different ways in which the raw EEG is processed, and numerous machines are commercially available. Whatever the choice of instrument or process, several very desirable features of the processed EEG should be taken into account before a machine is purchased (Table 29-2).

Detection of Fast Waves: Lifescan™

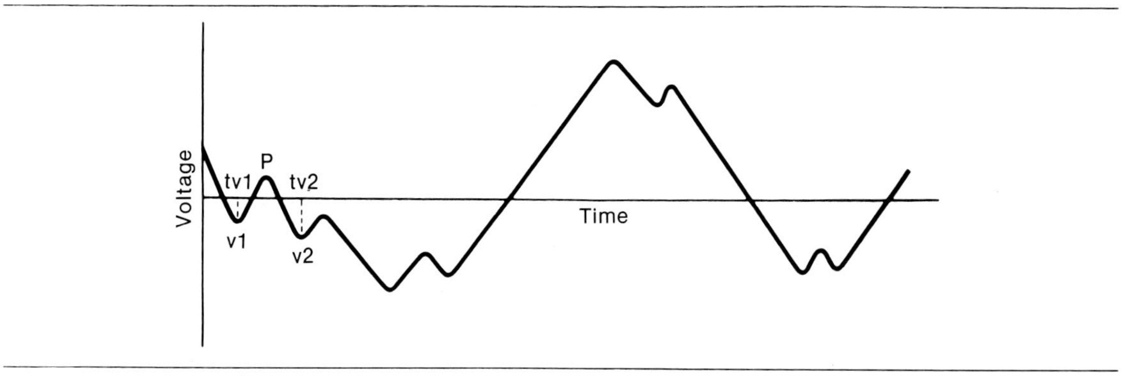

Figure 29–7 • The basic fast-wave detection procedure of the Lifescan analyzer. The algorithm used analyzes the signal for extremes in the waveform voltages. For each peak and valley, the voltage amplitude and the time of occurrence are measured. The computer then extracts wave amplitude and frequency from these data. A *wave* is defined as a fluctuation in voltage that occurs between two local minima in voltages (*v1–v2*). The algorithm then scans for the local maximum peak (*P*). The *amplitude* of the wave is defined as the average of the difference in voltage between P and v1 and the difference in voltage between P and v2. The *frequency* of the wave is then defined as the inverse of the in time (*tv1 and tv2*) between the occurrence of v1 and v2. (Gregory TK, Pettus DC. An electroencephalographic processing algorithm specifically intended for anlysis of cerebral electrical activity. J Clin Monit 2:190–197, 1986.)

1. The EEG system should have a minimum of two channels because ischemia may be unilateral, and two channels are required to help recognize such focal ischemia.
2. An impedance tester is needed to insure the status of electrode contact (see the section on electrode placement).
3. The EEG system must have a continuous hard copy or retrievable memory to facilitate comparisons of the EEG at different points in time.
4. The EEG system should have artifact rejection and flagging capabilities to reduce the intrusion of artifact into the output and to reduce the possibility of misinterpretation.
5. The raw EEG signal should be accessible for inspection (an important element for quality control).
6. The processed EEG algorithm should preserve both frequency and amplitude information. Excessive simplification of the data creates the potential for misrepresentation.

Detection of Slow Waves: Lifescan™

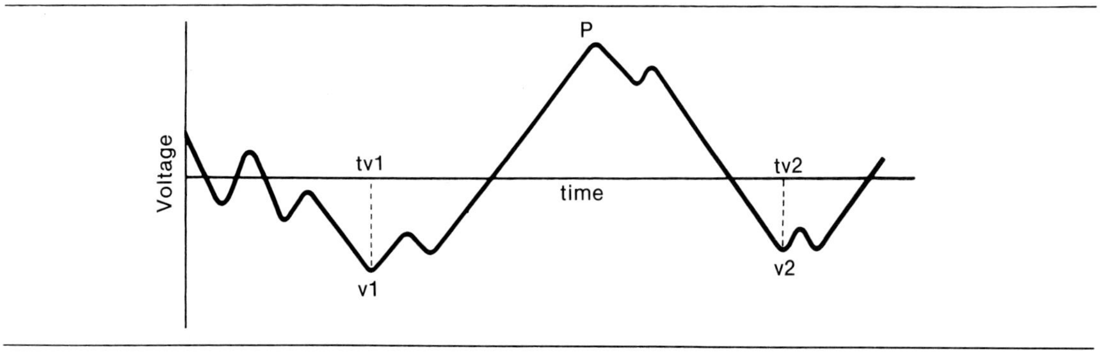

Figure 29–8 • Detection of slow waves by Lifescan analysis. This method is similar to the fast-wave detection except that it detects the largest valleys (*v1, v2*) and peaks (*P*) between zero voltage crossings. (Gregory TK, Pettus DC. An electroencephalographic processing algorithm specifically intended for analysis of cerebral electrical activity. J Clin Monit 2:190–197, 1986.)

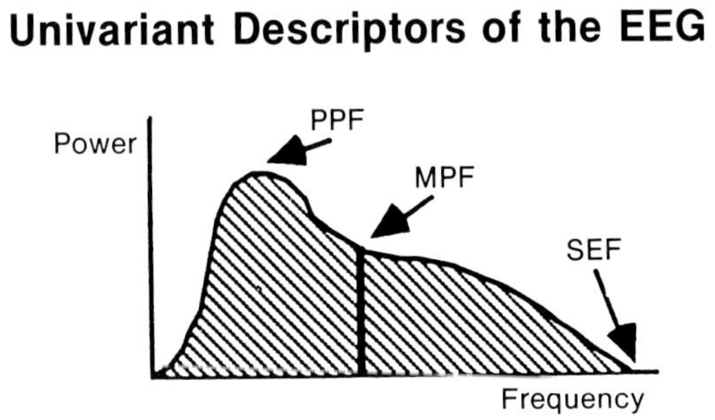

Figure 29–9 • The derivation of univariant descriptors. The information obtained from the computer-processed power-frequency spectrum is treated in a manner so that descriptive statistics and parameters such as peak power frequency (*PPF*), median power frequency (*MPF*), and spectral edge frequency (*SEF*) are defined. The SEF is the upper frequency limit of the statistical distribution of the frequency spectrum (ie, the +2 standard deviation point). The PPF is the frequency with the greatest power in the spectrum (ie, the mode of the spectrum). The MPF is the frequency that lies at the midpoint of the EEG power distribution. (Rampil IJ, et al. Procedures in anesthesia and intensive care. Int J Clin Monit Comput 4:85–98, 1987.)

II. Specific Indications for Processed EEG Monitoring

The specific indications for intraoperative monitoring of the EEG are not yet uniformly accepted so as to constitute the standard of practice. Use of the EEG to detect the intraoperative development of cerebral ischemia, no matter what the cause, is the most common indication. However, there are several applications of intraoperative EEG monitoring that may be useful, especially if the surgical procedure has the potential to put the cerebral circulation at risk (Table 29–3). These situations include cardiopulmonary bypass, carotid endarterectomy, and procedures in which deliberate hypotension is needed. Other indications for intraoperative monitoring of the EEG include the need to monitor the depth of anesthesia or maintain electrocerebral silence, as well as disaster prophylaxis and epilepsy surgery.

Table 29–2 • Desirable Features of Processed EEG Instruments

1. Minimum of two channels
2. Built-in impedance tester
3. Retrievable memory or hard copy
4. Artifact indication
5. Accessible raw EEG
6. Algorithm uses both frequency and amplitude data

Table 29–3 • Specific Indications for EEG Monitoring

1. Monitoring depth of anesthesia
2. Quantification of anesthetic potency
3. Cardiopulmonary bypass
4. Carotid artery surgery
5. Deliberate hypotension
6. Monitoring barbiturate coma
7. Disaster prophylaxis
8. Epilepsy surgery

Whatever the indication, the use of intraoperative EEG monitoring must be viewed with caution. The user must not base clinical decisions on the information from the EEG, no matter how well processed and presented that information is. Instead, EEG changes must be viewed in conjunction with other vital information such as blood pressure, temperature, depth of anesthesia, and surgical manipulation. It has been suggested that one of the reasons for the pessimism about the usefulness of intraoperative EEG monitoring has resulted from attempts to use the EEG by itself without consideration of the above factors.[17]

A. *Monitoring the Depth of Anesthesia*

The determination of the depth of anesthesia and, consequently, the lack of awareness during anesthesia was the original intraoperative application of the EEG. As early as 1890, the effects of chloroform anesthesia on the brain waves were noted.[18] These and other early studies led to the conclusion that the EEG was able to continuously measure the effect of drugs on the brain and had the potential to be an adequate physiologic indicator of anesthetic depth. It was clear that many broad generalizations could be applied to effects of anesthetic agents on the EEG. These included the characteristics of light anesthesia, which were thought to produce active synchronized activity, whereas increasing the depth of anesthesia was supposedly characterized by decreasing frequency and amplitude of waves. Unfortunately, there is tremendous variation in these classical effects depending on the specific agent or combination of agents being used. Also, there is a moderate degree of individual patient variation that occurs even if the same agent is used.

Despite these variations among agents and individual patients, several recent studies have looked at the EEG effects of the modern anesthetic agents such as the fentanyl analogues and inhalation agents.[19,20] These studies have described what appear to be consistent, predictable patterns of anesthetic effects on the EEG and have tried to correlate the EEG with lack of awareness and anesthetic depth.[19] An early effort to determine whether or not high-dose fentanyl was capable of producing a state of anesthesia (ie, lack of awareness) studied the effects of 30 to 70 μg/kg of fentanyl on the EEG of patients undergoing coronary artery bypass grafting.[20] This study recorded, analyzed, and classified the EEG according to clinical status of the patient and constructed "narcograms." These narcograms were based on the specific appearance of the raw EEG, which ranged from an awake state characterized by normal alpha high-frequency rhythm to continuous low-frequency delta activity of high amplitude. There was no incidence of awareness, and the authors concluded that fentanyl produced a characteristic EEG response.

Smith and coworkers, using the Lifescan monitor, compared the EEG produced by alfentanil with the EEG produced by fentanyl, sufentanil, and thiopental.[19] Effects of the high-dose fentanyl analogues on the EEG resulted in a characteristic pattern of high amplitude and low frequency (delta wave) that was easily discernible on the color display of the Lifescan monitor.[20] The increasing depth of anesthesia produced by these potent opiates was easily followed on the monitor.

In contrast to the fentanyl analogues, thiopental produced a different EEG effect, characterized by a pattern of concentrated power in the midfrequency theta range, that was also easily followed on the Lifescan display screen.[14] In addition to pattern recognition of anesthetic effects on the EEG, this study compared previously derived variables such as number of waves, percent of power, total power, mean power per wave, cumulative percent power (CP) for each of 30 one-Hz intervals, the total number of waves (TNW), total power (TP) at various frequencies, SEF-90, and mean power per wave for all frequencies. This study concluded that, in addition to the easily recognized patterns resulting from injectable anesthetics, certain derived parameters can be used to characterize individual anesthetics.

Other injectable agents such as the benzodiazepines produce an effect on the processed EEG that results in a "carpeting" of the entire display with low-amplitude, multiple-frequency "telephone poles," which make interpretation of the processed EEG difficult. A comparison of fentanyl and its analogues with morphine has also been made.[19] The inhalation agents halothane, enflurane, and isoflurane also produce characteristic patterns on the processed EEG.

B. *Quantification of Anesthetic Potency*

In addition to the characteristic patterns produced on the EEG by various injectable anesthetic agents, there have been several reports of the use of various derived parameters of the EEG to quantify and model the clinical pharmacology of intravenous anesthetics.[15,21] Hudson and coworkers used changes in the SEF-95 (derived from the power spectral analysis of the EEG) to study anesthetic depth and acute tolerance to thiopental following sequential doses of thiopental.[15] The model developed was believed to be an adequate pharmacodynamic model for thiopental anesthesia and led to the suggestion that by continually monitoring the spectral edge of the EEG, a continuous measure of the depth of anesthesia could be developed. Bowdle and Ward studied the EEG effects of various induction doses of fentanyl and sufentanil in an attempt to differentiate the pharmacologic potency of these agents.[21] They concluded that the EEG was able to distinguish differences in potency at higher doses. An earlier study attempted to correlate clinical changes in patient condition with both blood levels of fentanyl and alfentanil and the spectral edge.[11] As well as concluding that the EEG could be used to track narcotic anesthetic effect, this study demonstrated a significant lag between peak fentanyl and alfentanil plasma concentrations and peak spectral edge changes. This time lag between EEG changes and peak plasma drug levels was less for alfentanil than for fentanyl. It was concluded that the continual monitoring of the processed EEG is a valid tool for studying the pharmacodynamics of narcotic anesthetics.

The EEG has been suggested as a method of providing a closed-loop feedback control of anesthesia.[12] Using the MPF of the EEG power spectrum, Schwilden and associates suggested that not only can anesthesia depth be controlled by a servo feedback loop, but also that, of the derived EEG descriptors, the MPF is a valid choice to be used for control.[12]

Finally, any conclusion that the EEG is a totally reliable indicator of adequacy of narcotic-induced anesthesia, or of any anesthetic, must be tempered by the fact that EEG indicators of anesthetic depth may not indicate the presence of sympathetic response to surgical stimulation.[22] As an indicator of the depth of anesthesia, the processed EEG at present is, at best, a good means of confirming our clinical impressions and identifying anesthetic trends.

C. *Carotid Endarterectomy*

As mentioned earlier, changes in the nonprocessed EEG induced by critical events during carotid endarterectomy surgery may be separated by many inches of paper. An early report concluded that automating the raw EEG did not increase the sensitivity with which changes during carotid surgery were seen, but that the processed EEG provides simplicity of use and clarity of display that were advantages over the raw EEG.[1] Although there is not absolute agreement among vascular surgeons and anesthesiologists, the EEG is now widely used as one of the guidelines to help determine the necessity for a shunt during the time of carotid occlusion. Most surgeons will place a shunt if there is an EEG change during the period of test occlusion. However, there is no agreement as to what degree of change in the EEG must occur before a shunt is placed. Some groups prefer that a shunt be placed for any detectable ischemic change in the EEG.[23] Another view is that a profound change in the EEG indicative of ischemia must be present before a shunt is placed.[24]

Whether or not the processed EEG is a better monitor of cerebral ischemia is still a point of debate. Rampil and colleagues stated that the loss of high-frequency activity from a DSA of a single EEG channel analysis was not only easy to visualize, but was predictive of gross neurologic outcome following carotid surgery in patients who did not have preoperative neurologic deficits.[9] There is some controversy about whether or not a single univariant descriptor of the EEG (eg, SEF-95) can diagnose cerebral ischemia with certainty, and whether or not visual inspection of the real-time processed EEG reflected a neurologist's later interpretation of the ischemic events on the raw EEG.[25] These authors concluded that the processed EEG was able to serve as a trend monitor to reflect changes in cerebral blood flow that can result in recognized patterns of ischemia. Ischemic changes on the processed EEG record correlate with profound changes in cerebral blood flow during carotid occlusion and were able to be interpreted as ischemia by a nonneurologist.[26] However, in this study there were false negatives when cerebral blood flow was marginal. The conclusion of this study was that automated EEG such as the Lifescan analyzer is a useful monitor during carotid endarterectomy. Recently, Silbert and colleagues proposed that the processed EEG may not be an adequate monitor for cerebral ischemia during carotid surgery.[27]

Our experience with use of the processed EEG during carotid endarterectomy has resulted in the diagnosis of cerebral ischemia during carotid occlusion (Color Fig. 8). We have also been able to diagnose an instance is which the shunt was malpositioned, as evidenced by the failure of a change in the processed EEG to return to the preocclusion pattern. Indeed, we believe that the best way for the anesthesiologist to use the processed EEG instruments is by using pattern recognition. However, there are still many unanswered questions concerning the routine use of the EEG during carotid surgery, such as which lead systems are best and whether one or two lead systems are needed to monitor for ischemia. Finally, further work on quantification of changes in cerebral blood flow with single or multiply derived descriptors is needed.

The answer to the question of why the EEG may not be good for monitoring cerebral embolic events relates to the necessity for multiple montages; however, automatic trending with newer instruments may be an advantage to attempting to pick up these focal events. *Keep in mind that hypothermia and hypocapnia associated with coronary artery bypass grafting surgery may mimic the EEG effects of cerebral hypoxia.*

There are also reports of the changes induced in the EEG by changes in the position of the head due to insertion of central venous lines via the internal jugular vein, and to neck extension during intubation attempts.[28,29]

D. *Cardiac Surgery*

The routine use of EEG monitoring (processed or not) during cardiac surgery is still controversial.[29,30] Changes in EEG during cardiopulmonary bypass are confounded by changes of hypothermia and hypocapnia, as well as other events such as hypotension, particulate emboli, air emboli, and even cannula malposition or vascular clamp problems. Specific indications for routine EEG monitoring during cardiac surgery are few. However, monitoring for burst suppression during barbiturate-induced electrocerebral silence, especially during surgeries requiring deep hypothermia and circulatory arrest, necessitates

EEG monitoring. In addition, the administration of barbiturate for cerebral protection during the onset of cardiopulmonary bypass is another indication for continuous EEG monitoring during routine coronary artery bypass surgery.[31]

Several groups have found that postoperative EEG changes correlate well with intraoperative changes in the EEG.[27,32] These results support the experience from the Mayo Clinic with carotid surgery, in which no patient awoke with a new neurologic deficit who did not have intraoperative EEG changes. However, the many changes seen on the EEG during cardiac surgery that could be indicative of cerebral ischemia have not always resulted in postoperative neurologic deficits.

Since the EEG changes induced by hypothermia, hypocapnia, and hypoxia can appear to be similar, it has been suggested that one of the derived descriptors of the processed EEG be used during cardiopulmonary bypass to help separate changes due to hypoxia from those due to hypothermia.[33] During the cooling phase of bypass, changes in the EEG univariant descriptors followed a variable pattern of correlation with decreasing temperature. During rewarming, several descriptors such as total power and the peak power frequency of the high-frequency range showed a linear correlation with rewarming. On the other hand, spectral edge and average frequency did not correlate with temperature changes. However, it is believed that acute ischemic effects can be separated from temperature effects by observing the magnitude of frequency changes rather than the magnitude of amplitude changes.

In our experience the routine monitoring of the EEG during cardiac surgery is useful as a guide to administration of additional anesthetics, as an indicator of burst suppression during barbiturate administration, and as a guide to the adequacy of cerebral perfusion at the onset of cardiopulmonary bypass. One must interpret changes in the EEG as potentially diagnostic of a problem resulting in global changes, such as a misapplied aortic cross-clamp or embolic phenomena, especially if there are changes in the symmetry of the EEG recording. Bilateral EEG slowing on the initiation of bypass should be followed by a search for the cause. Often the simple raising of perfusion pressure is enough to return the EEG to prebypass levels. The EEG should be watched carefully during the institution of bypass, and the patient should not be made hypothermic before the EEG is deemed satisfactory. An example of a mechanical problem with bypass initiation is shown in Fig. 29–10. Although the search for a mechanical cause of EEG changes during cardiac surgery may not always be fruitful, the occasional positive EEG finding may prevent a potential adverse neurologic outcome.

E. *Induced Hypotension*

Although it is not an absolute indication for routine intraoperative EEG monitoring, the technique of induced hypotension can be facilitated by EEG monitoring. The EEG should be viewed as a guide to the adequacy of cerebral perfusion, and the blood pressure can be adjusted appropriately to maintain cerebral well-being. However, the EEG does not guarantee safety, since only one or, at most, four channels of the EEG are monitored with the computerized instruments. Any resultant EEG abnormality, such as loss of symmetry or bilateral slowing, should be viewed as an indication of inadequate cerebral perfusion, and the blood pressure should be raised accordingly.

F. *Disaster Prophylaxis*

There has been some suggestion that routine monitoring of the EEG would be useful in the early detection of cerebral hypoxia resulting from airway disconnections or inadvertent delivery of hypoxic gas mixtures. However, the changes induced by hypoxemia are relatively late, and there are other monitors such as pulse oximeters and capnographs that are better and earlier indicators of potential hypoxic problems.

G. *Maintenance of Electrocerebral Silence*

The administration of barbiturates to induce and maintain electrocerebral silence has been suggested as a modality to reduce cerebral metabolic oxygen usage. The usefulness of "barbiturate coma" or barbiturate-induced cerebral protection is still very controversial, and its therapeutic value has not been established. However, the EEG, whether or not it is processed, is the best available clinical monitor of the reduction of cerebral oxygen consumption.[34] One of the problems with the processed EEG during barbiturate administration is that the frequency and amplitude of the EEG approaches that of ambient noise; therefore, the gain of the EEG must be

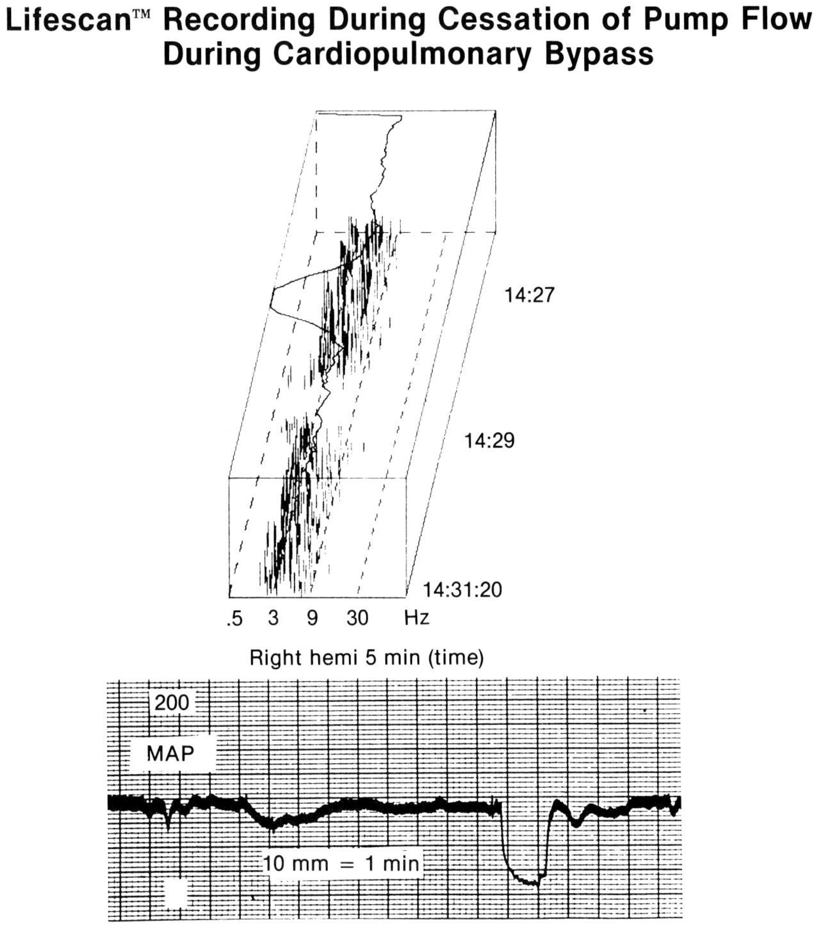

Figure 29–10 • A printout obtained from the Lifescan analyzer showing a mechanical problem during the initiation of cardiopulmonary bypass. The patient had already been begun on bypass when a mechanical problem necessitated the shutdown of the pump at 14:27. The resultant EEG demonstrated loss of frequency and amplitude as well as marked decreased in the spectral edge frequency (here the continuous black line). A tracing of the mean arterial pressure (*MAP*) is also included (lower panel) for comparison of the effects of acute loss of cerebral perfusion pressure. The mechanical problem was resolved, and the patient did not suffer any neurologic sequelae.

in the 50-mV range. An example of burst suppression induced by a large dose of barbiturates is shown in Fig. 29–11.

III. How to Monitor the EEG

A. *EEG Lead Placement*

The most important aspect of EEG monitoring begins with the ability to obtain and make adequate recordings of brain activity. According to one author, "The problem of recording the EEG is the electrical equivalent of finding a needle in a haystack."[17] The weakest point in recording electric activity from the brain is most likely to be in the type and application of electrodes used to pick up the electric signals from the surface of the scalp.

A small error in technique as well as an error in placement of a key electrode can significantly alter the ability of the clinician to interpret tracings correctly. The availability of EEG processors now allows the anesthetist to monitor at least two leads simultaneously. The montage (placement and set-up of electrodes) used should depend on the goal of the monitoring scheme. For instance, the montage used for monitoring depth of anesthesia may be different than that used to detect focal ischemia.

There are several very good methods for assuring adequate electric contact with the patient's scalp. These include use of small gold- or silver-plated cups, platinum or stainless-steel needles, or the common everyday pregelled adhesive silver–silver chloride electrodes used for EKG recording. The cuplike electrodes have the advantage of being relatively insensitive to motion artifact, and they do not dry out as quickly because their cup shape acts as a reservoir for the electrolyte gel. Needle electrodes are the easiest to apply but are very sensitive to motion and can break, as well as carrying a risk for infection and hematoma formation. They are also somewhat painful when placed because they have small surface areas and high electric impedance. However, needle

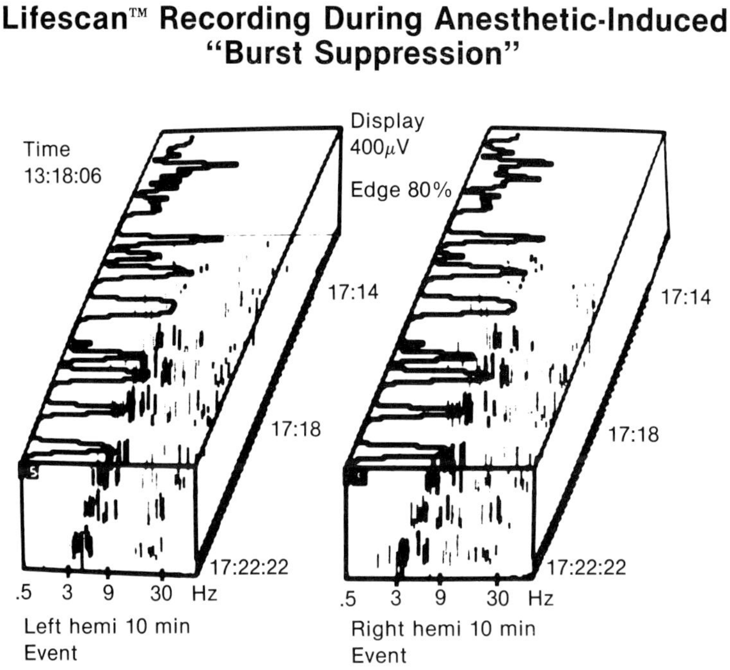

Figure 29-11 • A recording from the Lifescan™ analyzer of EEG showing a pattern of "burst suppression," easily recognized by its saw-tooth pattern and also can easily be seen by following the spectral edge frequency, if displayed. This tracing was obtained during a high-dose isoflurane anesthetic.

electrodes have an advantage in that they can be (or are already) sterilized and can be placed in a sterile operative field.

Actual placement of the electrodes onto the patient depends somewhat on the position of the patient during surgery. If the entire head is accessible, then electrode placement does not need to be particularly intricate. The easiest approach is to apply pre-gelled, self-adhesive pediatric electrocardiographic electrode leads. Probably the most accurate technique for actual lead placement uses gold or silver cup electrodes, which can be placed in a variety of ways. Use of needles or the precious metal cups requires that a strong mechanical connection be insured by gluing these electrodes to the scalp using a solution of collodion. Accurately and securely placing electrodes is time well spent, especially if the electrodes will not be readily available during surgery.

1. SITE PREPARATION

The scalp must be prepared before placement of electrodes. The proper site is first identified. Be sure to identify the site by anatomy and measurements rather than by where the hairline is. If there is hair in the area, a small patch can be shaved. Usually this will be quite inconspicuous, since only about 1 square cm need be shaved. Once the sites are identified, the skin is prepared with an abrasive degreaser such as Omniprep, which is a paste containing a fine pumice. This degreaser lowers the impedance of the skin by removing dead cells and oils. A lower impedance means that electrons (current) may move easier through a specific area. Since the signals to be recorded are on the order of microvolts, a low impedance between the skin and the electrode is necessary. The goal should be an impedance of less than 3000 ohms.

Once the skin has been thoroughly cleaned and abraded with the degreaser (care must be taken to remove all degreaser), the site can be swabbed with an alcohol sponge. For the best quality recordings, the following procedures can be used.

a. Electrode Placement Above the Hairline (Table 29-4)

Table 29-4 • How to Place EEG Leads Above the Hairline

1. Identify the proper sites.
2. Shave the sites if necessary.
3. Scrub with gauze pad and degreaser.
4. Wipe off excess degreaser preparation.
5. Make up several collodion-soaked gauze pads.
6. Place lead on prepared site; put collodion gauze over it.
7. Allow the collodion to dry.
8. Place a small amount of electrolyte gel under gauze.
9. Check impedances as soon as possible.

Table 29-5 • How to Place EEG Leads Below the Hairline

1. Identify the proper sites.
2. Shave the site if necessary.
3. Scrub with gauze pad and degreaser.
4. Wipe off excess degreaser preparation.
5. Apply gel-filled electrode—do not use too much gel.
6. Secure in place with occlusive dressing.
7. Check impedances as soon as possible.

1. If necessary, shave the electrode site.
2. Scrub the site with a gauze pad and Omniprep degreaser.
3. Carefully wipe off all the degreaser.
4. Soak some small squares of gauze in collodion (wear gloves).
5. Apply the electrode to the prepared site, and firmly press the collodion-soaked gauze over it.
6. Allow the collodion to dry (gently blowing on the gauze will help).
7. Using a blunt-tip needle on a 3-mL syringe filled with ultrasonic conduction gel, puncture the gauze, and gently abrade the skin under the electrode.
8. Inject a small amount (0.1 mL) of the gel before removing the needle.

b. Electrode Placement Below The Hairline (Table 29-5)

After the site has been prepared (steps 1–3 in Table 29-5), a gel-filled electrode may be applied and held in place with an occlusive dressing and benzoin. This may be punctured and an additional small amount of gel injected. If too much gel is used, the dressing will not stick.

A faster method is the use of the pediatric or adult ECG electrodes. Although this is the method we prefer for routine EEG monitoring, it has the disadvantage of being somewhat imprecise in terms of the actual area monitored. Following skin prep with Omniprep solution, the ECG pad is firmly applied to the scalp. It is important to frequently check impedances with this method because the electrodes often pull loose.

2. Montage Selection

Confusion surrounding locations for electrode placement existed until 1958, when a standard convention—the *International 10–20 System*—was adopted.[35] Although the designations may seem arbitrary, the International 10–20 System basically uses the following conventions (Table 29-6): F = frontal, C = coronal, T = temporal, O = occipital, Z = midline, FPZ = nasion. Any electrode placement on the right side of the cranium is identified with an even number, and odd numbers refer to the left side of the cranium.

Hundreds of combinations or patterns of electrode placement, known as *montages,* have been suggested. Montages vary among institutions and encephalographers. It must be understood that unlike a specific ECG lead, which monitors the direction of electric activity relative to the position of the electrode, the EEG recorded from a certain electrode represents the electric potential between two electrodes. The inference is that a specific EEG electrode may not be representative of the electric activity directly under that electrode. Therefore, the choice of specific EEG electrode must allow for gaps in coverage and that it is very possible that focal signs of change from specific areas may be missed.[10]

Different montages are used to monitor specific areas of the brain or specific events. The placement of the electrodes for the great majority of cases can be easily accomplished using bilateral frontal-mastoid leads $FP_1 - O_1$ and $FP_2 - O_2$ (Fig. 29-12). This gives the user the ability to assess activity in both hemispheres. Although this electrode system is not particularly sensitive, it is easy to set-up and will show both global and grossly focal (hemispheric) changes (such as during carotid artery surgery). To monitor the depth of anesthesia, a simple $FP_1 - O_1$ and $FP_2 - O_2$ (Fig. 29-13) montage should be sufficient. Note that the actual placement of the occipital lead is really on the mastoid process, since it is usually devoid of hair and is an easy place to clean and affix a pre-gelled lead. To monitor for signs of cerebral ischemia secondary to vascular compromise during carotid surgery, a more complex lead system is probably needed. For the most part, the standard $FP_1 - O_1$ and $FP_2 - O_2$ montage will pick up unilateral cerebral ische-

Table 29-6 • International 10-20 Montage Convention

F	= Frontal	Left side	= EVEN number
C	= Coronal	Right side	= ODD number
Z	= Midline		
O	= Occiput		
T	= Temporal		
FPZ	= Nasion		

Sequence for Placement of EEG Electrodes

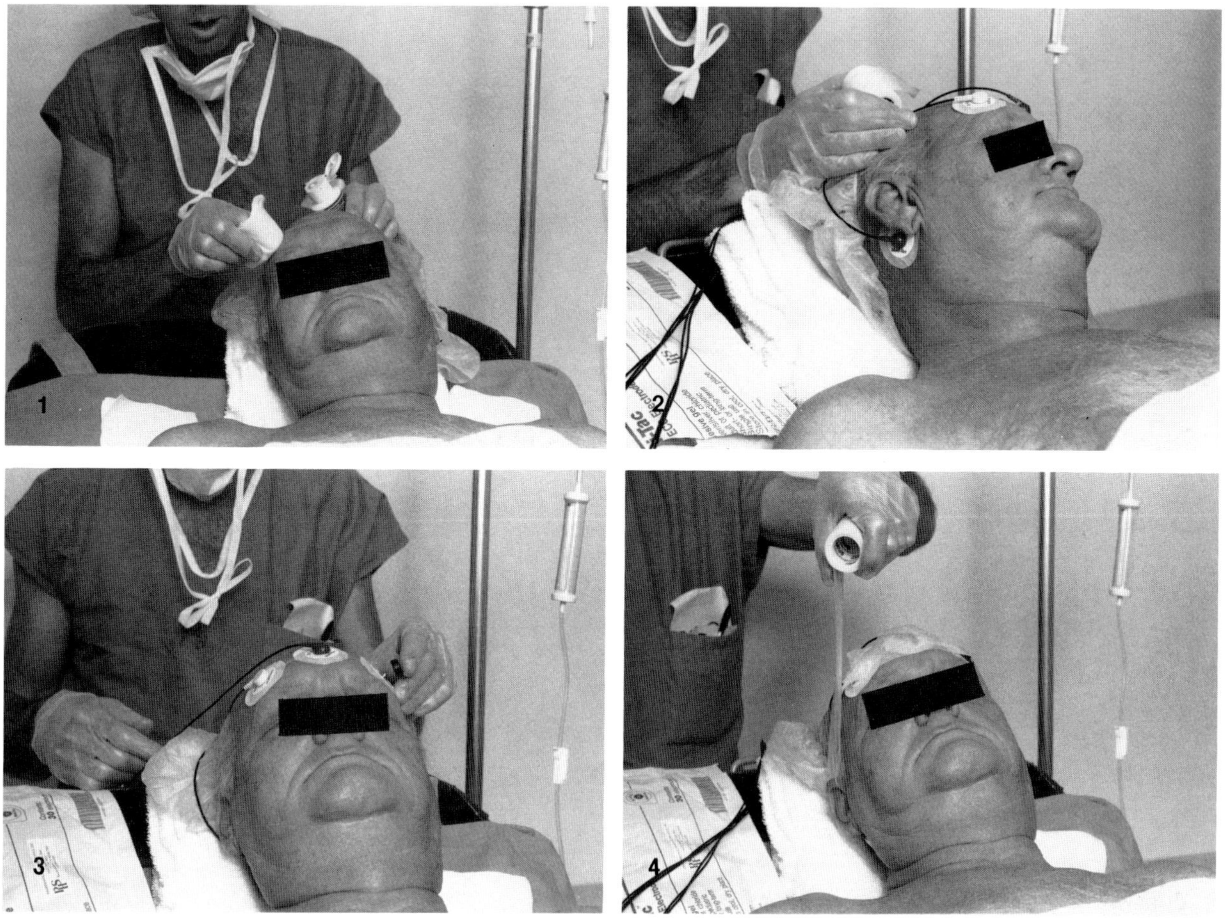

Figure 29–12 • EEG electrode placement for the montage FP_1–A_1 and FP_2–A_2 that is easiest to apply using ECG electrodes below the hair line. Sequence is as follows: (*1*) Following site identification the skin is cleaned using an abrasive degreaser such as Omniprep, and any residual prep is removed. (*2*) Some physicians or technicians use a small amount of benzoin to insure adequate electrode adhesion to the skin. (*3*) The electrodes are then applied to the prepared site. (*4*) Following application of all the electrodes, a strip of wide paper tape is placed over the electrode to insure continued skin contact and to prevent dislodgement of the wires from the electrodes.

mia. If a more specific coverage of the areas served by the middle cerebral artery is required, the montage should be constructed of an $F_3 - C_3$ and $F_4 - C_4$ (see Fig. 29–12) and should be secured with precious metal cups or needle scalp electrodes.

B. *How to Use the EEG in the Operating Room*

Whatever montage is chosen to perform intraoperative EEG monitoring, the basic set-up and guidelines for the application and interpretation of the EEG are the same. We recommend the following checklist for set-up and interpretation. Although some of the items on the list may sound simple, it is often the simple things that get omitted and delay or prevent adequate intraoperative EEG monitoring and interpretation (Table 29–7).

1. Once the electrodes have been placed on the patient, they must be connected to the EEG device. In the case of processed EEG machines, the scalp electrodes are connected via some sort of preamplifier. After lead placement, the next area of potential problem is malpositioning of the leads in the preamplifier. Care must be taken to insure that the proper lead is plugged into the corresponding connector slot. Crossed leads are one of the most common causes of EEG misinterpretation.

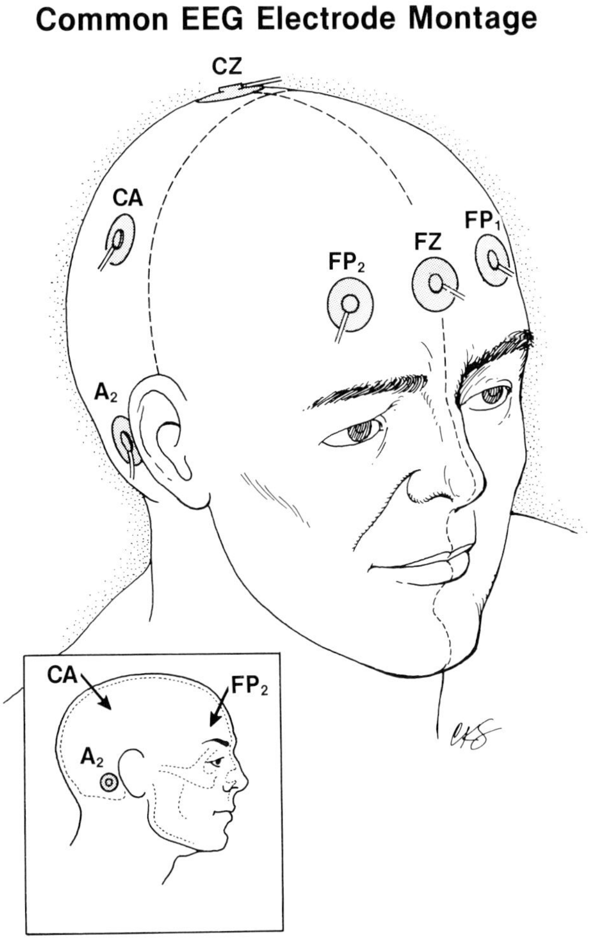

Figure 29–13 • An example of the commonly used bilateral montage FP_1–A_1 and FP_2–A_2 (right side) and other lead placement sites for EEG monitoring. Although the actual lead is placed very near the mastoid, there is no Standard International 10–20 System symbol for the mastoid lead. Instead, the closest accepted labelled site is the A lead site. Also shown is the common ground lead placed in the center of the forehead (Fz).

2. Connect the preamplifier cable to the EEG machine.
3. Turn on the machine. As simple as this may sound, it must be understood that almost all of the currently available processed EEG devices when turned on go through a certain period of warm-up and an automatic self-check of computer software. In addition, there is some initial check on the integrity of the cable connections.
4. Select various parameters such as time base, hemispheres to be displayed, spectral edge, and so forth. The operator must elect certain parameters, or most machines will default to predetermined settings. Minimally, this portion of the set-up procedure should include the following:
   a. Set the computer clock to the current time.
   b. Select a time base that allows for an updating of the screen that is neither too fast to show changes that occur gradually (ie, over several minutes) nor too slow to detect changes that occur rapidly. In other words, compressing the time scale to allow the viewing of an hour's worth of EEG on one screen will not allow for minor changes to be seen. Conversely, a short time scale will not allow for detection of gradual changes.
   c. Select an EEG display that at least begins with a display of both hemispheres.
   d. Make a copy of the baseline EEG. This can either be made on a paper write-out or more easily stored in the memory of the computer.
   e. Select a wave amplitude range, more correctly known as the *gain*. The selection is usually between 200 fV and 400 fV. We usually set the range at 400 fV because this enhances the ability to "see behind" the continuous recording of the processed EEG. However, if the EEG is to be monitored for burst suppression during hypothermia and barbiturate administration, the gain must be reduced to 50 fV.
   f. Select the SEF to be monitored. Most machines will present the option to set the SEF at any frequency. However, as discussed earlier, the minimum SEF should probably be 80%, and we often select 90%. Be aware that most machines will default the SEF at 80%.
5. Check the integrity of the electrode connection to the patient. This is done by checking the impedance of each individual electrode. This is usually done electronically and is either shown in some sort of color coding (red indicating no electrode contact; yellow, poor contact; and green, good contact) or as actual numeric values. These values should be low, and although they do not need to be identical, they should be in the same range. If the initial indica-

Table 29–7 • Checklist for Intraoperative Processed EEG

1. Turn on the instrument.
2. Verify proper electrode placement.
3. Connect electrodes to preamplifier.
4. Select parameters:
   a. Time base
   b. Spectral edge
   c. Number of channels
   d. Wave amplitude range
5. Check impedance.
6. Check raw EEG.
7. Make a hard copy of baseline, or store a baseline tracing.
8. *Begin recording before induction of anesthesia.*

tor of impedance is high, the electrode should be reapplied. It is important when reapplying an electrode that all the steps for applying the electrode are followed. One reason for early application of the electrodes (ie, in the hold area) is that the electrolyte gel has time to soak and establish good skin contact.

Electrode impedance should then be checked as often as every hour to insure that the electrodes have not lost their skin contact. If the impedance begins to go up, it usually indicates either that the electrolyte gel is drying out and needs to be replenished or that the entire electrode needs to be replaced.

6. Check the raw EEG, looking for such things as ECG artifact. If this is present, the processed EEG may interpret this artifact as a waveform and attempt to include it in the processed report. Unfortunately, there is very little that can be done if the ECG artifact shows up in the raw and subsequently in the processed display. With any luck, the ECG artifact may only be seen on one side. This means that some useful information can be derived from the side without the artifact; however, with unilateral artifacts, comparison of both sides for symmetry is made difficult.
7. Begin recording the EEG before induction of anesthesia.
8. Always have some way to compare a real-time EEG with a previous control (hard copy or computer stored baseline).

IV. DISCUSSION

A. *Interpretation of The Processed EEG*

Keep in mind that interpretation of the processed EEG, (no matter which format is chosen) requires some familiarity with the effects of various drugs and surgical events on the EEG. Becoming a "pattern reader" will help, and there are some general guidelines to be considered (Table 29–8). Train yourself to go through the same protocol for EEG interpretation each time you view either a raw or processed EEG:

Table 29–8 • Interpretation of the Processed EEG

1. Ask questions: Know the anesthetic and surgical course.
2. Look for changes in symmetry.
3. Look for changes in amplitude.
4. Look for shifts in spectral edge frequency.
5. Look for changes in frequency distribution.
6. Communicate with the surgeon.

1. Know what is occurring anesthetically and surgically at the time you are viewing the EEG record.
2. Look for symmetry: Are the changes bilateral?
3. Look for changes in amplitude of the waveform. Changes in amplitude can be caused by drugs, temperature, hypoxia, or hypoperfusion.
4. If you are using the spectral edge, look for shifts that occur bilaterally. If the changes are not bilateral, then look for focal causes, such as artery cross clamping or a malpositioned aortic cross clamp.
5. Look for changes in the frequency distribution of the EEG. Again remember that these changes can be drug or perfusion induced.

B. *Specific Changes of the Processed EEG*

1. CEREBRAL ISCHEMIC EFFECTS

Mild ischemia causes a decrease in the high frequency. Moderate ischemia causes a decrease in high-frequency activity and an increase in the low-frequency activity. Severe ischemia causes a decrease in the activity of all frequencies.

If the etiology of cerebral ischemia is due to hypotension, either deliberate or accidental, this decrease in activity is usually bilateral (see Fig. 29–10). If the changes are due to carotid artery cross clamping, then the changes are almost always unilateral on the same side as the cross clamp (see Color Fig. 8).

2. DRUG EFFECTS

Opiates, especially the fentanyl analogues, given in high doses result in loss of higher-frequency waves and the appearance of high-amplitude waves in lower frequencies (Fig. 29–14). There is characteristic increase of low-frequency delta waves and the spectral edge frequency shifts to the left (lower frequency). Lower doses of these opiates may not result in this characteristic shifting of the EEG to lower frequencies. Morphine, on the other hand, results in an EEG pattern that is very hard to differentiate from an awake pattern.

Inhalation anesthetics result in midrange frequencies (midalpha to subalpha range) of moderate amplitude. If looked for, a "dual pattern" of activity can be seen, especially on the Lifescan monitor. Spectral edge for the inhalation anesthetics is midrange.

Pentothal or other barbiturates usually result in a peak of activity in the 10- to 13-Hz range. High doses

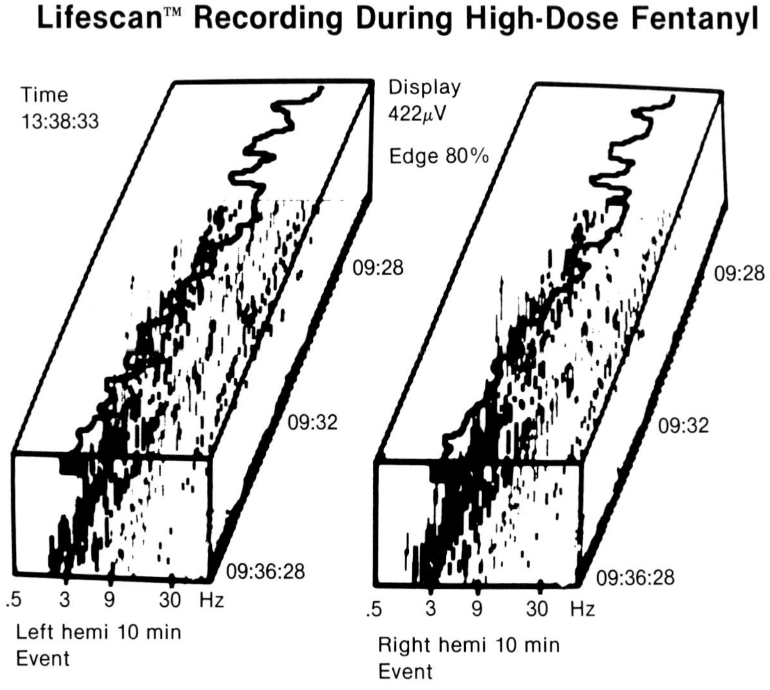

Figure 29–14 • An example of the changes seen on the Lifescan EEG analyzer during induction with high-dose fentanyl. Note the bilateral shift of the EEG to the left or lower frequencies as well as the characteristic marked increase in the delta-wave, indicated by very high-amplitude low-frequency waves. Again, by following the spectral edge frequency display, the marked changes during induction can be followed easily.

of barbiturates administered to induce barbiturate coma will result in burst suppression, which appears as a sawtooth pattern on the processed EEG. This can also be seen with very high doses of inhalation anesthetics (see Fig. 29–11).

Benzodiazepines produce a pattern of mid- to low amplitude on all frequencies.

Hypothermia frequently is seen as a marked decrease in amplitude and frequency, and in most cases of moderate hypothermia (28° C) there will be no discernible EEG activity. Therefore the EEG should be viewed before induction of deliberate hypothermia. Activity may return as the patient is warmed; however, there are occasions when the return of the EEG is not symmetric.

V. Complications of Interpretation and Other Pitfalls of Processed EEG Monitoring

Many of the pitfalls of EEG monitoring (especially the processed or computerized presentation of the raw EEG data) involve interpretation of what is on the screen. However, misinterpretation can occur if there is artifact contamination of the raw EEG. *Artifacts* are defined as all recorded features not of cerebral origin. Most of the modern processed EEG instruments have algorithms included in the software that attempt to eliminate artifacts. However, not recognizing artifact and relying on software to eliminate them can lead to misinterpretation of the EEG.

Artifacts can be of electrophysiologic origin or extracorporeal origin. Examples of the former include electrochardiographic, electromyographic, or even arterial pulsations, and examples of the latter include electrode displacement or malfunction. Although artifacts are problematic, they often provide useful information, such as muscle movement due to light anesthesia. Finally, whenever the EEG does not fit the clinical situation, a thorough search should be made for artifacts before major intervention is initiated.

A. *60-Cycle Interference*

1. Appearance

A 60-cycle electrical interference is usually seen on the raw EEG as a low-amplitude, regular sinusoidal pattern. Recent processed EEG machines have filters that usually prevent 60-cycle interference from appearing on the raw EEG.

2. CAUSE

If 60-cycle interference does appear, it is most frequently caused by poor electrode contact, a broken wire, or a short circuit due to water or electrode gel spilling over from one electrode to the next. A broken wire and a short circuit will often result in the appearance of 60-cycle interference on only one side of the EEG. Interference caused by fluorescent lighting, faulty ground, or an electric motor near the patient is usually seen on several electrodes. Also, large loops of cable may result in an antenna-like effect.

3. REMEDY

First, check the electrodes for skin contact and adequate impedance. If the impedance is poor, replace the electrodes after further degreasing of the skin. Second, make sure the skin around each electrode is dry and that there is no spillover of electrode gel. Finally, keep all the wires and cables together. This may help eliminate the problem. However, avoid large loops of cable since this may result in an antenna-like effect.

B. *Muscle Activity: Electromyographic Artifact*

1. APPEARANCE

Muscle activity usually appears as high-frequency waves of very irregular amplitude. The EEG resulting from marked muscle activity will frequently be illegible. Muscle activity can be differentiated from 60-cycle electric interference in that the former is irregular, whereas the latter presents as a regular pattern. However, respiratory muscle artifact is usually rhythmic, with slow waves occurring every 2 to 6 seconds.

2. CAUSE

Motor activity is usually the result of muscle activity nearby or directly underneath the electrode sites. Additional EMG artifact can result from respiratory motions. Observation of the patient may help differentiate respiratory artifact from other muscle artifact.

3. REMEDY

Making sure that the patient is adequately anesthetized and has adequate muscle relaxation may correct this artifact.

C. *Arterial Pulsations*

1. APPEARANCE

Arterial pulsations are usually slow waves that have a frequency of 1–2 Hz with variable amplitude. These waves may even take on a regular sawtooth appearance. Arterial pulsations can sometimes be seen during cardiopulmonary bypass; these are frequently unilateral.

2. CAUSE

Arterial pulsations are usually the result of placing one of the electrodes over an artery.

3. REMEDY

Reapply the lead slightly to one side of the original site.

D. *ECG Artifact*

Although a desirable feature of the processed EEG devices is an algorithm that recognizes artifact almost all of the currently available devices do not see the ECG signal that sometimes appears in the raw signal as an artifact. Therefore, if there are changes in the processed EEG that do not correlate with the clinical situation (ie, increased frequency in the face of very high doses of opiate), then there should be a high index of suspicion that the ECG signal is being picked up on the EEG.

1. APPEARANCE

There is very little confusion in diagnosis of ECG artifact. The appearance of regularly occurring spikes (1–2/sec) of low amplitude should result in a search of the raw EEG for the ECG signal. If artifact from the ECG is suspected, always check the raw EEG signal (Fig. 29–14).

2. CAUSE

The ECG will most likely contaminate the EEG in obese patients who have a bitemporal-lead EEG montage that is oriented close to and parallel with the cardiac axis. Electric activity from cardiac pacemakers will appear in the EEG recording from almost any montage.

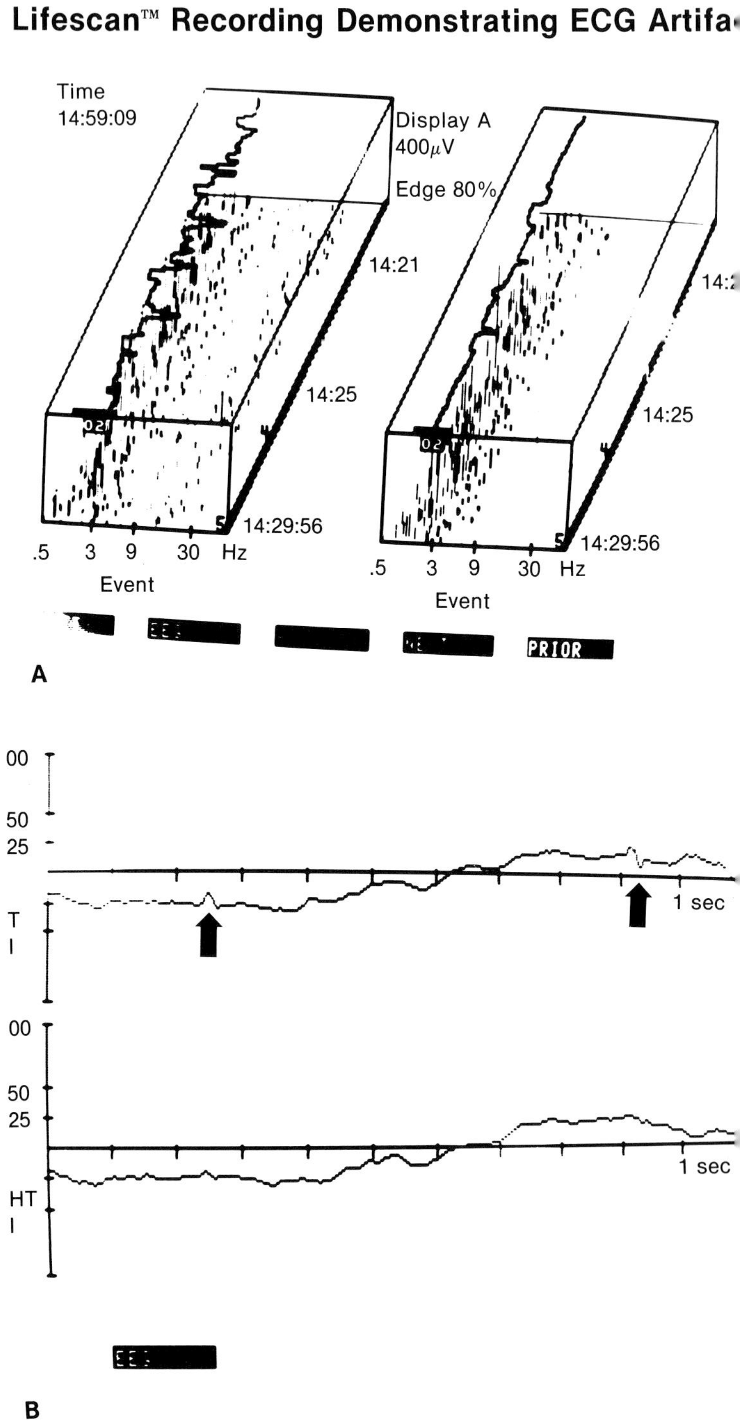

Figure 29-15 • (***A***) A Lifescan display that shows what appears to be a normal trace during a high-dose fentanyl anesthetic. However, there is more activity at a higher frequency than expected for the dose of opiate administered. (***B***) Examination of the raw EEG clearly shows the ECG spike in the raw trace (*arrows*).

3. REMEDY

The ECG artifact is probably the most difficult artifact to fix. Changing the position of the ground electrode has been suggested. Selecting a different montage with a different orientation to the cardiac axis may help. It is probably impossible to eliminate the artifact from a cardiac pacemaker.

E. *Electrocautery*

Although very easy to see on any EEG, raw or processed, electrocautery represents a significant problem. Not only can electrocautery interference damage the pens of the raw EEG machines, but if the surgical procedure involves the extensive use of cautery, monitoring of the intraoperative EEG will be difficult.

1. APPEARANCE

Electrocautery appears as sharp, very high-amplitude waves throughout the entire frequency range of the EEG.

2. CAUSE

The cause of this artifact is the high-frequency electric interference from the electrocautery.

3. REMEDY

There is really no good cure for the interference resulting from the use of electrocautery. Most modern machines will try to filter out this signal and indicate on the display that interference is occurring. If monitoring of the intraoperative EEG is critical then co-operation with the surgeon to limit the use of cautery is needed.

F. *Electrode Displacement or Malfunction*

Apart from the above-mentioned artifacts, nearly all other artifacts result from electrode problems. The extra time spent properly preparing the skin site and applying the electrode will save time and trouble intraoperatively.

1. APPEARANCE

There is really no characteristic pattern that will assist in diagnosing a bad electrode. The impedance will be above normal levels. A high index of suspicion will often lead to reapplication of an electrode or replacement of a wire.

2. CAUSE

Electrodes will dry out over time and lose adhesive contact with the skin. Wires will break if care is not exercised throughout the procedure.

3. REMEDY

Check electrode impedance frequently. Check that the leads are connected securely to the amplifiers and connected to the proper channels. Do not be hesitate to replace electrodes.

G. *Other Considerations of Intraoperative EEG Monitoring*

Avoid highly variable anesthetic situations. Keep the mixing of agents, inhalational and injectables, to a minimum. This may avoid the question of whether or not a change in the EEG was drug induced or due to an actual neurovascular event. Finally, do not be so concerned with the EEG that attention is directed away from actual patient care. As mentioned earlier, the processed EEG is only one of several available intraoperative monitors, and the clinical situation must always be correlated with changes in the EEG.

VI. REFERENCES

1. Levy WJ, Shapiro HM, Maruchak G, Meathe E. Automated EEG processing for intraoperative monitoring: A comparison of techniques. Anesthesiology 55:223–236, 1980.
2. Maynard DE, Prior PF, Scott DF. Device for continuous monitoring of cerebral activity in resuscitated patients. Br Med J 4:545–46, 1969.
3. Schwartz MS, Colvin MP, Prior PF, Strunin L, et al. The cerebral function monitor: Its value in predicting the neurological outcome in patients undergoing cardiopulmonary bypass. Anaesthesia 28:611–617, 1973.
4. Glaria AP, Murray A. Comparison of EEG monitoring techniques: An evaluation during cardiac surgery. Electroencephalogr Clin Neurophysiol 61:323–330, 1985.
5. Klein FF. A waveform analyzer applied to the human EEG. Trans Biomed Eng BME 23:246–252, 1976.
6. Demetrescu M. The aperiodic character of the electroencephalogram (EEG): New approach to data analysis and condensation. Physiologist 18:189, 1975.

7. Gregory TK, Pettus DC. An electroencephalographic processing algorithm specifically intended for analysis of cerebral electric activity. J Clin Monit 2:190–195, 1986.
8. Rampil IJ, Sasse FJ, Smith NT, Hoff BH, et al. Spectral edge frequency: A new correlate of anesthetic depth. Anesthesiology 53:S12, 1980.
9. Rampil IJ, Holzer JA, Quest DO, Rosenbaum SH, et al. Prognostic value of computerized EEG analysis during carotid endarterectomy. Anesth Analg 62:186–192, 1983.
10. Levy WJ. Processed EEG: A machine and a number are not enough. J Cardiovasc Anes 2:121–122, 1988.
11. Scott JC, Ponganis KV, Stanski DR. EEG quantification of narcotic effect: The comparative pharmacodynamics of fentanyl and alfentanil. Anesthesiology 62:234–241, 1985.
12. Schwilden H, Schutter J, Steckel H. Closed-loop feedback control of methohexital anesthesia by quantitative EEG analysis in humans. Anesthesiology 67:341–347, 1987.
13. Drummond JD, Perkins D, Wolfe D. A comparison of median frequency, spectral edge, frequency band ratios, total power, and dominance shifts in the determination of depth of anesthesia. Anesthesiology 65:A316, 1988.
14. Smith NT, Westover CJ, Quinn M, Benthuysen JL, et al. An encephalographic comparison of alfentanil with other narcotics and with thiopental. J Clin Monit 1:236–244, 1985.
15. Hudson RJ, Stanski DR, Saidman LJ, Meathe E. A model for studying depth of anesthesia and acute tolerance to thiopental. Anesthesiology 59:301–308, 1983.
16. Rampil IJ, Wesikopf RB, Brown JG, Eger EI, et al. I-653 and isoflurane produce similar dose-related changes in the electroencephalogram of pigs. Anesthesiology 69:298–302, 1988.
17. Levy WJ, Grundy BL, Smith NT. Monitoring the electroencephalogram and evoked potential during anesthesia. In Monitoring In Anesthesia. 2nd ed. Boston, Butterworths, 1987,227–267.
18. Von Marxow, EF. Mitteilung, betreffebd die Physiologie der Hirnrinde. Zentralbl f Physiol 4:537–540 (Dec) 1890.
19. Smith NT, Dec-Silver H, Sanford TJ, Westover CJ, et al. EEGs during high-dose fentanyl-, sufentanil-, or morphine-oxygen anesthesia. Anesth Analg 63:386–193, 1984.
20. Sebel PS, Bovill JG, Wauquier A, Pieternella R. Effects of high-dose fentanyl anesthesia on the electroencephalogram. Anesthesiology 55:203–211, 1981.
21. Bowdle TA, Ward RJ. Induction of anesthesia with small doses of sufentanil or fentanyl: Dose versus EEG response, speed of onset, and thiopental requirements. Anesthesiology 70: 26–30, 1989.
22. Hug CC. Lipid Solubility, pharmacokinetics, and the EEG: Are you better off today than you were four years ago? Anesthesiology 62: 221–226, 1985.
23. Sundt TM, Sharbrough FW, Piepgras DG, Kearns TP, et al. Correlation of cerebral blood flow and electroencephalographic changes during carotid endarterectomy. Mayo Clin Proc 56:533–543, 1981.
24. Ferguson GA. Carotid endarterectomy: To shunt or not to shunt? Archives of Neurol 43:615–618, 1986.
25. Young WL, Moberg RS, Ornstein E, Matteo RS, et al. Electroencephalographic monitoring for ischemia during carotid endarterectomy: Visual versus computer analysis. J Clin Monit 4:78–85, 1988.
26. Spackman TN, Faust RJ, Cucchira RF, Sharbrough FW. A comparison of aperiodic analysis of the EEG with the standard EEG and cerebral blood flow for detection of ischemia. Anesthesiology 66:229–231, 1987.
27. Silbert BS, Kluger R, Cronin KD, Koumoundouros E. The processed electroencephalogram may not detect neurologic ischemia during carotid endarterectomy. Anesthesiology 70:356–368, 1989.
28. Kim BY, Ngeow JY, Kitahata LM, Swift CA. EEG changes with lateral rotation of the head. Anesthesiology Rev 12:36–37, 1985.
29. Sablocki AD, Albin MS. Pro: The EEG should be monitored during cardiopulmonary bypass. J Cardiothorac Anesth 3:119–123, 1989.
30. Murray A, Glaria AP, Pearson DT. Monitoring EEG frequency and amplitude during cardiac surgery. Anaesthesia 41:173–177, 1986.
31. Nussmeier NA, Arlund C, Slogoff S. Neuropsychiatric complications after cardiopulmonary bypass: Cerebral protection by a barbiturate. Anesthesiology 64:165–170, 1986.
32. Sotaniemi KA, Sulg IA, Hokkanen TE. Quantitative EEG as a measure of cerebral dysfunction before and after open-heart surgery. Electroencephalogr Clin Neurophysiol 44:575–585, 1978.
33. Levy WJ. Quantitative analysis of EEG changes during hypothermia. Anesthesiology 60:294–297, 1984.
34. Quasha L, Tinker JH, Sharbrough FW. Hypothermia plus thiopental. Anesthesiology 55:636–640, 1981.
35. Jasper H. The 10–20 electrode system of the International Federation. Electroencephalogr Clin Neurophysiol 10:370–375, 1958.

Chapter 30

Mark H. Zornow, MD
John C. Drummond, MD, FRCPC

Monitoring Sensory Evoked Potentials in the Operating Room

OUTLINE

I. INTRODUCTION

Over the past ten years, the intraoperative monitoring of evoked potentials has spread from research institutions and academic medical centers to the operating rooms of community hospitals. This phenomenon has been stimulated by increased concern over liability for neurologic injury occurring during surgery and by the commercial availability of evoked potential monitoring systems. Because anesthesiologists monitor so many other physiologic parameters during anesthesia and surgery, the responsibility for acquiring and interpreting the evoked responses has often fallen on their shoulders. Even in those institutions where the anesthesiologist does not have the primary responsibility for this type of monitoring, a basic understanding of the way in which anesthetic agents influence the evoked responses is crucial to the successful use of this monitoring modality during surgery.

The goal of this chapter is to provide an introduction to the intraoperative monitoring of somatosensory and brainstem auditory evoked responses. Information regarding the use of visual evoked responses will not be presented because the high rate of false-positive and false-negative results has so far limited the usefulness of this technique in detecting intraoperative injury to the visual pathways.[1]

The topics discussed include the definition of an evoked response, acquisition of evoked responses, and the identification of pathologic changes in the evoked response. Only a limited description of each of these topics can be provided within a single chapter. Nonetheless, the following information will provide an appropriate introduction and reference for those who are just beginning to gain experience with this monitoring modality. However, no amount of reading can substitute for hands-on experience, which can be obtained only in the operating room in the course of acquiring, interpreting, and troubleshooting evoked responses.

A. *What Is an Evoked Potential?*

In general terms, an *evoked response* is an electrophysiologic event that occurs in the central nervous system in response to a brief sensory stimulus. The stimulus commonly takes the form of an electric current pulse applied to a peripheral nerve (*somatosensory evoked potentials [SSEPs]*) or an auditory stimulus such as a click or a tone (*brainstem auditory evoked responses [BAERs]*). The electric potentials produced by the nervous system in response to these stimuli may be recorded from surface electrodes and range from a few tenths of a microvolt in amplitude (for auditory brainstem potentials) to a few microvolts [μV] (for somatosensory potentials). To extract these small signals from background EEG activity, which has an amplitude in the range of 1 to 100 μV, it is necessary to average the nervous system's response to many repeated stimuli. The background EEG, which is continuously being produced but is temporally unrelated to the stimulus, can be considered random noise. The evoked potential signal-to-noise ratio increases in proportion to the square root of the number of responses that are averaged (ie, the more responses averaged, the "cleaner" the signal).[2] This allows the identification of the time-locked evoked response despite the presence of electric noise with an amplitude several orders of magnitude greater than the signal of interest.

II. Indications for Monitoring

A. *Somatosensory Evoked Potentials (SSEPs)*

1. Posterior Tibial Nerve SSEPs

Posterior tibial SSEPs may be used to monitor spinal cord function during procedures in which the cord is at risk for either mechanical or ischemic injury. These include scoliosis surgery, spinal stabilization procedures, resections of intraaxial tumors, correction of aortic coarctations, and repair of thoracic aortic aneurysms or dissections. Evoked potential monitoring permits continuous monitoring of cord function throughout the surgical procedure. This is in contrast to the wake-up test, which allows an assessment of cord function only at one time point during the operation. Furthermore, evoked potential monitoring can be performed during those procedures in which a wake-up test would be ill advised or impossible (ie, thoracotomy for vertebrectomy or resection of a thoracic aortic aneurysm). It should be noted that afferent SSEP impulses are carried predominantly by the posterior columns of the spinal cord. Therefore, there exists the possibility that injury may occur to the anterior (motor) portion of the cord without diagnostic changes in the SSEP.

Posterior tibial SSEP monitoring during aortic surgery entails some special considerations. Paraplegia following surgery on the thoracic aorta may occur as a result of spinal cord ischemia due to arterial hypotension distal to the aortic clamps or due to an interruption of flow through critical intercostal arteries arising from the occluded segment of aorta. If distal perfusion pressure is not maintained during aortic occlusion, intraoperative loss of the posterior tibial SSEP may be due either to cord ischemia (which may result in a postoperative deficit) or peripheral nerve ischemia. When distal perfusion is not maintained, the ability to interpret evoked potential changes is greatly limited. For a more thorough discussion of the role of evoked potentials in preventing spinal cord damage during aortic surgery, see the series of articles by Laschinger and colleagues.[3–7]

Posterior tibial SSEPs may also be used when there is a risk of ischemia in the distribution of the anterior cerebral artery (eg, during clipping of anterior circulation aneurysms or resection of arteriovenous malformations supplied by the anterior cerebral artery). Monitoring posterior tibial SSEPs may provide valuable information about the safety of sacrificing the anterior cerebral artery.[8]

2. MEDIAN NERVE SSEPs

Median nerve SSEPs may be used to monitor cortical function during procedures that place the portion of the brain supplied by the middle cerebral artery at risk. These include clipping of middle cerebral artery aneurysms and resection of parietal/temporal tumors or arteriovenous malformations. Intraoperative deterioration of the evoked response may allow surgeons to modify their procedure to minimize the chance of a postoperative deficit. Although median nerve SSEPs may also be used to monitor the integrity of the upper cervical cord, the waveforms obtained with stimulation of the posterior tibial nerve tend to be more robust and easier to obtain.

B. *Brainstem Auditory Evoked Responses (BAERs)*

Intraoperative monitoring of BAERs is useful during procedures that place the eighth cranial nerve at risk. These include microvascular decompression of the fifth (for tic douloureux) or seventh (for hemifacial spasm) cranial nerves, and resections of cerebellopontine angle tumors.[9-12] The loss or deterioration of BAERs during these procedures should prompt an assessment of retractor positioning, since an unnecessary degree of tension may be exerted on either the cranial nerves or the brainstem.

III. HOW TO MONITOR EVOKED POTENTIALS

A. *Acquisition of an Evoked Potential*

1. FILTERING, AMPLIFYING, AND AVERAGING

A better understanding of how a somatosensory evoked response is acquired may be achieved by examining what occurs after the delivery of a single stimulus. The evoked potential apparatus causes a current pulse of the selected strength (milliamps [mA], or less commonly, volts [V]) and duration (microseconds [μsec]) to be delivered to the stimulating electrodes. Beginning at the moment of stimulus delivery and continuing for a predetermined poststimulus interval (often referred to as the *timebase*), an analog-to-digital converter acquires data (analog voltage potentials) from the scalp. The analog signals (voltages) from these electrodes are filtered to eliminate frequencies outside the range of interest, amplified, and converted into a digital form that the evoked response apparatus can average with the data acquired from previous stimuli. This data acquisition and manipulation is repeated following each stimulus. The stimulus-acquisition sequence is repeated many times (eg, 200–400 repetitions for SSEPs) at frequencies ranging from 3 to 7 Hz. With each successive stimulus, increasing amounts of the background EEG activity (which is random with respect to the stimulus) are eliminated and what remains is the recurrent, time-locked electric response of the central nervous system to the stimuli (Fig. 30–1). Following each stimulus, the display may be updated with the new information. In addition, most evoked response apparatus allows the operator to examine the raw EEG signal as a means of quality control to insure that a valid signal is being obtained from the recording electrodes. Once the desired number of stimuli has been delivered, the final average may be compared with the amplitude and latencies of previously acquired averages.

2. WAVEFORM MORPHOLOGY AND NOMENCLATURE

An evoked response is commonly described by the latency and the amplitude of each of its component waves (Fig. 30–2). *Latency* (measured in milliseconds) is the interval between stimulus delivery and the peak amplitude of a particular wave. *Amplitude* (measured in microvolts) may be relative to the baseline or to an adjacent wave. Conventions regarding the naming of individual waves are not uniform. In the anesthesia literature, positive waves are usually presented as upward deflections and are identified as *P waves*. Negative waves or troughs are written as downward deflections and are designated as *N waves*. In some sources, the opposite is the case (ie, negative is up and positive is down). Associated with each P or N wave is a number. This number may represent the latency in milliseconds from the stimulus delivery to the peak of the wave, or it may represent the order of the wave in the evoked response. Hence P1 would be the first positive wave in a tracing. If P1 occurs at a mean latency of 67 msec in a normal population, it may also be referred to as P67. It is common to

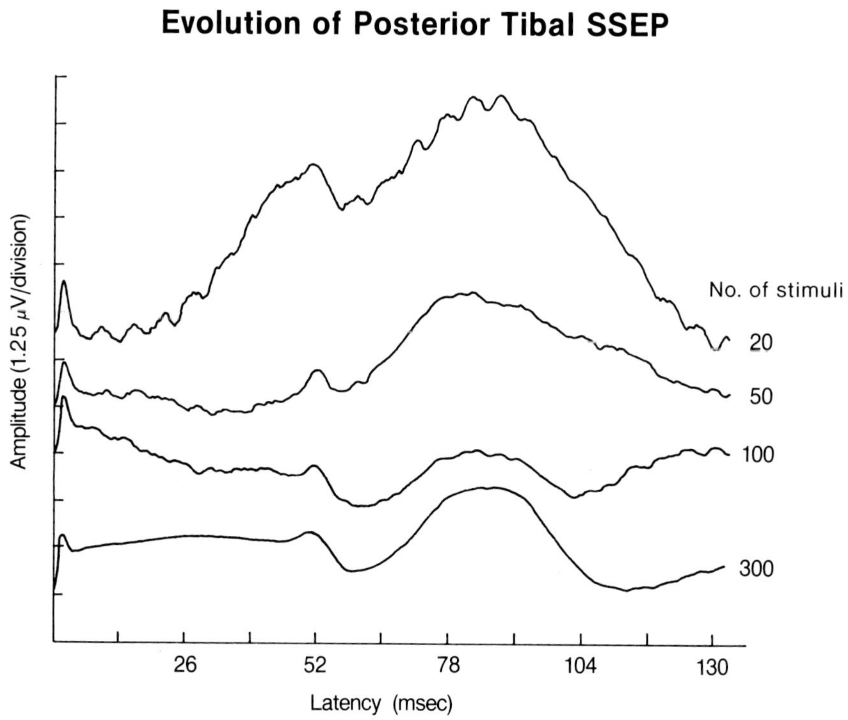

Figure 30-1 • Evolution of posterior tibial SSEP is shown following the averaging of the cortical response to 20, 50, 100, and 300 stimuli. The evoked response is clearest (greatest signal to noise ratio) after averaging the response to 300 stimuli.

continue to identify this wave as P67, even if its latency in an individual patient is quite different or changes during the monitoring period.

3. Application of Stimulating and Recording Electrodes

a. Stimulus Delivery: SSEPs

Stimulating electrodes for lower extremity somatosensory evoked potential monitoring are commonly placed over the posterior tibial nerve posterior to the medial malleolus, or over the peroneal nerve at the fibular neck. For upper extremity monitoring, the stimulating electrodes are usually placed over the median nerve at the wrist. In patients with spinal cord injury, it is desirable to test for preservation of proprioception before the induction of anesthesia. If proprioception is intact, it is almost always possible to obtain reproducible evoked responses. In those patients whose injury has caused a complete loss of position sense, attempts at intraopera-

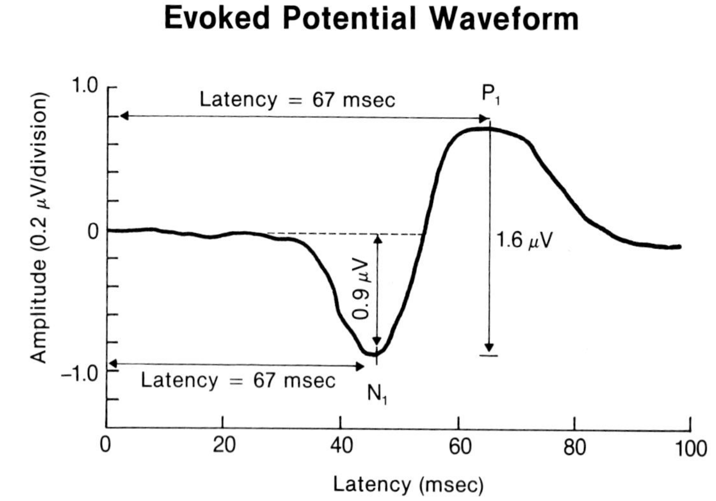

Figure 30-2 • Evoked response demonstrates labeling of major waves (*N1 and P1*), latencies (*46 and 67 msec*), and amplitudes (*0.6 and 0.9μV*).

tive monitoring may be futile. It is often desirable to place the stimulating electrodes prior to the induction of anesthesia. After the skin has been cleansed with a suitable abrasive electrode paste (eg, Omniprep™), a variable output nerve stimulator may be used to locate the desired peripheral nerve. A visible motor response can usually be elicited with a 5- to 10-mA current. Grass EEG needle electrodes (Model E2; Grass Instrument Co, Quincy, MA) are then bent to approximate a 60° angle and inserted percutaneously at the sites previously identified. These electrodes are securely taped to the patient's skin and the wires coiled to prevent dislodgement during positioning of the patient before sugery. Needle electrodes should not be reused because there is an increased risk of breakage and loss of the needle in the subcutaneous tissue. Retrieval of needle fragments is difficult and time consuming.

Before the induction of anesthesia, evoked responses can be obtained with minimal discomfort to the patient if the stimulus intensity is adjusted to approximately the threshold for a motor response. For intraoperative recording, the stimulus intensity should be increased to 15–20 mA. In those patients with normal spinal cord function, the stimuli may be delivered at a rate of 5.1 Hz. In patients who present with severe incomplete injuries to the spinal cord, the acquisition of adequate waveforms for intraoperative monitoring may be facilitated by the use of a slower stimulus rate (eg, 1.1–2.1 Hz).[13]

b. *Stimulus Delivery: BAERs*

The stimulus for brainstem auditory evoked responses consists of either short clicks or single-frequency tone bursts. These stimuli are delivered through small foam or plastic earpieces inserted into the external auditory canal. Before placing these devices, it is important to visually examine the auditory canal for the presence of wax or blood, which may act to insulate the tympanic membrane from the stimulus. After the earpieces have been positioned, a cotton ball is placed on top of the earpiece and both are firmly secured with tape or a transparent adhesive dressing. The auditory threshold is then determined by gradually increasing the intensity of the sound (in decibels [dB]) delivered through first one and then the other earpiece. Patients are instructed to raise a finger as soon as they can hear the sound. The auditory threshold in decibels for each ear is then recorded. For intraoperative monitoring, stimuli are delivered at 70 dB over the auditory threshold at a rate of 11.1 Hz.

c. *Recording Electrodes*

Recording electrodes are placed on the scalp according to the International 10–20 System (Fig. 30–3).[14] This system was devised to allow the reproducible placement of scalp electrodes. All electrode positions are referenced to the nasion (bridge of the nose), the inion (occipital protuberance), and the external auditory canals. The

Sites of Scalp Recording Electrodes for SSEPs and BAERs

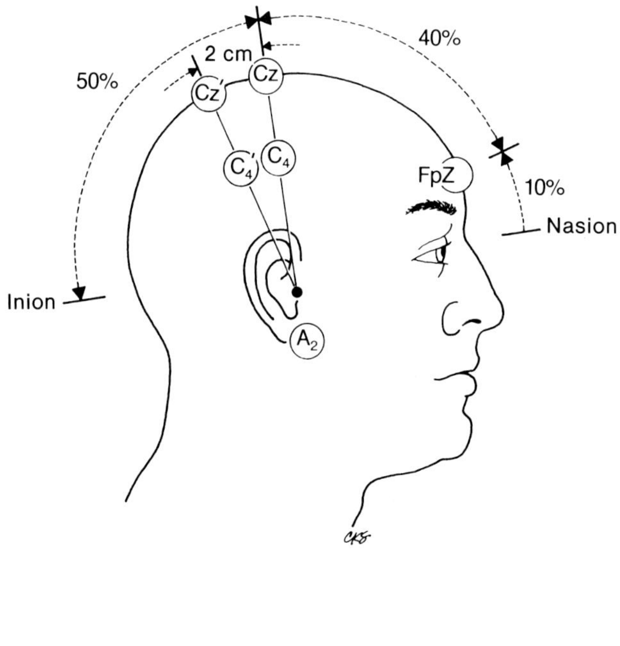

Figure 30–3 • The International 10–20 System (see text for explanation) and the commonly used scalp electrode positions are used to record evoked responses. Cz′ and FpZ are used to record posterior tibial SSEPs. C4′ (C3′ for left cortical responses) and FpZ are used when monitoring median nerve somatosensory evoked potentials (SSEPs). Cz′ with A2 (or A1 with left-sided stimulation) are used for recording brainstem auditory evoked responses (BAERs).

scalp is divided into quadrants by the lines connecting the auditory canals and the inion/nasion. Each electrode position is located at increments of 10% or 20% of the length of these lines. Electrodes placed over the right hemisphere are evenly numbered, whereas the corresponding positions for the left hemisphere are given odd numbers. Because the International 10–20 System locations are not optimal electrode positions for all evoked response monitoring applications, additional electrode positions have been designated. These are denoted by appending a prime sign (′) to the conventional 10–20 designation. These electrode locations are approximately 2 cm posterior to their corresponding International 10–20 System positions. Although numerous electrode positions can be designated, a limited number are of relevance to the recording of evoked potentials. The most commonly used scalp locations for evoked response monitoring are FpZ, Cz′, C3′, and C4′ (see Fig. 30–3). The location FpZ is on the midline of the forehead, 10% of the distance from nasion to inion. Cz′ is also a midline electrode position 2 cm posterior to the midpoint (Cz) of the nasion to inion line. The location Cz′ is situated over the primary sensory cortex for the lower extremities and accordingly is used to monitor lower extremity SSEPs. The location C3′ is over the left hemisphere at a point 40% of the distance from Cz′ to the external auditory canal. The corresponding position C4′ is over the right hemisphere (see Fig. 30–3). These locations, C3′ and C4′, are over those areas of the cortex that receive sensory input from the right and left upper extremities and are used in the monitoring of responses to median nerve stimulation.

For recording evoked responses during long surgical procedures, we have had good success using EEG-type gold cup electrodes (Type E5 GH; Grass Instrument Co, Quincy, MA) secured to the scalp with collodion. The electrodes are reusable gold-plated metal disks approximately 1 cm in diameter. After the proper scalp site has been identified, the hair is parted and the scalp prepared using a cotton swab and an abrasive electrode paste. A good skin preparation that removes oils and keratinized dead skin is essential to obtain the low impedances necessary for evoked potential recording. The cup electrode is then filled with a conductive gel, positioned on the scalp, and secured in place with a piece of gauze soaked in collodion. Use of a pressurized jet of air will speed the evaporation of the ether in the collodion, thereby reducing the time it takes to apply each electrode. After the collodion has dried, a syringe filled with conductive gel and tipped with an 18 gauge blunt needle may be inserted through the small hole in the top of the cup electrode. The underlying scalp can be gently abraded with the blunt needle, and a small additional amount of gel injected.

Once all of the recording electrodes have been applied, their impedances should be checked. Most evoked potential monitoring equipment has the built-in capability to measure electrode impedances; if not, a small hand-held impedance monitor may be used. Attempts should be made to reduce all electrode impedance to <3 kOhms.

4. Storage And Documentation

Good monitoring technique dictates that a permanent copy of representative responses be made during the various phases of the operative procedure. Responses are commonly stored on a magnetic disk or printed on paper. It is usually advisable to store examples of the evoked response at the following times: after induction of anesthesia but before positioning of the patient; after positioning has been completed; immediately before and during any surgical manipulation that has a risk of neurologic injury; and near the conclusion of the case. Storage of these responses along with their time of acquisition and a comment about the stage of the surgical procedure (ie, "distraction rods placed" or "start tumor resection") is essential not only for rational interpretation of changes in the evoked responses that may occur, but also should litigation ever arise concerning the operation. Documentation of changes in the evoked responses and evidence that these changes were discussed with the surgical team are appropriate.

B. *Interpretation of the Waveforms*

1. Identification of False-Positive Responses

The goal of evoked potential monitoring is to identify injury to the central nervous system before it becomes irreversible. Neural injury is evidenced in evoked response tracings by (1) a decrease in the amplitude of waveforms, (2) an increase in their latency, or (3) a complete loss of recognizable waveforms. Unfortunately, a decreased amplitude and increased latency may result from many factors other than neural injury. The person responsible for interpretation of intraoperative evoked responses must become adept at recognizing these *false-*

positive changes to avoid numerous and needless interruptions of the surgical procedure. Fortunately, as one gains experience with evoked potential monitoring, the incidence of false-positive interpretations decreases.

a. *Anesthetic Effects*

In modern clinical practice, the induction and maintenance of general anesthesia involves the administration of a wide variety of drugs (eg, barbiturates, narcotics, benzodiazepines, volatile anesthetics, nitrous oxide, local anesthetics). In general, all of these agents tend to decrease the amplitude while increasing the latency of the evoked response, although the volatile agents are much more potent in this respect than the intravenous drugs (Fig. 30–4).[15–17,19,20–22] Etomidate is unique in that it has actually been shown to increase the amplitude of median and posterior tibial nerve SSEPs.[15,21,23]

Evoked responses of cortical origin are more vulnerable to alterations in anesthetic depth than those arising in the brainstem, spinal cord, or peripheral nerve. This may be due to the fact that a greater number of synaptic events are involved in the generation of a cortical response. Hence, BAERs, which have latencies in the range of 2 to 10 msec and are generated in the brainstem, are unlikely to show significant changes with anything less than minimum alveolar concentration–(MAC–) level alterations in anesthetic depth.[24] Indeed, BAERs can be readily recorded during barbiturate-induced coma with an isoelectric EEG.[17,18]

In the early literature on intraoperative evoked response monitoring, it was stated that reproducible waveforms could not be recorded in the presence of a volatile agent such as halothane. More recent data has shown that when normal responses are present preoperatively, as much as 0.5 MAC of these agents may be used (see Fig. 30–4).[16]

There is an inverse relationship between the concentration of volatile anesthetic administered and the amplitude of the evoked response (eg, the more halothane administered, the smaller the amplitude of the evoked response). The anesthesiologist involved in evoked response monitoring must be cognizant of the effects of anesthetic agents and develop an anesthetic plan which will include

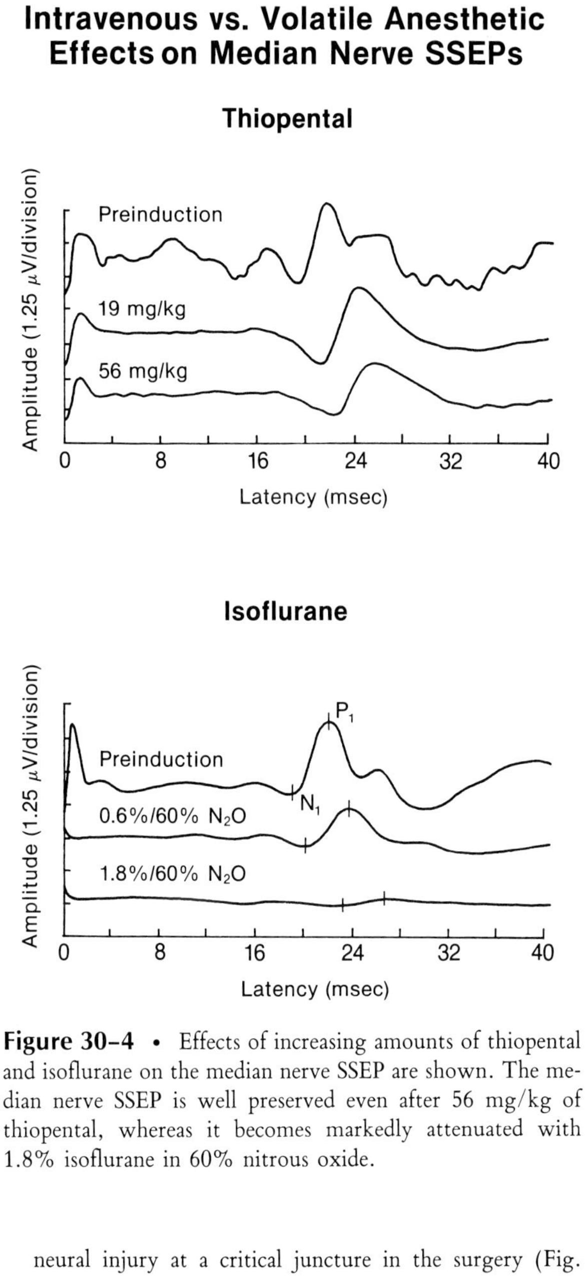

Figure 30–4 • Effects of increasing amounts of thiopental and isoflurane on the median nerve SSEP are shown. The median nerve SSEP is well preserved even after 56 mg/kg of thiopental, whereas it becomes markedly attenuated with 1.8% isoflurane in 60% nitrous oxide.

1. *A stable anesthetic state*. This is particularly important at times when critical surgical events may occur. Changes in the depth of anesthesia will result in alterations in the evoked responses that may be difficult to differentiate from neural injury at a critical juncture in the surgery (Fig. 30–5).
2. *Moderate to low concentrations of volatile anesthetics*. An appropriate level of anesthesia must be produced, with concentrations of volatile anesthetic less than those that have been shown to interfere with monitoring of the evoked response. We try to limit end-tidal volatile anesthetic concentrations to approximately 0.5 MAC. A nitrous/narcotic based anesthetic (70% nitrous oxide, 10–20 μg/kg of fentanyl loading dose followed by an infusion of 1–3 μg/kg/hr) seems to be suitable for many procedures in which evoked potentials are to be monitored. As much as 0.5% isoflurane is often added to help insure amnesia and maintain blood pressure in the normotensive range.

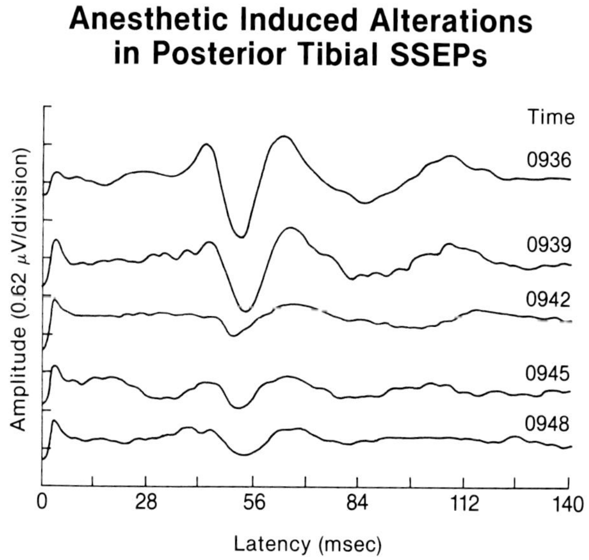

Figure 30–5 • Marked loss of amplitude of posterior tibial SSEP is caused by increasing the isoflurane concentration from 0.5% to 1.5% at 0940 to treat an episode of bronchospasm. The reduction in amplitude of the dominant waveform is due to this change in volatile anesthetic concentration and is indistinguishable from that caused by neural injury.

Muscle relaxants can reduce the amount of muscle artifact that may be seen in awake or lightly anesthetized patients and, accordingly, may improve the signal to noise ratio (Fig. 30–6)[25]

With the onset of paralysis, the irregular high-frequency activity associated with muscle activity is eliminated, thereby aiding the identification of SSEP waveforms. Unfortunately, muscle artifact is common in patients who are lightly anesthetized and incompletely paralyzed. It may be especially pronounced immediately prior to an intraoperative wake-up test.

b. Equipment Failure

A common cause of false-positive changes in the evoked response is the dislodgement of either recording or stimulating electrodes. Evoked potential monitoring commonly requires the application of 7 to 15 electrodes and their associated wire connectors. One or more of these may be pulled loose during the transfer of the patient from the gurney to the operating room table, during positioning, or during the surgical preparation prior to incision. The dislodgement of a recording electrode may be suspected whenever its impedance becomes extremely high. Disconnection or dislodgement of stimulating electrodes may be more difficult to detect. Some evoked potential monitoring devices have error indicators that signal a failure to deliver the preset stimulus. However, visual inspection of the electrodes under the drapes is often required. Optimal technique includes the recording of the afferent nerve impulse from a recording electrode in the popliteal fossa (posterior tibial SSEPs) or over the brachial plexus (Erb's point, median nerve SSEPs). Loss of this peripheral nerve action potential suggests a failure to deliver the stimulus to the nerve in question.

Evoked potential monitoring systems are complex devices. Although most systems are well designed and constructed, the operating room environment is a hostile one, and equipment failures may occur. For this reason, it may be advisable to have a back-up machine available should such a failure occur during a critical

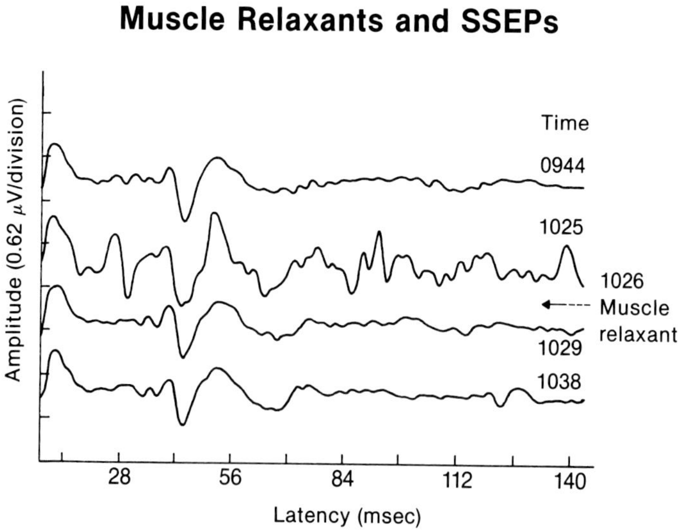

Figure 30–6 • Effect of pharmacologic paralysis on posterior tibial SSEPs is shown. 0944 = baseline recording soon after induction and paralysis with succinylcholine; 1025 = evoked response after full return of neuromuscular function; 1029 and 1038 = evoked response following administration of 10 mg of vecuronium at 1026.

monitoring situation. Frequently, the local neurology department will have the appropriate equipment should the need arise.

c. *Electric Noise*

The modern operating room is filled with electrically-powered devices. These devices may emit leakage currents or radio frequency signals that can interfere with the recording of evoked potentials. Some of the worst offenders include blood warmers, heating blankets, anesthesia circuit heater/humidifiers, and intravenous infusion pumps. Often this interference takes the form of a 60-Hz pattern that can be recognized by examining the raw signal coming from the recording electrodes. Strategies for eliminating this interference include turning the offending device off, moving the device and its power source away from the evoked potential apparatus, and eliminating loops in the leads coming from the recording electrodes. Loops in recording lead wires act as antennas that can receive the radio frequency signals generated by other devices located in the operating room.

Most evoked potential monitors have 60-cycle filters that will help minimize interference produced by these devices. Unfortunately, activity in the 60-Hz range may also be of interest in the recording of the evoked potential. These filters must therefore be used cautiously and consistently. No filtering is capable of eliminating the artifact induced by electrocautery. A single burst of monopolar electrocautery during the recording of a SSEP can obscure the entire average. For this reason, evoked potential monitoring may be blind during those parts of the procedure that require frequent use of the electrocautery.

d. *Miscellaneous Causes of Alterations in the Evoked Response*

Many factors other than surgically induced injury to the nervous system (and anesthetic drug equipment failure and electric noise) may result in the loss of the evoked response These include severe hypoxia,[26-28] hypotension[29-31] or hypothermia (either local or systemic).[32-34] An alert anesthesiologist should be able to detect these changes and recognize that they may cause increases in latency and decreases in amplitude of the evoked response. Other causes of altered responses may not be so obvious. Air accumulating under the calvaria during seated craniotomies has been reported to act as an insulator between the cortical generators of the evoked response and the recording electrodes (Fig. 30–7).[35] This has resulted in the complete loss of the evoked response with immediate return following repositioning of the head so that the cortex was again in contact with the calvaria.

2. CRITERIA FOR TRUE-POSITIVE CHANGES

It is generally accepted that an amplitude decrement of more than 50% of baseline values is sufficient to cause concern that there may be ongoing injury to the neural pathways being monitored. During long procedures, normal evoked response amplitude may vary by 10% to

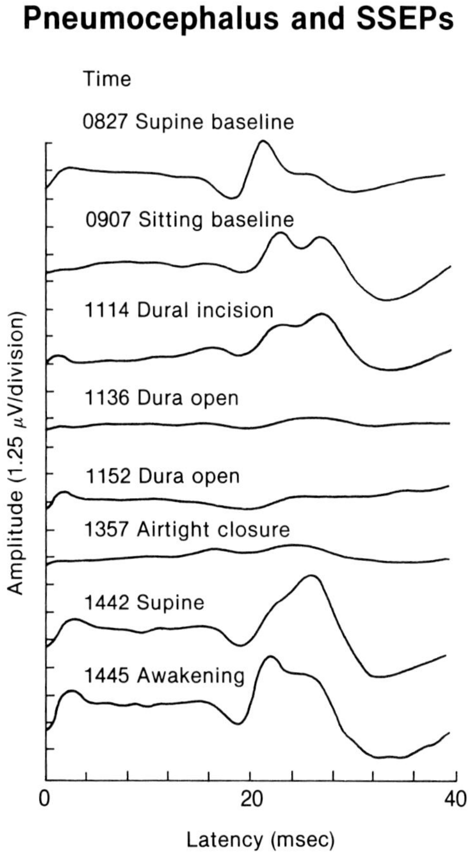

Figure 30–7 • Loss of median nerve SSEP is due to intracranial accumulation of air during posterior fossa craniectomy in the seated position. The evoked potential waveform was lost shortly after dural incision and cerebrospinal fluid drainage but prior to any surgical manipulation that might have caused neural injury. Note the prompt return of the cortical potential when the patient was placed in the supine position at the conclusion of the operation. This repositioning displaced intracranial air to the region of the frontal poles, allowing the somatosensory cortex to again come into approximation with the calvaria and recording electrodes.

30% even when there is no damage to neural structures.[36] For this reason, it is often desirable to take as the baseline response a tracing obtained shortly before the phase of the procedure during which injury is most likely to occur. For scoliosis surgery this would be shortly before placement of the distraction rods, whereas during aortic surgery it might be prior to cross clamping of the thoracic aorta. A reproducible 50% reduction of amplitude from this baseline warrants notification of the surgical team that there may be compromise of the neural pathway being monitored. Complete and sustained loss of the evoked response is an ominous sign that is associated with a high incidence of new postoperative deficits. The implications of a transient loss and subsequent recovery of the evoked potential are not as straightforward. Certainly, the recovery of an evoked response following a transient loss is an encouraging sign, although it does not guarantee normal neurologic function (Fig. 30–8).

C. *Stimulus and Recording Parameters*

Table 30–1 shows the parameters commonly employed in our institution when monitoring posterior tibial SSEPs, median nerve SSEPs, and BAERs in the operating room. These are intended to serve only as an initial guide and may be modified depending on the clinical situation. Typical posterior tibial and median nerve SSEPs and typical BAERs are also shown (Figs. 30–9 through 30–11).

IV. Discussion

A. *Response to an Intraoperative Change in the Evoked Potential*

When an intraoperative change occurs in the evoked response that is suggestive of neural injury, it is important to have a mental algorithm that will allow quick verification of the change so that prompt warning of impending or actual neural injury may be transmitted to the surgical team. A suggested approach to an observed loss of amplitude or increase in latency is as follows:

1. Check recording electrode impedances. A high impedance suggests electrode dislodgement.
2. Check stimulator settings and error indicators. Many evoked potential instruments provide a visual indicator that warns of failure to deliver the set stimulus.

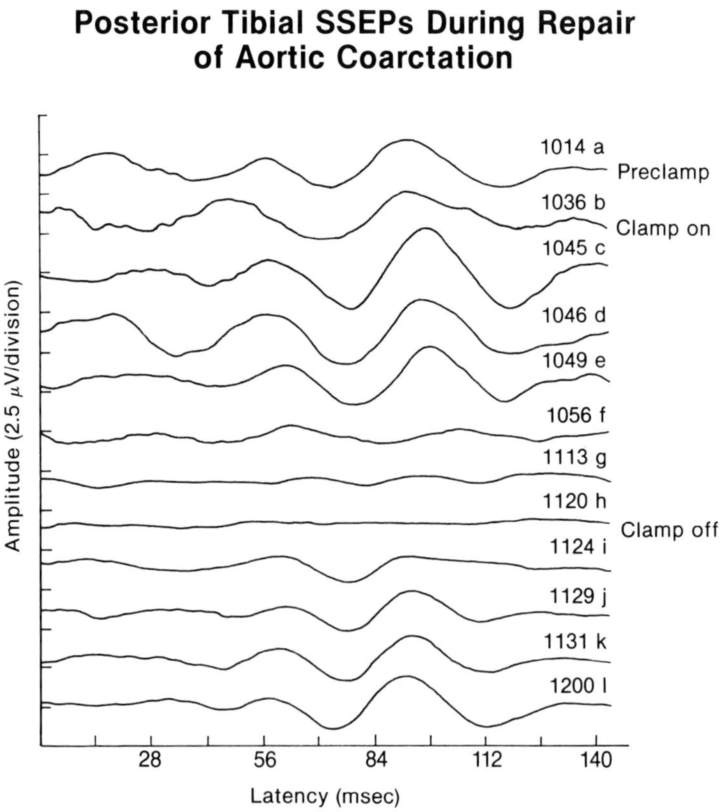

Figure 30–8 • Posterior tibial SSEPs were recorded during repair of aortic coarctation. (*A*) Prior to aortic cross clamping, 7 intercostal arteries were ligated. (*B*) Aortic clamps were placed at 1036. (*C–G*) At 9, 10, 13, 20, and 37 minutes postocclusion. (*H*) Aortic clamps released. (*I–L*) At 4, 9, 11, and 40 minutes following reperfusion. Despite the prompt return of the SSEP, the patient was left with a lower extremity paralysis due to an anterior spinal artery syndrome.

Table 30-1 • Stimulus and Recording Parameters for SSEPs and BAERs

Posterior Tibial SSEPs (Fig. 30-9)

Timebase = 140 ms
Repetitions = 200
Recording electrodes
Channel 1
FPz (−) to Cz′ (+): Cortical response
Channel 2
Medial thigh (−) to popliteal fossa (+): Nerve action potential for verification of stimulus delivery
Ground electrode
A1 or A2 (mastoid process or earlobe)
Filtering*
Low filter = 30 Hz
High filter = 250–500 Hz

Gain

Sensitivity = 50 μV

Stimulus parameters

Stimulus site = posterior tibial nerves at the ankle
Stimulus duraton = 100 μsec
Stimulus rate = 3.1 Hz for awake patients; 5.1 Hz post-
induction
Stimulus current = motor threshold + 30% for wake patients; 20 mA postinduction.

Median Nerve SSEPs (Fig. 30-10)

Timebase = 40 ms
Repetitions = 200
Recording electrodes
Channel 1
FPz (−) to C3′ (+): Cortical response to right median nerve stimulation
Channel 2
FPz (−) to C4′ (+): Cortical response to left median nerve stimulation
Channel 3
FPz (−) to Erbs point (+): Nerve action potential from brachial plexus for verification of stimulus delivery
Ground electrode
A1 or A2
Filtering
Low filter = 30 Hz
High filter = 250 Hz

Gain

Sensitivity = 50 μV

Stimulus parameters

Stimulus site = Right or left median nerve at the wrist
Stimulus duration = 100 μsec
Stimulus rate = 3.1 Hz for awake patients; 5.1 Hz post-
induction
Stimulus current = motor threshold + 30% for awake patients; 20 mA postinduction.

BAERs (Fig. 30-11)

Time base = 10 ms
Repetitions = 2000
Recording electrodes
Channel 1
Cz′ (+) to A1 (−)
Channel 2
Cz′ (+) to A2 (−)
Ground electrode
FPz
Filtering
Low filter = 150 Hz
High filter = 3000 Hz

Gain

Sensitivity = 20 μV

Stimulus parameters

Stimulus site = Right or left ear
Alternating rarefaction/condensation clicks with white noise (40 dB above threshold) into contralateral ear
Stimulus rate and intensity = 11.1 Hz at 70 dB above auditory threshold

*These settings are more restrictive than most other published values in an attempt to eliminate electrical interference in the "noisy" operating room environment.

SSEP, somatosensory evoked potential; BAER, brainstem auditory evoked response

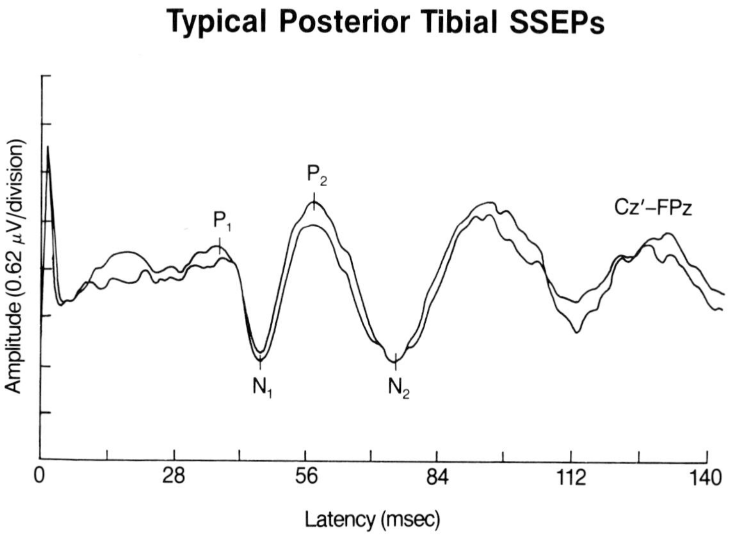

Figure 30-9 • Typical posterior tibial SSEP demonstrates reproducibility of waveform. Note the stimulus artifact spike at the extreme left margin of the waveform.

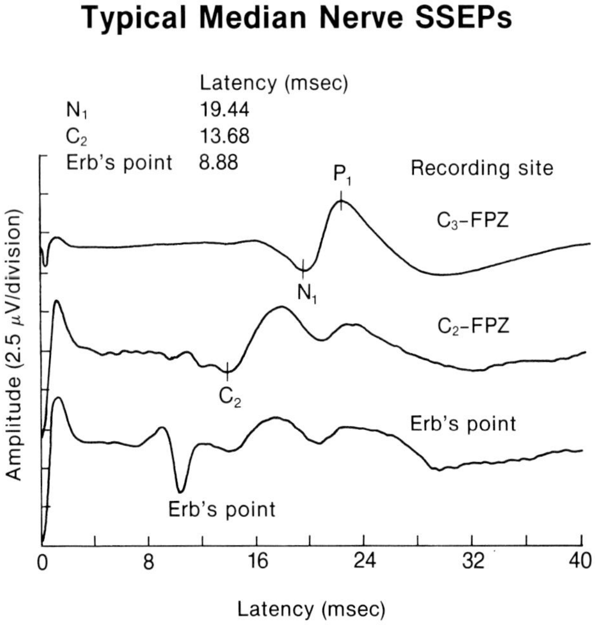

Figure 30–10 • Typical median nerve SSEPs show waveforms and latencies as recorded from electrodes over Erb's point (supraclavicular fossa over the brachial plexus), the cervical spinal cord (skin electrode over the posterior arch of the second cervical vertebra [*C2*]), and scalp electrodes.

3. Examine the evoked potential tracings for the presence of a stimulus artifact and the preservation of the peripheral nerve action potential. Loss of either of these suggests a failure to deliver the stimulus. An examination of the input signal may reveal the presence of 60-cycle interference or EMG activity.
4. Inquire as to any sudden changes in anesthetic depth or alterations of vital signs.
5. Start a new average.

All of the above can accomplished within 30 to 60 seconds of noting an ominous change in an evoked potential. If the repeat recording reproduces the changes, the surgeons should be notified that a change suggestive of neural injury has been observed. Averages should continue to be obtained and stored, and the surgical team should be notified of any further alterations in the responses, including a return toward the baseline configuration. At the conclusion of the procedure, a notation should be made in the patient's chart describing what, if any, significant changes were observed and that these were discussed with the surgeons.

B. *Efficacy*

There have been no controlled human trials comparing the incidence of new neurologic deficits with and without intraoperative evoked potential monitoring. Given the widespread acceptance of this monitoring modality and the ethical concerns that would be raised by studies including a control group in which there was no response to observed changes in the SSER, it is unlikely that conclusive evidence of the benefit of intraoperative evoked potential monitoring will ever be obtained. Nonetheless, there is a large body of human and animal data that supports the concept that evoked potential monitoring can provide early warning of neurologic injury. As early as 1982, Raudzens concluded that persistence of the BAER waveform "was associated with intact auditory acuity" and that "deterioration or loss of the BAER waveform was associated with minimal or profound postoperative hearing deficit."[37] In studies of patients undergoing procedures on the thoracoabdominal aorta, there appears to be a good correlation between

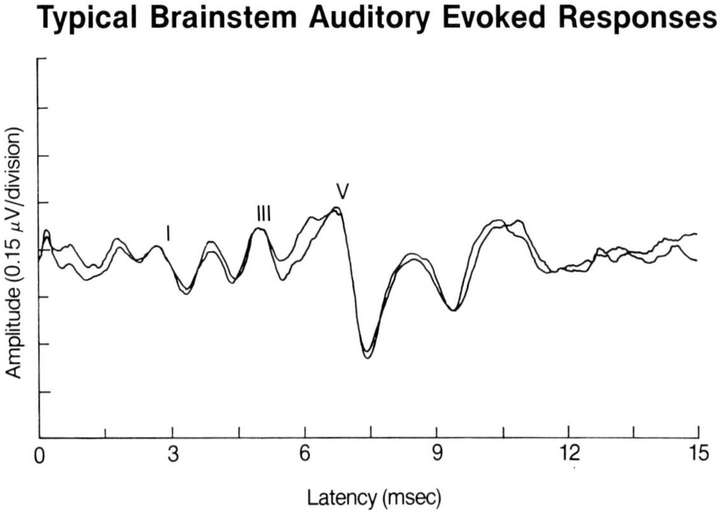

Figure 30–11 • Typical BAER is shown with waves I, III, and V identified.

duration of SSEP loss and incidence of postoperative neurologic deficit. Cunningham and associates found a 71% incidence of paraplegia in patients with an intraoperative SSEP loss lasting more than 30 minutes. This was in contrast to a 0% incidence of paraplegia in patients in whom the SSEP loss was prevented or limited to less than 30 minutes.[6] In animal models involving aortic occlusion, significant decreases in spinal cord blood flow have been shown to be temporally related to the loss of SSEPs.[3,38] Increasing the duration of SSEP loss from 5 to 10 minutes resulted in increasing the incidence of paraplegia from 0% to 67%.[3]

Despite the preponderance of evidence that intraoperative changes in evoked potentials correlate well with the postoperative neurologic status, there have been several case reports in which false-positive [39] and false-negative[40,41] results have been observed. These discrepancies may be due to the fact that SSEPs predominantly monitor posterior column function. Injury could conceivably occur to the motor pathways but leave the sensory tracts intact. These case reports do not invalidate the use of intraoperative SSEPs, but rather emphasize the need to be aware of the potential limitations of this monitoring modality.

V. COMPLICATIONS

There are few complications associated with SSEP monitoring. In our more than 8-year experience and 750 cases, there have been three patients in whom subcutaneous recording or stimulating needles have broken off under the skin. Attempts to recover the fragments were unsuccessful in all cases. In one case, a pressure sore of the forehead was caused by an FPz electrode on a patient in the prone position. This electrode rested for several hours against a Mayfield horseshoe headrest and resulted in an ischemic ulceration of the underlying skin.

Although we have not observed any cautery-induced burns at electrode sites, such a complication is always a possibility if there is improper patient grounding or isolation of the evoked potential machine's amplifiers. Finally, there is the remote possibility of peripheral nerve injury when stimulating needle electrodes are inserted in anesthetized patients.

VI. REFERENCES

1. Cedzich C, Schramm J, Fahlbusch R. Are flash evoked visual potentials useful for intraoperative monitoring of visual pathway function? Neurosurgery 21:709–715, 1987.
2. Grundy BL. Intraoperative monitoring of sensory evoked potentials. Anesthesiology 58:72–87, 1983.
3. Laschinger JC, Cunningham JN, Cooper MM, Baumann FG, et al. Monitoring of somatosensory evoked potentials during surgical procedures on the thoracoabdominal aorta. 1. Relationship of aortic cross-clamp duration, changes in somatosensory evoked potentials, and incidence of neurologic dysfunction. J Thorac Cardiovasc Surg 94:260–265, 1987.
4. Laschinger JC, Cunningham, JN, Baumann FG, Isom OW, et al. Monitoring of somatosensory evoked potentials during surgical procedures on the thoracoabdominal aorta. 2. Use of somatosensory evoked potentials to assess adequacy of distal aortic bypass and perfusion after thoracic aortic cross-clamping. J Thorac Cardiovasc Surg 94:266–270, 1987.
5. Laschinger JC, Cunningham JN, Baumann FG, Cooper MM, et al. Monitoring of somatosensory evoked potentials during surgical procedures on the thoracoabdominal aorta. 3. Intraoperative identification of vessels critical to spinal cord blood supply. J Thorac Cardiovasc Surg 94:271–274, 1987.
6. Cunningham JN, Laschinger JC, Spencer FC. Monitoring of somatosensory evoked potentials during surgical procedures on the thoracoabdominal aorta. 4. Clinical observations and results. J Thorac Cardiovasc Surg 94:260–265, 1987.
7. Laschinger JC, Cunningham JN, Catinella FC, Nathan IM, et al. Detection and prevention of intraoperative spinal cord ischemia after cross-clamping of the thoracic aorta: Use of somatosensory evoked potentials. Surgery 92:1109–1117, 1982.
8. Grundy BL, Nelson PB, Lina A, Heros RC. Monitoring of cortical somatosensory evoked potentials to determine the safety of sacrificing the anterior cerebral artery. Neurosurgery 11:64–67, 1982.
9. Friedman WA, Kaplan BJ, Gravenstein D, Rhoton AL. Intraoperative brain-stem auditory evoked potentials during posterior fossa microvascular decompression. J Neurosurg 62:552–557, 1985.
10. Raudzens PA, Shetter AG. Intraoperative monitoring of brainstem auditory evoked potentials. J Neurosurg 57:341–348, 1982.
11. Schramm J, Mokrusch T, Fahlbusch R, Hochstetter A. Detailed analysis of intraoperative changes in monitoring brain stem acoustic evoked potentials. Neurosurgery 22:694–702, 1988.
12. Linden RD, Tator CH, Benedict C, Charles D, et al. Electrophysiological monitoring during acoustic neuroma and other posterior fossa surgery. Canadian J Neurol Sc 15:73–81, 1988.
13. Schubert A, Drummond JC, Garfin SR. The influence of stimulus presentation rate on the cortical amplitude and latency of intraoperative somatosensory-evoked potential recordings in patients with varying degrees of spinal cord injury. Spine 12:969–973, 1987.
14. Jasper HH. The ten twenty electrode system of the International Federation. Electroencephalogr Clin Neurophysiol 10:371–375, 1958.
15. Koht A, Schutz W, Schmidt G, Schramm J, et al. Effects of etomidate, midazolam, and thiopental on median nerve somatosensory evoked potentials and the additive effects of fentanyl and nitrous oxide. Anesth Analg 67:435–441, 1988.
16. Peterson DO, Drummond JC, Todd MM. Effects of halothane, enflurane, isoflurane and nitrous oxide on somatosensory evoked potentials in humans. Anesthesiology 65:35–40, 1986.
17. Ganes T, Lundar T. The effect of thiopentone on somatosensory evoked responses and EEGs in comatose patients. J Neurol Neurosurg Psychiatr 46:509–514, 1983.
18. Sutton LN, Frewen T, Marsh R, Jaggi J, et al. The effects of deep barbiturate coma on multimodality evoked potentials. J Neurosurg 57:178–185, 1982.
19. Grundy BL, Brown RH, Berilla JA. Fentanyl alters somatosen-

sory cortical evoked potentials. Anesth Analg 59:544–545, 1980.
20. Pathak KS, Brown RH, Cascorbi HF, Nash CL. Effects of fentanyl and morphine on intraoperative somatosensory cortical-evoked potentials. Anesth Analg 63:833–837, 1984..
21. McPherson RW, Sell B, Traystman RJ. Effects of thiopental, fentanyl, and etomidate on upper extremity somatosensory evoked potentials in humans. Anesthesiology 65:584–589, 1986.
22. Drummond JC, Todd MM, U HS. The effect of high dose sodium thiopental on brain stem auditory and median nerve somatosensory evoked responses in humans. Anesthesiology 63:249–254, 1985.
23. Sloan TB, Ronai AK, Toleikis JR, Koht A. Improvement of intraoperative somatosensory evoked potentials by etomidate. Anesth Analg 67:582–585, 1988.
24. Schmidt JF, Chraemmer-Jorgensen B. Auditory evoked potentials during isoflurane anaesthesia. Acta Anaesth Scand 30:378–380, 1986.
25. Nuwer MR. Evoked Potential Monitoring in the Operating Room. New York, Raven Press, 1986, p 78.
26. Grundy BL, Heros RC, Tung AS, Doyle E: Intraoperative hypoxia detected by evoked potential monitoring. Anesth Analg 60:437–439, 1981.
27. McPherson RW, Zeger S, Traystman RJ. Relationship of somatosensory evoked potentials and cerebral oxygen consumption during hypoxic hypoxia in dogs. Stroke 17:30–36, 1986.
28. Pierelli F, Rizzo PA, Romano R, Mattiolo GL, et al. Early auditory evoked potential changes during hypoxic hypoxia in the rabbit. Experimental Neurology 94:479–488, 1986.
29. Brodkey JS, Richards DE, Blasingame JP, Nulsen FE. Reversible spinal cord trauma in cats: Additive effects of direct pressure and ischemia. J Neurosurg 37:591–593, 1972.
30. Lesnick JE, Coyer PE, Michele JJ, Welsh FA, et al. Comparison of the somatosensory evoked potential and the direct cortical response following severe incomplete global ischemia: Selective vulnerability of the white matter conduction pathways. Stroke 17:1247–1250, 1986.
31. Grundy BL, Nash CL, Brown RH. Arterial pressure manipulation alters spinal cord function during correction of scoliosis. Anesthesiology 54:249–253, 1981.
32. Stockard JJ, Sharbrough FW, Tinker JA. Effects of hypothermia on the human brainstem auditory response. Ann Neurol 3:368–370, 1978.
33. Van Rheineck Leyssius AT, Kalkman CJ, Bovill JG. Influence of moderate hypothermia on posterior tibial nerve somatosensory evoked potentials. Anesth Analg 65:475–480, 1986.
34. Russ W, Sticher J, Scheld H, Hempelmann G. Effects of hypothermia on somatosensory evoked responses in man. Br J Anaesth 59:1484–1491, 1987.
35. Schubert A, Zornow MH, Drummond JC, Luerssen TG. Loss of cortical evoked responses due to intracranial gas during posterior fossa craniectomy in the seated position. Anesth Analg 65:203–206, 1986.
36. Nuwer MR. Evoked Potential Monitoring in the Operating Room. New York, Raven Press, 1986, p 101.
37. Raudzens PA: Intraoperative monitoring of evoked potentials. Ann NY Acad Sci 388:308–326, 1982.
38. Kaplan BJ, Friedman WA, Gravenstein N, Richards R, et al. Effects of aortic occlusion on regional spinal cord blood flow and somatosensory evoked potentials in sheep. Neurosurgery 21:668–675, 1987.
39. Chatrian GE, Berger MS, Wirch AL. Discrepancy between intraoperative SSEP's and postoperative function. J Neurosurg 69:450–454, 1988.
40. Ginsburg HH, Shetter AG, Raudzens PA. Postoperative paraplegia with preserved intraoperative somatosensory evoked potentials. J Neurosurg 63:296–300, 1985.
41. Lesser RP, Raudzens P, Luders H, et al. Postoperative neurological deficits may occur despite unchanged intraoperative somatosensory evoked potentials. Ann Neurol 19:22–25, 1986.

Chapter 31

Gershon Levinson, MD

Spinal Anesthesia

OUTLINE

I. INTRODUCTION

Spinal anesthesia is one of the most frequently employed methods of regional anesthesia. Temporary interruption of nerve transmission is easily produced by injecting local anesthetic into the readily identified subarachnoid space. The ensuing anesthesia is predictable, occurs rapidly, and is associated with profound muscle relaxation and contraction of the gastrointestinal tract. The patient may be wide awake, or if preferred, the anesthetic may be supplemented with varying amounts of sedative-tranquilizers. The technique is particularly useful for surgery involving the lower extremities, pelvis, perineum, and lower abdomen. For upper abdominal and thoracic surgery, it may be combined with light general endotracheal anesthesia.

A. Anatomy

1. Vertebrae

The spinal column, which surrounds the spinal cord, is formed by a series of bony vetebrae separated by cartilaginous intervertebral disks and united by a series of ligaments. The vertebral column is usually composed of 33 vertebrae: 7 cervical, 12 thoracic, 5 lumbar, 5 fused sacral, and 4 fused coccygeal. A typical vertebra is shown in Fig. 31–1. The body of the vertebra bears the weight of the patient and forms the base of the neural arch. The arch, which surrounds the spinal cord, is made up of a pedicle and lamina on each side. Projecting from the arch are two transverse processes and one spinous process, which allow for the attachment of muscles and ligaments, and four articular processes (two upper and two lower), which allow for movement between vertebrae. The pedicles are not as deep as their respective vertebrae and are notched superiorly and inferiorly. The inferior notch of one vertebra and the superior notch of the contiguous vertebra form an intervertebral foramen through which a spinal nerve passes. Between the laminae of each vertebra there is a posterior opening in the vetebral canal. It is through this opening that a spinal needle is passed when performing a subarachnoid block.

2. Spinal Curves

The vertebral column has four anterior–posterior curves, which are shown in Fig. 31–2. In the supine position, the highest point of the lumbar curve is the third lumbar vertebra and the lowest point of the thoracic curve is the fifth thoracic vertebra. The thoracic concavity discourages spread of hyperbaric local anesthetic solution above the fourth thoracic vertebra. The lumbar convexity encourages sacral pooling, thereby limiting cephalad spread of solutions injected below the third lumbar vertebra. The lithotomy position usually eliminates the lumbar concavity and makes the lowest point approximately the tenth thoracic vertebra.

3. Intervertebral Ligaments

Individual vertebrae and their intervening disks are held together by a number of ligaments, each of which has a characteristic feel that helps the experienced anesthesiologist recognize the position of the advancing spinal needle. The three ligaments traversed in administering a spinal anesthetic are the *ligamentum flavum*, which unites the laminae; the *interspinous ligament*, which joins the spinous processes; and the *supraspinous ligament*, which connects the tips of the spinous processes (Fig. 31–3).

In the lumbar region, the supraspinous ligament may be almost half an inch wide. In the elderly, ossification of this ligament may make the midline insertion of a thin needle almost impossible. However, a needle placed just lateral to the supraspinous ligament can be directed toward the interlaminar space without meeting obstruction. The interspinous ligament is a thin, spongy structure, which does not afford much resistance to the advancing spinal needle. The ligamentum flavum is thick and strong in the lumbar region, and the loss of

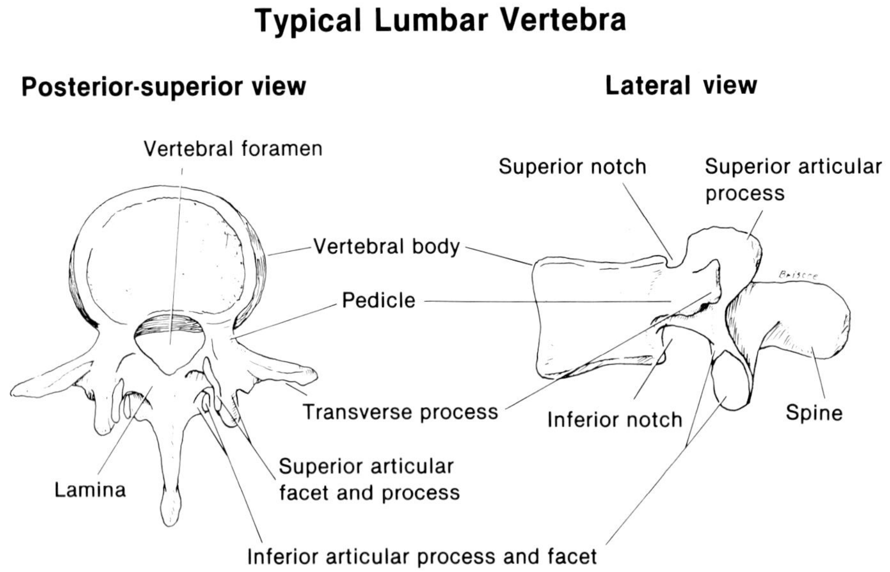

Figure 31–1 • Lateral and posterior–superior view of a typical lumbar vertebra.

The Vertebral Column Curves

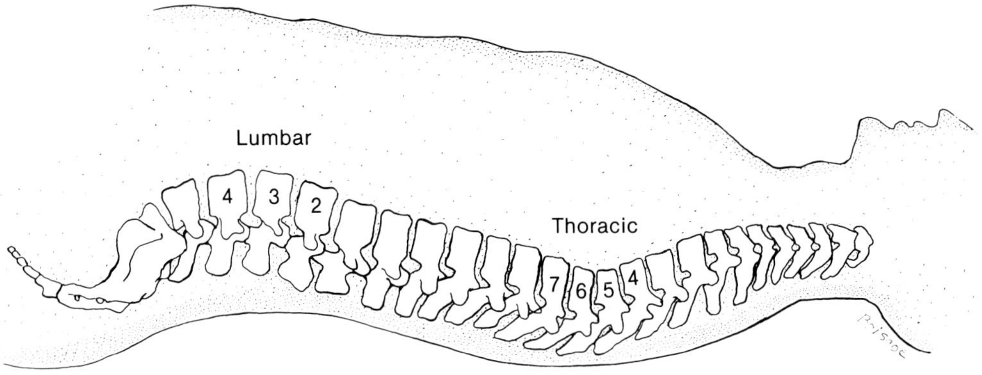

Figure 31–2 • Normal curvature of the vertebral column with the patient in the supine position. The lumbar lordosis produces a high point at the third lumbar vertebra, and the thoracic kyphosis produces a low point at the fifth thoracic vertebra.

resistance felt as the needle passes through it into the epidural space may be incorrectly perceived as a dural puncture. With further advancement of the needle, the next layer of resistance, the dura-arachnoid, is encountered. The piercing of this layer allows the free flow of cerebrospinal fluid.

4. SPINAL CORD

The cylindrical spinal cord varies in length from 40 to 45 cm. It is continuous with the medulla oblongata above it and ends below in the conus medullaris. The spinal cord ends at variable levels depending on the age of the pa-

The Intervertebral Ligaments

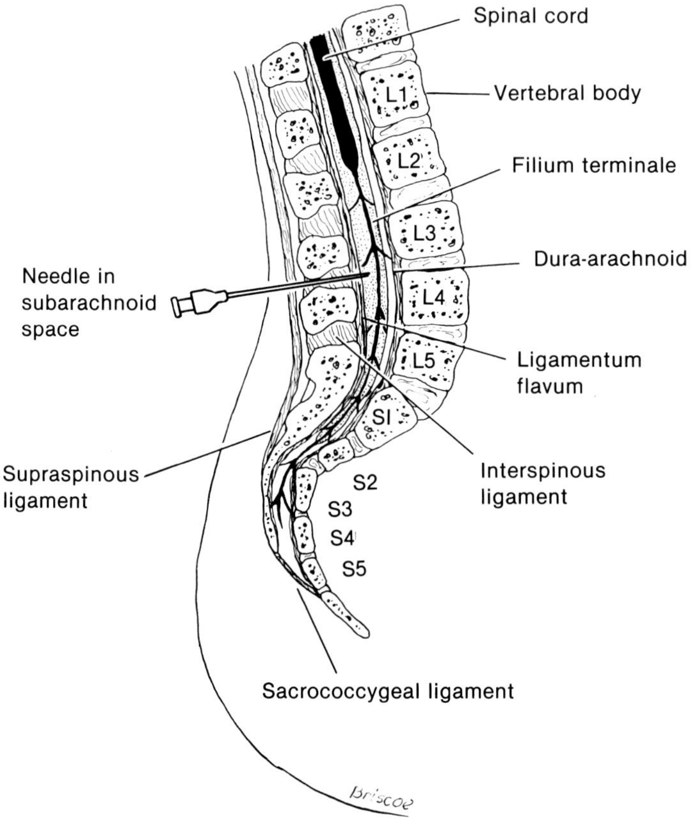

Figure 31–3 • Schematic diagram of lumbosacral anatomy showing the spinal cord and intervertebral ligaments (the supraspinous and interspinous ligaments and the ligamentum flavum).

tient. In the newborn, the cord extends to the third lumbar vertebra, but in the adult the cord usually ends at the lower border of the first lumbar vertebra because the spinal cord does not grow as much as the vertebral column. There is, however, considerable variation, and extension of the cord to the second or third lumbar vertebra is not uncommon.[1]

Thirty-one pairs of symmetrically arranged spinal nerves are each attached to the spinal cord by an anterior and posterior root. Because the spinal cord is shorter than the vertebral column, the spinal cord segments in adults do not lie opposite their corresponding vertebrae. The spinal nerve roots must travel obliquely in a caudad direction to reach their respective intervertebral foramina. The roots of the lumbar, sacral, and coccygeal nerves comprise the *cauda equina* and are necessarily the largest and longest in order to reach their intervertebral foramen. The individual nerve roots of the cauda equina are easily movable and are therefore seldom traumatized by an advancing spinal needle. The greater size of these nerve roots provides a larger surface area to be exposed to the action of local anesthetics, thus allowing more rapid onset of anesthesia.

5. Spinal Meninges

The spinal cord is covered by three membranes or meninges. The *dura mater* (the outermost membrane) is the downward continuation of the meningeal layer of the cranial dura mater. It extends from the foramen magnum to the lower border of the second sacral vertebra. Below this level it closely adheres to the filum terminale, which runs to the back of the base of the coccyx, where it fuses with the periosteum.

The middle of the three coverings, the *arachnoid*, is a thin membrane closely adherent to the dura mater. The dura and the arachnoid are in such close contact that usually it is not possible to puncture the dura without also piercing the arachnoid. Nevertheless, on rare occasions, the tip of an epidural or spinal needle may accidentally wind up in the subdural space. In a spinal anesthetic this should not present a problem because there would be no free flow of cerebrospinal fluid, and presumably the needle would be repositioned before local anesthetic is injected. Should the bevel of the spinal needle lie partially in both the subdural and the subarachnoid space, as may result from rotating the needle repeatedly, a considerable amount of the local anesthetic may enter the subdural space, where it would diffuse poorly and result in inadequate contact with the nerve roots. Poor or absent anesthesia may ensue.[2] Should subdural placement occur during an attempted epidural anesthetic, the improper position of the needle may not be recognized and the injection of an epidural dose of local anesthetic may result in a much higher block than anticipated.

The innermost membrane, the *pia mater*, is a thin, delicate, highly vascular membrane closely adherent to the spinal cord. It also covers each spinal nerve root as far as the intervertebral foramen and extends several ligamentous projections outward, helping to support the spinal cord. It has been suggested that these ligamentous structures may occasionally cause obstruction of small-gauge spinal needle orifices during aspiration.[3]

6. Subarachnoid Space

Filled with cerebrospinal fluid, the *subarachnoid space* is lined internally by the pia and externally by the arachnoid. It is continuous above with the cranial subarachnoid space and ends below at the second sacral vertebra. In addition to spinal fluid, the space contains the spinal nerve roots and the main blood vessels of the central nervous system. In the cervical and thoracic regions, the space is only about 3 mm deep, but below the lower border of the first lumbar vertebra, where the spinal cord usually ends, the space has a diameter of 14–15 mm.

7. Cerebrospinal Fluid

Cerebrospinal fluid (CSF) is a clear, colorless fluid. It is formed at the rate of about 400 mL/day. In the average adult, the total volume is about 120–150 mL, of which 20–35 mL are in the spinal portion of the subarachnoid space. In the lumbar region, the normal pressure of CSF is 60–100 mmH_2O with the patient in the lateral position, and 200–250 mmH_2O in the sitting position. At 37° C, its specific gravity is 1.007 (from 1.003 to 1.009) relative to water at the same temperature.

II. How to Perform Spinal Anesthesia and Lumbar Puncture

A. *Equipment*

A wide variety of commercially prepared disposable spinal trays are available, and anesthesiologists should have no difficulty in finding one containing the syringes, needles, skin preparation swabs, and drapes they prefer. A spinal needle 9 cm (3.5 inches) long is usually adequate, but longer ones (10–15 cm) should be available for the occasional obese patient or difficult paramedian approach. The needle should have a removable, close-fitting stylet to prevent coring of the skin.

Two sizes of spinal needle are commonly used: 22 gauge and 25 gauge. The more rigid, larger diameter 22 gauge needle is easier to direct and makes characteristic feel of the various ligaments easier to appreciate. With the larger needle, however, the incidence of postspinal headache is increased.[4] The standard spinal needle (Quincke) has a sharp point with a cutting bevel (Fig. 31–4). The pencil-point needle (Whitacre) has a solid tip and a completely rounded noncutting bevel.[5] This bevel spreads, rather than cuts, the predominantly longitudinal dural fibers, and on removal of the needle the resulting dural hole should be smaller. Indeed, the incidence of postspinal headache when a 22 gauge Whitacre needle is used is comparable to that following use of a 26 gauge Quincke needle.[6]

When using a thin 25 or 26 gauge spinal needle it is frequently helpful to use an introducer. The introducer eliminates contact of the spinal needle with the skin, properly directs it, and allows the relatively flimsy needle to avoid the tough supraspinous ligament. Various introducers are available, but the standard disposable thin-wall, 18 gauge, 1.5-inch needle is adequate.

B. Anesthetic Solutions

The components of a typical spinal anesthetic solution are a local anesthetic, a solution to produce the proper baricity, and if necessary, a vasoconstrictor to prolong the duration of the block. The choice of anesthetic solution is determined by the desired sensory level and duration of anesthesia for the planned surgical procedure. The approximate sensory level required for various surgical procedures is shown in Table 31–1.

1. DISTRIBUTION OF ANESTHESIA

Many factors influence the ultimate level of anesthesia achieved.[7] The most important factors are the dose and volume of anesthetic solution administered, the baricity of the solution, and the position of the patient. Other factors that affect distribution of local anesthetic in CSF, but are of less clinical significance, are patient age and height, volume of CSF, and anatomic configuration of the spinal column. Factors that have no clinically significant effects on distribution are patient weight, CSF pressure, and local anesthetic concentration.

2. DURATION OF ANESTHESIA

The factors that affect the duration of anesthesia are the type and dose of local anesthetic used, the level of anesthesia achieved, patient age, and the presence of vasoconstrictors.[8] Larger amounts of local anesthetic will produce blocks of longer duration. For a given dose of local anesthetic, a higher sensory level will have a shorter duration of action, since it provides a greater absorptive surface for elimination of local anesthetic. In elderly patients the duration of action is longer than in young patients, probably because there is less blood flow to the spinal cord and the subarachnoid space.

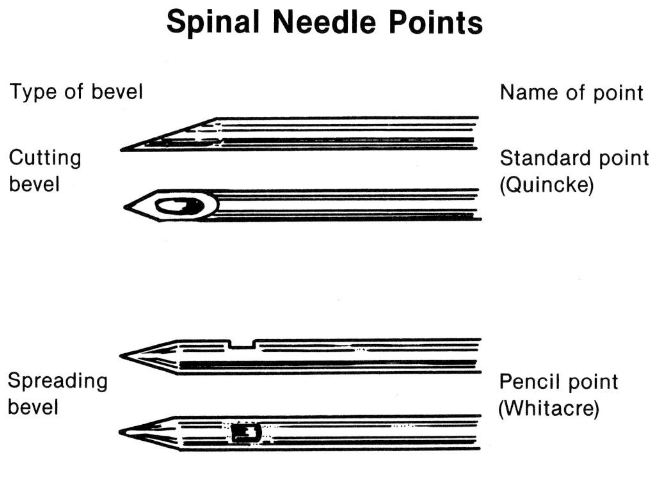

Figure 31–4 • The standard spinal needle bevel cuts tissue, whereas the pencil-point Whitacre needle bevel spreads tissue.

Table 31–1 • Approximate Sensory Levels Required for Various Surgical Procedures

Surgical Site	Anesthetic Level
Lower Extremity	
Knee and below	L-2 to L-3
(with tourniquet)	T-8 to T-10
Hip	T-10
Rectal Procedures	S-2 to S-5
Lower Intraabdominal	
Inguinal hernia	T-4 to T-6
Appendix	T-4 to T-6
Intestine	T-4 to T-6
Pelvis	T-4 to T-6
Genitourinary	
Vagina and uterus	T-10
Testes and ovaries	T-4
Transurethral resection, prostate	T-10
Obstetric	
Vaginal delivery	T-10
Cesarean section	T-4
Upper Abdominal	T-4

3. LOCAL ANESTHETICS

The local anesthetics commonly used for spinal anesthesia are procaine, lidocaine, tetracaine, and bupivacaine. The major clinical difference between them is the duration of action. Suggested doses of commonly used spinal anesthetic drugs and their approximate duration of action are shown in Table 31–2.

Procaine, with a duration of action of about 30 to 60 minutes, is used primarily for short procedures. It is available as a 10% solution that must be diluted before injection. It may be diluted with an equal volume of 10% glucose or CSF depending on whether a hyperbaric or an isobaric mixture is desired. Lidocaine has a slightly longer duration of action than procaine, 60 to 90 minutes. A premixed solution of 5% lidocaine and 7.5% glucose is usually used for spinal anesthesia. Tetracaine and bupivacaine produce anesthesia lasting 2 to 4 hours. Their usage is described below.

4. BARICITY

Density is the weight in grams of 1 mL of a solution (g/mL) at a specific temperature. *Specific gravity* is the ratio of the density of a solution to the density of water. Since density varies with temperature, accurate reporting of density and specific gravity requires that the respective temperatures of the solutions are stated. *Baricity* is the ratio of the density of the anesthetic solution at a specific temperature to the density of CSF at the same temperature, preferably 37° C. The usual volume of anesthetic solution injected reaches body temperature within 60 seconds, and it is the density at body temperature that determines baricity relative to CSF.

An *isobaric* solution has a baricity of 1.0. If the baricity is greater than 1.0, the solution is *hyperbaric*; if it is less, the solution is *hypobaric*. Since there are individual variations in the density of normal human CSF (0.9997 to 1.0009), the baricity of hyperbaric local anesthetic solutions should be greater than 1.0010 and hypobaric solutions less than 0.9990.[9] The baricities of some commonly used spinal anesthetic mixtures are shown in Table 31–3.

Spinal anesthetic solutions are usually made hyperbaric by the addition of glucose. Hyperbaric solutions of lidocaine and bupivacaine come premixed with 7.5% and 8.25% glucose, respectively. The commercially available solution of 1% tetracaine is made hyperbaric by mixing with an equal volume of 10% glucose. Hyperbaric spinal anesthetic solutions, being heavier than CSF, will gravitate to the most dependent portion of the subarachnoid space. The level of anesthesia achieved with these solutions is determined by the position of the

Table 31–2 • Suggested Doses of Commonly Used Anesthetic Solutions

	Dose (mg) at Desired Sensory Level			Duration (min)	
Anesthetic Solution	***L-1***	***T-10***	***T-4***	***Plain***	***With 0.2 mg epinephrine***
Procaine 5% and glucose 5%	50–75	100–150	150–200	30–45	60–75
Lidocaine 5% and glucose 7.5%	25–50	50–75	75–100	60–90	60–90
Bupivacaine 0.75% and glucose 8.25%	7–5	10–15	15–20	120–150	120–150
Tetracaine 0.5% and glucose 5%	4–6	8–10	12–15	120–180	180–240

Table 31-3 • Baricity of Commonly Used Spinal Anesthetic Mixtures

Solution	Baricity
Cerebrospinal fluid	1.0000
Procaine	
10%	1.0104
2.5% in distilled water	0.9983
Lidocaine 5% and glucose 7.5%	1.0265
Tetracaine	
0.33% in distilled water	0.9977
0.5% and 5% glucose	1.0133
Bupivacaine 0.75% and glucose 8.25%	1.0227

(Modified from Lambert DH, Covino BG: Hyperbaric, hypobaric and isobaric spinal anesthesia. Res Staff Phys 33:79, 1987.)

patient during and after injection. For example, anesthesia can be limited to the lumbar and sacral roots by injecting with the patient in the sitting position and allowing the patient to remain in this position for at least 10 minutes. Although attempts to produce unilateral anesthesia are not usually successful because spread occurs after surgical positioning, a more profound block usually occurs on the side initially kept dependent.[10]

Solutions of tetracaine and procaine are made hypobaric by diluting with distilled water. Concentrations of tetracaine from 0.1% to 0.33% provide good anesthesia and are reliably hypobaric.[11] These solutions will ascend to the least dependent portion of the subarachnoid space. They are commonly used for rectal procedures in the prone position or for hip and extremity surgery in the lateral position.

With isobaric anesthetic solutions, the position of the patient during and after injection does not affect the level of anesthesia.[10] The site of injection and the volume of the solution appear to be the important factors. The most commonly used isobaric solution is made by diluting the standard 1% tetracaine solution with equal volumes of either CSF or normal saline.

5. Vasoconstrictors

Epinephrine or phenylephrine may be added to spinal anesthetic solutions of tetracaine to prolong the duration of the block. The primary mechanism of block prolongation is believed to be vasoconstriction producing decreased vascular absorption of the local anesthetic and prolonging the time the anesthetic is in contact with neutral tissue. Epinephrine, however, has also been shown to block pain transmission by a direct effect on the spinal cord.[12]

The usual dose of epinephrine is 200–300 μg (0.2–0.3 mL of a 1:1000 solution) and of phenylephrine 2–5 mg (0.2–0.5 mL of a 1% solution). In equipotent doses, both drugs prolong the duration of tetracaine spinal anesthesia equally well.[13] The increase in duration is approximately 50% to 100%, depending on the dose of vasoconstrictor used and the endpoint for measuring duration.[13,14] Vasoconstrictors do not significantly prolong the duration of clinically useful spinal anesthesia with lidocaine and bupivacaine[15,16,17]

C. *Patient Selection*

The appropriateness of spinal anesthesia for a patient undergoing surgery depends on the site and duration of the planned surgical procedure, the surgical pathology, and the presence of coexisting disease. The anesthesiologist must consider the advantages and disadvantages of the various forms of anesthesia for each individual patient before recommending an anesthetic technique. Some of the factors to be considered are discussed below.

1. Indications and Advantages

Spinal anesthesia is most useful for operations performed below the level of the umbilicus. Upper abdominal surgery is usually better managed with a well-conducted general anesthetic, since even with a high spinal block the patient may experience pain, hiccoughs, nausea, and vomiting because of the unanesthetized vagus and phrenic nerves. A single-injection spinal anesthetic does not reliably produce surgical anesthesia for longer than 3 to 4 hours, and lengthy operations will therefore require either a continuous catheter technique or general anesthesia.

Surgical procedures in which low spinal anesthesia is particularly advantageous include procedures involving the lower extremities and perineal and perianal areas. For example, in rectal procedures in the prone position, a spinal block of the sacral segments provides excellent operating conditions with minimal physiologic alterations and without the need for endotracheal intubation. For urologic procedures such as transurethral prostatectomies, a low spinal block provides good anesthesia with little likelihood of exacerbating coexisting cardiovascular and pulmonary disorders. Elderly patients undergoing elective hip replacements or repair of hip fractures under spinal anesthesia have a lower frequency of postoperative deep vein thrombosis and improved mortality rate in the early postoperative period than comparable patients receiving general anesthesia.[18,19,20]

If the surgical procedure is appropriate, patients with potentially difficult airways and those with a full stomach may be better managed with a low spinal block than with general anesthesia. Although some physicians advocate spinal anesthesia for patients with coexisting pulmonary disease, Greene concluded after an extensive review of the literature that the frequency and type of postoperative respiratory complications are similar after spinal or general anesthesia in both normal patients and those with preexisting respiratory disease.[21] However, there are exceptions to this broad conclusion. A spinal block to the tenth thoracic dermatome has little effect on ventilation, but with progressively higher motor blockade the expiratory reserve volume falls sharply and is reduced to zero when all thoracic motor roots are blocked.[22] The ability to cough is similarly depressed.[23] Consequently, high spinal anesthesia may be deleterious in patients with pulmonary diseases associated with production of large amounts of sputum, since these patients may be unable to cough and clear their secretions during anesthesia.

In patients with cardiac disease, especially ischemic heart disease and congestive heart failure, the decrease in cardiac work and myocardial oxygen demand produced by spinal anesthesia is beneficial and easily compensates for the decreased perfusion produced by a moderate fall in blood pressure.[24-26] The good effects of spinal anesthesia are due to the combination of a decrease in heart rate both preload and afterload. In patients with cardiac lesions in which these decreases may not be salutary (ie, idiopathic hypertrophic subaortic stenosis, aortic stenosis, mitral stenosis), spinal anesthesia must be administered very cautiously.

2. Absolute Contraindications

There are relatively few *absolute* contraindications to spinal anesthesia. These include:

- Patient refusal
- Infection at the site of needle injection
- Septicemia
- Severe hypovolemia and other forms of shock
- Increased intracranial pressure
- Major coagulopathies

3. Relative Contraindications

Relative contraindications are conditions in which spinal anesthesia is appropriate if, in the medical judgment of the anesthesiologist, the potential benefits of the technique outweigh possible added hazards to the individual patient. These contraindications include:

- Preexisting disease of the spinal cord. Although there is no evidence that spinal anesthesia exacerbates conditions such as multiple sclerosis or old poliomyelitis, many anesthesiologists still prefer to avoid the technique in these circumstances. In chronic paraplegics, spinal anesthesia has the distinct advantage of preventing autonomic hyperreflexia and may be the anesthetic of choice.
- Chronic severe backache. In this condition there is also no evidence that lumbar puncture aggravates the problem, but the technique is often avoided lest the anesthesiologist be blamed for a coincidental exacerbation of the pain.
- Minor clotting abnormalities. If regional anesthesia is to be used in patients receiving minidose heparin or chronic aspirin therapy, it is probably prudent to establish that partial thromboplastin and bleeding times are in the normal range before performing the lumbar puncture.

4. Preoperative Management

Preoperative evaluation of the patient for spinal anesthesia is essentially the same as for general anesthesia and should include a thorough neurologic history and documentation of any preexisting neurologic deficits. If a possible coagulopathy is suspected, a prothrombin and partial thromboplastin time, platelet count, and bleeding time test may be indicated in addition to the usual laboratory studies appropriate to the patient's disease and physical status.

Prior to the administration of a spinal anesthetic, blood pressure and heart rate should be checked, and an intravenous line should be in place. Drugs and equipment for cardiovascular resuscitation, airway management, and administration of oxygen should be immediately available.

D. *Techniques*

Lumbar puncture may be accomplished using a variety of different approaches with the patient in the lateral, prone, or sitting position. A well-trained anesthesiologist should be proficient in a variety of techniques so that the patient position and approach selected will be the one most appropriate to the patient's pathology and planned surgery.

1. LATERAL POSITION AND MIDLINE APPROACH

The midline approach with the patient in the lateral decubitus position is the simplest technique for the anesthesiologist and the most comfortable for the patient. It is the position and approach most commonly used for spinal anesthesia and is therefore described in detail as follows:

1. The patient is placed in the lateral position at the edge of the table closest to the anesthesiologist (Fig. 31–5). An assistant should stand in front of the patient to assist with positioning and prevent the patient from falling. The lumbar vertebrae are then flexed as far as possible to increase the interlaminar spaces. This is accomplished by having the patient bring the knees up toward the stomach and the chin down toward the chest. The hips and shoulders should be perpendicular to the edge of the table. If the vertebral column is truly parallel to the edge of the table, a needle entering in the midline will remain in the midline as long as it is kept parallel to the top of the table.
2. The intercristal line, drawn between the highest points of the iliac crests, will cross either the fourth lumbar vertebra or the space between the third and fourth vertebrae. Other vertebral levels can then be easily identified from this point. The distances between the lumbar vertebrae vary, and usually the widest interspinous space is selected. The precise level is not important as long as it is below the second lumbar vertebra.
3. The patient's back is prepared with an appropriate antiseptic solution, which is allowed to dry, and sterile drapes are applied.
4. The selected interspace is palpated and straddled using the index and middle finger of the nondominant hand (Fig. 31–6). An intracutaneous skin wheal is made at the proposed puncture site using a 25 or 27 gauge needle and either 1% lidocaine or procaine. Using the same local anesthetic and a 2- or 3-cm, 22 gauge needle, the subcutaneous tissue and supraspinous and interspinous ligaments are infiltrated along the intended needle track.
5. Without moving the straddling fingers, the anesthesiologist inserts the spinal needle (Fig. 31–7) or introducer (Fig. 31–8) in the middle of the interspace parallel to the table and angled about 10° cephalad, since the interlaminar space is slightly cephalad to the interspinous space. If a spinal needle with a Quincke or similar point is used, the bevel is positioned laterally so that the longitudinal

Curled Lateral Decubitus Position for Spinal Anesthesia

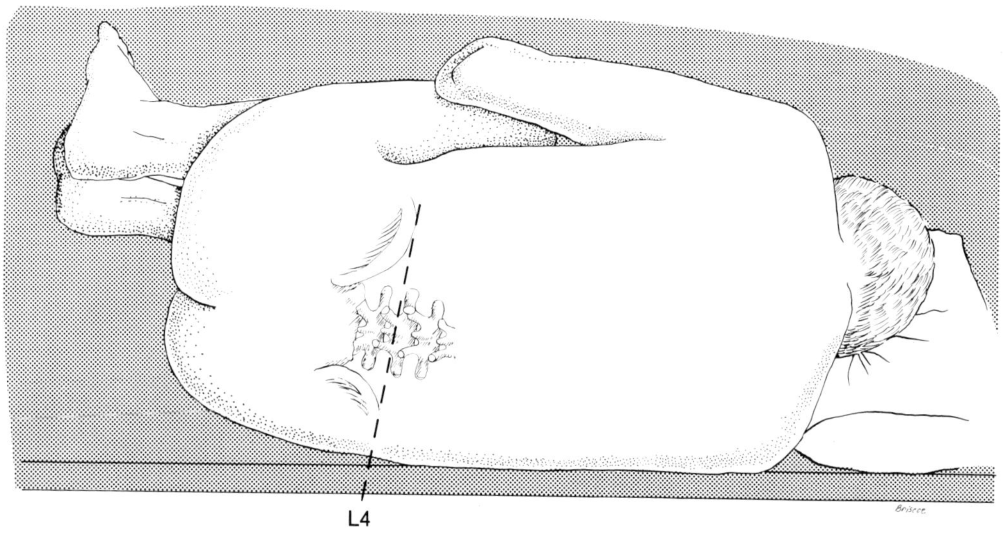

Figure 31–5 • Proper position for lumbar puncture in the lateral decubitus position. The knees are brought up toward the abdomen and the head flexed down on the chest. The hips and shoulders should be perpendicular to the edge of the table.

Local Anesthetic Infiltration Prior to Spinal Anesthesia

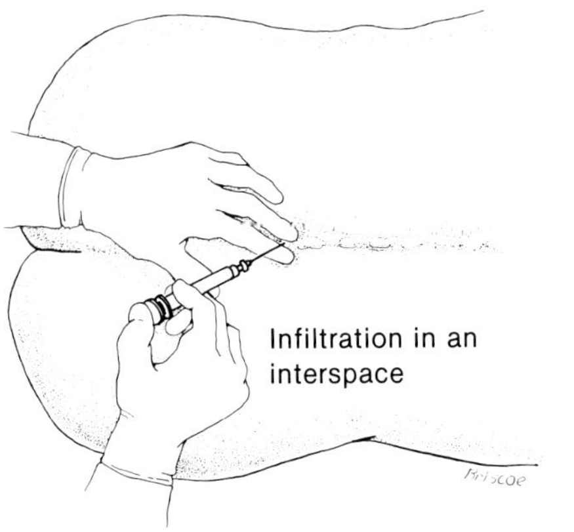

Figure 31–6 • The index and middle fingers of the left hand straddle the selected interspace while local anesthetic is slowly infiltrated along the intended needle track.

Insertion of Introducer Needle

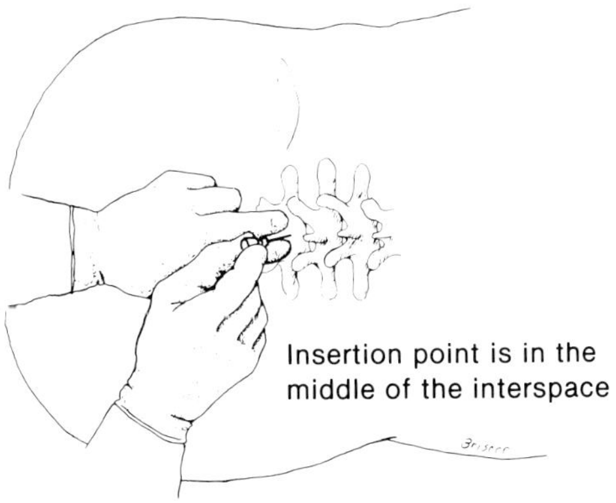

Figure 31–8 • When a 25 or 26 gauge needle is used, an introducer may be inserted into the supraspinous ligament. The straddling fingers remain in place, and the introducer is inserted midline and angled cephalad. The introducer is then held firmly in position and the spinal needle passed through it.

dural fibers are spread rather than cut. The palpating hand should remain in place until the needle or introducer is secure in the supraspinous or interspinous ligament.

6. The spinal needle is then slowly advanced toward the subarachnoid space. The two-handed position shown in Fig. 31-9 provides optimal control of a fine needle. As the needle pierces the ligamentum flavum and the dura-arachnoid, distinct changes in resistance and a characteristic pop will be felt.
7. The stylet should be removed and the hub observed for the free flow of CSF. With fine gauge needles, gentle aspiration with a small syringe may be necessary. If flow is still not obtained, and it is believed that the needle is in the subarachnoid space, the needle should be rotated 90° or 180° and gentle aspiration attempted again. If this is unsuccessful, the stylet should be replaced, the needle advanced, and the check for proper flow of spinal fluid repeated.
8. A transient paresthesia usually indicates that the needle is not in the midline and should be redirected accordingly. If a brief paresthesia has occurred during insertion of the needle and CSF subsequently flows readily, injection of anesthetic can proceed. If a paresthesia occurs during injection of solution, the needle must be repositioned before any further drug is injected.
9. If the initial CSF obtained is blood-stained, it should be allowed to clear before injecting local anesthetic. If it does not clear, the possibility of a recent subarachnoid hemorrhage should be considered, and the procedure abandoned.
10. When proper flow of CSF is obtained, the syringe containing the local anesthetic solution is firmly attached to the hub of the spinal needle. To prevent movement of the spinal needle, the hub should be firmly held between the thumb and forefinger while the back of the hand is placed against the patient's back (Figs. 31–10 and 31–11). A small amount of spinal fluid is aspirated, and if free flow is still present, the local anesthetic is slowly injected. At the end of the injection, aspiration is again performed to reconfirm the proper position of the needle tip. This final aspirate, which contains a high concentration of local anesthetic, should be reinjected.

Insertion of the Spinal Needle

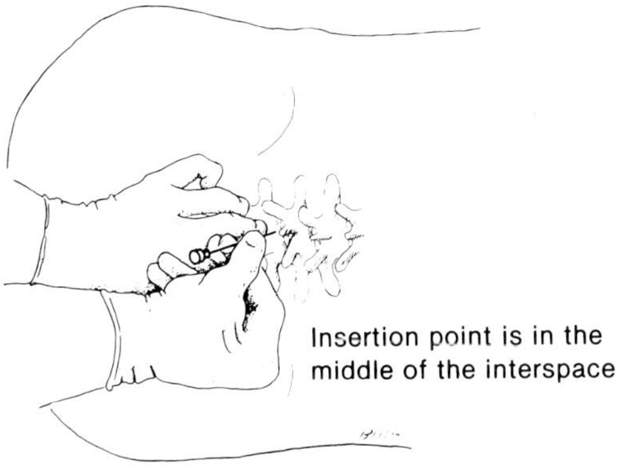

Figure 31–7 • The fingers of the left hand straddle the interspace while the spinal needle is inserted midline and slightly cephalad into the supsraspinous ligament.

Two-Handed Position for Insertion of Spinal Needle

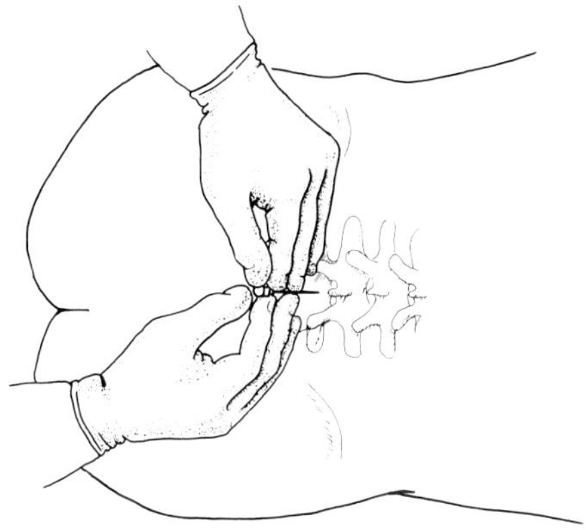

Figure 31–9 • The two-handed position is used to advance the needle slowly toward the subarachnoid space.

11. The needle is then withdrawn and the patient is placed in the appropriate position. Allowing the patient to remain in the lateral position for 5 to 10 minutes may produce a denser block on one side. The affected side is determined by the baricity of the local anesthetic solution.
12. The analgesic level is checked at 2 and 5 minutes. If it is higher or lower than anticipated, the operating table is adjusted as necessary according to the baricity of the local anesthetic solution. The level of anesthesia may continue to rise for 20 to 30 minutes.

Prevention of Spinal Needle Movement During Syringe Attachment

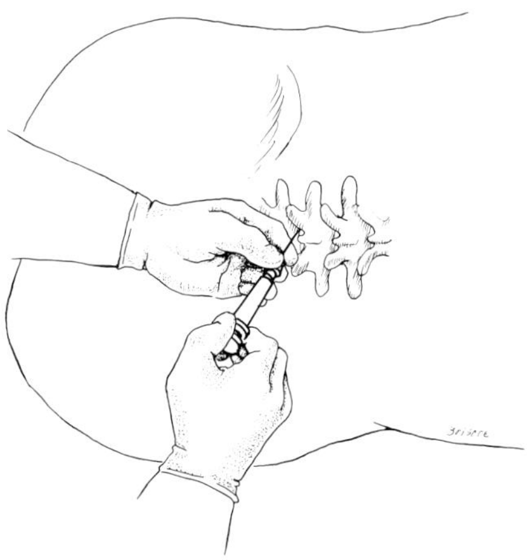

Figure 31–10 • Proper position for stabilizing the spinal needle during syringe attachment. The hub of the needle is held firmly between the thumb and forefinger, while the back of the hand is placed against the patient's back.

Prevention of Spinal Needle Movement During Injection of Spinal Anesthetic

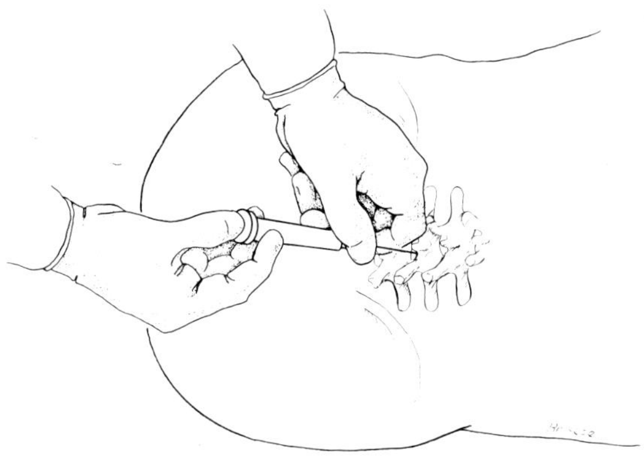

Figure 31–11 • Position for immobilizing the needle during injection of local anesthetic. The hub of the needle is firmly held while the back of the hand rests securely against the patient's back.

13. Following injection of the spinal anesthetic, blood pressure should be monitored frequently and ECG and oxygen saturation should be monitored continuously. Administration of supplemental oxygen may be beneficial.

2. Alternative Positions

a. Sitting Position

The sitting position is particularly useful (1) when anesthesia of only the sacral roots is desired; (2) in obstetric patients having vaginal delivery, for which a low spinal block is usually preferred; (3) in patients with pathology such as an intratrochanteric fracture that makes the sitting position more comfortable than the lateral; or (4) in situations in which it is difficult to palpate the spinous processes. The latter situation most commonly occurs in the very obese patient. When these patients lie in the lateral position, the midline furrow usually sags below the line joining the spinous processes, making palpation of the spines and identification of the midline very challenging. In the sitting position, the furrow remains central. When use of the sitting position is planned, minimal premedication should be used because narcotics and sedatives may produce postural hypotension when the patient is upright. The proper sitting position for spinal anesthesia is shown in Fig. 31–12 and described in detail as follows:

1. The patient sits at the midpoint of the operating table with legs over the side edge, knees bent, and feet supported by

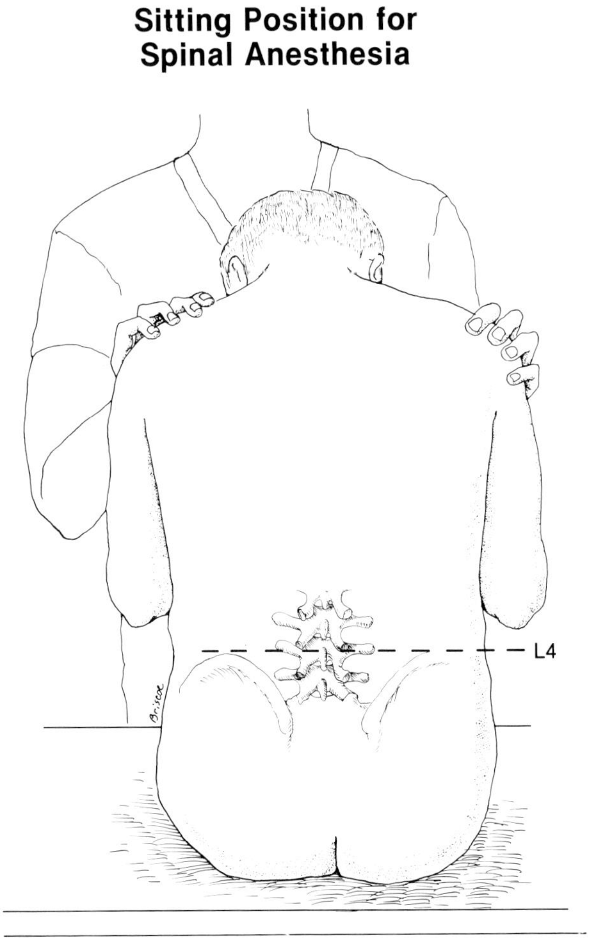

Figure 31–12 • Proper position for lumbar puncture in the sitting position.

a stool. The anesthesiologist stands on the opposite side, and the patient's buttocks should be as close as possible to this edge. The back and neck are flexed to produce the widest possible interlaminar opening. This is accomplished by having the patient lean forward on an assistant or other suitable support. In either case, an assistant should always stand in front of the patient to assist with positioning and supporting the patient.

2. Locating the appropriate interspace, performing the lumbar puncture, and administering the anesthetic drug is accomplished as described for the lateral decubitus position.
3. If only sacral anesthesia is required, and a hyperbaric local anesthetic has been used, the patient may remain in the sitting position until the block is established, usually about 5 minutes. If a higher block is needed, the patient should be immediately assisted back into the supine position following the injection of the local anesthetic.

b. Prone Position

The prone position is used mainly for surgical procedures involving the rectum, perineal area, sacrum, or lower vertebral area. Its major advantage is that the patient does not have to be repositioned after the spinal anesthetic is administered. The patient is usually placed in the jackknife position, and a hypobaric local anesthetic solution is used.

Proper positioning for a spinal anesthetic in the jackknife position is shown in Fig. 31–13 and described as follows:

1. The patient lies on his or her abdomen with the hip joints lying over the flexion point of the operating table. The table is flexed, lowering the head and legs and extending the lumbar curve. This maximizes the interlaminar space.
2. The anesthesiologist stands at the side of the table and performs a lumbar puncture in the usual manner. Aspiration may be necessary to insure free flow of spinal fluid, since in this position spinal fluid pressure in the lumbar area is often low. As the patient in this position cannot flex fully, a lateral or paramedian approach to the subarachnoid space may be easiest.
3. Before slowly injecting the hypobaric anesthetic solution, the table should be adjusted to insure that the desired level of anesthesia is at the highest point.

3. ALTERNATE APPROACHES TO THE SUBARACHNOID SPACE

a. Lateral and Paramedian (Sublaminar) Approaches

In these approaches the spinal needle is inserted lateral to the supraspinous and interspinous ligaments, and flexion of the spine is not required. These approaches are especially useful in elderly patients with heavily calcified supraspinous and interspinous ligaments and in patients with hip fractures or other pathologic conditions making spinal flexion painful. The sublaminar approach is also very helpful in obese patients because the correct depth of needle insertion can be established by first finding the vertebral lamina with the tip of the spinal needle. These approaches can be used with the patient in the lateral decubitus, sitting, or prone position. The procedure for the *lateral approach* is as follows:

1. An appropriate interspace is selected, the area prepped and draped, and subcutaneous anesthesia performed in the usual manner. The spinal needle is inserted 1.5–2.0 cm lateral to the midline opposite the *center of the selected inter-*

Prone Position for Spinal Anesthesia

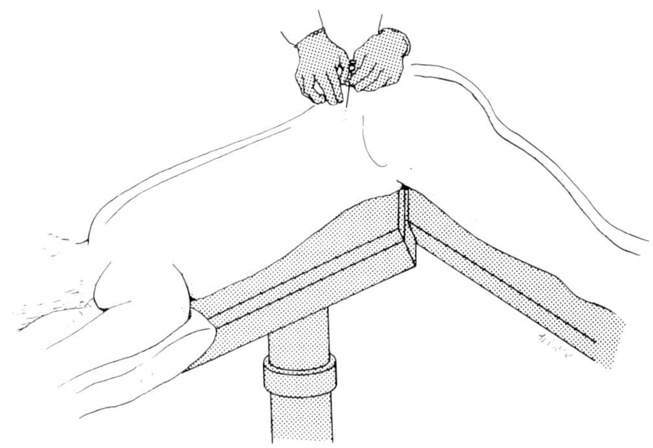

Figure 31-13 • Proper position for lumbar puncture in the prone position.

space (Fig. 31-14). If the patient is in the lateral decubitus position, the dependent side is usually chosen.

2. The needle is directed slightly cephalad and angled about 20° to the midline. It is slowly advanced through the paraspinal dorsal muscle mass, lateral to the interspinous ligament, until the characteristic sensation of the needle piercing the ligamentum flavum and dura-arachnoid is detected. If bone is encountered, the needle is withdrawn partially and redirected slightly cephalad.
3. Once the subarachnoid space is entered, spinal anesthesia is managed as previously described.

The procedure for the *sublaminar approach* is outlined as follows:

Alternate Approaches to the Subarachnoid Space

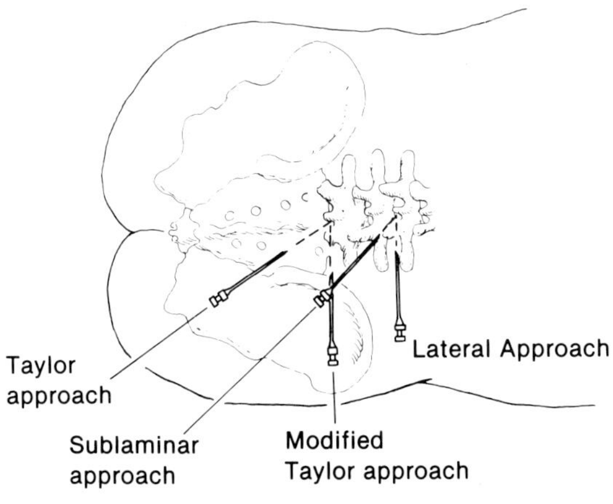

Figure 31-14 • Needle positions for performing lumbar puncture via the lateral, sublaminar, Taylor, and modified Taylor approaches. See text for full explanation.

1. An appropriate interspace is selected and prepared as in the lateral approach. The spinal needle is inserted 1.5–2.0 cm lateral to the midline *opposite the spinous process caudad to the selected interspace* (see Fig. 31-14).
2. The needle is initially advanced parallel to the spine (perpendicular to the skin) until the bony endpoint of the lamina is reached. This gives the anesthesiologist an estimation of the correct depth of the ligamentum flavum and allows more accurate redirection of the needle.
3. The needle is withdrawn partially, directed cephalad and medially at an angle of approximately 30° to 45° to the plane of the skin, and slowly advanced. If bone is again encountered, the needle is redirected slightly more cephalad and again advanced, thus walking off the lamina into the ligamentum flavum at the cephalic end of the lamina. With further advancement the subarachnoid space is entered.
4. Subsequent management of the spinal anesthetic is as previously described.

b. Taylor and Modified Taylor Approaches

The Taylor approach was originally developed by a urologist to provide low segmental anesthesia for urologic procedures, but it has since been used for rectal and perineal surgery.[27] The technique is similar to the sublaminar approach but uses the L-5 to S-1 interspace, the largest interspace in the vertebral column. The modified Taylor approach also uses the lumbosacral foramen but takes a direct lateral route.[28] Both approaches may be used with the patient in any position but are usually performed with the patient in the prone or lateral position. The procedure for the Taylor approach is as follows:

1. The oblique angle used in this approach requires that the spinal needle traverse a relatively long distance over the sacrum; therefore, a 10- to 15-cm spinal needle is recommended.
2. The spinal needle is inserted through a skin wheal raised 1 cm medial and 1 cm caudad to the lowest part of the posterior superior iliac spine (see Fig. 31–14).
3. The needle is advanced cephalad with an upward angle of about 55°, aiming for the middle of the lumbosacral interspace. If bone is encountered, the needle is partially withdrawn, redirected cephalad, and walked into the subarachnoid space.
4. Subsequent spinal anesthesia is managed in the usual manner.

The procedure for the modified Taylor approach is outlined below:

1. The spinal needle is inserted through a skin wheal raised 1.5 cm lateral to the lumbosacral interspace. If difficulty is encountered palpating this interspace, a point 1.0 cm medial and 2.5 cm cephalad to the medial superior aspect of the posterior iliac spine may be used (see Fig. 31–14).
2. The needle is advanced at an angle of about 25° to the midline until the subarachnoid space is entered. As with the lateral approach, little resistance will be encountered until the ligamentum flavum is reached.
3. Spinal anesthesia is then managed as previously described.

4. Continuous Spinal Anesthesia

Passing a catheter into the subarachnoid space has several advantages. Intermittent doses of small amounts of local anesthetic can be administered until the appropriate level of anesthesia is achieved. This is particularly useful for fragile patients in whom an unplanned high block may produce serious cardiovascular or respiratory problems. Repeated injections of anesthetic also allow the duration of the block to be prolonged as necessary. Short-acting local anesthetics may be repeatedly injected, as needed, for a long surgical procedure, but still permit a short recovery period. In patients with difficult anatomy, such as the morbidly obese, the definite endpoint of CSF flow makes continuous spinal anesthesia more likely to be successful than continuous epidural anesthesia.

Disadvantages of the technique include an increased risk for infection and nerve trauma, although this has not proven to be a significant problem. Concern that the large bore needle commonly used for continuous techniques would produce an unacceptably high incidence of postdural puncture headaches has also not been supported by clinical studies.[29–31] It has been postulated that the catheter produces an inflammatory reaction, which helps seal the hole in the dura and prevent CSF leakage, thereby reducing the incidence of headache. Recently a 32 gauge catheter that will pass through a standard 25 or 26 gauge spinal needle has become available. Experience with microcatheters is still limited, but if technical difficulties with insertion and maintenance of these catheters prove surmountable, the continuous technique may become much more popular. The procedure for continuous spinal anesthesia is described in detail below:

1. Lumbar puncture is performed in the usual manner. Any approach to the subarachnoid space may be used, although the paramedian approach provides the best angle for catheter insertion. A standard Touhy epidural needle with a Huber point is usually used. If use of a microcatheter is planned, a standard 25 or 26 gauge spinal needle may be used.
2. The level of the needle should be positioned laterally (ie, parallel to the longitudinal dural fibers) until the dura is pierced and then directed cephalad or caudad depending on the desired direction of catheter passage and level of anesthesia.
3. The catheter is passed only 2–3 cm beyond the tip of the needle. This distance is sufficient to prevent accidental dislodgement but short enough to prevent curling or passage of the catheter into a dural sleeve. If the catheter cannot be threaded into the subarachnoid space, the needle and catheter should be withdrawn together and the procedure repeated. A catheter should never be withdrawn through a needle because a portion of it may be sheared off.
4. After the catheter has been inserted, the needle is slowly withdrawn over the catheter, taking care not to simultaneously remove the catheter. The catheter is then secured to the patient's back as in epidural anesthesia (see Chapter 32).
5. Aspiration of CSF indicates proper placement of the catheter. With a 32 gauge microcatheter, aspiration of CSF may not be possible.
6. Any spinal anesthetic solution may be used, but if precise titration is desired, drugs with a rapid onset, such as procaine or lidocaine, are preferred. The volume of the typical epidural catheter is 0.25 mL, and when small volumes of solution are administered the catheter should be flushed after each injection.
7. Subsequent doses through the catheter are about 50% of the initial dose and are administered at a time equal to three-quarters of the expected duration of the original dose.

III. DISCUSSION AND COMPLICATIONS

A. *Hypotension*

Hypotension is one of the most common complications of spinal anesthesia. In normovolemic patients, total sympathectomy produces a decrease in total peripheral vascular resistance of only 12% to 15%, and only modest falls in blood pressure are due to this mechanism.[32] The etiology of greater falls in blood pressure is venous pooling resulting in decreased venous return to the heart and a consequent fall in cardiac output.

Before the administration of spinal anesthesia, any deficits in intravascular volume should be corrected and an additional volume of at least 500 mL of a balanced saline solution should be infused. This will usually prevent a precipitous fall in blood pressure following the establishment of a block.

In most patients, a fall in systolic blood pressure greater than 30% of baseline value should be treated. Therapy is aimed at increasing venous return. Elevating the legs or placing the table in a 5° to 10° Trendelenburg position will accomplish this without significantly increasing the cephalad spread of the local anesthetic. In patients with normal cardiac reserve, a rapid intravenous infusion of 1–2 L of a balanced saline solution may be helpful.

Small intravenous doses of a vasopressor may also be needed. Vasopressors such as ephedrine and mephentermine have mixed alpha- and beta-receptor activity and produce venoconstriction. These are the preferred drugs for most patients. When hypotension develops rapidly or does not respond adequately to fluid infusion, intravenous ephedrine in 5- to 10-mg increments is indicated. Alpha-receptor agonists such as phenylephrine and methoxamine produce an increase in afterload and may increase myocardial oxygen demand more than coronary blood flow and myocardial oxygen supply. Their use is seldom indicated.

B. *Bradycardia*

Spinal anesthesia typically produces a decrease in heart rate. Unopposed vagal tone due to interruption of the sympathetic cardiac acceleration fibers arising from T-1 to T-4 roots partially explains the bradycardia. However, even in the absence of a high sympathetic block, a decrease in venous return decreases atrial pressure and decreases activity of the intrinsic chronotropic stretch receptors in the right atrium. This mechanism accounts for the profound bradycardias that sometimes occur and the decreased heart rate that occurs with a low spinal block. Severe bradycardia progressing to cardiac asystole has been reported in young healthy subjects not premedicated with atropine[33,34,35] Decreases in heart rate to less than 60 beats per minute should be promptly treated by increasing venous return and, if necessary, by administering atropine and/or ephedrine. If conventional doses of atropine or ephedrine are not effective, intravenous epinephrine should be administered.

C. *Total Spinal Anesthesia*

On rare occasions, due to either the injection of an excessive dose of local anesthetic or to inappropriate positioning of the patient, very high or total spinal anesthesia may occur. This is usually accompanied by hypotension, bradycardia, apnea, and loss of consciousness. Therapy consists of ventilation, slight Trendelenburg position to insure good venous return, ephedrine, intravenous fluids to treat the hypotension, and if necessary, atropine to treat the bradycardia. If the patient has a full stomach, endotracheal intubation to prevent aspiration is necessary. A total spinal block will not produce relaxation of the jaw muscles, and succinylcholine may be required for intubation. After adequate ventilation and circulation has been restored, amnesic or anesthetic drugs may be administered.

In cases of cardiac arrest under high spinal anesthesia, comparatively poorer neurologic outcome has been reported with the usual cardiopulmonary resuscitation (CPR) techniques.[35] It is believed that a high sympathetic blockade allows increased peripheral blood flow during CPR and prevents the usual preferential perfusion of the brain. It is therefore recommended that on recognition of cardiac arrest during a spinal anesthetic, a full-resuscitation dose of epinephrine, a potent alpha-agonist, be given immediately.

1. *Postdural Puncture Headache*

A postdural puncture headache is the most common postoperative complication of spinal anesthesia. The incidence increases with larger spinal needles and decreases with increasing patient age. Postdural puncture headache occurs more commonly in women than in men, and more often in pregnant women than in nonpregnant women.[4] The headache is positional; it comes on in the upright position and is relieved or improved in the recumbent position. The mechanism is believed to be continuing leakage of CSF through the dural opening left by the spinal needle. The decrease in CSF pressure produces compensatory cerebral vasodilatation. The erect position results in traction on the pain-sensitive dilated blood vessels.[4] In severe cases, ocular or auditory symptoms may also occur. The ocular complaints, such as double vision, blurring, and difficulty in focusing, are thought to be due to pressure on the abducens nerve. Auditory complaints, which include decreased hearing, tinnitus, and popping noise, have been ascribed to either pressure on the auditory nerve or a fall in intralabyrinthine pressure.

A variety of preventive measures have been advocated. The common practice of keeping the patient supine for 4 to 24 hours after lumbar puncture has been shown to be ineffective.[36,37] Similarly, increased hydration after dural puncture has little or no effect on the incidence of subsequent headache. The smaller the spinal needle, the lower the incidence of headache. Insertion of the needle with the bevel parallel to the longitudinal fibers of the dura appears to produce a smaller rent in the dura and a lower incidence of headache.[38] Pencil-point needles (Whitacre) also have a lower incidence of headaches.[6]

If a postdural puncture headache does develop, conservative therapy consists of bed rest and analgesics. Increased hydration probably does not increase CSF production and probably does little to relieve the headache. In the patient without a urinary catheter, it may aggravate the situation by necessitating frequent ambulation to void. Intravenous caffeine sodium benzoate has been reported to be effective.[39] The mechanism is believed to be related to cerebral vasoconstriction. Epidural blood patch is the most efficacious therapy (see Chapter 32). The optimal volume of blood appears to be approximately 15 mL.[40]

E. *Neurologic Complications*

The incidence of neurologic sequelae following spinal anesthesia is extremely low. In a review of 582,190 spinal anesthetic cases, Lund could not find a single case of permanent motor paralysis.[41] Kane reviewed approximately 65,000 spinal anesthetic cases and noted 31 cases of neurologic complications.[42] The most likely causes of the majority of these complications were the use of local anesthetic concentrations higher than currently recommended, the inclusion of toxic additives, the use of obsolete liquid sterilization techniques, improper cleaning of syringes, or preexisting neurologic disease. With currently available local anesthetics, disposable spinal equipment, and the use of proper technique, the occurrence of neurologic injury due to spinal anesthesia is extremely unlikely.

Neurologic lesions related to regional anesthesia may occur from direct trauma by spinal needles or catheters. Pressure on the cord or spinal roots produces severe pain and is an indication to withdraw the needle or catheter immediately. Epidural hematoma or subarachnoid hemorrhage is extremely rare unless significant coagulopathy is present. Epidural abscess or subarachnoid infection is usually due to bacteremia or unrecognized infection at the site of needle insertion. Chemical contamination of the subarachnoid space producing prolonged nerve blocks, paraparesis, or adhesive arachnoiditis has been reported to result from a variety of substances including preservatives such as benzyl alcohol and antioxidants such as metabisulfite. Drugs used for spinal anesthesia should not contain these substances. Spinal cord ischemia (anterior spinal artery syndrome) may result from a low perfusion pressure secondary to prolonged hypotension during regional anesthesia.

If a neurologic problem develops following spinal anesthesia, a neurologist should be consulted as soon as possible. In a large retrospective study, it was found that of 482 cases of patients with neurologic problems first believed to be due to spinal anesthesia, 478 were actually due to concurrent and unrelated conditions.[43] A careful examination and mapping of sensory and motor deficits will often indicate if the lesion is segmental or peripheral. Prompt surgical evacuation of a hematoma or drainage of an abscess increases the chances of full neurologic recovery. Laboratory evaluation including computerized tomography, magnetic resonance imaging, and electromyography may be indicated. Electromyography can often be used to estimate the duration of injury and identify lesions that existed prior to the spinal anesthetic.

IV. References

1. Reimann AF, Anson BJ. Vertebral level of termination of the spinal cord with a report of a case of sacral cord. Anat Rec 88:127–138, 1944.

2. Sechzer PH. Subdural space in spinal anesthesia. Anesthesiology 24:869–870, 1963.
3. Lund PC. Principles and Practice of Spinal Anesthesia. Charles C. Thomas, Springfield, IL, 1971, 52.
4. Vandam LD, Dripps RD. Long-term follow-up of patients who received 10,098 spinal anesthetics: Syndrome of decreased intracranial pressure (headache, ocular and auditory difficulties). JAMA 161:586—591, 1956.
5. Hart JR, Whitacre RJ. Pencil needle in prevention of postspinal headache. JAMA 147:657–658, 1951.
6. Snyder GE, Person DL, Flor CE, Wilden RT. Headache in obstetrical patients: Comparison of Whitacre needle versus Quincke needle. Anesthesiology 71:A860, 1989.
7. Greene NM. Distribution of local anesthetic solutions within the subarachnoid space. Anesth Analg 64:715–730, 1985.
8. Greene NM. Uptake and elimination of local anesthetics during spinal anesthesia. Anesth Analg 62:1013–1024, 1983.
9. Levin E, Muravchick S, Gold MI. Density of normal human cerebrospinal fluid and tetracaine solutions. Anesth Analg 60:814–817, 1981.
10. Wildsmith JAW, McClure JH, Brown DT, Scott DB. Effects of posture on the spread of isobaric and hyperbaric amethocaine. Br J Anaesth 53:273–278, 1981.
11. Rosenberg H. Density of tetracaine–water mixtures and the effectiveness of 0.33 per cent tetracaine in hypobaric spinal anesthesia. Anesthesiology 45:682–684, 1976.
12. Collins JG, Kitahata LM, Matsumoto M, Homma E, et al. Spinally administered epinephrine suppresses noxiously evoked activity of WDR neurons in the dorsal horn of the spinal cord. Anesthesiology 60:269–275, 1984.
13. oncepcion M, Maddi R, Francis D, Rocco AG, et al. Vasoconstrictors in spinal anesthesia with tetracaine: A comparison of epinephrine and phenylephrine. Anesth Analg 63:134–138, 1984.
14. Armstrong IA, Littlewood DG, Chambers WA. Spinal anesthesia with tetracaine: The effect of added vasoconstrictors. Anesth Analg 62:793–795, 1983.
15. Chambers WA, Littlewood DG, Logan MR, Scott DB. Effect of added epinephrine on spinal anesthesia with lidocaine. Anesth Analg 60:417–420, 1981.
16. Chambers WA, Littlewood DG, Scott DB. Spinal anesthesia with bupivacaine: Effect of added vasoconstrictors. Anesth Analg 61:49–52, 1982.
17. Spivey DL. Epinephrine does not prolong lidocaine spinal anesthesia in term parturients. Anesth Analg 64:468–470, 1985.
18. Thorburn J, Louden JR, Vallance R. Spinal and general anesthesia in total hip replacement: Frequency of deep vein thrombosis. Br J Anaesth 52:1117–1125, 1980.
19. McKenzie PJ, Wishart HY, Dewar KMS, Gray I, et al. Comparison of the effects of spinal anesthesia and general anesthesia on post-operative oxygenation and perioperative mortality. Br J Anaesth 52:49–53, 1980.
20. McKenzie PJ, Wishart HY, Smith G. Long-term outcome after repair of fractured neck of femur. Comparison of subarachnoid and general anesthesia. Br J Anaesth 56:581–585, 1984.
21. Greene, NM. Physiology of Spinal Anesthesia. ed. 3. Baltimore, Williams and Wilkins, 1981, pp 161–163.
22. Freund F, Bonica JJ, Ward RJ, Akamatsu, TJ, et al. Ventilatory reserve and level of motor block during high spinal and epidural anesthesia. Anesthesiology 28:834–837, 1967.
23. Egbert LD, Tamersoy K, Deas TC. Pulmonary function during spinal anesthesia: The mechanism of cough depression. Anesthesiology 22:882–885, 1961.
24. Eckenhoff JE, Hafkenschiel JH, Foltz EL, Driver RL. Influence of hypotension on coronary blood flow, cardiac work, and cardiac efficiency. Am J Physiol 152:545-553, 1948.
25. Hackel DB, Sancetta, SM, Kleinerman J. Effect of hypotension due to spinal anesthesia on coronary blood flow and myocardial metabolism in man. Circulation 13:92–97, 1956.
26. Sivarajan M, Amory DW, Lindbloom LE, Schwettman RS. Systemic and regional blood-flow changes during spinal anesthesia in the Rhesus monkey, Anesthesiology 43:78–88, 1975.
27. Taylor JA. Lumbosacral subarachnoid tap. J Urol 43:561–564, 1940.
28. Surks SN, Wood PM, Lateral approach for subarachnoid puncture. Anesthesiology 12:239–243, 1951.
29. Peterson DO, Borup JL, Chestnut JS: Continuous spinal anesthesia, case review and discussion. Reg Anesth 8:109–113, 1983.
30. Kallos T, Smith TC. Continuous spinal anesthesia with hypobaric tetracaine for hip surgery in lateral decubitus. Anesth Analg 51:766–773, 1972.
31. Denny N, Masters R, Pearson D, Read J, et al. Postdural puncture headache after continuous spinal anesthesia. Anesth Analg 66:791–794, 1987.
32. Greene, NM. Physiology of Spinal Anesthesia. 3rd ed. Baltimore, Williams and Wilkins, 1981, 101–105.
33. Akamatsu TJ. Cardiovascular response to spinal anesthesia. In JJ Bonica (ed). Regional Anesthesia: Recent Advances and Current Status. Philadelphia, FA Davis, 1969.
34. Wetstone DL, Wong KC. Sinus bradycardia and asystole during spinal anesthesia. Anesthesiology 41:87–89, 1974.
35. Caplan RA, Ward RJ, Posner K, Cheney FW. Unexpected cardiac arrest during spinal anesthesia: A closed claims analysis of predisposing factors. Anesthesiology 68:5–11, 1988.
36. Carbaat PAT, van Crevel H. Lumbar puncture headache: Controlled study on the preventive effect of 24 hours' bed rest. Lancet 2:1133–1135, 1981.
37. Thornberry E, Thomas T. Posture and post-spinal headache. Br J Anaesth 60:195–197, 1988.
38. Mihic DN. Postspinal headache and relationship of needle bevel to longitudinal dural fibers. Reg Anesth 10:76–81, 1985.
39. Sechzer P, Abel L. Post-spinal analgesia headache treated with caffeine: Evaluation with the demand method. Curr Ther Res 24:307, 1978.
40. Szeinfeld M, Ihmeidan IH, Moser, MM, Machado R, et al. Epidural blood patch: Evaluation of the volume and spread of blood injected into the epidural space. Anesthesiology 64: 820–822, 1986.
41. Lund PC. Principles and Practice of Spinal Anesthesia. Springfield, IL, Charles C. Thomas, 1971, p 604.
42. Kane RE. Neurologic deficits following epidural or spinal anesthesia. Anesth Analg 60:150–161, 1981.
43. Marinacci AA, Courville CB. Electromyogram in evaluation of neurological complications of spinal anesthesia. JAMA 168:1337–1345, 1958.

Chapter 32

Laurence S. Reisner, MD
Jill Ellis, MD

Epidural and Caudal Puncture

OUTLINE

I. Introduction

The first administration of epidural anesthesia has been credited to Corning, who in 1885 injected cocaine between the spinous processes of a dog.[1] The first human experience occurred in 1901, when Sicard and Cathelin in independent reports described successful epidural anesthesia using the sacral hiatus as the entry point.[2,3] Since that time numerous physicians and scientists have expanded both the available techniques and our knowledge of this valuable means of providing anesthesia and pain relief. The use in this decade of epidural narcotics for postoperative pain prevention and relief and for cancer pain control has increased exponentially and piqued the interest of many anesthesiologists in mastering the techniques of epidural puncture, catheter insertion, and drug administration.

A. Anatomic Considerations

1. The Epidural Space

The *epidural space* is bounded dorsally by the *ligamentum flavum* (Fig. 32–1A). This ligament varies in thickness from individual to individual but is thickest in the lumbar region. It is actually a series of ligaments connecting the laminae of the vertebrae. A recent study by Zarzur and associates has defined the structure of this ligament in detail.[4] The ligament is somewhat triangular in shape when viewed from the cross section and is therefore thickest in the midline (see Fig. 32–1B). The ventral border of the epidural space is the posterior longitudinal ligament, which covers the posterior aspect of the vertebral bodies. Laterally the epidural space has as its boundary the pedicles of the vertebrae and the intervertebral foramina, which communicate with the paravertebral space. The rostral extreme of the spinal epidural space is the foramen magnum. The dura divides at this point into two leaves, one covering the inner table of cranial bone and the other covering the brain. This anatomically separates the spinal epidural space from the cranial epidural space. Caudally the epidural space ends at the sacral hiatus, where it is covered by the sacrococcygeal ligament membrane, a fused extension of the supraspinous and interspinous ligaments. The distance from the ligamentum flavum to the dura varies from as little as 3 mm in the cervical region to 6 mm in the midlumbar region. Because of this relative large volume, the lumbosacral region appears to act as a relative barrier to the spread of local anesthetic solutions in the adult, but not in children.

The *sacrum* is composed of the fused sacral vertebrae S1 to S5 (Fig. 32–2). The sacral hiatus is a U- or V-shaped defect resulting from a fusion failure of the lamina of the fifth sacral vertebra. The unfused lamina form bony prominences on each side; these are known as the *cornua*. There are numerous sacral variations and anomalies in the adult that may make caudal anesthesia difficult or impossible to perform. This is not true in children.

The contents of the epidural space are the spinal cord within its dura-arachnoid sac, the nerve roots covered with their dural investments, adipose tissue, and blood vessels including the internal vertebral plexus of veins (Batson's plexus) (Fig. 32–3). The epidural plexus of veins is quite extensive and is located in the anterolateral portion of the epidural space. It communicates freely with the external vertebral plexus by way of the intervertebral veins, which course through the intervertebral foramina. These plexuses are valveless and ultimately drain into the azygous system. This provides an alternate means of venous return to the heart for the lower extremities and pelvic organs. The epidural plexus becomes quite engorged during pregnancy as the enlarging uterus obstructs the inferior vena cava by compressing it against the midlumbar vertebral bodies. It also becomes enlarged with coughing or straining. This effectively reduces the volume in the epidural space.

Modern imaging techniques and epiduroscopy have identified either septae or supporting connective tissue structures that may divide the epidural space into compartments.[5,6] There appears to be a septum that divides the dorsal epidural space in the midline and, under some circumstances, a fold of dura mater referred to as a *dorsal mediana plicalis.* However, it is unclear if these dividing structures are completely intact as they traverse the length of the epidural space.

The spinal cord itself ends at the body of the first lumbar vertebra in approximately 90% of adults and at the second lumbar vertebra in another 4% (Fig. 32–4). The remaining 6% end at the level of the 12th thoracic vertebra or higher. The dural sac, on the other hand, extends to the level of the sacrum and is most commonly believed to end by the second sacral segment. The mean distance from the apex of the sacral hiatus to the tip of the dural sac is between 4 and 5 cm in adults. However, the dural sac may extend as low as the fourth sacral segment, a major concern when using a caudal entry to the epidural space.

2. The Spinal Column

The natural curvatures of the spinal column have much less effect on the achieved level of epidural anesthesia than they do on spinal anesthesia. However, the construction of the vertebrae at different levels will have a significant effect on the technique employed to enter the

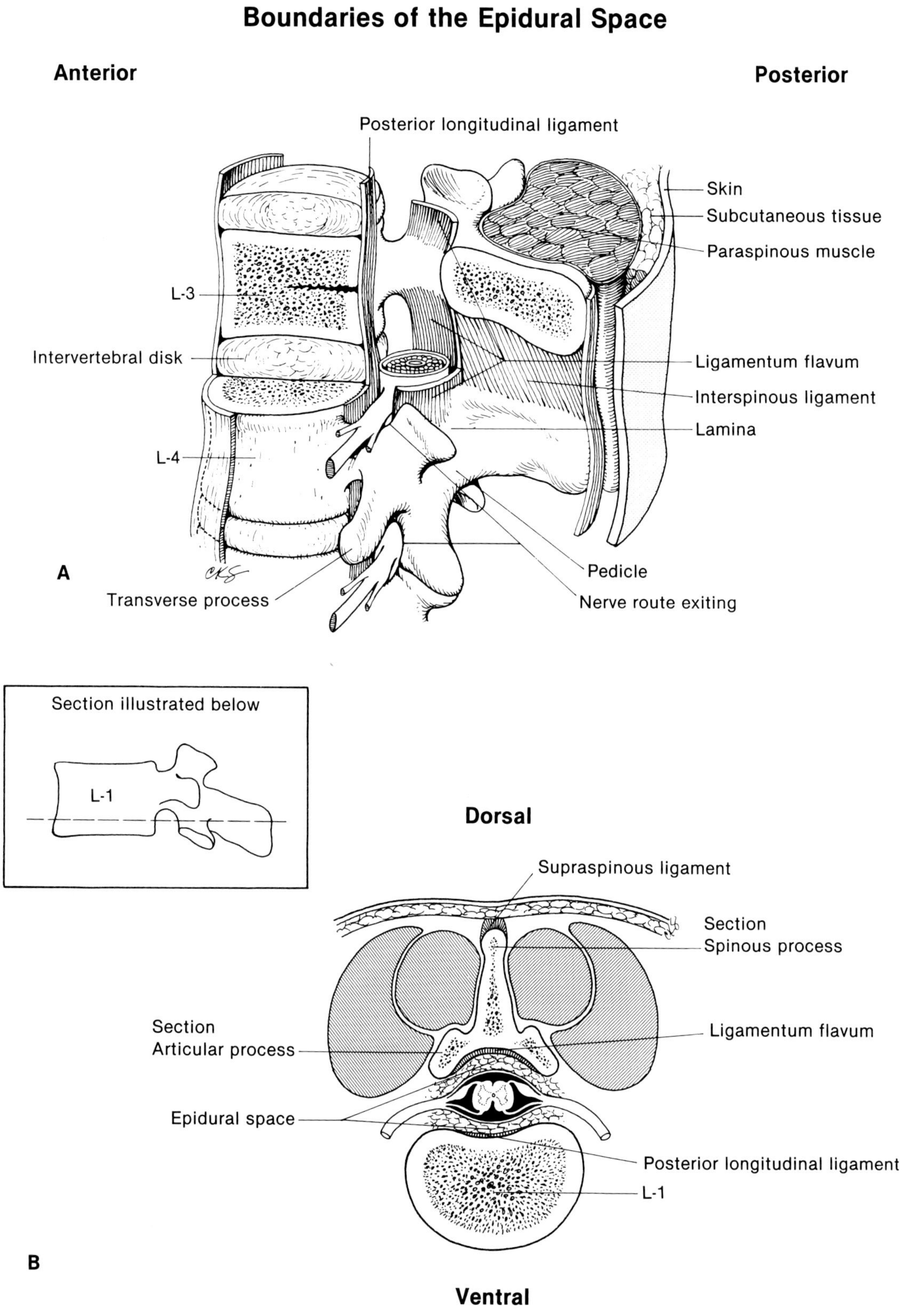

Figure 32–1 • Boundaries of the epidural space: anterior–posterior view (***A***) and dorsal–ventral view (***B***). The epidural space is bounded dorsally by the ligamentum flavum, ventrally by the posterior longitudinal ligament, and laterally by the pedicles and the intervertebral foramina.

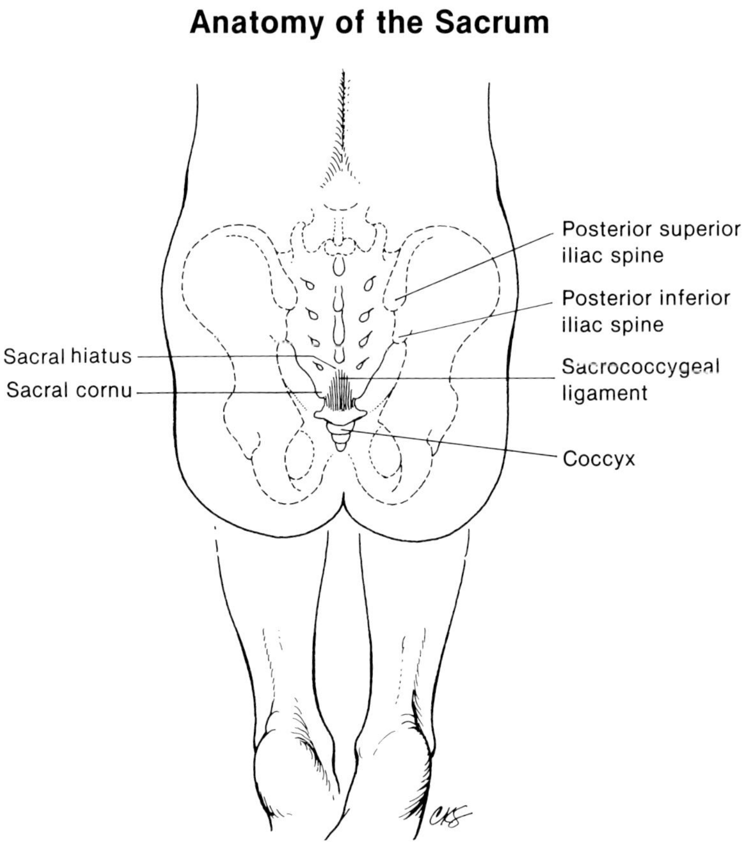

Figure 32–2 • Anatomy of the sacrum. The sacrococcygeal ligament extends from the sacral hiatus to the coccyx and is the most caudal of potential entry points into the epidural space.

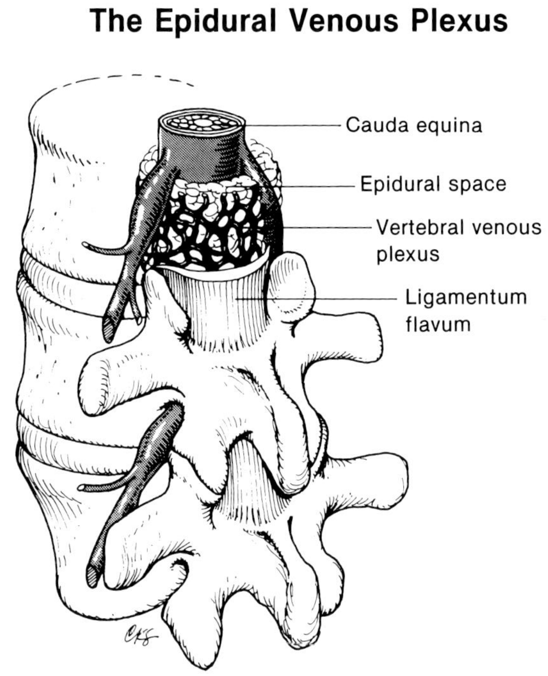

Figure 32–3 • The large epidural venous plexus may become quite engorged with increased intraabdominal pressure and pregnancy.

epidural space (Fig. 32–5). Epidural anesthesia or injection is commonly performed at the thoracic, lumbar, and caudal regions. The cervical region is infrequently used for anesthetic purposes but has proved useful for epidural steroid injections to treat cervical disk syndrome.[7] The thoracic region, particularly the midthoracic spine, has spinous processes that are quite angulated and overlapping, rendering a direct midline approach to the epidural space more difficult. The lumbar region is characterized by more bluntly formed spinous processes, which permit relatively easy midline access.

3. Layers and Ligaments of the Back

The structures usually encountered from the outside inward when performing a midline puncture are the skin and subcutaneous tissue, the supraspinous ligament, the interspinous ligament, and the ligamentum flavum. The supraspinous ligament is dense and fibrous; the interspinous ligament is more loosely constructed. The ligamentum flavum is quite dense in character. The depth from the skin to entry into the dorsal epidural space in

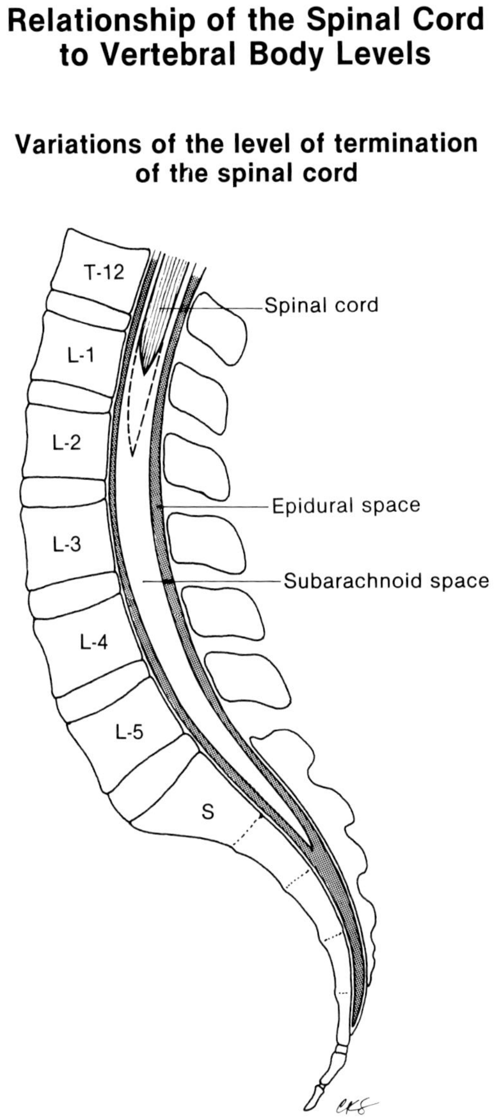

Figure 32–4 • Although the spinal cord ends at the body of L-1 in most adults, it may extend as low as L-2.

the lumbar region is from 4 to 6 cm in the average adult.[8]

4. PRESSURES IN THE EPIDURAL SPACE

The measurable pressure in the epidural space tends to vary with the location and the region. Pressures in the thoracic and cervical region tend to be negative and reflect the intrapleural pressure.[9] The pressure in the lumbar region is probably very slightly positive under most normal conditions and appears to be positive during term pregnancy.[10]

B. *Mechanisms of Action*

There are several modes by which epidurally placed local anesthetics may exert their action. Drugs may travel centrifugally to the paravertebral space and produce blockade at that level. They may also slowly diffuse through the dura and achieve a blocking concentration in the cerebrospinal fluid that will affect the nerve roots without dural sheaths as well as the spinal cord. The most significant mechanism may be the one described by Shantha and associates, who identified the existence of a variety of arachnoid villi, some of which penetrate the dura in the region of the dural root cuff (Fig. 32–6).[11] It is suggested that local anesthetics easily penetrate this flimsy barrier and gain direct access to the unsheathed nerve root at this level.

Epidural narcotics gain access to the subarachnoid space by methods similar to local anesthetics and bind to the opioid receptors on the spinal cord. They also are

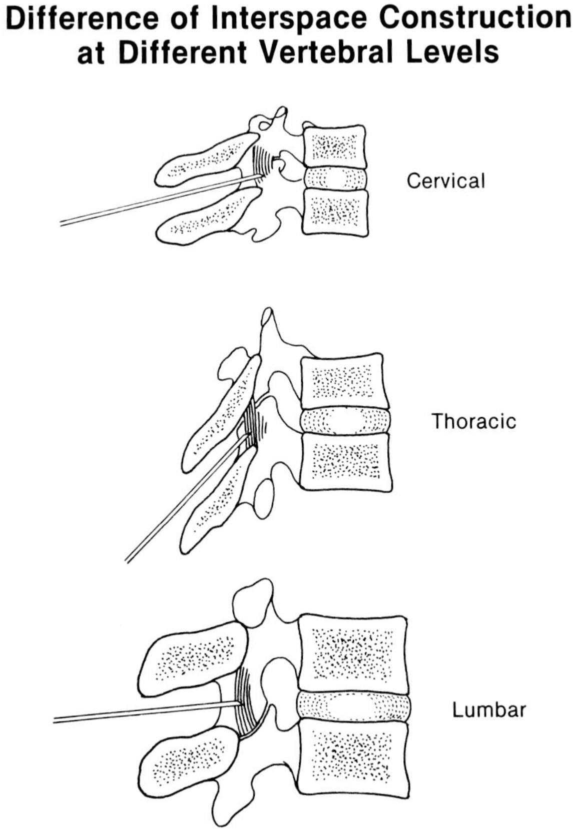

Figure 32–5 • The slope of the spinous processes at different levels will dictate the angle at which the needle should be advanced.

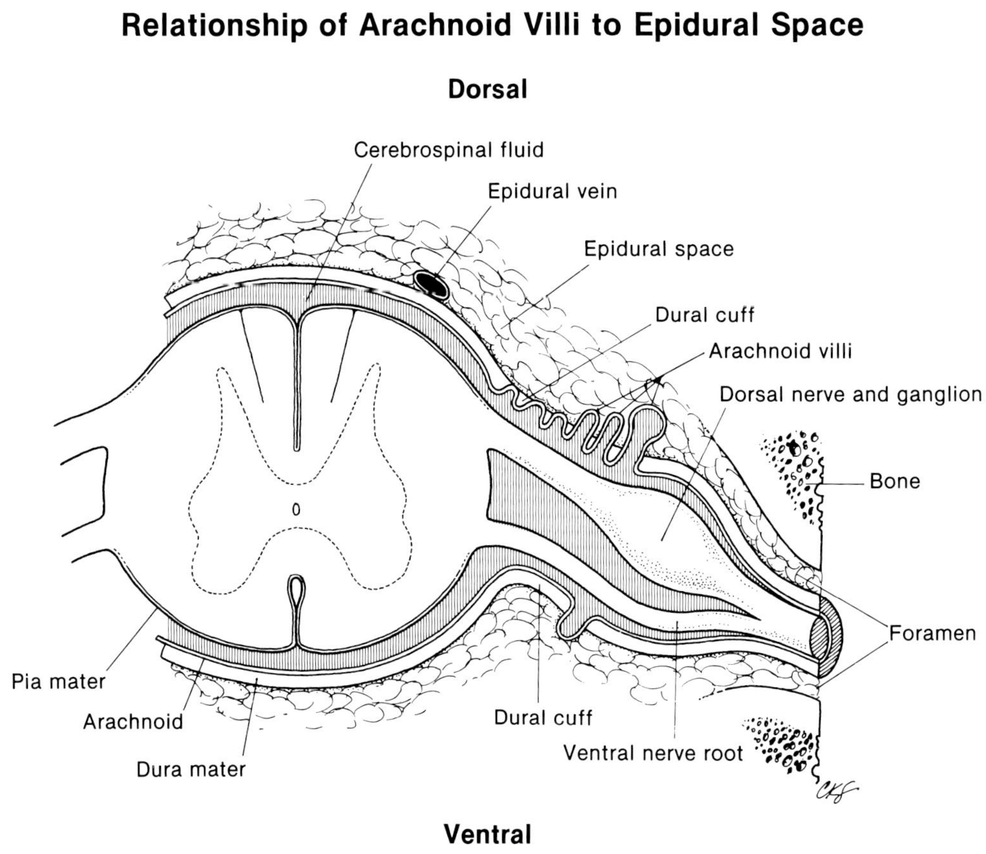

Figure 32-6 • The presence in the epidural space of penetrating arachnoid villi that can rapidly absorb local anesthetics and opioids helps explain a significant mechanism of epidural analgesia production.

taken up by the epidural veins and may have some central effect as well.

II. Indications and Contraindications

Lumbar epidural anesthesia is indicated for surgical procedures in the lower abdomen and on the extremities and perineum. This would include procedures such as cesarean section, aortofemoral bypass, and arthroscopy. Because it is suitable for a continuous technique (indwelling catheter), epidural anesthesia is also quite useful for extracorporeal shock wave lithotripsy for renal and gall bladder calculi as well as for invasive diagnostic/therapeutic radiologic procedures such as percutaneous nephrostomy. Thoracic epidural anesthesia is used for procedures in the upper abdomen and thorax. Caudal anesthesia is suitable for perineal procedures and anorectal operations as well as for childbirth.

Epidural analgesia with local anesthetics is indicated for labor and delivery, postoperative pain relief, and for multiple rib fractures. Epidural analgesia with opioids is indicated for the same procedures as well as for chronic pain management. Epidural steroids are indicated for the treatment of low back pain and sciatica as well as for symptoms of cervical nerve root compression after an appropriate evaluation. Epidural neurolysis with alcohol for the pain associated with cancer has been recently evaluated but is not yet a routine component of our armamentarium.[12] Finally, epidural puncture may be used to inject blood into the epidural space to treat postdural puncture headache.

Absolute contraindications to the use of epidural anesthesia are infection at the site of proposed injection, irreversible alteration in the hemostatic system, and hypovolemic shock. Absolute contraindications should also include the patient's informed refusal and lack of appropriate support equipment and drugs. Relative contraindications are the presence of an active neurologic disor-

Table 32-1 • Contraindications to Epidural Anesthesia

Absolute contraindications
1. Infection at the site of injection
2. Irreversible alteration of the coagulation system
3. Hypovolemic shock
4. Patient's informed refusal
5. Lack of appropriate support equipment and drugs

Relative contraindications
1. Active neurologic disorder
2. Symptoms associated with herniated disk
3. Systemic infection

der, symptoms associated with a herniated disk, and systemic infection (Table 32-1).

III. How to Do Epidural and Caudal Puncture

A. *Technical Considerations*

1. Equipment

A variety of epidural needles are available, each with specific advantages and disadvantages (Fig. 32-7). Several of these are relatively minor alterations of a basic type. The most popular needle is the Hustead modification of Tuohy's needle, which has a curved tip that helps avoid dural puncture and allows for the direction of a catheter. The Crawford needle has a blunt bevel and is designed primarily for use in the thoracic region both with and without a catheter, although many practitioners use it in the lumbar region. There may be a slightly higher incidence of dural puncture in the lumbar region when using this needle. The Cheng needle has a rounded blunt tip with a hole in the side of the shaft of the needle and requires a sharp introducer to penetrate the tissues and ligaments of the back. The addition of a pair of wings to the Tuohy needle at the hub results in greater user control and greatly aids in the use of negative pressure identification techniques. This modification is known as the Weiss needle (see Fig. 32-7). Other versions of winged needles are available including units that allow the operator to attach or detach the wings. Needles are available in gauges ranging from 20 gauge to 16 gauge. The 18 gauge thin-wall needle is currently among the most popular. Needle length is usually 9 cm (3.5 inches), although both longer and shorter needles are available.

A variety of epidural catheters are also available (Fig. 32-8). It is imperative that the operator confirm that the selected catheter fits through the bore of the needle and what the reference marks on the catheter indicate relative to the needle selected. Catheters are constructed of Teflon, polyvinylchloride, nylon, and polycarbamate. They are commonly available in gauges 18 to 21, although pediatric catheters in gauges 22 and 24 are being manufactured. A 20 gauge catheter easily passes through an 18 gauge thin-wall Tuohy needle, whereas a 19 gauge catheter passes through the 17 gauge

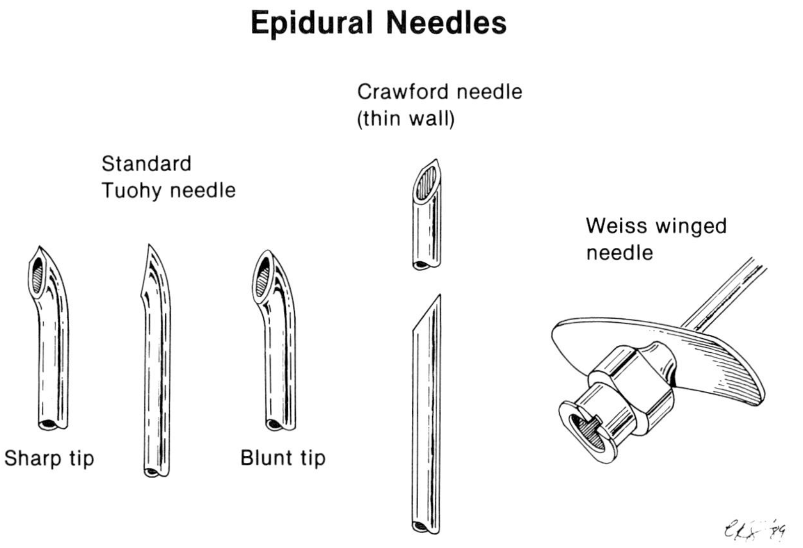

Figure 32-7 • Epidural needles. Note the rounded distal end of the Tuohy needles, designed to minimize dural puncture and direct the catheter. The Crawford needle is a straight, blunt-beveled needle designed primarily for the paramedian approach. The wings of the Weiss needle allow for smooth control of needle advancement without disturbing the "hanging drop."

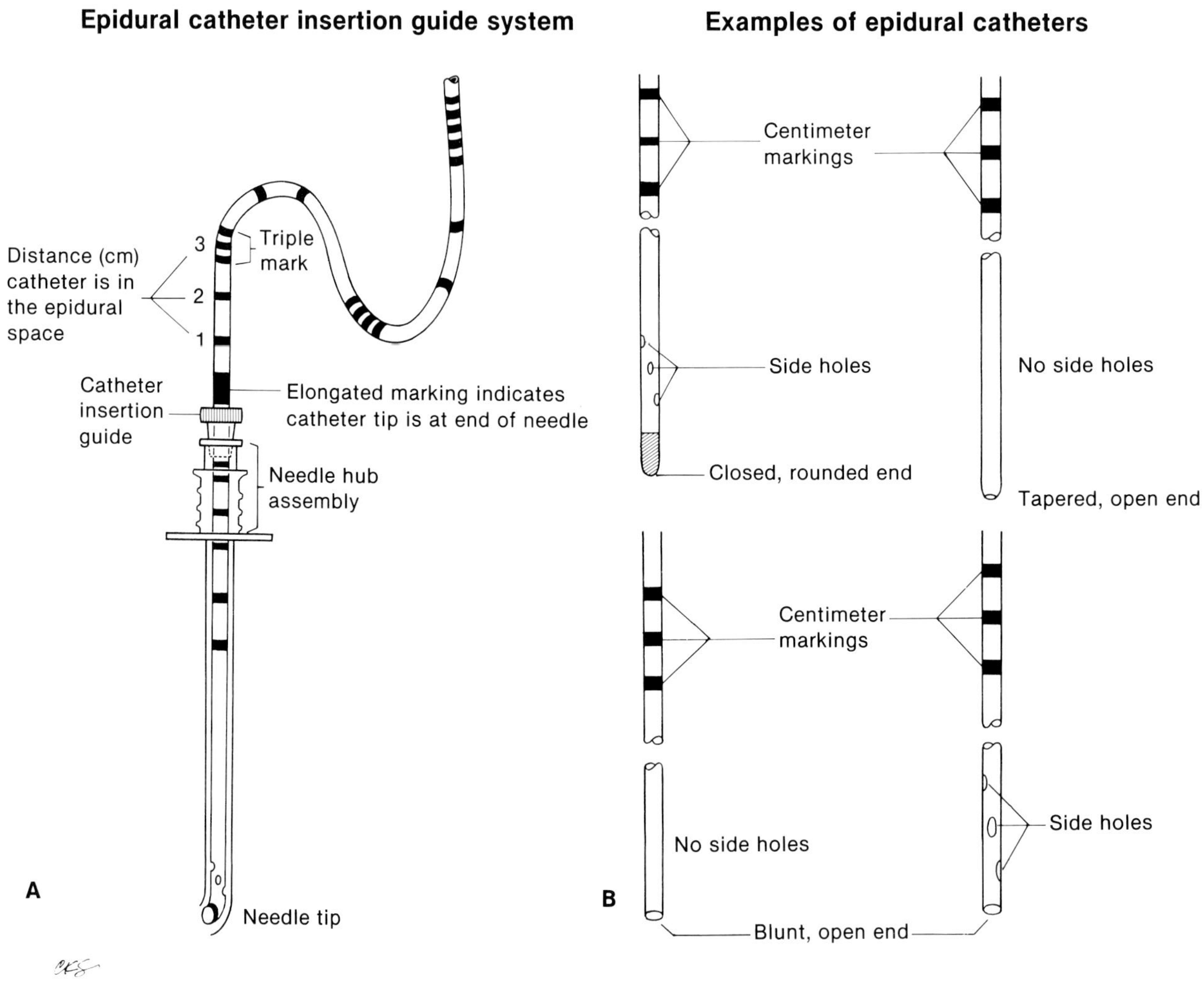

Figure 32–8 • (***A***) The epidural catheter insertion guide allows smooth introduction of the catheter into the needle without buckling at the hub and eliminates the need for a stylet. (***B***) There are a wide variety of epidural catheter tips available. Many clinicians prefer the blunt open-ended catheter without side holes because the injection can only be introduced into one location.

needle. A special catheter for long-term use and high kink resistance has been designed by Racz and employs a wire spiral coated with plastic, similar to an armored endotracheal tube. Some catheters have an open end, some have a tapered, rounded, and closed end with side holes, and some have an open end with side holes. The alleged advantage of side holes is the more even distribution of drug solution. A disadvantage is that one hole may lie in the epidural space, whereas another may be in the subarachnoid space or in a blood vessel. Some catheters contain a stylet of metal or plastic that gives extra rigidity for manipulation and when removed leaves a very soft and pliable catheter behind. The stylet should be backed up at least 1–2 cm prior to insertion to avoid perforating the dura or a blood vessel. The adapter at the end of the catheter will also vary, from blunt needles, which the operator must tease into the narrow lumen, to the self-sealing external adapters that are currently preferred (Fig. 32–9).

With the exception of special or unique circumstances, most anesthesiologists will be using a disposable kit that contains the majority of the components prepackaged. Most manufacturers offer some options, and a few allow the user to custom design the set.

2. Methods for Identifying the Epidural Space

There are two categories of techniques used to identify and confirm entrance into the epidural space: *loss-of-resistance techniques* and *negative pressure techniques.* Loss-of-resistance techniques take advantage of the fact that when a needle's bevel is well embedded in the ligamentum flavum, the contents of a fluid-filled syringe cannot be

Epidural Catheter Adapters

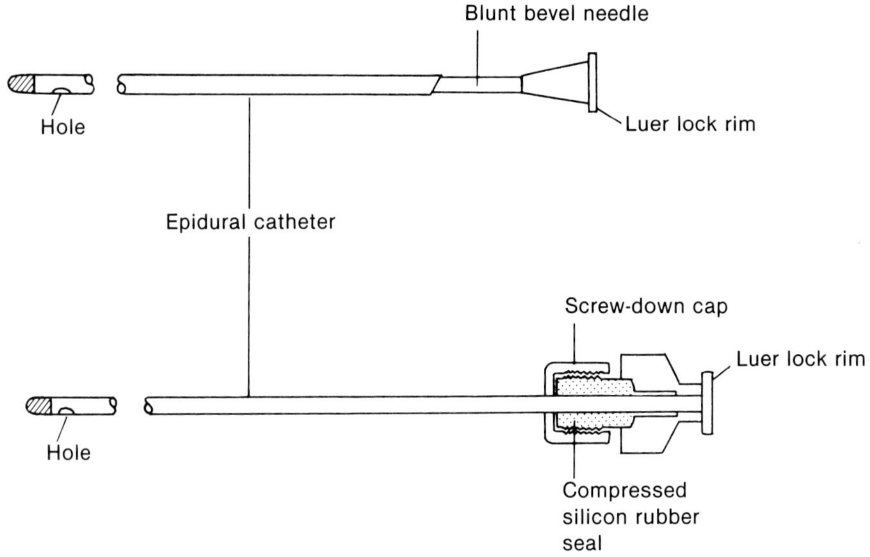

Figure 32–9 • The external type of catheter adapter is easier to apply and avoids catheter perforation by an adapter needle.

Identification of Epidural Space: Loss-of-Resistance Method

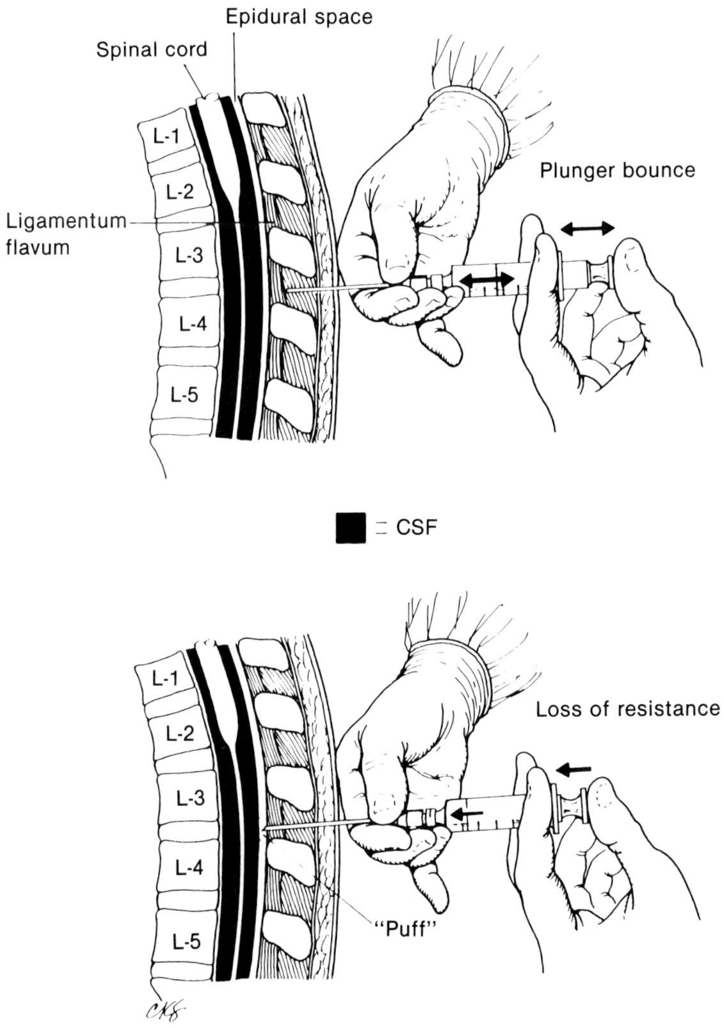

Figure 32–10 • The resistance to injection offered by the ligamentum flavum is promptly lost when the needle tip enters the epidural space. CSF = cerebrospinal fluid.

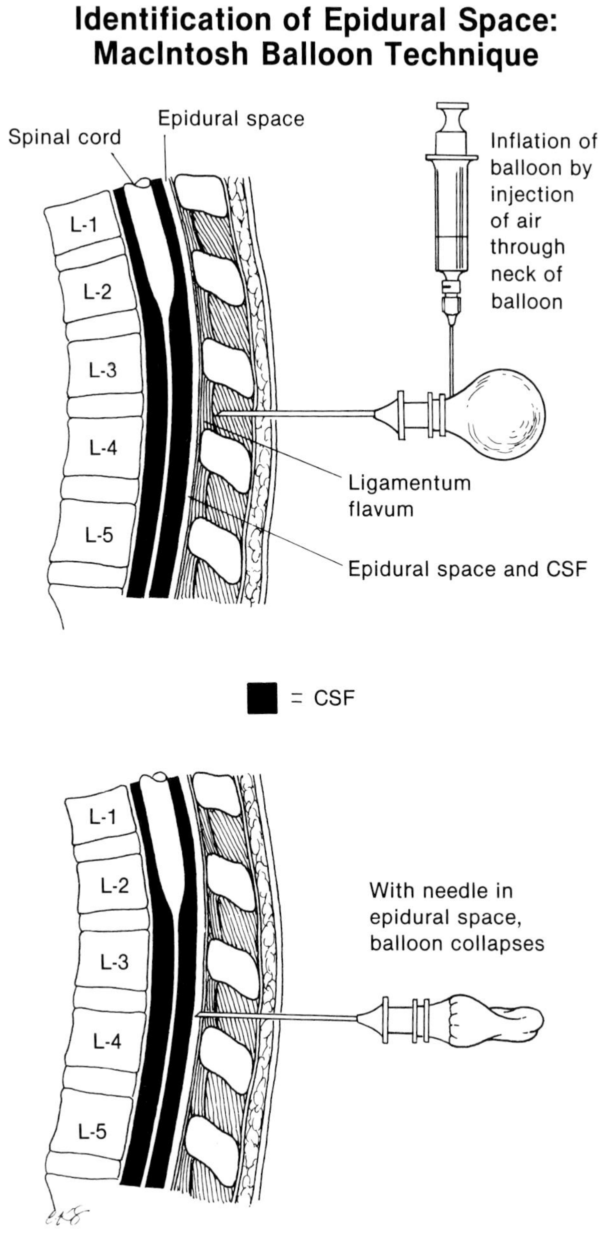

Figure 32–11 • The MacIntosh balloon technique combines the loss of resistance to air with the visual indicator of the collapsing balloon.

easily discharged and the plunger takes on a characteristic bounce to repeated gentle pressure. When it enters the epidural space, the contents of the syringe are easily injected (Fig. 32–10). Mechanical devices such as rubber bands and spring-loaded syringes have been developed, but most epiduralists prefer to feel the plunger with their own hand. MacIntosh described a similar technique using a small latex balloon attached to the needle hub. The balloon is inflated by puncturing it with a small needle and adding air with a syringe until it has attained its shape. The needle is then advanced until the balloon collapses (Fig. 32–11).

The medium used for the loss-of-resistance technique may be air, sterile saline, sterile saline with an air bubble, sterile water, or local anesthetic solution. The advantage of air is that it is readily available, avoids a solution error, and gives a characteristic bounce that is fairly reliable but is more compressible than fluid because it is a gas mixture. Disadvantages include the potential for air injection into the vascular system, pneumocephalus if injected into the subarachnoid space in quantity, a possibly greater incidence of catheter venipuncture, and subcutaneous emphysema. Saline provides a noncompressible fluid that will tend to keep the needle bore clean and potentially push the dura away from the needle tip as it enters the epidural space. An air bubble added to the fluid is a visual indicator, since the bubble compresses and changes shape when in tissue but maintains its shape when entering the epidural space. This is a recommended technique. Disadvantages of saline are that the user must be sure that it is preservative free and that when saline refluxes from the free needle (disconnected from the syringe) it must be distinguished from cerebrospinal fluid (CSF). This latter problem can be minimized by using modest volumes. Sterile water has the same fluid advantages as saline but causes nerve root irritation on contact. Although this may assure the operator that the epidural space has been entered, it is uncomfortable for the patient. The advantage of using a local anesthetic is that the test dose is administered simultaneously with epidural space identification. This may save a few minutes, but a subarachnoid block may be induced when it obviously would not be desired.

Negative pressure techniques rely on the existence or creation of negative pressure in the epidural space. A visual indicator of the pressure change is used. The simplest technique involves placing a drop of a liquid, usually saline or local anesthetic, in the hub of the needle, which has been situated in the ligamentum flavum. The needle is then slowly advanced until the negative pressure sucks the drop into the needle. This is referred to as the *hanging drop of Gutierrez* (Fig. 32–12). Precise and careful advancement of the needle is essential to avoid perforation of the dura. There are several techniques employing small manometric indicators of the negative pressure change as described by Dogliotti and Zelenka. Odom's indicator is a small fluid-filled capillary tube fitted to the hub of the needle. The fluid level moves to indicate a negative pressure when the epidural space is entered.

Paramount to any technique for identifying the epidural space is that all signs and observations should

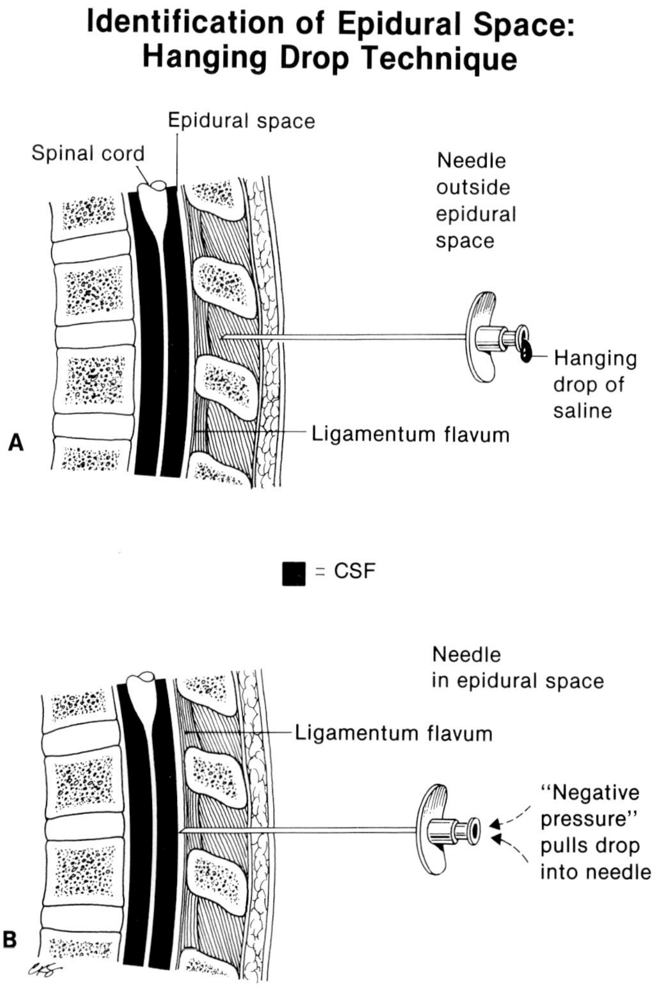

Figure 32–12 • Care must be taken when using the hanging drop technique to avoid displacing the drop with the operator's fingers.

be as expected. If there is any doubt, withdraw the needle and begin again.

B. *Technique of Midline Lumbar Epidural Puncture*

Lumbar epidural analgesia, anesthesia, and steroid injection are the most common epidural procedures performed. Since most lumbar epidural punctures are done performed below the body of L-2, there is little likelihood of the advancing needle encountering the spinal cord. Even if the operative procedure or desired analgesia is out of the usual range of lumbar epidural anesthesia, this route can still be used if the patient can tolerate the additional amount of drug required to extend the level. As discussed earlier, there are two basic classes of indicator methods used to identify the epidural space: loss-of-resistance and negative pressure. The loss-of-resistance method using saline is outlined below because this technique appears to minimize dural puncture in the lumbar region. The alternative techniques will be discussed as appropriate.

1. Examine the patient's back and determine the interspace of choice and an alternate. The L-3 to L-4 interspace is usually transected by a line drawn across the iliac crests (Fig. 32–13). Usually the L-2 to L-3 interspace gives one the most room; the dorsal epidural space is the deepest (~6 mm) and this interspace is below the conus medullaris of the spinal cord. However, any lumbar interspace may be selected.
2. Place the patient in either the lateral decubitus position or the sitting position. The decubitus position is often safer for the patient, particularly the premedicated patient, since venous pooling and fainting are prevented. Right-handed operators may find the left lateral decubitus the most comfortable position; left-handed persons may find the right lateral position more comfortable. The sitting position offers maximal flexion of the back and accurate midline determination, especially in obese patients. In either case, an assistant should be present to aid in maintaining the position and for patient support. The patient in the lateral position should have the knees flexed against the abdomen and the chin against the chest, and be encouraged to curve or push the middle of the back out like an angry cat. In the sitting position, the patient should have the elbows resting on the anterior thigh or knees, the head as in the lateral position, and an assistant for stabilization. A useful alternative for pregnant patients is the crossed-leg position. For cervical epidural injection, it is very useful to have the patient sit on a chair or stool.
3. The epidural tray should now be opened and additional equipment added as needed. Back preparation solution should be placed in the appropriate receptacle. The choice of preparation solutions varies considerably, but the usual solutions are alcohol or the povidone-iodine compounds.

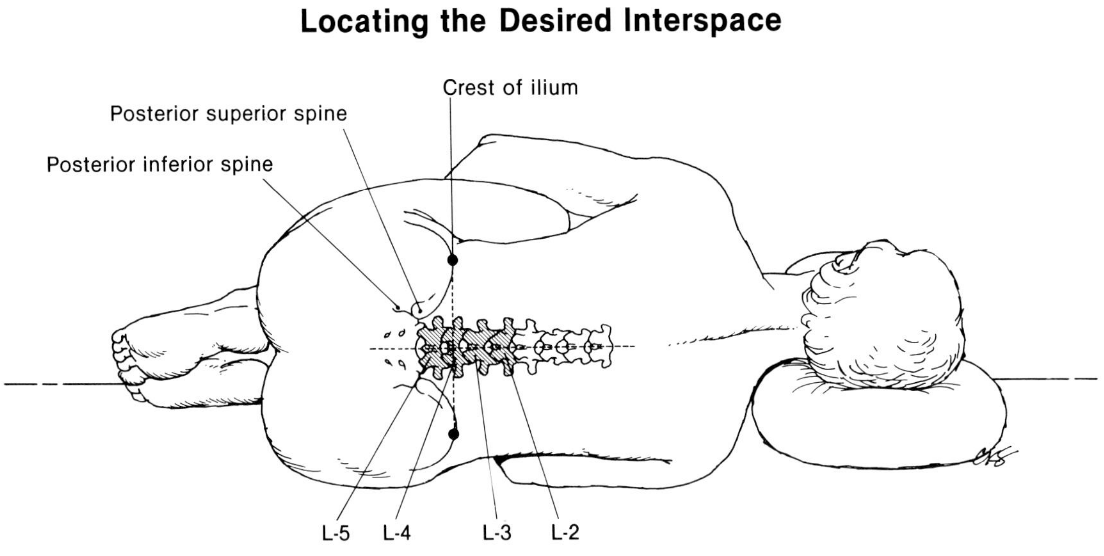

Figure 32–13 • A line drawn across the iliac crests usually identifies the fourth lumbar vertebra or the L-3 to L-4 interspace.

In all probability any of these used properly will cleanse the back sufficiently to avoid introducing infection.

4. The operator should now put on a surgical hat and mask (if not previously done) and a pair of surgical gloves. Examine the equipment in the tray, and if necessary insure that the catheter passes through the needle easily. Check the syringes for proper plunger fit and function. Ascertain that all drugs are present and that the ampules or vials are not outdated.
5. Prepare the patient's back, concentrating on the midline and allowing for the possibility of using an interspace both above and below the one initially selected. Repeat the cleansing procedure twice more and remove the excess with a folded dry 4 × 4 gauze, taking care not to get any on the gloves. This step removes the loose detritus and excess solution from the back, which could prove neurotoxic if carried to the central nervous system (CNS).
6. Create a skin wheal just caudal to the center of the selected interspace with 1% lidocaine or an equivalent local anesthetic, using a 25 gauge needle. Attach a 22 gauge 1.5-inch needle to the local anesthetic syringe and pass it through the skin wheal at the same angle as intended for the epidural needle. In the lumbar region this is usually perpendicular to the skin or with a slight cephalad angle. After aspirating, inject 2–3 mL of local anesthetic while withdrawing the needle. This anesthetizes the track intended for the epidural needle and allows the operator to gently probe the interspace and determine the most suitable angle of approach.
7. Pierce the skin in the center of the wheal with an 18 gauge needle to allow for easier passage of the relatively blunt epidural needle. Insert the Tuohy epidural needle into the skin and subcutaneous tissue. Insure that the bevel is oriented in a cephalad direction.
8. Advance the epidural needle with stylet in place through the supraspinous and interspinous ligaments until the needle tip is situated in the ligamentum flavum. This ligament has a much firmer feel than the other tissues, and if one releases the needle it remains situated as if placed in a piece of wood. If the needle is located in other tissues, the hub tends to fall and the needle appears insecure when released (Fig. 32–14).
9. Withdraw the stylet and examine the hub for the presence of CSF or blood. If neither is present, attach the seeking syringe with its fluid to the hub of the needle. A 5-mL glass syringe is recommended, but a 10-mL syringe may be acceptable. Newer plastics and silicone lubricants have led to the development of some plastic syringes that may prove suitable. If the negative pressure technique is to be used, attach either the balloon or the indicator, or insert the hanging drop, at this point.
10. Place one hand firmly against the back, using either the hypothenar eminence (heel of the hand) or the knuckles as the main support. Grasp the wings or the needle hub with the thumb and index finger (Fig. 32–15). If possible, use the second and third fingers for stability. The hand that grasps the needle hub can advance the needle by itself and is usually the left hand for right-handed persons. The other hand supports the syringe with the

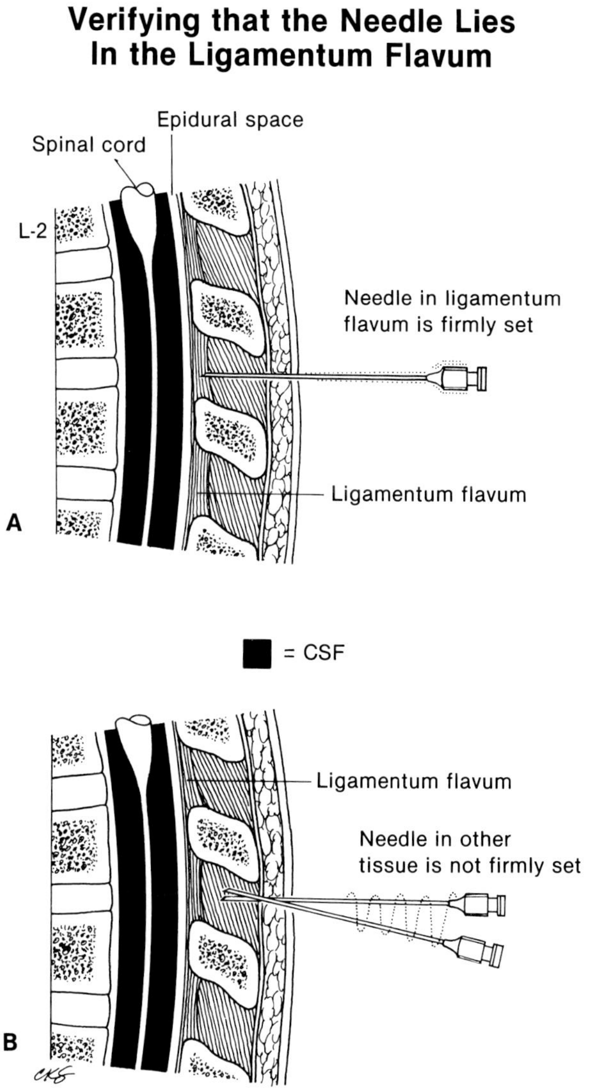

Figure 32–14 • When the needle lies in the ligamentum flavum, it feels as if it had been placed into a soft piece of wood. Releasing the hub results in the needle maintaining its position, whereas if it is superficial to this ligament, the hub and needle will move toward the floor.

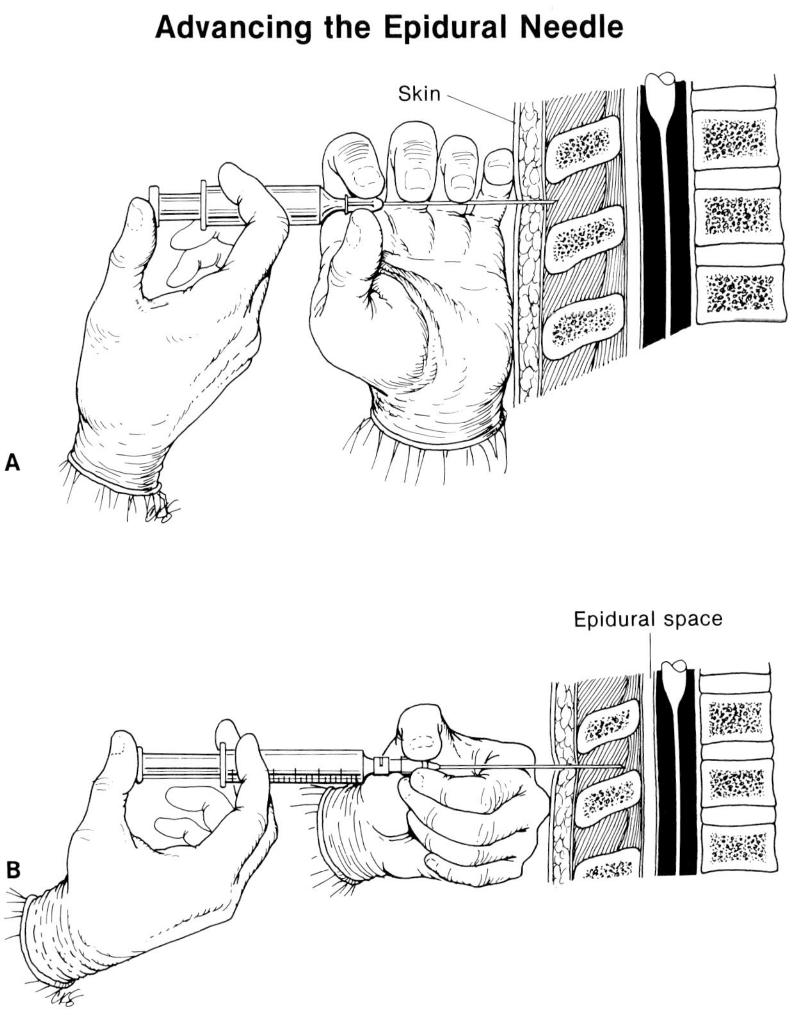

Figure 32–15 • Although we find that placing the hypothenar eminence firmly against the patient's back is the method of choice for stabilizing and advancing the needle syringe assembly, many prefer to use the knuckles as a cam on which to rotate.

thumb, constantly testing the plunger for the presence or absence of resistance. When using a negative pressure technique, place both hands firmly against the back and grasp a wing on each side of the needle (or on the lateral aspect of the hub if no wings are present).

11. Advance the needle slowly and steadily while constantly testing the plunger or observing the indicator. When the needle enters the epidural space there is a slight pop or give, and the contents of the syringe flow freely. The indicator with negative pressure techniques will move appropriately (ie, the balloon collapses, the indicator moves down, or the drop moves inward in the hub).
12. With the needle now presumably in the epidural space, remove the syringe or indicator and observe for the efflux of blood or CSF. If either is present, the needle must be removed and relocated in a different interspace.
13. If a catheter is to be used, insert the catheter so that no more than 5 cm lies in the epidural space. A reasonable distance under most circumstances is 3 cm. *Never* pull the catheter back through the needle, even for a short distance. This action may shear off the length of catheter remaining in the epidural space. The injection of air, saline, or a local anesthetic test dose has been recommended prior to catheter insertion to open the epidural space and facilitate catheter insertion. We do not recommend the use of air or the local anesthetic test dose because either may lead to additional complications. Hold the catheter steady, and back the needle out over the catheter approximately 1 cm at a time (Fig. 32–16). Once the needle is removed, check the markings on the catheter. Under most circumstances the catheter should be at 7–10 cm at the skin.
14. Attach the adapter to the end of the catheter (see Fig. 32–9). Flush the catheter with 1–2 mL of saline to be sure that the openings are patent and to assess the feel of the catheter. Then very gently aspirate the catheter using a 3-mL syringe and rotating the plunger. Observe carefully for blood or CSF. If blood or CSF is not found,

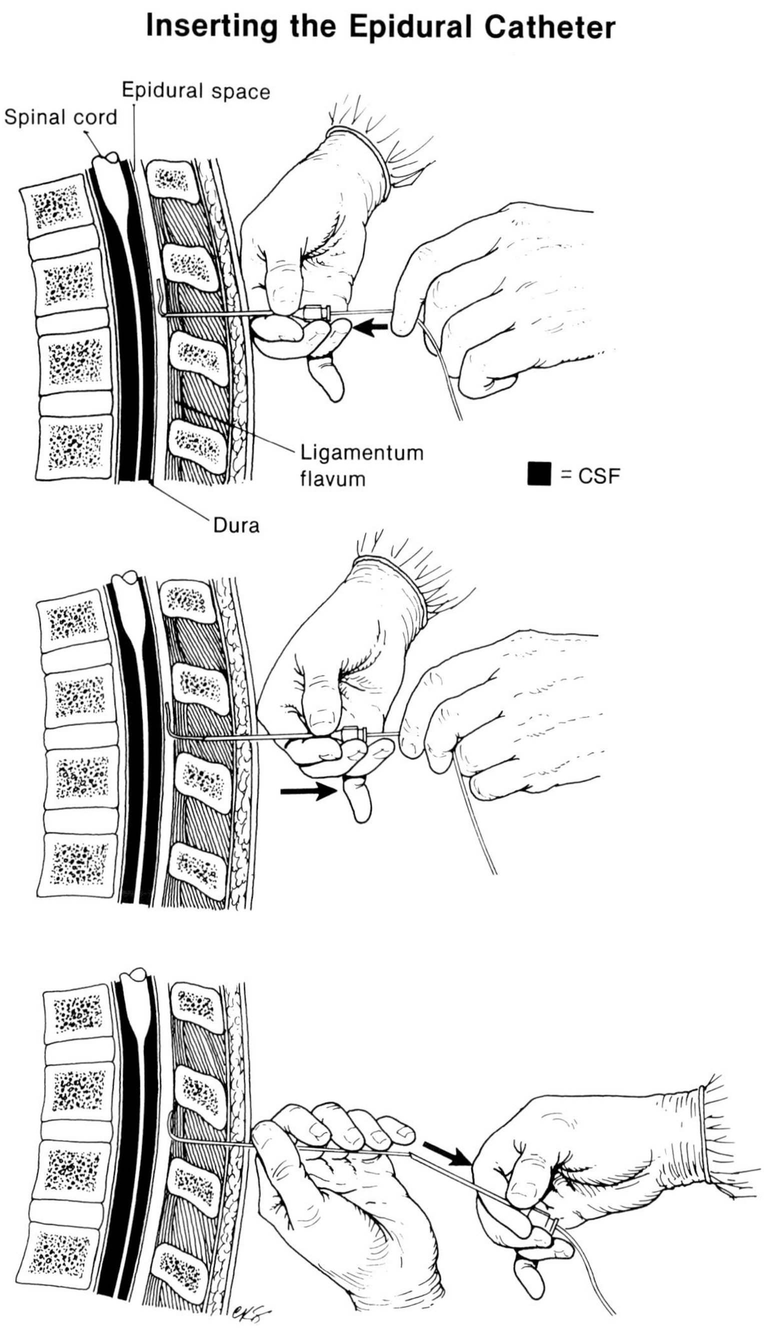

Figure 32–16 • The needle should be well stabilized during catheter insertion, and the catheter should pass easily with minimal resistance when in the epidural space. Needle removal should be cautious and at 1-cm intervals over a stabilized catheter.

remove the syringe, place the open end of the catheter below the puncture site, and observe carefully. This step is necessary because sometimes even the gentlest aspiration will collapse the epidural vessels or pull a flap of tissue over the opening and yield a false negative aspiration test.

15. Secure the catheter to the patient's back. An adhesive plastic drape of approximately 4 × 4 inches, placed over the puncture site with the catheter gently curved to form a J, works nicely and allows inspection of the puncture site, the catheter, and its markings. The remainder of the catheter is secured with 3-inch adhesive tape along the patient's back to the shoulder or off to one side just above the iliac crest. Avoid crossing the midline to minimize the likelihood of kinking the catheter (Fig. 32–17).
16. Administer a test dose through the catheter. The administration of the test dose at this point in time is advantageous because the technical aspects are now completed, the patient is in the supine or lateral position and can be observed more easily, and the operator is in a more

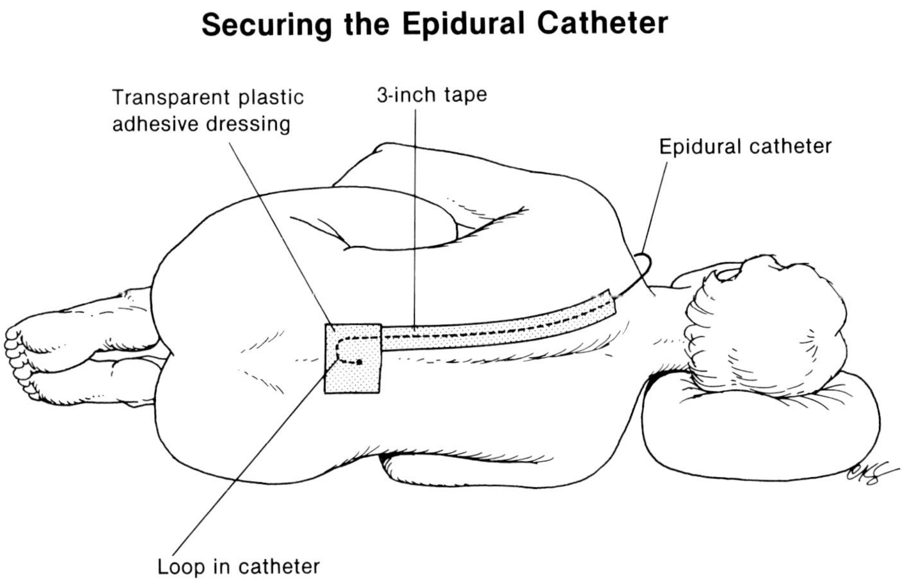

Figure 32–17 • Securing the catheter with a transparent plastic dressing allows a firm hold and a view of the catheter and the puncture site without removing the dressing.

appropriate position to evaluate the responses to the test dose and treat any undesirable responses.

17. If local anesthetic injected directly through the needle is to be used, administer a test dose of local anesthetic after gentle aspiration. The assistant should be qualified to assess the response to the test dose and to administer any corrective therapy if needed, because the operator must remain gloved until the catheter is inserted and secured, the "single shot" therapeutic dose administered, or the procedure abandoned.
18. After a negative response to the test dose has been obtained, incremental therapeutic doses of the selected local anesthetic or narcotic solution may be injected.

C. *Technique of Paramedian Lumbar Epidural Puncture*

The paramedian approach as described by Bonica allows the operator to avoid the narrow space present between spinous processes in patients who cannot flex their backs (as in pregnancy with a disproportionately large abdomen).[13] The needle avoids the spinous processes and thus does not pass through the supraspinous and interspinous ligaments. This alters the feel of the technique. The ligamentum flavum is also thinner laterally. When properly inserted, the needle enters the epidural space in the midline or quite close to it.

1. Identify the interspace to be used.
2. Proceed with positioning and back preparation.
3. Raise a skin wheal 1–1.5 cm lateral to the caudal aspect of the spinous process below the interspace.
4. Insert the epidural needle with an angle of approximately 15° to the midsagittal plane and 135° to the axis of the spinal canal. The needle will exhibit greater cephalad angulation than with the midline technique (Fig. 32–18).
5. The needle is advanced until the resistance of the ligamentum flavum is encountered. If contact with the lamina occurs, partially withdraw the needle and change the cephalad angulation slightly.
6. Proceed as for the midline approach.

D. *Technique of Midline Thoracic and Cervical Epidural Puncture*

The midline approach is best employed in the cervical and thoracic regions from C-7 to T-4. The thoracic vertebrae from T-5 to T-9 have long, acutely angulated overlapping spinous processes which make the paramedian approach more suitable (see Fig. 32–5). Since a true negative pressure exists in this region and the depth of the epidural space is small (flat), negative pressure techniques are preferred because they allow the operator to use both hands on the needle and advance very slowly. Using the sitting position leads to a greater negative pressure, as does an appropriately timed inspiration. Therefore, thoracic epidural puncture should be accomplished with the patient in the sitting position and the needle advanced during the inspiratory phase. Thoracic epidural anesthesia should only be attempted by an anes-

Epidural Puncture: Paramedian Approach

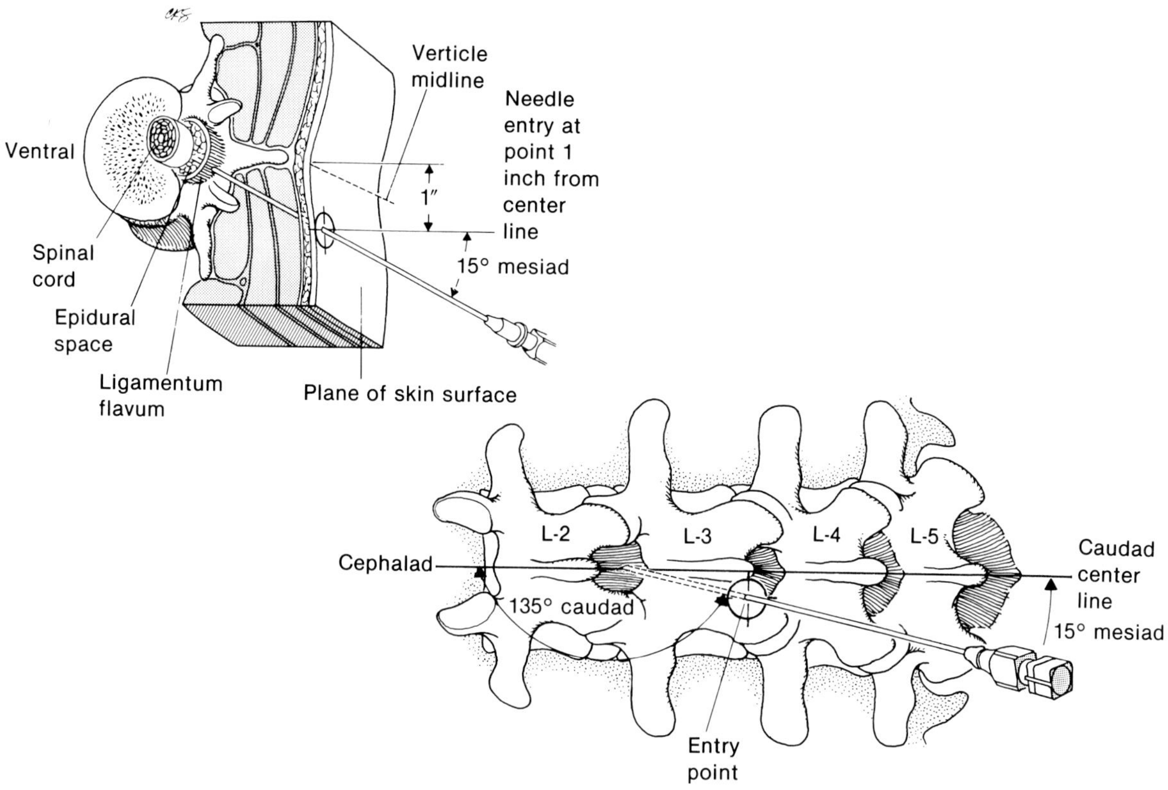

Figure 32–18 • The paramedian approach avoids overlapping of spinous processes but does not have the same feel as the midline approach because the supraspinous and interspinous ligaments are avoided.

thetist with considerable epidural anesthesia experience because the distances to traverse are quite small and the spinal cord lies in front of the advancing needle.

1. Place the patient in a chair or a low bed and have the subject lean forward with the support of an assistant. It is essential to reassure the patient and encourage him or her to remain as still as possible.
2. Identify the interspace to be used.
3. Proceed with equipment and back preparation as for lumbar midline approach.
4. Infiltrate the skin and subcutaneous tissues in the selected interspace.
5. Insert a Tuohy-style needle with its bevel oriented cephalad or a Crawford needle with the blunt edge toward the dura into the interspinous ligament or ligamentum flavum. This will be at a depth of 1.5–2.5 cm.
6. Remove the stylet and fill the hub of the needle with saline or local anesthetic solution.
7. Place both hypothenar eminences firmly against the patient's back, and grasp the wings, hub, and shaft of the needle with the thumb and three fingers of each hand (Fig. 32–19).
8. Advance the needle very slowly during the inspiratory phase of respiration, with eyes constantly on the hanging drop.
9. A sudden give or change in resistance will be felt as the needle passes through the ligamentum flavum into the epidural space. The drop in the hub will be sucked into the needle as a result of the negative pressure in the epidural space. Bromage reports that a fine stream of local anesthetic or other solution squirted into the hub will also be sucked in because negative pressure persists in the upper thoracic and cervical regions.[14] Advancement of the needle must completely stop at this time to avoid dural puncture.
10. If blood returns, promptly remove the needle and repeat the procedure in an adjacent interspace.
11. Proceed as above for test dose or catheter insertion.

The hanging drop method is recommended as the negative pressure technique of choice because it avoids

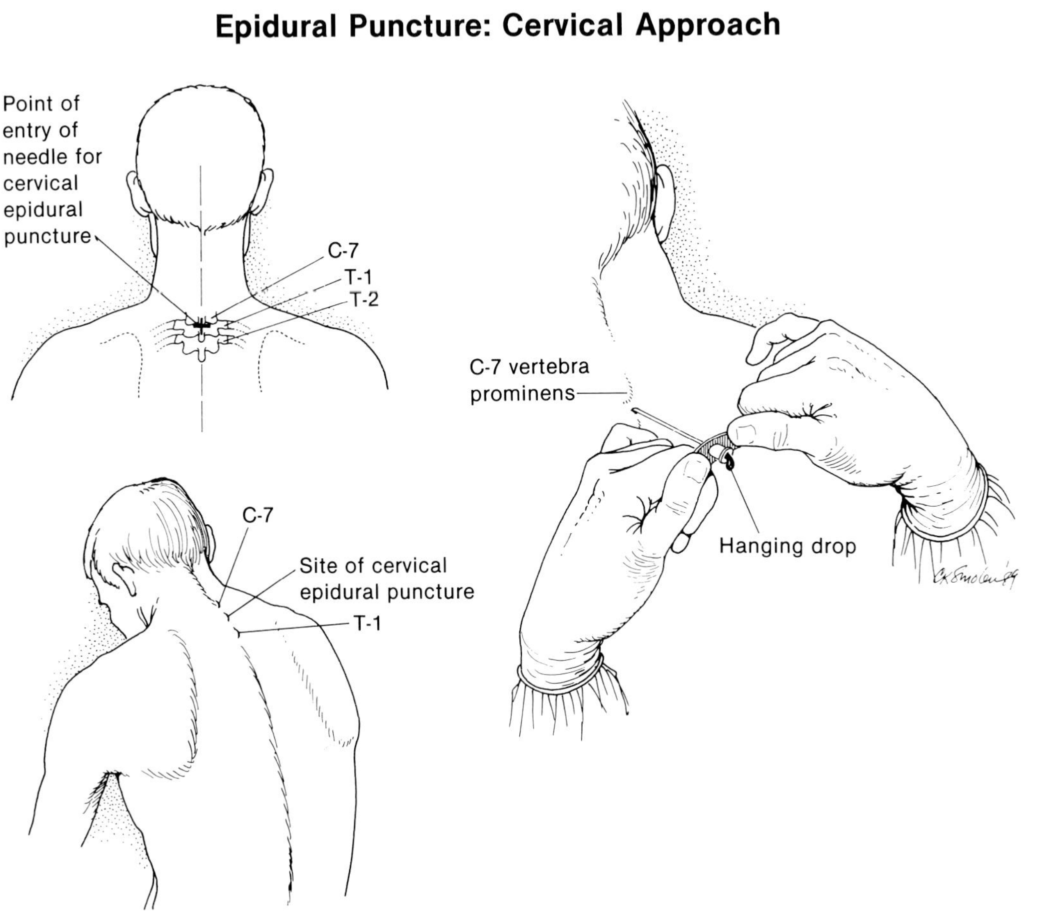

Figure 32–19 • Cervical epidural puncture is best performed with a winged needle and with both hands placed firmly against the patient's back to allow for very slow and precise advancement. The hanging drop method of identifying the cervical epidural space is recommended. The needle is inserted at the C7 to T1 interspace in the midline with a cephalad angle of approximately 30°. It is slowly advanced until the drop is sucked in by the negative pressure. This approach should only be attempted by those with substantial experience in administering epidural anesthetic.

the need for additional devices. However, if a manometric visual indicator is desired, it should be attached at the point where the hanging drop is inserted. The technique otherwise is identical.

E. *Technique of Paramedian Thoracic Epidural Puncture*

The severe angulation and overlapping of the vertebral spines and laminae in the midthoracic portion of the spine render the paramedian approach technically much easier, although the midline approach can be used successfully with extreme care. This approach requires the needle to be inserted lateral to the midline with both a mesiad and cephalad angle so that the needle will slide past the lamina and enter the epidural space close to the midline.

1. The patient is positioned and the back prepared after the desired interspace has been identified.
2. A skin wheal is raised with local anesthetic 1.5–2.0 cm lateral to the tip of the spinous process above the interspace (from the cephalad vertebra).
3. Locate the lamina with a 22 gauge, 1.5-inch needle. Inject a small amount of local anesthetic around the lamina and into the subcutaneous tissues on withdrawal.
4. Insert the epidural needle at an angle of 130° to the back and 15° to the axis of the spine until the lamina is encountered (Fig. 32–20).
5. Remove the stylet and insert the hanging drop.

Epidural Puncture: Thoracic Paramedian Approach

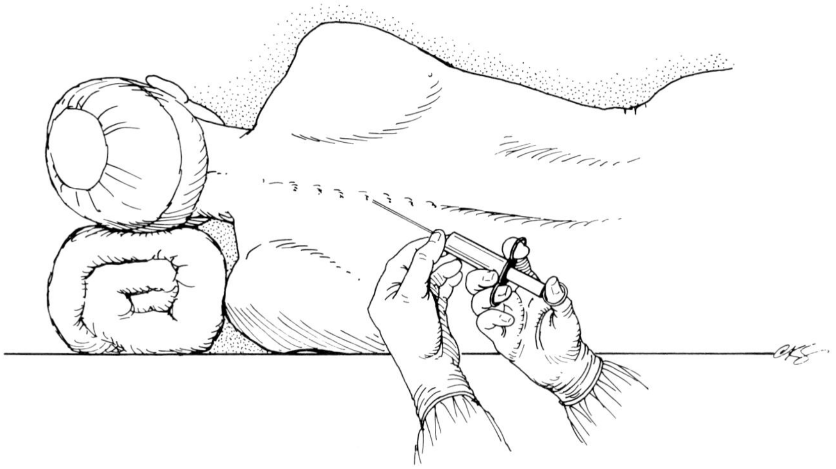

Figure 32–20 • The paramedian approach is often preferred for the midthoracic epidural anesthetic because it avoids the sharply angulated and overlapping spinous processes.

6. Gently walk the needle off the cephalad aspect of the lamina, and slowly advance the needle through the ligamentum flavum. As above, the needle should be under precise control by grasping it with the thumb and first three fingers of each hand. Avoid sudden or jerking movements. Advance during inspiration.
7. The remainder of the procedure is as for the thoracic midline approach.

It should be noted that the needle will be at a more acute angle than in the midline approach. Catheter passage may be facilitated by having the patient take a deep breath. This increase in negative pressure will momentarily decrease the size of the venous plexus and increase the amount of the epidural space.

F. *Technique of Caudal Puncture*

Entry into the epidural space was first made by the caudal approach. After the establishment of spinal approaches to the epidural space, the caudal approach lost favor and has failed to regain the popularity it enjoyed in the 1940s. A failure rate of 5% to 10% is expected in the best of hands because of the many variations of sacral anatomy. One should carefully select patients for caudal anesthesia by the ease of identifying their anatomic landmarks. Caudal anesthesia/analgesia may prove useful for surgical procedures in the anorectal region and in the perineum, and for some obstetric procedures. It has also proved useful for some pain control procedures and for diagnostic sympathetic blockade. Both single- and continuous-injection techniques may be used. The use of the caudal approach to the epidural space for anesthesia and pain control is becoming increasingly popular for use in children because of their relatively consistent landmarks and the ease of performing the procedure.[15]

The needle employed will depend on the age of the patient and the purpose of the procedure. A Tuohy or Crawford needle may be employed for either single-shot needle administration or standard catheter technique. A standard needle 1.5 inches long from 22 gauge to 18 gauge may also be used for single-injection techniques. A 25 gauge needle is suitable for small children. An intravenous over-the-needle cannula may be inserted and left in situ for a continuous technique.

1. The patient should be placed in the prone position with a pillow under the iliac crests and symphysis pubis to allow for some flexion of the hips. An alternative position is the lateral Sims position (Fig. 32–21).
2. Palpate and identify the sacral hiatus and the coccyx. Place the tip of the index finger over the tip of the coccyx, and palpate for the cornua with the thumb. They should lie 3–5 cm cephalad from the tip of the coccyx. If necessary, use a skin marker to retain the landmarks.
3. Prepare the site and equipment as for other epidural punctures.
4. Raise a small skin wheal of local anesthetic over the sacral hiatus.
5. At an angle of approximately 120° to the back, pass the needle through the skin, subcutaneous tissue, and sacrococcygeal membrane. A give or pop will be felt.

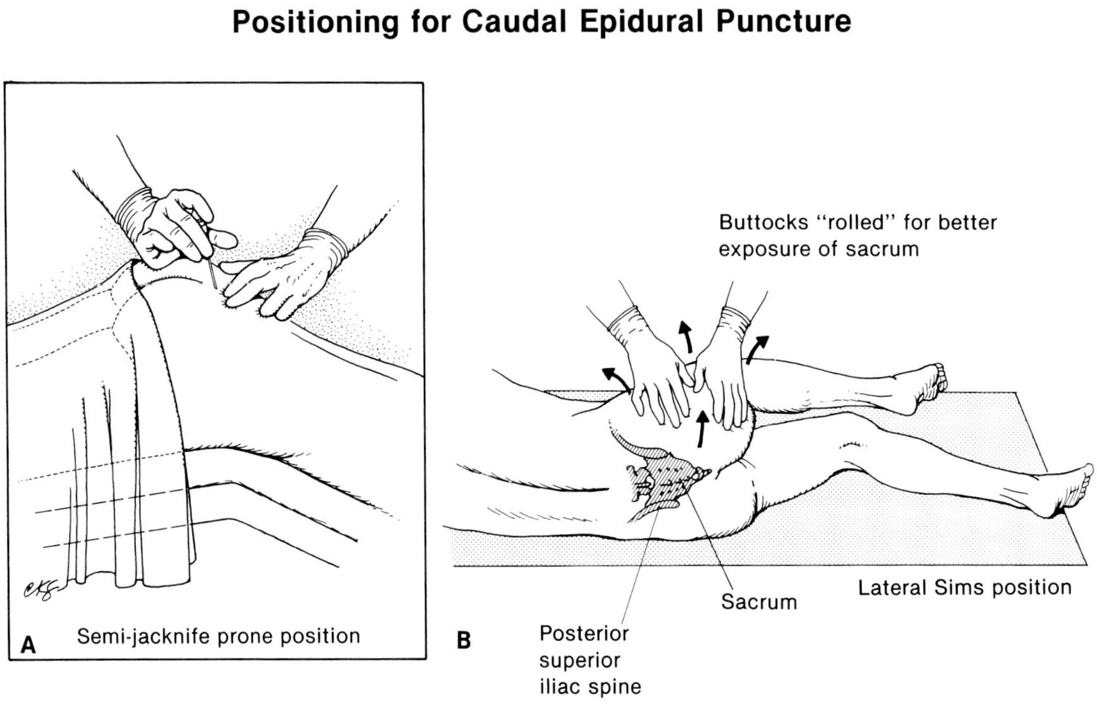

Figure 32–21 • Although either the prone (***A***) or the lateral (***B***) Sims position may be employed, the prone position provides for the easiest identification of anatomical landmarks.

6. Advance the needle a few millimeters further until the periosteum of the sacral canal is encountered. Avoid excessive force because the needle could easily enter the cancellous bone and the drugs could be injected into the marrow where they would act as intravenous agents. This is particularly of concern in children. In the pelvis of a parturient, the sacral wall could also be penetrated completely and the needle placed in the patient's rectum or the head of a fetus. If a single-injection technique is to be used, proceed to step 8.
7. Withdraw the needle 1–2 mm, and depress the needle hub and shaft so they are oriented parallel to the sacral canal. Advance the needle another 2–3 cm into the sacral canal (Fig. 32–22). An alternative method is to withdraw the needle 1–2 mm only, thus avoiding the potential problems of venipuncture or dural puncture with needle advancement in the sacral canal (Fig. 32–23).
8. Aspirate gently, and carefully observe for blood or CSF.
9. Inject 5 mL of saline solution or air while the opposite hand lies firmly over the lower sacrum. No bulge or crepitus should develop. If this does occur, the needle is most likely not in the sacral canal but in overlying tissue and must be withdrawn and redirected.
10. Inject the test dose of local anesthetic or insert the catheter, and secure and administer the test dose.
11. Proceed as for other epidural techniques.

G. *Drug Considerations*

1. The Test Dose

The test dose and its components have been given a great deal of attention during the last decade because of the identification of the potent cardiotoxicity of bupivacaine and the possible neurotoxicity of 2-chloroprocaine (Nesacaine). The elements of the test dose should alert the anesthetist to a subarachnoid injection, and, in some circumstances, to an intravenous injection. The dose of local anesthetic should therefore be sufficient to easily identify subarachnoid block without providing such extensive block as to compromise the patient or the situation. This can be achieved with 30–60 mg of lidocaine, 10 mg of bupivacaine, or 60–90 mg of 2-chloroprocaine (Nesacaine). This dosage can be administered and the patient carefully observed for 3–5 minutes for signs of subarachnoid block and for hemodynamic changes. If spinal blockade is not present, very careful assessment of the patient will usually reveal a partial segmental sensory alteration, which is a reassuring indicator of correct epidural placement. Some experts add glucose to their test dose to insure a hyperbaric solution.

The test dose is inadequate to identify intravenous placement in most subjects. When it is desirous and pos-

Caudal Puncture: Standard Approach

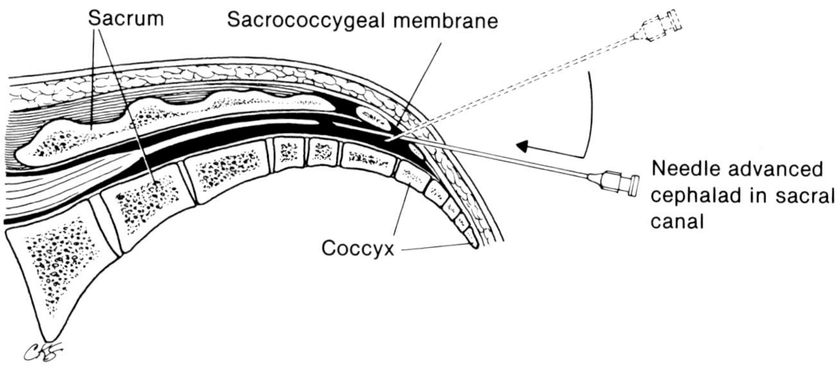

Figure 32–22 • Note that the needle is advanced along the sacral canal for 2–3 cm. Care must be taken not to advance further than this or the dural sac may be penetrated.

sible to rule out intravenous placement, epinephrine or another beta-adrenergic agonist can be added to the test dose and the patient carefully observed for increases in pulse rate and blood pressure. The use of 15 μg of epinephrine has been demonstrated to produce significant, but brief, heart rate elevations in humans.[16] This is the amount contained in 3 mL of a 1:200,000 solution of epinephrine. This is not particularly useful for the patient in active labor because pulse and blood pressure tend to change with the contraction cycle, and the use of epinephrine has been demonstrated to impair uterine blood flow, although this point remains controversial. Isoproterenol is currently under investigation as an alternative.

Lidocaine (40–60 mg) is recommended because of the rapidity of onset and limited duration of subarachnoid blockade. Epinephrine (15 μg) is employed except for patients in labor. It is important to recognize that each subsequent increment of the therapeutic dose should be treated as a test dose with the same degree of careful observation.

2. Therapeutic Dosages of Local Anesthetics

One of the most important lessons learned about epidural anesthesia during the past decade is that the administration of the full calculated therapeutic dose for a surgical procedure in a single rapidly administered bolus increases the risk associated with the technique. Nearly all of the case reports of neurotoxicity associated with 2-chloroprocaine (Nesacaine) were situations in which a full therapeutic epidural dose was unintentionally injected into the subarachnoid space. The first case reports

Caudal Puncture: Modified Approach

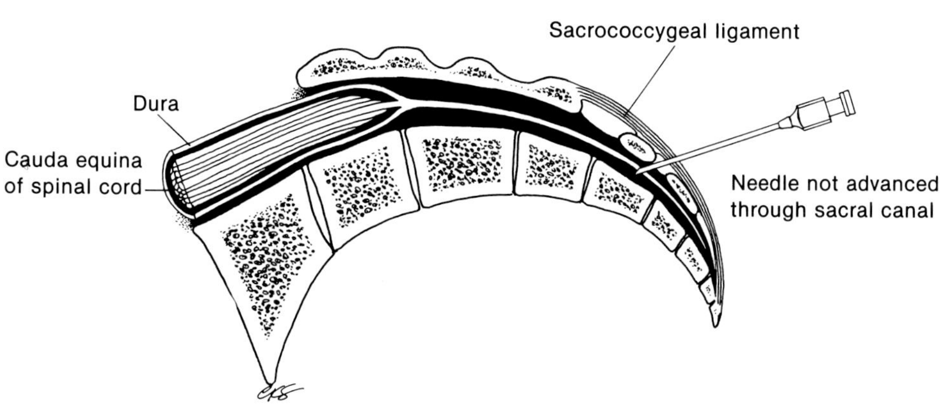

Figure 32–23 • This technique avoids the risk of dural puncture, but threading the catheter may be more difficult.

of profound bupivacaine cardiotoxicity were similarly associated with large single doses intended for the epidural space but unintentionally injected intravascularly. This has led the distributors of bupivacaine to issue a warning against the use of the 0.75% solution for pregnant patients and patients at high risk. Although the mechanisms of these problems have yet to be firmly elucidated, their clinical use continues with few mishaps because anesthetists now inject their therapeutic doses in a fractional manner. If the estimated dose is 28 mL of a solution, the prudent anesthetist administers 5–10 mL, then observes and evaluates the patient over the next few minutes. If all appears appropriate, subsequent aliquots are given, usually in a slightly larger amount and with only a minute or two between injections. If there is any doubt raised by any of the injections, careful reassessment of the catheter or needle is indicated and, if all appears well, incremental dosing should continue at a slower pace. Although interval dosing is essential to insure patient safety, if the time intervals are too long (eg, 10–15 minutes), the desired level may not be achieved. Although incremental dosing is quite simple with a catheter technique, it is a bit more difficult with a needle technique because the needle and patient must remain in the same place for a longer period of time. Some experts have recommended abandoning the needle approach in favor of the catheter technique.

The dose requirements for epidural block have been well derived by Bromage and others.[17] At age 18, these appear to be about 1.6 mL per segment of blockade desired, declining approximately 0.1 mL per decade of age. Pregnant patients require approximately one third less (ie, about 1.0 mL per segment), primarily as a result of progesterone's effect on the nerve's sensitivity to local anesthetics.[18]

The volume of the sacral canal varies considerably, as does the egress of local anesthetic solution from the sacral foramina. Consequently, the dosage of local anesthetic required for caudal anesthesia may vary. The average adult requires 2–3 mL of solution per segment of blockade. This translates to 15–20 mL for a block from L-5 down. Children have lower dosage requirements that seem to vary with age, at about 0.1 mL/segment/year of age.[15]

Reinforcing or "top up" doses will vary from between one third to one half the original dose. They may be administered as the upper level of the block declines by two segments or by a time schedule based on the average duration of the drug selected. Typically, the timed injection is made at the average duration less 1.5 standard deviations. Table 32–2 summarizes two-segment regression for some popular local anesthetics as determined by Bromage.[19] All solutions contain 1:200,000 epinephrine (5 μg/mL). It is important to recognize that epidural anesthesia dosing must be based on the individual patient's response to the anesthetic and on the surgical procedure being carried out. Tables and formulas only serve as a guide.

3. Epidural Narcotics

The use of epidural opioids for postoperative pain relief as well as for more chronic conditions has become very widespread. The water-soluble narcotics slowly diffuse into the subarachnoid space and bind to the opiate receptors in the spinal cord. Rostral movement of the drugs occurs, and respiratory depression has been demonstrated with the use of all of the mu-agonist narcotic drugs. The lipid-soluble drugs, such as fentanyl and sufentanil, tend to be absorbed by the lipid-containing tissues in the epidural and subarachnoid spaces and are less likely to cause severe respiratory depression. Morphine is among the least lipid-soluble agents and is much more likely to result in respiratory depression, particularly in

Table 32–2 • Duration of Epidural Local Anesthetic Action

Drug	Duration (min) of two-segment regression	Standard deviation (S.D.)	Duration (min) (1.5 × S.D.)
2-chloroprocaine (3%)	57	7	47
Lidocaine (2%)	98	19	70
Bupivacaine (0.5%)	196	31	150
Bupivacaine (0.75%)	201	40	141
Etidocaine (1%)	170	57	85

the presence of other CNS sedative drugs. Nausea, pruritus, and urinary retention are less threatening but more frequently observed side effects. Morphine has a duration of action significantly longer than the other available drugs. The narcotics may be given as single injections or as a continuous infusion. They may be added to local anesthetics for enhanced intraoperative analgesia. It essential that the preparation used is free of preservatives. Table 32-3 summarizes the epidural characteristics of some of the narcotics.

4. EPIDURAL STEROID INJECTIONS

Epidural steroid injection for back pain and sciatica has been used for nearly four decades. Cervical epidural steroid injection has also been used with success for cervical disk syndrome. The theory is that the steroids reduce nerve swelling and edema and thus reduce symptoms of an inflamed nerve in a compressed space (ie, the narrowed foramina as a result of disc compression or disc bulging). The effectiveness of therapy seems to be between 60% and 85%.[20] Careful patient selection tends to improve results. Relief from pain and symptoms may last from as little as a few days to as long as a year or more. It is often necessary to repeat the treatment 2 or 3 times. Some anesthetists use a large volume of diluent solution (30–50 mL) in the hopes of breaking up scar tissue or adhesions. Evidence to support this belief is lacking. Local anesthetic or narcotic may be used simultaneously for immediate relief of symptoms because it appears that the steroids may take as long as 72 hours to demonstrate an effect. The use of narcotics and local anesthetics will prolong the patient's stay at the clinic and, if local anesthetic is used, necessitate intravenous access for fluids and vasopressors if needed. It is important to remember that these steroids are absorbed and exert a systemic effect for 2–3 weeks.[21] Patients should be so informed and advised to notify their physician of the injection if any medical or surgical therapy is required within that time.

Personal experience suggests that the subjects who will receive the most relief for the longest time are those with new onset pain with sciatica. Such patients tend to receive 1 to 2 injections and will have significant relief for several months. Altering lifestyle and attending back care school also contribute to the duration of pain relief. The most frequently used steroids are methylprednisolone (Depomedrol) and triamcinolone (Aristocort). These preparations contain polyethylene glycol in a 2.8–3.0% concentration, which demyelinates nervous tissue. Therefore, these drugs should be diluted by at least a factor of 10 before injection into the epidural space. Vials should be used only once and any excess discarded. Although there are no cut-and-dried schemata for using epidural steroids, the following protocol using methylprednisolone has proved useful:

1. The patient should have been evaluated by a qualified back specialist and the level(s) of the lesion identified.
2. After obtaining informed consent, record the patient's pulse, blood pressure, and respiratory rate. Informed consent should include a discussion of the side effects of steroids, the possibility of no relief, the necessity for repeat injections, and the possibility of the pain and symptoms becoming worse, in addition to the usual risks of epidural therapy.
3. Insert an intravenous cannula if appropriate.
4. Insert a needle into the epidural space at the level of the lesion or as close as possible.
5. If a local anesthetic is to be used, administer a test dose and evaluate the patient over a 5-minute period.
6. Shake the vial containing the steroid, since it is a suspension. It is available as a 20-mg/mL, 40-mg/mL, and 80-mg/mL suspension.
7. Withdraw the desired dosage, which will range from 80

Table 32-3 • Characteristics of Epidural Opioids

Drug	Relative Lipid Solubility	Dosage (mg)	Onset (min)	Duration (hrs)
Morphine	1	4–10	60	12–18
Meperidine	27	50–100	30	4–12
Methadone	83	5–10	20	6–8
Fentanyl	572	0.05–0.10	15	2–4
Sufentanil	1252	0.03–0.075	15	2–4

to 160 mg. A reasonable dosage for the average patient is 80–120 mg.

8. Dilute the steroid in 10–20 mL of preservative-free saline or dilute concentration of local anesthetic. If saline alone is used to dilute the steroid, 50–100 μg of fentanyl may be added for immediate pain relief lasting up to 4 hours. This is often reassuring to the patient and avoids the sympathetic and sensory blockade of the local anesthetic.
10. Inject the solution slowly. The irritated nerve roots are quite sensitive to rapid injection.
11. Remove the needle. If steroid alone was used, the patient may be observed for 15 minutes and discharged. If fentanyl was added, observe the patient for 30–60 minutes and discharge with a responsible adult and a caution not to drive or use dangerous equipment for 12 hours. If a local anesthetic was used, the patient may be discharged in the company of a responsible adult when effects have dissipated to the point of stabilization and safety.
12. The patient should be advised that the pain may actually be enhanced for a day or two, but should then dissipate.
13. Reevaluate in 2 weeks. If symptoms have resolved, no further therapy is required until symptoms recur.
14. If symptoms are partially but not completely alleviated, a repeat injection or two is indicated.
15. Little additional benefit is gained after a series of three injections.

5. Epidural Neurolytic Block

The use of epidural alcohol to provide pain relief for patients with malignancy was introduced in 1930. Subsequent studies have reported on the efficacy of both epidural alcohol and phenol. Although neurolytic block is usually recommended only for malignant pain, a recent report has suggested its use for certain benign pain conditions as well.[22] The actual clinical applications for epidural neurolytic block are few, and it is a technique that may be attended by severe consequences, especially if an unintended subarachnoid injection occurs. It is recommended that this type of therapy be used only by those expert in pain management and regional anesthesia.

Epidural Blood Patch

The use of the autologous epidural blood patch for the treatment of postdural puncture headache has increased substantially since its reintroduction nearly two decades ago.[23] Success rates appear to be consistently greater than 90%. Although there is potential for introducing infection, producing neurologic compression injury, or inducing a meningismic syndrome from subarachnoid injection of blood, the actual incidence of these complications appears to be nil when proper precautions are taken. Expected side effects of low-grade fever and backache are relatively minor and well tolerated.

The mechanism of action appears to be twofold. First, a gelatinous tamponade of the CSF leak occurs, thus stopping the loss of CSF and allowing it to reaccumulate, as well as permitting the dura-arachnoid rent to heal in a normal fashion.[23] In addition, the injection of a 10- to 15-mL nondissipating mass results in an immediate rise in CSF pressure, promptly alleviating symptoms. The presence of blood in the epidural space does not appear to cause significant alterations in the area, as demonstrated in animal studies and in humans receiving epidural anesthesia subsequent to epidural blood patch.[23,24] As with any regional technique, it is important to inform the patient of the potential risks as well as benefits and to document this in the medical record. The following technique is recommended:

1. After confirming the diagnosis of postdural puncture headache, place the patient on his or her side or in the sitting position as tolerated.
2. Enter the epidural space with a standard epidural needle in the usual fashion at the level of the original dural puncture or as close as possible to it.
3. Have an assistant draw 10–15 mL of autologous blood from the patient in a sterile fashion into a plastic syringe. The region, usually the antecubital fossa, should be thoroughly prepared with povidone-iodine solution (Betadine) prior to drawing the blood. The assistant should be gloved and the syringe and needle handled in a sterile manner.
4. Slowly inject the blood (1 mL every 3–4 seconds). If the patient complains of pain, stop the injection immediately and reassess the needle location. The procedure should not produce pain.
5. Remove the needle and have the patient remain supine for 30 minutes.
6. The patient may now elevate the head gradually to evaluate the effectiveness of the block. Reassure the patient that symptoms will be reduced significantly, if not eliminated.
7. The patient may now be discharged with instructions to remain at bed rest as much as possible for the next 48 hours and to consume at least 8 glasses of water per day for this period to encourage CSF replacement.
8. If relief proves inadequate, a second, and on occasion a third, blood patch may be performed at 48-hour intervals.

A common cause of failure is misdiagnosis of the source of the headache!

H. *Special Technical Considerations of Epidural Puncture*

Several events can confound the operator during the performance of an epidural puncture or catheter insertion. Epidural anesthesia will be safer and more reliable if these are identified and managed effectively.

Glass syringes are generally preferred for loss-of-resistance techniques. However, they do have the drawback of becoming sticky on occasion so that the loss of resistance may not be perceived. The incidence of this problem may be reduced by taking care not to get any glove powder on the plunger. It also is wise to fill the syringe with liquid just prior to use. If filled earlier, some solution will seep around the plunger and form a thin film that eventually dries and makes the syringe lose its smoothness. Some have suggested that using air instead of a liquid will also minimize this problem.

The presence of blood in the needle or the catheter may indicate that it is within the lumen of an epidural vein. This will most certainly be the case if blood flows spontaneously or if blood aspiration is obvious. In this case, the device should be withdrawn and reinserted into another interspace. On occasion, blood will appear in a very small quantity initially and then stop. If aspiration on the needle or catheter is negative, a dilemma arises as to whether this blood is from vascular insertion or adjacent vessel injury. The dilemma may be resolved by gently flushing the device with sterile saline in a quantity sufficient to completely clear it. Gentle aspiration should now reveal if it is a vessel or not.

If free-flowing CSF is encountered, the needle or catheter should be removed and the procedure repeated at another interspace (Table 32–4). It has been suggested that the catheter could be slowly backed up until the flow of CSF ceases, but this maneuver is not recommended. Occasionally a small amount of clear fluid will flow back from the needle. It could be CSF, saline, or local anesthetic. Some confusion can be avoided by injecting only a milliliter or two of saline upon entry into the epidural space. If this situation cannot be resolved by observation and aspiration, one could resort to one of the numerous tests devised to make this distinction. A simple maneuver is to allow some of the solution to drop onto the back of the operator's arm or hand. The CSF should be warm, whereas other solutions should be cool. On occasion this is difficult to determine, particularly if the fluid return is slow, and one of a few simple chemical tests could prove useful.

The *pentothal test* is based on the fact that a 2.5% solution of sodium pentothal is quite alkaline and will yield a precipitate if local anesthetics are allowed to drip into a container or syringe containing this solution.[25] This occurs because the pH of the local anesthetic solution is increased well above its pKa, and thus the majority of the substance becomes the nonionized base form, which is relatively insoluble in water. This test would be useful if efflux of fluid were noted after the test dose or a reinforcing dose had been given. However, the test cannot easily distinguish between a mixture of spinal fluid and local anesthetic and a solution of local anesthetic alone.

Another test is the *glucose oxidase test.*[26,27] A glucose test strip for urine or blood can be exposed to the solution returning from the needle or catheter and will indicate the presence of glucose if the solution is CSF. Ackerman and associates have recently demonstrated the sensitivity of this test even in the presence of local anesthetic solutions.[27] A *urine multitest dipstick* may also prove

Table 32–4 • Methods to Determine the Presence of Cerebrospinal Fluid

	Cerebrospinal Fluid	Local Anesthetic
Temperature of solution	Warm	Cool
Pentothal test	No precipitation	Precipitation
Glucose oxidase test	Positive	Negative
Urine dipstick	Glucose +	Glucose –
	Protein +	Protein +
	pH Neutral	pH acidic

useful because it can detect glucose present in spinal fluid and gives a strongly positive protein test if local anesthetic is predominant, and the pH section will be acidic if the solution is a local anesthetic.[28] Although each test is capable of assisting the operator, experience has shown that meticulous technique, diligent and careful aspiration, and the appropriate use of test and therapeutic doses is what will avoid disaster.

A potential subdural extra-arachnoid space exists and is entered during attempted myelography in approximately 1% to 15% of adults.[11] This space may contain a small amount of fluid. It is possible to enter this space when performing epidural anesthesia and not be able to recognize it until the test dose or a subsequent dose of local anesthetic has been given. Although the block spreads relatively slowly when compared with spinal anesthesia, it becomes much more extensive than anticipated for the amount of drug given in the epidural space. The possibility of entering this space may be minimized by meticulous technique and by avoiding needle rotation. Diagnosis will be made by careful assessment of the distribution of the block. Since no clinically useful techniques exist for using this space, it is recommended that the needle or catheter be removed if it appears to have been inserted there.

IV. Discussion

A. *Physiologic Changes with Epidural Anesthesia*

This section will highlight the major physiologic changes observed in the clinical setting with epidural anesthesia. The reader desiring more in-depth or complete knowledge is referred to Bromage's excellent text.[29] The most significant physiologic changes occurring under epidural anesthesia are cardiovascular. These alterations are the net result of two different categories of modification: neural blockade and systemic absorption of substances placed in the epidural space.

1. Cardiovascular Effects

The sympathetic nervous system supports both vascular tone and heart rate. The parasympathetic system (vagus) slows the heart rate. The sympathetic tone of the vascular tree is decreased to a greater extent as the number of segments involved in the blockade increases, as well as in proportion to the intensity of blockade. The ability of the unblocked regions to compensate for changes induced by the blocked regions results in some degree of stability in the awake patient with functioning reflexes. The following have been noted to occur with epidural anesthesia:

1. Sympathetic blockade results in a 10% to 20% reduction in systemic vascular resistance when the level of blockade extends from T-4 to S-5.
2. Sympathetic blockade results in a very large increase in capacitance. This occurs because veins do not share the thick, smooth-muscle wall of the arterial system. Thus, the loss of tone from innervation leads to a vascular bed which may dilate to a greater degree. Since 80% of the blood volume already resides in the venous system, it is apparent that this effect is a very significant, if not the major, cause of hypotension.
3. Bradycardia can occur when sympathetic blockade extends above T-5, particularly when at T-2 or above. This is believed to be secondary to blockade of cardioaccelerator fibers residing in segments T-1 to T-5. The fibers in T-1 and T-2 seem to be most important.
4. Bradycardia may also occur as a result of decreased cardiac return from venodilation and a Bainbridge response. This is suggested to be due to changes in atrial baroreceptor stimulation.[30]
5. Hypotension is less frequent with plain local anesthetic solutions than with epinephrine-containing solutions, even at levels to T-5 or higher. Although significant local anesthetic absorption occurs, the blood levels seen with routine clinical doses of local anesthetic are not high enough to produce a negative inotropic effect or vasodilation.
6. A greater incidence and degree of hypotension and an increase in cardiac output and tachycardia are observed in patients receiving epinephrine-containing solutions. This may be due to systemic absorption of epinephrine with a predominant beta-adrenergic effect due to the low blood levels.[31] Another hypothesis suggests that this is the result of more intense sympathetic blockade because of the presence of epinephrine.[32] Proponents of this concept point out that the cardiovascular effects observed when epinephrine is added are much longer in duration than when the same amount of epinephrine is placed in the epidural space by itself.
7. If a local anesthetic solution is alkalinized, more rapid onset of blockade occurs, and hypotension is more frequent. This is probably due to the greater penetration of the local anesthetic and a more profound block.
8. If an excessive amount of local anesthetic is rapidly placed

in the epidural space, CNS or cardiovascular symptoms may occur due to vascular absorption.

2. VENTILATORY EFFECTS

The effect of epidural anesthesia on the ventilatory system are not extensive under ordinary conditions. The phrenic nerve is virtually never involved, unless a cervical epidural anesthetic is employed. The ability to maintain a normal tidal volume and vital capacity adequate to insure cough is not compromised even with a sensory block to T-1. However, conditions such as pregnancy with multiple gestation or tense ascites result in ventilatory impairment with epidural blockade to this level. Respiratory arrest during extensive epidural anesthesia, as with high spinal anesthesia, is probably not due to neural blockade of respiration or high medullary levels of local anesthetic, but rather to decreased cardiac output with reduced oxygenation of the respiratory center.

V. COMPLICATIONS OF EPIDURAL PUNCTURE AND ANESTHESIA

A. *Immediate Complications*

1. HYPOTENSION

Hypotension as a result of sympathetic blockade can be minimized by providing an adequate intravenous fluid load prior to initiating epidural blockade. One must always be alert for this common side effect because it may occur even with limited segmental involvement, depending on the patient's overall condition. This is particularly true during pregnancy, when aortocaval compression due to supine positioning will complicate the problem. The pregnant patient should never remain in the supine position without adequate left uterine displacement.

Hypotension with surgical levels of epidural anesthesia may be minimized by infusing between 15 and 30 mL/kg of balanced saline solution prior to the anesthetic. The administration of prophylactic intramuscular ephedrine in a dose of approximately 0.7 mg/kg will provide further protection, although this is rarely needed. Hypotension does not usually occur after the administration of epidural narcotics.

Hypotension is treated by increasing the rate of intravenous fluid administration, intravenous ephedrine (5–15 mg), and improving cardiac return by Trendelenberg positioning (Table 32–5). Other vasopressors may be selected, although the pure alpha-adrenergic agonists are relatively contraindicated during pregnancy. If persistent bradycardia should occur, atropine (0.5–1.5 mg) may be necessary. If the patient is in the third trimester of pregnancy, additional left uterine displacement is mandatory.

Table 32–5 • Management of Hypotension

1. Administer intravenous fluids rapidly.
2. Raise the legs to increase central blood volume.
3. Place the patient in a modest degree of Trendelenburg position.
4. Administer a vasopressor (eg, ephedrine or phenylephrine).
5. Anticipate nausea and vomiting.
6. Anticipate loss of consciousness.

2. HIGH SPINAL ANESTHESIA

High spinal anesthesia will occur if a significant epidural dose is unintentionally injected in the subarachnoid space. This is usually avoided by using an appropriate test dose and incremental dosing with careful observation. If this problem should occur, the essence of the therapy is to secure the airway and ventilate the patient with oxygen (if respiration appears grossly impaired) and to support the blood pressure and the cardiovascular system. Once the patient is stable, the administration of an amnestic drug such as diazepam or midazolam should be considered to decrease awareness until the block dissipates, although total deafferentation from massive spinal anesthesia is thought to eliminate most sensory input (Table 32–6).

Table 32–6 • Management of High Spinal Anesthesia

1. Establish and secure the airway, and ventilate with oxygen.
2. Maintain perfusion pressure with intravenous fluids and/or vasopressors.
3. Provide amnesia after hemodynamic stability is obtained.

3. SYSTEMIC LOCAL ANESTHETIC TOXICITY

If local anesthetic is injected intravenously, or if a large dose of local anesthetic is placed in the epidural space, systemic local anesthetic toxicity will result because of vascular absorption. Symptoms will vary from mild CNS involvement to seizure activity to cardiac arrest, depending on the amount admitted to the bloodstream.

a. Central Nervous System Effects

The symptoms most commonly seen with mildly toxic blood levels include numbness of the lips and tongue, a strange, metallic taste, restlessness, talkativeness, and tinnitus. As the blood level rises, further nausea, visual disturbances, and disorientation occur. Twitching may be observed. The most severe form is heralded by tonic-clonic convulsions followed by systematic CNS depression. The seemingly paradoxical stimulation of the CNS followed by depression is explained by the fact that the local anesthetics first depress cortical or subcortical inhibitory pathways, leading to seizures. At higher blood levels, all pathways are depressed. Laboratory studies suggest that inhibition of the release of the neurotransmitter gamma-aminobutyric acid (GABA) may be the mechanism by which local anesthetics induce seizures. A particular local anesthetic's ability to inhibit GABA release and to induce seizures is positively correlated with its potency.

b. Cardiovascular Effects

The cardiovascular system is more resistant to local anesthetics than the CNS, as demonstrated by the higher doses required to produce significant effects. Large doses of local anesthetics are generally depressant to all components of the cardiovascular system. They produce a decrease in myocardial contractility, a decrease in conduction and excitability, and vasodilation. All of the local anesthetics decrease myocardial contractility, which, in turn, causes a decrease in stroke volume and cardiac output.

This depression is the result of the same mechanism of action involved in nerve conduction blockade and inhibition of sodium conductance. The ability to depress the myocardium and the conduction system parallels a local anesthetic's potency. The hypotension which occurs with local anesthetic toxicity is caused by the decrease in stroke volume and cardiac output. Vasodilation and a fall in systemic vascular resistance occurs only with massive overdosage. The more potent agents, bupivacaine and etidocaine, may produce a cardiovascular collapse that is rapid and profound and does not respond to the usual measures for resuscitation. Ventricular arrhythmias, AV dissociation, and electromechanical dissociation have been reported. Their physicochemical characteristics allow them to enter a cell rapidly but leave it slowly, thus perpetuating the effect.

Table 32-7 • Prevention of Local Anesthetic Systemic Reactions

1. Observe proper maximum dose guidelines for size and age of patient.
2. Add epinephrine whenever appropriate.
3. Aspirate before and during injection.
4. Use a test dose with "tracer" to detect intravascular injection.
5. If premonitory signs occur, stop the injection and reassess the situation.

c. Prevention of Local Anesthetic Toxicity

Do not administer more than the recommended maximum dose for the site of the block. This dose will be greater for peripheral nerve block than for peridural anesthesia. Add epinephrine to the local anesthetic solution in a concentration of 5 μg/mL or less (1:200,000 or less). This will delay the absorption and decrease the peak level attained in the bloodstream. It may also afford protection from myocardial depression in the event of an intravascular injection. Careful aspiration should be carried out prior to and during the injection (Table 32–7).

d. Treatment of Local Anesthetic Toxicity

Stop the injection, administer oxygen, and encourage hyperventilation (Table 32–8). This will decrease the carbon dioxide tension in the blood and elevate the seizure threshold. Support the airway. Seizures often abate in a minute or less. If the patient is not breathing, then ventilate the patient. If control of the airway cannot be obtained due to tonic-clonic seizures that persist, admin-

Table 32-8 • Treatment of Mild Central Nervous System Reactions

1. Stop the injection.
2. Administer oxygen.
3. Encourage hyperventilation.
4. Administer a small dose of a short-acting barbiturate or benzodiazepine, if needed.
5. Anticipate a severe reaction.

ister an appropriate intravenous dose of short-acting barbiturate or succinylcholine. Intubation is often indicated if this is necessary (Table 32–9). If the patient is hypotensive, administer a vasopressor such as ephedrine (15–25 mg IV). If the patient has bradycardia, administer atropine (0.5–1.0 mg for adults). If profound cardiovascular collapse occurs, particularly with etidocaine or bupivacaine, administer epinephrine (0.1–0.2 mg). Cardiopulmonary resuscitation should be instituted and maintained as appropriate (Table 32–10).

B. *Delayed Complications*

1. POSTDURAL PUNCTURE HEADACHE

Postdural puncture headache should be an infrequent occurrence subsequent to epidural anesthesia because the incidence of unintentional dural puncture should be 1/200–500 attempts. The syndrome and its management are thoroughly discussed in this chapter (see the section on epidural blood patch) and in Chapter 31, "Spinal Anesthesia."

2. BACKACHE

Backache following epidural anesthesia is difficult to distinguish from back discomfort as a result of the surgical procedure or positioning on the table. The incidence of backache ranges from 1% to 2% for surgical patients to as high as 3% to 40% for the obstetric population. Although the incidence seems no different from that of similar groups of patients who received no epidural anesthesia for their operations, the possibility that trauma to the tissues, periosteum, or ligaments could lead to some discomfort remains. Bleeding from vessel trauma may also cause a small hematoma in the subcutaneous tissues. In addition, the injection of a large volume of saline or local anesthetic in a site other than the epidural space could also cause some discomfort. Reassurance and local measures are usually all that is required, and symptoms resolve within a few days.

Table 32–9 • Treatment of Severe Central Nervous System Reactions

1. Support and protect the airway.
2. Ventilate with oxygen.
3. Stop convulsions if they do not cease spontaneously. Use:
   a. Short-acting barbiturate
   b. Benzodiazepine
   c. Succinylcholine
4. Anticipate cardiovascular depression.

Table 32–10 • Treatment of Severe Cardiovascular Reaction

1. Secure the airway and ventilate with oxygen.
2. Position the patient to improve cardiac venous return (eg, head down).
3. Rapidly infuse IV fluids.
4. Administer a vasopressor such as 15–25 mg ephedrine IV.
   a. Administer 0.2–0.5 mg epinephrine, if there is severe depression from bupivacaine or etidocaine.
5. Treat persistent bradycardia with 0.5–1.0 mg atropine IV.
6. Correct acidosis with sodium bicarbonate.
7. Administer antiarrhythmic agents as needed.
   a. Bretylium may be useful for polymorphic ventricular tachycardia.
8. Perform CPR as indicated. This may be necessary for some time with bupivacaine or etidocaine toxicity.

3. EPIDURAL ABSCESS

Epidural abscess is rarely associated with epidural anesthesia. In fact the epidural space seems fairly resistant to outside bacterial contamination if there is not a concentrated inoculum. Local anesthetics have been demonstrated to be bacteriostatic.[33] Most cases are spontaneous and occur in patients with severe systemic infection who have not had epidural anesthesia. There are, however, reports of epidural abscess that appear to be directly linked to epidural anesthesia. The prevention is to practice meticulous technique in both equipment and drug handling. It might be advisable to avoid epidural anesthesia in patients who have a systemic bacterial infection and who have not yet been treated with a sufficient course of antibiotics.

Epidural abscess is a devastating problem because it leads to extensive neural damage from compression of the tissue of the spinal cord or nerve roots or both. Early diagnosis is paramount to successful treatment (ie, laminectomy and drainage). The most common presenting symptoms are backache exacerbated by movement, local tenderness, and fever. The typical length of time from onset of back pain to the complaint of nerve root pain is 2–3 days. A high level of suspicion must be entertained, since by the time neurologic symptoms are apparent it is unlikely that they can be reversed. The definitive diagnosis can be established by myelogram, CT scan, or ultrasonography, and immediate surgical decompression should follow. Epidural abscess takes some time to develop; therefore, one needs to exercise judgment if the symptoms appear shortly after the block (eg, in the recovery room).

4. Epidural Hematoma

Epidural hematoma has a much more rapid onset of symptoms than epidural abscess, which tends to be insidious. The presenting symptoms are usually back pain and neurologic deficit. Prompt neurosurgical intervention is necessary to prevent permanent damage resulting from spinal cord and nerve root compression as well as vascular compromise.

As with epidural abscess, this condition is often seen in patients who develop it spontaneously after trauma or who are receiving anticoagulant therapy. Hematomas have been associated with epidural anesthesia in patients who are receiving anticoagulant therapy, presumably due to laceration of one of the veins in the epidural plexus. This has led many anesthetists to avoid using epidural anesthesia when anticoagulants are to be administered intraoperatively (ie, in major vascular surgery). However, many such patients would benefit from receiving epidural anesthesia. Rao and associates, after careful study of patients who underwent vascular procedures and were anticoagulated intraoperatively, concluded that symptomatic hematomas following anticoagulation occur very rarely in patients with epidural or subarachnoid catheters, assuming proper patient selection, an atraumatic technique, and appropriate monitoring of anticoagulant activity.[34] They reported no epidural hematomas. These patients were maintained on intravenous heparin at 6-hour intervals.

Epidural catheter insertion should take place prior to anticoagulation. Any manipulation or removal of the catheter should be made just prior to the next scheduled dose of heparin, and only after determining that this patient's coagulation profile is acceptable at this interval. A large study conducted by Odoom and Sih suggests that epidural anesthesia may be safe for patients on oral anticoagulants (eg, coumarin derivatives) as well.[35] One thousand epidural injections were performed in patients who received oral anticoagulants preoperatively and heparin intraoperatively and underwent vascular surgery. The study found no occurrence of epidural hematoma. Despite these studies, which represent an important step in the right direction, prudence dictates careful assessment of risks and benefits before proceeding with epidural anesthesia in these patients.

5. Neurologic Injury

Neurologic injury from direct trauma should be easily avoided by withdrawing the needle if pain is reported and by discontinuing injection upon report of pain. Long-term or permanent neurologic injury is quite rare, having been estimated at approximately 1 in 11,000 cases.[12] The etiology of such unfortunate problems is multiple and includes anterior spinal artery syndrome secondary to hypotension, neurolytic action of preservatives, contamination of local anesthetic solution with other chemicals, and possibly neurotoxicity of some local anesthetic preparations.

The local anesthetic 2-chloroprocaine (Nesacaine) has been suspected of having greater neurotoxic potential in humans.[36,37] The clinical toxic syndrome has been almost exclusively confined to unintentional intrathecal injections with near-maximal doses for epidural anesthesia. High or total spinal anesthesia ensued in several cases, with a prolonged dissipation. Residua were varied but, as could be expected, primarily involved the cauda equina. Adhesive arachnoiditis was documented in one patient.[36] A very important discovery has been that sodium bisulfite and sodium metabisulfite have consistently produced neural damage in rabbits when injected in the subarachnoid space, but that pure 2-chloroprocaine did not.[38] This effect was further evaluated by another group using an isolated vagus nerve trunk model from adult rabbits. They found that permanent impairment of nerve conduction could be induced when sodium bisulfite was placed in the bathing solution at a low pH. They attributed the dysfunction to the diffusion of sulfur dioxide into the cell at this low pH with subsequent hydration to sulfurous acid.[39] Clearly, antioxidant sodium bisulfite in a low pH environment may be wholly or partially involved in the clinically observed syndromes, although other animal studies suggest that the agent 2-chloroprocaine may also have an effect. Perhaps the clinical problem is a result of a combination of effects. Measures to eliminate bisulfite from the 2-chloroprocaine solutions and to elevate the effect of varying pH have been taken by the current manufacturer. The commercially available solution of 2-chloroprocaine (Nesacaine) now uses ethylenediame tetraacetic acid (EDTA) as the antioxidant. Available evidence indicates that this substance is not neurotoxic in the concentration used.

VI. REFERENCES

1. Corning JL. Spinal anesthesia and local medication of the cord. NY Med J 42:483, 1885.
2. Sicard A. Extradural injection of medication by way of the sacrococcygeal canal. CR Soc Biol (Paris) 53:396, 1901.
3. Cathelin, F. A new route of spinal injection: A method of epidural injections by way of the sacral canal: Application to man. CR Soc Biol (Paris) 53:452, 1901.
4. Zarzur E. Anatomic studies of the human lumbar ligamentum flavum. Anesth Analg 63:499–502, 1984.
5. Blomberg R. The dorsomedian connective tissue band in the lumbar epidural space of humans: An anatomical study using epiduroscopy in autopsy cases. Anesth Analg 65:747–752, 1986.
6. Savolaine ER, Pandya JB, Greenblatt SH, Conover SR: Anatomy of the human lumbar epidural space: New insights using CT-epidurography. Anesthesiology 68:217–220, 1988.
7. Shulman M. Treatment of neck pain with cervical epidural steroid injection. Regional Anesth 11:92–94, 1986.
8. Rosenberg H, Keykhak MM. Distance to the epidural space in nonobstetric patients. Anesth Analg 63:539–540, 1984.
9. Usubiaga JE, Wikinski JA, Usubiaga LE. Epidural pressure and its relation to spread of anesthetic solutions in the epidural space. Anesth Analg 46:440–446, 1967.
10. Galbert MW, Marx GW. Extradural pressures in the parturient patient. Anesthesiology 40:499–502, 1974.
11. Shantha TR, Evans JA. The relationship of epidural anesthesia to neural membranes and archnoid villi. Anesthesiology 37:543–557, 1972.
12. Bromage PR. Epidural Analgesia. Philadelphia, WB Saunders, 1978, 927–636.
13. Bonica JJ. Continuous peridural block. Anesthesiology 17:626–630, 1956.
14. Bromage PR. Epidural Analgesia. Philadelphia, WB Saunders, 1978, p 187.
15. Yaster M, Maxwell LG. Pediatric regional anesthesia. Anesthesiology 70:324–338, 1989.
16. Moore DC, Batra MS. The components of an effective test dose prior to epidural block. Anesthesiology 55:693–696, 1981.
17. Bromage PR. Physiology and pharmacology of epidural analgesia. Anesthesiology 28:592–622, 1967.
18. Flanagan HL, Datta S, Lambert DH, Gissen AJ, et al. Effect of pregnancy on bupivacaine-induced conduction blockade in the isolated rabbit vagus nerve. Anesth Analg 66;123–126, 1987.
19. Bromage PR. Epidural Analgesia. Philadelphia, WB Saunders, 1978, 239.
20. Kepes ER, Duncalf D. Treatment of backache with spinal injections of local anesthetics, spinal and systemic steroids: A review. Pain 22:33–47, 1985.
21. Benzon HT. Epidural steroid injections for low back pain and lumbosacral radiculopathy. Pain 24:277–295, 1986.
22. Korevaar WC. Transcatheter thoracic epidural neurolysis using ethyl alcohol. Anesthesiology 69:989–992, 1988.
23. DiGiovanni AJ, Galbert MW, Wahle WM. Epidural injection of autologous blood for postlumbar puncture headache. II. Additional clinical experiences and laboratory investigation. Anesth Analg 51:226–232, 1972.
24. Abouleish E, de la Vega S, Blendinger I, Tio TO. Long-term follow-up of epidural blood patch. Anesth Analg 54:459–463, 1975.
25. Catterberg J. Local anesthetic vs. spinal fluid. Anesthesiology 46:309, 1977.
26. Berry A. Test for spinal fluid. Anaesthesia 13:100–101, 1958.
27. Ackerman WE, Juneja MM, Kaczorowski DM, Denson DD, et al. The accuracy of using thiopental or test strips to detect dural puncture during continuous epidural analgesia. Regional Anesth 13:169–173, 1988.
28. Reisner LS. Epidural test solution or spinal fluid? Anesthesiology 44:451, 1976.
29. Bromage PR. Epidural Analgesia. Philadelphia, WB Saunders, 1978, 347–442.
30. Greene NM. Physiology of Spinal Anesthesia. 3rd ed. Baltimore, Williams & Wilkins, 1981, 95–99.
31. Bonica JJ, Akamatsu TJ, Berges PU, Morikawa K, et al. Circulatory effects of peridural block. II. Effects of epinephrine. Anesthesiology 34:514–522, 1971.
32. Scott DB, Littlewood DG, Drummond GB, Buckley BF, et al. Modification of the circulatory effects of epidural block combined with general anesthesia by the addition of adrenalin to lidocaine solutions. Br J Anesth 49:917–925, 1977.
33. Rosenberg PH, Renkonen OV: Antimicrobial activity of bupivacaine and morphine. Anesthesiology 62:178–179, 1985.
34. Rao TL, El-Etr AA. Anticoagulation following placement of epidural and subarachnoid catheters: An evaluation of neurologic sequelae. Anesthesiology 55:618–620, 1981.
35. Odoom JA, Sih IL. Epidural analgesia and anticoagulant therapy. Experience with one thousand cases of continuous epidurals. Anesthesia 38:254–259, 1983.
36. Reisner LS, Hochman BN, Plumer MH. Persistent neurologic deficit and adhesive arachnoiditis following intrathecal 2-chloroprocaine injection. Anesth Analg 59:452–454, 1980.
37. Ravindran RS, Bond VK, Tasch MD, et al. Prolonged neural blockade following regional analgesia with 2-chloroprocaine. Anesth Analg 59:447–451, 1980.
38. Wang BJ, Hilman DE, Spielholz NI, Turndorf H: Chronic neurologic deficits and Nesacaine-CE: An effect of the anesthetic, 2-chloroprocaine, or the antioxidant, sodium bisulfite? Anesth Analg 63:445–447, 1984.
39. Gissen AJ, Datta S, Lambert D. The chloroprocaine controversy. II. Is chloroprocaine neurotoxic? Regional Anesth. 9:135–145, 1984.

Chapter 33

Randall M. Chesnut, MD
Lawrence F. Marshall, MD

Intracranial Pressure Monitoring and Cerebrospinal Fluid Drainage

OUTLINE

I. INTRODUCTION

Intracranial pressure (ICP) monitoring and cerebrospinal fluid (CSF) drainage play an important role in the diagnostic and therapeutic armamentarium of present neurosurgical and intensive care practice. The necessity and utility of manipulating the volume of CSF has been recognized for some time, although many of the currently used techniques are of recent development. One of the most important developments in neurosurgery is the availability of stable, biologically inert, implantable tubing for indwelling CSF shunting. This tubing is particularly useful in pediatric neurosurgery. The ability to drain or shunt CSF, both acutely and chronically, has become a commonly employed therapeutic and diagnostic maneuver. Anyone involved in anesthetic or intensive care management of neurologic patients must be familiar with CSF drainage application and instrumentation.

The monitoring of ICP is a relatively new procedure and, in many instances, is still coming into its own. Although there are still a few who believe that the efficacy of ICP monitoring is unproven, the vast majority of centers with the available technology routinely employ ICP measurement. Particularly in the setting of acute brain injury, it is now reasonably well established that intracranial hypertension is associated with a poorer prognosis and that managing ICP improves outcome. There are now legal precedents in the United States and abroad stating that failure to monitor ICP in the setting of acute brain injury may be presented as inadequate patient care in a court of law. It is therefore anticipated that the use of ICP monitoring will continue to increase and be routinely encountered by the anesthesiologist and intensivist. It is thus necessary for these specialists to become familiar with the techniques and management strategies involved.

Although ICP monitoring and CSF drainage have some theoretical and practical differences, they exhibit significant technical and conceptual overlap and will be discussed together in this chapter.

II. Indications

A. *Intracranial Pressure (ICP) Monitoring*

Indications for ICP monitoring are outlined in Table 33–1 and discussed in detail below.

Table 33–1 • Indications for Intracranial Pressure Monitoring

Trauma
Intracerebral hemorrhage
Intracerebral neoplasm
Metabolic encephalitis
Anoxic encephalitis
Selective arteriovenous malformation surgeries

1. Trauma

An often encountered situation in which ICP monitoring and CSF drainage are vitally intertwined is the treatment of the traumatized brain. As the understanding of the role of ICP in influencing the global and regional cerebral perfusion pressure has evolved, reasonably well-accepted indications for monitoring ICP have been developed. It is now recognized that over 50% of patients with severe head injuries, defined as Glasgow Coma Scale (GCS) scores of 8 or less, will have at least one episode of ICP greater than 30 mmHg during their course. Although such elevation is more common in those patients with lower GCS scores, it is frequent and ominous enough in patients with scores of 7 and 8 to generally indicate a need for monitoring the entire group of patients scoring 8 or less following resuscitation. Certainly this is the case in patients whose level of consciousness precludes the sensitive following of the clinical neurologic examination as an indicator of their progress. The inability to follow the neurologic status may be due to the trauma itself or to the need for anesthesia during an operative procedure. Although the period of monitoring may be brief in such patients, its use can provide early detection and treatment of potentially disastrous alterations in intracranial dynamics.

In addition to the above group, there are select patients with GCS scores of 9 to 12 who may also benefit from ICP monitoring. A correlation has been demonstrated between compressed or absent mesencephalic cisterns on CT scan and increased mortality (Fig. 33–1A–B).[1,2] Patients with a history of shock have an increased likelihood of increased ICP and increased morbidity and mortality.[3] Finally, in patients with significant cerebral contusions, the tendency to deteriorate due to enlargement of the contusion and the development of surrounding edema is well known. Patients presenting with such findings or history are often restless and agitated. This diminishes the ability to follow them clinically, particularly if they require sedation for management. Therefore, although their GCS scores may be greater than 8, such patients should be considered for ICP monitoring for the initial 24–48 hours. In patients who lack such mandatory indications for monitoring, we normally use the accurate but less invasive Camino Fiberoptic ICP monitoring system (Camino Laboratories, San Diego, CA) to minimize the risk of potential complications.

In contradistinction to the above group, there are patients with GCS scores of 7 or 8 who selectively may

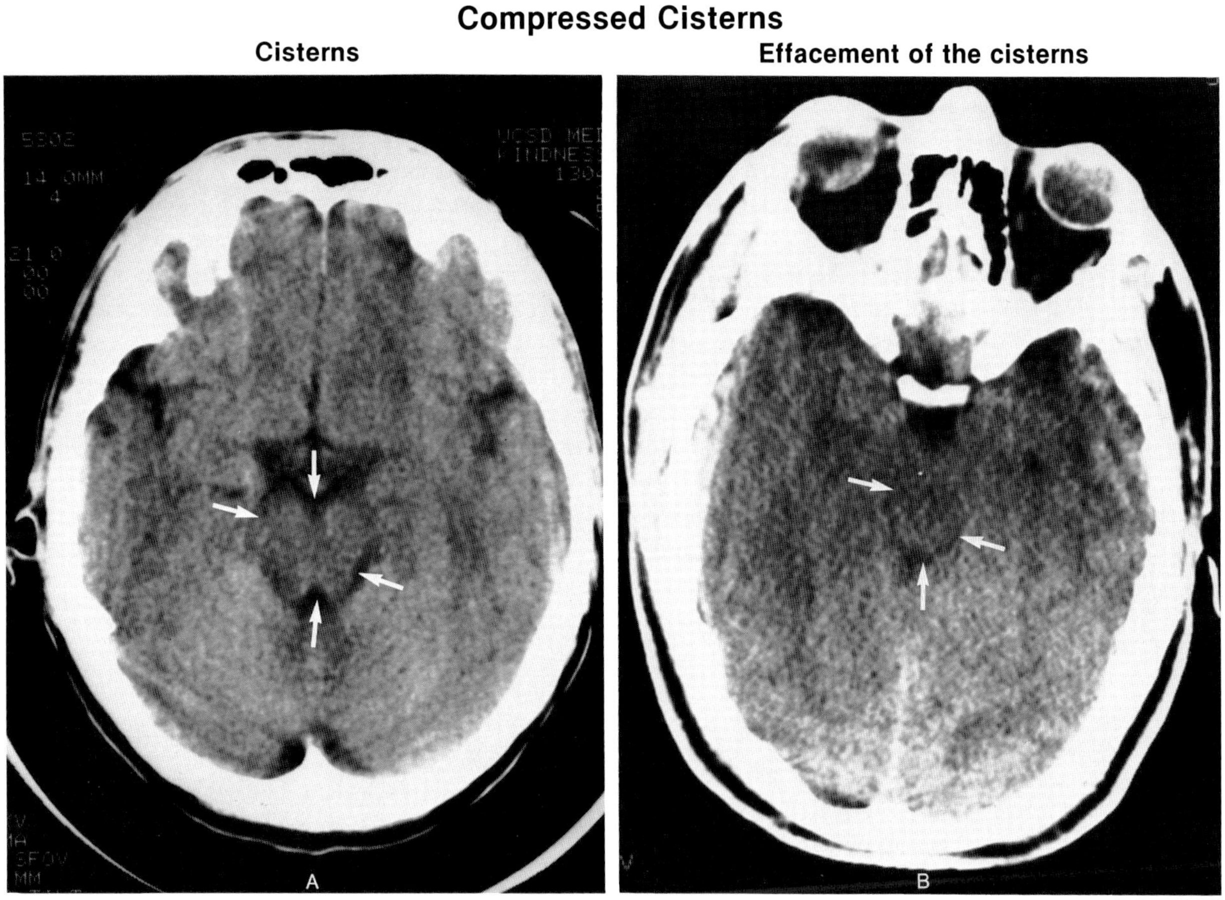

Figure 33–1 • (***A***) The cerebrospinal fluid (*CSF*) spaces surrounding the brainstem, called *cisterns,* are shown as they appear in a computed tomography (*CT*) scan of a normal brain. (***B***) A CT scan through the midbrain of a patient shortly following a severe head injury, demonstrates effacement of these cisterns. Such effacement is indicative of intracranial hypertension and predictive of transtentorial herniation.

not be monitored if high-quality, vigilant patient observation is available. These are patients whose histories are complete and reliable and exclude hypoxia and hypotension, and whose CT scans reveal no lesions, shifts, or compression of their basilar cisterns. In this carefully selected group of patients, the risk of raised ICP is less than 5%; nevertheless, they all require expectant management in a neurosurgically oriented ICU environment.

2. INTRACEREBRAL HEMORRHAGE

The neurosurgical treatment of intracerebral hemorrhage is presently in a state of flux. The location of the intracerebral hemorrhage, the age of the patient, and the underlying pathology are also important factors in determining the course of therapy. In light of these factors, there exist groups of patients (1) who are unsalvageable; (2) who are statistically not surgical candidates due to their age or the location of their lesion; (3) who require immediate surgery owing to deterioration or shift on their CT scan, with the appropriate lesion location; or (4) who are minimally impacted by the hemorrhage and therefore do not require surgery. A large number of patients, however, lie in a zone of uncertainty. In these patients, there is a significant correlation between ICP and clinical status, and ICP monitoring can be quite useful in guiding management decisions.[4] These patients often have relatively large masses with intermediate shifts of 3–6 mm and comparatively good clinical states. If their ICP remains at less than 20 mmHg, they may be managed nonoperatively in the absence of other surgical indications. Conversely, ICP elevations above 20 mmHg should immediately initiate reevaluation of the need for surgical intervention.

3. Intracranial Neoplasm

Removal of intracranial neoplasms is a procedure for which ICP monitoring has become less important. Armed with anesthetic agents and systemic pressors that minimize undesirable augmentation of cerebral blood flow, hyperventilation and muscle relaxant during intubation and the early stages of resection, and preoperative CT data, the neuroanesthesiologist has played an important role in lessening the need for ICP monitoring in these cases. At present, fewer than 10% of patients undergoing supratentorial tumor resections will develop intracranial hypertension, and these patients characteristically manifest prominent midline shift and peritumoral edema on their preoperative studies. In those patients who develop brain swelling during operation or during closure, ICP monitoring is often useful and may be initiated at closure. With modern anesthetic and neurosurgical techniques, these instances are becoming relatively infrequent.

4. Metabolic Encephalitis

The monitoring of ICP in metabolic encephalopathy remains controversial. The general consensus among neurologic surgeons is that ICP monitoring is indicated in Reye's syndrome to guide therapeutic decisions that would otherwise be based solely and much less sensitively on clinical grounds. This is particularly true in patients with a GCS score of 7 or less, or those falling into National Institutes of Health categories II to IV.[5] In other metabolic encephalopathies, such as hepatic failure or heavy metal poisoning, the role of ICP monitoring is less clear. In liver disease, it appears that elevations of ICP do occur but that the primary treatment is correction of the hepatic abnormalities themselves.

5. Anoxic Encephalitis

The role of ICP monitoring in anoxic encephalopathy as exemplified by drowning is another controversial area. Although intracranial hypertension does occur in drowning patients, it appears that it is more of an indicator of the severity of the insult and the gravity of the prognosis than a treatable component of the pathology, since attempts at lowering the ICP do not result in improved outcome.[6–9] In this light, we do not routinely monitor these patients at our institution.

6. Arteriovenous Malformations (AVM)

Small malformations that have hemorrhaged, particularly those on the cortical surface, are usually straightforward problems and should be surgically removed if the patient has survived the bleed in good condition. If there has been intraparenchymal bleeding, the indications for ICP monitoring are those for intracerebral hemorrhage. There is generally no need for ICP monitoring in simple AVM cases.

Recent major improvements in surgical technique, as well as in nonsurgical methods such as radiographically guided embolization of AVMs, have made the large lesions somewhat less formidable than before. The intraoperative and postoperative management of patients undergoing surgery for large AVMs, however, is critical. Catastrophic intraoperative as well as postoperative hemorrhages can occur. The pathophysiology of such hemorrhages lies in the redistribution of increased flow into vessels unused to such forces and that often evidence abnormalities in their wall structure. This bleeding, which Spetzler has called *perfusion pressure breakthrough bleeding*, is a major problem in surgery on deep AVMs[10]. Hemorrhage or malignant brain swelling can occur at a distance from the malformation, in an area where the vasculature is normal, indicating that tremendous shifts in brain blood flow can occur in such patients.

A number of surgical approaches have evolved to deal with this problem. Depending on the size and complexity of the AVM, surgery for removal may be done in multiple stages to distribute the flow redistribution over several surgeries. In addition, deep barbiturate anesthesia may be used. In these instances, ICP is monitored intraoperatively and postoperatively to provide early warning of possible deterioration.

The combination of a large bed or recently divided and cauterized vascular elements and the risk of perfusion pressure breakthrough bleeding makes the postoperative management of patients undergoing resection of large AVMs a potentially hazardous period. It is crucial that rapid increases in blood pressure during emergence from anesthesia be avoided. When large AVM resections are done under deep barbiturate anesthesia, the goal of a smooth awakening is aided by the slow metabolism of pentobarbital. If this is not the case, sedation must be maintained to the extent of relaxing the patient without interfering with extubation. In either instance, the patient's level of consciousness is pharmacologically depressed postoperatively, and the ICP monitor is the most sensitive method of detecting neurologic deterioration during this period.

B. *Cerebrospinal Fluid (CSF) Drainage*

Some indications for CSF drainage are outlined in Table 33-2 and discussed in detail in the following sections.

1. INTRAVENTRICULAR HEMORRHAGE

There are numerous situations in which CSF drainage is indicated in the absence of ICP monitoring. Intraventricular hemorrhage characteristically results in deficits in absorption of CSF by the arachnoid granulations with resultant communicating hydrocephalus. As this will often not spontaneously resolve, these patients will frequently require shunting. Unfortunately, the semiclotted blood in the ventricular system predisposes early shunts to obstruction; indeed, during the early course, it is not uncommon for even the interventricular communication to become obstructed, requiring bilateral ventriculostomies. We generally drain these patients externally during their early course and use the quality of the CSF, the response of the patients, and CT data to determine the need for and timing of subsequent shunting.

2. SHUNT INFECTION

The treatment of an infected ventricular or lumbar shunt requires removal of the infected hardware followed by replacement with a sterile system. Optimally, this includes an intervening period in which the patient can be maintained without a drain. Unfortunately, many patients are shunt dependent or require intraventricular antibiotics. These patients are best treated by externalizing their initial system to a drainage bag for the first several days of therapy, followed by replacement with an intermediate external drain/antibiotic port for the duration of the interval before insertion of a new, indwelling shunt system.

Table 33-2 • Indications for Cerebrospinal Fluid Drainage

Intraventricular hemorrhage
Shunt infection
Infratentorial tumors
Cerebrospinal fluid leak
Normal pressure hydrocephalus
Intraoperative brain relaxation

3. INFRATENTORIAL TUMORS

In some patients with hydrocephalus secondary to obstruction of CSF pathways by neoplastic, infectious, or parasitic tissue, the necessity of ventricular shunting depends on the outcome of therapy. This is particularly true for large infratentorial tumors. A good example is the pediatric patient with medulloblastoma. These patients, particularly those whose age precludes their complaining of symptomatic difficulties, often have significant obstructive hydrocephalus at the time of initial evaluation. Although some believe these patients should be shunted ab initio, there is up to a 19% incidence of shunt-mediated metastasis and, with careful perioperative management, two thirds of these patients may be treated without shunting.[11] In light of these statistics, many pediatric neurosurgeons do not shunt these patients directly. Instead, these patients are treated with high-dose steroids for several days preoperatively, and a supratentorial ventriculostomy is placed at surgery prior to craniotomy. This is used for brain relaxation at surgery and is maintained for 48 to 72 hours postoperatively, during which time the ICP is measured (often intermittently) and the response to ventriculostomy clamping is assessed. If the patient's ICP is high and clamping is not tolerated, the ventricular drain can be internalized to a filtered ventriculoperitoneal shunt.[12] If not, the drain is removed and the child is monitored clinically and radiographically. Similar logic applies to other neoplastic obstructive hydrocephalics as well to infectious or inflammatory disorders in which the obstruction may be relieved by satisfactory response to surgical or pharmacologic therapy.

4. CSF LEAK

Patients may present with a CSF leak following trauma, craniotomy, or spinal surgery. This leak may be external or result in a pseudomeningocele. Although many instances require primary repair, transient external CSF drainage may allow some patients to avoid surgery. In the absence of suspected craniospinal compartmentalization, this is generally best accomplished using a lumbar drain.

5. Normal Pressure Hydrocephalus

Use of a lumbar drain as a therapeutic trial in patients with suspected normal pressure hydrocephalus who are being considered for shunting has been recently suggested.[13] The clinical response to 5 days of external lumbar drainage in selected patients was found to be highly predictive of benefit from permanent shunting.

6. Brain Relaxation

A common role for CSF drainage in the operating theater is brain relaxation during craniotomy. We routinely use lumbar drainage to facilitate exposure during aneurysm surgery, thereby minimizing retraction pressures on a brain that is often hyperemic, congested, and perhaps inflamed. This drain is removed at the close of the procedure.

C. Contraindications

Absolute contraindications to ICP monitoring or CSF drainage are few. Certainly, the placement of a monitor in a patient whose prognosis is hopeless or in whom no therapy is planned is perfidy. As with any invasive monitoring system or life-support device, the appropriateness of the application must be addressed for each individual case prior to the initiation of therapy and never post facto.

The placement of an intraventricular catheter in a patient with thrombocytopenia (platelet count less than 100,000/mm^3) or significant dysfunction of the coagulation cascade (prothombin time [PT] or partial thromboplastin time [PTT] greater than twice normal) is attended by a high risk of hemorrhage. This is often the situation in the head-injured patient owing to the release of tissue thromboplastin from damaged brain parenchyma. In such cases, ventricular catheterization should be delayed until the coagulation defects can be corrected. This may require interval use of a less invasive monitor, which, although not allowing therapeutic CSF drainage, will place the patient at less risk for a hemorrhagic complication.

Another relative contraindication to ICP monitoring or CSF drainage is immunosuppression. Patients whose immunologic status is impaired by disease (eg, AIDS, leukemia) or iatrogenically (eg, steroids or cytotoxic agents) have a substantially increased risk for infection. Given the potentially disastrous consequences of intracranial infection in these patients, particularly because they may be polymicrobial or involve odd and difficult-to-treat agents, these patients should be managed on the basis of clinical and radiologic data if possible.

The placement of a lumbar catheter in any situation in which there may be embarrassment of the normal communication between or within the supratentorial, infratentorial, or spinal compartments is also contraindicated because there is a risk of herniation due to the induction of pressure gradients.

III. How to Do ICP Monitoring and CSF Drainage

Under normal circumstances, ventricular puncture is facilitated by the principle that the external surface of the lateral ventricular system lies parallel to the skull. This allows ventricular puncture to be accomplished from virtually any point on the skull above the external markers of the tentorium, as long as the needle track is perpendicular to the skull. Based on this principle, numerous sites have been used for diagnostic and therapeutic ventricular cannulation (Fig. 33–2A–F.)[14–18] Despite this plethora of possibilities, we believe it is best to limit the puncture site armamentarium to gain familiarity and facility by repeated use of one or two techniques. Because ventriculostomy is a blind procedure not infrequently performed on injured brains with small and shifted ventricles, a well-worn routine is highly valuable. We employ the frontal, parasagittal approach almost exclusively because it gives us good access to the frontal horn of the lateral ventricular system (even if it is shifted toward the midline), while minimizing the chance of involving eloquent cerebral tissue in the passage of the catheter. In addition, this location facilitates nursing access to the system and places it in a location where it is less likely to be damaged during patient turning or transfer. Such considerations are particularly important when using the Camino catheter system or the Richmond bolt, which project some distance from the head and are sensitive to being broken or dislodged from their purchase in the skull.

We take a similarly parsimonious view with respect to ICP monitoring devices. There are presently a large number of devices available and several in develop-

Approaches for Ventricular Puncture

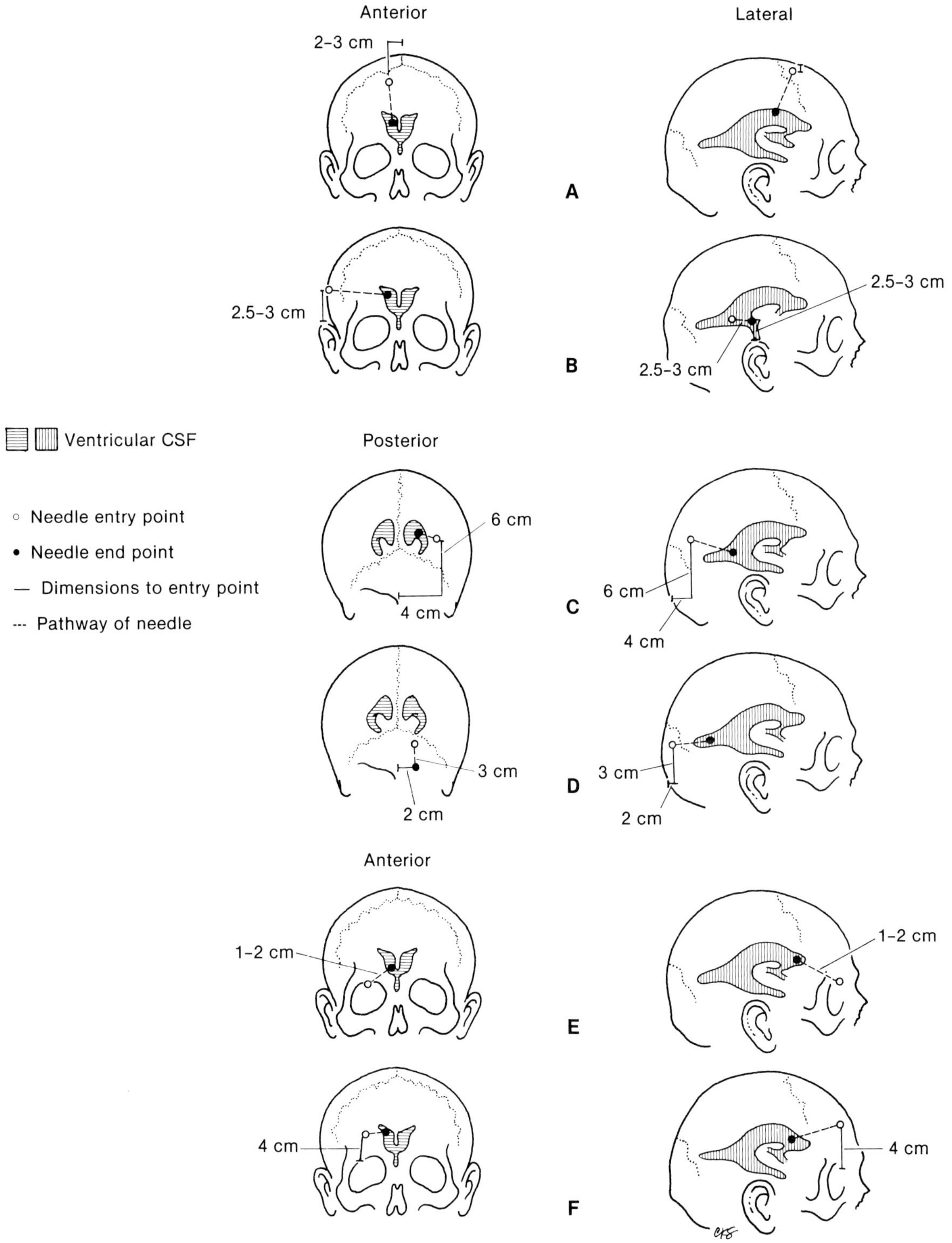

Figure 33–2 • Six approaches for accessing the cerebral ventricles through trephines in the skull are shown in this figure. The ventricles are represented by the shaded areas, and the path of the ventricular cannula is shown as a dashed line. (***A***) Kocher's point; 2–3 cm from the midline, just anterior to the coronal suture. (***B***) Keen's point; 2.5–3 cm posterior and superior to the top of the ear. (***C***) Occipital parietal; 4 cm from the midline and 6 cm above the inion (external occipital protuberance). (***D***) Dandy's point; 2 cm from the midline and 3 cm above the inion. (***E***) Orbital; 1–2 cm behind the orbital rim. (***F***) Supraorbital; 4 cm above the orbital rim in the plane of the pupil. CSF = cerebrospinal fluid.

ment. Rather than attempting to cover this myriad of technology, we have chosen three ICP monitoring systems to present in some detail. The *Richmond bolt* is a simple, widely available, and popular subarachnoid system. The *ventriculostomy*, the present gold standard, is simple, and although the most invasive of the three systems, it is the only device that allows therapeutic withdrawal of CSF or measurement of the intracranial pressure-volume index. The *Camino Fiberoptic* ICP monitoring system, albeit somewhat fragile and requiring a dedicated transducer, is only slightly more invasive than the Richmond bolt and is the only system presently widely available that actually monitors parenchymal pressures directly.

We have not included an epidural pressure monitoring system here. It has been argued that this technique minimizes infectious complications by not violating the dura mater, thereby remaining separate from the CSF compartment. Unfortunately, this leaves a very noncompliant, relatively thick membrane interposed between the monitor and the region of interest; this membrane has been shown to produce considerable artifact in some systems.[19–22] Such considerations have led us to abandon epidural monitoring at present.

Due to its utility as a drainage procedure, placement and use of the lumbar catheter are also described.

A. *Trephination and Durotomy*

The initial steps of ICP monitor placement are common to all three techniques. The midline is located by inspection and the coronal suture by palpation. For ventricular cannulation or insertion of a Camino fiberoptic catheter, the placement is generally on the right side to avoid the usually dominant left hemisphere (unless left-sided placement is indicated by the specific pathology). With the Richmond bolt, however, it is necessary to place the monitor ipsilateral to the major injury to avoid measurement error.[23] The puncture site is located 3 cm lateral to the midline (sagittal sinus) and over (or 1–2 cm anterior to) the coronal suture (see Fig. 33–2A). This area is shaved and sterilely prepped, and the skin is anesthetized with 1% lidocaine with 1:100,000 epinephrine. A No. 15 scalpel blade is used to make a small (1-cm or less) incision parallel with the midline and carried down through the pericranium.

A twist drill is then used to trephine the skull. The bit chosen should be chucked so as to project only the thickness of the skin plus 1 cm to avoid plunging upon penetrating the inner table of the skull. The bit size is $^{11}/_{64}$ for the ventriculostomy, $^{1}/_{4}$ for the Richmond bolt, and $^{7}/_{64}$ for the Camino fiberoptic ICP monitoring system. It is important to maintain a perpendicular drilling axis and to avoid "walking" the bit on the skull when starting to drill. This will misalign the incision and the hole and make passing the catheter more difficult. It is also important to feel the bit catch as it bites into the inner table of the skull; this signifies that the bit is beginning to thread into the new opening and will plunge into the brain if drilling pressure is not slackened. At this point, carefully rotating the bit an additional 360° will usually finish the trephination without damaging the dura. Copiously irrigating the wound at this point will remove any bone debris and prevent it from being introduced into the brain during subsequent steps.

The size of the durotomy is important. For the ventriculostomy, it must allow the catheter passage without providing egress for CSF, which could then reach and potentially permeate the incision line and lead to meningitis. We use a No. 11 blade and make a cruciate durotomy just large enough to pass the catheter without causing it to hang up on the dura.

In contrast, for the Richmond bolt, it is important that the dura not underlie the inner orifice of the lumen because this increases the likelihood of obstruction. Furthermore, the arachnoid membrane should not be penetrated during the durotomy because this may allow the underlying brain to herniate into the lumen and occlude it.[24] We therefore use a No. 11 blade to carefully perform a cruciate durotomy that encompasses the entire area of the trephination. Adequate lighting is required during this process to avoid incising the underlying arachnoid.

The durotomy used in placing the Camino fiberoptic ICP monitoring system is described later.

B. *Ventriculostomy*

A graphic overview of ventriculostomy placement is presented in Fig. 33–3A–F. Once the durotomy has been made, the stylet is inserted fully into the catheter. The catheter is passed into the lateral ventricle, using the inner canthus of the ipsilateral eye as a guide and remaining perpendicular to the skull. A slight pop will be felt as the ependyma of the ventricle is violated, and CSF

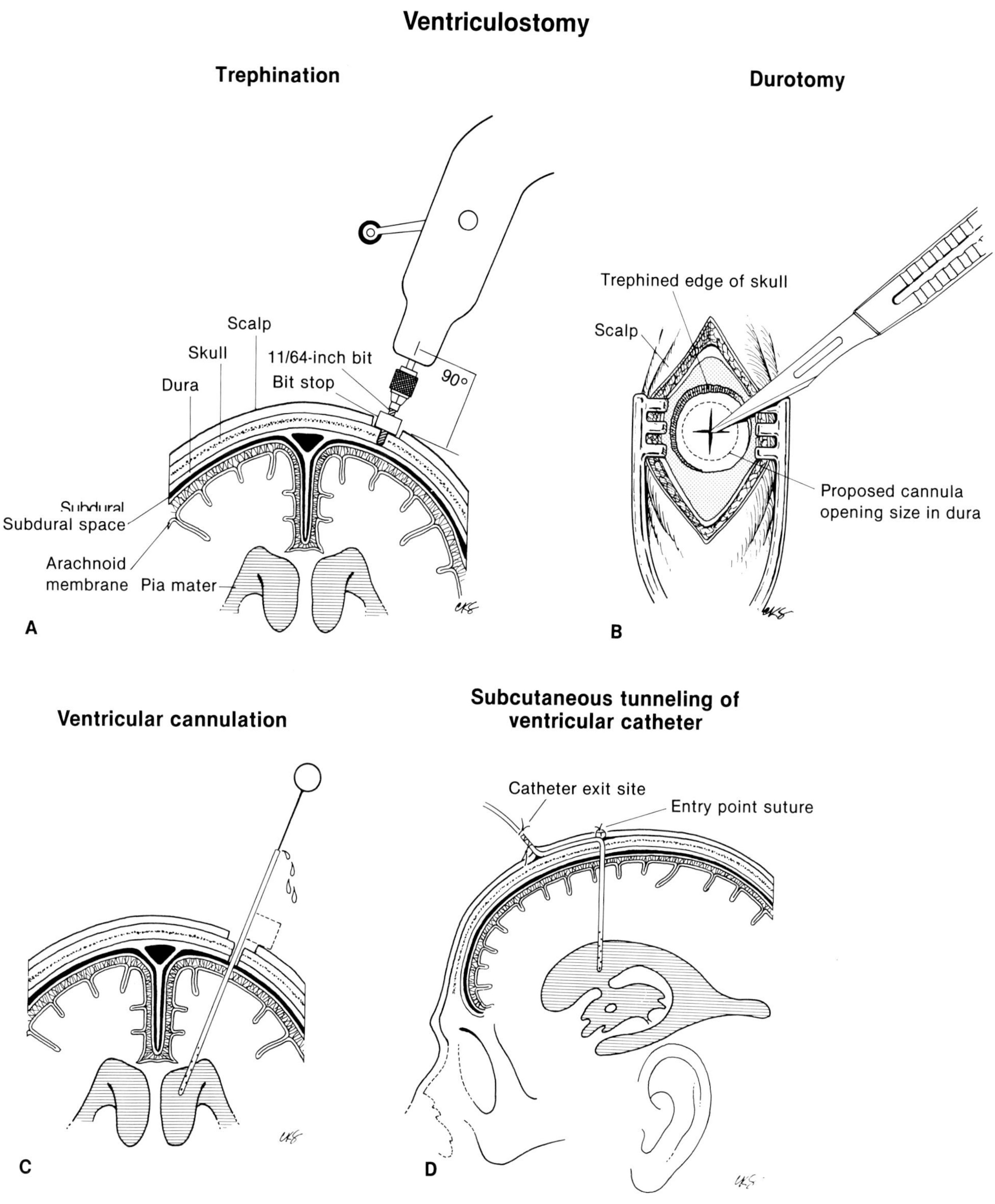

Figure 33–3 • Ventriculostomy. (***A***) Trephination. Trephination is accomplished with an 11/64-inch bit, care being taken not to lacerate the dura or plunge into the brain. Following trephination, the wound is thoroughly irrigated to remove all debris. (***B***) Durotomy. A cruciate durotomy is performed using a No. 11 blade. The size of the durotomy is limited so that the catheter will just pass through the opening, thereby avoiding a CSF leak. Care is taken to avoid lacerating the underlying brain. (***C***) Ventricular cannulation. The ventricle is cannulated at no more than 5 cm from the dura, keeping the catheter at a right angle to the skull. (***D***) Tunnelling the catheter. The ventricular catheter is tunnelled subcutaneously (external to the galea aponeurotica) and brought out through a separate wound. It is well secured at its point of exit.

(continued)

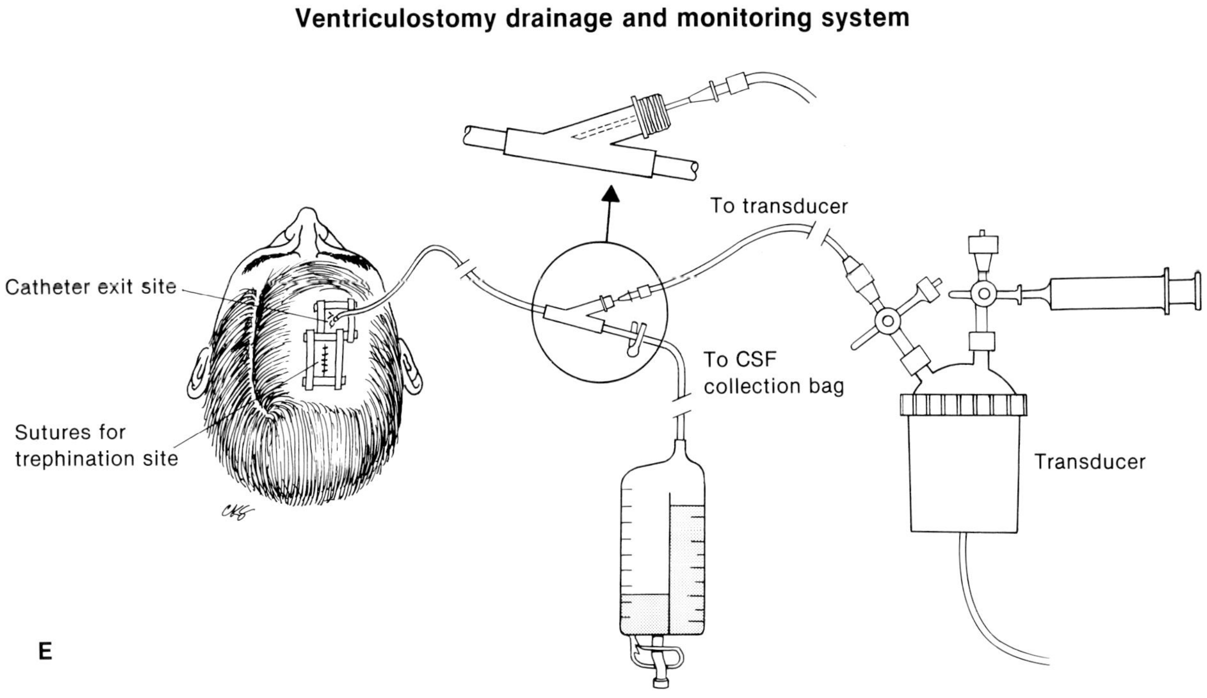

Figure 33–3 *(continued)*
(***E***) Ventriculostomy drainage and monitoring system. See text for details.

will then flow into the catheter tubing. If this has not occurred by the time that the catheter has passed 6 cm beyond the dura, the catheter must not be passed further but rather withdrawn and another attempt made. Slight variation in angulation of the catheter toward or away from the midline may compensate for shift if a current CT scan is available. If the ventricle is not cannulated by the third attempt, another technique should be used to monitor ICP because the risk of a complication increases with each passage.[25] Based on our large clinical experience, if the ventricle is not entered by the third pass, it is unlikely that one will succeed with further attempts.

Once the ventricle is cannulated, the stylet should be removed and the ICP approximated before any CSF drains from the tubing. This can be done by holding the catheter tubing up and measuring the pressure-head manometrically by varying the catheter height. This serves to insure that the system is functional and allows immediate initiation of treatment if indicated. When this has been done, the catheter should be passed subcutaneously (superficial to the galea aponeurotica) and brought out through a separate stab wound a minimum of 5 cm from the trephine. It may then be securely attached to the closed drainage bag and connected to the transducer. The system should be quickly zeroed and the pressure and waveform confirmed before closure of the wounds. If all is satisfactory, the catheter must be securely attached to the scalp at the point of exit to avoid dislodgement by inadvertent traction. The primary incision should be closed in one layer with nylon suture securely enough to prevent egress of CSF from the wound. The wounds should then be dressed in a sterile, occlusive fashion.

The method of connection to the transducer is worthy of comment. Because this is a fluid-coupled system, the goal is a stable, continuous fluid column that will not introduce infection or air into the system and will not result in disaster if inadvertently uncoupled. We have met these demands by incorporating a Silastic injection port into the tubing running from the ventriculostomy catheter to the drainage bag. We then attach a 23 gauge needle to the end of the fluid-filled tubing leading to the transducer and couple it to the ventricular fluid column by passing the needle through the Silastic injection port (see Fig. 33–3). The junction is securely taped together to minimize the risk of disconnection. This method provides a stable coupling but, due to the presence of the Silastic injection seal, will not open the system to contamination in the instance of a disconnection.

C. *Richmond Bolt*

The components of the Richmond bolt ICP monitoring system are shown in Fig. 33–4. A graphic overview of Richmond bolt placement is presented in Fig. 33–5. After the durotomy has been made, the distance from the outer table of the skull and the underlying arachnoid–brain surface should be approximated. Using the special driver (see Fig. 33–4), the bolt should then be threaded into the skull at a right angle and advanced to the previously approximated depth so that it projects 1 mm or so below the inner table of the skull and is juxtaposed to the arachnoid covering the brain surface. If it is not seated deeply enough, there is increased likelihood of loss of pressure or dislodgement. If it is seated too deeply, it will damage the brain surface and brain may herniate into the lumen, plugging the system. This is more likely with high ICP and, under this condition, may occur even with placement at the proper depth if the arachnoid membrane was inadvertently violated during durotomy.

Once properly placed, the lumen should be carefully flushed with sterile saline (without preservative) introduced using a blunt 22 gauge needle. The system should then be coupled to the previously zeroed transducer, and the ICP and waveform confirmed. The incision should be securely closed in a single layer with nylon suture, taking care that there are no gaps where the bolt exits the skin. This can be facilitated if the trephine is placed at one end of the incision so that the wound only needs to be closed on one side of the bolt. The wound is then dressed in a sterile, occlusive fashion.

A significant drawback of the Richmond bolt is its tendency to become occluded by wound debris, the dura, or blood. Wound debris can be removed by scrupulous irrigation of the trephine prior to durotomy to remove bone particles. The risk of occlusion by dura is minimized by an adequate durotomy. Occlusion by blood is lessened by careful hemostasis but may recur and may require irrigation of the bolt.

Richmond Bolt

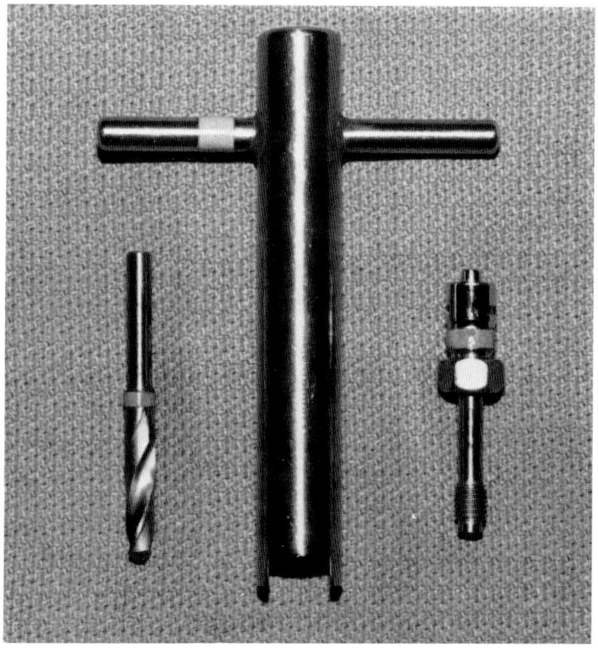

Figure 33–4 • The Richmond bolt is shown on the right. The special driver used to thread the bolt into a trephination in the skull is in the center, and the 1/4-inch bit used for trephination is on the left. Figure 33–5 (*C*) illustrates the use of the driver in inserting the bolt.

D. *Camino Fiberoptic ICP Monitoring System*

The components of the Camino fiberoptic ICP monitoring system are shown in Fig. 33–6. A graphic overview of its placement is presented in Fig. 33–7. Owing to the small size of the Camino barrel, the incision size may be limited to 4–5 mm. A $\frac{7}{64}$ bit is supplied with the catheter and used to trephine the skull. Care should be taken to avoid plunging, since the small bit does not catch on the inner table of the skull. For this reason, a stop is provided on the bit and should be adjusted to serve as a backup safety device. Following the trephination, the barrel is threaded into the skull until it comes up against the plastic stop (which leaves it projecting approximately 1–2 mm below the inner table). A 20 gauge needle is then passed through the lumen until the dura is penetrated. This needle is withdrawn, and the blunt trochar supplied with the catheter is passed into the brain until it stops (set at 15 mm), thereby forming the cavity for the fiberoptic sensor. At this point, the fiberoptic bundle preamplifier is attached to the transducer, and the system is zeroed to atmospheric pressure by turning the biasing screw on the preamplifier. The fiberoptic catheter is then passed through the lumen of the barrel into the brain until the 5-cm mark is the top

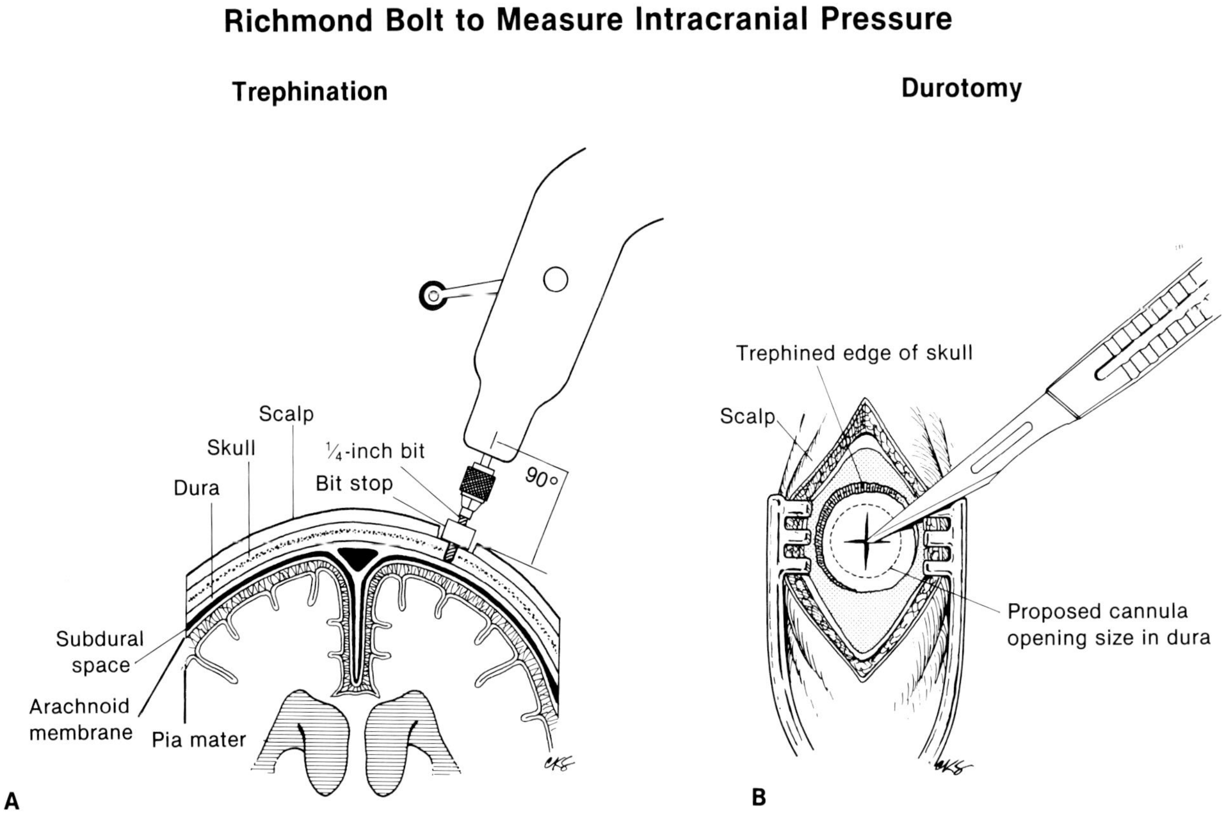

Figure 33–5 • Richmond bolt. (***A***) Trephination. Trephination is accomplished with a 1/4-inch bit, care being taken not to lacerate the dura or plunge into the brain. Following trephination, the wound is thoroughly irrigated to remove all debris. (***B***) Durotomy. A cruciate durotomy is performed using a No. 11 blade. The two arms of the durotomy completely cross the orifice in the skull so that the resulting opening in the dura is of maximal size. Care is taken to leave the underlying arachnoid membrane intact.

(continued)

of the barrel. At this point, the catheter projects 13–14 mm beyond the tip of the barrel, leaving 1–2 mm between the tip and the end of the cavity in the parenchyma. (If this gap does not exist, the system will generally display a factitiously elevated ICP reading.) The ICP and waveform are confirmed on the monitor and, if satisfactory, the knurled lock nut is gently tightened to secure the catheter in place. A stitch is then placed into the wound, if required, and the dressing applied.

E. Lumbar Drain

The essentials of insertion of a lumbar intrathecal catheter are addressed elsewhere in this volume, and the reader is referred to the chapter on spinal puncture/anesthesia for details. A graphic representation of a lumbar drainage system in situ and the method of determining the drainage pressure is presented in Fig. 33–8. For drainage, we use a Spetzler lumbar catheter that has been cut off at an angle at the intrathecal end. Briefly, the area of the L-3 to L-4 interspace is prepped and draped, and a 14 gauge Tuohy needle is introduced into the subarachnoid space, care being taken to avoid excessive loss of CSF. The bevel is then directed cephalad, and the catheter is introduced through the needle. It is important that this be done gently and slowly to avoid hanging the catheter up in the axillae of the exiting nerve roots. If the catheter will not advance, it is sometimes helpful to twist it gently to alter the position of the catheter tip. If it cannot be advanced, the catheter must not be withdrawn through the needle because this risks amputating the tip and stranding it in the lumbar intrathecal space. Instead, the needle and catheter must be withdrawn together and separated only after the needle has exited the skin.

When successful passage has been accomplished, the catheter should be advanced so that 10–15 cm lie within the subarachnoid space. The Tuohy needle should be carefully withdrawn over the other end of the catheter. The catheter is then attached to the drainage bag (a platelet transfer pack or bile bag may be used) and

Bolt insertion **Filling the lumen of the bolt**

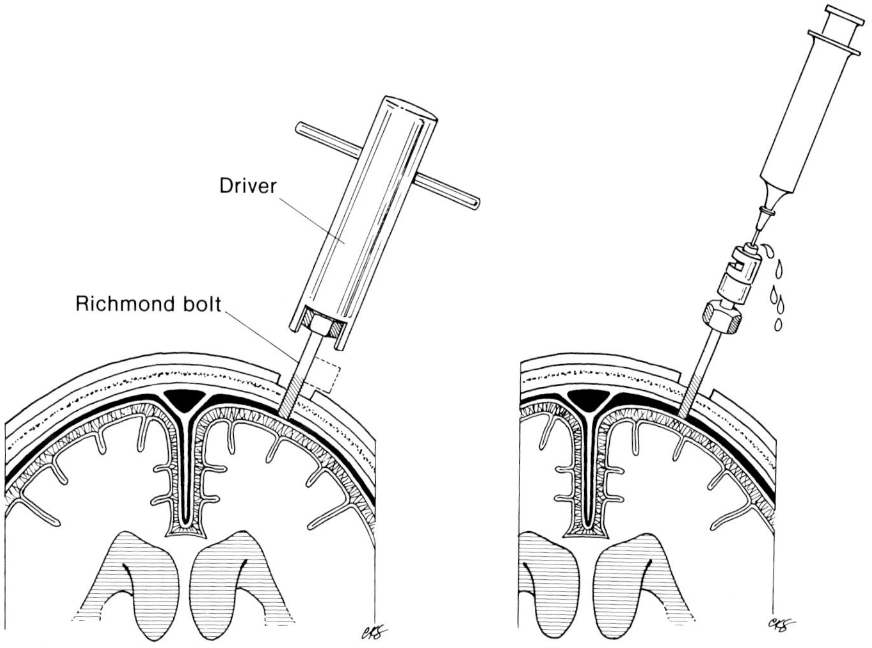

C D

Richmond bolt

Richmond bolt monitoring system

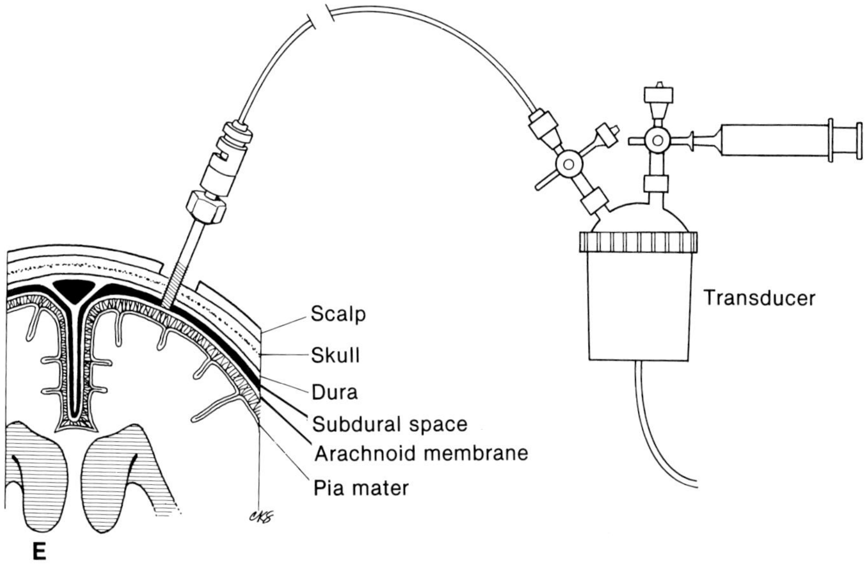

E

Figure 33–5 *(continued)*
(***C***) Bolt insertion. Using the special driver, the bolt is screwed into the skull at a right angle so that the tip projects 1–2 mm below the inner table. (***D***) Filling the lumen of the bolt. The lumen of the bolt is gently filled with nonbacteriostatic normal saline solution so that no air bubbles remain. (***E***) Richmond bolt monitoring system. See text for details.

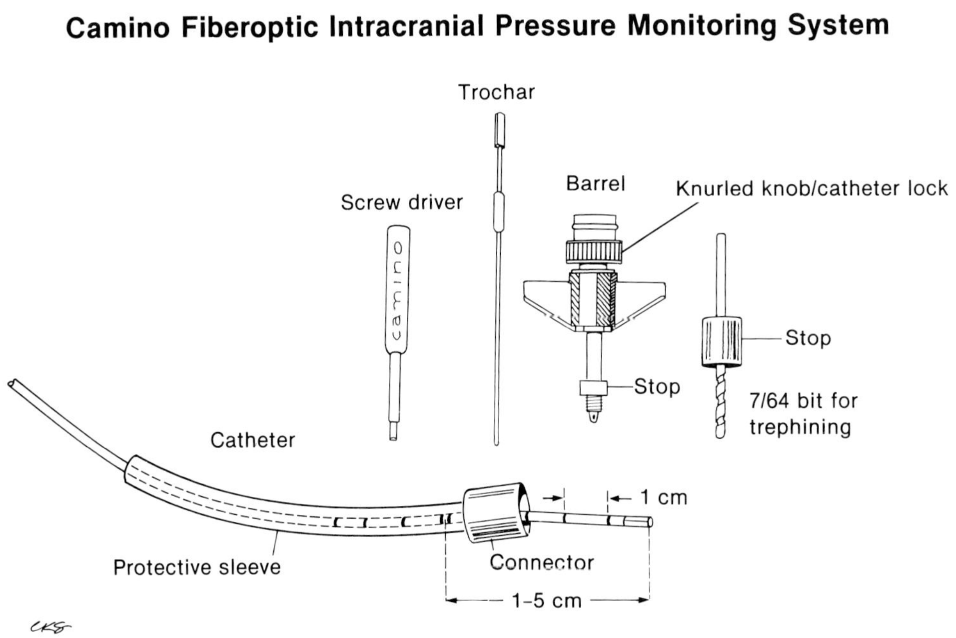

Figure 33–6 • The components of the Camino Intracranial Pressure (ICP) monitoring system. The barrel is second from the right. The lower end is threaded into the trephine until limited by the white plastic stop. The top of the barrel comprises the knurled knob (which locks the catheter in place) and the male aspect of the joint between the catheter sleeve and the barrel (which closes the system). To the left of the barrel is the trochar, which is used to form the cavity in the brain into which the catheter is inserted. On the far left is the small screwdriver supplied to set the transducer to zero. On the far right is the 7/64-inch bit for trephining the skull with the attached stop to prevent plunging. Below are the catheter itself and its protective sleeve, which connects to the barrel by sliding the white connector over the top of the barrel. The catheter is marked in 1-cm intervals. The use of the various components of this system is illustrated in Fig. 33–7.

the dressing applied. It is important that the dressing be sufficiently thick where the catheter exits the skin to prevent kinking at this point when the patient is supine. It is also important to secure the catheter to prevent accidental dislodgement.

If the drainage system is being used intraoperatively for brain relaxation, the drainage bag and flow control is brought out under the patient and arranged at the convenience of the anesthesiologist. It will be opened after the craniotomy has been accomplished, usually during the durotomy. If the drainage is used at the patient's bedside, the tubing is arranged so that the drip point of the siphon system (*not* the highest point of the siphon tubing) is the required distance above the thecal sac so that the drainage pressure head is determined and overdrainage prevented (see Fig. 33–8). If the patient is ambulatory, the patient or nurse must clamp the drain before arising and change the height of the bed or raise the patient's head, ensuring that the correct pressure dynamics are restored before the drain is reopened.

When the catheter has served its purpose, the patient should return to the lateral decubitus position and reassume the fetal position to minimize resistance to catheter removal. The tubing should be pulled out slowly and steadily, and the intact nature of the catheter should be confirmed on removal. The exit site should be dressed and the patient maintained in a flat for several hours to minimize the potential for further CSF leakage through the dural rent.

F. Drain Care

In view of the potential for infection or patient injury involved in ICP monitoring (discussed in Section V), several aspects are worthy of mention. Because it is important to maintain a sterile, closed system, we do not routinely change the collection bag unless it becomes

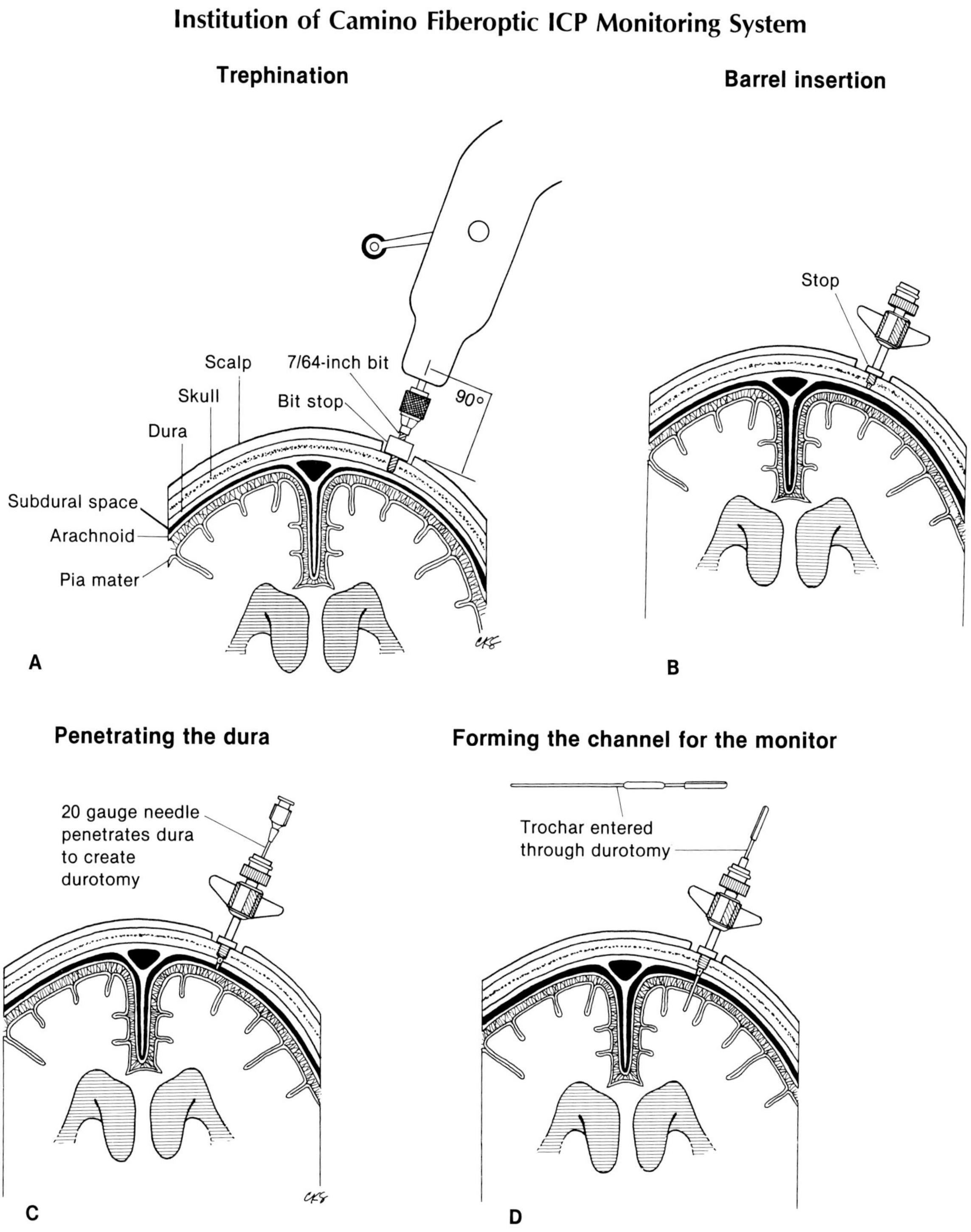

Figure 33–7 • Institution of the Camino fiberoptic ICP monitoring system. (***A***) Trephination. Trephination is accomplished with a 7/64-inch bit, with care not to lacerate the dura or plunge into the brain. Following trephination, the wound is thoroughly irrigated to remove all debris. (***B***) Barrel insertion. The barrel is screwed into the skull until it comes up on the stop mounted on the device to control the depth of insertion. (***C***) Penetrating the dura. The dura is penetrated with a 20 gauge needle passed only deep enough to create a small durotomy. (***D***) Forming the channel for the monitor. The trochar is passed through the barrel and the durotomy as far as possible, being limited by the design of the trochar. This forms a cavity for the monitor, which extends 15 mm beyond the tip of the barrel. The trochar is illustrated on the right.

(continued)

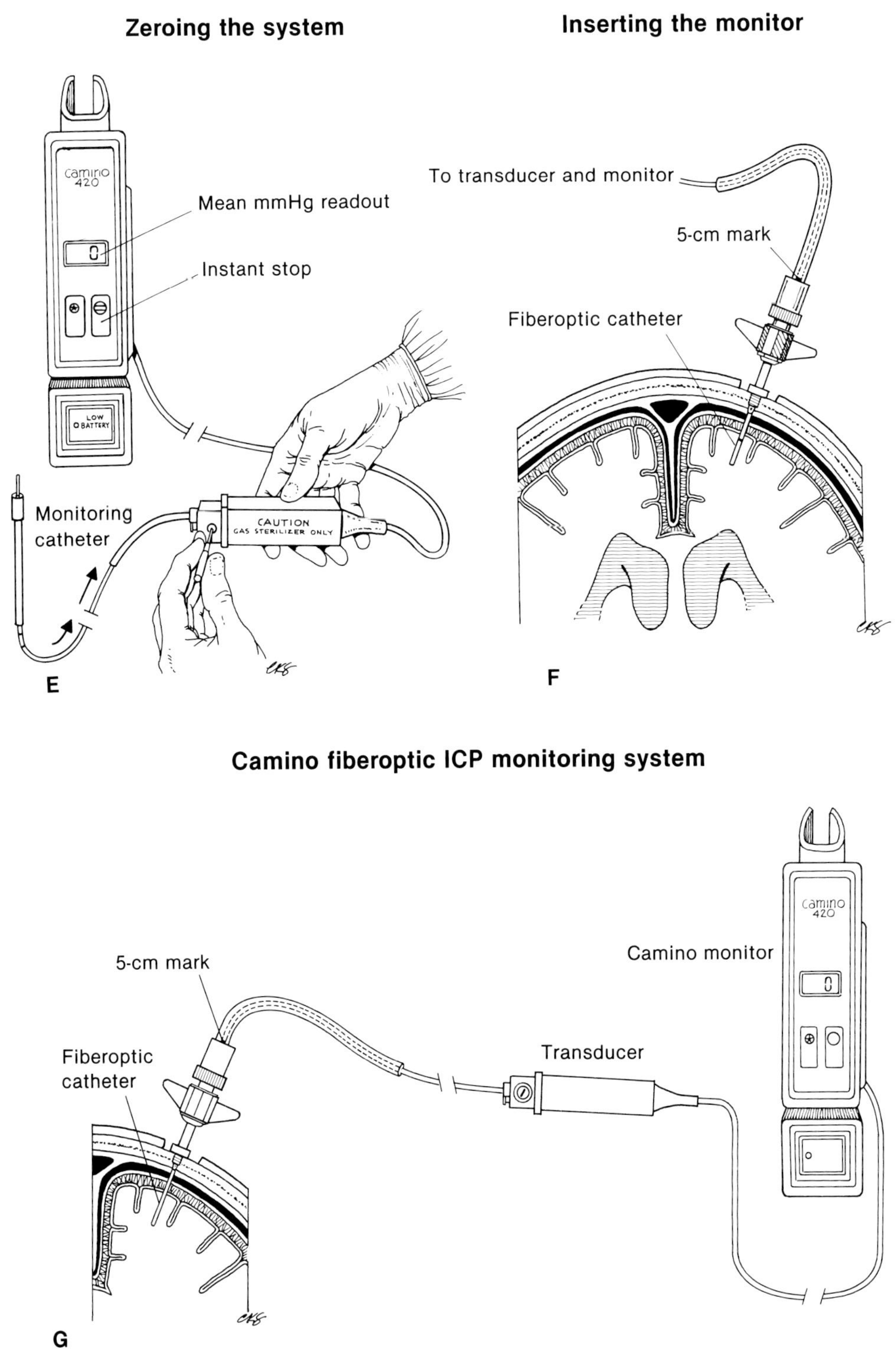

Figure 33–7 *(continued)*
(***E***) Zeroing the system. Prior to insertion of the monitor, the system is connected to the transducer and the small slotted knob is adjusted with the supplied screwdriver until the system is set to zero. (***F***) Inserting the monitor. Once at zero, the monitor is passed through the barrel until the 5-cm mark is at the top. At this point, the catheter tip will project 13 mm beyond the tip of the barrel and will *not* touch the tip of the tissue cavity. The knurled knob is gently tightened to secure the fiberoptic catheter in place, and the collar is slid down over the top of the barrel, sealing the system. (**G**) Camino fiberoptic ICP monitoring system. See text for details.

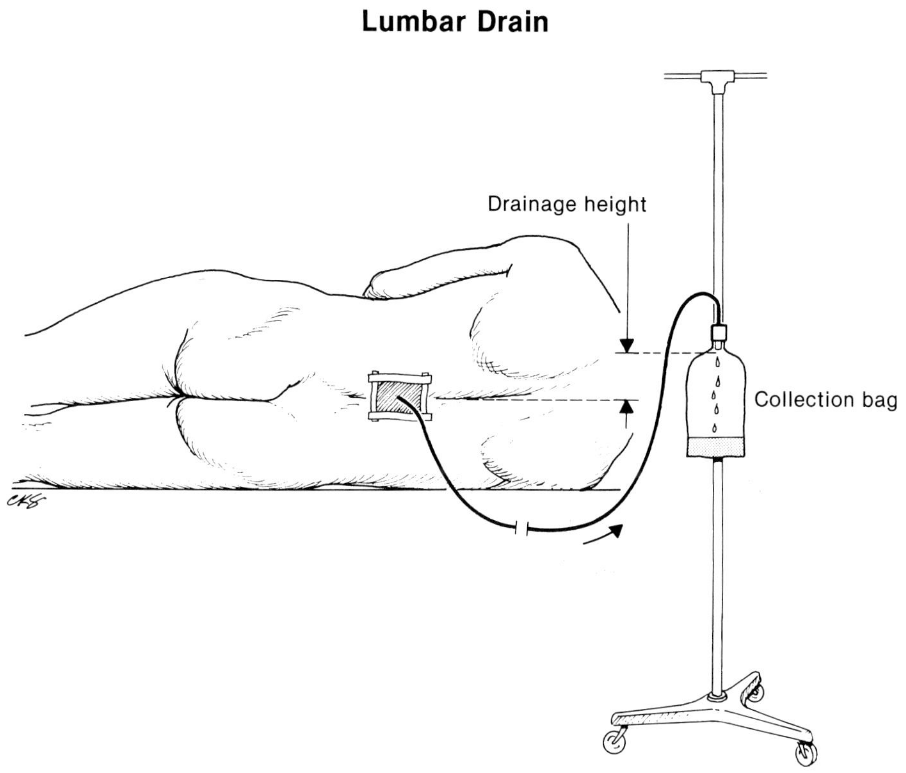

Figure 33–8 • Diagram of the lumbar drainage system in situ. The drainage pressure is determined by the distance between the spinal axis of the patient and the "drip point" of the drainage system (*not* the top of the draining tubing).

disconnected or contaminated. It is emptied under sterile conditions via the Silastic aspiration port only when it becomes full. For similar reasons, open manometers are never used to measure ICP.

All wounds or catheter exit sites are cleansed, swabbed with povidone-iodine (Betadine) ointment, and redressed in an occlusive fashion every 24 hours. Any irregularity in the appearance of any site is reported to the physician and must be readily evaluated.

Finally, no fluid reservoirs (such as used for purging the monitoring system of air) are hung above the level of the transducer if they are attached in any way to the system. This prevents inadvertent instillation of fluid volume into the intracranial space.

IV. DISCUSSION OF ICP MONITORING AND CSF DRAINAGE

A. *Background*

The roots of ICP monitoring are found in the Monro-Kellie doctrine, which holds that, due to the inelastic nature of the coverings of the CNS, small changes in the contents of this space will result in large changes in ICP.[26,27] Elaborating on this principle, Burrows concluded that the volume of blood in the brain does change under various conditions and that reciprocal changes in the remaining two intracerebral components, brain and CSF, must occur as a result.[28]

In the early 1900s, Quincke, Queckenstedt, Ayala, and Ayer, using the technique of lumbar puncture, outlined the basic clinical physiology of ICP and rooted the tenets of Monro, Kellie, and Burrows in clinical data.[29–33] The applicability of ICP monitoring to head injury was suggested in the 1930s by Browder and Meyers, who, using lumbar puncture and being naive of the gravity of potential craniospinal compartmentalization, stated that variations in ICP were not accurately correlated with or predicted by variations in the clinical state of the patient and were best monitored directly.[34,35]

Although ventricular puncture was sporadically described during the late nineteenth and early twentieth centuries,[36–38] it remained for the seminal reports of Guillaume and Janny[39] and Lundberg[40] to establish the feasibility and utility of continuous ICP monitoring in humans for diagnosing and treating a variety of intracranial disorders. Guillaume and Janny demonstrated that head-injured patients could benefit from direct monitoring of ICP, and they also confirmed the assertion of Browder and Meyers that clinical neurologic examination is an unreliable indicator of ICP.[39]

Lundberg, in his classic 1960 monograph, reported the results of direct ICP monitoring by means of ventriculostomy in 143 patients.[40] In this report, he outlined the pathophysiology and clinical significance of the three basic ICP waveforms: A (plateau) waves, B waves, and C waves. The *A waves,* also called *plateau waves*, are characterized by a steep ICP ramp in which the pressure may rise to 50–80 mmHg and remain there for 2–15 minutes (Fig. 33–9). Thereafter, there is an abrupt fall back toward the initial pressure but the new baseline is reset at a slightly higher level. These A waves repeat with increasing frequency, duration, and amplitude, resetting at a new and higher baseline with each wave. Lundberg recognized that these waves heralded impending uncontrollable ICP and believed that they indicated that the intracranial dynamics had reached a point in the pressure-volume relationship where further small increases in intracranial volume would raise the ICP asymptotically.

Lundberg's *B waves* are ICP pressure pulses of 10–20 mmHg and generally occur at ½ to 2 waves per minute (Fig. 33–10.) They are ICP reflections of respiration and are pathologic in that they are more frequently seen with increased ICP and decreased intracranial compliance. However, they are inconsistent in this relationship and are a more qualitative than quantitative indicator of intracranial dynamics. Lundberg's *C waves* reflect arterial Traube-Hering waves and, similar to B waves, are suggestive but not pathognomonic of increased ICP (Fig. 33–11).

Since the feasibility and utility of ICP monitoring was established by these pioneers, its role has burgeoned, particularly in the field of head injury. Clinical studies over the past decade have established a firm correlation between ICP and outcome, and most neurosurgeons involved in the treatment of trauma have advocated aggressive therapy of increased ICP.[25,41–43] Although protocols and techniques vary from center to

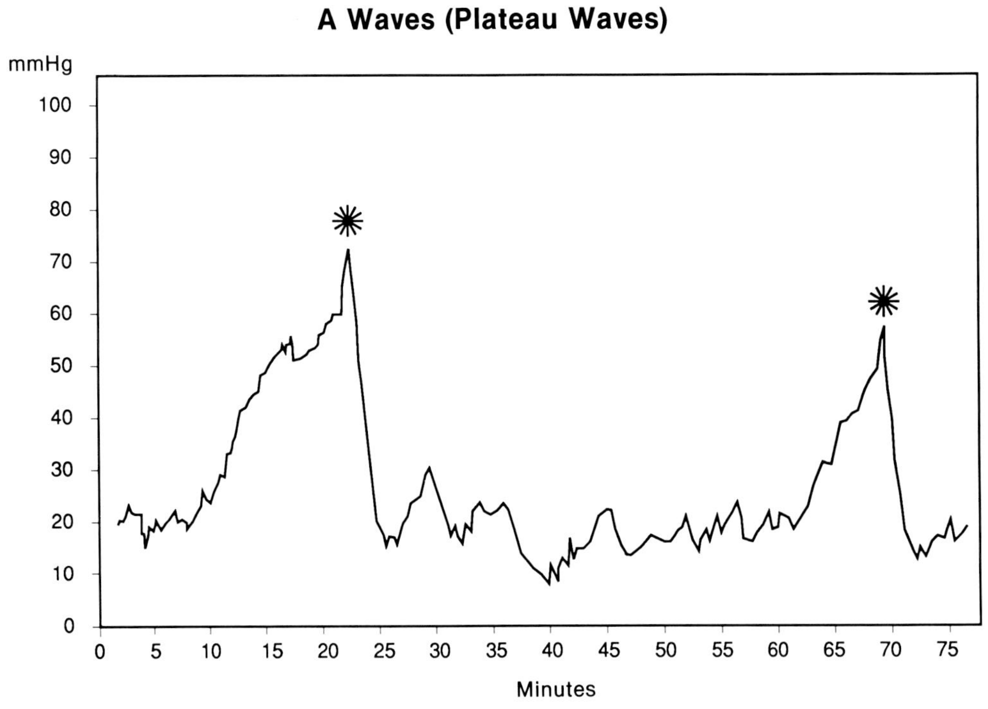

Figure 33–9 • Lundberg's A or plateau waves are ICP waveforms characterized by a steep ramp to pressures of up to 50–80 mmHg and a duration of 2 to 15 minutes. There is then an abrupt fall to a new baseline slightly higher than the initial pressure. The ICP waveforms tend to recur at increasing frequencies, durations, and amplitudes with progressively higher baselines. A waves reflect extreme compromise of intracranial compliance and are incontrovertible harbingers of uncontrollable ICP.

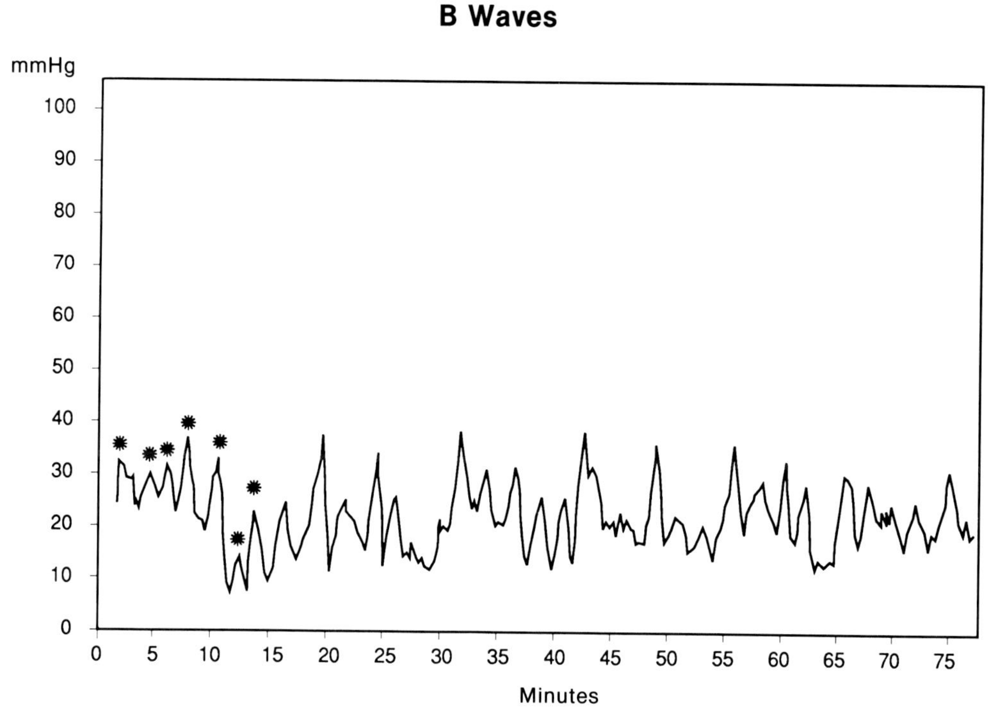

Figure 33–10 • Lundberg's B waves are pressure pulses of 10–20 mmHg that occur at 1/2 to 2 waves per minute. They reflect respiration. B waves illustrated in this figure are highlighted with asterisks. They usually occur in the setting of increased ICP and generally indicate decreased intracranial compliance, although in a less consistent manner than A waves.

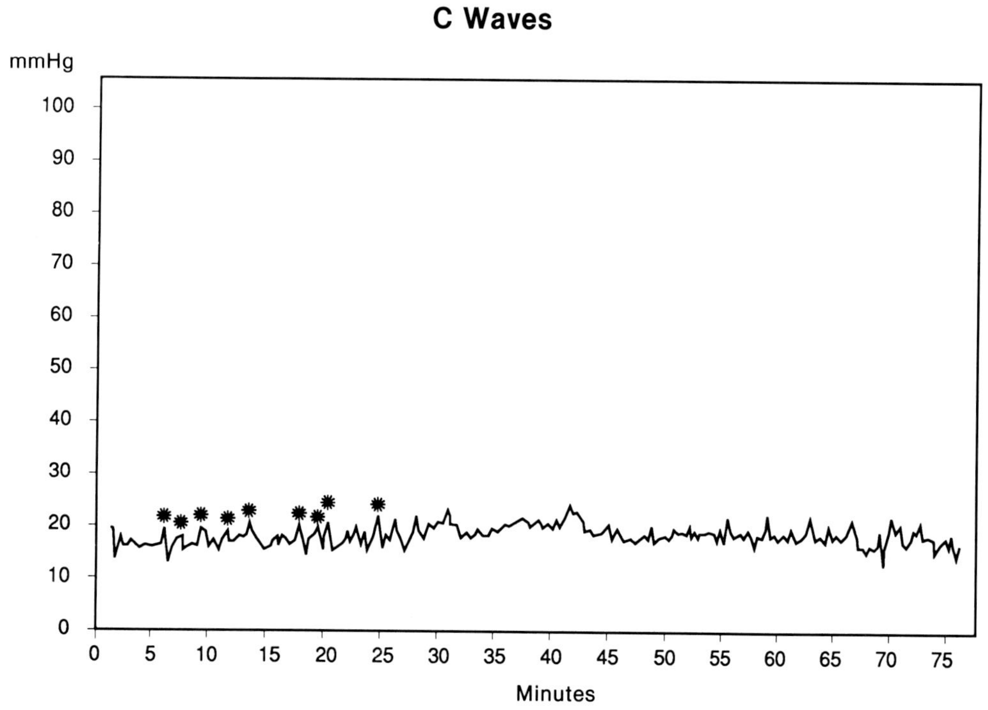

Figure 33–11 • Lundberg's C waves are ICP waveforms reflecting arterial Traube-Hering waves. They suggest of diminished intracranial compliance in a qualitative fashion similar to B waves. C waves illustrated in this figure are highlighted with asterisks.

center, the basic goals of maintaining ICP below 20 mmHg and cerebral perfusion pressure (CPP) above 50 mmHg are well accepted. The basic steps in ICP control and a suggested protocol are outlined later in this chapter.

B. Compliance

Combining experimental investigations into intracranial dynamics with clinical observations in head-injured patients, Miller[44–48] and Marmarou[49–52] have laid the groundwork for quantification of the pressure–volume relationships in normal and abnormal states. They have evolved the concept of *intracranial compliance,* which is reflected in the pressure–volume index (PVI). The PVI describes the change in ICP resulting from addition or withdrawal of a small volume of intraventricular fluid and is proportional to the amount of compliance in the intracranial compartment. Quantitatively, the relationship can be described as

$$\mathrm{PVI} = \frac{\mathrm{V}}{\log \dfrac{\mathrm{P_0}}{\mathrm{P_\Delta}}}$$

where V = volume of fluid added or withdrawn; P_0 = baseline ICP prior to manipulation; and P_Δ = ICP following manipulation (minimum ICP following fluid withdrawal or peak ICP following fluid addition). Measuring the PVI in 34 severely head-injured patients, Marmarou reported that patients with values of 20 mL or greater required no or minimal ICP therapy, patients whose PVIs ranged from 15 to 20 mL tended to have significant ICP elevations that were controllable with moderate therapy, and patients with PVI values below 15 mL required intensive ICP therapy and were at risk for developing uncontrollable ICP.[51]

These studies reinforce the belief that ICP, although a static measurement, reflects a dynamic process and that patients with the same ICP values may differ significantly in their intracerebral compliance. The presence of intracerebral hemorrhage, edema, loss of autoregulation, extraaxial fluid collections, neoplastic tissue, and so forth all make demands on the intracerebral volume-buffering capacity and are reflected in the PVI. Although the clinical measurement of the PVI is not without risks and is not yet to be generally recommended, the concept is critical and indirect indices of intracranial compliance should be attended to. The presence of Lundberg's pathological ICP waves, particularly A waves, indicates marginal compliance. In addition, the sensitivity of the patient's ICP to nursing maneuvers and, in particular, the intensity of therapy required to keep the ICP under control are good indicators of the volume-buffering capacity of the brain. Patients requiring frequent ventricular drainage, mannitol administration, or barbiturate therapy in addition to hyperventilation and sedation generally have minimal intracranial compliance and are at significant risk of intracranial disaster even if their ICP is under 20 mmHg with such therapy. In such patients, further attempts at increasing volume-buffering capacity outside of ICP control may be required.

C. Management

The concepts outlined earlier, such as the Monroe-Kellie doctrine, are the fundamentals guiding ICP therapy. Simply put, the basic contents of the brain are blood, CSF, and tissue. An increase in one component will result in increased ICP unless counterbalanced by compensatory decrease in the volume of one or both of the other two components. The size of the blood compartment, particularly in the brain with a dysfunctional autoregulatory system, is sensitive to arterial inflow pressure, venous outflow resistance, and orthostatic influences, as well as to local microenvironmental factors affecting regional blood flow such as tissue pH, prostoglandins, free radicals, and adenosine. The size of the CSF compartment reflects production, reabsorption, and communication between the various CSF spaces. The tissue component may be composed of brain, inflammatory or neoplastic tissue, or clot (eg, subdural hematoma). The brain volume may be increased by cellular swelling or edema, both hydrostatic and cytotoxic. Addition of any noncerebral tissue to the intracerebral compartment will obviously severely stress the compensatory systems, and even a small mass may lead to decompensation in a tight brain. This gives rise to the principle that any time intracranial hypertension becomes problematic, the possibility that a surgically extirpable mass exists should be immediately entertained. Not infrequently, removing a relatively small volume of tissue can normalize ICP and profoundly ease a patient's course.

A diagrammatic summary of the above principles is presented in Fig. 33–12. The fundamental concept illustrated in this figure is that ICP alone can be quite misleading if not considered within the framework of intracranial compliance. It is therefore very important

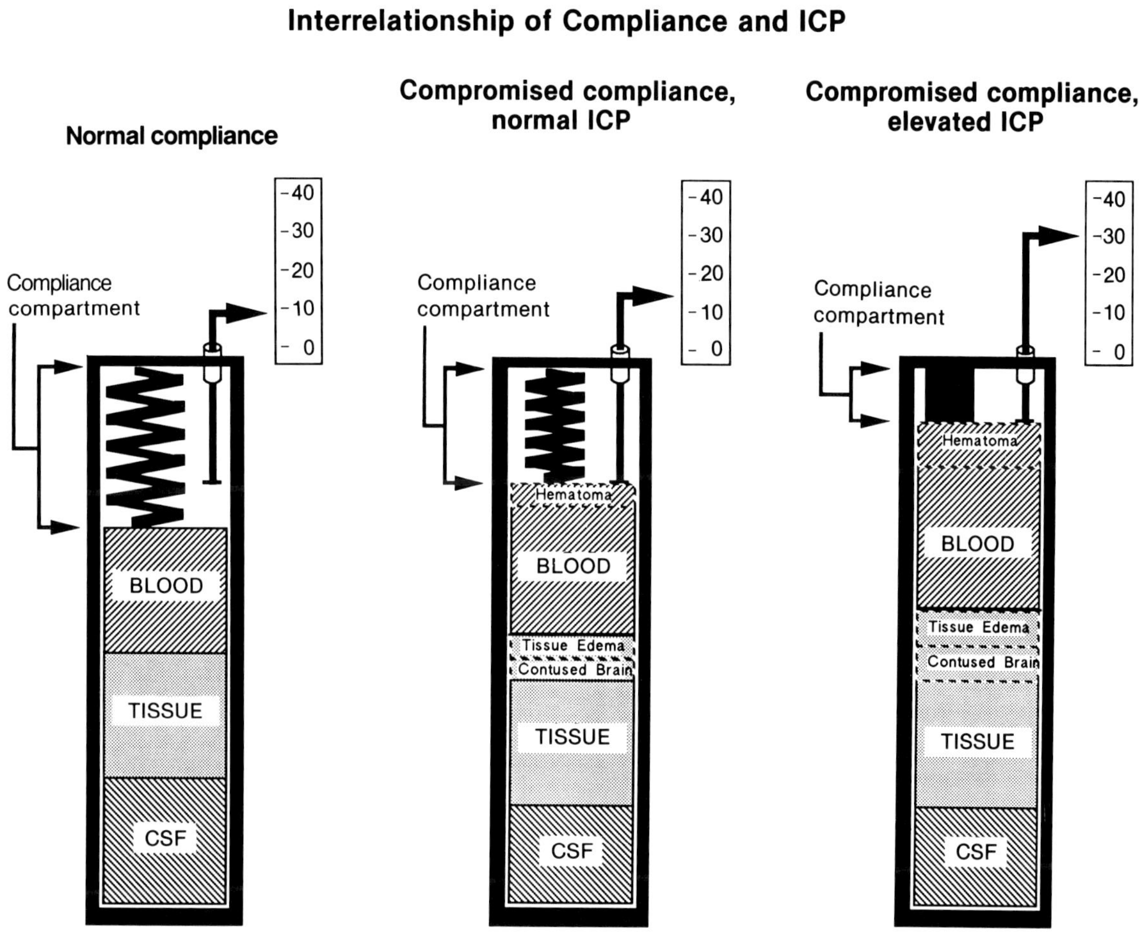

Figure 33–12 • The interrelationship of compliance and ICP. In this figure, compliance is represented by the spring, and ICP by the sliding indicator. The three components of the intracranial volume are shown as boxes. The left shows the representation of the normal situation, in which compliance is maximal and ICP is within the normal range. The center shows the situation in which a postulated brain injury has resulted in an intracranial hematoma with contused and edematous brain. The resultant expansion of intracranial volume has used up the intracranial compliance (eg, compressed the spring), but the ICP has not risen beyond the normal range. The right shows the situation in which the lesions have expanded further, expending the intracranial compliance and raising the ICP. It is important to note that in the left and center figures the ICP is within the normal range despite critically different intracranial dynamics.

to interpret static ICP measurements in light of the patient's ICP history, knowledge of the intracranial pathology as revealed in the CT scan, the amount of therapy required to produce the present ICP value, and the sensitivity of the ICP reading to external stimuli (such as nasotracheal suctioning or turning). All of these factors reflect intracranial dynamics and trends and are vital indicators of the implications of the static ICP value.

A suggested protocol for the management of increased ICP is presented in Fig. 33–13. The individual steps in this protocol are discussed below.

The basic supportive measures of restoring and maintaining normotension, normal arterial oxygenation, and normothermia, although a standard part of medical care, are vitally important in the patient suspected of intracranial hypertension, because alterations in these homeostatic parameters are associated with increased ICP. The hyperdynamic state often seen in the trauma patient who is compensating for hypovolemia will make ICP control difficult until adequate volume status is restored. Frank hypotension is itself associated with a higher probability of increased ICP[3] and, in the setting of trauma, is associated with a doubling of the mortality due to brain injury.[1,52A,52B] Hypoxia will exac-

Unpublished data, 1988.

Treatment of Intracranial Hypertension

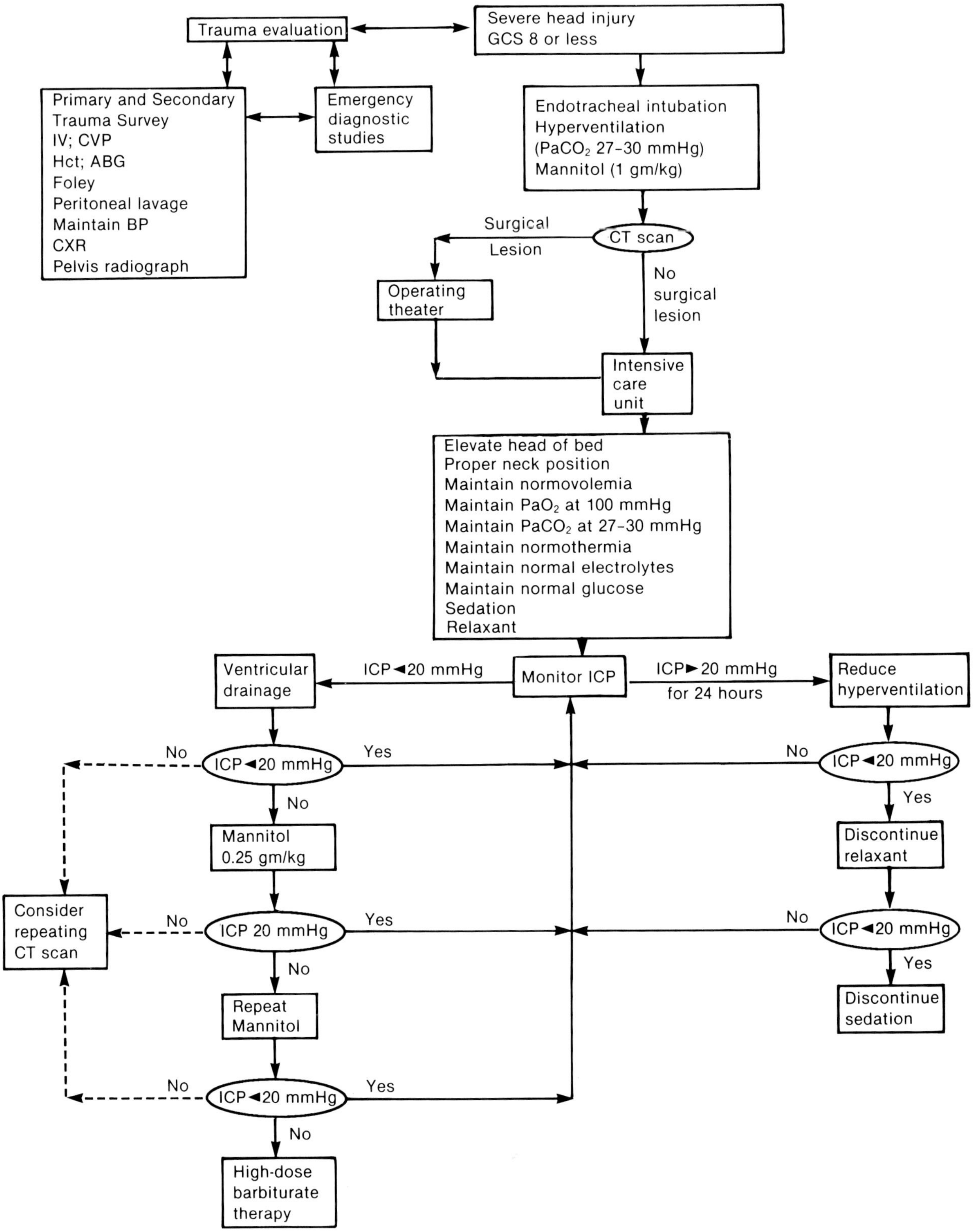

Figure 33–13 • Treatment of intracranial hypertension. This flowchart illustrates a systematic approach to medical management of intracranial hypertension in the severely head-injured patient (Glasgow Coma Scale [*GCS*] of 8 or less), although this approach may be modified and applied to elevated ICP of any etiology. It is important, in all situations, to keep in mind that *medical* management of elevated ICP in the face of a *surgical* lesion is improper and to consider repeating CT or magnetic resonance imaging of the brain whenever management becomes difficult or unexpected developments occur. See text for details.

erbate neuronal injury and, if significant, will increase cerebral blood flow (CBF) and therefore ICP. Hyperthermia will increase ICP by several points for each degree centigrade and should be treated in the head-injured patient.

In addition to the general supportive measures outlined above, increased ICP can be treated by raising the head of the bed and avoiding venous outflow obstruction such as may be caused by head rotation or an overly tight cervical orthosis.[53] When possible, these measures should be instituted expectantly in any patient suspected of increased ICP.

Seizures also will raise ICP and should be investigated if suspected and aggressively treated if present. Although the value of prophylactic anticonvulsant therapy in preventing the development of a posttraumatic seizure disorder has not been definitively established, the risk of posttraumatic seizures, particularly when masked by unconsciousness or pharmacologic paralysis, is sufficiently high that we treat all such patients with anticonvulsants in addition to monitoring a processed EEG in selected cases.

Because pain and agitation also exacerbate intracranial hypertension, judicious use of analgesics and sedatives may be considered. Of course, obscuring the neurologic examination by altering mental status, the earliest indicator of intracranial mischief, should be avoided. In the patients with an ICP monitor and established intracranial hypertension, however, analgesia with or without sedation is very useful, and we routinely treat all such patients who are pharmacologically relaxed with intravenous narcotic analgesics.

In the treatment of established intracranial hypertension, hyperventilation is an effective method of decreasing CSF and lowering ICP. Because "bucking" the ventilator will increase intrathoracic pressure and raise ICP by interfering with venous outflow, pharmacologic paralysis and analgesia/sedation is generally combined with hyperventilation. Under such conditions, the neurologic status of the patient is accessible only through examination of the pupils and the monitored ICP, so expectant management and prompt investigation and treatment of alterations in these parameters is critical.

In the patient with a functioning ventricular catheter, drainage of CSF is an effective and rapid method of lowering ICP. We characteristically employ drainage before administering mannitol. It is not possible to monitor ICP with a ventriculostomy while it is left open to drain. The probability of clogging the ventricular catheter increases dramatically if it is left open in a collapsed ventricle. We therefore limit drainage periods to 1 or 2 minutes at one time and reclamp the catheter if no CSF is draining.

Osmotic agents play a major role in treating intracranial hypertension and, at present, the agent of choice is mannitol. Present dosing schedules suggest 0.25 to 1.0 gm/kg by bolus injection. Repeated, frequent administration of mannitol, however, may induce hyperosmolar states, which render mannitol ineffective and have been associated with acute renal failure.[54] In addition, continuously high serum mannitol levels may increase the penetration of mannitol into the injured brain.[55] Since it has been shown that doses of 0.25 gm/kg are as effective in lowering ICP as larger doses, it is recommended that this dosage schedule be employed initially.[56] In any patient requiring repeated mannitol infusions, serum electrolytes and osmolarity should be periodically monitored.

The efficacy of nonosmotic diuretics in treating increased ICP is controversial. Although furosemide is often administered, it appears to be less reliable than mannitol in reducing ICP.[57] In addition, it exacerbates the dehydrating effects of mannitol and induces potassium wasting. We do not believe that it adds significantly to the actions of mannitol and do not recommend its use in head injury. Although acetazolamide causes a significant reduction in CSF production, its cerebral vasodilator effect may transiently exacerbate intracranial hypertension. For this reason, it is contraindicated in head-injured patients.

Steroids are often administered to the head-injured patient despite the lack of evidence of their efficacy. There are now a number of well-designed studies that have failed to support early hopes that steroids could improve intracranial dynamics and outcome from brain injury.[58-63] In view of their suppression of the immune response and their significant effects on metabolism, the administration of steroids in the setting of head injury is to be discouraged.

In contrast, steroids do play a significant role in treating cytotoxic edema arising in other disease situations. The most notable of these is intracranial neoplasm, for which steroids probably represent the single most notable therapeutic advance in the last 30 years.[64-67] Steroids have also been shown to decrease the ICP of patients with supratentorial tumors.[68] Indeed, it appears that the steroid responsiveness of intracranial tumors may parallel their cytosolic glucocorticoid receptor concentration.[69]

The role of anesthetic doses of barbiturates in the

treatment of refractory intracranial hypertension is also controversial. Nonrandomized series from San Diego and Minnesota have demonstrated that high-dose barbiturate therapy administered to patients who failed in conventional treatment was associated with improved ICP control and improved outcome in responders.[70,71] Two randomized trials, however, in which barbiturates were administered prophylactically to patients felt to be at high risk for uncontrollable ICP[72] or in lieu of mannitol[73] failed to find beneficial effects of barbiturates. The first randomized multicenter barbiturate trial was recently concluded and reported that the ability to control ICP was significantly improved by the administration of barbiturates to patients who had failed conventional therapy.[74] Relying on the strong association between elevated ICP and increased mortality, these authors believed that their data supported the administration of high-dose barbiturates to patients with sustained intracranial hypertension despite maximal therapy.

In light of these studies, it appears that patients with sustained, refractory intracranial hypertension should be considered for barbiturate therapy, with the constraint that they lack contraindications to steroid treatment and will be closely attended in well-staffed intensive care units by neurosurgically trained caregivers. These patients are at significant risk for hypotension, cardiac depression, hypothermia, and pneumonia, all of which may quickly eclipse the benefits of improved ICP control. There does not appear to be a role for barbiturates used prophylactically or in substitution for other established ICP treatment methods.

Barbiturates used for ICP control are administered in addition to continued conventional therapy. After the insertion of a pulmonary artery catheter and the confirmation of adequate intravascular volume and cardiac output, pentobarbital loading is accomplished with a dose of 10 mg/kg over 30 minutes followed by 5 mg/kg/hr for the next 3 hours. Maintenance dosage is initiated at 1 mg/kg/hr and adjusted to burst suppression on bedside processed EEG. The serum pentobarbital level is checked at 4, 12, and 24 hours and then every 24 hours; it is characteristically maintained in the range of 3 to 4 mg%. Cardiac depression is treated with dobutamine; dopamine is used to treat hypotension due to low systemic vascular resistance in the face of adequate intravascular volume.

At all points during the care of a patient with intracranial hypertension, surgical treatment must be considered. Extraaxial or intracerebral hematomas, coalescense of parenchymal contusion, or swelling of severely contused tissue may produce sufficient mass effect to overcome the volume-buffering capacity of the intracranial compartment. Certainly, in the case of extraaxial or large intracerebral hematomas, the role of surgery is straightforward. In the instances of contused brain or coalescence of hemorrhagic tissue, the indications and surgical margins are less distinct. The decision to operate must be predicated on the difficulty of ICP control and an estimate of the "tightness" of the brain. Nevertheless, it is improper to escalate the medical management of increasing intracranial hypertension in the presence of a surgical lesion.

D. *Choice of Monitoring Device*

The choice of a monitoring device should be based on the clinical, radiographic, and logistical status of the patient. We believe that the Richmond bolt system and the Camino fiberoptic ICP monitoring system are theoretically comparable. Given the increased accuracy and reliability of the fiberoptic system and the exceptionally low complication rate with this device, we now employ the Camino system exclusively.[75] This requires the availability of sufficient transducers and familiarity with the device among the physicians and nurses involved in its use. Certainly, in most cases, the Richmond bolt device may be freely substituted for the Camino system if the technical differences between the two systems can be accepted.

V. COMPLICATIONS

A. *Medical Complications*

1. INFECTION

The most incident and commonly discussed complication of ICP monitoring or CSF drainage is infection. The range of infection varies from local wound infection to meningitis, ventriculitis, and brain abscess. The type of infection varies with the monitoring system. Although numerous studies have attempted to determine the risk of infection and proper preventive measures for the various monitoring systems, they have varied significantly in monitoring procedures and technology, study design, definition of infection, and variables addressed. As a result, there remains significant controversy in this area and, although the opinion expressed here is the product of a wide experience in ICP monitoring at our institution, the existence of equally valid alternatives is recognized.

Published estimates of the rate of infection resulting from monitoring with the Richmond bolt range from 0% to 11.6%.[25,76–78] These infections include meningitis, osteomyelitis, and local wound infection. The risk of meningitis can be minimized by avoiding CSF leakage around the wound, preventing disconnections in the system, and minimizing manipulations such as irrigation. The rate of local infection appears to be higher for the Richmond bolt than for the ventricular catheter, in part because osteomyelitis appears to be somewhat unique to the bolt.[76] Such risks may be minimized by careful, repeated local wound care by the nursing staff and by removing the system as soon as medically feasible. Antibiotic prophylaxis has not been directly studied but did not alter the rate of infection in the two reports in which it was addressed.[76,77] However, it did appear to increase the percentage of infections caused by gram-negative organisms.[76]

Although the risk of wound infection may be lower with the ventriculostomy, the risk of meningitis or ventriculitis is greater, ranging from 0% to 26.8%.[25,40,76,79,80] Figure 33–14 illustrates some of the complications of ventriculostomy. Given the frequency and serious nature of this complication, a number of factors have been addressed and found to contribute to the likelihood of infection. Daily wound care at the incision and catheter exit site has been shown to be important in long-term hyperalimentation catheter care.[81] Irregularities in performing such routine care has been associated with increased infection incidence.[82] As in central venous catheters, tunnelling the catheter subcutaneously and bringing it out through a separate, removed stab wound appears to lessen the risk of infection.[83] Irrigation and other manipulations of the system (such as ventriculography) increase the chance of infection.[79,80,84] The existence of a CSF leak (evidenced by otorrhea or rhinorrhea) or intraventricular hemorrhage also makes infection more likely.[76,79,85]

The influence of the duration of ventricular catheterization is less clear. Several studies have reported that the rate of infection increased significantly if the catheter remained in place for 5 or more days.[76,79,86] Other studies have reported no influence of duration on risk of infection.[40,78,84] A recent analysis of cumulative infection data using life-table methods found that the risk of subsequent infection, from the monitor or other causes, diminished after 6 days; this group suggested that the majority of infections are introduced at the time of monitor insertion.[87] Although the situation is far from clear, we do not replace monitors by protocol unless there is another significant risk factor present (such as a CSF leak), the monitor malfunctions, or surveillance CSF cultures or cytologies suggest infection.

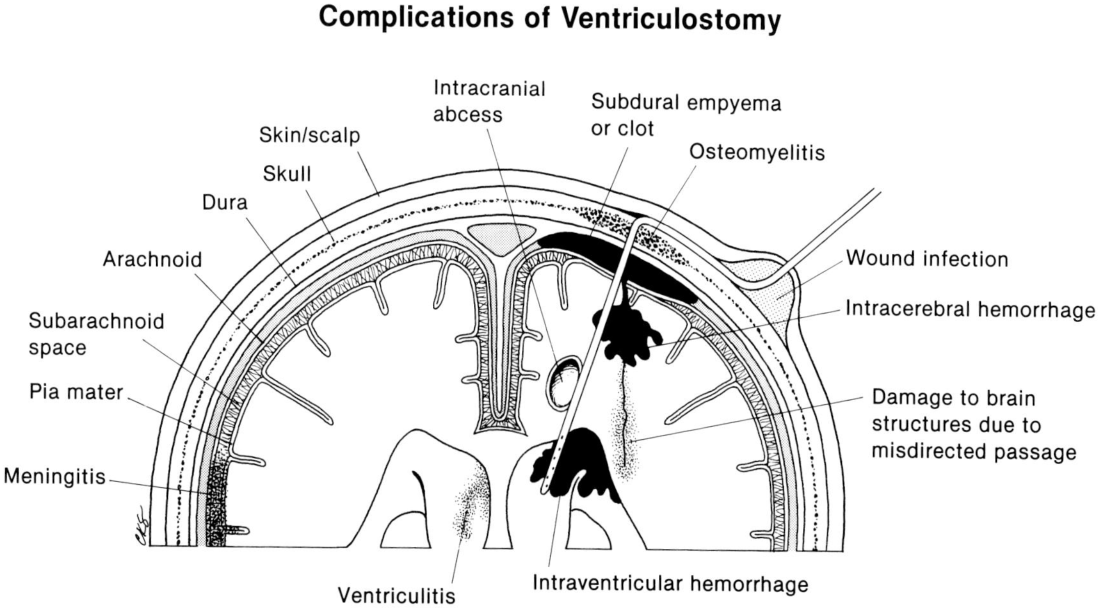

Figure 33–14 • The various intracranial complications of ICP monitoring are demonstrated using the ventricular drainage system as an example.

The role of prophylactic antibiotics is also controversial. In his ground-breaking study, Lundberg reported no infections in 130 patients, all of whom were on prophylactic antibiotics.[40] In their continuation of this series to over 1000 patients, Sundbärg and associates reported an infection rate of 1.1% but denied continued use of prophylactic antibiotics.[80] Wyler and Kelly reported that one third as many infections occurred with prophylactic ampicillin coverage than with no antibiotics.[84] Others have found no effect.[76,77,79] Importantly, the type of antibiotics used appears to significantly influence the infectious organism. Using ampicillin, Wyler and Kelly found a predominance of coagulase-positive, gram-positive organisms in their antibiotic-treated group, whereas they found coagulase-negative organisms in their controls.[81] The use of nafcillin by Mayhall and associates, nafcillin or cephalothin by Aucoin and associates, and ampicillin or methicillin by Smith and Alksne markedly increased the predominance of gram-negative organisms such as *Pseudomonas, Enterobacter,* or *Klebsiella* in their series.[76,78,79] In light of the increased virulence and antibiotic resistance of many nosocomial gram-negative pathogens and our apparent low rate of infection using the methods outlined earlier, we do not administer prophylactic antibiotics for routine ICP monitor placement in our institution. We prefer to approach monitor-related infection by early diagnosis and rapid, organism-specific antibiotic treatment of bacteria not selected for by prophylactic antibiotic usage.

Due to its recent availability, the Camino fiberoptic ICP monitoring system has not been widely studied with respect to infectious complications. In the initial clinical trial, there were no infections in 120 cases.[88] A follow-up to that study reporting on 250 patients again found no infections related to the monitor.[75]

2. HEMORRHAGE

Hemorrhage is the most dreaded complication of ICP monitoring. Its incidence is directly related to the method of monitoring, being negligible with extradual devices and occurring more often with intraventricular than with intraparenchymal monitors, although conclusive data are not available on this. The actual incidence of hemorrhage appears small. Sundbärg and associates reported two small, asymptomatic intraventricular clots and one intracerebral hemorrhage (which required surgical evacuation) in report on over 1000 patients without CT scan.[80] Narayan and coworkers, with the benefit of CT scanning, reported three intracranial hemorrhages in 207 patients (1.4%), one of whom required surgery.[25] They noted a correlation of hemorrhage with coagulopathy or multiple passes during placement. It is anticipated that with the increased use of ICP monitoring and CSF drainage, the occurrence of hemorrhage as a complication of ICP monitoring will become increasingly recognized but will remain infrequent.

Hemorrhage may result from direct trauma caused by the monitoring device or from overdrainage of CSF. In the first instance, hemorrhage may be intraventricular or intracerebral. The occurrence of intraventricular hemorrhage is a complication of ventricular puncture and is evidenced by returning bloody CSF through the ventriculostomy. Recognition of this complication can be confounded by bloody CSF resulting from the pathology underlying the need for monitoring (eg, trauma or hypertensive hemorrhage with ventricular extension). Differentiating between these possibilities must be individualized to the case at hand, including knowledge of the preexisting CT or MRI pathology, and may require reimaging for clarification. Because such bleeding is self-limited in the absence of a bleeding diathesis, management involves close observation for ICP elevation, with drainage as necessary.

Intracranial hemorrhage may occur with either intraparenchymal or intraventricular monitoring. Although it may be evidenced by return of blood, it is characteristically unrecognized until manifested by elevated ICP or clinical neurologic deterioration. Again, although recognition of this complication may be confounded by the underlying neurologic pathology, clinical deterioration or unanticipated difficulty with control of intracranial hypertension following placement of an ICP-monitoring device should raise the possibility of a hemorrhagic complication and prompt a CT scan. Management of such intracranial hemorrhage is a neurosurgical decision and varies from careful observation to surgical evacuation.

Hemorrhage resulting from overdrainage of CSF characteristically results in subdural hemorrhage. This may occur with drainage from the ventricular system or the spinal intrathecal space. Although often silent, subdural hemorrhage in this setting may manifest as clinical deterioration or intracranial hypertension.

Hemorrhagic complications can be avoided by preventive methodology and technique. As noted above, the presence of a clotting abnormality requires correction of the abnormal bleeding tendency prior to instrumentation of the brain. This is particularly important in the case of trauma, both because there is a high concentration of tissue thromboplastin in the brain and because it is easily overlooked in the hectic resuscitation setting. The technical constraints are abstaining from repeated passages of monitoring devices and ensuring that the drainage of CSF is neither overly rapid nor set to an inappropriately low pressure. In the setting of CSF drainage in the awake patient, it is important that the patient not inadvertently alter his or her own drainage parameters (eg, by raising the head of the bed or arising without occlusion of the drainage system).

3. IATROGENIC INTRACRANIAL HYPERTENSION

Inadvertently elevating the ICP through the addition of intracranial volume is a potential complication with both the ventricular catheter and the Richmond bolt. This may occur as a technical mistake if the tubing system is accidentally flushed into the intracranial space or attached to an infusion system. In the presence of diminished compliance, ICP will increase by over 5 cm/H_2O/ added mL of intracranial volume, with potentially disastrous effects.[47,48] It is imperative that careful labelling of tubing involved in ICP monitoring and diligence in nursing management of the system be maintained. In addition, fluid reservoirs should never remain connected to the system in a position in which gravity will result in intracranial infusion if they are inadvertently opened.

The second manner by which ICP can be iatrogenically elevated is during testing of intracranial compliance. It has been recommended that the fluid withdrawal method be employed in patients with known or suspected low compliance.[51] Although this runs the risk of occluding the catheter by collapsing the ventricular walls against it or by aspirating the choroid plexus through its ports, it avoids the risk of elevating the ICP. It is notable that measuring intracranial compliance remains a primarily experimental exercise and must be clearly indicated in cases in which it involves significant risk to the patient.

B. *Technical Complications*

In the modern age of medical care, the barrage of technical information originating from a patient in the intensive care unit presents the risk of isolating the patient from the medical team. As a result, *technical errors* arising from any monitoring system may be translated into *management errors* if they are uncritically relied upon in the absence of careful patient examination. With ICP monitoring, an artifactually elevated ICP will result in the patient receiving costly and potentially harmful unneeded therapy, whereas an incorrectly measured low ICP can result in serious deterioration in the patient's neurologic status before the error is noted. Even a correctly recorded ICP in the normal range may be misleading if it is not noted that vigorous medical therapy is being required to maintain such a value, suggesting marginal intracranial compliance. It is very important that the ''ICP number'' not be substituted for a thorough neurologic assessment, even when such examination is limited by coma or muscular paralysis.

1. MEASUREMENT ERROR

Errors in measurement due to baseline drift or loss of accuracy are inherent in any monitoring system. They may arise from the electronic transducer or from alterations in the coupling system such as microleaks in the tubing from the ventricular catheter or Richmond bolt.[89] Systems using fluid coupling and external transducers can be rezeroed and recalibrated externally by using atmospheric pressure as the zero and a fluid column of known height as the calibration signal. For ventriculostomy, a simple and rapid accuracy check can be easily performed at the bedside by *slowly* raising the drainage tube from the ventricular catheter and using the height of the meniscus as a manometer. The zero calibration and accuracy, as well as the height of the transducer, should be checked whenever a value arises that is inconsistent with other aspects of the patient's course.

Implanted electronic systems such as the Camino fiberoptic ICP monitor rely on their minimal drift and ability to maintain accuracy and stability in situ. The Camino catheter is stable to no more than 1 mmHg/ day of baseline drift, and this drift appears to occur toward higher pressures.[88] If it is believed that the Camino catheter is reading incorrectly, it must be removed and, in the interest of sterility, a new catheter should be inserted (although the same site and housing device may be used if sterility is maintained).

Signal loss may occur due to damping of the fluid coupling. Damping may occur due to bubbles of air in the system (the most common source), leaks, occlusion of the catheter or bolt, or breakage of the Camino fiberoptic catheter. All air must be purged from the system, and the tubing connections must be secure. Occlusion may often be irrigated free, but because this involves risk to the patient, irrigation must be cautiously performed by a physician using sterile technique, and only as a last resort. Unresolved occlusion or breakage of the fiberoptic catheter requires replacement. Unfortunately, the Richmond bolt has a disturbing tendency to occlude or dampen. This may occur even in the face of an adequately large dural opening and careful insertion perpendicular to the surface of the brain. Under conditions of high ICP, the brain may herniate into the lumen and occlude it, even if the arachnoid is left intact.[24] In other instances, such a system may read inaccurately without satisfactory explanation, particularly in underreporting ICP under conditions of intracranial hypertension.[90,91] This is one of the major reasons why we prefer to employ ventriculostomy for ICP monitoring and tend to employ the Camino catheter system when ventricular puncture is not recommended.

In the setting of trauma, when the ICP is increased and the ventricles are compressed, it is not uncommon to penetrate the ventricle and observe a transient, subtle flow of CSF that quickly ceases and does not reappear. This signifies collapse of the ventricle around the catheter. If this is not recognized and the catheter is withdrawn, it will be impossible to recannulate the ventricle at that time. Although the catheter will not accurately reflect ICP as long as the ventricle is collapsed, it should be left in place, tunnelled out, clamped, and connected to a drainage bag and monitor. In addition, a second, nonventricular monitor should be placed to monitor ICP. Using this system, raised ICP can often be significantly lowered by unclamping the ventricular catheter and draining the small amount of CSF that will collect while the catheter is closed. In the instance of a very low PVI, this can often make a significant difference in ICP. In the instance of acceptable ICP levels not requiring drainage, CSF will accumulate and the ventricular catheter monitor will begin to show a normal waveform. At this point, one of the two functioning monitors may be removed.

2. Damage to Parenchymal Structures

The other major technical error that can potentially result in major pathology is damage to brain parenchymal structures due to misdirected or overly deep placement of monitoring devices. This is certainly a risk of ventricular cannulation and an undocumented but potential complication of the Camino system. Misdirected attempts at ventricular puncture can result in damage to the caudate nucleus, lenticular nuclei, internal capsule, or anterior thalamic nuclear groups. Overly deep passage can damage the hypothalamus, and we have seen one case in which a large anterior communicating aneurysm was punctured.

The likelihood of such misadventures is increased by distortion of anatomic structures such as those that occur with brain injury or neoplasia with edema. It is therefore important to limit the number of punctures and the depth of catheter passage, as well as to recognize situations in which successful ventricular puncture is unlikely and an alternate monitoring system is indicated. We believe that if successful cannulation is not accomplished by the third pass, ICP should be monitored with a Richmond bolt or Camino catheter. There is never any reason to pass the catheter more than 6 cm beyond the dura, and lack of flow by this depth is indication of a misdirected passage. If ventricular drainage is deemed necessary despite three unsuccessful attempts at cannulation, ventriculostomy may be attempted on the other side with a similar limit on the number of allowable passes.

VI. References

1. Toutant, S, Klauber M, Marshall L, Toole B, et al. Absent or compressed basal cisterns on first CT scan: Ominous predictors of outcome in severe head injury. J Neurosurg 61:691–694, 1984.
2. van Dongen K, Braakman R, GJ G. The prognostic value of computerized tomography in comatose head-injured patients. J Neurosurg 59:951–957, 1983.
3. Seelig J, Klauber M, Toole B, Bowers-Marshall S. Increased ICP and systemic hypotension during the first 72 hours following severe head injury. In Miller J, Teasdale G, Rowan J, Galbraith S, Mendelow A (eds). Intracranial Pressure VI. Berlin, Springer-Verlag, 1986, 675–679.
4. Papo I, Janny P, Caruselli G, Colnet G, Luongo A. Intracranial pressure time course in primary intracerebral hemorrhage. Neurosurgery 4:504–511, 1979.
5. Consensus Development Conference Summary. The diagnosis and treatment of Reye's syndrome. Baltimore, National Institute of Health, 1981.
6. Jacobsen WK, Mason LJ, Briggs BA, Schneider S, et al. Correlation of spontaneous respiration and neurologic damage in near-drowning. Crit Care Med 11:487–489, 1983.
7. Nussbaum E, Galant SP. Intracranial pressure monitoring as a guide to prognosis in the nearly-drowned, severely-comatose child. J Pediatr 102:215–218, 1983.
8. Nussbaum E, Maggi JC. Pentobarbital therapy does not improve neurologic outcome in nearly drowned, flaccid-comatose children. Pediatrics 81:630–634, 1988.
9. Oakes DD, Sherck JP, Maloney JP, Charters AC. Prognosis and management of victims of near-drowning. J Trauma 22:544–549, 1982.
10. Spetzler RF, Wilson CB, Weinstein P, Mehdorn M, et al. Normal perfusion pressure breakthrough theory. Clin Neurosurg 25:651–672, 1974.
11. Hoffman H. Management of medulloblastoma. Austral Pediatr J 15:55–56, 1979.

12. Bruce D, Schut L. Cerebellar medulloblastoma, sarcoma, and hemangioblastoma. In American Association of Neurological Surgeons; Section of Pediatric Neurosurgey (eds). Pediatric Neurosurgery. New York, Grune & Stratton, 1982, 375–381.
13. Haan J, Thomeer R. Predictive value of temporary external lumbar drainage in normal pressure hydrocephalus. Neurosurgery 22:388–391, 1988.
14. Dandy W. Ventriculography following the injection of air into the cerebral ventricles. Ann Surg 68:5–11, 1918.
15. Kaufmann G, Clark K. Emergency frontal twist drill ventriculostomy: Technical note. J Neurosurg 33:226–227, 1970.
16. Keen W. Surgery of the lateral ventricles of the brain. Medical News 57:275–278,1890.
17. Navarro I, Renteria J, Peralta V, Castilli M. Trans-orbital ventricular puncture for emergency ventricular decompression. J Neurosurg 54:273–274, 1981.
18. Robertson J, Denton IJ. Surgical considerations of ventriculography. In Youmans J (ed). Neurological Surgery. Philadelphia, WB Saunders, 1982, 375–381.
19. Coroneos N, McDowall D, Gibson R, Pickerodt V, et al. Measurement of extradural pressure and its relationship to other intracranial pressures. J Neurol Neurosurg Psychiatry 36:514–522, 1973.
20. Coroneos N, Turner J, Gibson R, McDowall D, et al. Comparison of extradural with intraventricular pressure in patients after head injury. In Brock M, Dietz H (eds). Intracranial Pressure: Experimental and Clinical Aspects. Berlin, Springer-Verlag, 1972, 51–58.
21. McGraw C. Epidural intracranial pressure monitoring. In Lundberg N, Ponten U, Brock M (eds). Intracranial Pressure II. Berlin, Springer-Verlag, 1974, 394–396.
22. Sundbärg G, Nornes H. Simultaneous recording of the ventricular fluid pressure and the epidural pressures. Acta Neurol Scand 46:634–635, 1970.
23. Weaver D, Winn H, Jane J. Differential intracranial pressure in patients with unilateral mass lesions. J Neurosurg 56:660–665, 1982.
24. Wilkinson H. Intracranial pressure monitoring: Techniques and pitfalls. In Cooper P (ed). Head Injury. Baltimore, Williams & Wilkins, 1982, 147–184.
25. Narayan R, Kishore P, Becker D, Ward J, et al. Intracranial pressure: To monitor or not to monitor? A review of our experience with head injury. J Neurosurg 56:650–659, 1982.
26. Kellie G. An account of the appearance observed in the dissection of two of the three individuals presumed to have perished in the storm of the 3rd, and whose bodies were discovered in the vicinity of Leith on the morning of the 4th November 1921 with some reflections on the pathology of the brain. Trans Med Chirurgical Sci (Edinburgh) 1:84–169, 1824.
27. Monro A. Observations on the structure and function of the nervous system. Edinburgh, Creech & Johnson, 1783.
28. Burrows G. Disorders of the cerebral circulation. London, Longman, 1846.
29. Quincke H. Die diagnostiche und therpeutische bedeutung der lumbalpunktion. Klinishcher Vortrag Deutsch Med Wochnschr 31:1825–1828, 1905.
30. Quincke H. Lumbar puncture. In Church A (ed). Modern Clinical Medicine: Diseases of the Nervous System. New York, Appleton, 1911.
31. Queckenstedt H. Zur diagnose der ruckenmarkkompression. Duetsch Ztschr Nerveh 55:325–333, 1916.
32. Ayala G. Uber den diagnostichen wert des liquordruckes und einenapparat zu seiner messung. Zeitschrift fr Neurologie und Psychiatrie 84:42–95, 1923.
33. Ayer J. Analysis of the lumbar cerebrospinal fluid in 67 cases of tumours and cysts of the brain. Association for Research in Nervous and Mental Disease 8:189–199, 1929.
34. Browder J, Meyers R. Observations on behavior of the systemic blood pressure, pulse, and spinal fluid pressure following craniocerebral injury. Am J Surg 31:403–426, 1936.
35. Browder J, Meyers R. Behavior of the systemic blood pressure, pulse rate, and spinal fluid pressure associated with acute changes in intracranial pressure artificially produced. Arch Surg 36:1–19, 1938.
36. Adson A, Lillie W. The relationship of intracranial pressure, choked disc, and intraocular tension. Trans Am Acad Ophthalmol 30:138–154, 1927.
37. Hill B. American Electric System of Surgery. Cincinnati, W Phillips, 1850.
38. Ingraham F, Campbell J. An apparatus for closed drainage of the ventricular system. Ann Surg 114:1096–1098, 1941.
39. Guillaume J, Janny P. Monometrie intracranienne continué; Intért physio-pathologique et clinique de la methode. La Presse Medicale 59:953–955, 1951.
40. Lundberg N. Continuous recording and control of ventricular fluid pressure in neurosurgical practice. Acta Psychiatr Neurol Scand 149(Suppl):1–193, 1960.
41. Becker D, Miller J, Ward J, Greenberg R, et al. The outcome from severe head injury with early diagnosis and intensive management. J Neurosurg 47:491–502, 1977.
42. Marshall L, Smith R, Shapiro H. The outcome with aggressive treatment in severe head injuries. Part I. The significance of intracranial pressure monitoring. J Neurosurg 50:20–25, 1979.
43. Saul T, Ducker T. Effect of intracranial pressure monitoring and aggressive treatment on mortality in severe head injury. J Neurosurg, 56:498–503, 1982.
44. Leech P, Miller J. Intracranial volume-pressure relationships during experimental brain compression in primates. J Neurol Neurosurg Psychiatry 37a:1093–1098, 1974.
45. Leech P, Miller J. Intracranial volume-pressure relationships during experimental brain compression in primates. 2. Effect of induced changes in systemic arterial pressure and cerebral blood flow. J Neurol Neurosurg Psychiatry 37b:1099–1104, 1974.
46. Leech P, Miller J. Intracranial volume-pressure relationships during experimental brain compression in primates. 3. Effect of mannitol and hyperventilation. J Neurol Neurosurg Psychiatry 37c:1015–1111, 1974.
47. Miller J, Pickard J. Intracranial volume/pressure studies in patients with head injury. Injury 5:265–268, 1974.
48. Sullivan H, Miller J, Griffith R, Becker D. CSF pressure-volume dynamics is neurosurgical patients: a preliminary evaluation in six patients. Surg Neurol 9:47–54, 1978.
49. Marmarou A, Shulman K, LaMorgese J. Compartmental analysis of compliance and outflow resistance of the cerebrospinal fluid system. J Neurosurg 43:523–534, 1975.
50. Marmarou, A Shulman K, Rosende R. A nonlinear analysis of the cerebrospinal fluid system and intracranial pressure dynamics. J Neurosurg 48:332–334, 1978.
51. Maset A, Marmarou A, Ward J, Choi S, et al. Pressure-volume index in head injury. J Neurosurg 67:832–840, 1987.
52. Shapiro K, Marmarou A. Clinical applications of the pressure-volume index in treatment of pediatric head injuries. J Neurosurg 56:819–825, 1982.
53. Hulme A, Cooper R. The effects of head position and jugular vein compression on intracranial pressure. In Beks J, Bosch D, Brock M (eds). Intracranial Pressure III. Berlin, Springer-Verlag, 1976, 259–263.
54. Stuart F, Torres E, Fletcher R, Crocker D, et al. Effects of

single, repeated, and massive mannitol infusion in the dog: Structural and functional changes in kidney and brain. Ann Surg 172:190–204, 1970.
55. Wise B, Perkins R, Stevenson E, Scott K. Penetration of 14C-labelled mannitol from serum into cerebrospinal fluid and brain. Exp Neurol 10:264–270, 1964.
56. Marshall L, Smith R, Rauscher L, Shapiro H. Mannitol dose requirements in brain-injured patients. J Neurosurg 48: 169–172, 1978.
57. Levin A. Treatment of increased intracranial pressure: A comparison of different hyperosmotic agents and the use of thiopental. Paper presented at the meeting of the American Association of Neurological Surgeons Annual Meeting, New Orleans, 1978.
58. Cooper P, Moody S, Clark W, Kirkpatrick J, et al. Dexamethasone and severe head injury: A prospective double blind study. J Neurosurg 51:307–316, 1979.
59. Gudeman S, Miller J, Becker D. Failure of high-dose steroid therapy to influence intracranial pressure in patients with severe head injury. J Neurosurg 51:301–306, 1979.
60. Marshall L, King J, Langfitt T. The complications of high-dose corticosteroid therapy in neurosurgical patients: A prospective study. Ann Neurol 1:201–203, 1977.
61. Miller J, Leech P. Effects of mannitol and steroid therapy on intracranial volume pressure relationships in patients. J Neurosurg 42:275–281, 1975.
62. Pitts E, Katkis J. Effect of megadose steroids on ICP in traumatic coma. In Shulman K, Marmarou A, Miller A (eds). Intracranial Pressure IV. New York, Springer-Verlag, 1972, 638–642.
63. Saul T, Ducker T, Saleman M, Carro E. Steroids in severe head injury: A prospective, randomized clinical trial. J Neurosurg 54:596–600, 1981.
64. Cairncross J, Macdonald D, Pexman J, Ives F. Steroid-induced CT changes in patients with recurrent malignant glioma. Neurology 38:724–726, 1988.
65. French L. The use of steroids in the treatment of cerebral edema. Bull NY Acad Med 42:301–311, 1966.
66. Galicich J, French L, Melby J. Use of dexamethasone in treatment of cerebral edema associated with brain tumors. Lancet 81:46–53, 1961.
67. Renaudin J, Fewer D, Wilson C, Boldrey E, et al. Dose dependency of Decadron in patients with partially excised brain tumors. J Neurosurg 39:302–305, 1973.
68. Brock M, Wiegand H, Zillig C, et al. The effect of dexamethasone in intracranial pressure in patients with supratentorial tumors. In Pappius H, Feindel W (eds). Dynamics of Brain Edema. New York, Springer-Verlag, 1976, 330–336.
69. Yu Z, Boöthius J, Hatam A, Granholm L, et al. A study of glucocorticoid receptors in intracranial tumors. J Neurosurg 55:757–760, 1981.
70. Rea G, Rockswold G. Barbiturate therapy in uncontrolled intracranial hypertension. Neurosurgery 12:401–404, 1983.
71. Rockoff M, Marshall L, Shapiro M. High-dose barbiturate therapy in humans: A clinical review of 60 patients. Ann Neurol 6:194–199, 1979.
72. Schwartz M, Tator C, Towed D, Reid S, et al. The University of Toronto Head Injury Treatment Study: A prospective, randomized comparison of pentobarbital and mannitol. Can J Neurol Sci 11:434–440, 1984.
73. Ward J, Becker D, Miller J, Choi S, et al. Failure of prophylactic barbiturate coma in the treatment of severe head injury. J Neurosurg 62:383–388, 1985.
74. Eisenberg H, Frankowski R, Contant C, Marshall L, et al. Comprehensive central nervous system trauma centers. High-dose barbiturate control of elevated intracranial pressure in patients with severe head injury. J Neurosurg 69:15–213, 1988.
75. Luerssen T, Shields P, Vos H, Marshall L. Clinical experience with a fiberoptic parenchymal pressure monitor. In Hoff J (ed). Intracranial Pressure VI. New York, Springer-Verlag, 1989, (in press).
76. Aucoin P, Kotilainen H, Gantz N, Davidson R, et al. Intracranial pressure monitors: Epidemiologic study of risk factors and infections. Am J Med 80:369–376, 1986.
77. Rosner M, Becker D. ICP monitoring: Complications and associated factors. Clin Neurosurg 23:494–519, 1976.
78. Smith R, Alksne J. Infections complicating the use of external ventriculostomy. J Neurosurg 44:567–570, 1976.
79. Mayhall C, Archer N, Lamb A, Spadora A, et al. Ventriculostomy related infections: A prospective epidemiologic study. N Engl J Med 310:553–559, 1984.
80. Sundbärg G, Kjällquist A, Lundberg N, Ponten U. Complications due to prolonged ventricular fluid recording in clinical practice. In Brock M, Dietz H (eds). Intracranial Pressure: Experimental and Clinical Aspects. Berlin, Springer-Verlag, 1972, 348–352.
81. Filler R, Coran A. Total parenteral nutrition in infants and children: Central and peripheral approaches. Surg Clin North Am 56:395–412, 1976.
82. Franges E, Beidman M. Infections related to intracranial pressure monitoring. J Neurosci Nurs 20:94–103, 1988.
83. Friedman W, Vries J. Percutaneous tunnel ventriculostomy: Summary of 100 procedures. J Neurosurg 53:662–665, 1980.
84. Wyler A, Kelly W. Use of antibiotics with external ventriculostomies. J Neurosurg 37:185–187, 1972.
85. Smith K. Head Trauma: Comparison of infection rates for different methods of intracranial pressure monitoring. J Neurosci Nurs 19:310–314, 1987.
86. Levin A. Physiological monitoring of the head injured patient. Clin Neurosurg 29:240–287, 1982.
87. Kanter R, Weiner L, Patti A, Robson L. Infectious complications and duration of intracranial pressure monitoring. Crit Care Med 13:837–839, 1985.
88. Ostrup R, Luerssen T, Marshall L, Zornow M. Continuous monitoring of intracranial pressure with a miniaturized fiberoptic device. J Neurosurg 67:206–209, 1987.
89. Shields D, McGraw P, Garretson H. Accurate intracranial pressure monitoring: Technical note. Neurosurgery 14:592–593, 1984.
90. Mendelow A, Rowan J, Murray L, Kerr A. A clinical comparison of subdural screw pressure measurements with ventricular pressure. J Neurosurg 58:45–50, 1983.
91. Miller J, Bobo H, Kapp J. Inaccurate pressure readings for subarachnoid bolts. Neurosurgery 19:253–255, 1986.

Section V

•

Peripheral Nerve Procedures

Chapter 34

•

Isaac Azar, MD

Monitoring of Neuromuscular Transmission

OUTLINE

I. INTRODUCTION

A. *Why Monitor Neuromuscular (NM) Transmission?*

Muscle relaxants are an essential component of modern anesthesia. They greatly enhance patient care by facilitating tracheal intubation, control of ventilation, and performance of surgery. Postoperatively, however, muscle relaxants may compromise respiratory function. A high incidence of partial paralysis has been observed in postanesthesia care units.[1,2] These patients may develop ventilatory failure and suffer hypoxia and hypercapnia. It is vital, therefore, to limit the doses of muscle relaxants to the minimum necessary, and to insure that their effect is completely reversed at the conclusion of surgery. This can be reliably accomplished by monitoring neuromuscular (NM) transmission.

Because of the great variation in patient response to muscle relaxants, it is difficult to determine the optimal dose for a particular patient. A dose that would hardly produce relaxation in one patient may cause intense paralysis in another. Also, patients with renal or liver insufficiency often need smaller doses than usual. Monitoring NM transmission in these patients is particularly useful because it allows precise titration of the NM blockade.

The introduction of the intermediate-acting muscle relaxants, atracurium and vecuronium, has increased the need for NM transmission monitoring because of the rapid changes in blood level of these agents. Their administration by infusion, as advocated by some authors, is practically impossible without monitoring.

In addition to the above, NM transmission monitoring provides answers to the following questions:

- Is the patient ready for tracheal intubation? If not totally paralyzed, some patients react strenuously to tracheal intubation and may sustain injuries.
- Is the patient's sensitivity to muscle relaxants normal? Altered sensitivity to muscle relaxants is not uncommon. Patients with atypical pseudocholinesterase sustain prolonged apnea following usual doses of succinylcholine. Also, patients with various NM disorders often exhibit increased or decreased sensitivity to nondepolarizing muscle relaxants.[3] NM transmission monitoring can identify these patients and provide important information for future surgery.
- Is the patient adequately relaxed for the proposed surgery? Adequate muscle relaxation facilitates surgery. However, surgeons occasionally misinterpret surgical difficulties as insufficient paralysis. Monitoring NM transmission can determine whether an additional dose of a muscle relaxant is indeed necessary.
- Is the NM blockade reversible? Intense NM blockade may not be reversible at the conclusion of surgery. If nerve stimulation elicits no response, reversal is not recommended. Persistent attempts to reverse the blockade may further intensify it, rather than reversing it.
- If a patient is not breathing adequately postoperatively, is it due to the residual effect of anesthetics or muscle relaxants? Monitoring NM transmission can determine whether a residual effect of muscle relaxants is contributing to postoperative ventilatory failure.

B. *Normal NM Transmission*

Skeletal muscles are made up of many thousands of motor units. Each unit is composed of a nerve axon, a muscle fiber, and an NM junction. The junction consists of a presynaptic membrane (the ending of the nerve axon), a postsynaptic membrane, and a synaptic cleft (Fig. 34–1). The *postsynaptic membrane* (the endplate) is a modified section of the muscle fiber membrane, densely covered with acetylcholine receptors. Similar receptors, although not identical, are also found on the *presynaptic membrane.*

The nerve ending at the NM junction contains minute vesicles filled with acetylcholine molecules. When a nerve action potential arrives at the junction, the vesicles burst and thousands of acetylcholine molecules pour into the *synaptic cleft.* There the acetylcholine molecules interact with special recognition sites on the acetylcholine receptors.

The *acetylcholine receptor* consists of an ion channel surrounded by a rosette of several large protein molecules. The channel serves as a conduit for electrolytes between the inside and the outside of the muscle fiber. At rest, the ion channels are closed and the endplate is polarized (*membrane resting potential*).

When acetylcholine molecules interact with the recognition sites of the receptors, the ion channels open. This allows rapid flow of sodium ions into, and potassium ions out of, the muscle fiber. The rush of electrolytes across the postsynaptic membrane causes depolarization of the membrane and generates an action potential. The endplate action potential propagates throughout the muscle fiber and provokes muscle contraction.

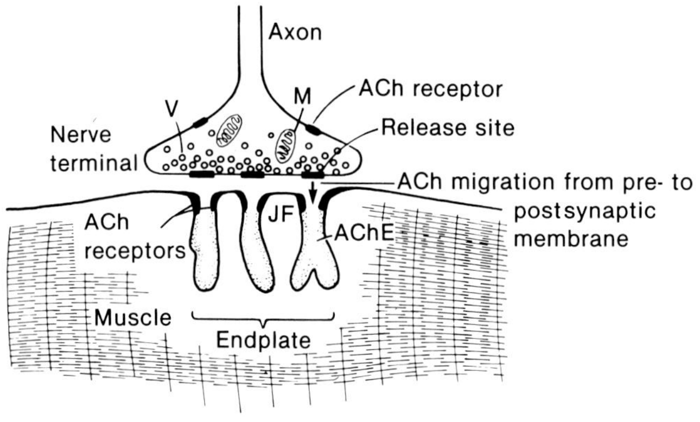

Figure 34–1 • A schematic illustration of the neuromuscular junction: the nerve terminal, the pre- and postsynaptic membranes, the synaptic cleft, and the motor endplate. See text for full explanation of the junctional anatomy. V = acetylcholine vesicles; M = mitochondria; Ach = acetylcholine; AchE = acetylcholinesterase; JF = junctional fold. (Redrawn from Drachman DB. Myasthenia gravis. N Engl J Med 298:136, 1978; with permission.)

Acetylcholine molecules also interact with presynaptic acetylcholine receptors. This apparently facilitates acetylcholine release during high-frequency tetanic stimulation, and thus sustains the tetanic response of the muscle.

The effect of acetylcholine at the NM junction is short-lived because it is rapidly metabolized by the local acetylcholinesterase. This permits rapid closure of the ion channels and restoration of the muscle membrane resting potential.

Normal NM transmission has a large margin of safety. Depending on the muscle, as little as 5% to 25% of the acetylcholine receptor population is needed to maintain normal NM transmission.[4,5] Transmission, therefore, persists even when as many as 75% to 95% of the receptors are occupied by a muscle relaxant.

C. *Modes of Action of Muscle Relaxants*

Muscle relaxants block NM transmission primarily by interacting with acetylcholine receptors at the NM junction. The depolarizing muscle relaxants, such as succinylcholine, interact with acetylcholine receptors in a fashion similar to that of acetylcholine, and cause depolarization of the endplate. However, unlike acetylcholine, succinylcholine is not metabolized by the local acetylcholinesterase. As a result, the endplate remains depolarized (and the muscle paralyzed) until succinylcholine diffuses out of the NM junction.

The nondepolarizing muscle relaxants block NM transmission by competing with acetylcholine for acetylcholine receptors. The more molecules of a muscle relaxant that reach the NM junction, the higher the receptor occupancy by the muscle relaxant, and the greater the likelihood of NM blockade. Conversely, an increase in the number of acetylcholine molecules at the NM junction (caused by a reversal agent such as neostigmine) would decrease receptor occupancy by the muscle relaxant and reverse the blockade. Reversal of the blockade would occur despite the presence of molecules of the muscle relaxant at the NM junction.

In addition to binding postsynaptic acetylcholine receptors, the nondepolarizing relaxants also bind presynaptic acetylcholine receptors. This apparently inhibits acetylcholine release during tetanic stimulation and causes tetanic fade. Some muscle relaxants have greater affinity than others for the presynaptic receptors, and thus cause greater tetanic fade with an earlier onset. For example, curare causes greater fade, with an earlier onset, than pancuronium.

In addition to binding the recognition sites of acetylcholine receptors, the molecules of a muscle relaxant may enter the ion channels of the receptors. When given in excessive doses, muscle relaxants block the channels and prevent the movement of ions across the membrane. This causes NM blockade that is unresponsive to anticholinesterases.

D. *Principles of NM Transmission Monitoring*

In awake and cooperative patients, NM transmission can be assessed by asking the patient to open the eyes, protrude the tongue, swallow, cough, and sustain handgrip and head-lift. Bedside pulmonary function tests, such as tidal volume, vital capacity, inspiratory pressure, and peak expiratory flow rates are also useful. In the anesthetized patient, monitoring can be accomplished only by nerve stimulation.

In general, NM transmission monitoring is achieved by assessing the mechanical or electrical response of a muscle to nerve stimulation. The mechanical response can be assessed either visually and tactually, or by a pressure monitoring system. The electrical response is measured by an electromyograph.

II. How to Monitor NM Transmission

A. *The Hardware of NM Transmission Monitoring*

1. Nerve Stimulators

A variety of nerve stimulators are available for clinical use (Figs. 34–2 through 34–4).[6,7] All are battery-operated and deliver impulses of direct current at adjustable voltage and frequency. Each impulse forms a perfect rectangle that lasts 0.1–0.2 msec (Fig. 34–5).

In accordance with Ohm's laws of electricity, the current output of a nerve stimulator is directly proportional to its voltage output and inversely proportional to the electric resistance of the patient's skin. When the voltage output is constant, the greater the skin resistance the smaller the current that reaches the nerve.

For reliable monitoring, the current output of the nerve stimulator should be sufficiently high to activate all functional (unblocked) motor units of the muscle (maximal stimulation). Since the electric resistance of the patient's skin often increases with time (usually due to drying out of the stimulating electrodes), the current that reaches the nerve gradually decreases, resulting in artificially reduced muscle response. This may mislead the clinician to believe that the patient is adequately relaxed.

To maintain maximal nerve stimulation at all times, the nerve stimulator is set to deliver voltage 20% higher than maximal stimulation (supramaximal stimulation). This insures maximal stimulation as long as skin resistance does not increase by more than 20%.[8]

When using surface electrodes, a current of 30–60 milliamperes (mA) is necessary to produce supramaximal stimulation.[7,9] The thicker the patient's skin, the more current is needed. Most nerve stimulators can deliver supramaximal stimulation even when skin resistance is as high as 5,000 ohms.[7,10] Normal skin resistance is about 1000 ohms.

If surface electrodes fail to deliver supramaximal stimulation, needle electrodes can be used instead.[7] Since the needles are embedded in interstitial fluid, they bypass skin resistance, and therefore require lower voltage to produce supramaximal stimulation.

Advanced nerve stimulators automatically adjust the current output to compensate for changes in skin electric resistance. These constant-current stimulators maintain maximal stimulation as long as skin resistance is not greater than 5000 ohms.[6,7] Some nerve stimulators are equipped with a digital display that indicates the current output in milliamperes (see Fig. 34–4). Although they do not automatically maintain constant current, their digital display facilitates manual adjustment of the output.

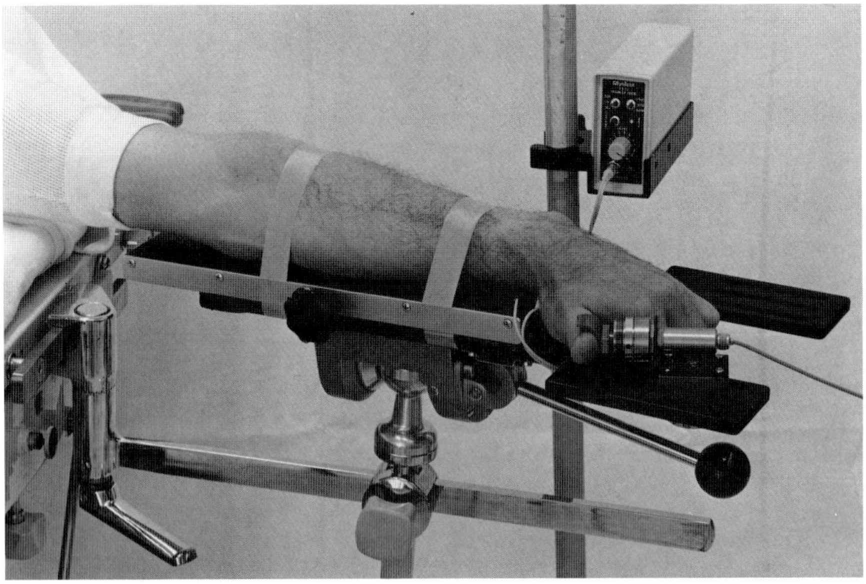

Figure 34–2 • Monitoring of the mechanical response of the thumb with force displacement transducer. The nerve stimulator causes contraction of the thumb, which presses against the transducer and generates a written record of the contraction. (Courtesy of Dr J. Viby-Mogensen and Biometer International, Inc, Denmark.)

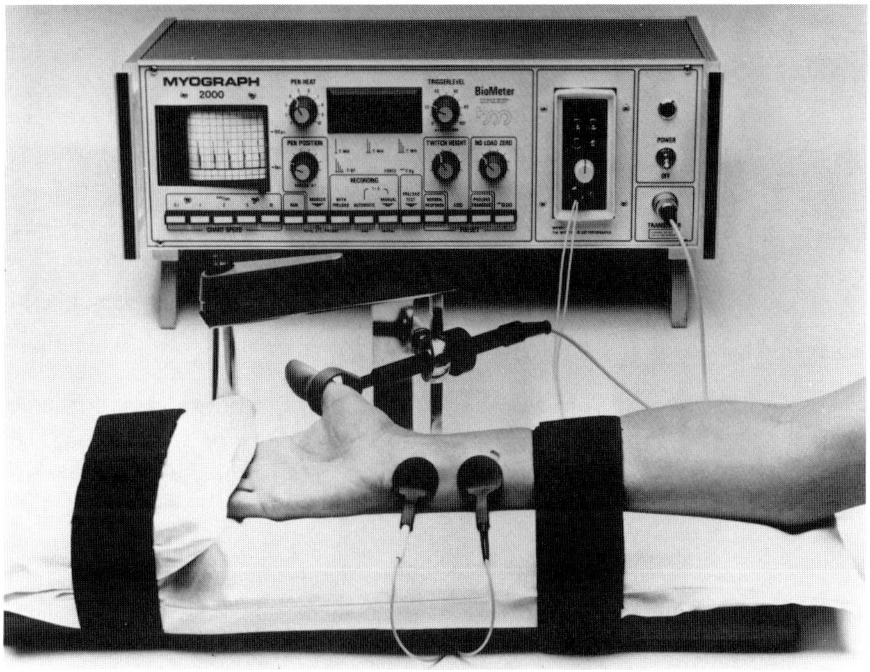

Figure 34–3 • The Myograph 2000, a complete monitoring system of the mechanical response of the thumb, contains all the components shown in Fig. 34–2. The pulling force of the thumb is measured. (Courtesy of Dr J Viby-Mogensen and Biometer International, Inc, Denmark.)

Nerve stimulators can deliver impulses at various frequencies. The most commonly used frequencies are single stimuli delivered at 0.1 or 0.15 Hz (one stimulus every 10 or 6 seconds, respectively); trains of stimuli delivered at 50 Hz and 100 Hz; and train-of-four (TOF) delivered at 2 Hz. Recently, a nerve stimulator with double burst stimulation (DBS) capability has been introduced.

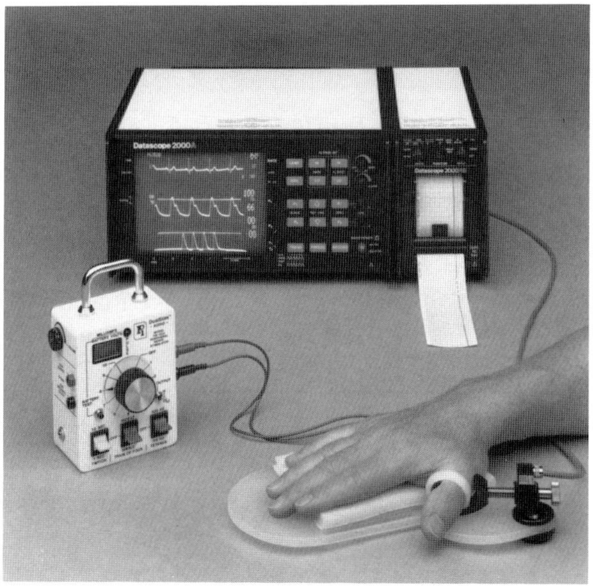

Figure 34–4 • The Myotrace, a complete monitoring system of the mechanical response of the thumb. (Courtesy of Dr A. Stanec.)

Occasionally, nerve stimulators malfunction. The more common causes are exhausted batteries, defective leads, excessive skin resistance, and poor electrode–skin contact.

2. MONITORS OF THE MECHANICAL RESPONSE OF A MUSCLE

Since visual and tactile assessment of NM transmission is often inaccurate,[11] various devices have been developed to measure the mechanical response of the muscle to nerve stimulation.[12,13] However, most are cumbersome and often suffer from baseline drift. The following devices for monitoring the mechanical response of a muscle are easy to use and are considered reliable.

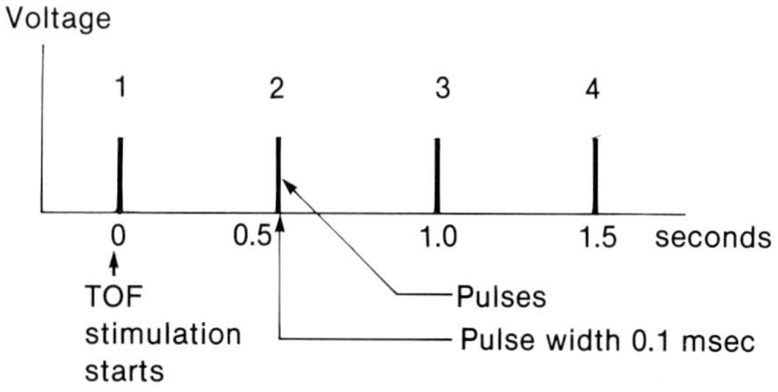

Figure 34–5 • Simulation of train-of-four (TOF) output of a nerve stimulator. Notice the sharp rise and decline of each narrow rectangular impulse.

a. *Force Displacement Transducer*

The *transducer* measures the force generated by the muscle in response to nerve stimulation and generates an electronic signal that is quantitated, displayed, and recorded by a monitor (see Figs. 34–2 through 34–4).[14,15] Force displacement transducers are susceptible to overloading and to changes in orientation of the force measured.[16,17] Since the commonly monitored contractions of the thumb may develop a force of 8–10 kg, only transducers with an 8- to 10-kg capacity shou ld be used. This avoids transducer overloading.[17] Changes in the orientation of the force of contraction can be minimized by firmly attaching the transducer to the patient's hand and splinting the arm.

b. *Acceleration Transducer*

Accelography is a new method of monitoring the mechanical response of a muscle to nerve stimulation.[18] It is based on Newton's second law of motion, which states that a moving object accelerates at a rate directly proportional to the magnitude of the force that is moving it. Accordingly, during NM transmission monitoring, the thumb accelerates at a rate directly proportional to the force of contraction of the adductor pollicis. The acceleration of the thumb can be measured by a specially designed piezoelectric transducer. When this transducer is attached to the thumb, it generates an electronic signal that is directly proportional to the force of contraction of the adductor pollicis. The signal is quantitated, displayed, and recorded by a monitor (Fig. 34–6).[19]

Accelography is easy to use because it requires minimal fixation of the hand. However, this method is particularly prone to baseline drift.*† For unknown reasons, the baseline TOF response shows reverse fade (the first response is smaller than the fourth one).[2] However, in general, there is good correlation between force displacement monitoring and accelography, except during recovery from muscle relaxants.[18]

c. *The Myoscan*

The Myoscan is a simple device that stretches the thumb and enhances the response to nerve stimulation (Fig. 34–7).[20] Weak twitches that might otherwise be overlooked are augmented and visually detected. The Myoscan was found to be as useful as a force displacement transducer for clinical monitoring.[20]

3. Monitors of the Electric Response of a Muscle

The electric response of a muscle to nerve stimulation can be monitored with an electromyograph. In the past, electromyographs were too cumbersome and expensive for routine operating room use. Presently, however, small portable units are available and regularly used.[21,22]

A typical electromyographic monitor is the Datex Relaxograph (Datex, Wilmington, MA) (Fig. 34–8). It includes a nerve stimulator, a chart recorder, and a digital display. The monitor integrates individual muscle action potentials and then quantitates and prints the re-

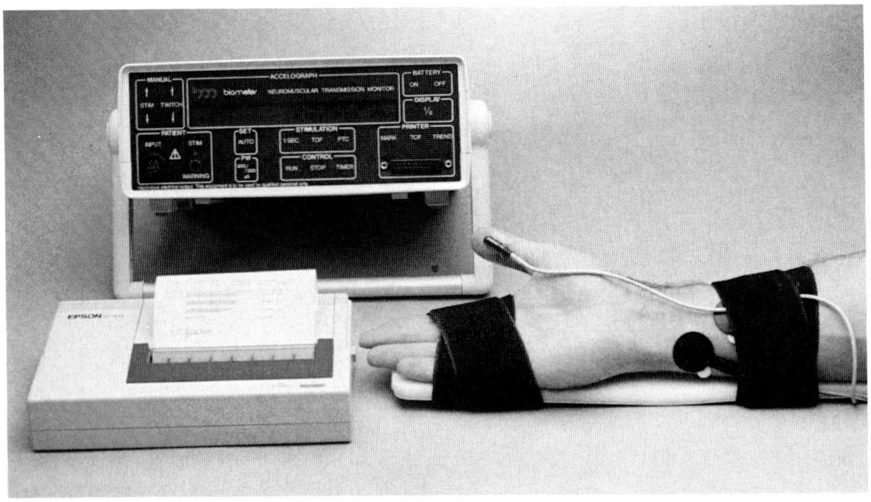

Figure 34–6 • A complete system for accelographic monitoring of the mechanical response of the thumb. The nerve stimulator causes contraction of the thumb, which then activates the acceleration transducer, resulting in a digital readout, and generates a written record of the transaction. (Courtesy of Dr J. Viby-Mogensen and Biometer International, Inc, Denmark.)

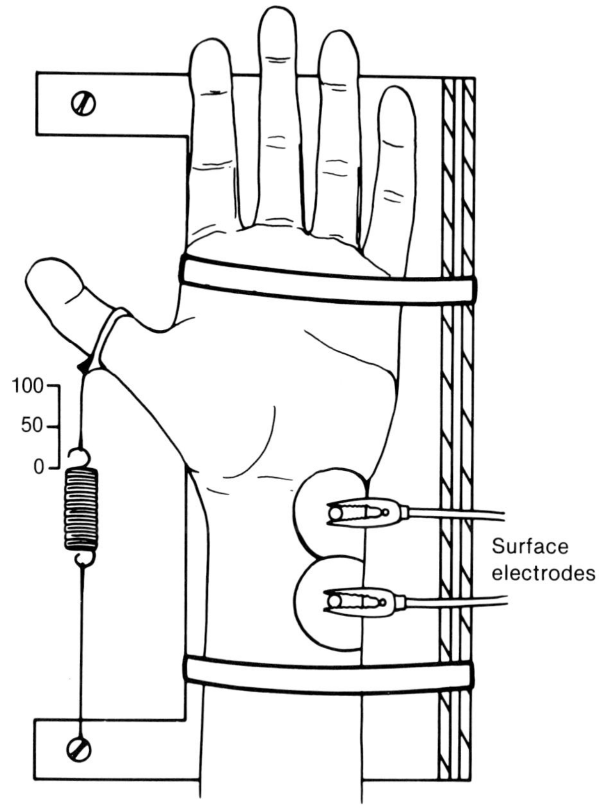

Figure 34-7 • The Myoscan, a device that stretches the thumb and augments the response to nerve stimulation. (Courtesy of Dr H. Nagashima.)

sults. Also, percent twitch depression and TOF fade ratio (see later) are calculated and displayed.

In contrast to force displacement monitoring, electromyographic is not vulnerable to overloading. However, the response often fails to return to baseline, despite complete reversal of the NM blockade.[23-25] Some believe that this is due to a change in orientation of the electric vector of the muscle.[23] Others suggest that stretching of the thumb is necessary for reproducible results.[24,25]

B. *The Procedure for Monitoring NM Transmission*

1. How to Apply Nerve Stimulation

a. *Selecting a Site*

A convenient and easy-to-reach site should be selected for nerve stimulation. This will depend primarily on the patient's position during surgery. The monitored muscle and the corresponding nerve should be free of disease, and the skin at the site of stimulation should be free of lesions and oily lotions.

The most popular and convenient site for nerve stimulation is the wrist. The stimulating electrodes are

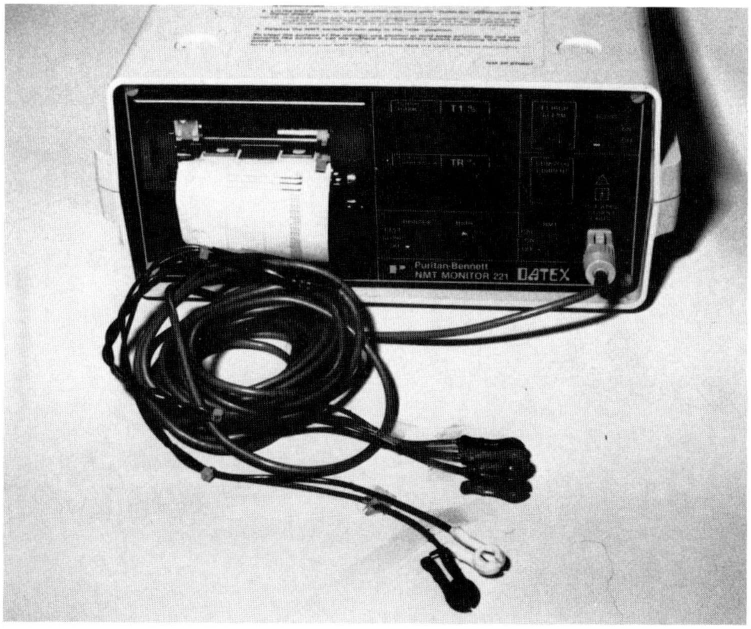

Figure 34-8 • The Datex Relaxograph, a complete system for monitoring the electrical response of a muscle. The monitor integrates individual muscle action potentials that are evoked by nerve stimulation and received by the recording electrodes. (Courtesy of Datex Inc, Wilmington, MA)

applied to the anteromedial aspect of the wrist, in the groove between the tendons of the flexor carpi ulnaris and the flexor digitorum superficialis (see Fig. 34–3). There the ulnar nerve travels superficially before it enters the hand (Fig. 34–9).

Other less commonly used sites for nerve stimulation are

- The medial-posterior aspect of the elbow, where the ulnar nerve travels superficially behind the medial epicondyle (see Fig. 34–9).
- The medial aspect of the ankle, where stimulating the tibialis posterior nerve behind the medial malleolus causes contraction of the flexor hallucis brevis and plantar flexion of the foot (Fig. 34–10).[26]
- The lateral aspect of the knee, where stimulating the peroneal nerve behind the head of the fibula causes contraction of the extensor hallucis brevis and dorsiflexion of the foot (Fig. 34–11).
- The lateral aspect of the face, where stimulating the ophthalmic branch of the facial nerve causes contraction of the orbicularis oculi and wincing of the corresponding side of the face (Fig. 34–12).

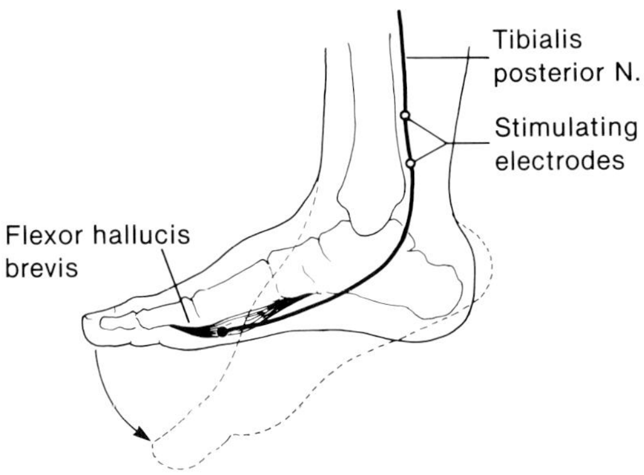

Figure 34–10 • A schematic drawing of the anatomy of the medial side of the ankle and foot, with a site for nerve stimulation. Contraction of the flexor hallucis brevis causes plantar flexion of the foot.

b. *Placing the Stimulating Electrodes*

Nerve stimulators are equipped with two electrodes, an *anode* (positive polarity) and a *cathode* (negative polarity). The electrode closer to the nerve serves as the active, or stimulating, electrode. Stimulation is most efficient (ie, less current is needed to generate supramaximal stimulation) when the cathode is the active electrode. Therefore, the cathode should be placed closer to the nerve than the anode.[27,28] When both electrodes are placed at the same distance from the nerve (as is usually the case when the ulnar nerve is stimulated at the wrist), the

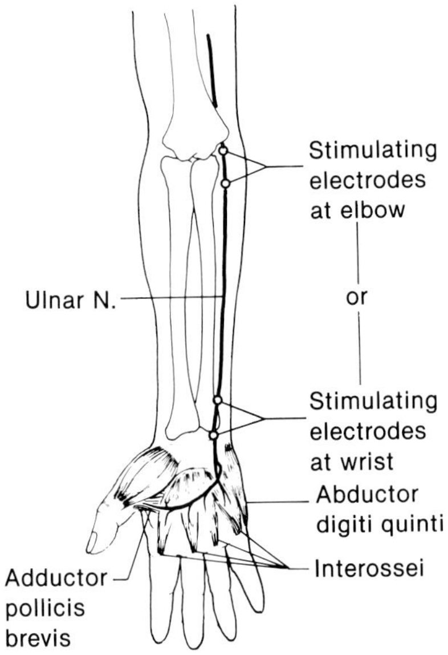

Figure 34–9 • A schematic drawing of the anatomy of the arm and hand, with optional sites for nerve stimulation. (See Fig. 34–3 for a photograph of the position of the stimulating electrodes at the wrist.) The site at the elbow is behind the medial epicondyle.

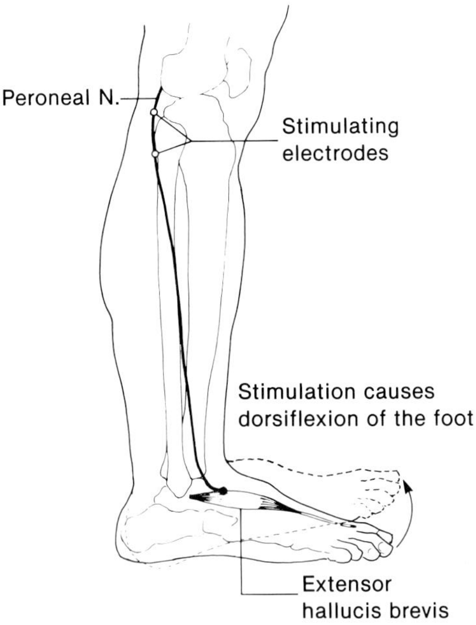

Figure 34–11 • A schematic drawing of the anatomy of the lateral aspect of the knee and foot, with a site for nerve stimulation. Contraction of the extensor hallucis brevis causes dorsiflexion of the foot.

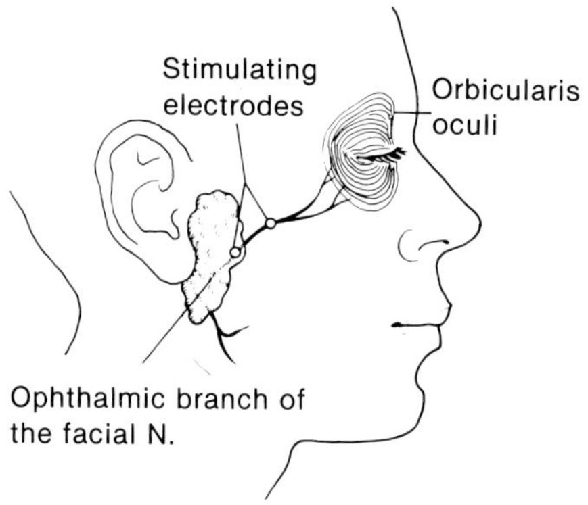

Figure 34–12 • A schematic drawing of the anatomy of the lateral aspect of the face, with a site for nerve stimulation. Contraction of the orbicularis oculi causes ipsilateral facial wincing.

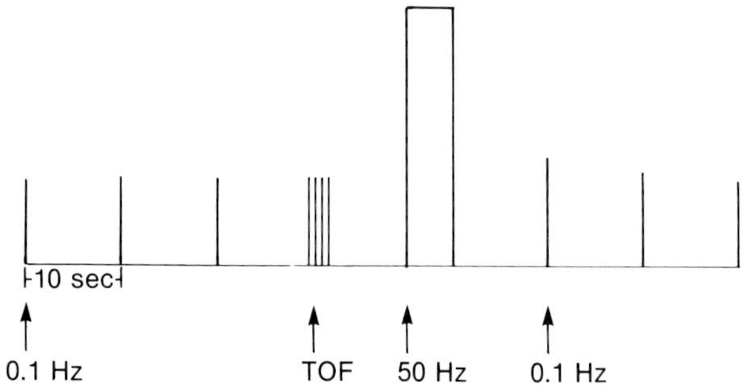

Figure 34–13 • Simulation of baseline response of a muscle-to-nerve stimulation. The response to single stimuli, TOF stimulation, 50-Hz tetanic stimulation, and posttetanic stimulation is illustrated. The immediate posttetanic response is greater than the pretetanic response.

cathode functions as the active electrode, and stimulation is most efficient.

In the operating room, skin surface electrodes are usually used for nerve stimulation. Although needles and bananalike metal probes are occasionally also used, they are not as convenient and may be fraught with complications.[29]

c. *Setting Supramaximal Stimulation*

After the patient is anesthetized (but before muscle relaxants are given), the nerve stimulator is turned on. The voltage output is gradually increased, and the response of the muscle is observed. At first, with each increment in output, the response of the muscle increases. Eventually, increasing the output causes no further increase in the response. This indicates than maximal stimulation has been reached (see earlier).

After reaching maximal stimulation, the stimulator's output is further increased by 20% to deliver supramaximal stimulation. This insures maximal stimulation at all times, even if the skin's electric resistance increases during surgery.

d. *Setting the Frequency of Stimulation*

The most commonly used stimulation frequencies are single stimuli, train-of-four (TOF), and 50-Hz tetanic stimulation (Figs. 34–13 and 34–14). The single stimuli are delivered at a frequency no greater than 0.15 Hz (one every 6 seconds). Higher frequencies may reduce the amount of acetylcholine that is released per stimulus and diminish the response of the muscle. This may mislead the clinician into believing the blockade is more intense that it really is.[30]

Train-of-four stimulation is presently the most popular mode of nerve stimulation. It allows simple quantitation of the NM blockade by counting muscle twitches. Also, unlike tetanic stimulation, it causes only moderate discomfort to the awake patient. Monitoring TOF is based on the response of the muscle to four stimuli administered at a 2-Hz frequency. This frequency was selected because higher frequencies cause fusion of individual muscle twitches (making twitch counting impossible), and lower frequencies cause no fade (in the presence of nondepolarizing NM blockade the fade provides essential information on the quality and intensity of the blockade).[31,32] The duration of each TOF stimulus is 1.5 seconds. This duration was selected because a longer duration would provide no additional information, and a shorter one would miss part of the fade (Fig. 34–15).

For tetanic stimulation, a 50-Hz frequency is often used because it is physiologic (the frequency observed

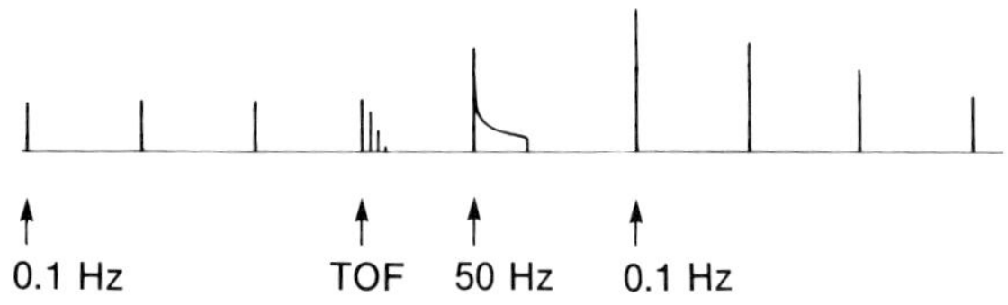

Figure 34–14 • Simulation of the response of a muscle to nerve stimulation in the presence of partial nondepolarizing neruomuscular blockade. The responses to single stimuli, TOF stimulation, 50-Hz tetanic stimulation, and posttetanic response to single stimuli are illustrated. Compare the amplitude of responses with those in Fig. 34–13.

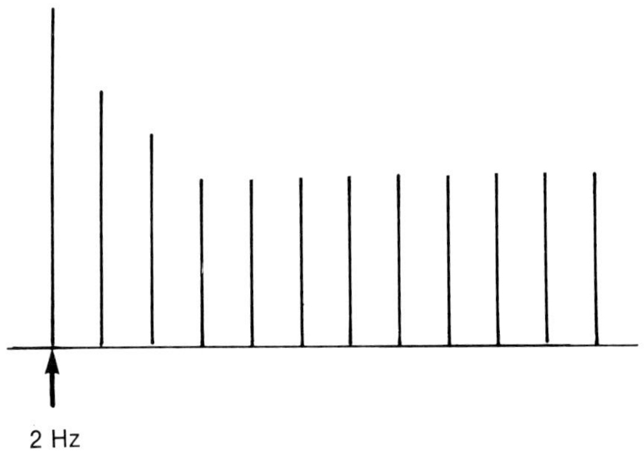

Figure 34–15 • Simulation of mechanical response of a muscle to 2-Hz nerve stimulation (as is used in train-of-four monitoring) in the presence of partial nondepolarizing neuromuscular blockade. Note that the fade in the response reaches its nadir on the fourth twitch, and that no additional information is gained beyond that.

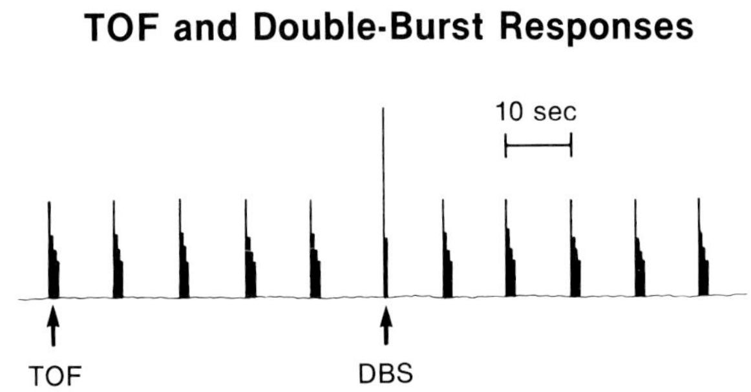

Figure 34–17 • A comparison of double-burst stimulation (DBS) and TOF responses. Note the greater initial response and the greater difference between the first and last response during double burst stimulation. (Redrawn from Engback J, Ostergaard D, Viby-Mogensen J. Double burst stimulation (DBS): A new pattern of nerve stimulation to identify neuromuscular blockade. Br J Anesth 62:274–278, 1989; with permission.)

during voluntary muscle contraction).[33] Some authors recommend higher frequencies for detection of subliminal NM blockades.[34] However, higher frequencies may cause tetanic fade even when no muscle relaxants have been given.

Recently, the use of double burst stimulation (DBS) has been described (Fig. 34–16).[36] It is comprised of two 50-Hz bursts of three stimuli each, separated by a 750-msec time interval (Fig. 34–17). Double burst stimulation has been shown to facilitate visual assessment of NM transmission; however, experience with this modality is still limited.

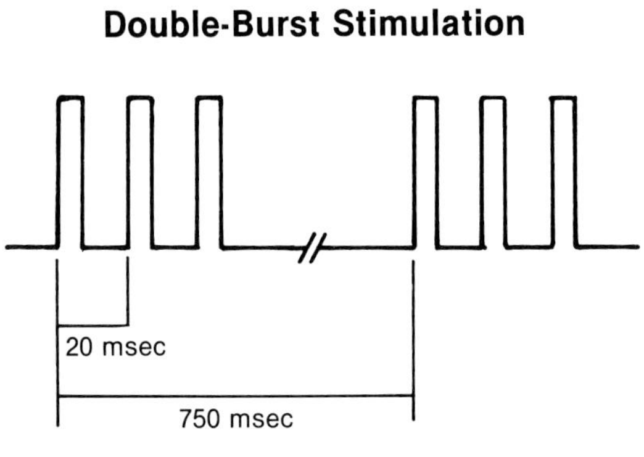

Figure 34–16 • Double-burst output of a nerve stimulator. Each burst comprises three impulses delivered at a 50-Hz frequency. The two bursts are separated by a 750-msec time lag. See text for further explanation. (Redrawn from Engback J, Ostergaard D, Viby-Mogensen J. Double burst stimulator (DBS): A new pattern of nerve stimulation to identify neuromuscular blockade. Br J Anaesth 62:274–278, 1989; with permission.)

2. How to Monitor the Mechanical Response of a Muscle

a. *Visual and Tactile Assessment*

Visual and tactile assessment of the mechanical response of a muscle is simple and, therefore, most commonly used in the operating room. For tactile assessment, the clinician places his or her fingers over the patient's thumb and feels the response to nerve stimulation. This provides qualitative and quantitative information on the blockade. If the clinician sees or feels tetanic fade, nondepolarizing blockade exists. The intensity of the blockade can be determined by counting TOF twitches. The fewer twitches perceived, the more intense the blockade.

Visual and tactile assessment of NM transmission is often inaccurate, particularly postoperatively, when residual NM blockade is being assessed.[11] The Myoscan facilitates visual assessment by stretching the monitored muscle and thus augmenting its response to nerve stimulation (see Fig. 34–7).[20]

b. *Monitoring Force Displacement*

A force displacement transducer is usually attached to the patient's hand in a manner that permits the thumb to exert pressure or pull on the transducer (see Figs.

34–2 through 34–4). The hand and forearm are firmly strapped to a special arm board, and the thumb is stretched with a 200- to 300-g force. This insures maximal and consistent response to nerve stimulation.[37]

c. *Accelography*

A thin, 1-inch acceleration transducer is taped to the palmar side of the thumb (see Fig. 34–6). The thumb is allowed to move freely, but the hand is strapped to reduce baseline drift.

3. How to Monitor the Electric Response of a Muscle

The muscles most commonly used for electromyography are the adductor pollicis (thenar), the abductor minimi digitti (hypothenar), and the first interosseous muscle of the hand.[38] Because of its thin skin, the hypothenar is particularly well suited for recording muscle action potentials (Fig. 34–18).[39] If the patient's hands are not accessible, the muscles of the feet can be monitored instead (see Figs. 34–10 and 34–11).[26]

A popular portable electromyograph, the Datex Relaxograph, includes a nerve stimulator and three sets of electrodes: one to stimulate the nerve, another to record the electric response of the muscle, and yet another for grounding (see Fig. 34–8). Supramaximal TOF stimulation is automatically set immediately after the monitor is turned on.

III. Discussion of NM Transmission Monitoring

A. *Interpretation of NM Transmission Monitoring*

1. General Considerations

Perioperative monitoring of respiratory and abdominal muscles would be useful because their function is closely related to respiratory function and surgical relaxation. However, monitoring these muscles in the operating room is not practical.[40] Instead, the hand muscles are usually monitored.

Significant differences exist in the response of various groups of muscles to muscle relaxants. Compared with muscles of the extremities, the respiratory, laryngeal, and facial muscles are resistant to muscle relaxants.[5,10,26,41–43] Therefore, monitoring of hand muscles tends to overestimate the NM blockade in more centrally located muscles. It is not unusual for a patient with minimal or no response of hand muscles to nerve stimulation to exhibit significant spontaneous respiratory effort and facial grimaces.

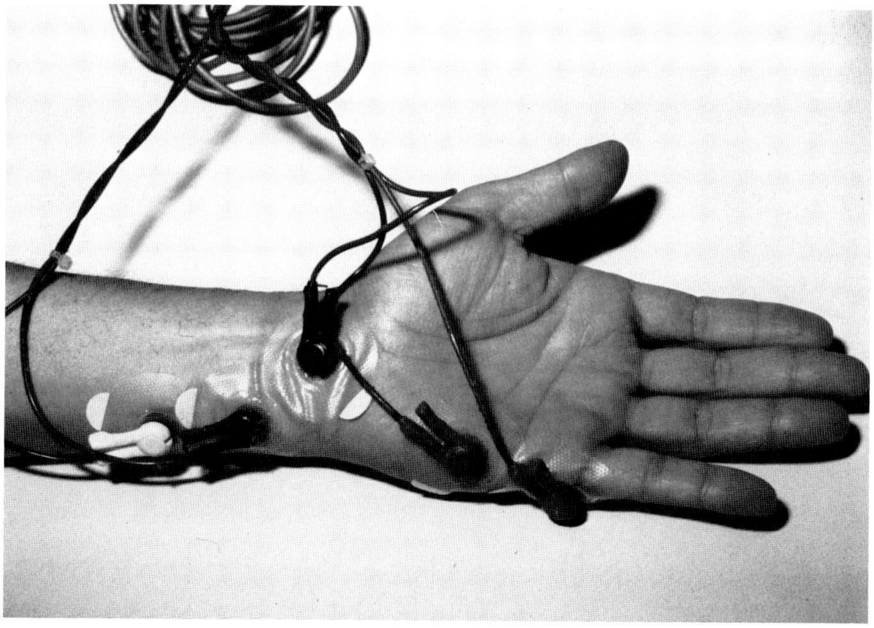

Figure 34–18 • Placement of electrodes for ulnar nerve stimulation and for electromyography of the hypothenar muscles. One set of electrodes is for electrical stimulation, another for recording the electrical response, and yet another for grounding.

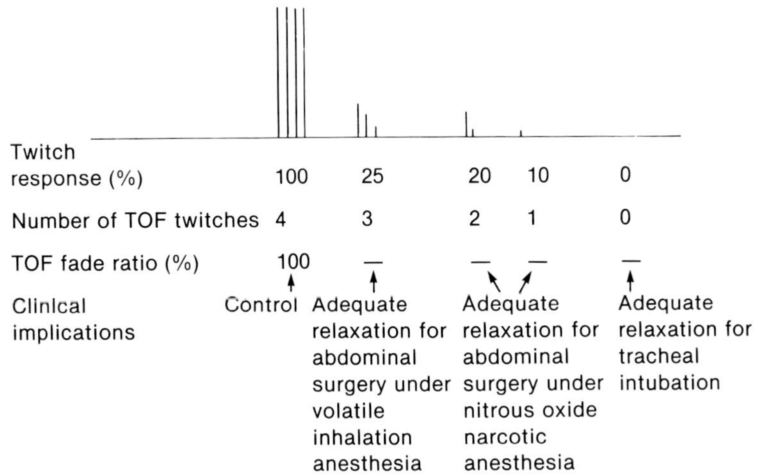

Figure 34–19 • The relationship between single-twitch depression, TOF response, TOF fade ratio, and clinical implications during onset of nondepolarizing neuromuscular blockade. (After Viby-Mogensen J Clinical assessment of neuromuscular transmission. Br J Anaesth 54:209, 1982.)

2. THE SINGLE-TWITCH RESPONSE

The single-twitch response is used to compare potencies, onset times, and durations of action of various muscle relaxants.[44] It is also used to determine important clinical endpoints of muscle relaxation. For example, 75% to 90% twitch depression provides adequate relaxation for abdominal surgery, and 95% to 100% for tracheal intubation (Fig. 34–19).[44] The single-twitch response, however, is a poor indicator of adequate NM blockade reversal; when it returns to its baseline size, the receptor occupancy rate at the NM junction may still be as high as 80%.[5,45,46]

3. THE TETANIC RESPONSE

Tetanic stimulation is used to determine the quality of the NM blockade (whether it is depolarizing or nondepolarizing), as well as to detect residual NM blockade. Tetanic stimulation causes fusion of individual muscle twitches into a single tetanic contraction. This occurs because the time interval between stimuli is very short and does not allow complete muscle relaxation (see Fig. 34–13).

All NM blockades reduce the response to tetanic stimulation; however, only nondepolarizing and phase II blockades cause tetanic fade. The fade is a result of a decrease in acetylcholine release at the NM junction during tetanic stimulation. The higher the tetanic frequency, the smaller the amount of acetylcholine released per stimulus.

Normally, NM transmission is fully maintained at tetanic frequencies as high as 100 Hz (Fig. 34–20). However, in the presence of a nondepolarizing muscle relaxant, the margin of safety decreases (a larger amount of acetylcholine is needed to maintain NM transmission), and therefore, the tetanic response fades (Fig. 34–21). The more intense the NM blockade and the

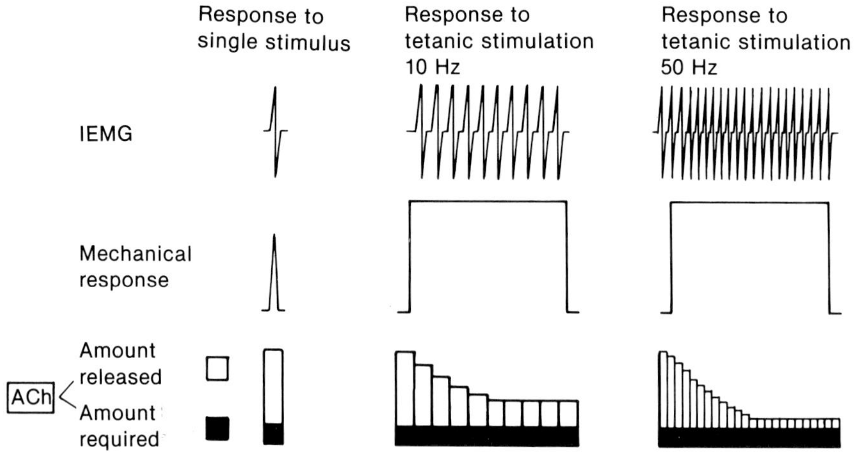

Figure 34–20 • A schematic representation of putative events at the neuromuscular junction in response to nerve stimulation before administration of muscle relaxants. (Top) integrated electromyography (IEMG); (middle) mechanical response; (bottom) quantities of acetylcholine (Ach) required and released. Note that although acetylcholine release per impulse decreases during tetanic stimulation, the tetanic response is sustained. The quantitative parameters in this figure are not necessarily authentic.

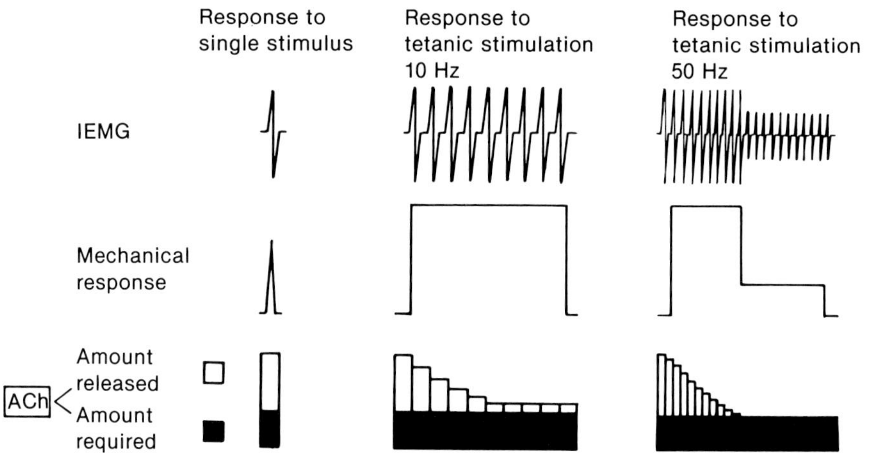

Figure 34–21 • A schematic representation of putative events at the neuromuscular junction in response to nerve stimulation in the presence of partial nondepolarizing neuromuscular blockade. (Top) Integrated electromyography (IEMG); (middle) mechanical response; (bottom) the quantities of acetylcholine (ACh) required and released. Note that a higher level of acetylcholine is required to sustain the tetanic response in the presence of nondepolarizing NM blockade. During high-frequency (50-Hz) tetanic stimulation, acetylcholine release falls below the critical level required to sustain tetanic response. The quantitative parameters in this figure are not necessarily authentic.

higher the tetanic frequency, the greater the tetanic fade (Fig. 34–22).

High-frequency nerve stimulation is used to detect subliminal NM blockade. The frequency is gradually increased while the tetanic response is observed. The lower the frequency that causes tetanic fade, the higher the receptor occupancy rate (see Fig. 34–22).

Tetanic stimulation has several drawbacks. It is painful and, therefore, poorly tolerated by conscious patients. Also, when frequently repeated, it increases blood flow to the monitored muscle and accelerates its recovery from muscle relaxants. This may lead to underestimation of the overall NM blockade. In addition, frequently repeated tetanic stimulation may cause skin injuries.[47]

4. THE POSTTETANIC RESPONSE

One of the hallmarks of nondepolarizing NM blockade is post-tetanic potentiation (PTP). The response to single-nerve stimuli, administered shortly after tetanic stimulation, is temporarily enhanced by at least 50% (see Fig. 34–14). This is apparently a result of a transient increase in acetylcholine release induced by the tetanic stimulation. In addition to distinguishing between depolarizing and nondepolarizing blockades, the post-tetanic

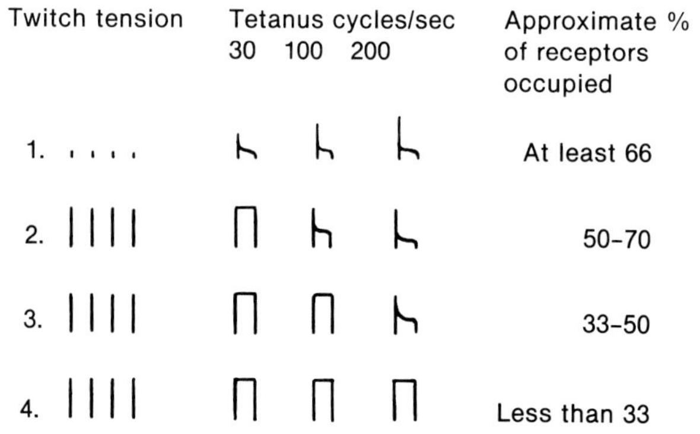

Figure 34–22 • The response of a muscle-to-tetanic-nerve stimulation in the presence of various rates of receptor occupancy. The higher the receptor occupancy rate, the lower the frequency that will cause fade. (Redrawn from Miller RD. Monitoring of neuromuscular transmission. In: Saidman LT, Smith NT (eds). Monitoring in Anesthesia. (2nd ed.) Boston: Butterworth, 1984, p. 196. Data from Waud BE, Waud DR. The relation between tetanic fade and receptor occlusion in the presence of competitive neuromuscular block. Anesthesiology 35:456–464, 1971; with permission.)

response can also be used to estimate the recovery time from intense NM blockade. Some degree of PTP is often observed during the baseline monitoring, before muscle relaxants have been given. However, it is minimal and significantly smaller than that seen in the presence of nondepolarizing NM blocking agents.[48]

5. The Train-of-Four Response

Train-of-four monitoring is used to titrate the NM blockade during surgery, to distinguish between depolarizing and nondepolarizing NM blockades, and to assess reversal of the NM blockade. The baseline response to TOF stimulation is made of four equal muscle twitches. Shortly after the administration of a nondepolarizing muscle relaxant, the TOF response starts to fade. As the blockade further intensifies,the number of TOF twitches decreases to three, two, one, and then none. This corresponds to 75%, 80%, 90%, and 100% single-twitch depression, respectively (see Fig. 34–19).[49] Depending on the anesthetic agent, adequate muscle relaxation for abdominal surgery is achieved when the TOF response is reduced to one to two twitches (80%–90% twitch depression). Tracheal intubation usually requires complete abolishment of the TOF response (100% twitch depression) (see Fig. 34–19).

When assessing reversal of NM blockade, TOF monitoring has been shown to be more informative than either single-twitch or 50-Hz tetanic response monitoring.[50] At the time when the single twitch and tetanic response return to baseline, the TOF response still shows fade.[45,46] When all four twitches of the TOF response are present, the intensity of the NM blockade can be quantitated by calculating the ratio between the fourth and first twitches. This is the *TOF fade ratio* (Fig. 34–23). This ratio is inversely related to the intensity of the residual blockade. The greater the intensity of the blockade, the smaller the fade ratio. A fade ratio of 0.7 or greater indicates adequate reversal of the blockade.

Train-of-four monitoring can also be used to distinguish between the two phases of succinylcholine-induced NM blockade. Phase I reduces the TOF response, but causes no significant fade. When it appears, the blockade is considered to be in Phase II if the fade ratio is 0.4 or less.[51]

6. Differences Between the Mechanical and Electric Responses of Muscles

The mechanical response of a muscle to nerve stimulation is significantly slower than its electric response.

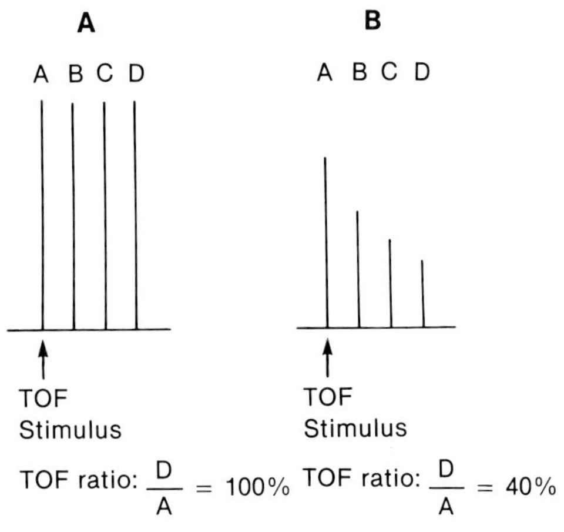

Figure 34–23 • The response to TOF stimulation and the TOF fade ratio before (***A***) and after (***B***) administration of a nondepolarizing muscle relaxant.

This is particularly obvious during tetanic stimulation. The electric response consists of distinct individual muscle action potentials, whereas the mechanical response consists of one tetanic contraction.

There is no consensus as to whether muscle relaxants equally depress the electric and mechanical responses of a muscle. Most authors believe the effect is similar.[22,38,40,48,52] However, during recovery from nondepolarizing blockade, the mechanical response lags behind the electric response: When the mechanical TOF fade ratio reaches 0.7, the concurrent electric fade ratio is 0.9.[39] Since a mechanical fade ratio of 0.7 is widely accepted as an indicator of adequate blockade reversal, a fade ratio of 0.9 should be achieved for equivalent reversal when using electromyography.[53]

In contrast to nondepolarizing muscle relaxants, succinylcholine has a greater depressant effect on the electric response than on the mechanical response of a muscle.[19,48,54]

B. *Clinical Applications of Monitoring NM Transmission*

1. Determining Whether the Patient Is Ready for Tracheal Intubation

This determination is most important in patients with vascular aneurysms, increased intracranial pressure, pulmonary blebs, increased intraocular pressure, and open eye. If not totally paralyzed, these patients may react strenuously to tracheal intubation and sustain irreversible injury.

2. ASSESSING SENSITIVITY TO MUSCLE RELAXANTS

Because of great variability in response to muscle relaxants, patients occasionally receive excessive or inadequate doses. Monitoring the effect of a test dose before surgery starts should reduce the incidence of prolonged paralysis or inadequate surgical relaxation.

3. TITRATING NM BLOCKADE

Neuromuscular transmission monitoring during surgery permits precise titration of NM blockade. This allows maintenance of adequate muscle relaxation and reduces the risk of postoperative ventilatory failure.

4. ASSESSING REVERSIBILITY OF INTENSE NONDEPOLARIZING NM BLOCKADE

When nerve stimulation elicits no response, intense NM blockade exists. Persistent attempts to reverse such a blockade are usually futile, and may even potentiate it. Instead, the patient should be mechanically ventilated until there is response to nerve stimulation. When this occurs, reversal may be attempted, and is usually successful.

In the presence of intense NM blockade, the first nerve-stimulation response to return is the post-tetanic response (PTR).[55,56] Although the tetanic stimulation fails to elicit response, it transiently increases acetylcholine release, and thus allows post-tetanic response to single nerve stimuli (Fig. 34–24). The return of PTR during intense NM blockade is an indicator of time-to-return of the first TOF response. In the presence of pancuronium-induced intense NM blockade, the first TOF response returns about 36 minutes after the first PTR has returned.[55] Similarly, in the presence of vecuronium-induced intense NM blockade, the first TOF response returns 18 minutes after the first PTR has returned.[56]

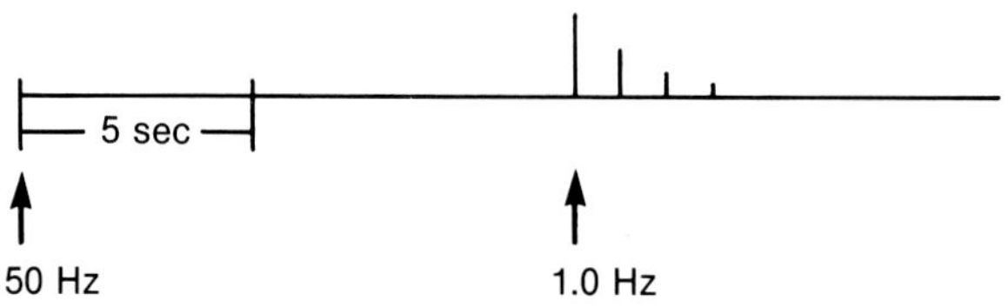

Figure 34–24 • Simulation of a posttetanic response (PTR) in the presence of an intense nondepolarizing neuromuscular blockade. Note the lack of response to 50-Hz tetanic stimulation and the transient posttetanic response to single stimuli. The posttetanic count (PTC) is 4.

Since the return of the first TOF response signals that the blockade is ready for reversal, monitoring the PTR can be used to determined the recovery time from intense NM blockade.

As the intense NM blockade gradually wears off, the number of twitches in the PTR, known as the *PTR count (PTC),* increases. The greater the PTC, the shorter the time-to-return of the first TOF response.[55,56] In the presence of pancuronium-induced intense NM blockade, a PTC of 2, 4, or 8 correlates with 25, 18, or 5 minutes of time-to-return of the first TOF response, respectively (Fig. 34–25).[55] Similarly, in the presence of vecuronium-induced intense NM blockade, a PTC of 2, 4, or 8 correlates with 7, 5, or 1 minutes of time-to-return of the first TOF response, respectively (Fig. 34–26).[56] With either muscle relaxant, a PTC of 10 signals the return of the first TOF response.[55,56]

5. ASSESSING REVERSIBILITY OF PHASE II BLOCKADE

Succinylcholine-induced phase II NM blockade poses a particular clinical problem. Although it is caused by a depolarizing muscle relaxant, it has features of nondepolarizing NM blockade (tetanic fade and PTP). On occasion, phase II blockade can be reversed with an anticholinesterase.[51,57,58] However, indiscriminate administration of a reversal agent may intensify the blockade, rather than reversing it.

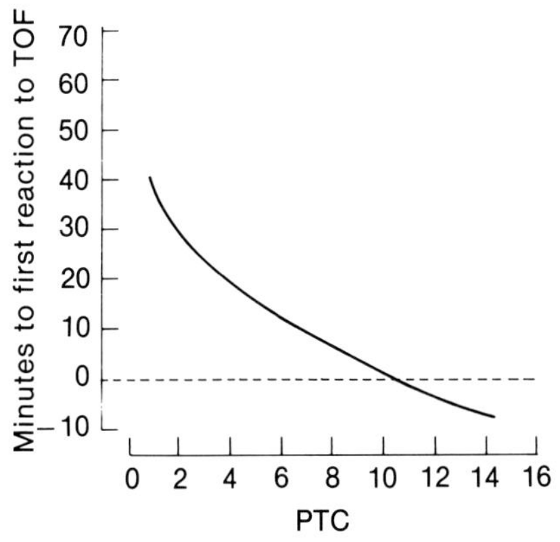

Figure 34–25 • The posttetanic count (PTC) and the time to return of TOF response during recovery from intense pancuronium-induced neuromuscular blockade. (Redrawn from Viby-Mogensen J, Howardy-Hansen P, Chraemmer-Jorgensen B, Ording H, et al. Post-tetanic count [PTC]: A new method of evaluating an intense non-depolarizing neuromuscular blockade. Anesthesiology 55:458–461, 1981; with permission.)

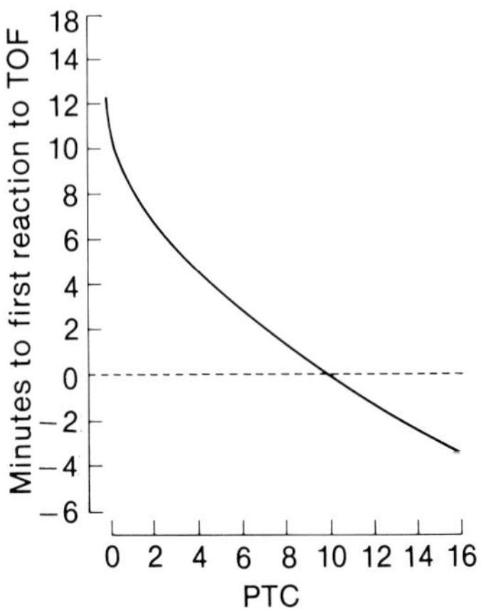

Figure 34–26 • The posttetanic count (PTC) and the time to return of TOF response during recovery from intense vecuronium-induced neuromuscular blockade. (Redrawn from Muchhal KK, Viby-Mogensen J, Fernando PUE, Tamilarsen A, et al. Evaluation of intense neuromuscular blockade caused by vecuronium using post-tetanic count [PTC]. Anesthesiology 66:846–849, 1987; with permission.)

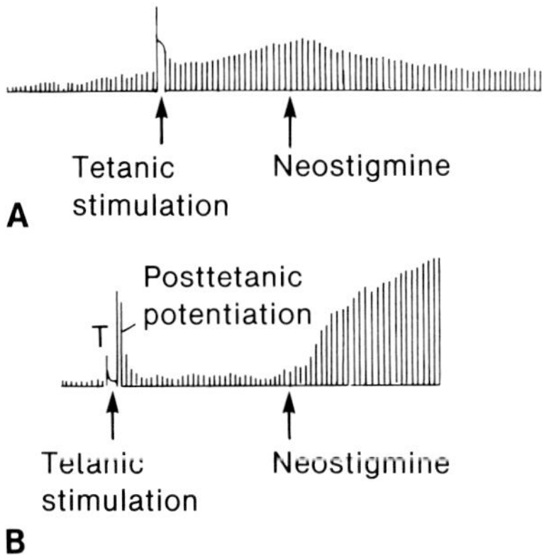

Figure 34–27 • The response of phase II NM blockade to neostigmine. Note that when the tetanic stimulation is not followed by posttetanic potentiation (***A***) the administration of neostigmine intensifies the NM blockade. In contrast, when the tetanic stimulation is followed by post-tetanic potentiation (***B***) the administration of neostigmine reverses the NM blockade. (Redrawn from Baraka A. Post-tetanic facilitation as an index for antagonism of phase II block of succinylcholine in participants with a typical cholinesterase. Anesth Analg 60:911–912, 1981; with permission.)

To determine whether phase II blockade is reversible, it is useful to test the response to tetanic stimulation. If tetanic stimulation causes no fade or PTP, the administration of an anticholinesterase is unlikely to reverse the blockade and may even intensify it. Conversely, if tetanic stimulation causes fade and PTP, the administration of an anticholinesterase is likely to reverse the blockade (Fig. 34–27).

6. Determining the Cause of Postoperative Ventilatory Failure

Common causes of postoperative ventilatory failure are residual effects of general anesthetics on the respiratory center, or residual effects of muscle relaxants at the NM junction. The use of nerve stimulation can determine whether a residual NM blockade exists.

7. Correlating Residual NM Blockade with Ventilatory Reserve

A correlation exists between the TOF fade ratio and pulmonary function. During recovery from NM blockade, when the fade ratio reaches a value of 0.7, the vital capacity and inspiratory force return to normal.[59,60] This fade ratio value, therefore, is commonly considered an indicator of adequate reversal of the NM blockade.

In volunteers,[61] a TOF fade ratio of 0.6 was associated with a 30% decrease in inspiratory pressure and 9% decrease in vital capacity. When the TOF fade ratio rose above 0.6, the tidal volume, vital capacity, and peak expiratory flow rates returned to normal[61] (Fig. 34–28). However, the return of pulmonary function tests to normal is not necessarily accompanied by the return of protective airway reflexes.[62] Inadequate cough and glottic closure might expose patients to pulmonary aspiration.

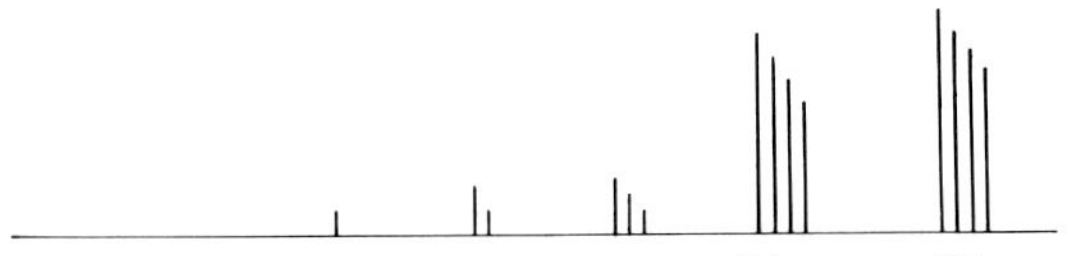

TWITCH RESPONSE (%)	10	20	25	90	100
No of TOF TWITCHES	1	2	3	4	4
TOF FADE RATIO (%)	–	–	–	60	75
CLINICAL IMPLICATIONS	Reversal requires 10-30 min	Reversal requires 8-18 min	Reversal requires 6-8 min	Headlift-3 sec VC ↓ PEFR ↓ IF ->25 cm/H_2O V_T - Normal	Headlift-5 sec VC-Normal PEFR-Normal IF ->25 cm/H_2O V_T - Normal

Figure 34–28 • The relationship between single-twitch depression, TOF response, TOF fade ratio, and clinical implications during recovery from nondepolarizing neuromuscular blockade. IF = Inspiratory force; VT = tidal volume; VC = vital capacity; PEFR = peak expiratory rate. (After Viby-Mogensen J Clinical assessment of neuromuscular transmission. Br J Anaesth 54:209–223, 1982; with permission.)

IV. COMPLICATIONS OF MONITORING NM TRANSMISSION

A. *Skin Burns*

Monitoring of NM transmission rarely causes serious complications. Occasionally, surface electrodes cause skin erythema due either to hypersensitivity to the conductive jelly or to irritation from repeatedly administered high-frequency nerve stimulation. If needle electrodes are used, tiny skin blisters may appear at the site of stimulation.[‡] This is probably due to high-density current at the tips of the needles.

Skin burns have been observed with the Block-Aid nerve stimulator, using bananalike stimulating probes.[47] A single 5-second tetanic stimulation was sufficient to cause an injury. This is probably due to the biphasic and wide impulses of this nerve stimulator. Other contributing factors could possibly be high-density current at the tips of the stimulating probes, and repeated maximal output tetanic stimulation. The skin lesions healed completely within 3 days.

B. *Electrocution*

Theoretically, the electrodes of a nerve stimulator could accidentally become grounded and conduct stray currents from faulty electric equipment in the operating room. This would cause severe skin burns, and even death. Such an incident, however, has not been reported.

The author wishes to express his gratitude to Drs. Aaron Kopman and James Eisenkraft for reviewing the manuscript and making many useful suggestions.

V. REFERENCES

1. Bevan DR, Smith CE, Donati F. Postoperative neuromuscular blockade: A comparison between atracurium, vecuronium, and pancuronium. Anesthesiology 69:272–276, 1988.
2. Viby-Mogensen J, Jorgensen BC, Ording H. Residual curarization in the recovery room. Anesthesiology 50:539–541, 1979.
3. Azar I. The response of patients with neuromuscular disorders to muscle relaxants: A review. Anesthesiology 65:173–187, 1984.
4. Paton WDW, Waud DR. The margin of safety of neuromuscular transmission. J Physiol 191:59–90, 1967.
5. Waud BE, Waud DR. The margin of safety of neuromuscular transmission in the muscle of the diaphragm. Anesthesiology 37:417–422, 1972.
6. Viby-Mogensen J, Hansen PH, Jorgensen BC, Ording H, et al. A new nerve stimulator (Myotest). Br J Anaesth 52:547–549, 1980.
7. Pollmaecher T, Steiert H, Buzello W. A constant current peripheral nerve stimulator (Neurostim T4): Description, and evaluation in volunteers. Br J Anaesth 58:1443–1446, 1986.
8. Mylrea KC, Hameroff SR, Calkins JM, Blitt CD, et al. Evaluation of peripheral nerve stimulators and relationship to possible errors in assessing neuromuscular block. Anesthesiology 60: 464–466, 1984.
9. Kopman AF, Lawson D. Milliamperage requirement for supramaximal stimulation of the ulnar nerve with surface electrodes. Anesthesiology 61:83–85, 1984.
10. Stiffel P, Hameroff SR, Blitt CD, Cork RC. Variability in assessment of neuromuscular blockade. Anesthesiology 52:436–437, 1980.
11. Viby-Mogensen J, Jensen NH, Engbaek J, Ording H, et al. Tactile and visual evaluation of the response to train-of-four stimulation. Anesthesiology 63:440–445, 1985.
12. Azar I, Wen W, Turndorf H. Twitch Box: A new device to monitor neuromuscular blockade. Med Inst 12:92–93, 1978.
13. Baraka A. Monitoring of neuromuscular transmission in anaesthetized man by a bulb transduced assembly. Anesth Analg 52:36–38, 1973.
14. Sokoll MD. A new transducer and holder for recording of thumb adduction. Anesthesiology 40:80–82, 1974.
15. Walts LF, Lebowitz M, Dillon JB. A means of recording force of thumb adduction. Anesthesiology 29:1054–1055, 1968.
16. Gissen AJ. Standardized technique for transmission studies. Anesthesiology 39:567–568, 1973 (letter).
17. Freund FG, Merati JK. A source of errors in assessing neuoromuscular blockade. Anesthesiology 39:540–542, 1973.
18. Viby-Mogensen J, Jensen E, Werner M, Nielsen HK. Measurement of acceleration: A new method of monitoring neuromuscular function. Acta Anaesth Scand 32:45–48, 1988.
19. Jensen E, Viby-Mogensen J, Bang U. The Accelograph: a new neuromuscular transmission monitor. Acta Anaesthesiol Scand 32:49–52, 1988.
20. Nagashima H, Nguyen HD, Comforti M, Duncalf D, et al. A simple method for monitoring muscle relaxation during continuous infusion of vecuronium. Can Anaesth Soc J 35:134–138, 1988.
21. Windsor JPW, Sebel PS, Flynn PS. The neuromuscular transmission monitor: A clinical assessment and comparison with a force transducer. Anaesthesia 40:146–151, 1985.
22. Harper NJN, Bradshaw EG, Healy TEJ. Evoked electromyographic and mechanical responses of the adductor pollicis compared during onset of neuromuscular blockade by atracurium or alcuronium and during antagonism by neostigmine. Br J Anaesth 58:1278–1284, 1986.
23. Kosek PS, Sears DH, Rubinstein EH. Minimizing movement-induced changes in twitch response during integrated electromyography. Anesthesiology 69:142–143, 1988.
24. Paloheimo M, Edmonds HL Jr. In reply (letter). Anesthesiology 69:143, 1988.
25. Kopman AF. The effect of resting muscle tension on dose-effect relationship of d-tubocurarine: Does preload influence the evoked EMG? Anesthesiology 69:1003–1005, 1988.
26. Sopher MJ, Sears DH, Walts LF. Neuromuscular function mon-

[*]Personal communication: Kopman AF, March 1989.

[†]Personal communication: Eisenkraft JB, March 1989.

[‡]Author's unpublished observation.

itoring comparing the flexor hallucis brevis and adductor pollicis muscles. Anesthesiology 69:129–131, 1988.
27. Berger JJ, Gravenstein JS, Munson ES. Electrode polarity and peripheral nerve stimulation. Anesthesiology 56:402–404, 1982.
28. Rosenberg H, Greenhow DE. Peripheral nerve stimulator performance: The influence of output polarity and electrode placement. Can Anaesth Soc J 25:424–426, 1978.
29. Kopman AF. A safe surface electrode for peripheral nerve stimulation. Anesthesiology 44:343–345, 1976.
30. Ali HH, Savarese JJ. Stimulus frequency and the dose response to d-tubocurarine in man. Anesthesiology 52:36–39, 1980.
31. Ali HH, Utting JE, Gray CT. Quantitative assessment of residual antidepolarizing block (Part I). Br J Anaesth 43:473–477, 1971.
32. Lee C, Katz RL. Fade of neurally evoked compound electromyogram during neuromuscular block by d-tubocurarine. Anesth Analg 56:271–275, 1976.
33. Merton PA. Voluntary strength and fatigue. J Physiol (London) 123:553–564, 1954.
34. Gissen AJ, Katz RL. Twitch, tetanus, and post-tetanic potentiation as indices of nerve-muscle block in man. Anesthesiology 30:481–487, 1969.
35. Stanec A, Heyduk J, Stanec G, Orkin LR. Tetanic fade and post-tetanic tension in the absence of neuromuscular block in anesthetized man. Anesth Analg 57:102–107, 1978.
36. Engbaek J, Ostergaard D, Viby-Mogensen J. Double burst stimulation (DBS): A new pattern of nerve stimulation to identify residual neuromuscular blockade. Br J Anaesth 62:274–278, 1989.
37. Donlon JV, Savarese JJ, Ali HH. Cumulative dose-response curves for gallamine: Effect of altered resting thumb tension and mode of stimulation. Anesth Analg 58:377–381, 1979.
38. Kopman AF. The dose-effect relationship of metocurine: The integrated electromyogram of the first dorsal interosseous muscle and the mechanomyogram of the adductor pollicis compared. Anesthesiology 68:604–607, 1988.
39. Weber S, Muravchick S. Electrical and mechanical train-of-four responses during depolarizing and non-depolarizing neuromuscular blockade. Anesth Analg 65:771–776, 1986.
40. Katz RL. Comparison of Electrical and mechanical recordings of spontaneous and evoked muscle activity: The clinical value of continuous recording as an aid to the rational use of muscle relaxants during anesthesia. Anesthesiology 26:204–211, 1965.
41. Caffrey RR, Warren ML, Becker KE. Neuromuscular blockade comparing the orbicularis oculi and adductor pollicis muscles. Anesthesiology 65:95–97, 1986.
42. Pansard JL, Chauvin M, Lebrault C, Gauneau P, et al. Effect of an intubating dose of succinylcholine and atracurium on the diaphragm and the adductor pollicis muscle in humans. Anesthesiology 67:326–330, 1987.
43. Wymore ML, Eisele JH. Differential effects of d-tubocurarine on inspiratory muscles and two peripheral muscle groups in anesthetized man. Anesthesiology 48:360–362, 1978.
44. Donlon JV, Ali HH, Savarese JJ. A new approach to the study of four non-depolarizing relaxants in man. Anesth Analg 53:934–939, 1974.
45. Waud BE, Waud DR. The relation between tetanic fade and receptor occlusion in the presence of competitive neuromuscular block. Anesthesiology 35:456–464, 1971.
46. Waud BE, Waud DR. The relation between the response to "train-of-four" stimulation and receptor occlusion during competitive neuromuscular block. Anesthesiology 37:413–416, 1972.
47. Lippman M, Fields WA. Burns of the skin caused by a peripheral nerve stimulator. Anesthesiology 40:82–84, 1974.
48. Epstein RA, Epstein RM. The electromyogram and the mechanical response of indirectly stimulated muscle in anesthetized man following curarization. Anesthesiology 38:212–223, 1973.
49. Lee C. Train-of-4 quantitation of competitive neuromuscular blockade. Anesth Analg 54:649–653, 1975.
50. Ali HH, Savarese JJ, Lebowitz PW, Ramsey FM. Twitch, tetanus, and train-of-four as indices of recovery from non-depolarizing neuromuscular blockade. Anesthesiology 54:294–297, 1981.
51. Lee C. Dose relationships of phase II, tachyphylaxis and train-of-four fade in suxamethonium-induced dual neuromuscular block in man. Br J Anaesth 47:841–845, 1975.
52. Carter JA, Arnold R, Yate PM, Flynn PJ. Assessment of the Datex relaxograph during anaesthesia and atracurium induced neuromuscular blockade. Br J Anaesth 58:1447–1452, 1986.
53. Kopman AF. The relationship of evoked electromyographic and mechanical response following atracurium in humans. Anesthesiology 63:208-211, 1985.
54. Donati F, Bevan DR. Muscle electromechanical correlations during succinylcholine infusion. Anesth Analg 63:891–894, 1984.
55. Viby-Mogensen J, Howardy-Hansen P, Chraemmer-Jorgensen B, Ording H, et al. Post-tetanic count (PTC): A new method of evaluating an intense non-depolarizing neuromuscular blockade. Anesthesiology 55:458–461, 1981.
56. Muchhal KK, Viby-Mogensen J, Fernando PUE, Tamilarasan A, et al. Evaluation of intense neuromuscular blockade caused by vecuronium using post-tetanic count (PTC). Anesthesiology 66:846–849, 1987.
57. Baraka A. Post-tetanic facilitation as index for antagonism of phase II block of succinylcholine in patients with atypical cholinesterase. Anesth Analg 60:911–912, 1981.
58. Savarese JJ, Ali HH, Murphy JD, Padget C, et al. Train-of-four nerve stimulation in the management of prolonged neuromuscular blockade following succinylcholine. Anesthesiology 42:106–111, 1975.
59. Ali HH, Wilson RS, Savarese JJ, Kitz RJ. The effects of tubocurarine on indirectly elicited train-of-four muscle response and respiratory measurements in humans. Br J Anaesth 47:570–574, 1975.
60. Ali HH, Kitz RJ. Evaluation of recovery from non-depolarizing neuromuscular block, using a digital neuromuscular transmission analyzer: preliminary report. Anesth Analg 52:740–745, 1973.
61. Brand JB, Cullen, DJ, Wilson NE, Ali HH. Spontaneous recovery from non-depolarizing neuromuscular blockade: Correlation between clinical and evoked responses. Anesth Analg 56:55–58, 1977.
62. Pavlin EG, Holle RH, Schoene RB. Recovery of airway protection compared with ventilation in humans after paralysis with curare. Anesthesiology 70:381–385, 1989.

Chapter 35

Janna Blanchard, MD
Somayaji Ramamurthy, MD

Brachial Plexus

OUTLINE

I. INTRODUCTION

A. *History*

The first brachial plexus block was performed by Halsted in 1884, when he applied a solution of cocaine directly to the surgically exposed plexus.[1,2] In the first decade of this century, Kulenkampf and Hirschel blocked the brachial plexus percutaneously through a supraclavicular approach, and Hirschel later described a plexus block via an axillary approach.[1,3,4] Many investigators subsequently improved on these methods and developed various techniques for plexus blockade. These include the classic supraclavicular, interscalene, parascalene, subclavian perivascular, infraclavicular, and axillary blocks.

B. *Anatomy*

The brachial plexus is composed of a group of nerves responsible for the sensory and motor innervation of almost the entire upper extremity. In order to successfully perform a brachial plexus block, it is essential to understand the formation of the plexus and its anatomic relationship to other structures as it descends from the cervical region in the neck to the proximal arm in the axilla.

The brachial plexus is formed from the union of the anterior rami of the lower cervical spinal nerves (C-5, C-6, C-7, C-8) and the first thoracic spinal nerve (T-1) (Fig. 35–1). It may also receive contributions from the fourth cervical and second thoracic nerves.

The ventral (motor) and dorsal (sensory) roots from the spinal cord combine beyond the dorsal root ganglion to form the mixed spinal nerve. This nerve then divides into the dorsal (posterior) and ventral (anterior) rami.

The anterior rami of C-5 through T-1 exit the intervertebral foramina and lie in the bony gutter between the anterior and posterior tubercles of the transverse processes of the cervical vertebrae; these are the *roots* of the brachial plexus. As they pass inferiorly and anterolaterally between the middle and anterior scalene muscles, they combine to form the three *trunks*—superior, middle, and inferior—of the brachial plexus.

The middle scalene muscle is attached to the posterior tubercles of the transverse processes of C-2 through C-7 and inserts on the first rib. The anterior scalene muscle is attached to the anterior tubercles of the transverse processes of C-3 through C-6 and inserts on the scalene tubercle of the first rib. These muscles are invested with a fascial covering that is an extension of the prevertebral fascia. As the trunks of the brachial plexus emerge from this interscalene space in between the muscles at their lateral margin, they carry an investing sheath of fascia with them as they descend toward the first rib. At this level, above the rib, the subclavian artery joins the trunks of the plexus within the "fascial sandwich" and forms the subclavian perivascular space.

As the three trunks pass over the first rib and under the clavicle, they each split into *divisions* (anterior and posterior), which then recombine to form the *cords* (lateral, medial and posterior) of the brachial plexus. As the cords pass downward to enter the axillary fossa behind the lateral border of the pectoralis minor muscle, they divide into the *terminal branches* of the brachial plexus: the median, musculocutaneous, ulnar, axillary, radial, medial brachial cutaneous, and medial antebrachial cutaneous nerves. In this region, the nerves are accompanied by the axillary artery in the axillary neurovascular space.

The terminal nerves of the brachial plexus provide all of the cutaneous innervation of the upper extremity,

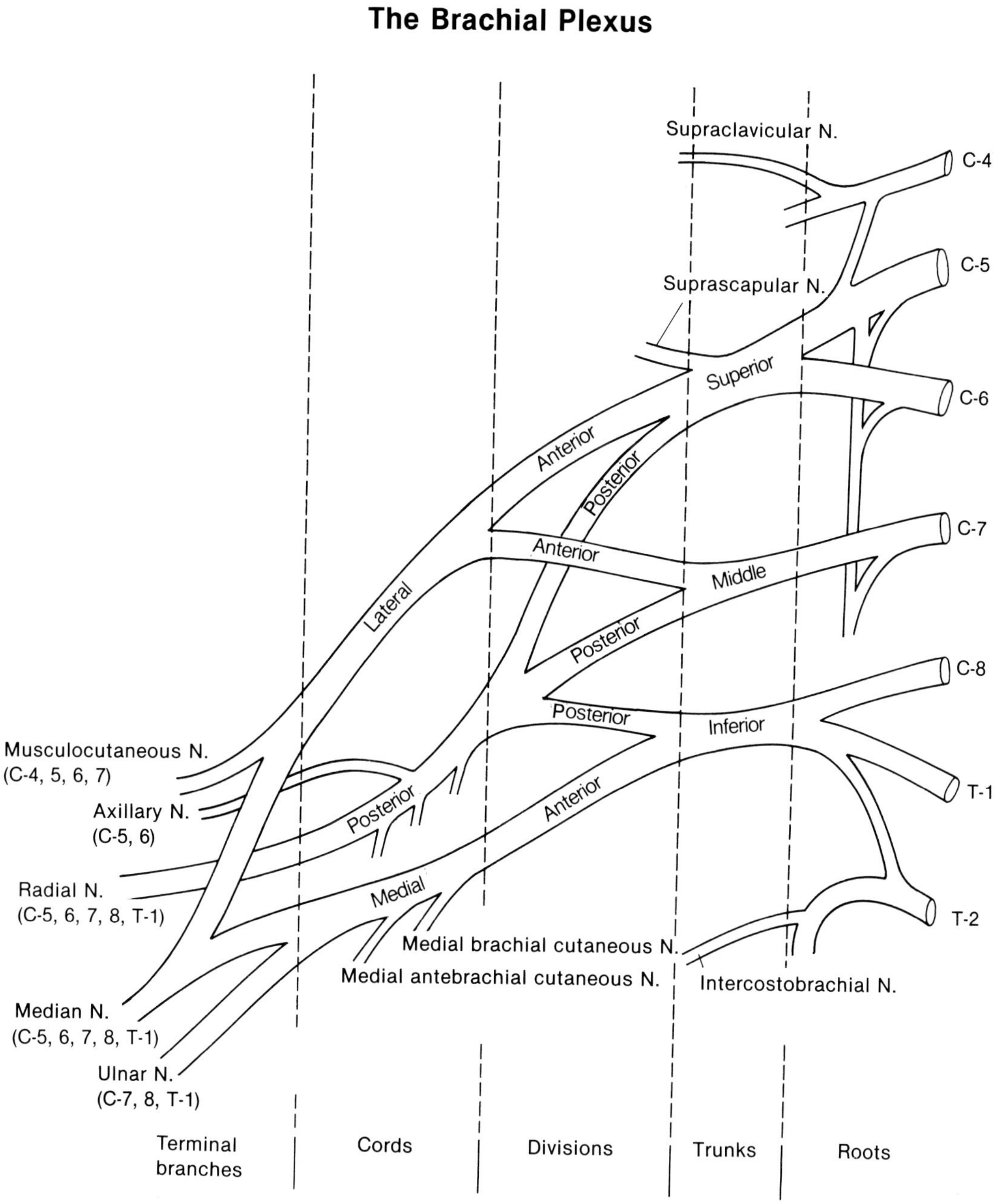

Figure 35–1 • The formation of the brachial plexus from C-4 to T-2 showing the roots, trunks, divisions, cords, and terminal branches.

except for areas of skin over the shoulder and the inner aspect of the upper arm, which are innervated by the supraclavicular and intercostobrachial nerves, respectively. Because the brachial plexus is contained in a continuous fascial sheath from the cervical vertebrae to the distal axilla, for the purpose of blockade, this perineural and perivascular space can be entered at different levels; virtually complete anesthesia of the arm can be provided with a single injection.[5-8] Recent studies, however, suggest that the sheath may contain fascial compartments and that the local anesthetic solution that is injected may be impeded in its spread.[9] Some investigators therefore recommend a multiple-injection technique.

The approaches to the brachial plexus discussed in this chapter include the axillary, the infraclavicular, and the supraclavicular (which can be subdivided into classical, interscalene, subclavian perivascular, and parascalene).

II. Indications for Brachial Plexus Blockade

Brachial plexus blockade is used to provide regional anesthesia of the upper extremity in many different situations. General, vascular, neurologic, and orthopedic surgical procedures and manipulations of the shoulder, arm, forearm, and hand can be performed with this technique as a result of the sensory and motor block that it provides. For patients with reflex sympathetic dystrophy, causalgia, or Raynaud's phenomenon, therapeutic benefits can be derived from the block of the sympathetic nerve fibers. Brachial plexus blockade can also be of diagnostic benefit to help determine whether a patient's pain is central or peripheral in origin. Performance of this block can relieve many painful conditions, including postoperative pain problems, traumatic pain conditions, and painful neuropathies. The many perioperative advantages to brachial plexus blockade include the following:[3,4,10]

1. A surgical patient with a full stomach is less likely to aspirate the stomach contents, because protective reflexes remain intact with a regional anesthetic.
2. High-risk patients can have surgery with minimal physiologic trespass.
3. The occasional postoperative side-effects of general anesthesia, such as nausea and vomiting, mental status changes, and pulmonary complications, can be avoided.
4. Prolonged postoperative pain relief can be provided by either a long-acting local anesthetic or a continuous block technique.
5. Patients with a fear of being put to sleep can remain awake and still have surgical anesthesia.
6. There are infrequent complications associated with these blocks, which are therefore well suited for outpatient procedures because they can allow early ambulation and discharge.
7. Vasodilation secondary to the sympathetic block can benefit a traumatized extremity.

III. How to Do Brachial Plexus Blockade

A. *General Preparation*

In preparation for performing any of the blocks of the brachial plexus, the anesthesiologist must have a thorough understanding of the anatomy of the neck and upper extremity (Figs. 35–2 to 35–4).

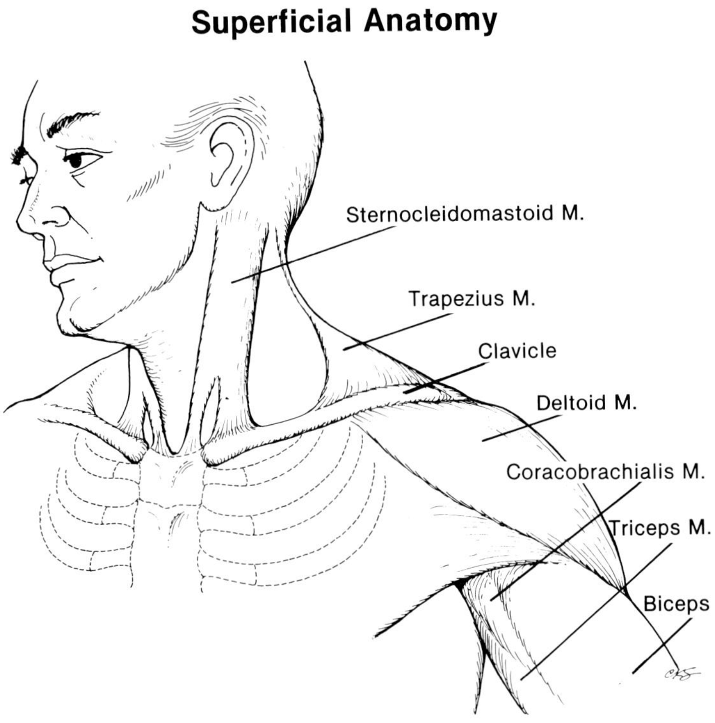

Figure 35–2 • The superficial anatomy of the neck and upper extremity showing the muscular and bony landmarks.

Superficial and Deep Anatomy

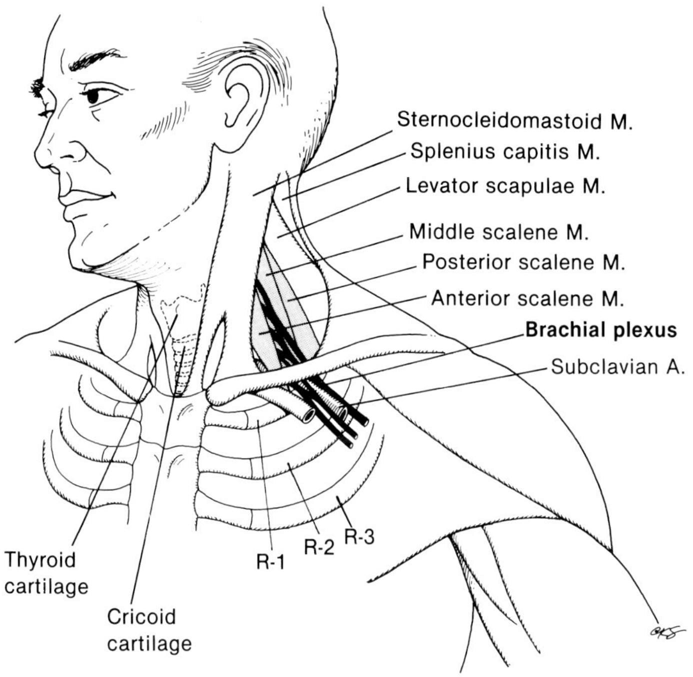

Figure 35–3 • The superficial and deep anatomy of the neck and upper extremity showing the brachial plexus in relation to the muscular, bony, and vascular landmarks.

Brachial Plexus—Deep Anatomy

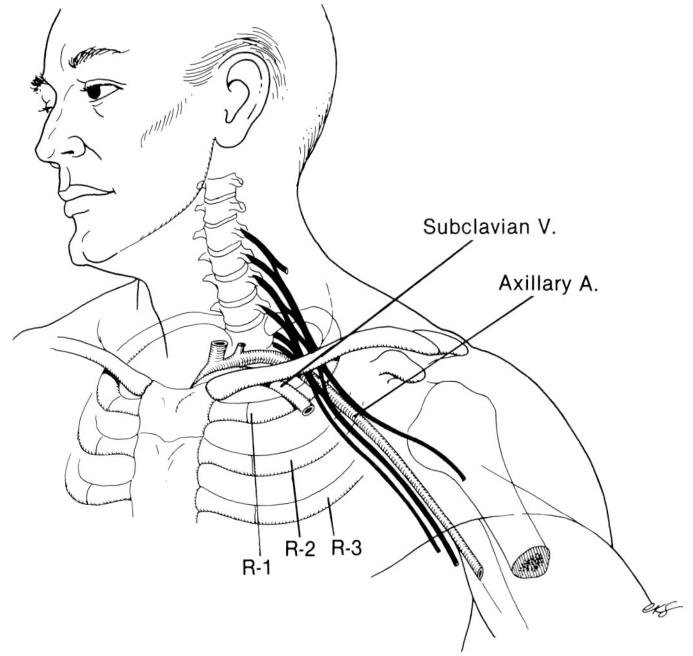

Figure 35–4 • The brachial plexus extending from the neck to the proximal arm in relation to deeper anatomic structures.

For complete patient preparation, it is imperative that resuscitation equipment be made available for the management of any possible adverse side effects that result from the procedure or the drugs administered. The patient should have an intravenous drip started, routine and any additional appropriate monitors applied, and baseline values obtained. It is advisable to perform a neurologic exam of the extremity before the block is placed. The procedure should be explained to the patient so that informed consent can be obtained and the patient understands what to expect in order to cooperate more fully. Obviously, it is also necessary for the surgeon to understand and agree with the anesthetic plan.

Preoperative and intraoperative sedation is given as is appropriate to the patient's age, general health, and situation. Additional comfort may be provided to the patient by putting the operating room table in a flexed position or by placing a pillow under the knees, so that there is less stress on the patient's back while lying supine during the surgery.

B. *Approaches To The Brachial Plexus*

1. Axillary Block

a. *Techniques*

The axillary approach to blockade of the brachial plexus is one of the most popular and commonly used. Four techniques will be discussed: the arterial puncture, paresthesia, infiltration, and perivascular techniques.

For each of these, the anesthesiologist stands or sits next to the patient on the side to be blocked. The patient is placed in a comfortable supine position with the arm abducted to approximately 90° and the forearm flexed to 90° and externally rotated so that the dorsum of the hand lies on the table proximal to but not underneath the patient's head (Fig. 35–5). Hyperabduction of the arm should be avoided, because this may obscure the arterial pulsations and also interfere with the spread of the local anesthetic. The axillary artery is the most important landmark for all of the techniques; it should be

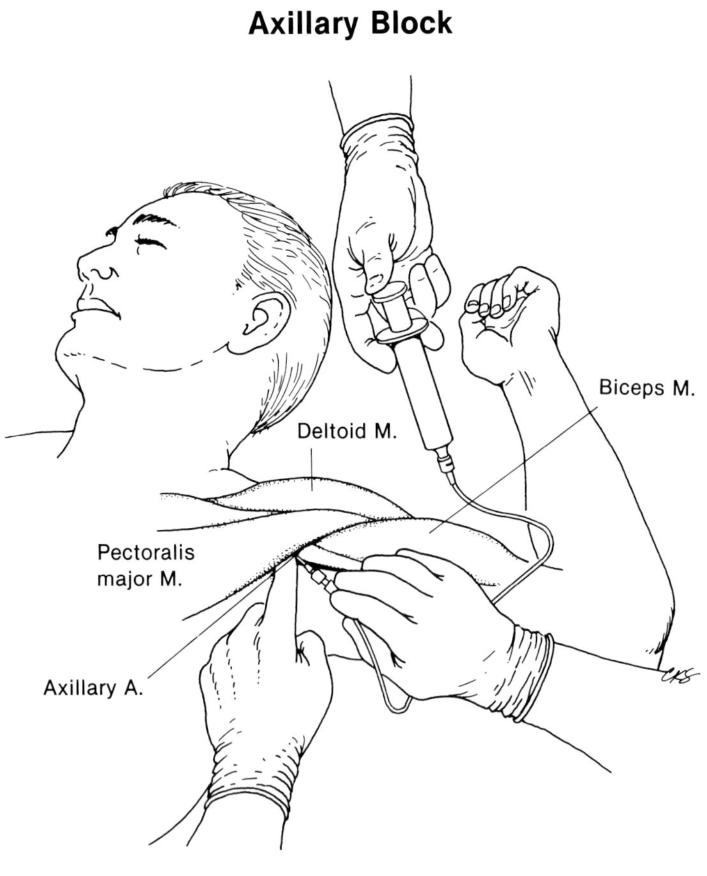

Figure 35–5 • Axillary block—hand position. In the technique of needle insertion, the nondominant hand palpates the axillary artery pulse as proximal as possible. An assistant can aspirate and inject from the syringe via the extension tubing.

palpated high into the proximal axilla, ideally up to or under the lateral margin of the pectoralis major muscle.

All the techniques for brachial plexus blockade in the axilla take advantage of the anatomy of the neurovascular bundle, which, at this level, contains the axillary artery and the three major nerves (Fig. 35–6). The axillary vein may or may not be in the neurovascular sheath. The median nerve lies in front of and slightly above the artery; the ulnar nerve lies in front and slightly below it; and the radial nerve lies behind it. The musculocutaneous and axillary nerves leave the fascial sheath of the plexus at the level of the coracoid process of the scapula, and these two nerves may not be anesthetized if a small volume of local anesthetic is used.

i. Arterial Puncture Technique. For this technique,[11,10] the palpating index finger of the nondominant hand follows the arterial pulse high into the axilla, where a skin wheal is raised just superior to the tip of the finger. The artery is deliberately punctured by the slowly advancing 3.8-cm, 22 gauge short-bevel block needle. When arterial blood is aspirated, the needle is slowly *withdrawn* just until blood can no longer be aspirated. At this point, the needle should be in a position outside of the artery but within the axillary sheath; 40–50 mL of local anesthetic can be injected with repeated aspirations performed intermittently to insure that the local anesthetic is not injected intravascularly.

Escaping blood from the arterial puncture can interfere with the quality of anesthesia owing to dilution or hydrolysis of the local anesthetic agent or hematoma formation, which may prevent the drug from contacting the nerves. For this reason, it is generally preferable to

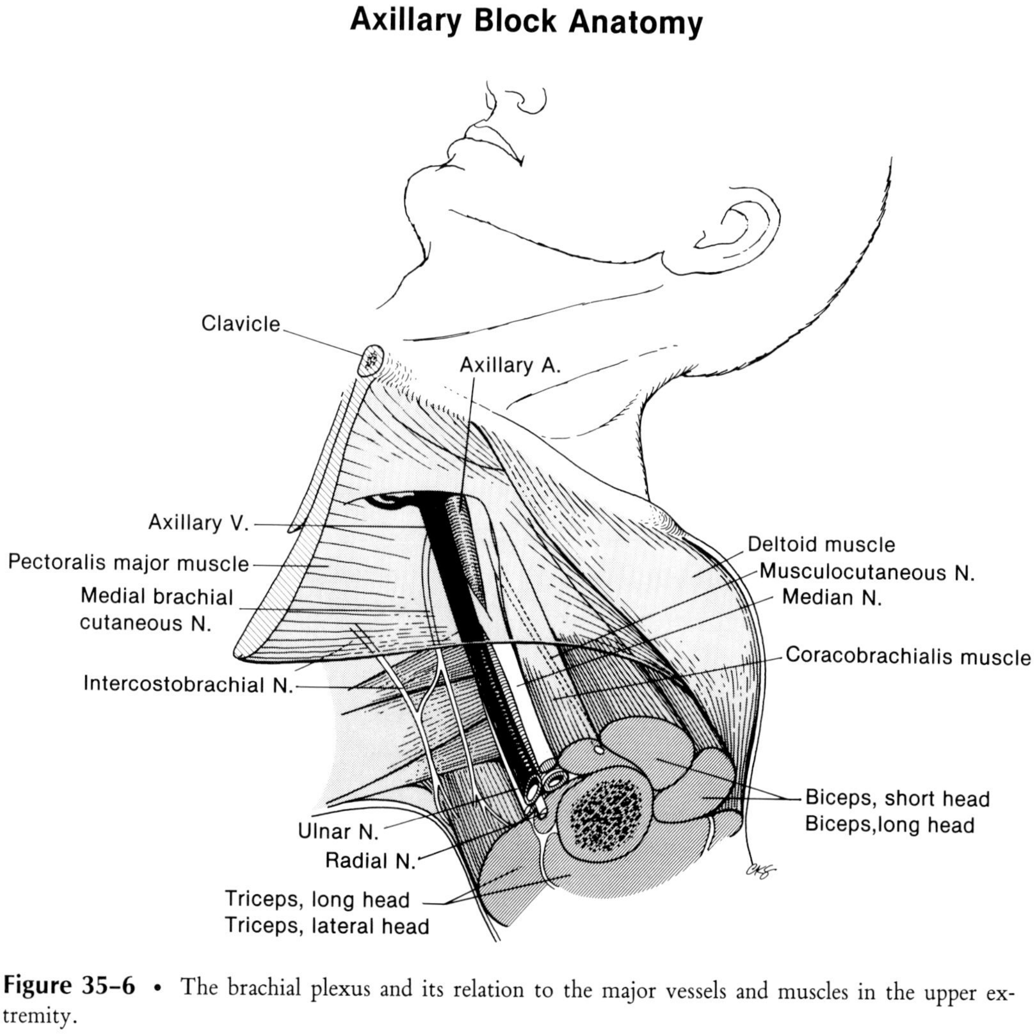

Figure 35–6 • The brachial plexus and its relation to the major vessels and muscles in the upper extremity.

puncture the artery, aspirate blood, slowly *advance* the needle through to the other side of the artery, and stop and inject the local anesthetic when blood can no longer be aspirated. Again, at this point the tip of the needle should be outside of the artery but still within the axillary sheath. There should be very little leakage of blood while the needle is in this position; if digital pressure is applied immediately after the needle is withdrawn, bleeding into the sheath should be minimal. Some clinicians deposit one half of the anesthetic behind the artery and the other half in front of it in an attempt to hasten the onset of the block.

ii. Paresthesia Technique. For this technique,[11,10] the palpating index finger of the nondominant hand follows the arterial pulse high into the axilla, where a skin wheal is raised just superior to the tip of the finger. A 3.8-cm, 22 gauge short-bevel block needle is slowly advanced toward the artery, but the direction is adjusted so that the needle will pass to one side of the vessel to avoid penetration. A paresthesia in the distribution of one of the various nerves is elicited by the advancing needle. A paresthesia is a spontaneous sensation such as electric tingling, prickling, or burning that occurs when the block needle comes into contact with a nerve. Before performing any of the blocks of the brachial plexus, if possible, the patient should be instructed that he or she may feel a paresthesia and should tell the anesthesiologist immediately when it occurs and describe its location without moving the extremity. When a paresthesia occurs, 40–50 mL of local anesthetic solution should be injected with repeated aspirations performed intermittently to insure that the local anesthetic is not injected intravascularly. The force of the local anesthetic solution as it is injected normally pushes the nerve safely away from the tip of the needle. If the patient describes *severe* pain when the needle is advanced or the solution is injected, it must be considered that the needle tip may be intraneural and the injection must be stopped. The needle should be withdrawn and repositioned before proceeding, so as to avoid nerve damage.

By intentionally passing the block needle above or below the artery, a paresthesia in the distribution of the median or ulnar nerves, respectively, may be elicited. Paresthesias in the radial distribution can be difficult to obtain because the nerve is usually located behind the axillary artery.[11] Ten to twenty mL of local anesthetic can be injected incrementally when each paresthesia is obtained.

If paresthesias are not easily obtained, a nerve stimulator can be used to elicit muscular contractions and paresthesias for confirmation of correct needle placement. The exploring electrode is attached with an alligator clip to the metal hub or proximal shaft of the block needle, and the ground electrode is attached to an electrocardiograph (ECG) pad placed on the opposite shoulder (see Section V, "Use of Nerve Stimulator," in this chapter).

iii. Infiltration Technique. For this technique,[10,11] the palpating index finger of the nondominant hand follows the arterial pulse high into the axilla, where a skin wheal is raised just superior to the tip of the finger. A 3.8-cm, 22 gauge needle is advanced toward the artery, but the direction is changed so that it just passes over the superior aspect of the vessel to avoid penetration. The advancement continues until the humerus is contacted, and then 5–16 mL of the local anesthetic is injected as the needle is withdrawn slowly to a subcutaneous position. This procedure is repeated two or three times as the direction of the needle is changed in a fanlike manner. The same steps are repeated after the needle is reinserted from a subcutaneous position to pass just beneath the inferior aspect of the artery. With this technique, the tissues between the humerus and the skin on either side of the artery are infiltrated with a total of 40–50 mL of local anesthetic with multiple-needle insertions. This is an especially useful method if landmarks are difficult to palpate.

iv. Perivascular Technique. For this technique,[10,12-14] the local anesthetic is intentionally deposited within the perivascular axillary sheath. Arterial puncture, production of paresthesias or muscle contractions from nerve stimulation, or identification of a fascial click can be used to confirm correct needle placement. The fascial click is a sound that may be heard or a sensation that may be felt when using a short-bevel block needle as it pierces the fascial sheath of the neurovascular bundle.

Winnie's perivascular technique consists of entering the sheath superiorly and tangentially to the artery, thus avoiding the axillary vein.[10,12,15] The palpating index finger of the nondominant hand follows the arterial pulse high into the axilla, where a skin wheal is raised just superior to the tip of the finger. A 3.8-cm, 22 gauge, short-bevel block needle is held at an angle of 10° to 20° to the skin and advanced cephalad toward the apex of the axilla. When the needle passes into the fascial compartment, one of three confirmatory signs should indicate that it is in correct position: (1) the fascial click may be felt or heard, (2) a paresthesia will be elicited, or (3) bright red blood will be seen in the needle hub.

Winnie suggests that when blood appears, the needle be advanced quickly and carefully, with continued aspiration until the flow of blood stops just as the needle is passed through the posterior wall of the vessel.[12] After negative aspiration, the total volume of 40–50 mL local anesthetic is injected with repeated aspirations performed intermittently to insure that the local anesthetic is not injected intravascularly. Digital pressure distal to the needle during and after the injection promotes the central spread of the solution and may impede retrograde (peripheral) flow.[12]

When performing any of the blocks of the plexus, if a tourniquet is to be used or if the surgical procedure will involve the area of the arm innervated by the intercostobrachial nerve (T-2) or the medial brachial cutaneous nerve, then these must be blocked separately. T-2 is never contained in the axillary sheath, and the medial brachial cutaneous nerve may not be in the sheath at this level because it is a branch of the medial cord and leaves the neurovascular bundle very high in the axilla. Blockade of these nerves can be accomplished after the major injection by withdrawing the needle to a subcutaneous position directly over the arterial pulse and injecting 5–10 mL of local anesthetic in a fanlike manner from this position to make a ring of solution around half of the proximal arm.

The arm should be adducted and placed at the patient's side immediately after injecting the local anesthetic for the axillary block, so that proximal spread of the anesthetic solution is not impeded by the head of the humerus in the abducted position.

Winnie recommends using the "immobile needle" technique when performing any of the blocks of the brachial plexus (see Fig. 35–5).[12,16] Instead of connecting and disconnecting a syringe directly to the block needle, intravenous extension tubing is attached between the needle and syringe and the entire system is filled with the local anesthetic solution before the procedure is started (see Fig. 35–5). With this method, there is stability when aspirating and injecting, and the needle remains immobile with less possibility of displacement of the tip from its proper position. The total volume of local anesthetic solution can be placed in a single syringe and attached to the extension tubing. It is also possible to use a three-way stopcock at the end of the tubing so that two syringes can be attached simultaneously and no disconnections will be necessary.

Some authors believe that there are compartments in the axillary sheath that may inhibit the spread of local anesthetic that is deposited as a single injection.[9] They therefore recommend depositing 10–15 mL of local anesthetic above and below the artery with a 25 gauge, 5/8-inch needle redirected three times in a fan-like manner on each side of the artery. If a paresthesia occurs, 3–5 mL of local anesthetic is injected, with a total injected of 20–30 mL. Other authors have confirmed the presence of septae within the sheath, but their tests have shown the septae to be functionally incomplete and not a barrier to the spread of local anesthetics.[5,8]

b. *Advantages*

The axillary technique of brachial plexus blockade is easy to perform because of the superficial and palpable anatomic landmarks. The complications of other approaches—pneumothorax, phrenic nerve block, stellate ganglion block, subarachnoid or epidural injection—are virtually impossible. This technique is suitable for children, uncooperative patients, or patients with respiratory problems. It is also the method of choice for outpatient anesthesia in which the development of a pneumothorax or a phrenic nerve block could produce serious problems.

c. *Disadvantages*

The axillary technique cannot be used if the arm cannot be passively abducted to expose the axilla. The musculocutaneous and axillary nerves leave the plexus sheath at the level of the coracoid process of the scapula, and they may not be blocked when the volume of local anesthetic used does not spread a sufficient distance proximally. In the axilla, the musculocutaneous nerve lies within the substance of the coracobrachialis muscle; it can be blocked by injecting 5 mL of local anesthetic into the substance of the muscle. This muscle is small, but is located just superior to the axillary artery; its fascial covering confines the solution so that the nerve will be blocked without having to identify it by eliciting paresthesias or muscle contractions.

d. *Contraindications*

This block is contraindicated when there is active infection or malignancy in the proximity of where the injection is to be given. It may also be relatively contraindicated in a patient with a bleeding diathesis, owing to an increased risk of hematoma formation if the vein or artery is punctured. However, of all of the techniques for blockade of the brachial plexus, this approach would be the most safe because the pressure needed to tamponade a bleed can be applied most effectively in the axilla.

e. Complications and Treatment

i. Hematoma. Puncture of the artery or vein often occurs with the axillary approach of brachial plexus block. A hematoma can result but is usually of little clinical significance if firm pressure is applied for a sufficient duration. Escaping blood from the arterial puncture can interfere with the quality of anesthesia, owing to dilution or hydrolysis of the local anesthetic agent or hematoma formation, which may prevent the drug from contacting the nerves.

ii. Local Anesthetic Toxicity. The maximum allowable safe dose of each local anesthetic that is used must be known so that an excessive amount is not given. This is true for all the blocks of the brachial plexus, but it is particularly true for some techniques of axillary blockade when larger volumes of agent are used. If an absolute overdose does occur, it may result in high plasma levels of local anesthetic that can cause immediate rapid or delayed serious systemic effects. Reaction to an overdose usually develops approximately 20 minutes after the injection, when the peak blood levels are reached. Early symptoms are ringing in the ears, lightheadedness, dysphoria, numbness of the tongue or mouth, metallic taste, slurred speech, twitching of facial muscles, restlessness, or somnolence. There may be progression to generalized convulsions, respiratory arrest, and cardiovascular depression and compromise.

If the patient becomes unconscious or has a convulsion, the steps in the treatment are the basic steps of cardiopulmonary resuscitation (CPR) as they are always applied. First, oxygenation must be maintained in spite of convulsions or vomiting. Convulsions are not lethal, but the hypoxia and metabolic acidosis that they produce may be. During convulsions, oxygen is being consumed at a high rate and, because respiration is usually inadequate, hypoxia and acidosis quickly develop. Therefore, every effort should be made to establish and maintain a patent airway. One hundred percent O_2 with a positive-pressure breathing apparatus for controlled or assisted ventilation is essential. At times ventilating the unparalyzed, convulsing patient may be difficult, and it may be necessary to paralyze the patient with 60–80 mg/kg of IV *succinylcholine*. *Tracheal intubation* with a cuffed endotracheal (ET) tube to facilitate ventilation and protect the airway from aspiration may also be necessary.

Second, *persistent convulsions* may be controlled by the IV administration of 1–2 mg/kg of *sodium thiopental* (a small dose is used to avoid additional cardiovascular depression). *Diazepam,* 0.05 mg/kg, may also be used. Convulsions, being more visible, tend to obscure the insidious and potentially more threatening fall in cerebral perfusion that may occur due to *hypotension* as a direct result of simultaneous cardiovascular toxicity.

Third, the *circulation* must be supported. Lowering the head and raising the feet will increase blood supply to the brain. Hypotension will respond to *IV fluids* and the use of *vasopressors.*

Fourth, *cardiac arrest* may develop after the above-mentioned initial sequelae. Marked hypercapnia, acidosis, and hypoxia occur very rapidly in some patients—especially obese or pregnant patients—following seizure activity due to local anesthetic toxicity, and this in turn potentiates the negative chronotropic and inotropic action of these anesthetic agents. Cardiopulmonary resuscitation is apparently more difficult in patients in whom cardiotoxicity has occurred following the administration of bupivacaine. With cardiac arrest, immediate institution of *CPR* is imperative and consists of external cardiac massage, defibrillation if necessary (high-energy levels may be necessary to restore sinus rhythm), and appropriate drugs with inotropic, chronotropic, and vasopressor effects.

iii. Intravascular Injection. Injection of local anesthetic in the axillary vein can occur with this technique and result in serious systemic effects. With the rapid development of a high plasma concentration of local anesthetic, adverse central nervous system (CNS), respiratory, and cardiovascular effects may manifest suddenly.

Prevention is always more desirable than treatment, and may be promoted in three ways. First, *aspirate* before injecting, but realize that an aspiration test that does not produce blood does not preclude an intravascular injection, and so one must be constantly vigilant. Second, always give a *test dose* and the remainder of the anesthetic agent in small incremental amounts. *Epinephrine*, 5 μg/mL (1:200,000), if not clinically contraindicated, should be freshly added to the local anesthetic. If an intravascular injection is occurring, the signs and symptoms of systemic epinephrine (tachycardia, headache, palpitations, hypertension) usually will alert the clinician within 30 seconds of injection. Third, *early recognition* of a reaction is possible through constant observation of the patient. By monitoring the vital signs closely and communicating with the patient, it is possible to be aware of an impending toxic reaction and to take steps to prevent it from becoming serious. If the patient complains of ringing in the ears, a vague sense of light-headedness, nystagmus, dysphoria, shivering, twitching, and somnolence, the administration of the local anesthetic agent should be stopped. Often, administering O_2 and asking the patient to breathe deeply suffices. No further treatment may be necessary because the blood level is rapidly reduced by redistribution of the anesthetic.

If the patient becomes unconscious or has a convulsion following an intravascular injection, the steps in the treatment are the basic steps of *CPR* as they are always applied (see earlier).

2. INFRACLAVICULAR BLOCK

a. Technique

For the infraclavicular approach to the brachial plexus, the local anesthetic is deposited at the level of the cords and branches of the plexus.[18] The patient is placed in the supine position with the affected arm abducted to 90 degrees. A line is drawn along the entire length of the clavicle, and the midpoint clavicle is identified and marked (Fig. 35–7A). If the subclavian artery can be palpated, the midpoint is when the artery dips under the clavicle. The brachial artery is palpated high into the axilla of the abducted arm and marked. A line is also drawn from Chassaignac's tubercle (C-6) in the neck across the midpoint of the clavicle and to trace the brachial artery in the upper extremity.[26] This line serves as a surface marker for the brachial plexus as it passes distally beyond the clavicle to the axilla (see Fig. 35–7A).

A nerve stimulator must be used for this block in order to identify the brachial plexus, which lies deep within the infraclavicular region.[18,26] The exploring electrode is attached with an alligator clip to the metal hub or proximal shaft of the block needle, and the ground electrode is attached to an ECG pad placed on the opposite shoulder.

A skin wheal is raised approximately 2.5 cm below the midpoint of the clavicle on the chest wall. A standard 22 gauge, 8-cm, unsheathed spinal needle is inserted through the skin wheal and directed in a lateral direction toward the line that has marked the course of the brachial plexus distal to the clavicle (Fig. 35–7B). The needle is advanced slowly at an angle of 45° to the skin. The nerve stimulator should be set to deliver approximately 6–8 volts at 1 to 2 impulses per second so that muscle contractions can be observed as the tip of the needle approaches the nerves in the brachial plexus.[26] When flexion or extension of the elbow, wrist, or digits is elicited, the needle advancement is stopped and the voltage should be decreased to the lowest level that will still produce a visible muscle contraction. The needle is then advanced or withdrawn slightly to find the point of maximal muscle contraction, which should indicate correct needle placement.[18]

To further confirm correct needle placement, 2–3 mL of 2% lidocaine solution is injected after a negative aspiration test, while the stimulator is still turned on so that a decrease in muscle contractions can be observed within 30 seconds from the effect of the local anesthetic. All 20–30 mL of the solution is then injected in 5-mL incremental doses with regular aspiration tests between injections. The immobile needle technique (see "Axillary Block—Perivascular Technique") will best allow for injection without displacing the needle tip. Digital pressure can be applied in the axilla to encourage the central flow of the local anesthetic.[17]

b. Advantages

This technique, which deposits the local anesthetic solution at a higher level in the neurovascular bundle than that of the axillary approach, can provide a good block of the nerves of the brachial plexus and provide anesthesia from the shoulder to the hand.

The needle is directed laterally from the midpoint of the clavicle, and the risk of pneumothorax is less than with some of the supraclavicular approaches.[18]

Catheters that are inserted infraclavicularly, such as with this approach, are more easily secured for continuous blockade.

Subarachnoid and epidural injections, sympathetic block, and recurrent laryngeal and phrenic nerve blocks are virtually impossible with this technique.

c. Disadvantages

A nerve stimulator must be used for this technique, and the paresthesias produced may be perceived as very unpleasant by some patients. There may be considerable discomfort as the long needle is passed through the pectoralis major and minor muscles to reach the brachial plexus cords, which are deep to these muscles. The landmarks of the plexus are not palpable, as they are with the other techniques. Because a long needle is used, there may be more difficulty with accurate placement

Infraclavicular Block

Landmarks

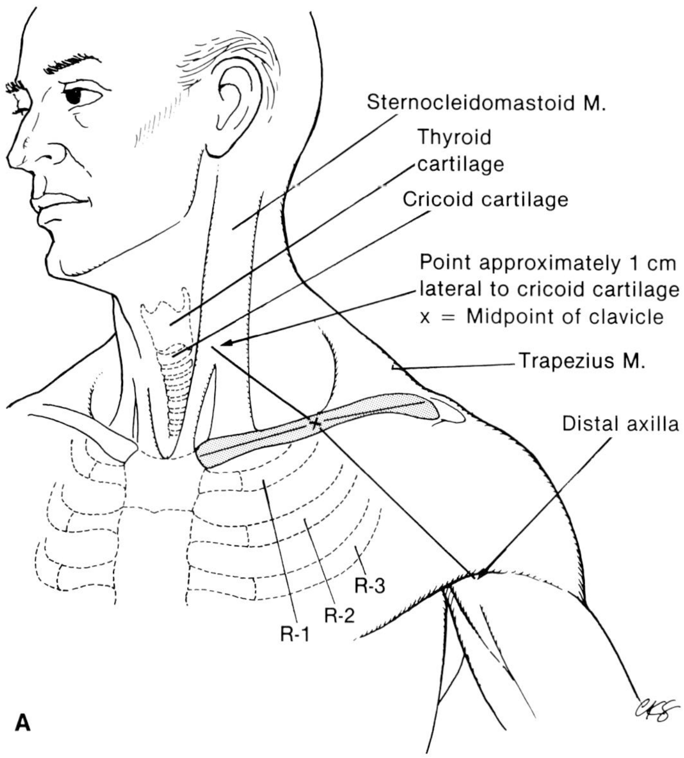

Technique: needle position and the brachial plexus

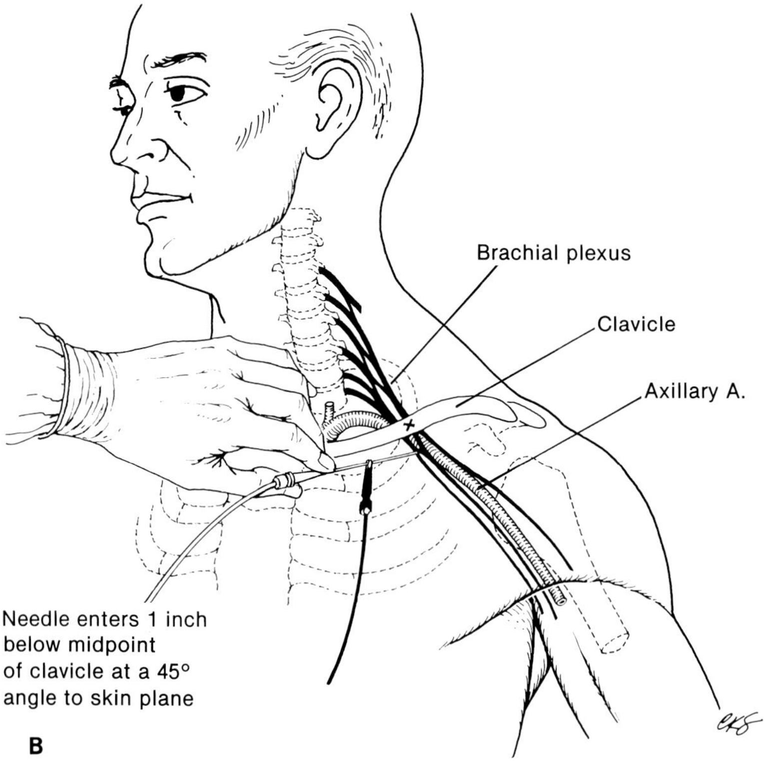

Figure 35–7 • (***A***) The superficial anatomic landmarks for the infraclavicular block. (***B***) The deeper anatomy: the brachial plexus extending from the neck and passing under the clavicle. The technique of needle insertion is shown along with the nerve stimulator attached to the shaft of the needle.

because the tissues may deflect the needle tip.[18] If the needle is placed distal to the coracoid process, the local anesthetic solution may spread distally, and the axillary and musculocutaneous nerves will not be blocked.[10,18]

d. *Contraindications*

This block should not be performed in patients with infections of the chest wall or distorted anatomy secondary to previous surgery or trauma.

It may also be a relative contraindication to do this block in a patient who is anticoagulated. If the subclavian vein is punctured, it may not be easy to apply pressure under the clavicle in order to prevent hematoma formation.

e. *Complications and Treatment*

i. Hematoma. If the subclavian vein is punctured, a hematoma may develop because it is not easy to tamponade this vessel if bleeding occurs.

ii. Intravascular Injection. The intravascular injection of local anesthetic into the subclavian vein may result in a convulsion. This is usually self-limited and of short duration but should be managed aggressively. The steps in the management of this complication are as outlined on page 18.

iii. Pneumothorax. A serious but rare complication that can result from this technique is the development of a pneumothorax if the needle is placed too far medially. The patient initially may have no symptoms at all, or he or she may develop a cough and some shortness of breath with or without complaints of chest pain that is accentuated with deep breathing. The chest radiograph may not reveal any abnormality.[10,17] Most pneumothoraces may take up to 24 hours to develop fully and usually do not get any larger after 24 hours. These are often small, less than 20%, and no treatment is necessary because the lung will reexpand on its own.[10] If the pneumothorax exceeds 20%, the patient should be given supplemental oxygen to breathe, appropriate analgesics, and the air should be aspirated from the pleural cavity. If the patient is symptomatic and has an extensive pneumothorax of greater than 50%, a chest tube should be placed. With a lesser degree of pneumothorax in a patient with symptoms, simple aspiration may be all that is required. Reexpansion must be confirmed by radiograph, and the patient must be followed until complete resolution of the problem. Because of the potential for this complication, this block should not be performed in any patient who, because of underlying pulmonary disease, would be severely compromised.

3. CLASSIC SUPRACLAVICULAR BLOCK

a. *Technique*

For the classical supraclavicular approach to the brachial plexus, the local anesthetic is deposited around the plexus, where it crosses the first rib (Fig. 35–8A).

The technique originally described by Kulenkampf involved a single injection above the midpoint of the clavicle after paresthesias were obtained.[19–21] The many modifications to this approach have included multiple injections; the insertion of multiple needles; and multiple injections that "walk" along the first rib. One of the most commonly used methods of supraclavicular block has been a combination of the techniques popularized by Moore and Bonica.[1,11]

The patient is placed in a comfortable supine position with the head turned slightly away from the side to be blocked. A small pillow can be placed under the patient's upper back to allow the head and neck to hyperextend and the shoulders to fall back.

The anesthesiologist stands on the side to be blocked or at the head of the table. The lateral border of the clavicular head of the sternocleidomastoid muscle is located by having the patient elevate his or her head slightly. For additional muscle definition, the patient can attempt to elevate his or her head while the anesthesiologist places a hand on the patient's forehead to provide resistance to head lift. First, the muscle is palpated with the index and middle fingers; the fingers are rolled laterally to palpate the anterior scalene muscle. If this muscle cannot be palpated, it may be brought into prominence by having the patient inhale deeply, which will cause it to contract because it is an accessory muscle of respiration. The brachial plexus passes at the distal or lateral edge of this muscle.[11] A skin wheal is raised 1 cm above the clavicle at this point, which is approximately 2 cm from the lateral border of the clavicular head of the sternocleidomastoid muscle (Fig. 35–8B). This point of needle insertion usually corresponds to the midpoint of the clavicle and serves as the landmark in patients in whom the anatomy is more difficult to define.[22,23] A 3.8-cm, 22 gauge, short-bevel block needle is advanced slowly and directed caudad and slightly mesiad. This discretion has also been described as vertically inward and downward.[24] The needle is advanced until a paresthesia is elicited.[25] Before performing the block, the patient

Supraclavicular Block

Anatomy: needle position and the brachial plexus

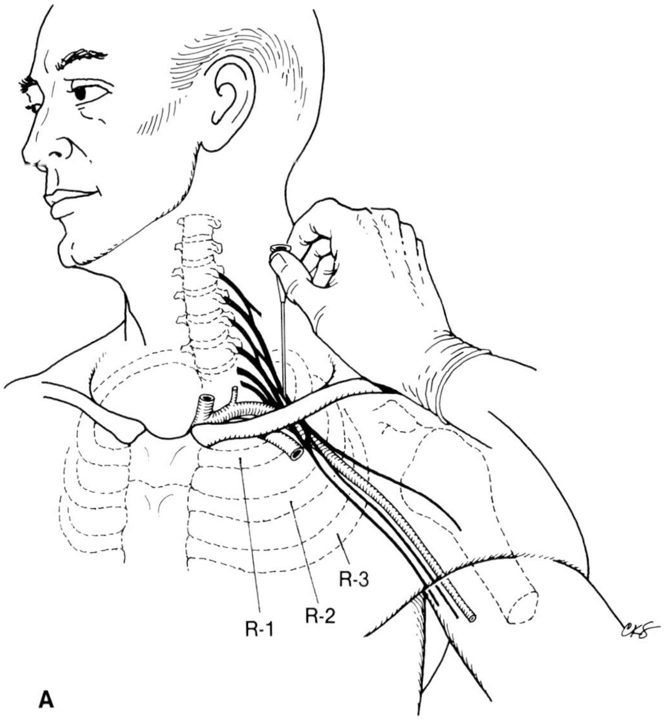

Supraclavicular Block

Technique: needle insertion and hand position

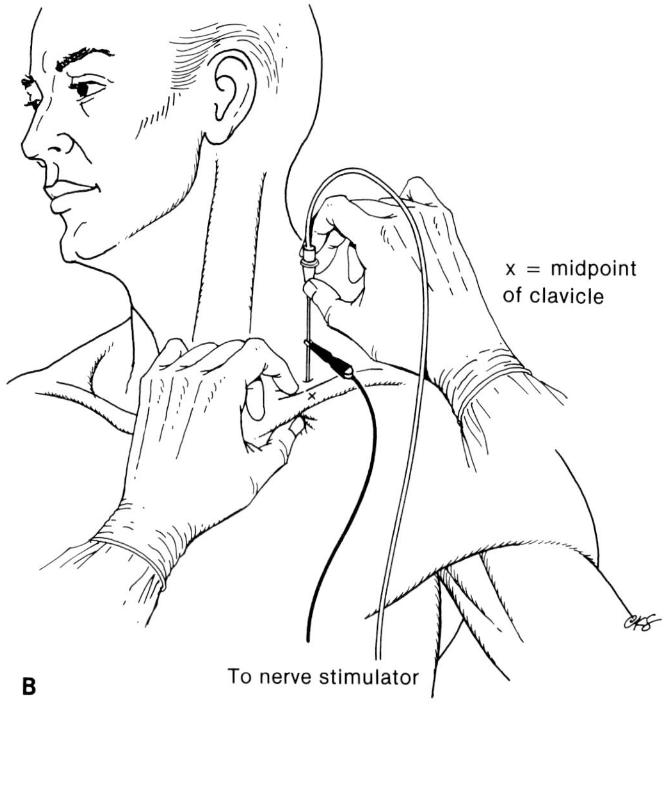

Figure 35–8 • Supraclavicular block. (***A***) Anatomy: the brachial plexus along with the position of the needle. (***B***) Needle insertion: the superficial anatomic landmarks along with the technique of needle insertion and hand position.

should be instructed to tell the anesthesiologist immediately, without moving, when and where the paresthesia is felt.

When a paresthesia to the arm below the elbow is obtained, the needle advancement is stopped, because this indicates correct needle placement. A paresthesia to the shoulder may result from stimulation of the suprascapular nerve, which may or may not be inside the sheath at this level, and therefore should not be relied on as confirmation of correct needle placement.

After the desired paresthesia is obtained, aspiration is performed, which should be negative for blood, 15–20 mL of local anesthetic is injected in incremental doses.[11] The needle is then advanced without changing direction, usually no more than 3 cm, until the needle point contacts the first rib. Ten mL of solution is injected after negative aspiration, while the needle is withdrawn slowly to subcutaneous tissue.[24] The needle is reinserted and redirected twice so as to touch the rib 1 cm closer to its sternal end and then 1 cm posterolateral to the first injection. Ten mL of solution is injected, after negative aspiration, in each location while withdrawing the needle slowly to a subcutaneous position. If a paresthesia is elicited with either the second or third needle insertions, advancement is stopped and 8–10 mL of anesthetic agent is injected. It is also possible to walk the needle 1 cm anteriorly and posteriorly along the length, not the width, of the first rib to seek additional paresthesias. If the initial plane of the needle direction is maintained while visualizing the anatomy of the first rib and walking the rib from the lateral border of the anterior scalene muscle to the anterior border of the medial scalene muscle, paresthesias should be obtained and the pleura avoided. If the needle is directed too medially or caudally, the first rib may not be contacted and instead the pleura may be touched.

If the needle direction is correct and the patient is not too obese, the first rib should be contacted at a depth of 3 cm or less from the skin. In a patient with a thick neck, the tissues can be depressed with the index finger of the nondominant hand to decrease the distance between the skin and the plexus.

For this block, paresthesias must be elicited and a total volume of 40–50 mL is injected. If no paresthesias are obtained when the first rib is touched, it should be carefully walked and the needle direction changed slightly to obtain paresthesias.[11]

If paresthesias are not produced and the first rib is not encountered at a depth of 3 cm, the needle should be withdrawn, the anatomy reassessed, and the block carefully reattempted or another approach considered.

b. Advantages

The supraclavicular block can provide reliable anesthesia for most manipulations and surgeries of the upper extremity. For this block, the patient's arm remains at his or her side and does not require movement in painful conditions. The injection of local anesthetic into the subarachnoid or epidural space is almost impossible.

c. Disadvantages

This technique depends on the relationship of the brachial plexus and subclavian artery to the midpoint of the clavicle and the first rib; anatomic dissections have shown that these structures do not have a constant relationship. Therefore, the landmarks for this block, especially in an obese patient or a patient with a thick neck, can be difficult to find and, in addition, may not provide for correct needle placement.

It is advisable to try to elicit paresthesias to confirm correct needle placement with this block; this may be perceived as a very unpleasant sensation by some patients, which may be considered a minor disadvantage.

d. Contraindications

This block should not be performed in patients who have infections in the head or neck area or if the anatomy has been distorted by trauma or previous surgery.

It may also be a relative contraindication to do this block in a patient who is anticoagulated or has a bleeding diathesis, because if the subclavian artery or vein is punctured, it may be difficult to apply pressure under the clavicle over these vessels to tamponade the bleeding and prevent hematoma formation.

This approach should not be used in patients who have severe emphysema or who are very tall and thin, because the apex of the lung may be high and the risk of entering the pleura would be increased.[23] In addition, bilateral blocks should not be performed because of the risk of pneumothorax.

e. Complications and Treatment

i. Pneumothorax. The most serious complication that can result from this approach is a pneumothorax. One author quotes the incidence as being 0.5% to 4%, which may decrease as the individual anesthesiologist develops more skill.[11,25]

If the needle is directed too far medially or laterally, or if the rib is not encountered with needle advancement, the dome of the pleura may be pierced by the needle. The management of pneumothorax associated with a supraclavicular block is the same as with an infraclavicular block.

ii. Phrenic Nerve Block. This sequela can occur in 40% to 60% of patients.[11] This nerve may be blocked by the spread of the local anesthetic in front of the anterior scalene muscle, where the nerve passes beneath the prevertebral fascia.[12] The patient may be asymptomatic or may complain of difficulty breathing secondary to decreased afferent impulses from the diaphragm. Treatment may require no more than reassurance or, in the case of respiratory embarrassment, assistance with ventilation. Bilateral block in an emphysematous patient may produce difficulty in breathing that warrants ventilatory assistance. The onset of any symptoms from motor block of the diaphragm parallels the time course for the local anesthetic to take effect. A definitive diagnosis can be made with a chest radiograph. A double-exposure technique, in which inspiration and expiration are displayed on the same film, is useful to determine if the hemidiaphragm ipsilateral to the block has little or no movement, indicating the presence of phrenic nerve block.[27] The symptoms will disappear as the action of the local anesthetic wears off.

iii. Sympathetic Nerve Block. A sympathetic block may also result from spread of the local anesthetic through the fascial barrier of the interscalene space to the cervical sympathetic chain.[12] If the sympathetic innervation to the head is affected, the patient may develop ptosis, miosis, and anhidrosis (Horner's syndrome). The patient should experience no compromise from the Horner's syndrome, but should have the symptoms explained in advance. The symptoms will disappear after the block dissipates and, if necessary, the ocular manifestations can be reversed with a drop of ophthalmic phenylephrine.[10] This sequela may occur in 70% to 90% of the patients who have a block using this approach.[11]

iv. Intravascular Injection. The subclavian artery and vein lie in close anatomic proximity to where the needle is placed for this block. The intravascular injection of local anesthetic may result in a convulsion. This is usually self-limited and of short duration, but should be managed aggressively. The steps in the management of this complication are as outlined under "Axillary Block—Complications and Treatments."[18]

4. Interscalene Block

a. Technique

For the interscalene approach to brachial plexus block, the local anesthetic is deposited at the level of the roots of the plexus, where they exit the intervertebral foramina and lie in the gutters of the cervical transverse processes before passing between the anterior and middle scalene muscles (Fig. 35–9A). There is a fascial covering enveloping these muscles that forms an interscalene space through which the roots pass.[28,29] The groove between the anterior and middle scalene muscles is the landmark for performing this block.

The anesthesiologist stands on the side to be blocked. The patient is placed in a comfortable supine position with the arm on the affected side gently extending toward the ipsilateral knee. The patient's head is then turned slightly to face away from the side to be blocked. The patient is asked to extend his or her neck slightly so that the cricoid cartilage can be identified. The level of the sixth cervical vertebra is found by extending a line laterally from the level of the cricoid cartilage to the posterior border of the sternocleidomastoid muscle (Fig. 35–9B). If this muscle is not easily palpated, it can be accentuated by having the patient elevate his or her head slightly.[12] For additional muscle definition, the patient can attempt to elevate his or her head while the anesthesiologist places a hand on the forehead to provide resistance to head lift. When the posterior border of the muscle is found, the palpating index and middle fingers are placed behind the muscle belly; the patient can then relax his or her head, and the fingers are rolled laterally over the anterior scalene muscle until the groove is palpated between the anterior and middle scalene muscles (Fig. 35–9C). If the groove is not palpated, it may be brought into prominence by asking the patient to inhale deeply, because the scalene muscles may contract when acting as accessory muscles of respiration.[30,31]

Often, the external jugular vein crosses the interscalene groove at the level of the sixth cervical vertebra; it can serve as a landmark to guide the needle placement.[31] A skin wheal is raised between the two palpating fingers in the groove, and a 3.8-cm, 22 gauge, short-bevel block needle is introduced. The direction of the needle is perpendicular to the skin in all planes.[29] The

Interscalene Block

Superficial anatomy: needle position and the brachial plexus

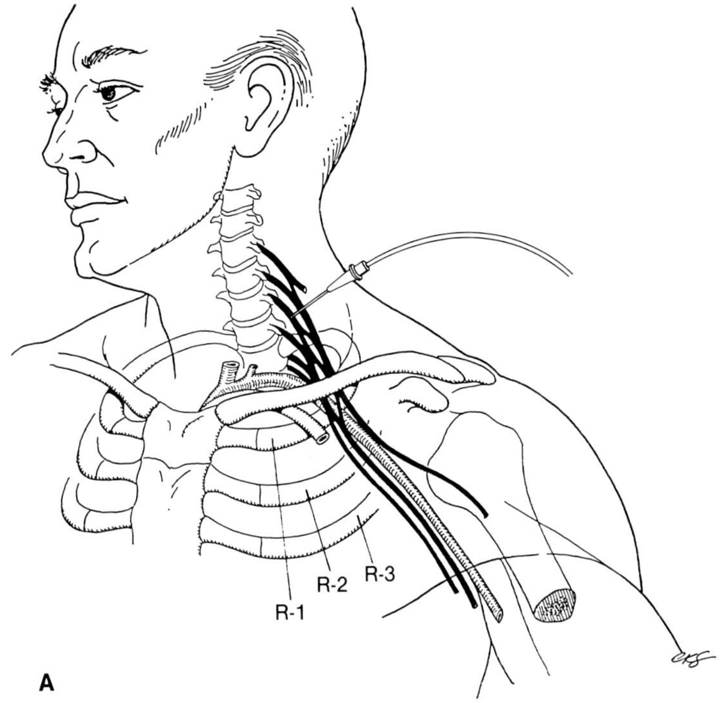

Deeper anatomy: needle position and the brachial plexus

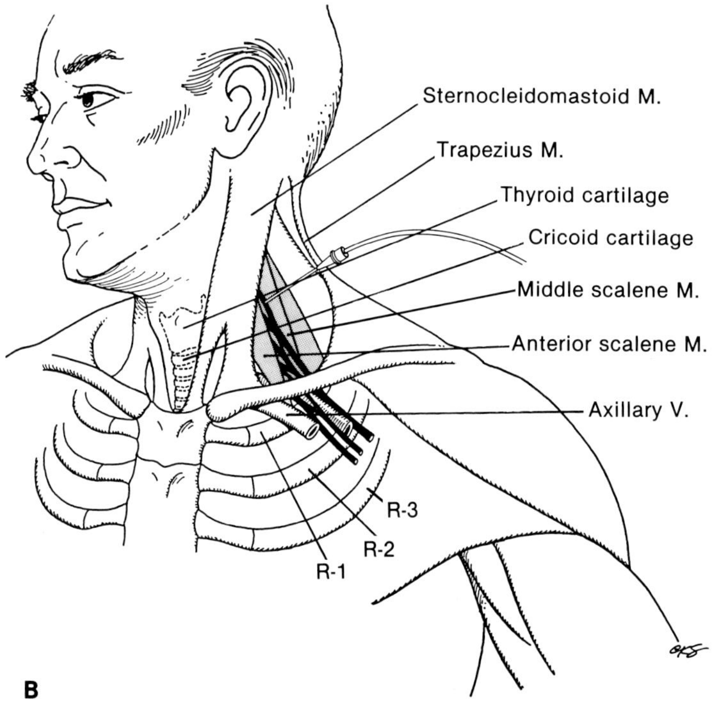

Figure 35-9 • Interscalene block. (***A***) Superficial anatomy: the brachial plexus along with the position of the needle approaching the roots. (***B***) Deeper anatomy: the brachial plexus and its relation to the major vessels and muscular landmarks in the neck along with the position of the needle.

(continued)

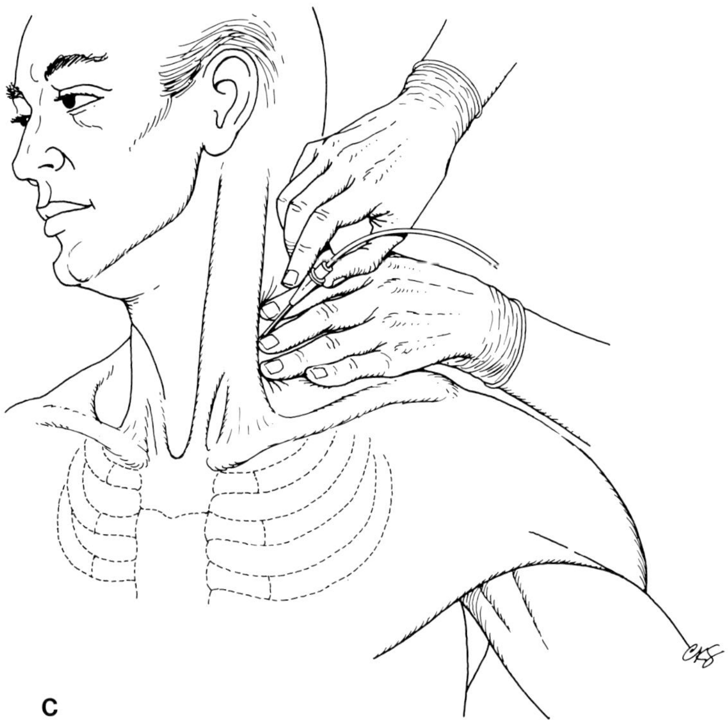

Figure 35-9 *(continued)*
(**C**) Technique: the superficial anatomic landmarks along with the technique of needle insertion and hand position. The nondominant hand palpates the groove between the anterior and middle scalene muscles.

immobile needle technique is used (see "Axillary Block—Perivascular Technique"), and the needle is then slowly advanced until a paresthesia is elicited or the periosteum of the cervical vertebra is encountered.[16] Before performing the block, the patient should be instructed to tell the anesthesiologist immediately, without moving, when he or she feels a paresthesia and where it is felt.[12,28,29]

When a paresthesia to the arm below the elbow is obtained, the needle advancement is stopped, because this indicates correct needle placement. A paresthesia to the shoulder may result from stimulation of the suprascapular nerve, which may or may not be inside the sheath at this level, and therefore should not be relied on as confirmation of correct needle placement.[12]

After the needle is in the correct position, aspiration is performed and should be negative for blood or cerebrospinal fluid. Two to three mL of local anesthetic can then be injected rapidly to try to elicit a "pressure paresthesia," which is additional confirmation that the needle is correctly positioned. According to Winnie, the pressure paresthesia is due to a sudden increase in pressure from the local anesthetic solution as it distends the perivascular space.[12] The patient may describe a dull aching sensation in the same dermatomal distribution in which he or she felt the "electrical paresthesia."[12]

The remainder of the local anesthetic is then injected, with negative aspiration attempts after each 5-mL incremental dose. The needle is then withdrawn, and the groove may be massaged to enhance the spread of the local anesthetic, or a palpating finger may be held in place in an attempt to influence the spread as appropriate.

Twenty mL of local anesthetic solution injected into the fascia-enclosed interscalene space results in anesthesia of the lower cervical plexus, as well as most of the brachial plexus. However, with this small volume, the blockade of the C-8 and T-1 nerve roots may be slow to develop and anesthesia in the ulnar distribution may be incomplete or absent. By using 40 mL of solution, one is more likely to block all of the brachial plexus.[12]

A nerve stimulator can be used if it is difficult to elicit or interpret paresthesias. The exploring electrode is attached with an alligator clip to the metal hub or proximal shaft of the block needle, and the ground electrode is attached to an ECG pad on the opposite shoulder. With stimulation of nerves in the interscalene space, contraction of muscles of the arm, forearm, or hand will be noted. If the diaphragm contracts, the needle is stimulating the phrenic nerve on the anterior surface of the anterior scalene muscle; the needle should be repositioned more laterally and posteriorly to lie within the groove.[26] In the neck of most patients, if the needle is advanced in the correct, slightly caudad direction, it will contact the transverse process of the cervical vertebra at a depth of no more than 1.5–2 cm. If no paresthesias are obtained, the needle can be walked across the U-shaped end of the transverse process until a paresthesia is elicited from contacting the nerve as it lies in the "gutter."[17,28] When periosteum is encountered only after deep insertion and no paresthesias are obtained, the needle is probably in contact with the vertebral body from being placed too far anteriorly; it should be repositioned more posteriorly after redefining the patient's anatomic landmarks. If a tourniquet is to be used or if the surgical procedure will involve the area of the arm innervated by the intercostobrachial nerve (T-2) or the medial brachial cutaneous nerve, these must be blocked separately. This blockade can be accomplished after the major injection by palpating directly over the axillary artery pulse high in the axilla. Five mL of local anesthetic is injected in a fanlike manner from this position to make a ring of solution around half of the proximal arm.

b. Advantages

The interscalene block is relatively easy to perform even in the obese or uncooperative patient.[28] It is the technique of choice for surgical manipulation of the upper arm or shoulder when it may also be necessary to block the lower cervical plexus. It can be used in patients who have malignancy or infection of the arm, because the needle is placed proximal to the level of any lymph nodes. Because it is highly improbable that a pneumothorax will result from the level of needle insertion with this block, it is ideal for any patient in whom this complication would best be avoided. For this block, the arm remains at the patient's side and does not require movement in painful conditions.

c. Disadvantages

There may be absence of anesthesia in the distribution of the ulnar nerve if the volume of local anesthetic used is too small and it therefore does not spread to reach the C-8 or T-1 nerve roots.[28]

In performing this block, it is advised that paresthesias be sought to confirm correct needle placement; this may be perceived as a very unpleasant sensation by some patients.

d. Contraindications

This technique should probably be avoided if the anatomy of the neck is distorted secondary to previous surgery or trauma or if there is malignancy or infection in the neck. It also may be relatively contraindicated in a patient who is anticoagulated or has a bleeding diathesis because of the inability to tamponade the vertebral artery if it is punctured.

e. Complications and Treatment

i. Subarachnoid or Epidural Block. Subarachnoid or epidural injections can occur with this block. Depending on the amount of resultant patient compromise, these complications are managed with therapy as appropriate and include airway management with intubation, fluids, vasopressors, and CPR. The steps in the management of these complications are as outlined under "Axillary Block—Complications and Treatment."

ii. Phrenic Nerve Block. The phrenic nerve may be blocked secondary to spread of local anesthetic to the cervical roots C-3, C-4, or C-5, or to spread in front of the anterior scalene muscle, where the nerve passes beneath the prevertebral fascia.[12] The patient may be asymptomatic or may complain of difficulty in breathing secondary to decreased afferent impulses from the diaphragm. Treatment may require no more than reassurance or, in the case of respiratory embarrassment, assistance with ventilation. Bilateral block in an emphysematous patient may produce difficulty in breathing and cyanosis that warrants ventilatory assistance. The onset of any symptoms from motor block of the diaphragm parallels the time course for the local anesthetic to take effect. A definitive diagnosis can be made with a chest radiograph. A double-exposure technique, in which inspiration and expiration are displayed on the same film, is useful to determine if the hemidiaphragm ipsilateral to the block has little or no movement, indicating the presence of phrenic nerve block.[27] The symptoms will disappear as the action of the local anesthetic wears off.

iii. Vagus or Recurrent Laryngeal Nerve Block. The patient may develop hoarseness secondary to unilateral vocal cord paralysis if the vagus or the re-

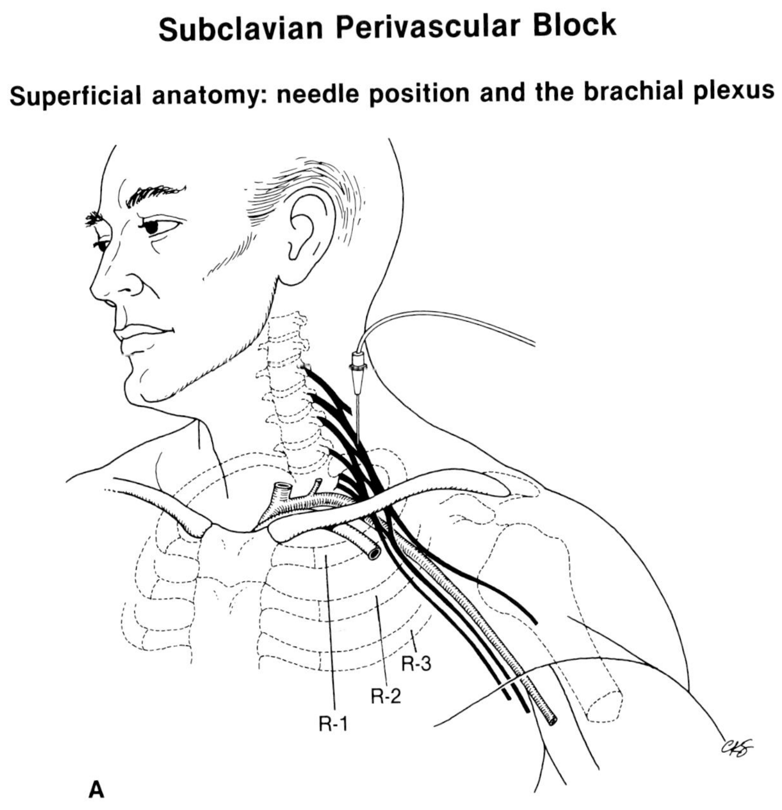

Figure 35–10 • Subclavian perivascular block. (***A***) Superficial anatomy: the brachial plexus along with the position of the needle approaching the trunks.

(continued)

current laryngeal nerve is blocked. The patient may only need reassurance but should also be cautioned to avoid oral intake until the hoarseness resolves and small sips of water can be tolerated. These complications are considered to be theoretical contraindications to the performance of bilateral blocks.[12] The block should also be avoided in patients who have unilateral vocal cord paralysis on the side opposite that to be blocked.

iv. Sympathetic Nerve Block. A sympathetic block may also result from spread of the local anesthetic through the fascial barrier of the interscalene space to the cervical sympathetic chain.[12] If the sympathetic innervation to the head is affected, the patient may develop Horner's syndrome. The patient should experience no compromise from the development of Horner's syndrome, but should have the symptoms explained in advance. The symptoms will disappear when the block dissipates and, if necessary, the ocular manifestations can be reversed with a drop of ophthalmic phenylephrine.[10]

v. Intravascular Injection. The vertebral artery lies in close anatomic proximity to the roots of the brachial plexus and can be penetrated while performing this block.[32] The intravascular injection of a very small volume of local anesthetic may result in an almost immediate convulsion. This is usually self-limited and of short duration, but should be managed aggressively. The steps in the management of this complication are outlined under "Axillary Block—Complications and Treatment."

5. Subclavian Perivascular Block

a. *Technique*

For the subclavian perivascular approach to the brachial plexus, the local anesthetic is deposited at the level of the trunks of the plexus, where they lie in the groove between the anterior and middle scalene muscles, superior to the clavicle (Fig. 35–10A and B).

The anesthesiologist may stand on the side to be blocked and hold the needle in the right hand for a block on the left and in the left hand for a block on the right. It is also possible to stand at the head of the bed, above the patient, and use the dominant hand to hold the needle. The patient is placed in a comfortable supine position with the arm on the affected side gently extending toward the ipsilateral knee. The patient's head is then turned slightly to face away from the side to be blocked. The sternocleidomastoid muscle is identified; if this muscle is not easily palpated, it can be accentuated by having the patient elevate his or her head slightly.[12]

Subclavian Perivascular Block

Deeper anatomy: needle position and brachial plexus

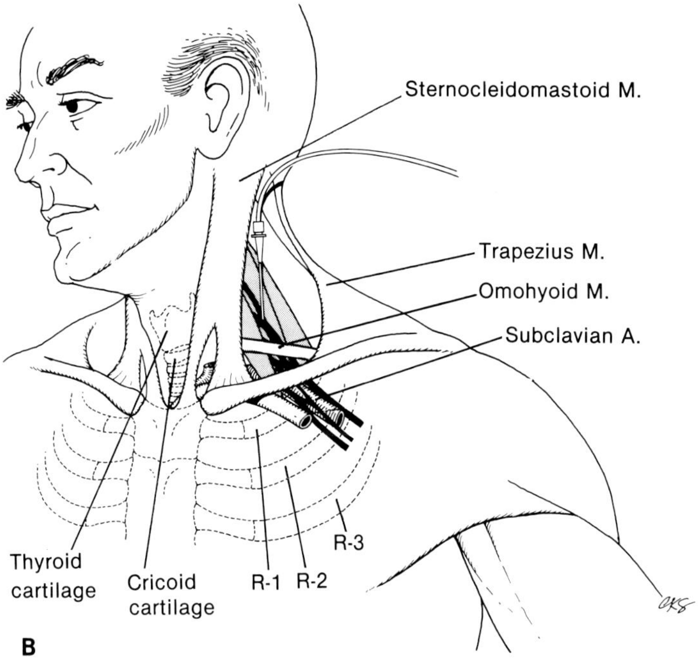

B

Technique

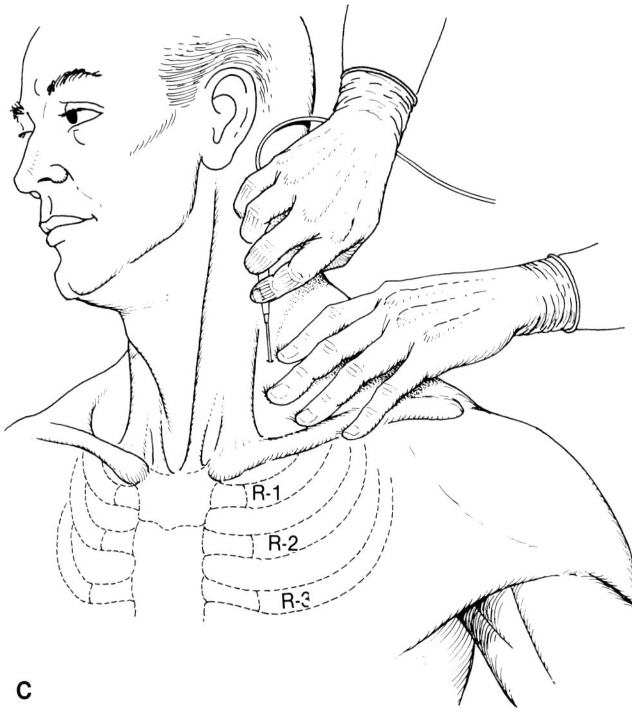

C

Figure 35–10 *(continued)*
(***B***) Deeper anatomy: the brachial plexus and its relation to the major vessels and muscular landmarks in the neck along with the position of the needle. (***C***) Technique: the superficial anatomic landmarks along with the technique of needle insertion and hand positions. The nondominant hand palpates the groove between the anterior and middle scalene muscles.

For additional muscle definition, the patient can attempt to elevate his or her head while the anesthesiologist places a hand on the forehead to provide resistance to head lift.

When the posterior border of the muscle is found, the palpating index and middle fingers are placed behind the muscle belly, the patient can then relax his or her head, and the fingers are rolled laterally over the anterior scalene muscle until the groove is felt between the anterior and middle scalene muscles. When the interscalene groove is identified, the physician uses one palpating finger and slides it inferiorly, following down along the groove toward the clavicle (Fig. 35-10C). It may not be possible to follow the groove very far inferiorly owing to the presence of the omohyoid muscle, which may obscure the groove.[12] In some patients, it will be possible to palpate the subclavian artery as it emerges between the anterior and middle scalene muscles above the clavicle; this can guide needle placement. Arterial puncture or transarterial technique should not be used as the sole indicator of correct needle placement, because this might result in a high failure rate of the block.[33] A skin wheal is raised at the tip of the palpating finger that lies at the most inferior level of the groove, and a 3.8-cm, 22 gauge, short-bevel block needle is inserted directly caudad along the anterior surface of the middle scalene muscle. The needle shaft may actually lie up against the skin of the neck, so it may not be possible to grasp the needle in the usual pencil-grip fashion, but it should be held between the thumb and forefingers.[12] Again, the immobile needle technique is used (see Axillary Block—Perivascular Technique) and the needle is slowly advanced until a paresthesia is elicited by touching one of the three trunks in the neurovascular space.[16] Before the block is performed, the patient should be instructed to tell the anesthesiologist immediately and without moving when he or she feels a paresthesia and where it is felt. A paresthesia that travels beyond the shoulder indicates correct needle placement, and needle advancement then is stopped.

The suprascapular nerve can be encountered and cause a paresthesia to be felt in the shoulder, but because this nerve may or may not be within the sheath at this level, this paresthesia cannot be accepted as confirming correct needle placement.[26] When the needle is in the correct position, aspiration is performed and should be negative for blood. Two to three mL of local anesthetic can then be injected rapidly to elicit a pressure paresthesia, which is additional confirmation that the needle is correctly positioned. The remainder of the local anesthetic is then injected with negative aspiration attempts after each incremental dose. The needle is withdrawn, and the groove may be massaged to enhance the spread of the local anesthetic. Twenty mL of local anesthetic solution should result in anesthesia of the entire brachial plexus. If the injection is made high in the subclavian perivascular space, there may be delay of onset or absence of anesthesia in the distribution of the inferior trunk, and therefore a volume of 40 mL of local anesthetic may be preferable.[12]

If no paresthesias are obtained by the advancing needle when performing this block, the needle will come into contact with the first rib and can then be withdrawn to a subcutaneous position and be redirected approximately 1 cm posteriorly along the length of the rib. If the subclavian artery is punctured, the needle should be reinserted slightly posterolaterally, closer to the middle scalene muscle to elicit paresthesias.[10] Because the artery lies within the perivascular space in front of the trunks, it serves as a valuable landmark for redirection. If a tourniquet is to be used or if the surgical procedure will involve the area of the arm innervated by the intercostobrachial (T-2) or the medial brachial cutaneous nerves, then these must be blocked separately. This blockade can be accomplished after the major injection by placing the needle directly over the axillary artery pulse high in the axilla. Five mL of local anesthetic is injected in a fan-like manner from this position to make a ring of solution around half of the proximal arm.

b. Advantages

The subclavian perivascular block is relatively easy to perform and can be used for most upper extremity surgery. The brachial plexus is contracted down to its fewest component parts in the neck, where this block is performed so that complete anesthesia is often obtained with smaller volumes of local anesthetic.[12] For this block, the arm remains at the patient's side and does not require movement in painful conditions.

The injection of local anesthetic into the subarachnoid or epidural space or the vertebral artery is almost impossible with this block.[10]

c. Disadvantages

This technique may fail to anesthetize the inferior trunk of the brachial plexus, with the resulting absence of anesthesia in the distribution of the inferior trunk, particularly if only a superior trunk paresthesia is elicited. This may be prevented by using a larger volume of local anesthetic or eliciting a middle or inferior trunk paresthesia.[34]

It is advised that paresthesias be sought to confirm correct needle placement with this block, and this may be perceived as a very unpleasant sensation by some patients.

d. Contraindications

This block should not be performed in patients who have infections in the head or neck area or if the anatomy has been distorted by trauma or previous surgery.[15]

It may also be a relative contraindication to do this block in a patient who is anticoagulated or has a bleeding diathesis. If the subclavian artery or vein is punctured, it may not be easy to apply pressure under the clavicle to prevent hematoma formation.

e. Complications and Treatment

i. Pneumothorax. The most serious complication that can result from this approach is a pneumothorax. If the needle is diverted too far medially or laterally instead of directly caudad along the interscalene groove, it may touch the dome of the pleura instead of the rib, which should serve as a backstop. The incidence of pneumothorax is 0.5% to 6%. The management of pneumothorax with this block is the same as with the other blocks (see "Infraclavicular Block—Complications and Treatment").

ii. Phrenic Nerve Block. Phrenic nerve block is rare with this technique and occurs in less than 2% of patients.[10] The nerve may be blocked by the spread of the local anesthetic in front of the anterior scalene muscle, where the nerve passes beneath the prevertebral fascia.[12] The management of this complication is the same as with the other blocks (see Classic Supraclavicular Block—Complications and Treatment).

iii. Vagus or Recurrent Laryngeal Nerve Block. The patient may develop hoarseness secondary to unilateral vocal cord paralysis if the vagus or the recurrent laryngeal nerve is blocked. The patient may only need reassurance but should also be cautioned to avoid oral intake until the hoarseness resolves and small sips of water can be tolerated. These complications are considered to be theoretical contraindications to the performance of bilateral blocks.[12] The block should also be avoided in patients who have unilateral vocal cord paralysis on the side opposite that to be blocked.

This complication can be seen in 1% of cases when the block is done on the patient's right side. Because the recurrent laryngeal nerve passes under the subclavian artery on the right side, hoarseness may occur more frequently when a right-sided block is performed.

iv. Sympathetic Nerve Block. A sympathetic block may also occur with the spread of the local anesthetic through the fascial barriers affecting the cervical sympathetic chain.[12]

If the sympathetic innervation to the head is affected, the patient may develop Horner's syndrome. The patient should experience no compromise from the development of Horner's syndrome, but should have the symptoms explained in advance. The symptoms will disappear when the block dissipates and, if necessary, the ocular changes can be reversed with a drop of ophthalmic phenylephrine.

v. Intravascular Injection. The subclavian artery and vein lie in close anatomic proximity to the subclavian perivascular space. The intravascular injection of local anesthetic may result in a convulsion. This is usually self-limited and of short duration, but should be managed aggressively. The steps in the management of this complication are as outlined under "Axillary Block—Complications and Treatment.

6. PARASCALENE BLOCK

a. Technique

For the parascalene approach to the brachial plexus, the local anesthetic is deposited at the level of the trunks of the brachial plexus at the lateral border of the anterior scalene muscle, which is the landmark for this block (Fig. 35-11A).

The anesthesiologist stands on the side to be blocked. The patient is placed in a comfortable supine position with the arm on the affected side gently extended toward the ipsilateral knee. The patient's head is then turned slightly to face away from the affected side. The patient is instructed to lift his or her head to identify the sternocleidomastoid muscle. A palpating finger is placed at the posterior edge of this muscle, just above the clavicle. The patient relaxes his or her head, and the palpating finger is rolled laterally to palpate the anterior scalene muscle. This muscle may be brought into prominence by asking the patient to inhale deeply, because it contracts as an accessory muscle of respiration. A skin wheal is raised on the lateral edge of the anterior scalene muscle at a point 1.5–2 cm above the clavicle[35] (Fig.

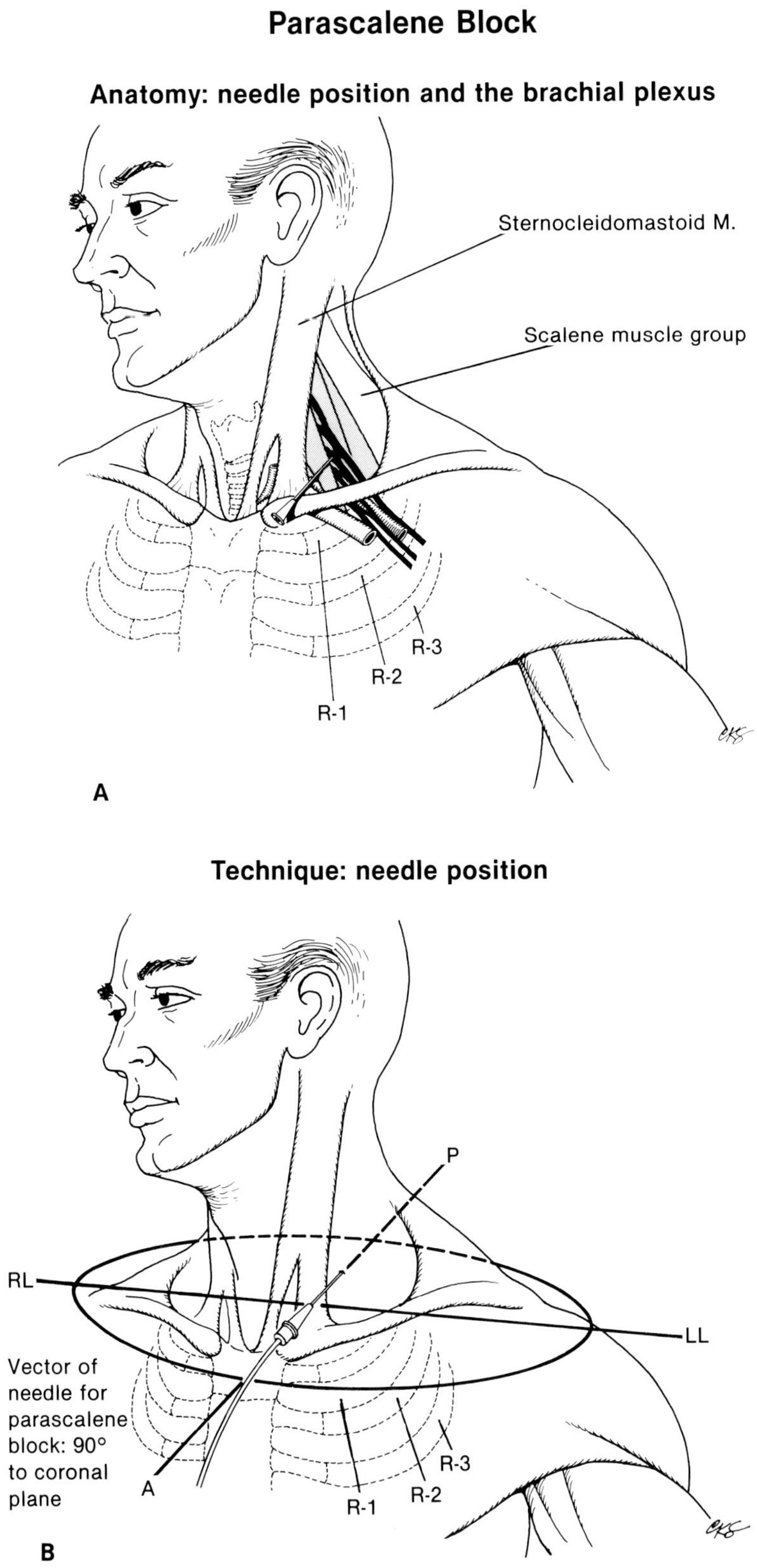

Figure 35–11 • Parascalene block. (***A***) Anatomy: the brachial plexus along with the position of the needle just lateral to the edge of the anterior scalene muscle. (***B***) Technique: the superficial anatomic landmarks along with the position of the needle.

35–11B). If the subclavian artery is palpable and the external jugular vein is visualized, the needle insertion point should lie superior and medial to these landmarks, respectively. The immobile needle technique (see "Axillary Block—Perivascular Technique") can be used with a 3.8-cm, 22 gauge, short-bevel block needle introduced at a 90° angle to the skin in an anteroposterior plane.[36] The needle is advanced slowly until a paresthesia is elicited. If no paresthesias are elicited, the needle is withdrawn to the subcutaneous position and redirected slightly laterally, and walked in a cephalad or caudal direction along the side of the muscle. The needle should not be inserted medial to the lateral margin of the anterior scalene, to avoid the cupola of the lung and possible pneumothorax. A nerve stimulator can be used if it is difficult to elicit paresthesias. The exploring electrode is attached with an alligator clip to the hub or proximal shaft of the block needle, and the ground electrode is attached to an ECG pad placed on the opposite shoulder. After the needle is in the correct position and aspiration test is negative for heme, the total volume of 40 mL of local anesthetic is injected in incremental doses with intermittent aspiration to insure that the solution is not injected intravascularly.

b. Advantages

The parascalene block can be used for most upper limb surgery. Complete anesthesia is often obtained because the local anesthetic is deposited at the level of the brachial plexus, where the trunks are most compact in the perineural sheath. For this block, the patient's arm remains at his or her side and does not require movement in painful conditions.

With a strictly anteroposterior insertion of the needle, it will encounter only muscular structure as it advances into the interscalene space (sternocleidomastoid, anterior scalene, and omohyoid muscles) or beyond the posterior aspect of the space (middle scalene and trapezius muscles).[36] If properly positioned, the needle should avoid the subarachnoid and epidural spaces and the major vessels of the neck.

c. Disadvantages

It is advised that paresthesias be sought with this technique to confirm correct needle placement; this may be perceived as a very unpleasant sensation by some patients. In certain patients it may not be possible to palpate the lateral border of the anterior scalene muscle owing to adiposity or poor muscle tone.

d. Contraindications

This block should not be performed in patients with infections in the head or neck region, or if the anatomy of the neck is distorted secondary to previous surgery or trauma.

e. Complications and Treatment

i. Pneumothorax. A rare but serious complication that can result from this approach is pneumothorax. If the needle is inserted medial to the lateral border of the anterior scalene muscles, the cupola of the lung, especially on the right side, may be penetrated. The management of pneumothorax associated with this block is the same as with the other blocks (see "Infraclavicular Block—Complications and Treatment.")

ii. Sympathetic Nerve Block. This complication may occur with the spread of local anesthetic through fascial barriers, affecting the cervical sympathetic chain.[12] The management of this complication is the same as with the other blocks (see "Classic Supraclavicular Block—Complications and Treatment.")

7. CONTINUOUS TECHNIQUES FOR BLOCKADE OF THE BRACHIAL PLEXUS

Continuous brachial plexus blockade by intermittent injection or continuous infusion of local anesthetic through a catheter has been described for various approaches to the brachial plexus to include the interscalene,[37,38] supraclavicular,[39,40] subclavian perivascular,[41] and axillary techniques.[42–46]

a. Technique

Patient preparation and positioning for continuous techniques is no different from those described previously for noncontinuous techniques. It is helpful to make a nick in the skin with an 18 gauge needle after the skin wheal is raised so that the catheter will advance easily. When the needle has been correctly positioned, 3–5 mL of local anesthetic or normal saline can be injected to expand the perineural space. If one is using a catheter over the needle, the plastic catheter can then be advanced off the needle and secured. The remainder of the local anesthetic is then carefully injected, either directly into the plastic catheter or through attached extension tubing.

Some authors have suggested threading a flexible guide wire through a 19 gauge needle positioned within the sheath, then withdrawing the needle and passing an 18 gauge flexible catheter over the guide wire.[44]

There are trays available for placing continuous catheters that contain all of the necessary equipment (Contiplex Continuous Brachial Plexus Anesthesia Tray, Burron Medical Inc., Bethlehem, PA).

b. *Advantages*

The continuous technique is especially useful for prolonged surgical procedures that may outlast the duration of a single dose of local anesthetic. It is also of benefit to leave a catheter in place for treatment of painful conditions such as reflex sympathetic dystrophy or postreimplantation pain. The catheter may be dosed periodically or a continuous infusion may be administered.[47]

c. *Disadvantages*

There is always a risk of infection when an indwelling catheter is placed; therefore, it must be checked daily.

The catheter may migrate out of the sheath or into a blood vessel and so it must be well secured and tested carefully before injection.

d. *Contraindications*

These are the same depending on the approach used; see the appropriate section.

e. *Complications and Treatments*

These are the same depending on the approach used; see the appropriate section.

IV. Determination of Quality of Block

After the local anesthetic has been injected, it is important to assess the completeness and adequacy of the block; this is usually manifested as progressively developing weakness and anesthesia in a proximal-to-distal distribution.

The onset of the sensory block may be slow for any of the approaches to the plexus that are used. Therefore, sensory testing should be done only after waiting at least 10 to 15 minutes after injection. Because the motor fibers are located more peripherally in the nerve bundle, motor blockade usually precedes sensory blockade and, therefore, one of the earliest signs of a successful block will be the onset of motor weakness. Motor testing can be done soon after injection.[12]

The patient who has received one of the brachial plexus blocks above the clavicle will not be able to elevate his or her arm off the table owing to blockade of the flexors and abductors of the shoulder.[15] If the patient is blocked distal to the level of the clavicle, the extensors of the forearm are initially blocked.

An understanding of the cutaneous innervation of the upper extremity and the sensory innervation of the hand by the median, ulnar, and radial nerves will guide both block assessment and supplementation.

V. Use of Nerve Stimulator

More accurate needle placement can be obtained by the objective observation of stimulated contractions of muscles that are innervated by the nerves in the plexus.[12,17] This can be accomplished by using a commercially available nerve stimulator that delivers pulses of current ranging from 0.1–10 mA.[17]

When using a peripheral nerve stimulator, the ground electrode is attached to an ECG pad, which is placed on the shoulder or chest opposite the side being blocked; the exploring electrode is attached to the needle with an alligator clip to the hub or proximal shaft. The needle is advanced through the skin, and then the stimulator is turned on to 3–5 mA. At this level of current, muscle contractions can be elicited if the nerve is a motor or mixed nerve, and a paresthesia will be elicited if the nerve is purely sensory. These responses can be obtained when the needle is still 1–2 cm away from the nerve, so the current should be reduced to 0.5–1 mA, and then the needle is very slowly advanced to find the point of maximum contraction.[48] It may be necessary to advance or withdraw the needle very slowly a few millimeters at a time to insure the most accurate needle placement by eliciting the maximum contraction or paresthesia with the lowest current.[26] After the needle is properly positioned, 2–3 mL of 2% lidocaine solution can be injected as a test dose. The muscle contraction or paresthesia should be abolished with this injection, and then the appropriate total dose of local anesthetic is carefully administered.[48]

VI. NEUROLOGIC COMPLICATIONS

Neurologic complications following brachial plexus blockade are very rare. Nerve damage from chemical toxicity can occur if the local anesthetic solution contains contaminants such as phenol, alcohol, sterilizing agents, or excessively high concentrations of epinephrine.[10] Errors can be avoided by carefully reading all container labels and the package inserts and then labeling the syringes into which the drugs are drawn up. The concentrations of local anesthetics that are used clinically do not result in nerve damage.

Nerve damage from mechanical trauma can occur secondary to the needle itself or via an intraneural injection.[5,49] When performing the various blocks of the brachial plexus, paresthesias are often actively sought to confirm correct needle placement, or they occur spontaneously as the needle is positioned. In a prospective study, Selander reported a 2% incidence of painful paresthesias in the postoperative period in patients in whom paresthesias were elicited during the block.[50] If paresthesias are elicited with gentle care and without rough probing, the incidence of complications will be decreased. Selander also determined in animal studies that there was greater risk of nerve damage with sharper needles.[51] A 45° beveled needle produces damage less frequently than a sharper, 14° needle, and the damage can be minimized if the bevel is oriented parallel to the nerve bundle fibers. It has also been shown that intrafascicular injections can result in axonal degeneration and a damaged blood–nerve barrier.[49] This problem can be avoided if the injection is stopped and the needle repositioned when the patient complains of pain on injection.

It is advisible to perform a neurologic examination of the involved extremity before placing a block. If the patient develops sensory or motor dysfunction after the procedure, electromyelographic and nerve conduction studies should be performed as soon as possible. These studies can define whether the neurologic sequela is the result of a preexisting lesion or a concomitant disease, and also can help determine the level of the lesion.[12] These studies and examinations should then be repeated 3 weeks after the block.

There is a tendency for the anesthesia technique to be blamed for any postoperative neurologic sequelae, but it must be remembered that there are a multiplicity of factors that might be responsible. These may include malpositioning of the patient or extremity during surgery, causing excessive pressure or stretching; direct surgical trauma pressure from surgical retractors; damage from the tourniquet or improperly applied casts; and trauma to the anesthetized and unprotected extremity after surgery, while the block is wearing off.

The risk of postblock nerve lesions can be greatly reduced if precautions are taken, the blocks are performed carefully and gently, and any postoperative symptoms or complaints are investigated quickly and thoroughly.

VII. REFERENCES

1. Bonica JJ. Regional anesthesia. Recent advances and current status. Clin Anesth 2:199–204, 1969.
2. Matas R. In Memoriam—William Stewart Halsted, An Appreciation. Bull John Hopkins Hosp 36:2–27, 1925.
3. Earle AS, Blanchard JM. Regional anesthesia in the upper extremity. Clin Plast Surg 12:97–114, 1985.
4. Bryce-Smith R, Lee JA (eds.). Local analgesia of the limbs. In Practical Regional Analgesia. American Elsevier Publishing, 1976, pp 51–60.
5. Selander D. Axillary plexus block: Parenthetic or perivascular. Anesthesiology 66:726–728, 1987.
6. Eriksson E, Schultz. Illustrated Handbook in Local Anesthesia. Chicago, Year Book Medical, 1979, pp 82–83.
7. Winnie AP, Radonjic R, Akkinemi S, Durrani Z. Factors influencing the distribution of local anesthetic injected into the brachial plexus sheath. Anesth Analg 58:225–234, 1979.
8. Partridge BL, Katz J, Benirschke K. Functional anatomy of the brachial plexus sheath. Implications for anesthesia. Anesthesiology 66:743–747, 1987.
9. Thompson GE, Rorie DK. Functional anatomy of the brachial plexus sheaths. Anesthesiology 59:117–122, 1983.
10. Ramamurthy S. Operative hand surgery. In Greene DP (ed): Anesthesia. 2nd ed. New York, Churchill Livingstone, 1988, 1:27–60.
11. Moore DC (ed). Supraclavicular approach for block of the brachial plexus. In Regional Block, A Handbook for Use in Clinical Practice of Medicine and Surgery. 4th ed. Springfield, IL, Charles C Thomas, 1953, pp 221–242.
12. Winnie AP. Plexus Anesthesia: Perivascular Techniques of Brachial Plexus Block. Philadelphia, W. B. Saunders, 1983.
13. Burnham P. Regional block of the great nerves of the upper arm. Anesthesiology 19:281, 1958.
14. Burnham P. Simple regional nerve block for surgery of the hand and forearm. JAMA 169:941–943, 1959.
15. Winnie AP. Regional anesthesia. Surg Clin North Am 55:861–892, 1975.
16. Winnie AP. An "immobile needle" for nerve blocks. Anesthesiology 31:577–578, 1969.
17. Bridenbaugh LD. The upper extremity: Somatic blockade. In

Cousins MJ, Bridenbaugh PO (eds): Neural Blockade in Clinical Anesthesia and Management of Pain. Philadelphia, JB Lippincott, 1988, pp 387–416.
18. Raj PR, Montgomery SJ, Nettles D, Jenkins MT. Infraclavicular brachial plexus block—a new approach. Anesth Analg 52: 897–904, 1973.
19. Kulenkampff D, Persky MA. Brachial plexus anesthesia. Ann Surg 87:883–891, 1928.
20. Patrick J. The technique of brachial plexus block anaesthesia. Br J Surg 27:734–739, 1939–1940.
21. Van Kleef JW, Burm AGL, Spierdijk J. Current Concepts in Regional Anesthesia. Boston, Martinus Nijhoff, 1984, pp 37–90.
22. Adriani J (ed). Blocks of peripheral nerves. In Nerve Blocks, a Manual of Regional Anesthesia for Practitioners of Medicine. Springfield, IL, Charles C Thomas, 1954, pp 112–120.
23. Eriksson E. Brachial plexus block—supraclavicular approach. In Illustrated Handbook in Local Anaesthesia. Chicago, Year Book Medical, 1969, pp 75–80.
24. Macintosh R, Mushin WW. Brachial plexus. In Local Analgesia. Edinburgh, ES Livingstone, 1967, pp 8–62.
25. Yamano Y. Safe method of supraclavicular brachial-plexus anesthesia. Arch Orthop Trauma Surg 102:92–94, 1983.
26. Murphy TM, Raj PR, Stanton-Hicks M. Techniques of nerve block—spinal nerves. In Raj PR (ed): Practical Management of Pain. Yearbook Medical, 1986, pp 597–636.
27. Hickey R, Ramamurthy S. The diagnosis of phrenic nerve block on chest x-ray by a double exposure technique. Anesthesiology 70:704–707, 1989.
28. Winnie AP. Interscalene brachial plexus block. Anesth Analg 49:455--466, 1970.
29. Winnie AP, Ramamurthy S, Durrani Z, Radonjic R. Interscalene cervical plexus block: A single-injection technic. Anesth Analg 54:370–375, 1975.
30. Sharrock NE, Bruce G. An improved technique for locating the interscalene groove. Anesthesiology 44:431–433, 1976.
31. Lombard TP. The interscalene approach to block of the brachial plexus. S Afr Med J 62:871, 1982.
32. Wildsmith JAW, Tucker GT, Cooper S, et al. Plasma concentrations of local anaesthetics after interscalene brachial plexus block. Br J Anesth 49:461–466, 1977.
33. Hickey R, Hoffman J, Ramamurthy S. Transarterial techniques are not effective for subclavian perivascular block. Reg Anaesth 15:245–249, 1990.
34. Hickey R, Garland TA, Ramamurthy S. Subclavian perivascular block: Influence of location of paresthesia. Anesth Analg 68:767–771, 1989.
35. Vongvises P, Panijayanond T. A parascalene technique of brachial plexus anesthesia. Anesth Analg 58:267–273, 1979.
36. Dalens B, Vanneuville G, Tanguy A. A new parascalene approach to the brachial plexus in children: Comparison with the supraclavicular approach. Anesth Analg 66:1264–1271, 1987.
37. Manriquez R, Pallares V. Continuous brachial plexus block for prolonged sympathectomy and control of pain. Anesth Analg 57:128–130, 1978.
38. Kirkpatrick AF, Bednarczyk LR, Hime GW, et al. Bupivacaine blood levels during continuous interscalene block. Anesthesiology 62:65–67, 1985.
39. Matsuda M, Kato Hosoi M. Continuous brachial plexus block for replantation in the upper extremity. Hand 14:129–134, 1982.
40. Ansbro F. A method of continuous brachial plexus block. Am J Surg 71:716, 1946.
41. DeKrey JA, Schroeder CF, Buechel DR. Continous brachial plexus block. Anesthesiology 30:332, 1969.
42. Sada T, Kobayashi T, Murakami S. Continuous axillary brachial plexus block. Can Anaesth Society J 30:201–205, 1983.
43. Gaumann D, Lennon R, Wedel D. Continuous axillary block for postoperative pain management. Reg Anaesth 13:77–82, 1988.
44. Ang ET, Lassale B, Goldfarb G. Continuous axillary brachial plexus block—a clinical and anatomical study. Anesth Analg 63:680–684, 1984.
45. Neimkin RJ, May JW, Roberts J, Sunder N. Continuous axillary block through an indwelling teflon catheter. J Hand Surg 9:830–833, 1984.
46. Selander D. Catheter technique in axillary plexus block; presentation of a new method. Acta Anaesthesiol Scand 21:324–329, 1977.
47. Tuominen M, Rosenberg PH, Kalso E. Blood levels of bupivacaine after single dose, supplement and during continuous infusion in axillary plexus block. Acta Anaesthesiol Scand 27:303–306, 1983.
48. Raj PR. Regional anesthesia for upper extremity surgery symposium: Ancillary measures to assure success. Reg Anaesth 5:9–12, 1980.
49. Bridenbaugh PO. Regional anesthesia for upper extremity surgery symposium: Complications. Reg Anaesth 5:6–8, 1980.
50. Selander D, Edshage S, Wolff T. Paresthesiae or no paresthesiae? Nerve lesions after axillary blocks. Acta Anaesthesiol Scand 23:27–33, 1979.
51. Selander D, Dhuner KG, Lundborg G. Peripheral nerve injury due to injection needles used for regional anesthesia. Acta Anaesthesiol Scand 21:812–188, 1977.

Chapter 36

•

H. Blane Howell, CDR, MC, USNR

Major Peripheral Nerve Blocks

OUTLINE

I. Introduction

This chapter describes how to block the major individual nerves of the upper extremity (the medial, radial, and ulnar nerves), as well as the major nerves of the leg (the sciatic, femoral, lateral femoral cutaneous, and obturator nerves). Because the major arm nerves supply sensation only to the hand, there is little advantage to blocking them at a site other than the wrist if hand area anesthesia is all that is desired.[1] Wrist blocks are reliable, successful, easy techniques, and use less volume of local anesthetic than do plexus blocks.[2] However, different locations for blocking those nerves as well as the sciatic nerve will be described for alternative approaches in case local conditions (eg, edematous, inflamed, or infected) at the preferred injection site cause that site to be unsatisfactory.

II. Indications and Contraindications

One may desire to block the individual major nerves of the upper extremity to solidify a brachial plexus block that is incomplete and has left the proposed surgical site with partial sensation, or to selectively block only the nerve that supplies sensation to that part of the hand where anesthesia is desired (Fig. 36–1).

Lower extremity blocks are most often done in groups. A "four-poster block" (sciatic, femoral, lateral femoral cutaneous, obturator) provides the lower extremity with anesthesia for surgical procedures that require the use of a thigh tourniquet for better control of blood loss. Also, the sciatic nerve can be blocked in conjunction with the femoral nerve for closed manipulations of fractures in the lower leg or for procedures during which a calf tourniquet can be used (Fig. 36–2).

Regional anesthesia of the extremities is contraindicated in those patients who are not willing or able to cooperate with the procedure, have infection in the area through which the block must be placed, have excessive interstitial pressure in the muscular compartments through which the block is to be placed, have a known bleeding diathesis, or are psychotic. Caution should also be exercised in blocking nerves that are known to be or have the potential to be involved in any sort of disease process or trauma, lest the physician performing the block exacerbate that process, worsen the injury, or be accused of doing either.

Obtaining a paresthesia in the body area supplied by the nerve when probing for the nerve to be blocked, or using a nerve stimulator to cause a motor response from the target nerve, is most helpful in ensuring that the block will indeed occur and will have a quick onset. However, the injection must be stopped if pain or an ongoing paresthesia occurs during injection of the local anesthetic, because these indicate that the injection is intraneural and, if continued, could result in permanent injury to the nerve.

Motor fibers of a nerve are stimulated at a threshold lower than that necessary to stimulate sensory fibers.[3] Obtaining a motor response by stimulating a nerve with 0.2 mA of electrical current allows discrete identification of individual peripheral nerves in those patients who are cooperative but unable to describe paresthesias because they are heavily sedated, inebriated, comatose, senile, or under general anesthesia.[4]

Ester local anesthetics are contraindicated in those known to be allergic to them.

III. How to Block the Major Peripheral Nerves

A. *Blocks of the Major Nerves of the Upper Extremity*

1. Arm

a. *Radial Nerve*

The radial nerve can be blocked on the lateral aspect of the arm at the junction of the lower and middle thirds of the arm, where the nerve emerges from wrapping posteriorly around the humerus.[5] Place a 22 to 23 gauge,

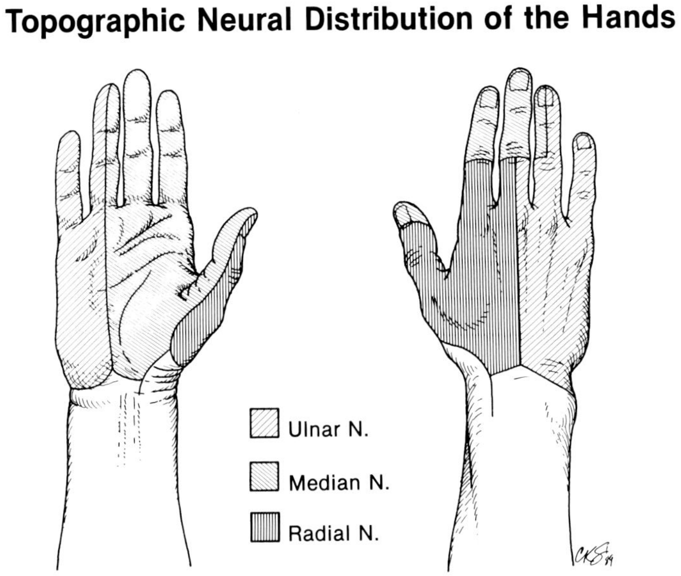

Figure 36–1 • Topographic neural distribution of the hands. The sensory distribution of the individual nerves is shown by different shadings.

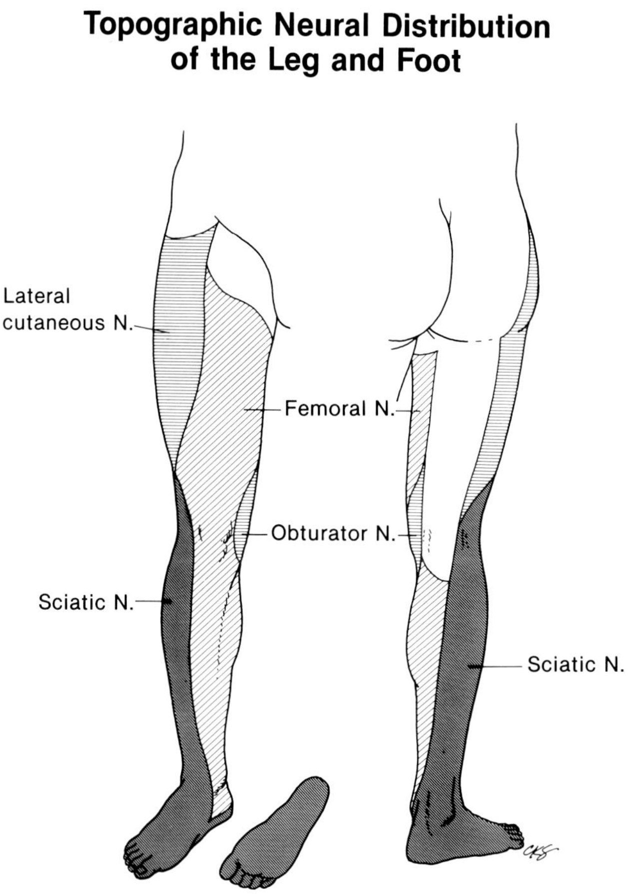

Figure 36–2 • Topographic neural distribution of the leg and foot. The sensory distribution of the individual nerves is shown by different shadings.

B-bevel (blunt tip) needle perpendicular to the skin at a point on the lateral aspect of the arm approximately 8–9 cm proximal to the lateral epicondyle of the humerus (Fig. 36–3), and advance the needle until a paresthesia to the dorsum of the thumb or first finger is obtained or bone is encountered. Although the nerve can sometimes be palpated at that spot in thin individuals, it is the better part of valor to inject 10 mL of anesthetic solution horizontally in a fanlike pattern in the general target area near the humerus if no paresthesia is obtained.

2. ELBOW

As a general rule, anesthesia is quicker in onset and more reliable if paresthesias are obtained when blocking the median and ulnar nerves at either the elbow or the wrist.[6]

a. *Median Nerve*

The elbow should be extended and the forearm supinated. Palpate the brachial artery just under a line from the medial epicondyle to the lateral epicondyle; this imaginary line usually is the same as the flexor crease of the elbow. On this line and just medial to the artery, place a short, 22 to 23 gauge, B-bevel needle perpendicularly through the skin until a paresthesia is elicited, and then inject 5 mL of anesthetic solution (Fig. 36–4).

b. *Radial Nerve*

This block is a hard one to obtain consistently, and a paresthesia is a welcome finding. The elbow should be extended and the forearm suppinated. On an imaginary line joining the epicondyles, place a long (4–5 cm), 22 to 23 gauge, B-bevel needle between the insertion of the biceps tendon and the brachioradialis muscle (see Fig. 36-4), advance it until contact is made with the bone of the anterior aspect of the lateral epicondyle, and place 3–4 mL of local anesthetic solution; inject another 5 mL as the needle is withdrawn toward the skin. The procedure should be repeated twice more, with the needle redirected so as to hit bone a little more medially each time.

c. *Ulnar Nerve*

The elbow is flexed 90°, and the nerve palpated in the groove on the posterior aspect of the medial epicondyle. Insert a short, 22 to 23 gauge, B-bevel needle toward the nerve; only after eliciting a paresthesia, place 3–5 mL of local anesthetic (Fig. 36–5). This block should be avoided in cases of ulnar nerve neuritis. It is also best to block the nerve 1–2 cm proximal to the ulnar sulcus to lessen the chance of neuritis.[7]

3. WRIST

a. *Median Nerve*

The elbow is extended, the forearm supinated, and the wrist slightly extended. Between the palmaris longus tendon and the flexor carpi radialis, at the proximal palmar flexor crease, place a 25 gauge needle through the skin a right angle, and advance it up and down in a fanlike fashion perpendicular to the longitudinal axis un-

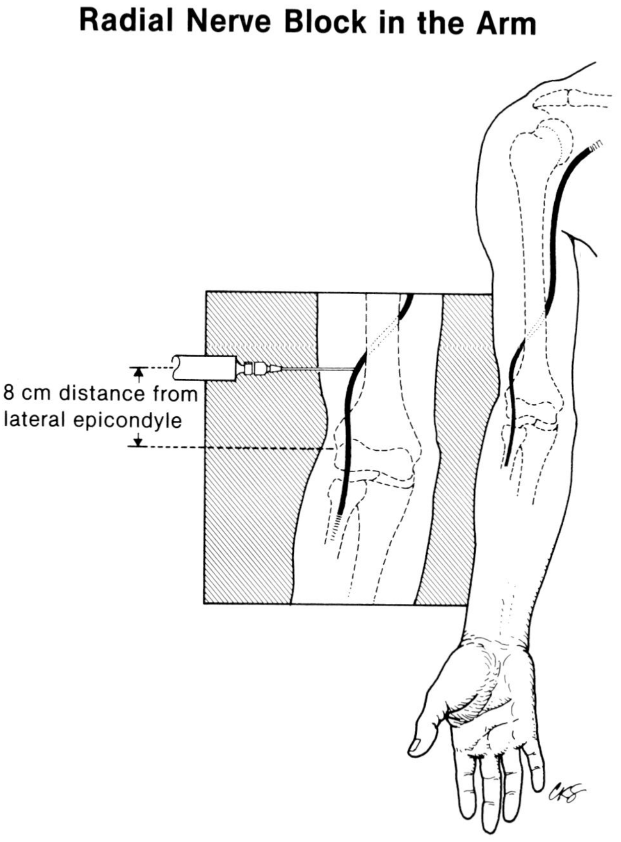

Figure 36–3 • Radial nerve block in the arm. The point of needle insertion is 8 cm proximal to the lateral epicondyle. The needle is advanced until a thumb or first finger paresthesia is obtained or the humerus is encountered.

til the desired paresthesia is obtained. Inject 2–5 mL of local anesthetic (Fig. 36–6).

b. Ulnar Nerve

At the proximal flexor crease of the wrist, the ulnar nerve has already divided into its palmar and dorsal branches.

The palmar branch may be blocked in one of two ways. In both approaches the elbow is extended, the forearm supinated, and the wrist slightly extended.

Approach 1. Place a 25 gauge needle at a right angle through the skin at the proximal flexor crease, medial to the flexor carpi ulnaris and lateral to the ulnar artery (see Fig. 36–6), and advance it until a paresthesia is obtained; then place 3–5 mL of local anesthetic there. If bone is encountered instead, place 7–10 mL of solution while the needle is withdrawn into the subcutaneous tissue.

Approach 2. Approach the nerve from the ulnar side of the wrist by placing the needle just under the flexor carpi ulnaris and advancing the tip approximately 1–2 cm until a paresthesia is obtained; there place 3–5 mL of local anesthetic (Fig. 36–7).

The dorsal branch is blocked by infiltrating the subcutaneous tissue of the ulnar border of the wrist from the flexor carpi ulnaris to the styloid process of the ulna with 3–5 mL of local solution.

c. Radial Nerve

The elbow is extended, the forearm supinated, and the wrist slightly flexed. Palpate the radial artery at the level of the proximal flexor crease, and place 3 mL of local anesthetic solution just lateral to the artery; pronate the forearm 90°, and place a 5-mL cuff of anesthetic solution in the subcutaneous tissue over the radial–dorsal aspect of the wrist from the site of the first injection to the styloid process of the ulna (Fig. 36–8).

B. *Blocks of the Major Nerves of the Lower Extremity*

1. Sciatic Nerve

The sciatic nerve may be blocked from the usual posterior approach, and also by an anterior approach.[6a]

Median and Radial Nerve Block at the Elbow

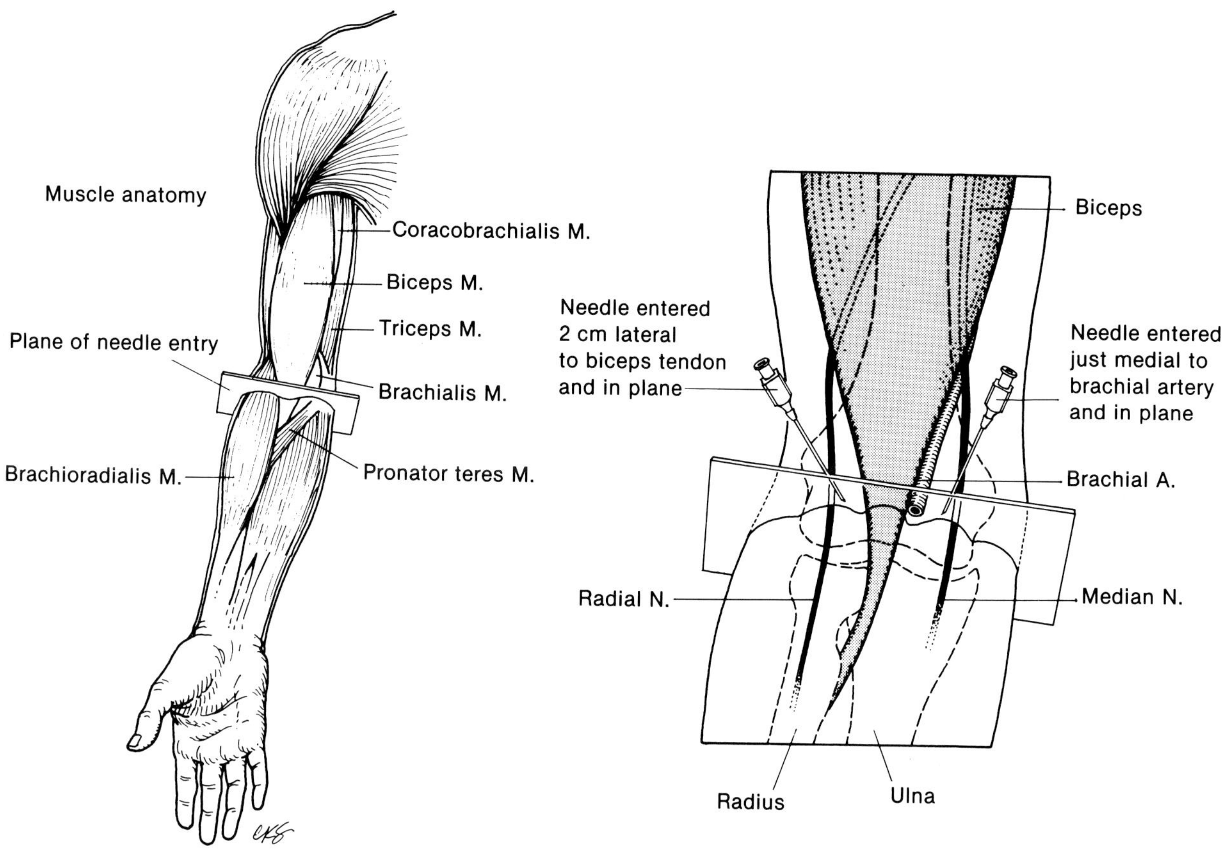

Figure 36–4 • Median and radial nerve block at the elbow. The left panel shows a plane that connects the medial to the lateral epicondyle and is perpendicular to the extended arm. The right panel shows the points of needle insertion for radial nerve and medial nerve block.

Ulnar Nerve Block at the Elbow

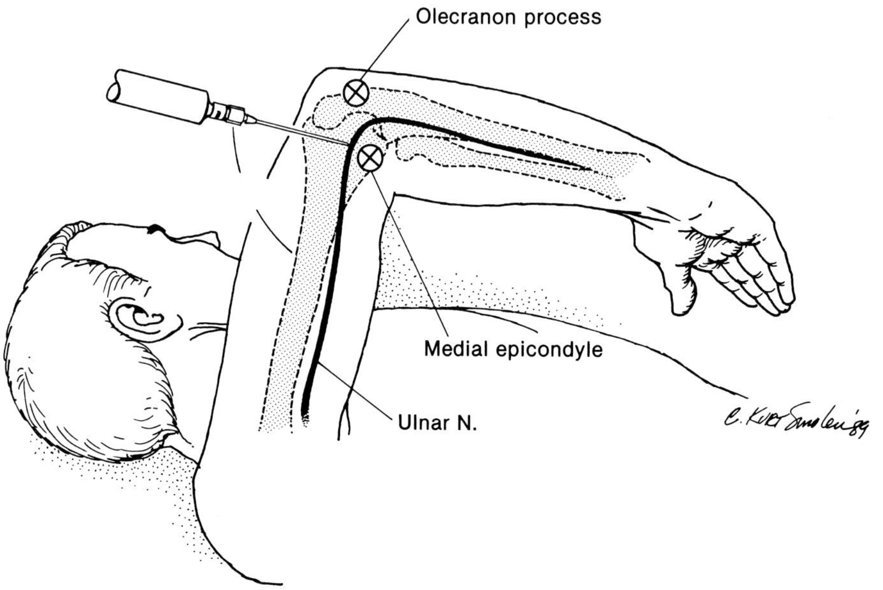

Figure 36–5 • Ulnar nerve block at the elbow. The point of needle insertion is the groove between the olecranon process and the medial epicondyle.

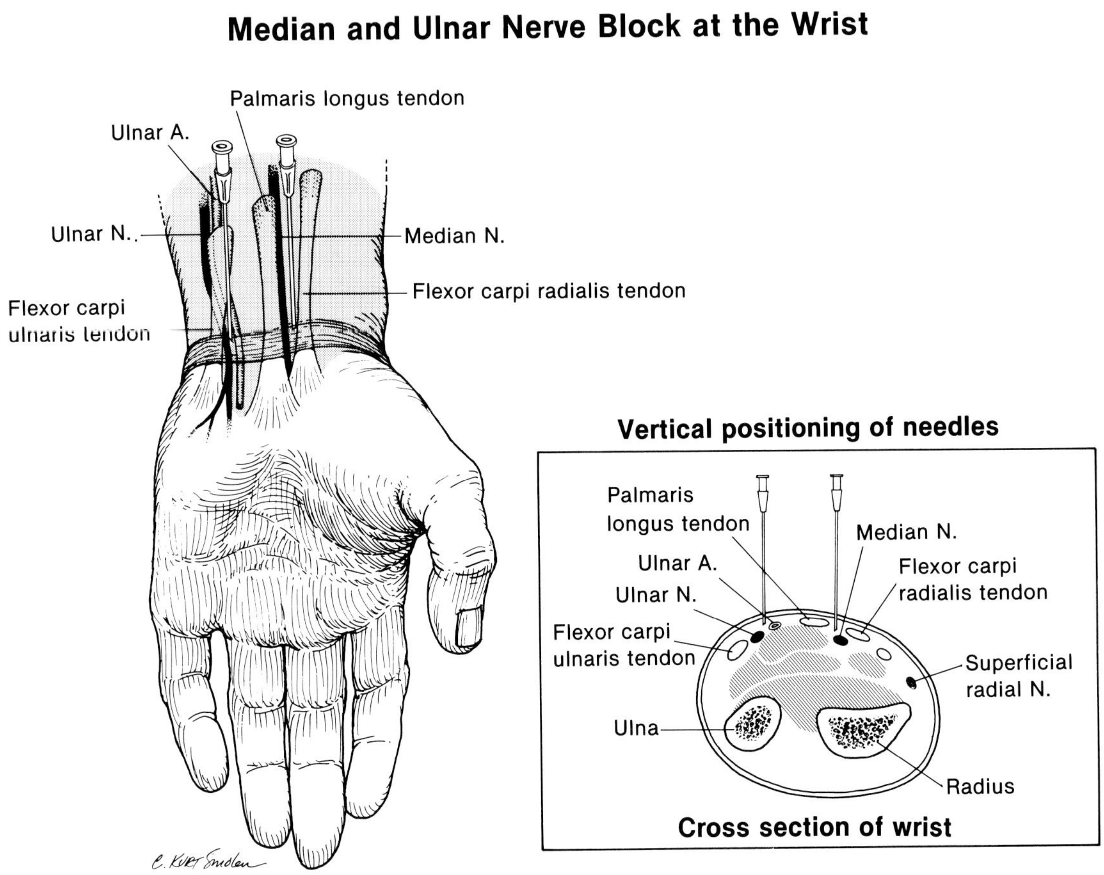

Figure 36–6 • Median and ulnar nerve block at the wrist. The left panel shows the points of needle insertion for medial and ulnar nerve block at the wrist. The inset, a cross section of the wrist, shows the relation of the vertical needles to the tendons, nerves, and arteries.

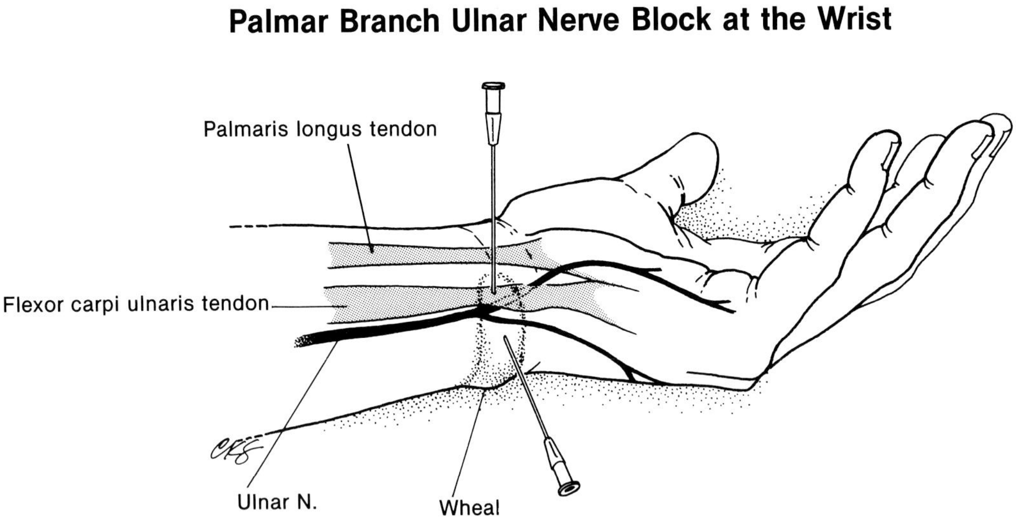

Figure 36–7 • Palmar branch ulnar nerve block at the wrist. This block is done in addition to the block of the ulnar nerve shown in Fig. 36–6.

Radial Nerve Block at the Wrist

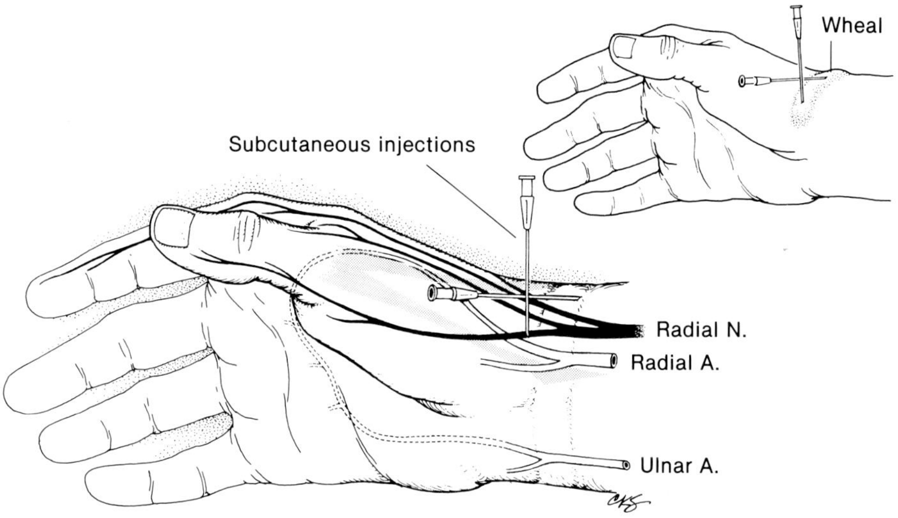

Figure 36–8 • Radial nerve block at the wrist. Local anesthetic is placed just lateral to the radial artery at the proximal flexor crease and as a cuff or wheal in subcutaneous tissue of the radial dorsal aspect of the wrist.

a. Posterior Approach

The patient is positioned on the side not to be blocked, with the knee and hip of the side to be blocked flexed such that the bell of that side lies in the opposite popliteal fossa. A line is drawn from the greater trochanter of the femur to the posterior superior iliac spine; that line is bisected, and another line extended inferiorly for 3 cm perpendicular to the first line to mark the point of injection, where a skin wheal of 0.5–1.0 mL of 1% lidocaine is placed (Fig. 36–9). This point can be verified by bisecting a line drawn from the greater trochanter to a point just below the sacral cornua. If unsuccessful in finding the nerve deep below the skin wheal, it should lie slightly more distally, just medial to the midpoint of a line drawn from the greater tuberosity to the ischial tuberosity. A long, 10- to 12-cm, 21 gauge needle is used to probe the nerve until a paresthesia is obtained that extends all the way to the toes or foot; after the needle tip is withdrawn 2 mm, 20–30 mL of local anesthetic solution is placed to block this large nerve.

b. Anterior Approach

The patient is placed supine. Draw a line (Fig. 36–10) from the anterior superior iliac spine to the pubic tubercle, corresponding to the inguinal ligament (line No. 1). At the junction of the middle and medial thirds of this line, draw a perpendicular line extending toward the lateral upper thigh (line No. 2). From the greater trochanter of the femur, draw a line (line No. 3) extending medially, parallel to line No. 1. The intersection of line No. 2 with line No. 3 marks the point of needle insertion, and a skin wheal of 0.5–1.0 mL of 1% lidocaine is placed there. A 10- to 12-cm-long, 21 gauge needle is inserted through the skin wheal with the needle angled just lateral to perpendicular to the skin, and advanced until bone (the femur) is touched. The needle is then withdrawn to just below the skin, redirected medially to just miss the femur, and advanced 5 cm beyond where bone contact was originally made. A test injection of a small amount of local anesthetic is given. If the injection requires an excess amount of firm pressure, the tip of the needle probably lies in a muscle bundle rather than close beside the nerve, so the tip of the needle should be advanced until there is minimal or loss of resistance to injection.[8] This indicates that the tip of the needle is in the fascial plane, investing the neurovascular bundle of which the sciatic nerve is a part. A paresthesia is welcomed, but not searched for. After aspirating to make sure the needle tip is not intravascular, 20–30 mL of local anesthetic solution is injected.

Sciatic Nerve Block: Posterior Approach and Point of Insertion

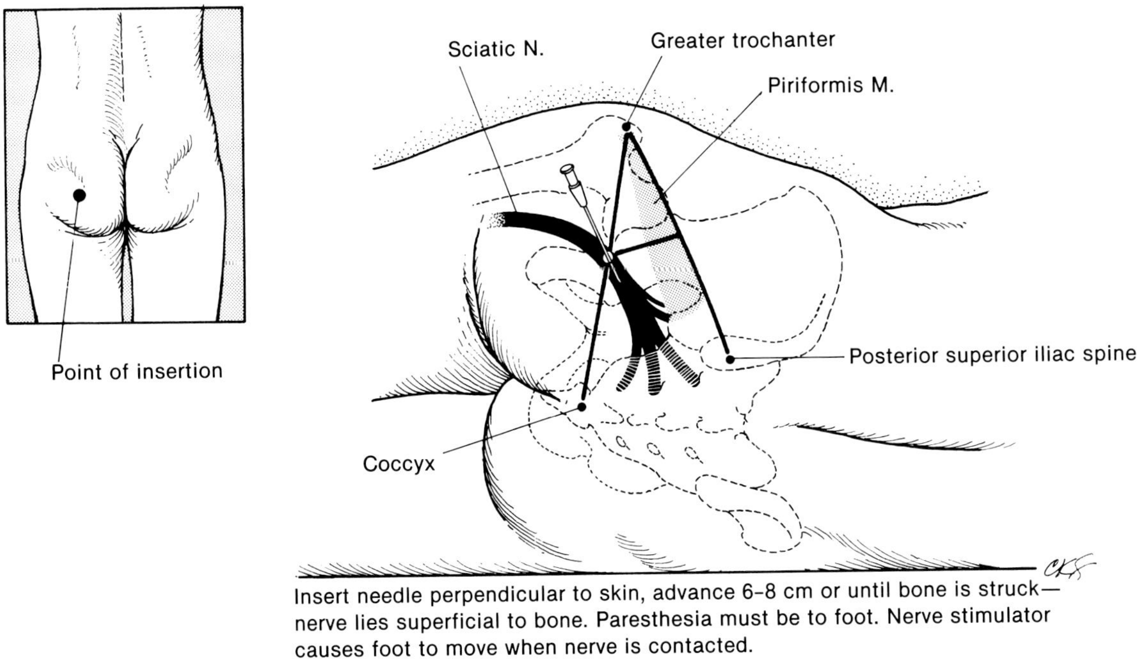

Figure 36–9 • Sciatic nerve block: posterior approach and point of insertion. See text for full explanation.

Sciatic Nerve Block: Anterior Approach and Point of Insertion

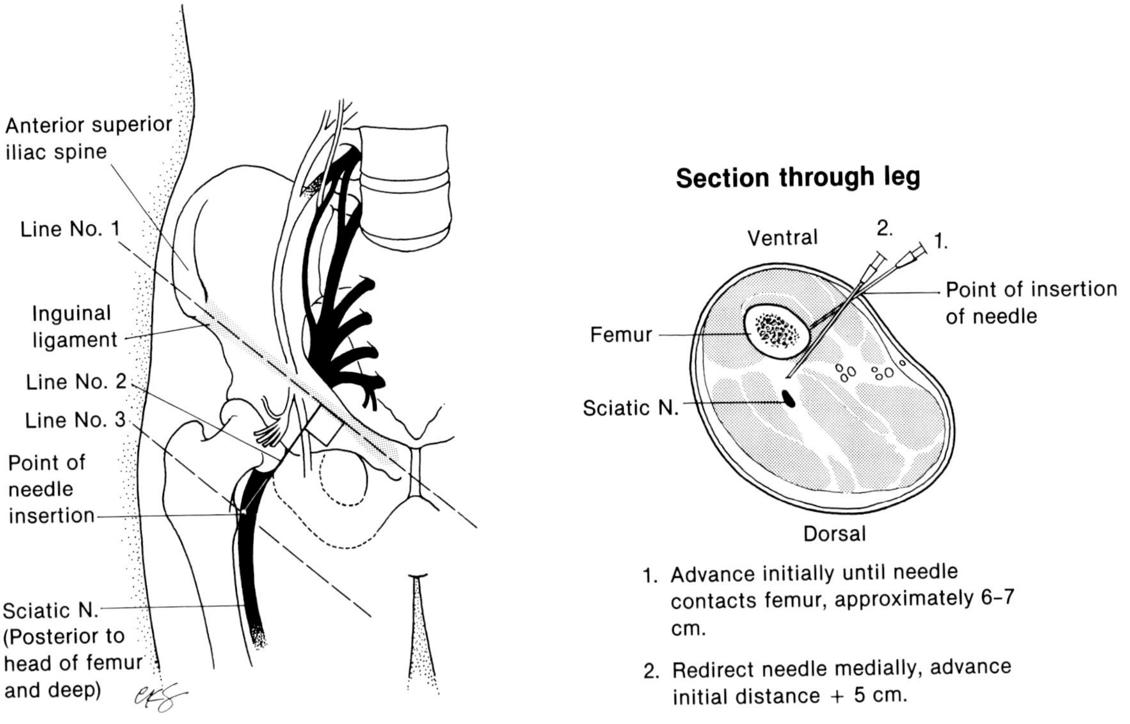

Figure 36–10 • Sciatic nerve block: anterior approach and point of insertion. See the text for full explanation.

2. FEMORAL NERVE

The femoral nerve supplies sensation to the anterior surface of the thigh and the medial side of the calf to the medial malleolus (see Fig. 36–2). It lies immediately lateral to the femoral artery, where both cross under the inguinal ligament; that is where the nerve is blocked (Fig. 36–11). The artery is palpated, and a nerve stimulator is used to locate the nerve by attaching the stimulator to a blunt-tip, 22 gauge needle, and choosing 0.2 mA of electrical current for the stimulator; the needle is placed lateral to the arterial pulsations and advanced perpendicularly through the skin 3–5 cm until the nerve is encountered, with resulting jerking of the quadriceps femoris muscle. After a negative aspiration, local anesthetic is injected and the muscle response stops. Because the nerve often has branched prior to reaching the inguinal ligament area, it often is necessary to search for all of the nerve's divisions to obtain an effective block. Approximately 15–20 mL of anesthetic solution usually is required to achieve a total block.

3. LATERAL FEMORAL CUTANEOUS NERVE

This nerve supplies sensation over the lateral aspect of the thigh (see Fig. 36–2). It is blocked where it runs superficially and near the anterior superior iliac spine and inguinal ligament (Fig. 36–12). Place a 22 gauge blunt needle at a point approximately 2 cm below and 2 cm medial to the anterior superior iliac spine, and advance the needle perpendicular to the skin 2–3 cm until the needle is felt to "pop" through the fascia lata. After negative aspirations, injections are given in a fanlike manner, perpendicular to the direction of the inguinal ligament. Usually 5–10 mL of anesthetic is sufficient.

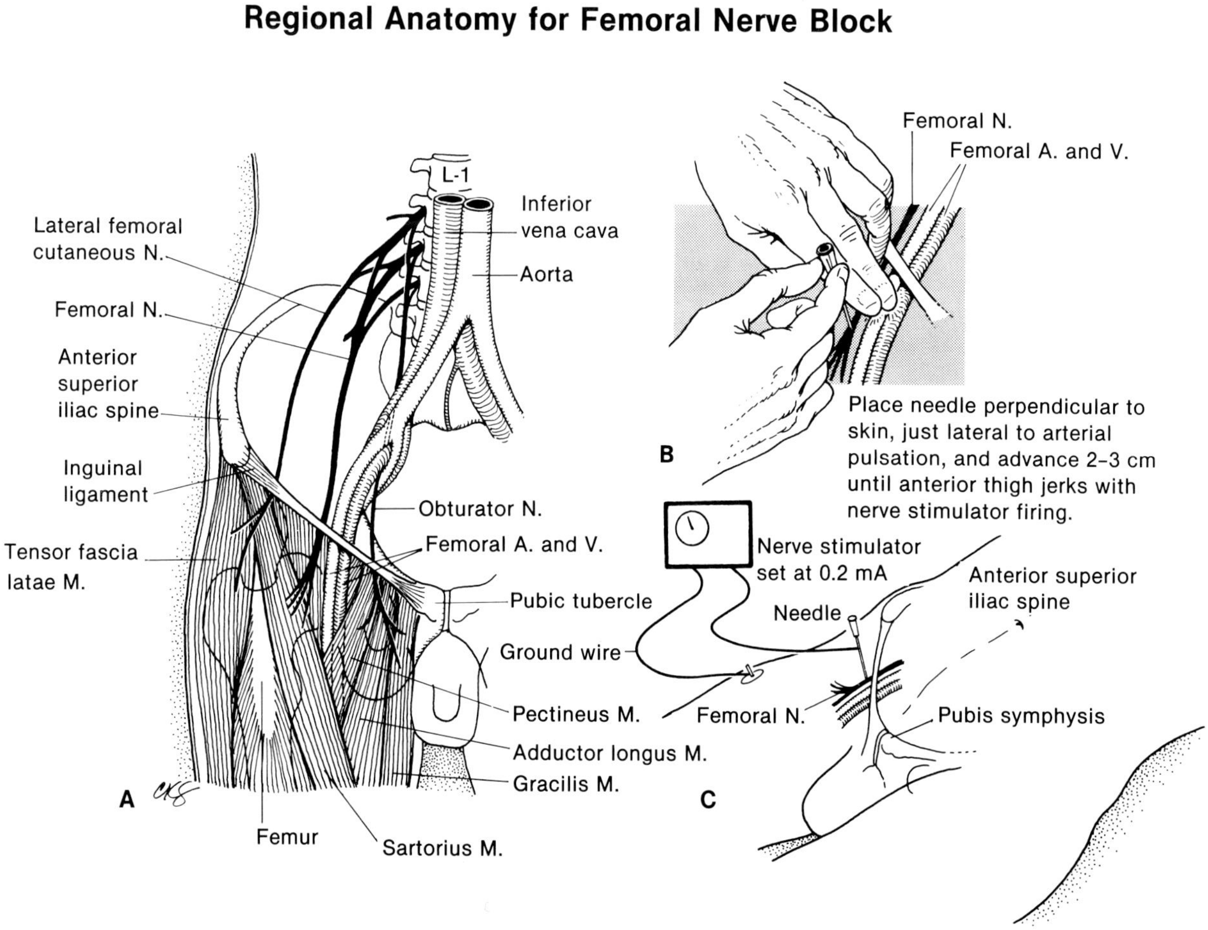

Figure 36–11 • Femoral nerve block. (***A***) Regional anatomy. (***B***) Point of needle insertion. (***C***) Use of nerve stimulator. See the text for full explanation.

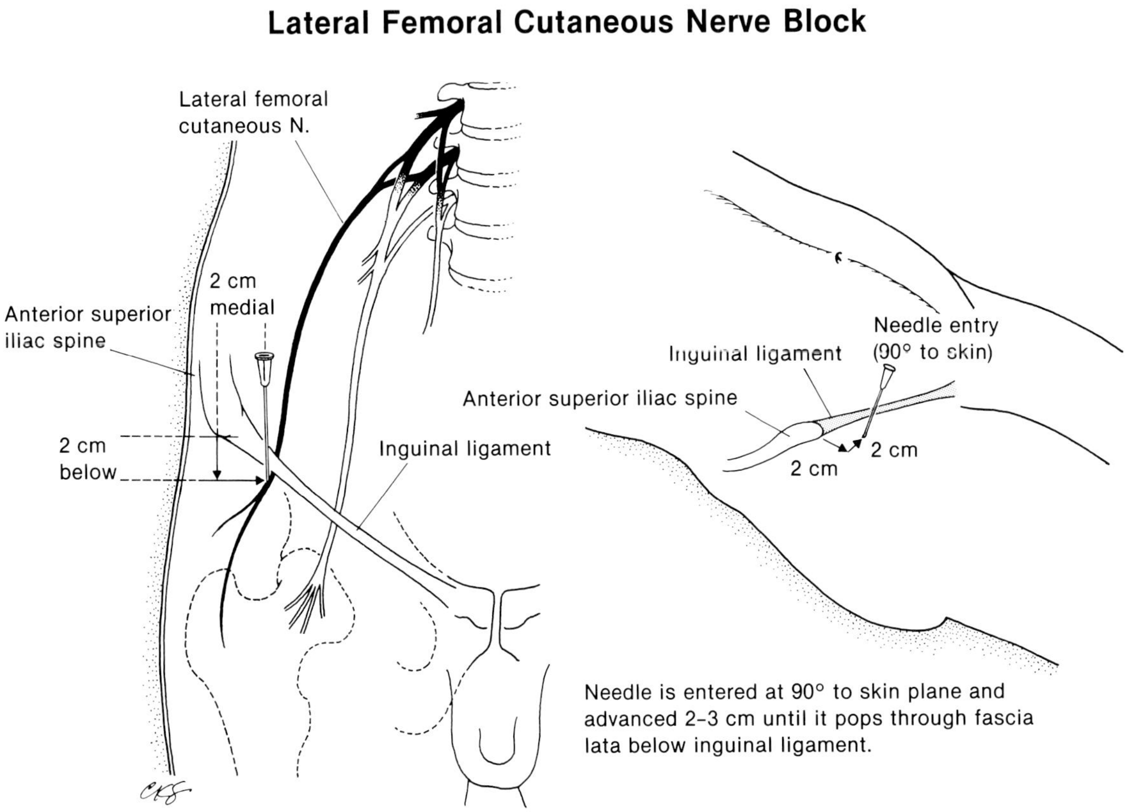

Figure 36–12 • Lateral femoral cutaneous nerve block. Point of needle insertion is 2 cm below and 2 cm medial to the anterior superior iliac spine. (***A***) Anterior view. (***B***) Lateral view.

4. Obturator Nerve

This nerve supplies sensation to an area on the medial side of the thigh (see Fig. 36–2) and exits the bony pelvis via the deep obturator canal, where it is blocked (Fig. 36–13). To do so, place the leg in slight abduction. At a point 1 cm lateral and 2 cm caudad to the pubic tubercle on the side to be blocked, insert a 7-cm, 22 gauge needle at a right angle to the skin until it comes in contact with bone (the inferior pubic ramus). Reposition the needle tip laterally and cephalad in steps until it misses bone and enters the obturator canal and can be advanced 2–3 cm further than when it hit bone on previous attempts (see Fig. 36–12). After a negative aspiration to insure that the obturator artery and vein have been missed, deposit 6–10 mL of anesthetic.

5. The "Three-in-One" Block

By varying the technique for the femoral nerve block slightly, it often is possible to block the femoral, lateral femoral cutaneous, and obturator nerves at the same time.[9] The variation is this: after locating the femoral nerve, apply firm pressure with all four fingers of one hand across the femoral canal area immediately distal to the site of injection, and maintain this pressure while injecting 30 mL of anesthetic solution after a negative aspiration. The distal pressure can help force the large volume of local anesthetic up the fascial envelope covering the nerve and into the area of the lumbar plexus, effecting blockade of all three major nerves that have lumbar roots (femoral, lateral femoral cutaneous, and obturator). It should be noted that the sacral roots that make up the sciatic nerve are missed with this technique.

IV. Discussion

A. *How to Tell if the Block is Working*

Loss of sensation to heat and pain in the desired area is the ultimate goal of regional anesthesia, but the onset of sensory loss may be delayed, and it may not be com-

Obturator Nerve Block

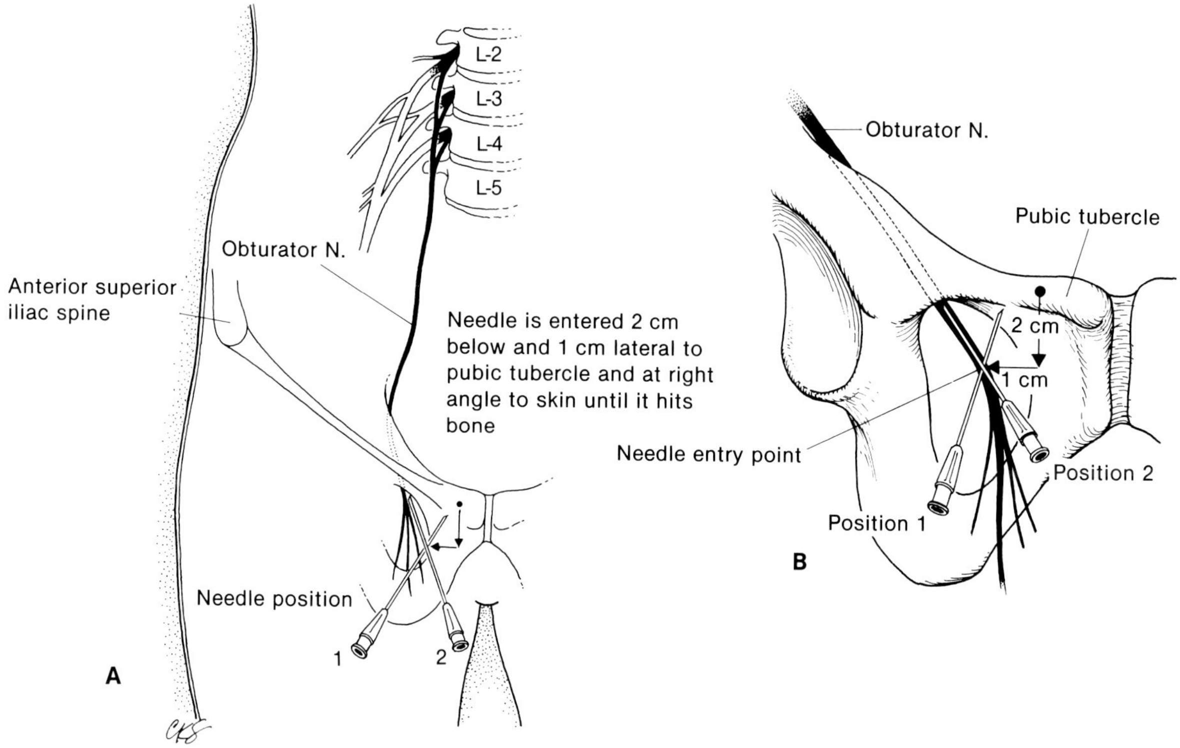

Figure 36–13 • Obturator nerve block. The point of needle insertion is 2 cm below and 1 cm lateral to the pubic tubercle. The needle is angled perpendicular to the skin until it hits the pubic tubercle (needle position 1). The needle is then walked off the bone laterally until it enters the obturator canal (needle position 2). (***A***) Anterior superficial view. (***B***) Frontal deep view.

plete for 15–20 minutes, even with the more rapidly acting local anesthetics. Evidence of blockade of the sympathetic and motor nerve fibers that run along with the sensory nerves gives a quicker indication that the sensory nerve block will eventually be successful. Evidence of sympathetic nerve blockade usually is noticed first, manifested by venodilation and increased skin temperature in the area supplied by the nerve.

Blockade of motor fibers gives the best estimate of how successful the sensory blockade will be. Total paralysis indicates that total blockade of pain fibers also will occur. Muscles that are getting weaker with time indicate that the degree of sensory blockade is increasing in the nerves that supply those muscles.

The following are good motor tests to evaluate specific nerve blocks (Fig. 36–14):

Median nerve: (A) Opposition of middle finger and/or index finger to thumb; flexion of medial three digits.
Radial nerve: (B) Extension of the fingers, wrist.
Ulnar nerve: (C) Flexion of the lateral two fingers.
Sciatic nerve: (D) Plantar and dorsal flexion of the foot and toes.
Femoral nerve: (E) Flexion of the thigh.
Obturator nerve: (F) Adduction of the thigh.

B. *Local Anesthetics for the Block*

Many combinations of local anesthetics have been and can be used for peripheral nerve blockade. The following solutions give varying anesthetic times and can be used to tailor the anesthesia to the procedure, or for prolonged postoperative analgesia.

1. Xylocaine 1.5% with 1:200,000 epinephrine: usually effective for 1.5–2 hours.
2. Carbocaine 2.0%: usually effective for 4 hours.
3. Marcaine 0.5% with 1:200,000 epinephrine: usually effective for 12–20 hours.

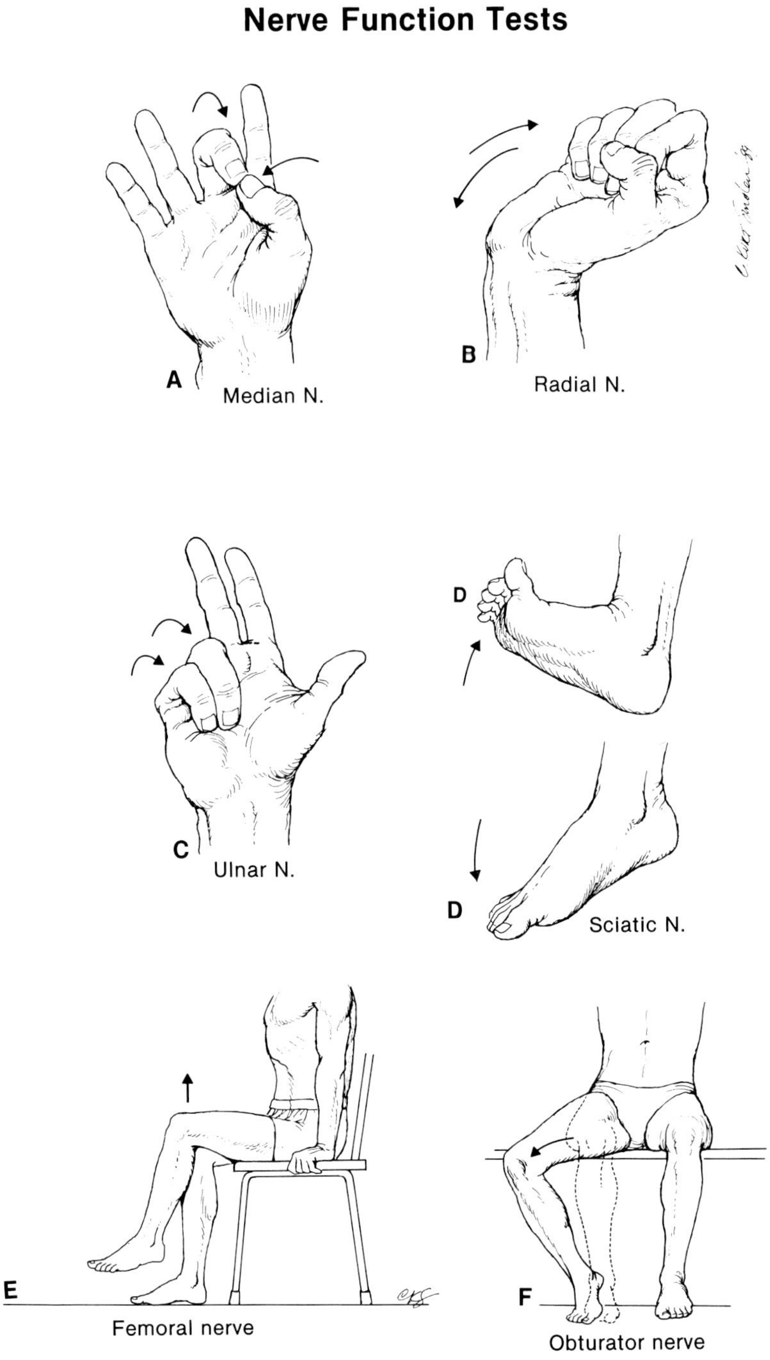

Figure 36–14 • Nerve function tests. The failure of these motor tests gives the best estimate of successful sensory blockade.

V. Complications

Many of the major peripheral nerves run in close proximity to larger arteries and veins, and there is always the possibility of an intravascular injection, with its subsequent central nervous system and cardiovascular toxic effects. Always aspirate prior to injection, and be sure that the aspiration is negative for blood or lymph. One should be absolutely prepared to treat convulsions and cardiorespiratory arrest by having adequate training and the necessary equipment close at hand.

Care should be taken to not inject medication if it causes pain or an increasing paresthesia in the distribution of the nerve to be blocked; this may indicate an intraneural injection, which could cause a permanent neurologic deficit.

Allergic reactions are extremely uncommon if the ester group of local anesthetics is avoided.

All blocks should be done aseptically to lessen the chance of introducing infection into the deeper tissues of the body. Of course, the needle should never be advanced through infected or inflamed tissue while performing the block.

VI. REFERENCES

1. Earle AS, Blanchard JM. Regional anesthesia in the upper extremity. Clin Plast Surg 12:87, 1985.
2. Raggi PR. Balanced regional anesthesia for hand surgery. Orthop Clin North Am 17:473, 1986.
3. Sarnof SJ, Sarnof IC. Prolonged peripheral nerve block by means of indwelling plastic catheter. Treatment of hiccup. Note on the electrical localization of peripheral nerve. Anesthesiology 12:270, 1951.
4. Reese CA. Conduction anesthesia of the lower extremity; a technique and literature review. J Am Assoc Nurse Anes June:237, 1978.
5. Miller RD (ed). Anesthesia. 2nd ed. Chapter 30. New York, Churchill Livingston, 1986.
6. The upper extremity: Somatic blockade. In: Cousins MJ, Bridenbaugh PO (eds). Neural Blockade and Pain Management. 2nd edition. Philadelphia, JB Lippincott, 1988.

6a. The lower extremity: Somatic blockade. In: Cousins MJ, Bridenbaugh PO (eds). Neural Blockade and Pain Management. 2nd edition. Philadelphia, JB Lippincott, 1988.

7. Eriksson E (ed). Illustrated Handbook in Local Anesthesia. London, Lloyd-Luke Medical Books, 1979, pp 86–93, 101–110.
8. McNicol LR. Anterior approach to sciatic nerve block in children: Loss of resistance or nerve stimulator for identifying the neurovascular compartment. Anesth Analg 66:1196, 1987.
9. Winnie AP, Ramamurthy S, Durrani Z. The inguinal paravascular technic of lumbar plexus anesthesia. ''The 3-in-1 block.'' Anesth Analg 52:989, 1973.

Chapter 37

•

Stephen E. Abram, MD
Robert A. Boas, MBChB, FFARACS

Sympathetic and Visceral Nerve Blocks

OUTLINE

I. Sympathetic Nerve Blocks

A. Introduction

Sympathetic nerve activity to the upper extremities may be interrupted by cervicothoracic sympathetic (or stellate ganglion) block, while interruption of sympathetic outflow to the lower limbs is accomplished by paravertebral block of the lumbar sympathetic chain. In addition to blocking sympathetic outflow, these procedures block afferent fibers traveling in the sympathetic chain. These include visceral afferents innervating thoracic viscera in stellate ganglion block, and afferents from pelvic viscera in lumbar sympathetic block. It is likely that the sympathetic chain contains some afferent fibers that innervate somatic structures as well (eg, deep midline somatic structures such as intervertebral disk, vertebral periosteum, and ligaments). There is some controversy about the existence of afferent fibers from the extremities in the chain. Some evidence indicates that there are afferents in the sympathetic chain that supply large vessels in the proximal portions of the limbs.

B. Indications

1. Sympathetically Maintained Pain

There are several painful disorders in which the sympathetic nervous system plays an important pathophysiologic role. Sympathetic blocks are important treatment modalities in the management of these conditions.

Reflex sympathetic dystrophy (RSD) is a painful condition affecting the upper or lower extremities that is characterized by burning pain; pain evoked by light touch or cold (mechanical allodynia, cold allodynia); and autonomic dysfunction, consisting of warm, flushed skin (often seen early) or very cool skin, hyperhidrosis, mottled cyanosis, and edema. With time, particularly in the absence of appropriate treatment, dystrophic changes appear. These consist of smooth, glossy skin, changes in hair and nail growth patterns, bone demineralization (Sudek's atrophy), muscle atrophy, and joint dysfunction. Usually, RSD follows trauma or surgery. Fractures, crush injuries, lacerations, and sprains are common antecedents. Postsurgical cases often follow surgery involving the median or tibial nerve distribution of the hand or foot (carpal or tarsal tunnel release, palmar fasciectomy).[1]

Sympathetic blockade is useful in confirming the diagnosis of RSD and should produce complete or nearly complete relief of pain. The analgesia usually far outlasts the duration of local anesthetic block. Treatment consists of repeated sympathetic blocks, usually carried out daily or every other day. Generally, the pain returns to less severe levels following each block. A series of 3 to 10 blocks is usually needed. Treatment is continued until symptoms subside completely or until no further benefit is noted. Physical therapy, consisting of active and active-assisted range-of-motion exercises, is an important adjunct to blocks and should be performed after each block, when analgesia is maximal. If treatment is initiated early in the course of the disease, long-term success is likely, reaching as high as 90% in some series.[1,2] When symptoms have persisted without appropriate treatment for many months, success with sympathetic blocks is substantially reduced.[3]

Causalgia is a term that has been used synonymously with reflex sympathetic dystrophy. Recently, however, it has generally been reserved for a specific condition consisting of burning pain, hypersensitivity, and autonomic dysfunction associated with major nerve trunk injury. Most cases are associated with gunshot wounds. Most involve injury proximal to the elbow or knee, and most are associated with trauma to the brachial plexus, median nerve, or tibial division of the sciatic nerve.[1] The extremity is often warm and vasodilated. Surgical sympathectomy has generally been considered the treatment of choice for causalgia, with success rates as high as 91% reported.[4] Sympathetic blocks should be performed before considering surgery, which should be undertaken only if local anesthetic blocks are repeatedly beneficial. Aggressive management of causalgia with repeated or continuous sympathetic blocks is sometimes effective and should generally be tried before surgical interruption of the sympathetic chain.[1]

The sympathetic nervous system appears to have important modulating effects in certain neuropathic states. Spontaneous firing has been shown to originate from experimentally induced neuromas, and such firing is dramatically enhanced by sympathetic stimulation.[5] Such mechanisms are probably responsible for at least a portion of the pain in some neuralgias. Such patients have few symptoms of RSD but obtain temporary benefit from sympathetic blocks. Repeated blocks do not generally produce lasting benefit in such conditions.

2. Acute Herpes Zoster

Bonica[6] suggested that sympathetic blocks relieve the pain of acute herpes zoster and may shorten the duration of symptoms and reduce the incidence of postherpetic neuralgia. Sympathetic blocks have been shown to be significantly more effective than placebos in resolving acute herpetic neuralgia.[7] It has been postulated that perineural vasculitis and vasospasm are important pathophysiologic factors in the development of neuralgic pain associated with herpes zoster eruption and that sympathetic blocks may improve blood flow in the vasa nervorum during the acute process. Little benefit is derived from blocks when treatment is instituted more than a month following the acute eruption. No convincing data have been published to demonstrate a significant reduction in the incidence of postherpetic neuralgia associated with the use of sympathetic blocks. The appropriate controlled studies are lacking.

3. POSTAMPUTATION PAIN

Pain following limb amputation has a complex etiology. Phantom limb pain is primarily central in origin. Neuroma formation is common. Some patients develop a diffuse burning pain often experienced in the phantom hand or foot, accompanied by hyperpathia and allodynia. Sympathetic blocks usually provide at least temporary relief of these symptoms and occasionally produce lasting improvement. Neurolytic sympathetic block or surgical sympathectomy may be indicated.[8] Evidence is accumulating that aggressive management of limb pain prior to amputation will reduce the incidence of postamputation pain syndromes.

4. COLD INJURY

Frostbite and trenchfoot are characterized by an initial vasospastic phase, often followed by a period of hyperemia. In severe cases, chronic vascular insufficiency may ensue. Sympathetic blocks performed in the early vasospastic phase may reduce the degree of tissue damage. A dramatic example treated by the author was that of a 2-year-old child brought in following exposure to subzero temperatures, with a core temperature of 15°C and some freezing of the digits. After resuscitation by cardiopulmonary bypass, sympathetic blocks to all four extremities were performed daily for several days, resulting in salvage of all limbs except for the tips of a few digits.

Sympathetic blocks performed during the phase of chronic vascular insufficiency may produce temporary improvement in pain and increase in blood flow but rarely provides lasting benefit. If local anesthetic blocks are transiently effective, neurolytic sympathetic block or surgical sympathectomy may be helpful.[8] Many of these cases, however, are unresponsive to changes in sympathetic tone.

5. VASOSPASTIC DISEASE

Sympathetic blocks produce variable changes in blood flow in patients with Raynaud's disease and Raynaud's phenomenon. Some patients with these vasospastic disorders improve dramatically; others apparently have no autonomic contribution to their vasoconstriction. In severe cases, in which sympathectomy is being considered as a therapeutic option, sympathetic blocks should be performed prognostically on several occasions.

Acrocyanosis is a disease characterized by intense cyanosis and very cool skin. Symptoms are generally responsive to sympathetic interruption, and repeated sympathetic blocks may be effective. Sympathectomy may be considered for resistant cases.[8]

Erythromelalgia is a condition in which patients experience burning pain and flushing in the involved extremities.

Sympathetic interruption was reported by Bonica to produce considerable benefit despite the fact that cutaneous vasodilation is a hallmark of the disorder.[8] However, Boas reported that five of nine patients with this disorder who were treated with sympathetic blocks experienced worsening of the burning pain,[9] and he considers this condition a possible contraindication to sympathetic blockade.

Patients with atherosclerotic peripheral vascular disease occasionally have a vasospastic component to their arterial insufficiency. Sympathectomy may benefit some patients with nonhealing ulceration of the skin and is occasionally of symptomatic benefit in patients with claudication. Temporary sympathetic blockade allows the physician to predict the potential benefit from surgical or chemical (neurolytic) sympathectomy. It is helpful to perform flow studies before and after the prognostic block.

6. VISCERAL PAIN

Prior to the introduction of coronary artery bypass surgery, relief of angina was reported with cervicothoracic sympathetic blockade. Following prognostic stellate ganglion blocks, cardiac afferent fibers were interrupted by either neurolytic thoracic sympathetic blocks or surgical sympathectomy. Success rates ranged from 75% to 85%.[8] Much of the relief of anginal pain achieved by coronary bypass grafting may be caused by related deafferentation of the heart by stripping of the cardiac afferents from the aorta.

C. *How to Do Cervicothoracic Sympathetic Block (Stellate Ganglion Block)*

1. Anatomic Considerations

The preganglionic sympathetic fibers that supply the upper extremities, head, and neck arise from cell bodies in the intermediolateral column of the spinal cord from T-1 through T-6. These fibers pass via the ventral roots and white rami communicantes to the thoracic paravertebral sympathetic chain, where they synapse with postganglionic fibers in the upper thoracic and cervical sympathetic ganglia (Fig. 37–1). The postganglionics pass to the brachial plexus via the gray rami communicantes of the midcervical and upper two thoracic roots. Some postganglionics enter the limb by passing from the stellate ganglion and T-2 and T-3 ganglia directly to a perivascular plexus that surrounds the subclavian artery (see Fig. 37–1). The cervical portion of the sympathetic chain lies in front of the prevertebral fascia and posterior to the carotid sheath. The stellate ganglion, formed by the fusion of the inferior cervical and first thoracic ganglia, lies posterior to the dome of the pleura, in close proximity to the vertebral artery. The middle cervical ganglion lies over the C-6 anterior tubercle (Fig. 37–2).

The cervical sympathetic chain may be injected at the level of the C-6 or the C-7 transverse process. The C-7 approach is favored by some practitioners because less anesthetic is required for spread to the level of T-3, blockade of which is needed for complete denervation of the upper extremity. Others favor a C-6 approach for the following reasons:

1. The C-6 anterior tubercle is easily palpable in most patients.
2. There is little likelihood of trauma to the pleura at C-6.
3. The vertebral artery lies in a foramen behind the C-6 anterior tubercle but in front of the C-7 transverse process just behind the sympathetic chain.

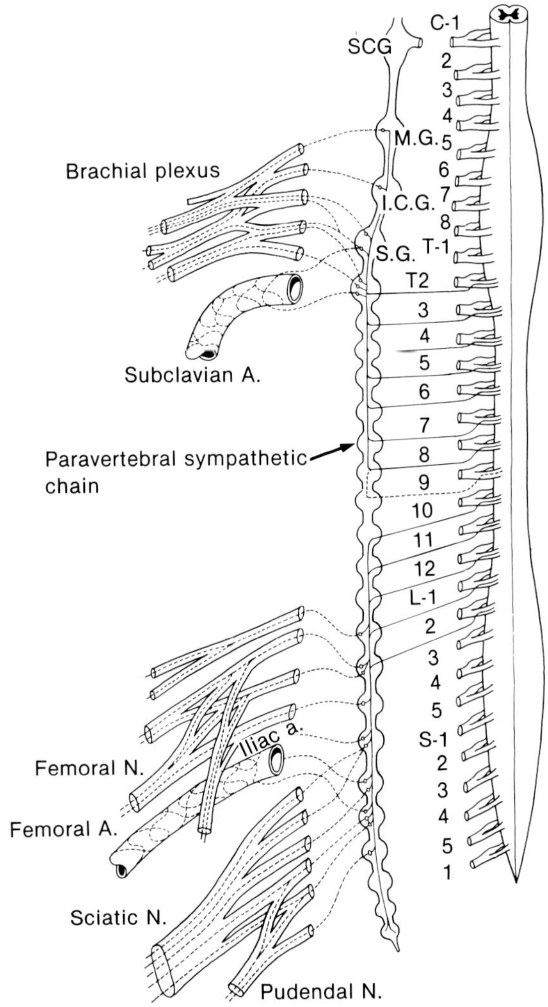

Figure 37–1 • Pre- and post-ganglionic sympathetic fibers to the upper and lower extremities. SCG = superior cervical ganglion; MG = middle ganglion; ICG = inferior cervical ganglion; SG = stellate ganglion. (From Bonica JJ. Clinical Applications of Diagnostic and Therapeutic Nerve Blocks. Springfield, IL: Charles C. Thomas, 1959, 146; with permission.)

2. Techniques of Cervicothoracic Sympathetic Block

a. *C-6 Paratracheal Approach*

The patient is placed supine, without a pillow, with the head in a neutral position. If the anterior neck muscles are tense, the patient is asked to open the mouth slightly to relax them. Standing on the side to be blocked, the physician palpates for the tip of the C-6 anterior tubercle just lateral to the cricoid cartilage. The neck is then prepared with antiseptic. It is prudent to wear a sterile glove on the palpating hand, since the needle will be in close proximity to the palpating fingers. The anterior tubercle is again sought, using the second and third fingers of the nondominant hand, just medial to the sternocleidomastoid. The fingertips are placed slightly apart and are positioned to straddle the tip of the anterior tubercle while retracting the sternocleidomastoid and ca-

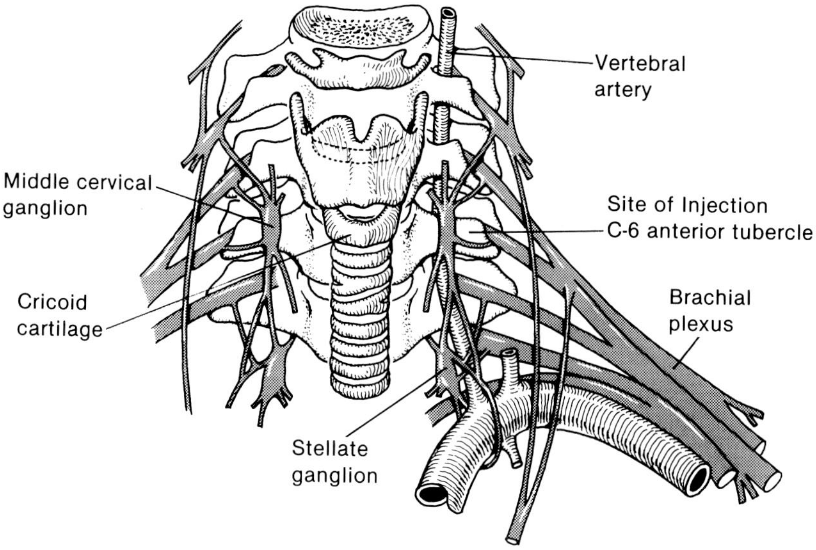

Figure 37–2 • Site of injection for the C-6 paratracheal approach to the stellate ganglion block. Note the relationship of the C-6 anterior tubercle to the cricoid cartilage. The vertebral artery passes anterior to the C-7 transverse process and behind the C-6 anterior tubercle. The lateral portion of the C-7 transverse process lies deep to the prevertebral fascia, adjacent to the C-7 nerve root and the dome of the pleura.

rotid sheath laterally (Fig. 37–3). The carotid pulsation should be felt on the volar aspect of the fingertips. Using a ring control syringe, a 1.5-inch, 22 gauge needle is placed through the skin between the tips of the palpating fingers and advanced to the tip of the anterior tubercle, which should lie within 1–1.5 cm of the skin in a nonobese patient. If bone is not contacted within 2 cm of the skin, the needle is retracted to the shallow subcutaneous tissue and contact is sought just superior or just inferior to the original site. When bone is contacted, careful aspiration is carried out, and 1 mL of local anesthetic is injected. If there is no adverse reaction, aspiration is repeated, and a total of 10 mL of local anesthetic (1% lidocaine or equivalent) is slowly injected, with frequent repeated aspiration. Although there is little chance of vertebral artery injection when the needle tip is in front of the anterior tubercle, continued care must be exercised, as the needle can slip off the tubercle. In addition, the vertebral artery runs in front of the anterior tubercle rather than behind it in about 6% of patients.[10] If there is some resistance to injection, the needle tip is slightly medial to the tip of the transverse process, within the longus colli muscle. The needle should then be withdrawn slightly before aspiration and

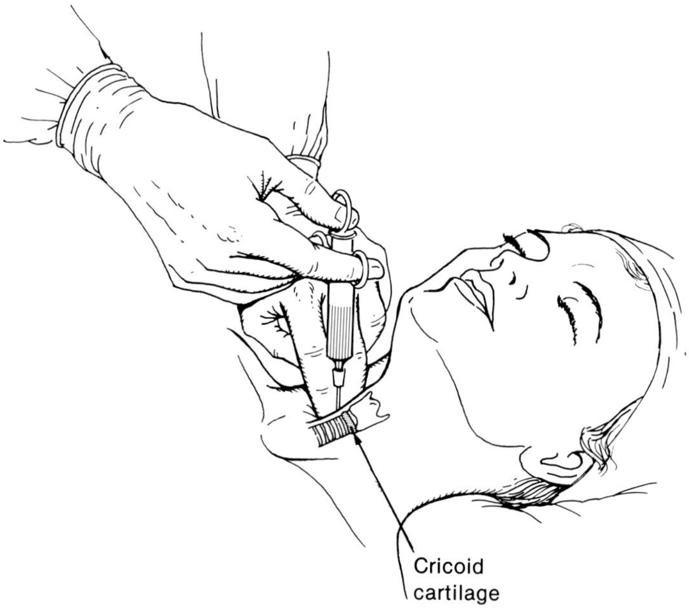

Figure 37–3 • Technique for the C-6 paratracheal approach to stellate ganglion block. The fingertips of the palpating hand straddle the tip of the C-6 anterior tubercle while retracting the carotid sheath laterally. The needle is introduced directly downward onto the tip of the anterior tubercle.

injection. When injection is completed, the patient is asked to sit up or the back of the table is raised to improve caudad spread of the anesthetic.

If a paresthesia to the upper extremity is elicited during needle placement, the needle has missed the anterior tubercle and has contacted a nerve root. The needle should be withdrawn and repositioned. In obese patients or patients with a short, muscular neck, it may be impossible to palpate the anterior tubercle. In that case, the needle should be inserted just lateral to the cricoid cartilage while retracting the sternocleidomastoid and carotid sheath. Slight medial angulation of the needle allows the needle to approach the broader portion of the transverse process adjacent to the vertebral body, minimizing the chance of missing the bony target.

An alternative to the use of a ring control syringe is the immobile needle technique. The needle is placed at the end of an intravenous extension set attached to a 10-mL syringe. Once the needle has been positioned, an assistant aspirates and injects intermittently.

b. C-7 Paratracheal Approach

The C-7 transverse process is located about 3.5 cm lateral and 3.5 cm superior to the sternal notch. It can be located by measuring those distances with the width of two fingers. The point so measured should lie at the anterior border of the sternocleidomastoid and lies about 1.5 cm below the tip of the C-6 anterior tubercle. The sternocleidomastoid and carotid sheath are retracted laterally with the index and middle fingers as in the C-6 approach. The needle is placed through the skin between the fingertips and advanced in a slightly mesiad direction until bone is contacted, usually at a depth of 1.5–2 cm in an average-sized nonobese patient. If the needle is directed straight downward or slightly laterally instead of in a slightly mesiad direction, it will contact the posteriorly sloping transverse process at a deeper level, behind the sympathetic chain and closer to the vertebral artery. As in the C-6 paratracheal approach, if bone is not contacted within 2 cm, the needle should be withdrawn, angled slightly cephalad or caudad, and readvanced. Following bony contact, the needle is withdrawn slightly, careful aspiration is carried out, and 1 mL local anesthetic is injected. If no adverse reaction occurs, a total of 10 mL of local anesthetic is injected in 1- to 2-mL increments, aspirating intermittently. Great care must be taken to avoid vertebral artery injection at this level, as the artery lies in front of the transverse process, just posterior to the sympathetic chain.

D. Complications

1. Recurrent Laryngeal Nerve Block

A hoarse voice following stellate ganglion block is generally attributed to recurrent laryngeal nerve block, but in some cases may be related to dilation of vessels to the vocal cords. It is often encountered when high anesthetic volumes (× 15 mL) are used. It seems prudent to keep the patient NPO until the block resolves to minimize the risk of aspiration caused by inability to close the glottis. The use of short-acting local anesthetics minimizes the duration of this inconvenience.

2. Brachial Plexus Block

Placement of the needle deep to the anterior tubercle may result in block of the adjacent nerve root and, frequently, spread of the drug to much of the brachial plexus. A partial sympathetic block usually ensues, often with sparing of blockade of sympathetic fibers to the ulnar aspect of the hand.

3. Subarachnoid Block

Introduction of local anesthetic into the dural cuff of a cervical nerve root may result in subarachnoid spread of the drug. A total spinal, with profound hypotension and apnea, will very likely occur. Treatment consists of Trendelenburg's position, positive pressure ventilation with oxygen, vasopressors, and intravenous fluid loading.

4. Vertebral Artery Injection

Injection of even minute quantities of local anesthetic into the vertebral artery will result in acute central nervous system toxicity (grand mal seizure). Seizures are usually short-lived, although prolonged or recurrent seizures may be anticipated if bupivacaine or etidocaine is used. The patient should be ventilated with oxygen. If convulsions do not stop promptly, they should be treated with a benzodiazepine or a barbiturate. A hematoma may develop subsequently.

5. Pneumothorax

Pneumothorax is encountered occasionally following the C-7 approach but is very rare with the C-6 technique. If it is less than 20% and is not expanding, no treatment is necessary. If it is relatively large, reexpansion by aspiration of air using an interpleural large-bore intravenous catheter may be sufficient treatment. Reappearance necessitates the use of a chest tube.

6. PHRENIC NERVE BLOCK

Phrenic block is unusual, particularly if lower anesthetic concentrations are used. It is usually accompanied by dyspnea, which improves in the sitting position. Unilateral phrenic block is of little consequence except in patients with severely compromised respiratory function.

E. *How to Do Lumbar Sympathetic Block*

1. ANATOMIC CONSIDERATIONS

The preganglionic sympathetic fibers that supply the lower extremity have their cell bodies in levels T-10 through L-2 of the spinal cord.[8] They enter the paravertebral sympathetic chain via the white rami communicantes. The postganglionic fibers to the limb leave the chain from the level of L-2 and below (see Fig. 37–1). Afferent fibers from the pelvic viscera enter the lumbar and sacral portions of the chain from prevertebral plexuses. They pass through the chain without synapsing, back to the dorsal root ganglia and dorsal horns of the lower thoracic and upper lumbar segments. The lumbar sympathetic chain lies over the anterolateral aspect of the lumbar vertebral bodies (Fig. 37–4). It is separated from the lumbar somatic nerve roots by the psoas major muscle and the psoas fascia. The sympathetic rami pass from the lumbar roots to the chain beneath a fibrous arch that attaches to the upper and lower aspects of the concave lateral portions of the vertebral bodies.

2. SINGLE-NEEDLE PARAVERTEBRAL APPROACH

Since the preganglionic fibers from the spinal cord to the lower extremity reach the sympathetic chain at or above the L-2 level, and the postganglionic fibers from the chain to the limb leave the chain at or below L-2 (see Fig. 37–1), interruption of impulses in the sympathetic chain at the L-2 level will effectively denervate the sympathetic supply of the lower extremity. It is important, however, that the needle tip be positioned on the sympathetic chain, at the anterolateral aspect of the L-2 vertebral body. This requires that the needle be introduced well lateral to the midline. A technique de-

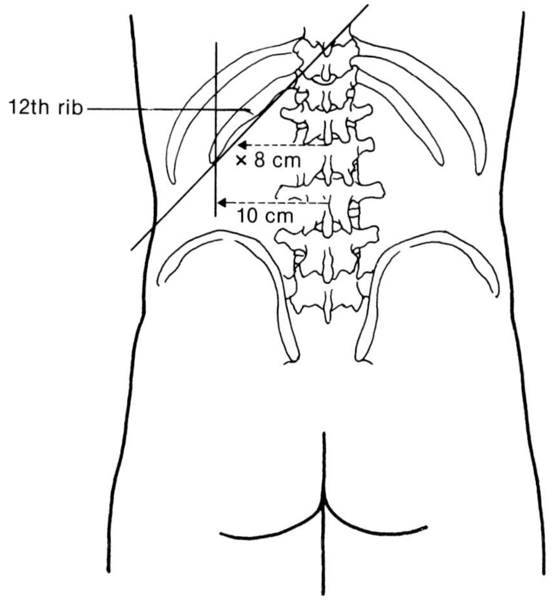

Figure 37–4 • Superficial landmarks for the lumbar sympathetic block. The needle may be inserted at the intersection of the line demarcating the lower border of the twelfth rib and the line 10 cm from the midline. To insure that the kidney is not punctured, needle insertion may be done two cm medial to that point, marked by an "X." (From Stanton-Hicks M, Abram SE, Nolte H. Sympathetic Blocks. In Raj PP (ed) Practical Management of Pain. Chicago; Year Book, 1986, p 674; with permission.)

scribed by Carron[11] is presented along with a slight modification that should minimize renal trauma.

The patient is placed in the prone position. If an operating room table is used, it is flexed slightly. Otherwise a pillow is placed under the patient's hips. The procedure may be done in the lateral decubitus position if the patient is unable to lie prone. The 12th rib is palpated in the upper lumbar region, and a line is drawn along the lower border of the rib (see Fig. 37–4). A second line is drawn 10 cm from the midline, parallel to the spine. Where these lines intersect is the point of insertion of the needle. This point should lie directly lateral to (and perhaps just inferior to) the L-2 spinous process (see Fig. 37–4). This position may be confirmed by locating the L-4 spine, which should be roughly even with the top of the iliac crest, and counting up two segments. To minimize risk of puncture of the kidney, ureter, or renal pelvis, the point of needle insertion may be moved 2 cm medially without appreciably compromising the technique (see x in Fig. 37–4 together with Fig. 37–5).

A skin wheal is raised at the needle entry point.

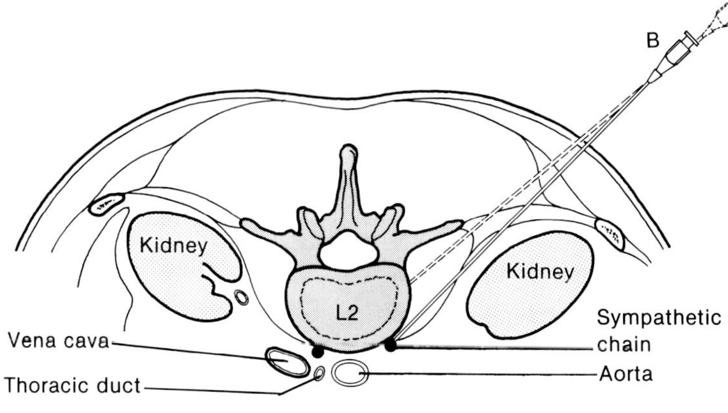

Figure 37–5 • Initial needle position (*A*) and final needle position (*B*) for single-needle lumbar sympathetic block. Initial bony contact is made at a depth of 3 1/2–4 inches (8–10 cm) in a normal-sized patient. Final needle position is generally at a depth to 4–5 inches (10–12.5 cm). (From Stanton-Hicks M, Abram SE, Nolte H: Sympathetic Blocks. In Raj PP (ed) Practical Management of Pain. Year Book, Chicago, 1986, p 674; with permission.)

The underlying muscles may be anesthetized by infiltrating in the coronal plane with the needle directed about 45° inward. A 20 or 22 gauge, 5-inch (13-cm) needle (6-inch [15-cm] in a large patient) is placed through the skin and held perpendicular to the skin of the back. The angle of the needle is then reduced by 30° by dropping the hub of the needle laterally while keeping it in the coronal plane. The needle is advanced until it contacts the midportion of the vertebral body (see Fig. 37–5, needle position *A*), usually at a depth of about 3 in (7.5 cm). If bony contact is made at 1.5–2 inches, it is most likely a transverse process, in which case the needle should be withdrawn and reinserted about 1 cm below the original insertion point. If dense elastic tissue is felt rather than bone, a disk has been contacted and the needle should be withdrawn and angled slightly cephalad or slightly caudad to the coronal plane. After vertebral body is contacted, the needle is then withdrawn to the subcutaneous tissue and is readvanced at a slightly steeper angle until it again contacts the body. If no bony contact is made at a depth of 4–4.5 in, the needle angle is reduced slightly. After the body is recontacted, the needle is "walked" down to deeper portions of the body. This is accomplished by withdrawing the needle slightly (2–3 cm) and advancing it at slightly steeper angles until the needle can be felt to slide along the anterolateral surface of the body (see Fig. 37–5, needle position *B*). It is advanced no more than a few millimeters once this sensation is felt. Aspiration is carried out in two planes and 5 mL 1% lidocaine is injected. There should be little resistance to injection if the needle is correctly placed.

Following initial injection, the skin temperature of the plantar aspect of the foot should be monitored. (The underside of the great toe is a reasonable site.) If the needle is adjacent to the sympathetic chain, the temperature on the blocked side will begin to rise within 3 minutes. (It may take considerably longer in a patient with peripheral vascular disease.) Complete sympathetic block to the limb is documented by a final temperature above 34°C. (The change in temperature is not important. If the initial skin temperature is very low, the change will be great. If the initial temperature is high, the change will be slight.) Again in patients with peripheral vascular disease, the final skin temperature may not reach 34° even with complete sympathetic denervation. Once the skin temperature begins to rise, 5–7 mL 0.5% bupivacaine may be injected to prolong the duration of the block. Neurologic examination of the lower extremities should be undertaken following the block to determine whether any somatic blockade has occurred. This is particularly important when the procedure is being done as a diagnostic or prognostic procedure.

The single-needle paravertebral lumbar sympathetic block may be expedited by the use of fluoroscopy, and fluoroscopic control is essential if neurolytic agents are used. When using C-arm fluoroscopy, the patient is positioned prone and a posteroanterior view of the lumbar spine is projected. A site 8 cm lateral to the midline and just below the level of the L-2 spinous process is selected as the needle insertion point. The procedure is carried out as noted earlier. When the final position is achieved, the spine is viewed in both the PA and lateral projections. The needle should lie against the vertebral body of L-2 in the posteroanterior projection and should lie at the anterior border of the body in the lateral projection. Injecting 1–2 mL of radiopaque dye in the lateral view should reveal spread of the dye in a thin longitudinal streak along the anterior border of the body. If the dye spreads in a fluffy, more spherical pattern, the needle tip is probably in the psoas muscle and should be advanced slightly.

If neurolytic sympathetic blockade is to be performed, radiographic documentation of needle position and dye spread should be carried out as noted earlier. Subsequently, 5 mL 1% lidocaine is injected, and skin temperature is monitored. If an appropriate temperature rise is noted, an additional 20 minutes is allowed to elapse with the needle still in position, and the patient is questioned carefully about pain relief and possible somatic blockade. If there is an appropriate response to the block and no sensory or motor block is detected, 5 mL 6% aqueous phenol is injected, providing a block of several weeks' duration. The needle is then cleared with 0.5 mL local anesthetic or saline and withdrawn. It is important to document a lack of somatic block, since spread of drug posteriorly along the sympathetic rami as they pass beneath a fibrous arch has been documented.[12] An alternate, longer-duration technique involves positioning the needle under fluoroscopic control and then injecting 0.25–0.5 mL 7% phenol in Conray 420 (70% sodium iothalamate in water) under ''live'' fluoroscopy.[13] If the material does not begin to spread in a longitudinal fashion along the vertebrae, injection is stopped and the needle is repositioned. If the spread of phenol in dye is appropriate, a total of 8–12 mL injected at a single level will spread over two or three vertebrae.[14] Again, the needle should be cleared before removal.

3. MULTIPLE-NEEDLE TECHNIQUE

The multiple-needle technique, popularized by Moore,[15] involves positioning needles in proximity to the lumbar sympathetic chain at three levels. Moore recommends placement at the L-1, L-2, and L-3 levels. The patient is placed prone, with a pillow under the abdomen. The L-4 spinous process is identified at the level of a line between the iliac crests, and the L-3, L-2, and L-1 spinous processes are identified (see Fig. 37–4) and marked. Horizontal lines are drawn through the middle of the spinous processes of L-1 through L-3. A vertical line is drawn 4.5–5 cm (depending on the patient's size) from the midline. This line should lie just lateral to the edges of the vertebral bodies. The intersection of the vertical line with the three horizontal lines marks the points of needle insertion.

Skin wheals are raised at the needle insertion points. The following procedure is carried out at each level: A 20 gauge, 4-inch needle is advanced through the skin inclined cephalad at a 45° angle. It is advanced until transverse process is encountered, usually at a depth of 1.5–2 inches, depending on the patient's physique (Fig. 37–6). A distance of 1.75–2 inches (depending on the patient's size) is measured along the shaft of the needle from the skin toward the hub, and this point is remembered or marked with a marker. The needle is then withdrawn to the skin and redirected in the coronal plane in a slightly mesiad direction (85° to the skin). It is advanced to the predetermined depth, and 10 mL local anesthetic is injected after careful aspiration (see Fig. 37–6). It should not be necessary to locate the transverse processes at the remaining two levels, as the depth of the chain should be approximately the same at all three segments.

This technique has the disadvantage of requiring multiple needle insertions. In addition, the needle lies somewhat lateral to the chain (Fig. 37–7), and larger anesthetic volumes must be used. It would seem reasonable when employing this method to begin at the L-2 level. If skin temperature monitoring demonstrates a

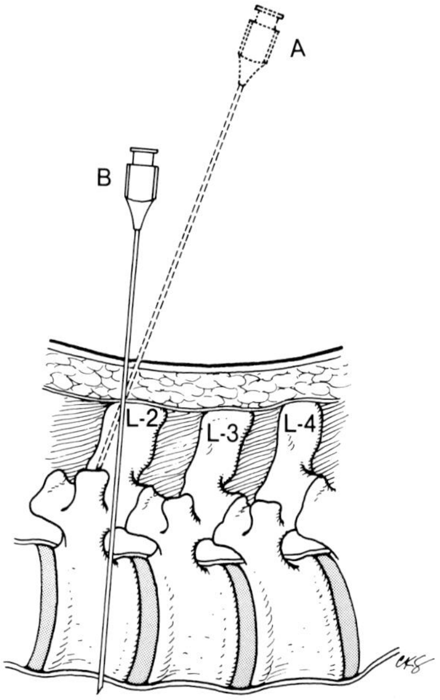

Figure 37–6 • Initial needle position (*A*) and final needle position (*B*) for the three-needle technique of lumbar sympathetic block (only one level is shown). The transverse process is contacted initially. The needle is withdrawn to the subcutaneous tissue and redirected straight inward. It is advanced 1.75–2 inches beyond the depth required to contact transverse process.

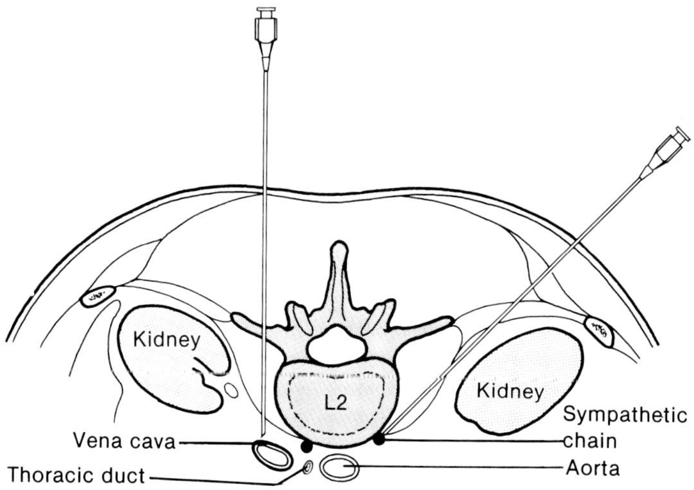

Figure 37–7 • Comparison of final needle positions for the single-needle technique initiated 8 cm from the midline and the multiple-needle technique initiated 4.5–5 cm from the midline.

prompt rise in skin temperature with a final temperature above 34°C, blockade of the other two segments is not necessary.

F. *Complications*

Complications from lumbar sympathetic block with local anesthetics are rare. Neurolytic sympathetic blockade is potentially more hazardous, the principal risk being spread of neurolytic agent to somatic nerves.

1. Intravascular Injection

Injection into the aorta, vena cava, or small vessels adjacent to the sympathetic chain is possible. Local anesthetic-induced seizures occurring with the patient prone are particularly hazardous. Local anesthetic should be injected in small increments.

2. Hematoma Formation

Substantial retroperitoneal bleeding can occur if the aorta or vena cava is punctured in a patient who is anticoagulated or who has a coagulation defect. There is little risk in patients with normal coagulation function.

3. Somatic Blockade

If there is no fluoroscopic documentation of needle position, it is possible for the needle to be advanced into the neural foramen. Injection there may result in epidural or subarachnoid blockade. Injection into the psoas muscle may result in block of lumbar nerve roots. These complications are serious only when neurolytic agents are used.

4. Genitofemoral Neuralgia

Neuralgic pain in the groin or upper anterior thigh is a fairly common problem following neurolytic lumbar sympathetic block. It has been postulated that the pain is the result of spread of neurolytic agent to adjacent somatic roots or branches of the lumbar plexus. Another theory is that it is a deafferentation phenomenon caused by destruction of sympathetic chain afferents.[16] The pain usually continues for 2–5 weeks.[12] Mild transient nerve root irritation may occur from needle trauma to the nerve root.

5. Perforation of Kidney, Ureter

Perforation of a kidney during lumbar sympathetic block occurs occasionally but is of little clinical significance unless neurolytic agent is injected into the kidney itself. At the levels of L-3 and L-4, the ureter lies fairly close to the sympathetic chain. Care must be exercised during the performance of neurolytic blocks at those levels to ensure that needle placement is not too far lateral.

II. Celiac-Splanchnic Nerve Blocks

A. *Introduction*

Visceral nerve block of the celiac plexus or splanchnic nerves interrupts all upper abdominal nociceptive transmission without interfering with normal somatic or peripheral nerve function. Such separation of sensory function lends itself to the treatment of chronic visceral pain with little serious risk when undertaken with due care. Even so, with recent advances in precision of needle and drug placement, plus supportive literature on long-term outcome, these nerve block techniques remain surprisingly underused. To some extent this is due to a perception that visceral blocks are difficult to perform, promoted by unfamiliarity with the anatomy and radiologic monitoring required, compounded further by the lack of experience suffered by most anesthesiologists in the use of these techniques in training and later clinical practice. Clinical reality indicates these procedures to be simple, safe, effective, and cost efficient, amply justifying their wider use.

B. *Indications*

Abdominal pain is not provoked by the same set of nociceptive stimuli that cause somatic pain. Extensive tissue destruction or visceral injury may occur without conscious perception, yet the distention of hollow visceral organs develops a clear stimulus intensity pattern of nerve discharge and pain perception.[17] Perhaps one of the greatest enigmas is the basis for continuing incapacitating pain associated with chronic pancreatitis. In principle, however, we can attribute abdominal pain to visceral stimulation consequent to obstruction and distention of a hollow viscus, capsular distention of solid organs, inflammation about vessels and parietal peritoneum, and infiltration or scarring within visceral nerves of the abdomen. The greatest single application of visceral nerve blocks is in the treatment of cancer pain, especially that due to carcinoma of the pancreas, gall bladder, or invasive tumor in the upper abdomen. Some surgeons are performing intraabdominal neurolytic injections at the time of surgery,[17] with apparent good effect in patients with upper abdominal cancer. More recently, there has also been renewed advocacy for use of celiac blocks in the treatment of pancreatitis (acute and chronic) and for pain control during hepatic embolization. A case can also be presented for the use of these blocks as diagnostic aids in patients with obscure abdominal pains. On the other hand, increasing familiarization with opiate infusion techniques and epidural opiates has diminished use of celiac blocks in anesthesia and in the less severe pain cases, lessening opportunities for teaching these blocks in other than critical cases. An important element in the use of these more difficult procedures is for the practitioner to maintain technical skills and experience in their use by performing them several times a year. The more common applications of splanchnic--celiac blocks are given in Table 37–1 with breakdown into those amenable to temporary local anesthetic blockade or those requiring permanent neurolysis.

Table 37–1 • Indications for Splanchnic/Celiac Blocks

Temporary	**Diagnosis**
Local anesthetic blocks	Acute pancreatitis Visceral embolizations Surgical anesthesia
Permanent	
Neurolytic blocks	Cancer pain Chronic pancreatitis

When used for local anesthetic or steroid block, there are few serious long-term complications if properly conducted, requiring only that patients have the usual precautions and monitoring standards that apply to major operative procedures. Ideally, needle placement in such cases would be done with radiologic control, but when surface markings and tactile control are used for the placement of nondestructive solutions, a high accuracy rate approaching 90% can be obtained by those experienced with performing these procedures. When the operator is inexperienced, or the outcome of a block is important to the patient's welfare or diagnosis, especially for those undergoing neurolytic solution injection, close radiologic screening is a critical adjunct to obtaining accuracy. Neurolytic injections are indicated when the diagnosis confirms inoperable disease and when pain control is no longer effective or feasible by conventional use of opiates. The efficacy of visceral nerve block is then good enough to allow almost all cancer patients so treated to live out a relatively comfortable life requiring only mild to moderate analgesics until their life's end. Because well-conducted and complete block is so effective, sustained, and safe, the cost benefit and convenience of these procedures justifies their use on a wider basis than is currently practiced.

C. *How to Do Celiac–Splanchnic Nerve Blocks*

1. ANATOMY

The celiac plexus is a diffuse aggregation of pre- and postganglionic sympathetic fibers and ganglia, together with parasympathetic vagal fibers, all dispersed about the great vessels within the retroperitoneal space. Their confines extend variably over a length of three vertebral levels centered at L-1, in a crescentic band from near the renal pedicles on either side to the celiac axis and superior mesenteric vessels ventrally. Complete dispersion of solution within this poorly delineated compartment is difficult to accomplish without multidimensional radiologic monitoring, while the risk of paravertebral or intravascular spread is also ever-present, given the anatomy and needle insertion techniques in current use. A lateral anatomic projection in Fig. 37–8 shows four alternative posterior approaches to sympathetic visceral blockade, two at the supradiaphragmatic level for blockade of the splanchnic nerves and two at the level of the intraabdominal celiac plexus. While an anterior approach to the celiac plexus using Doppler projection and echography has been reported, only posterior variants of the classic regional block are described in this section.

Critical to the use of splanchnic nerve blocks is the understanding that all visceral nociceptive fibers, arising from T-5–T-12 segmental levels, are carried in three splanchnic nerves bilaterally. These nerves, at their point of passing from the chest into the abdomen, traverse a narrow compartment as they penetrate the diaphragm. At this level the compartment is about 3 mm in depth, lying between the vertebral bodies of T-11–T-12 and the parietal pleura, bounded ventrally by structures in the posterior mediastinum and dorsally by an apparent attachment of pleura and veins to the dorsal edge of the vertebral bodies. Diaphragmatic crura form caudad limits to this compartment, bounding a potential space of about 10 mL on either side in the average adult. Upper cephalad limits can be extended with larger volumes,

Anatomy and Two Approaches to Celiac and Splanchnic Nerve Block

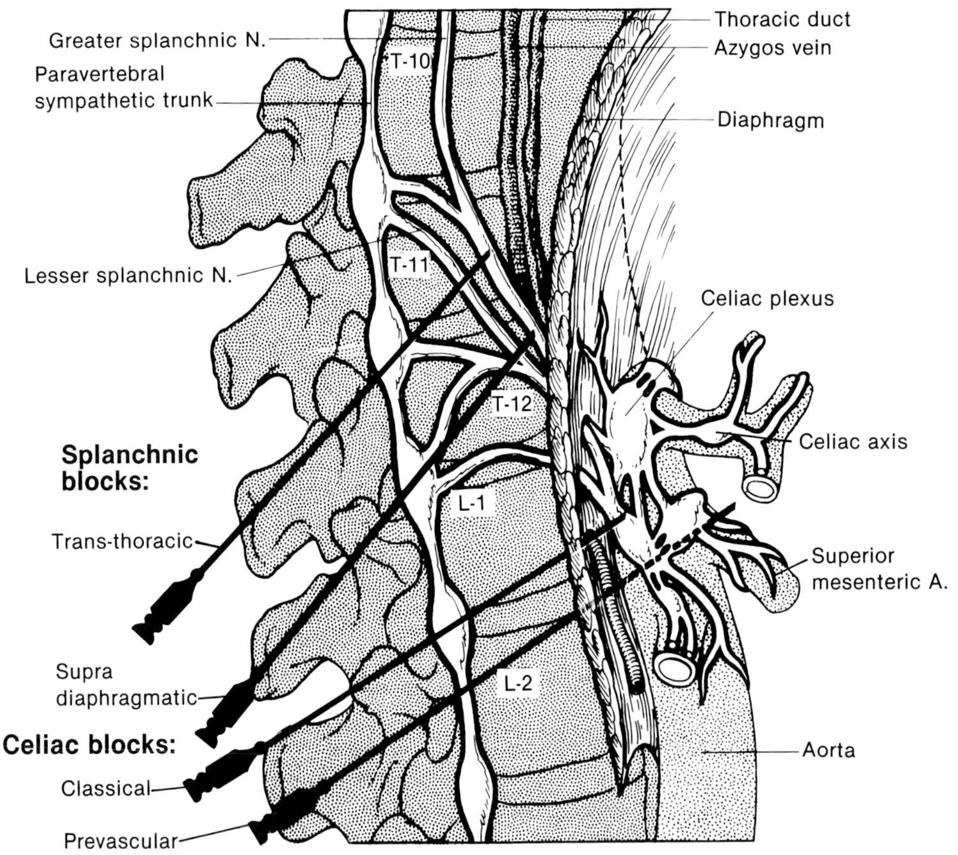

Figure 37–8 • Lateral projection showing the splanchnic nerves and celiac plexus in relation to the diaphragm vertebrae and aortic vessels. Placement of needles for two approaches to the celiac plexus and two approaches to the splanchnic nerves. See text for anatomic details.

but no advantage is gained by extending solution spread to higher levels.

2. THE PROCEDURES

Patients are required to lie prone, best supported with soft pillows and under light sedation. Caution is advised in those who are debilitated or receiving high-dose opiates, because drug-induced depression can arise during the procedure or following relief of pain with successful block. Those receiving alcohol injections may experience severe pain and should be given stronger analgesic cover, such as alfentanil, for this brief period. Intravenous volume loading of up to 2 L may also be needed to compensate for visceral vasodilation and hypotension associated with these autonomic blocks. Patients undergoing all forms of visceral block, whether temporary or permanent, require close monitoring and observation by somebody separate from the operator.

a. Landmarks

Surface markings use the spinous processes of T-12 and L-1, the 12th rib, and the transverse process of L-1 as identified by radiographic screening to determine the point of needle entry and direction of insertion for each of the splanchnic and celiac approaches as depicted in Fig. 37–9. A line is drawn connecting points just lateral to the tips of the transverse processes of L-1, about 1–2 cm inferior to the edge of the 12th rib on either side. Markings for the bodies of T-12 and L-1 vertebrae and for the 12th rib are also drawn to give some three-dimensional concept of the area, as well as the angles needed for needle insertion. Distinctions can now be made for each of the four optional placement techniques in performing variants on these blocks.

b. Needle Placement

i. Celiac Block—Classic (Paravascular) Approach. The classic (paravascular) method is essentially the updated technique of Moore and others,[18] with the improvements derived from computed tomographic (CT) studies. Skin entry is made on either side after local anesthetic infiltration, at a point about 7 cm from the midline, along the line through L-1. Using 12–15-cm, 20 gauge styletted needles, insertion continues at an angle of 45° to 60° to the midline (depending on body

Landmarks for Needle Insertion for Splanchnic and Celiac Blocks

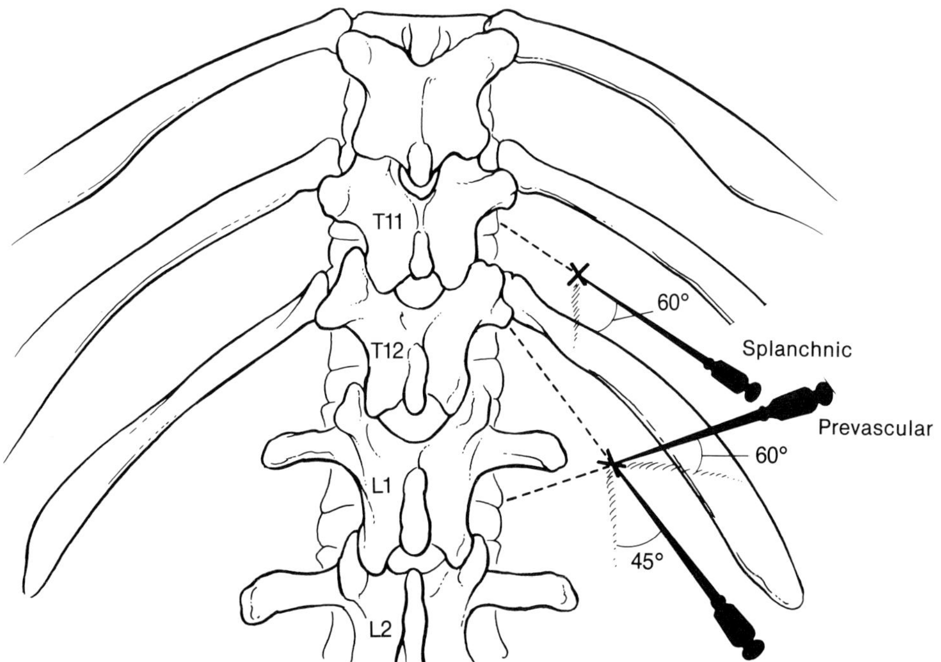

Figure 37–9 • Landmarks for needle insertion for splanchnic and celiac blocks show entry points and angulation in relation to vertebral bodies, spinous and lateral processes, and the 12th rib.

size and laterality of needle placement), until the side of the vertebral body of L-1 is encountered. If the needle has been inserted just above and lateral to the transverse process, neither the process itself nor any segmental nerve will be encountered. Withdrawal of the needle to subcutaneous levels and reinsertion to just glance off the side of the midlevel of the same vertebral body will then allow the needle to be advanced a further 2–3 cm, so as to lie just anterior to the vertebra and just behind the great vessels on either side. No clear endpoint is evident, although resistance to injection is minimal and aortic pulsation may be felt on the left at a depth of 9–12 cm in the average patient. For this reason it is often easier to commence with the left needle to determine depth and angulation, following in a mirror pattern with insertion of the right-sided needle. Single-needle techniques have been advocated, but radiographic monitoring indicates incomplete solution spread occurs in many such instances. Another option has suggested a slightly more medial point of insertion and vertical needle placement on the left so as to lessen inadvertent aortic puncture. In each of these approaches, solution deposition is usually lateral and dorsal to the large vessels, between them and the side of the vertebral bodies of T-12–L-1 on either side. A volume of 25 mL bilaterally was found effective clinically and subsequently verified by CT scanning.

ii. Celiac Block–Transvascular Approach. The transvascular approach uses a two-needle technique modified from that described by Ischia and associates,[19] with insertion slightly more lateral, at about 8 cm from the midline, to ultimately bring the needle points closer to the midline and deeper by about 3 cm, to lie within the retroperitoneal compartment between the pancreas ventrally and the aorta and inferior vena cava dorsally (Fig. 37–10). An angulation of about 45° to the midline is usually needed to keep the needle lying between vertebral body and the kidneys on either side, but the greater depth necessitates longer needles of 15 cm or more. Aspiration of blood and its cessation, associated with the slight click of vessel exit with the needle tip, gives a distinct endpoint for needle placement, although some form of imaging monitor is strongly advocated for this method. Block with this technique allows solution to be injected directly at the level of the celiac plexus rather than at the precrural level of preganglionic fibers that follows the classic approach.

iii. Splanchnic Nerve Blocks. Each of the splanchnic nerve block techniques is intended to reach the supracrural (or retrocrural) compartment at T-11–L-1, where the three splanchnic nerves converge before piercing the crura to enter the abdomen. This compartment is very narrow in its lateral extent, requiring abutment of the needles immediately against the bodies of T-11 or T-12 vertebrae. Two approaches are described, one being technically demanding, but carrying 10 years of experience and widespread use,[20] the second being new and easier to perform, but hitherto unpublished in

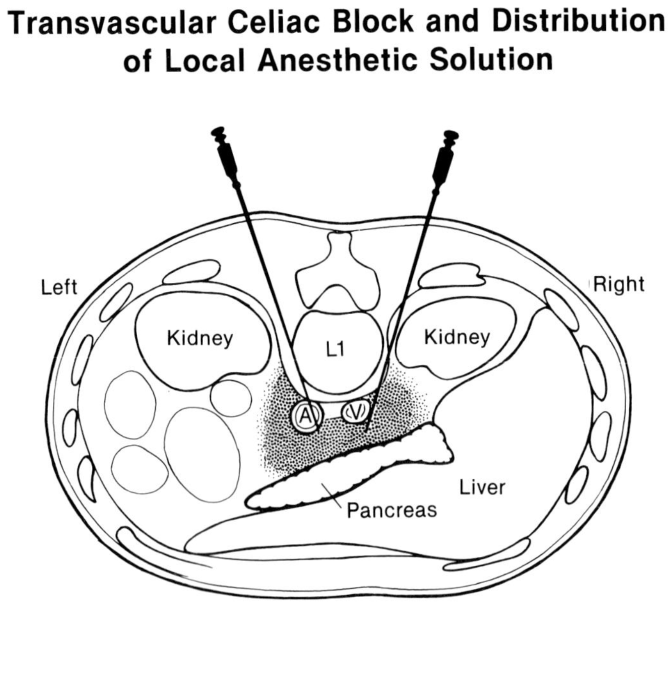

Figure 37–10 • Transvascular celiac block. Needle placement and solution spread following 25-mL injections on either side. A = aorta; V = vena cava.

detail and limited in patient numbers. In each case a volume of about 10 mL is required on either side to achieve the desired nerve block, irrespective of the type of solution to be employed.

(a) Transcrural Approach. In the transcrural approach, needle entry is commenced at almost the same point as that for the transvascular celiac approach, though this is dictated more by the space between the L-1 transverse process and the edge of the 12th rib. If insertion is at the midpoint between these bony landmarks, just cephalad to the tip of the process (a 45° angulation medial, ventral, and cephalad to the entry side) then the needle will be directed parallel to the rib until the body of T-12 vertebra is struck. At this level the needle usually rests near the intervertebral disk at the midpoint of the body. Furthermore, cephalad and ventral positioning requires an often difficult manipulation of the tip of the needle beyond the head of the 12th rib to bring it hard against the vertebral body, approximately 1 cm behind its anterior edge in its midlength (see Fig. 37–8). A 12-cm, 20 gauge styletted needle is recommended because finer gauges are more difficult to insert and manipulate. Placement under fluoroscopic control will greatly assist correct angulation and final placement, also lessening risks of pneumothorax by avoiding too cephalad an angulation.

(b) Transthoracic Approach. The transthoracic method uses a paravertebral entry with standard 22 gauge spinal needles, approximately 6 cm from the midline in the 11th intercostal space. Needle insertion is unimpeded by other structures, being quick and easy to perform, reaching almost the same vertebral level as the transcrural approach seeking the body of T-11. Its risk is clearly one of pneumothorax, though this has not yet occurred in 10 cases concluded to date. When undertaken with the patient breathing quietly under fluoroscopic imaging, lower limits of the lung are seen to lie one segmental level higher in the costophrenic angle, allowing the needle to traverse pleural spaces safely at this point. However, it is also important to keep needle insertion medial from the outset.

c. Monitoring for Accuracy

Regional blocks have long been the domain of the entrepreneurs in anesthesia, relying on tactile skill, good judgment, and a profound knowledge of anatomy. In most instances this suffices, but occasional mishaps occur that are not tolerated in present-day practice, where the medicolegal climate virtually demands precision and perfection without complication for even the most difficult procedures. Visceral block techniques are a case in point; their difficulty is compounded by the often distorted anatomy consequent to disease, and their risk is as great as that for any procedure in current use. Technologic advances have enhanced our capacity to monitor the conduct of these blocks, perhaps the most notable being the ability to define and control solution spread, the ultimate goal of all regional anesthesia techniques. Such monitoring is also educational and a salutary experience in the vagaries of clinical practice. Several options are available in modern hospital facilities, where these procedures should be conducted on an inpatient basis, with all the care usually accorded major surgical cases.

1. Tactile control of needle placement using surface and bony landmarks, with careful probing by gentle and experienced fingers, served as the basis for celiac and virtually all other blocks until relatively recent times. Skilled practitioners achieve success rates of around 90%, and in some cases even more, resulting in commendable time and cost reduction, provided local anesthetic solutions are the agents injected. When performed by skilled operators, these tactile skills are probably sufficient for safe and effective use in the classic paravascular celiac block technique, especially for those cases receiving only temporary blockade. However, in our increasingly litigious society and in cases with abnormal anatomy or those having destructive neurolysis, alternative graphically recordable monitoring and documentation are highly recommended. Patients undergoing any of the approaches to visceral blockade (transvascular celiac, transcural, and transthoracic splanchnic) usually require these measures to perform them both safely and effectively.
2. Fluoroscopic visualization of real-time needle placement is one of the modern advances in the conduct of these more difficult blocks, far exceeding the use of periodic radiographs. Low-radiation mobile C-arm units, capable of multiplane screening, image storage, and full film exposures, offer little hindrance to the conduct of these procedures and facilitate the rapid and accurate insertion of needles to almost any site in the body. Perhaps their greatest attribute is their ability to observe the dispersion of radiopaque contrast solutions at the time of injection, immediately alerting one to aberrant solution spread. Such compounds are safe, stable, and easily made up by any hospital pharmacy or by the operator at the time.[20] Use of these radiopaque contrast solutions under fluoroscopic screening virtually obviates risk of inadvertent injection

into other vital structures. Additional benefit derives from provision for hard-copy documentation of the procedure as part of each patient's permanent record. A composite picture in Fig. 37–11, showing disposition of contrast solutions in anteroposterior and lateral projections, gives an example of the information that can be provided. This artistic depiction offers distinction between compartmental spread of solution in the techniques of splanchnic and celiac block.

3. Computerized tomography and magnetic resonance imaging afford three-dimensional projection that is unsurpassed in terms of visual documentation. Figure 37–10 depicts a representation of the type of information CT imaging yields, showing needle position in relation to kidneys, vertebrae, vessels, and pancreas while also displaying the extent of alcohol spread following injection with a transvascular block. On the other hand, such scans are cumbersome and slow by comparison, yielding pictures after the event as opposed to the immediacy allowed by fluoroscopic screening, and are expensive and time consuming for routine cases. Their use is appropriate for investigational purposes and for those cases of particular difficulty due to anatomic abnormality.

d. Choice of Agents

There are not many drug options for injection. The procedure and nature of the disease process provide the determinants of drug choice and volume requirements.

1. *Local anesthetic agents* should use concentrations applicable to nerve block at other sites, toxicity limits often constraining the total dose if large-volume (50-mL) injections are needed for celiac block, for instance. Lidocaine 1% with epinephrine will suffice for all those receiving diagnostic procedures, steroid injection, or pretreatment for neurolytic block. Surgical or embolization cases requiring longer duration of reversible blockade are better done with bupivacaine 0.25% also with epinephrine. Clinical experience and radiologic confirmation indicate that volumes of 25 mL are needed on either side for celiac blocks and that volumes of 10 mL are needed bilaterally for splanchnic blocks.
2. *Steroid injections* have traditionally used insoluble formulations such as methyl prednisolone acetate (Depo-Medrol) or triamcinolone diacetate (Aristocort Intralesional) without trial of comparison against other agents. Their use is

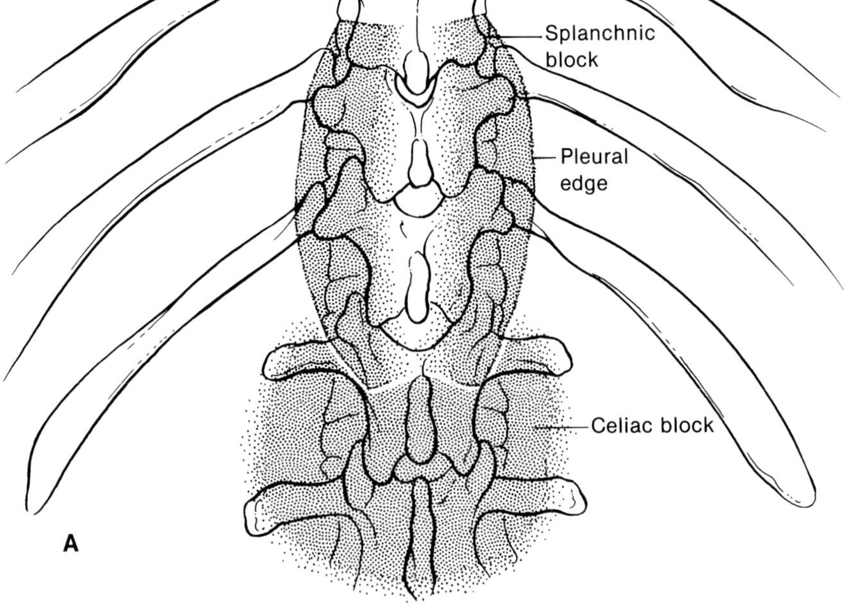

Figure 37–11 • Disposition of solution spread with either splanchnic or celiac block presented to show the different spread for each of the techniques. (***A***) A composite posteroanterior projection.

(continued)

confined to celiac blocks for either pancreatitis or cancer pain management. Doses of 40–80 mg are injected together with the required volume of local anesthetic. Brief mild irritation may follow, but systemic uptake from single dosing at these levels is usually insufficient to produce significant steroid effects. Used in this manner, they usually provide a benefit for several weeks.

3. *Phenol* should be used in concentrations of 12% or higher, dissolved in contrast solutions, where they remain stable for periods of at least 3 months. Lesser concentrations probably lead to incomplete neurolysis with partial neural regeneration over time. At this dosing level, toxicity in the form of cardiac irritation and heavy sedation has been encountered in debilitated patients at doses of 2 g or less, suggesting that, because of the volume required, this option is probably best limited to use for splanchnic rather than celiac procedures. Phenol injections are rarely painful, causing only a brief period of slight burning or a strong sensation of heat at the site.
4. *Ethyl alcohol* has been the standard neurolytic drug for celiac block, using either 50% or absolute alcohol, protagonists for each claiming sustained benefits. Greater intoxication from systemic absorption is evident in those receiving large doses with the absolute (95%) concentration. Intuitively, however, it is hard to ignore the maxim that if a little is good, a lot must be better. Unfortunately, the issue as to which concentration is best is one unlikely to be resolved by traditional clinical trials because of the small number of cases involved. Alcohol injections are invariably painful, necessitating heavy but brief medication for 1 or 2 minutes after the injection. Another option that may reduce the concentration of subsequent neurolytic solution is to inject local anesthetic prior to the alcohol. Injection of 12–15 mL local anesthetic on each side may be carried out prior to alcohol injection. After confirming analgesic effect and lack of somatic block, similar volumes of absolute alcohol may then be injected without changing needle position. The alcohol will presumably be diluted somewhat by the previously injected local anesthetic.

e. *Choice of Technique*

For those patients with relatively normal anatomy, such as those with confined tumors or those with pancreatitis

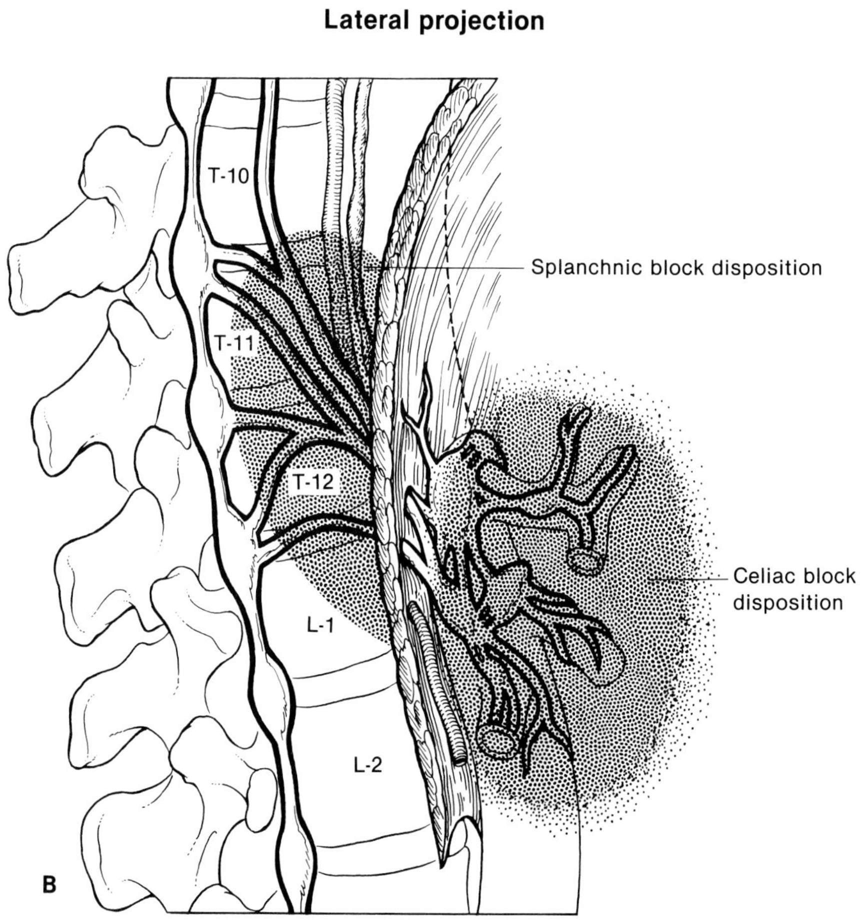

Figure 37–11 *(continued)*
(***B***) The spread as seen on lateral projection.

and peritoneal scarring or inflammation, the transvascular double-needle method offers complete diffusion of solution through the region of the celiac plexus itself. More vagal fibers are probably caught with this block, but it is not apparent whether this has any consequence. However, it is probably better, from the standpoint of safety and efficacy, to use the classic technique in cases where tumor has distorted retroperitoneal structures, or in situations requiring tactile rather than radiologic control. Intraoperative block, performed by the surgeon with an anterior approach to the plexus under direct visualization, should be encouraged for all cases presenting operatively with unresectable tumor even if pain is not the main presenting complaint. If done carefully, with aspiration and close observation of placement, alcohol or phenol solutions can be used to great effect, diminishing later discomfort. Solutions should be kept in the operating rooms for this purpose. Patients with extensive abdominal tumor spread are probably best treated with splanchnic blocks. They are less subject to aberrant solution spread and can be treated quickly and with lessened discomfort. Theoretically at least, these blocks may also be capable of a more complete neurolytic destruction. Their drawback is the need for fluoroscopic monitoring in all cases. Long-term outcome results have been fairly consistent over the years, with 75% of cancer patients sustaining major symptom relief.[21] Benefit for those with chronic pancreatitis has been less encouraging and an ongoing follow-up for those having combined splanchnic–celiac blocks shows less than 50% with effective relief.

D. Complications

It is no surprise that the literature is replete with examples of many types of complications with these techniques. The combination of deep needling into an area of vital structures lends itself to such consequences. Discussion of the almost endless variety of untoward events serves little in this context but to remind one of the potentially dramatic complications that may ensue. Patients should be counseled that there may be serious risks and that they almost invariably will have diarrhea for a few days, a few being also inconvenienced with postural hypotension until their blood volume is increased. They may also experience some degree of pain or discomfort from the needling and from pleural or diaphragmatic irritation due to the agents injected. A compilation of those problems encountered to date plus those reported in the literature is included in Table 37–2. Those categorized as being physiologic or pharmacologic are for the most part an expected consequence of these procedures and are probably unavoidable in most instances. Drug toxicity can be reduced by careful dosing considerations if patients are very ill. Postblock overdosing of narcotics or problems of withdrawal after opiate dose reduction are issues that can be anticipated and adequately addressed at the time. Technical complications that ensue from incorrect needle placement or from aberrant solution spread are feared by all. Their incidence can be reduced and almost completely avoided by use of the monitoring techniques outlined. Perhaps the one complication not amenable to total control with these measures is necrosis of the spinal radicular arteries arising from the aorta and traversing the bodies of lower thoracic or lumbar vertebrae to reach the anterior spinal artery. However, given the precautions and procedures as outlined, these visceral block techniques can be used with confidence in anesthesia and in acute and chronic pain control.

Table 37–2 • Complications of Splanchnic/Celiac Blocks

Physiologic	Hypotension Diarrhea Impotence Hiccough Pleuritic pain
Pharmacologic	Systemic drug toxicity Drug allergy Postblock sedation/withdrawal Postneurolysis regeneration/scarring
Technical	Paralysis/neuralgia Pneumothorax/chylothorax Hematuria/thrombosis

III. References

1. Bonica JJ. Causalgia and other reflex sympathetic dystrophies. In Bonica JJ et al (eds). Advances in Pain Research and Therapy. Vol. 3. New York, Raven Press, 1979, 141–166.
2. Carron H, Weller RM. Treatment of post-traumatic sympathetic dystrophy. In Advances in Neurology. Vol. 4. New York, Raven Press, 1974, 485–490.
3. Wang JK, Johnson KA, Ilstrup DM. Sympathetic blocks for reflex sympathetic dystrophy. Pain 23:13–17, 1985.

4. Mayfield FH. Causalgia. Springfield, IL, Charles C Thomas, 1951.
5. Devor M, Janig W. Activation of myelinated afferents ending in a neuroma by stimulation of the sympathetic supply in the rat. Neurosci Lett 24:43–47, 1981.
6. Bonica JJ. Management of Pain. Philadelphia, Lea and Febiger, 1953, 861–865.
7. Tenicela R, Lovasik D, Eaglstein W. Treatment of herpes zoster with sympathetic blocks. Clin J Pain 1:63–67, 1985.
8. Bonica JJ. Clinical Applications of Diagnostic and Therapeutic Nerve Blocks. Springfield, IL, Charles C Thomas, 1959, 142–187.
9. Boas RA. The sympathetic nervous system and pain relief. In Swerdlow M (ed). Relief of Intractable Pain. Amsterdam, Elsevier, 1983, 215–237.
10. Grant JCB. An Atlas of Anatomy, 5th ed. Baltimore, Williams & Wilkins, 1962, 567.
11. Carron H, Korbon GA, Rowlingson JC. Regional Anesthesia. New York, Grune and Stratton, 1984, 132–141.
12. Lofstrom JB, Cousins MJ. Sympathetic neural blockade of upper and lower extremity. In Cousins MJ, Bridenbaugh PO (eds). Neural Blockade. 2nd ed. Philadelphia, JB Lippincott, 1988, 461–496.
13. Boas RA, Hatangdi VS, Richards EG. Lumbar sympathectomy—a percutaneous chemical technique. In Bonica JJ, Albe-Fessard D (eds). Advances in Pain Research and Therapy. Vol. 1. New York, Raven Press, 1976, 685–689.
14. Hatangdi VS, Boas RA. Lumbar sympathectomy: A single needle technique. Br J Anaesth 57:285–289, 1985.
15. Moore DC. Regional Block. Springfield, IL, Charles C Thomas, 1961, 172–180.
16. Boas RA. Sympathetic blocks in clinical practice. Int Anesth Clin :149–182, 1978.
17. Cervero, F. Visceral pain. In Dubner R, Gebhart GF, Bond MR. Pain Research and Clinical Management. Vol. 3. Proceedings of the 5th World Congress on Pain. Amsterdam, Elsevier, 1988, 216–226.
18. Moore DC, Bush WH, Burnett LL. Celiac Plexus Block: A roentgenographic, anatomic study of technique and spread of solution in patients and corpses. Anesth Analg 60:369–379, 1981.
19. Ischia S, Luzzani A, Ischia A, Faggion, S. A new approach to the neurolytic block of the celiac plexus: The transaortic technique. Pain 16:333–341, 1983.
20. Boas RA. Sympathetic blocks in clinical practice. Int Anesthesiol Clin 16:149–182, 1978.
21. Brown DL, Bulley CK, Quiel EL. Neurolytic celiac plexus block for pancreatic cancer pain. Anesth Analg 66:869–873, 1987.

Chapter 38

H. Blane Howell, CDR, MC, USNR

Intravenous Regional Block (Bier Block)

OUTLINE

I. INTRODUCTION

Intravenous regional anesthesia (IVRA) produces excellent analgesia and motor paralysis with a high percentage of success when properly administered and has a good record of safety when used appropriately by well-trained and properly equipped personnel. However, like all anesthetic techniques that involve injecting directly into the vascular system a quantity of drug that could, if released in an uncontrolled fashion, cause a severe toxic reaction and possibly even death, this technique requires meticulous attention to detail. The person administering the agent must (1) understand the pharmacologic mechanisms of toxicity, (2) be aware of the mechanical factors that contribute to release of the drug into the systematic circulation, and (3) most of all, be qualified and equipped to quickly and skillfully treat any serious toxic reaction that may occur.[1–4]

In 1908, August Bier described a method of ''venous anesthesia'' in 134 patients, with good anesthesia and no single ''bad effect'' complication.[5,6] Adams, in a 1944 review article, cited Bier as well as Alms, who in 1886 had described intravenous injection of local anesthetic with subsequent analgesia in the area of the body drained by the vein.[7] The technique was little used beyond these early reports until reintroduced by Holmes in 1936.[8] Since then many reports have touted its simplicity and benefits.[9-24] The procedure has gained great popularity and is now used in emergency rooms, operating rooms, and office settings and has widespread use for minor surgery, as well as closed fracture realignment in the forearm and leg.

Occasional reports of cardiac arrest following intravenous lidocaine (Xylocaine),[25] etidocaine (Duranest), and bupivacaine (Marcaine)[26,27] caused questions to be raised about the inherent safety of the IVRA technique, and whether the technique should be used at all.[28, 29] It was well understood that toxic doses of local anesthetics could cause seizures and cardiac depression. Since the procedure was so fast and easy to perform, it was often administered by nonanesthetists and nonqualified medical personnel.[2] That lack of preparation, skill, and experience in caring for a patient who developed convulsions and apnea could have contributed to the degree of anoxia, which in turn could have contributed significantly to the onset and irreversibility of a cardiac arrest.[30] This emphasized the importance of having the person administering the block be skillful in airway management and resuscitation. As the mechanisms of direct and indirect cardiotoxicity of local anesthetic agents became better understood,[31,37] attention focused further on the safety of those agents and limited the drugs that could safely be used.[18,23,38] Finally, an appreciation of the possible mechanisms whereby the anesthetic drug can be injected directly into the systemic circulation from under a constricting tourniquet despite tourniquet gauge pressures of 400 mmHg[22,39,47] (the combination of a deep collateral circulation and too high an injection pressure) also added greatly to the safety of the technique.

Although the technique of IVRA has been used as a means of injecting reserpine, guanethidine, and bretylium into an extremity for treatment of reflex sympathetic dystrophy,[3,4] this chapter is limited to a discussion of using IVRA to produce surgical analgesia. The chapter ends with a simple but inclusive check-off list to help the busy practitioner perform the block expeditiously and with little risk of systemic toxicity.

II. Indications and Contraindications

Regional anesthesia is well suited for operations on a patient with a full stomach; that is, an adult who has eaten in the 8 hours prior to the anticipated start of surgery or in the 8 hours prior to the trauma that precipitated the need for surgery. Awake patients, unless too deeply sedated, generally retain control of airway reflexes and are better able to handle unanticipated vomiting by clearing their own airways. Some patients simply prefer to be awake during surgery, as they either feel more in control of the situation or are very frightened at the prospect of undergoing general anesthesia.

Intravenous regional anesthesia is appropriate for minor procedures on the distal upper and lower extremities that will take less than 1.5 hours, such as reducing and setting dislocations and fractures, debriding wounds, removing foreign bodies, wrist and ankle arthroscopy, carpal tunnel decompression, repair of ruptured tendons, incision and drainage of abscesses and paronychia, excision of ganglia, microsurgical repair of limbs, podiatric surgery, suturing extensive lacerations that would otherwise require a large and possibly toxic dose of local anesthetic infiltrated into the wound edges, excision of palmar neuromas, finger and toe amputation, excision of painful scars, and skin grafting.[3,9,11-14,16,21,23,38,40,48,49] IVRA has been used in patients from 2 years old to the elderly with satisfactory and safe results.[9,13,18,20] Since the need for supplemental medication is ordinarily minimal, the technique is particularly suitable for short procedures in an ambulatory surgery center.[94]

The major factors that limit the use of IVRA for peripheral surgery are two: (1) the operation must take no longer than 60–90 minutes or else discomfort from the tourniquet becomes bothersome, and possibly intolerable; (2) the site of the surgery must be distal enough on the extremity that a proper-sized double tourniquet can be safely placed proximal to it.[11] On the lower extremity this means placing the tourniquet at least 7.5 cm below the head of the fibula to avoid compression of the peroneal nerve.[21] On the upper extremity the tourniquet should not be placed over the humeral epicondyles to avoid soft tissue necrosis.[50]

Regional anesthetic techniques are contraindicated in those patients who are unable to cooperate with the anesthetist because of psychosis and dementia, as well as in patients with progressive neurologic disease or neurologic injury, coagulation disorders, sepsis, infection at the proposed site of injection, or a known sensitivity to the local anesthetic selected for use. In a patient with scleroderma the large volume of intravenous anesthetic injected distal to a tourniquet could cause an increase in interstitial tissue pressure sufficient to obliterate arterial perfusion of the extremity.[51,52] Sickle cell disease is an absolute contraindication because of the necessity of using a tourniquet. Calcified peripheral arteries may not be sufficiently compressed by an occluding tourniquet to stop all normal ingress of blood into the extremity, and the resulting venous congestion may cause the IVRA anesthetic to be forced out of the limb and into the general circulation.[28,39,40,44] Other relative contraindications to IVRA include pregnancy, seizure disorder, hepatic dysfunction, and myocardial disease with decreased cardiac output or arrhythmias, because of the large volume of local anesthetic that must be used.

As a general principle, no tourniquet should be used on a limb showing signs of hypoviability or acute or chronic trophic deficiency, as in arteriosclerosis, diabetes mellitus, polyneuropathy, Berger's disease, Raynaud's disease, any peripheral arteriopathy, or gangrene. The block cannot be used if infection or tumor is present in the extremity beneath the tourniquet.

Although not contraindications, the following disadvantages of the technique should also be considered: (1) The possibility of systemic toxicity may be greater than with other methods of regional anesthesia. (2) The acceptable duration of operating time is limited by tourniquet time and tourniquet pain. (3) Motor block may be incomplete. (4) When the tourniquet is released the patient experiences postoperative pain in a matter of minutes, without the delayed and slow return of sensation conferred by nerve block. (5) A disadvantage for the surgeon is that it is not possible to have the tourniquet released during the surgery.[38] Local anesthetics do not diffuse well through edematous or inflamed tissue, and IVRA should be avoided with those tissue conditions.

It is also suggested that the procedure not be performed on an obese extremity with a circumference larger than 32 cm because of problems with inadequate tourniquet occlusion of the artery enclosed in folds of adipose tissue.[44,53]

III. How to Do an Intravenous Regional Block

A. *Qualifications of the Person Administering the Block*

Local anesthetics can cause serious morbidity and mortality in small amounts through allergic reactions, and in the large amounts used in IVRA by direct toxic effects on the brain and heart. Although with IVRA great care is taken to insure that this large and toxic volume of anesthetic is sequestered away from the brain and heart, the person administering the anesthetic must be trained and qualified to handle convulsions, respiratory arrest, myocardial depression, and cardiac arrhythmia and arrest decisively and appropriately.[2] A current Advanced Cardiac Life Support (ACLS) or comparable certification, a facility with rapid endotracheal intubation and artificial ventilation, and familiarity with cardiac arrest and seizure treatment protocols should be the minimal acceptable qualifications.

Serious toxic reactions occur with dramatic, sudden swiftness and must be recognized and treated immediately as they occur. The person administering the anesthetic should be involved only in monitoring the patient and should not have his or her attention diverted from these duties by performing or assisting at the surgical procedure.

B. *Necessary Equipment*

Each patient should have a current weight recorded, be monitored with a continuous ECG readout and a blood pressure cuff, and have a free-flowing, large-bore intercatheter IV in place in one of the nonoperated extremities for use in administering fluids and emergency drugs if needed.

A double tourniquet set-up with appropriately sized cuffs (see later) is mandatory on the operated extremity. It is imperative that the tourniquet be free of leaks and be able to hold constant pressure in the system for at least 90 minutes.

Oxygen; a positive pressure bag–mask ventilation system; suction apparatus and tubing with Yankauer suction tip; a laryngoscope with charged batteries, functioning light, and blades of choice; appropriately sized and styletted endotracheal tubes; oropharyngeal and nasopharyngeal airways; and anticonvulsant medications of choice must be immediately accessible at the bedside.

The standard resuscitation equipment, including a defibrillator, ACLS drugs, and vasopressors must be readily available.

Finally, a temperature monitor and pulse oximeter are recommended. Both could be considered standard of care for administering any anesthetic.

C. *Technique*

1. PREMEDICATION

If the patient appears anxious or uncomfortable, an anxiolytic premedication can be given. Diazepam (Valium), 0.1 mg/kg total dose increases the seizure threshold almost twofold, in addition to decreasing anxiety levels. Midazolam (Versed), 0.05 mg/kg total dose, should be equally effective, causes neither burning on intravenous injection nor thrombophlebitis, and has a much shorter half-life. Fentanyl (Sublimaze), 0.5–2.0 fg/kg total dose, can also be used for premedication, sedation, and pain relief during the procedure. Butorphanol (Stadol), 0.5–2.0 mg total dose (for adults) is also effective. Dosage requirements for sedation of children, the elderly, the chronically ill, those with liver disease, and the pregnant will be decreased. Care must be taken not to obtund airway reflexes or depress the respiratory center by giving too much premedication. Incremental small doses given IV every 5 minutes will allow adequate titration to the desired effect. The same considerations apply during the surgery when giving sedation for anxiety, and/or analgesics for tourniquet pain if the procedure goes on beyond the optimal anesthetic time.

2. INSERTION OF THE CATHETER FOR IVRA

The IV for injecting the local anesthetic medication into the extremity to be operated on can be a catheter or a needle, but a catheter is much more stable and has much less chance of infiltrating (Fig. 38–1). The IV should be placed in a vein as far distal from the tourniquet site as is reasonably possible. If the anesthetic medication is injected into a vein close to the tourniquet, it is easier to raise the intravenous pressure in veins located beneath and just distal to the tourniquet to a level that exceeds the occluding pressure of the tourniquet, and result in a bolus of anesthetic entering the central vascular system, even if the tourniquet pressure is 400 mmHg.[41] It is desirable, but not necessary, to place the IV distal to the proposed surgical site. By injecting distal to the surgical site one can be more assured that concentrated anesthetic will bathe the nerve endings that supply the surgical site. An IV extension tubing going from a single large syringe to the intercatheter can be very helpful in injecting the required large volume of anesthetic medication without dislodging the intercatheter.

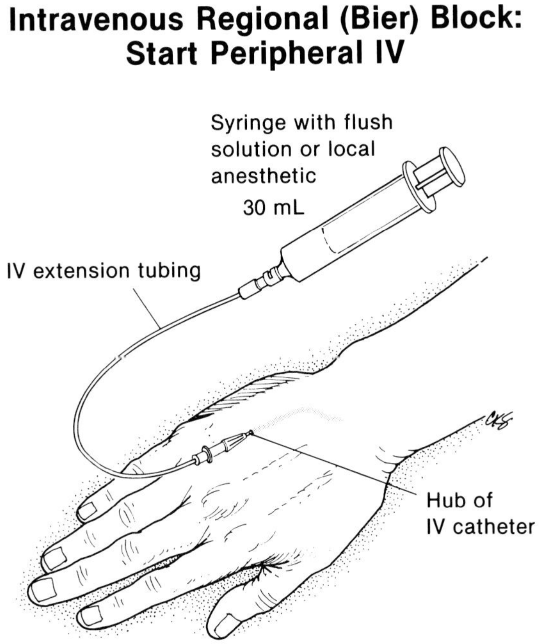

Figure 38–1 • Intravenous regional (Bier) block. Start the peripheral IV. The IV should be placed as far from the tourniquet and as close to the lesion as possible.

3. TOURNIQUET

A double tourniquet setup connected to a pneumatic pressure gauge should be placed on the extremity over a thin wrap of felt padding to protect against skin pinches (Fig. 38–2). The pressure in each tourniquet should be systematically increased, and the pressure at which the palpated pulse disappears should be noted[44] for each tourniquet. This is the occlusion pressure. When in use, each tourniquet should be inflated to 100 mmHg higher than the occlusion pressure obtained with that particular tourniquet in order to negate any errors from possible discrepancies in cuff sizes, or placement on the extremity, or between actual cuff pressures and indicated gauge pressure.[40]

An understanding of those factors that can cause a marked disparity between tourniquet pressure gauge readings and the actual pressure in the vessels, both venous and arterial, under the tourniquet is essential for safety. Proper width of the tourniquet compared with the circumference of the extremity is of critical importance. The tourniquet width should be 40% of the extremity circumference for the gauge pressure to accurately reflect arterial intraluminal pressure under the cuff.[57–59] If the cuff is narrower, the pressure read will be artifactually high, and if larger, artifactually low.

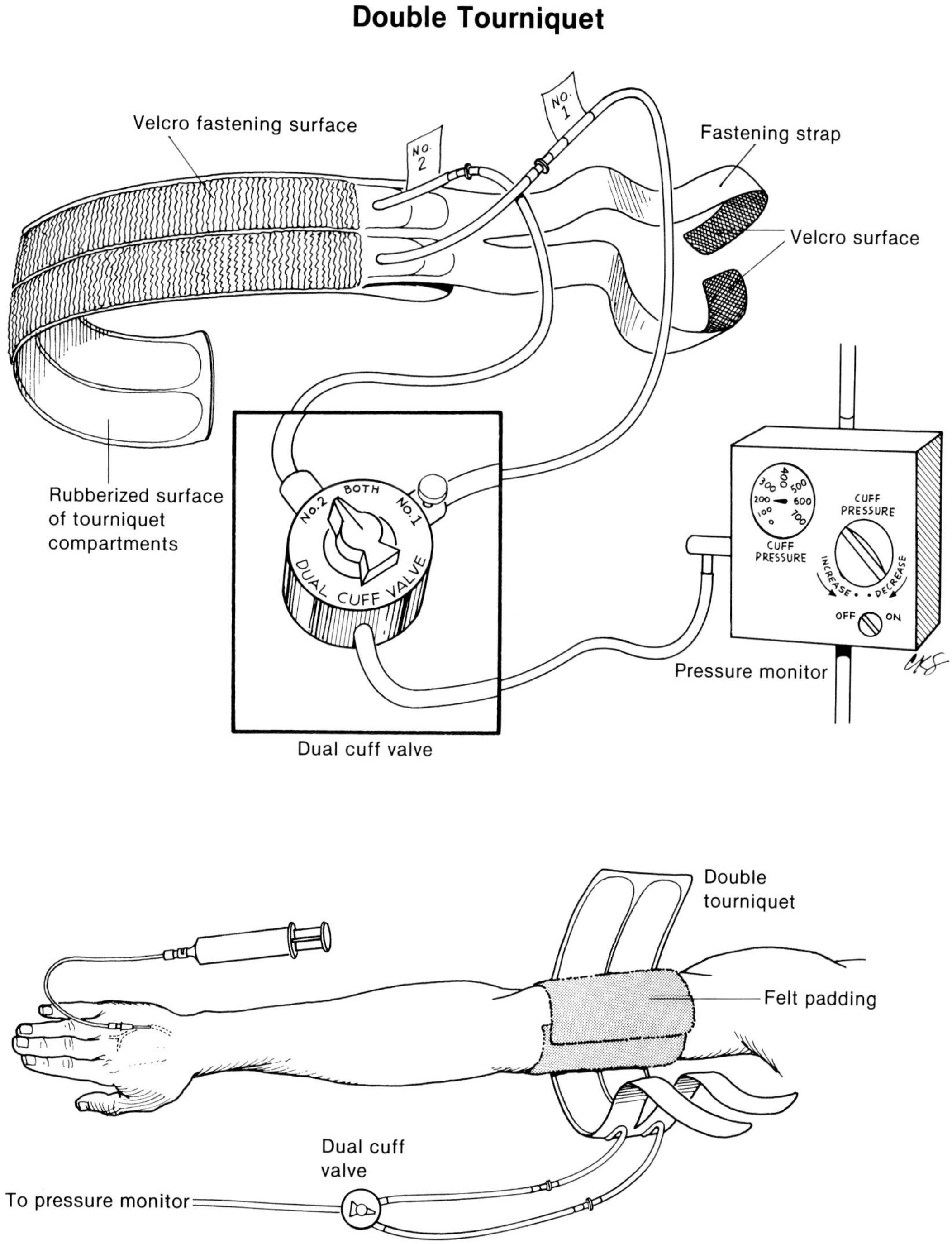

Figure 38–2 • Intravenous regional (Bier) block. Apply the double tourniquet over the felt padding. Check each tourniquet independently.

Complications with leakage of medication under the cuff and with arm congestion are more common with narrow cuffs.[41] A wider cuff can occlude the tubing from the machine going into the cuff, giving a higher pressure reading than is actually present in the cuff.[60] A common error is to assume that the pneumatic cuff pressure gauge shows the cuff pressure, when with some setups it actually shows the pressure inside the machine[1] and may be inaccurate.[39] Inadequate compression of the arm has been noted despite manometric readings of a pressure well above the systolic pressure of the arm.[47,61] Calibration of the pneumatic cuff–pressure gauge combination against a mercury manometer has shown wide discrepancies[47] and should be done on a regular maintenance schedule. Luer lock fittings should be used on all tourniquet connections to guard against possible blowout disconnections of the fittings under pressure.[20]

Determining occlusion pressure for each particular patient-extremity–cuff-tourniquet combination and making sure that the pressure in the cuff during the procedure is 100 mmHg higher than the occlusion pressure is a very safe way to avoid numerous pitfalls.

It is imperative to assure that the tourniquet system does not leak and will maintain the set pressure for the entire length of the procedure. Once the tourniquet is inflated, it is generally accepted that it can be left up for 1.5–2 hours without danger of causing ischemic damage to anatomic structures under the tourniquet or the tissues distal to it.[53,62–66]

4. Exsanguinating the Extremity

If it can be done without causing the patient pain, the extremity should be elevated for several minutes, and then while still elevated have an Esmarch (rubber or elastic) bandage wrapped tightly around it from the most distal part to over but not above the already applied but still deflated tourniquet (Fig. 38–3). A considerate technique is to slip a stockinette over the extremity prior to wrapping it, to keep the Esmarch bandage from pulling

Intravenous Regional Bier Block: Wrap Esmarch's Bandage

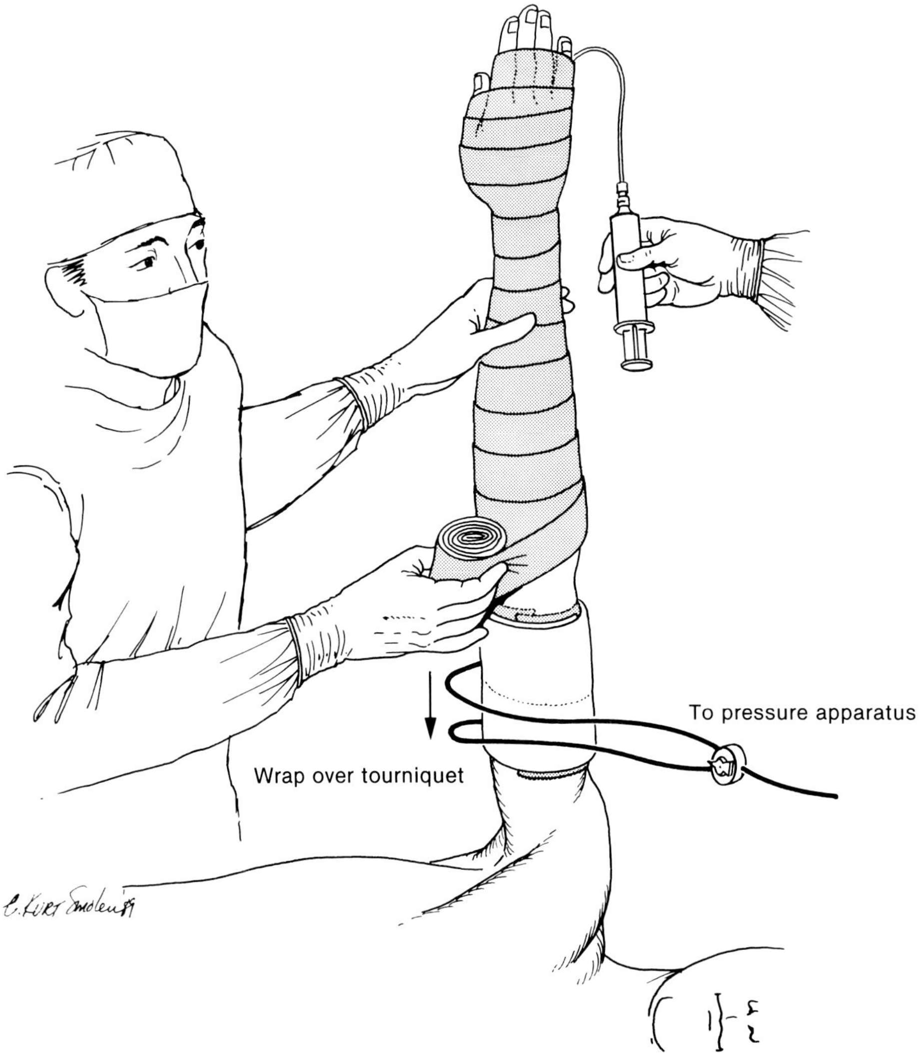

Figure 38–3 • Intravenous regional (Bier) block. Wrap the Esmarch's bandage while the extremity is elevated to exsanguinate the extremity.

on the extremity hairs and pinching the skin as it is being wrapped.[95] Both elevation and wrapping help exsanguinate the extremity of as much blood as possible. A volume of anesthetic agent injected into an exsanguinated extremity will be relatively more concentrated in that extremity than the same amount of agent injected into the same extremity full of blood.[67] Onset of IVRA anesthetic action should be quicker, and intensity of effect should be greater, within an exsanguinated extremity. Inadequate exsanguination and an inadequate tourniquet are the two main causes of failure of the technique.[11]

5. Injecting the Anesthetic Solution

After the proximal tourniquet cuff is inflated to 100 mmHg higher than the occlusion pressure (Fig. 38–4), the Esmarch bandage is removed. The extremity should appear ischemic and be pulseless.[40] The extremity is then placed horizontally, and the anesthetic is injected steadily (Fig. 38–5), less than 3 mL/second for a distal injection site, or less than 2 mL/second if the injection site is near the tourniquet.[41] Higher injection rates can easily raise the intraluminal venous pressure above the tourniquet occluding pressure.[36–38,40,42,43,63,64]

The injection should be stopped if it is apparent that the extremity is becoming congested by appearing pink or swollen or by developing petechiae. This indicates that the tourniquet is not completely occluding the flow of blood into the extremity, and there is a distinct possibility that continued injection will cause leakage of anesthetic into the general circulation, with possible serious toxic effects. To avoid causing an injection pressure higher than the tourniquet pressure the following principles should be kept in mind: the smallest appropriate amount of anesthetic should be injected slowly, from a distal injection site, and into an exsanguinated, noncongested extremity.[36,37,40,43]

After the medication is injected, the intravenous catheter or needle is removed if desired and pressure is applied to the venipuncture site until bleeding stops.

6. Characteristics of the Onset of the Anesthetic

As the anesthetic is injected, the patient may notice the onset of warmth in the extremity, followed by an awareness of tingling. Blotchy discoloration may appear near superficial veins. After 3–5 minutes, patches of numbness appear that gradually spread and coalesce until

Intravenous Regional (Bier) Block: Inflate Proximal Tourniquet

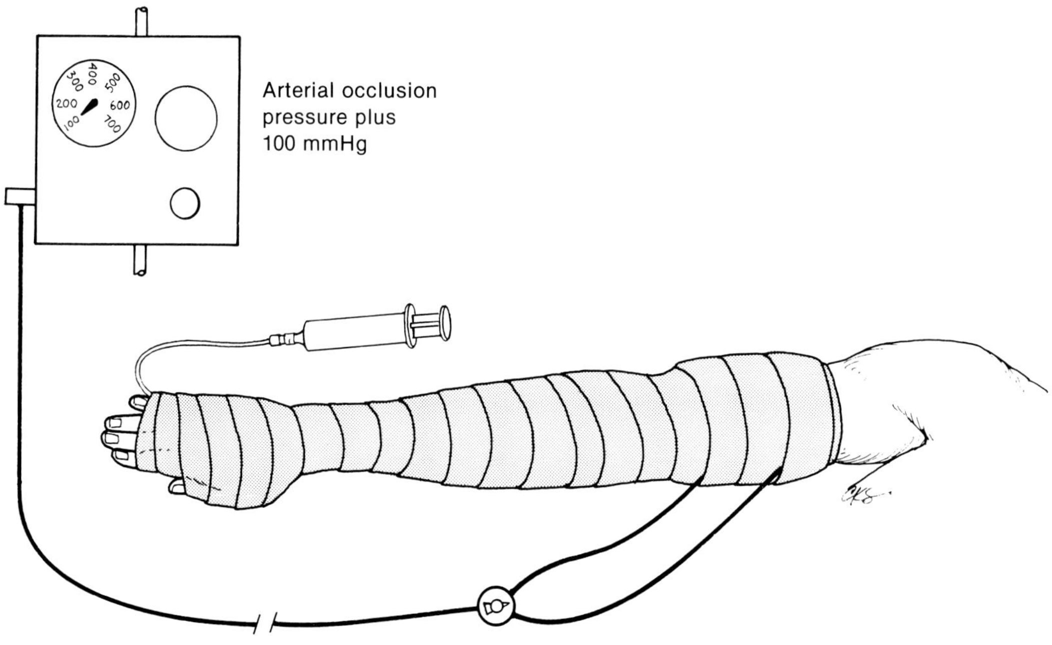

Figure 38–4 • Intravenous regional (Bier) block. Inflate proximal tourniquet to a pressure that is 100 mmHg greater than the arterial occlusion pressure. Then remove the Esmarch's bandage.

Intravenous Regional (Bier) Block: Inject Drug

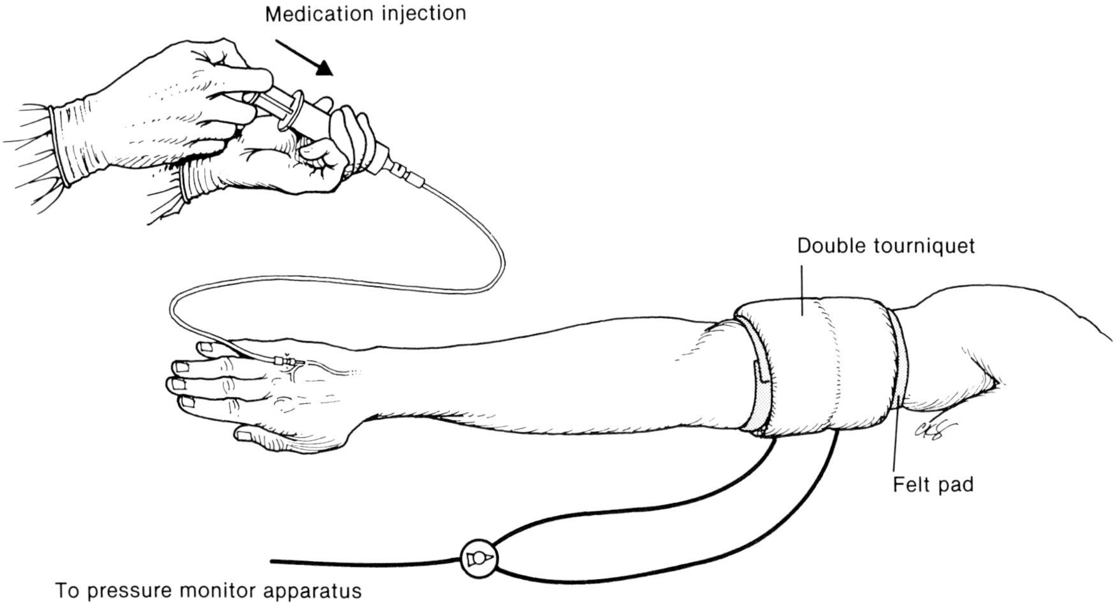

Figure 38–5 • Intravenous regional (Bier) block. Inject drug steadily at approximately 2–3 mL/second.

the whole extremity distal to the tourniquet is analgesic. In the upper extremity the area immediately around the olecranon is often not as well anesthetized as the rest of the forearm.[48,67] Paralysis is usually present, although it may be incomplete. After onset of anesthesia the skin of the extremity is prepared.

7. Duration of Effective Analgesia

After a time, usually about 45 minutes after tourniquet inflation, discomfort from the tourniquet becomes bothersome. The anesthetist can then inflate the distal tourniquet cuff, and when assured that satisfactory occlusion pressure for that tourniquet plus 100 mmHg is present and stable in the cuff, can deflate the proximal tourniquet cuff. This will give some relief and allow another 15–30 minutes before tourniquet pain again becomes relatively bothersome. Continued switching from proximal to distal tourniquet, and vice versa, will allow often another half hour of pain-free IVRA. Judicious use of small doses of intravenous sedatives, anxiolytics, and/or narcotics will also contribute to extending the time the tourniquet will be tolerated. If the surgical procedure extends beyond 1.5 hours, a light general anesthesia such as nitrous oxide and oxygen is almost always necessary.

The effectiveness of the anesthetic can be markedly enhanced by inflating the tourniquet 10–20 minutes prior to injecting the anesthetic. Only about half the dose of the anesthetic is needed for satisfactory analgesia if this is done.[9,18,79] However, this may be because of direct ischemic effects of the tourniquet on the nerves and does decrease the amount of time the tourniquet can be left inflated before tourniquet pain is a consideration.

8. Tourniquet Release

Controversy exists as to just how the tourniquet should be let down. If the surgery has lasted less than 30 minutes, it is suggested that the tourniquet be deflated for only 15 seconds and reinflated for 30 seconds to 2 minutes[68,69] and that this cycle be repeated several times before the cuff is let down permanently. If the tourniquet has been inflated for over 30 minutes, it is generally safe to let the tourniquet down all at once.[15] During the procedure there is a constant leakage of anesthetic out of the extremity[42,70] via intramedullary bone channels;[22,48] and it may be that after 30 minutes a nontoxic amount of anesthetic remains in the extremity. Some sources have shown that it is safe to deflate the tourniquet all at once even if the surgery has taken as little as 5–15 minutes.[71,72]

9. Analgesia After Tourniquet Release

Sensation (and pain) and motor strength return quickly to the extremity following tourniquet release, often in 2–5 minutes.[7] After 10 minutes there should be no remaining neurologic deficit.[16] This enables the surgeon to rapidly assess the postoperative condition of the extremity but does not permit any further surgical manipulation.

D. *Choice of Anesthetic Agent*

1. Site of Action

There is controversy as to whether the site of action of the local anesthetics is at the peripheral nerve endings, on the major nerve trunks, or even at the neuromuscular junction.[73] Carbon 14–labeled 1% lidocaine readily permeates tissues by direct migration through the walls of vascular beds.[74] Support for the view that the anesthetics act on the nerve trunks comes from intravenous injection of radiopaque dyes, and the observation that the more distal parts of the extremity are innervated by the core fibers of the nerve trunk. Since the core is well supplied with abundant vascular channels that could carry the anesthetic to the core fibers, the more distal parts of the extremity should become anesthetized first, as has been noted clinically.[75] Other studies—with radioisotopes,[76] radiographic visualization of the spread of contrast medium injected intravenously distal to an extremity tourniquet and the spread of anesthesia following the injection of the anesthetic into the dorsum of the hand,[77] and the observation that a swollen finger may not become anesthetized completely while the rest of the same hand is very well anesthetized—support the contention that the site of action is more peripheral than the major nerve trunks. Impulse transmission studies indicate that the site of action is at the branching points of the nerve fibers.[78]

2. Choice of Drug

Excellent regional anesthesia can be produced using lidocaine, prilocaine, chloroprocaine, and bupivacaine. Lidocaine is the most common anesthetic used for IVRA. Prilocaine used in the recommended dose will not cause clinically significant methemoglobinemia and is proposed by some as the drug of choice, because it is the most rapidly metabolized, gives blood concentrations 20% to 50% those of lidocaine, and will not cause cyanosis as long as the total dose is less than 600 mg in adults.[12,30,80–85] Because of the high incidence of thrombophlebitis with chloroprocaine, it is contraindicated.[79] Bupivacaine should not be used because of the marked danger of cardiac toxicity and irreversible cardiac arrest.[18,20,23,33,35–38,86–89]

Recommended dosages are:

1. Lidocaine (0.25% to 0.50%) 3–4 mg/kg.
2. Prilocaine (0.50–1.0%) 3 mg/kg.[15]
   The least concentrated solutions give a lower incidence of toxic reactions even if the same dose is injected. Anesthetic drug solutions must be preservative free.

3. Reinjection

After the tourniquet is deflated and the anesthetic is released into the general circulation, the lungs act as a giant reservoir and clear a large amount of the anesthetic as it first passes through them, releasing it over subsequent circulation times. Peak levels of the anesthetic are 20% to 80% less than if the same amount of local anesthetic had been given intravenously. Approximately 30% of the drug is released from the extremity at first, and 50% still remains in the arm after 30 minutes. Consequently, it is possible to reinject one half of the original dose of the anesthetic 30 minutes after tourniquet release and to achieve adequate analgesia for an additional 30–45 minutes of surgery without raising the intravascular anesthetic concentration to toxic levels.[90–92]

E. *Special Considerations*

1. Lower Extremity

Excellent anesthesia has been obtained for foot and ankle surgery when the tourniquet has been placed on the calf, although loss of anesthesia often occurs when attempting to inflate the distal cuff and deflate the proximal cuff for relief of tourniquet pain.[21,39] The tourniquet should be placed at least 7.5 cm below the head of the fibula to avoid pressure on the peroneal nerve. In general, less satisfactory results are obtained with a double-cuff system on the thigh, and a less concentrated solution is required to fill all the venous system of the entire leg and still avoid toxic reactions on cuff release. Lidocaine 3.3 mg/kg diluted to 0.25% is recommended for a sufficient volume of anesthetic, and a judicious premedication is usually needed to avoid tourniquet discomfort during the procedure.[93] Venous access in the lower extremity is poorer than in the upper extremity. Other forms of regional anesthesia or a preinjection ischemic period might be appropriate if a thigh tourniquet is mandated.

2. Age-Related Factors

Intravenous regional anesthesia can be safe, effective, and convenient even in very small children, particularly if time is taken to explain to the child and the parents what is going to happen, and if a parent is allowed to stay with the child during the procedure.[13] Elderly patients are more sensitive to the toxic effects of local anesthetics, and the lower drug concentrations should be used. Elderly patients are in general also more sensitive to the mind-altering and respiratory-depressing effects of the commonly used premedicants and analgesics, and these should be carefully titrated to effect.

IV. Complications

Toxic reactions during IVRA will usually become manifest either during the injection of the local anesthetic medication or soon after the tourniquet is released at the end of the procedure. Any mechanical malfunction that decreases the effective barrier of the tourniquet and allows the sudden release of large amounts of medication into the systemic circulation can also cause toxic reactions at any time during the procedure.

Minor reactions are characterized by circumoral numbness, tinnitus, blurred vision, an unusual or strange feeling, giddiness, dizziness, or even an autistic state, and may be noted on careful questioning in up to 50% of patients who receive IVRA. These minor reactions seldom progress to more serious reactions.[9] Slurred speech, shivering, muscle twitching, and tremors of the face and extremities appear to be immediate precursors of a generalized convulsion.[53]

Major reactions include convulsions, apnea, and nonperfusing dysrhythmias including sinus bradycardia, ventricular fibrillation, and asystole.

Paralysis of the hand following pneumatic tourniquet use in IVRA has been reported, but it is rare and recovery is usually complete, although prolonged.[54] A case of loss of the forearm and hand following IVRA has also been reported, but it was postulated that this was caused by erroneous injection of alcohol rather than by local anesthetic into the venous system.[55]

Allergic reactions have been well discussed elsewhere.[56]

V. Technique Check-off Lists

A. *Preblock*

Some preblock considerations follow:

1. Appropriate patient
2. Appropriate procedure
3. Current weight known
4. Monitors:
   a. ECG
   b. Blood pressure cuff
   c. Pulse oximeter—optional, but excellent
   d. Continuous temperature monitor—optional
5. Large-bore intercatheter in nonaffected extremity, with IV of balanced salt solution for emergency medication access
6. Double tourniquet set-up:
   a. Place on patient over thin wrap of felt padding
   b. Luer lock connections checked
   c. No tourniquet leaks
   d. Determine occlusion pressure for each cuff, and record
7. Emergency equipment at hand:
   a. Oxygen
   b. Positive pressure bag-mask ventilator
   c. Suction, with Yankauer tip
   d. Laryngoscope checked for function
   e. Styletted endotracheal tubes
   f. Oropharyngeal and nasopharyngeal airways
   g. Anticonvulsant medication of choice
   h. Standard cardiovascular resuscitation equipment and medications readily available
8. Premedication titrated to desired patient condition

B. *Performance of the Block*

While performing the block

1. Draw up appropriate medication in large plastic syringe, attach IV extension tubing, and fill tubing with the medication in the syringe.
2. Insert intercatheter into a vein in the affected extremity:
   a. Preferably distal to lesion

b. As far from tourniquet as possible
3. Elevate affected extremity for 3 minutes, if possible.
4. Wrap affected extremity with Esmarch bandage, if possible (wrap over but not above tourniquet).
5. Inflate proximal tourniquet to pressure of occlusion pressure plus 100 mmHg.
6. Remove Esmarch bandage.
7. Lower extremity to the horizontal position.
8. Observe extremity to appear ischemic and to be pulseless.
9. Inject medication:
   a. 3 mL/second for distal injection site
   b. 2 mL/second for proximal injection site (near tourniquet)
10. Stop injection if the extremity appears to be becoming congested or swollen, if petechiae develop, or if the extremity becomes pink.
11. After all medication is injected, remove intercatheter if desired.
12. Apply pressure to puncture site until bleeding stops.
13. Observe for toxic reactions:
   a. Visual changes, tinnitus
   b. Circumoral paresthesias
   c. Unusual feelings (giddiness)
   d. Agitation
   e. Convulsions
   f. Myocardial depression, with bradycardia and/or arrest
14. *Do not participate in the surgery (ie, watch the patient).*

C. *Intraoperative Considerations*

The following are some intraoperative considerations:

1. Continue observation throughout the entire procedure.
2. If tourniquet pain develops and is intolerable
   a. Inflate distal tourniquet to occlusion pressure + 100 mmHg.
   b. Deflate proximal tourniquet.
   c. Alternate having proximal or distal tourniquet inflated, but do not deflate one until the other is inflated.
   d. Use judicious amounts of analgesics.

D. *Postoperative Considerations*

1. Observe closely for toxic reactions at time of tourniquet release.
2. Continue to observe in postanesthetic area for 30 minutes following release of tourniquet.

VI. REFERENCES

1. Heath ML. Deaths after intravenous regional anesthesia. Br Med J 285:913, 1982.
2. Casey WF. Bupivacaine intravenous anaesthesia and resuscitation (letter). Anaesthesiology 39:612, 1984.
3. Bird TM, Strunin L. Anesthetic considerations for microsurgical repair of limbs. Can Anesth Soc J 31:51, 1984.
4. Ford SR, Forrest WH, Eltherington L. The treatment of reflex sympathetic dystrophy with intravenous regional bretylium. Anesthesiology 68:137, 1988.
5. Bier A. Ueber einen neuen Weg Local anasthesie an den Gliedmasses zu erzeugen. Arch Klin Chir 86:1007, 1908.
6. Bier A. A new method of local anesthesia in the extremities. Ann Surg 48:780.
7. Adams RC. Intravenous Anaesthesia. New York, Hoeber, 1944, 9111 pp.
8. Bell HM, Slater EM, Harris WH. Regional anesthesia with intravenous lidocaine. JAMA 186:544, 1963.
9. Brown LL. Anesthesia in the geriatric patient. Clin Plast Surg 12:51, 1985.
10. Adams JP, Dealy EJ, Kenmore PI. Intravenous regional anesthesia in hand surgery. J Bone Joint Surg 46A:811, 1964.
11. Atkinson MB, Modell J, Moya F. Intravenous regional anesthesia. Anesth Analg 44:313, 1965.
12. Thorn-Alquist A. Intravenous regional anaesthesia: A seven year survey. Acta Anaesth Scand 15:23, 1971.
13. Fitzgerald B. Intravenous regional anaesthesia in children. Br J Anaesth 48:485, 1976.
14. Schiller MG. Intravenous regional anesthesia for closed treatment of fractures and dislocations of the upper extremities. Clin Orthop 118:25, 1976.
15. Katz J. Intravenous regional anesthesia. Sem Anesth 11, March 1983.
16. Francis RI. Intravenous regional anaesthesia. Anaesthesia 38:290, 1983.
17. Pattison CW. A review of the Bier's block technique. The Prac 22:235, 1984.
18. Farrell RG, Swanson SL, Walter JR. Safe and effective IV regional anesthesia for use in the emergency department. Ann Emerg Med 14:288, 1985.
19. Cobb AG, Houghton GR. Local anaesthetic infiltration versus Bier's block for Colles fractures. Br Med J (Clin Res) 291:1683, 1985.
20. Turner PL, Batten JB, Hjorth D, et al. Intravenous regional anaesthesia for the treatment of upper limb injuries in childhood. Aust NZ J Surg 56:153, 1986.
21. Nusbaum LA, Hamelberg W. Intravenous regional anesthesia for surgery on the foot and ankle. Anesthesiology 64:91, 1986.
22. Davies JAH, Walford AJ. Intravenous regional anaesthesia for foot surgery. Acta Anesth Scand 30:145, 1986.
23. Raggi RP. Balanced regional anesthesia for hand surgery. Orthop Clin N Am 17:473 1986.
24. Raj PP. Intravenous regional anesthesia: Past, present, future. ASA Ref Course 422, 1988.

25. Kennedy BR, Duthie AM, Parbrook GD, Carr TL. Intravenous regional anaesthesia: An appraisal. Br Med J 1:954, 1965.
26. Albright GA. Cardiac arrest following regional anesthesia with etidocaine or bupivacaine. Anesthesiology 51:285, 1979.
27. Prentiss JE. Cardiac arrest following caudal anesthesia. Anesthesiology 50:51, 1986.
28. Mather SP. Intravenous regional analgesia or axillary block. Anaesthesia 39:946, 1984.
29. Hardy PAJ. Intravenous regional anesthesia or axillary block. Anaesthesia 39:946, 1984.
30. Reynolds F. Bupivacaine and intravenous regional anesthesia. Anaesthesia 39:105, 1984.
31. Scott DB. Toxicity caused by local anaesthetic agents. Br J Anaesth 56:435, 1984.
32. Wegrzynowicz ES. Comparison of equi-myocardial depressant doses of lidocaine vs bupivacaine on cardiac toxicity duration. Anesthesiology 63:A222, 1985.
33. Moller RA, Covino BG. Toxic cardiac electrophysiologic effects of bupivacaine and lidocaine at high concentrations. Anesthesiology 63:A223, 1985.
34. Clarkson CW, Hondeghem LM. Mechanism of bupivacaine depression of cardiac conduction: Fast block of sodium channels during the action potential with slow recovery from block during diastole. Anesthesiology 62:396, 1985.
35. Klasten GW. Amide local anesthetic alterations of effective refractory period temporal dispersion: Relationship to ventricular arrhythmias. Anesthesiology 65:61, 1986.
36. Rosenberg PH, Eija AK, Marjatta KT, Linden HB. Acute bupivacaine toxicity as a result of venous leakage under the tourniquet cuff during a Bier block. Anesthesiology 58:95, 1983.
37. Thomas RD, Behbehani MM, Coyle DE, Denson DD. Cardiovascular system toxicity with local anesthetics: An alternative hypothesis. Anesthesiology 63:A228, 1985.
38. Earle AS, Blanchard JM. Regional anesthesia in the upper extremity. Clin Plast Surg 12:97, 1985.
39. Jeyaseelan TM, Stevenson TM, Pfitzner J. Tourniquet failure and arterial calcification. Anaesthesia 36:48, 1981.
40. Davies JAH, Haall ID, Wilkey AD, et al. Intravenous regional anesthesia—the danger of the congested arm and the value of occlusion pressure. Anaesthesia 39:416, 1983.
41. El-hassan KM, Hutton P, Black MS. Venous pressure and arm volume changes during simulated Bier's block. Anesthesiology 39:229, 1984.
42. Davies JAH, Wilkey AD, Hall ID. Bupivacaine leak past inflated tourniquets during intravenous regional analgesia. Anaesthesia 39:996, 1984.
43. Finnegan BA, Bukht D, Strunin L. Venous pressure in simulated Bier's block (letter). Anaesthesia 39:1149, 1984.
44. Ogden PN. Failure of intravenous regional analgesia using a double cuff tourniquet. Anaesthesia 39:456, 1984.
45. Grice SC, Morell RC, Balestrieri FJ, et al. Intravenous regional anesthesia: Evaluation and prevention of leakage under the tourniquet. Anesthesiology 62:A221, 1985.
46. Grice SC, Morrell RC, Balestrieri FJ. Confusion regarding experimental studies of intravenous regional anesthesia. Anesthesiology 674:526, 1986.
47. Flatt AE. Tourniquet time in hand surgery. Arch Surg 104:190, 1972.
48. Sorbie C, Chaca P. Regional anaesthesia by the intravenous route. Br Med J 1:957, 1965.
49. Valli H, Rosenberg PH. Intravenous regional anaesthesia below the knee. Anaesthesia 41:1196, 1986.
50. Furlow LT. Cause and prevention of tourniquet ooze. Surg Gynecol Obstet :1069, 1971.
51. Sweeney B. Anaesthesia and scleroderma. Anaesthesia 39:1145, 1984.
52. Smith GB, Shribman AJ. Anesthesia and scleroderma—A reply to a letter. Anaesthesia 39:1145, 1984.
53. Covino BG. Criteria for selecting the best local anesthetic agent. ASA annual refresher course lectures, 432, 1985.
54. Larsen UT, Hommelgaard P. Pneumatic tourniquet paralysis following intravenous regional analgesia. Anaesthesia 42:526, 1987.
55. Luce EA, Mangubat E. Loss of hand and forearm following Bier block: A case report. J Hand Surg 8:280, 1983.
56. Cousins MJ, Bridenbaugh PO. Neural Blockade in Clinical Anesthesia and Management of Pain. 2nd ed. Philadelphia, JB Lippincott.
57. Geddes LA, Whistler SJ. The error in indirect blood pressure measurement with the incorrect size of cuff. Am Heart J 96:4, 1978.
58. Kirkendall WM, Burton AC, Epstein FH, Fries ED. American Heart Association report Recommendations for human blood pressure determination by sphygmomanometers. Circulation 36:980, 1967.
59. Kirkendall WM, Feinleib M, Fries ED, Mark AL. Subcommittee of the American Heart Association postgraduate education committee report. Circulation 62:1146A, 1980.
60. Emmet C. More trouble with Bier's block. Anaesthesia 38:390, 1983.
61. Henderson A, Sujitkumar P. Successful resuscitation after cardiac arrest following IV regional anaesthesia (IVRA). Br J Anaesth 58:362, 1986.
62. Dery R, Pelletier J, Jacques A, et al. Metabolic changes induced in the limb during tourniquet ischaemia. Can Anaesth Soc J 12:367, 1965.
63. Kalso EA, Lalla ML, Rosenberg PH, et al. Evaluation of the myotoxicity of bupivacaine in Bier blocks—a biochemical and electron microscope study. Anesth Analg 62:796, 1983.
64. Solonen KA, Hjelt L. Morphological changes in striated muscles during ischaemia. Acta Orthop Scand 39:13, 1968.
65. Solonen KA, Tarkkanen L, Narvanen S, Gordin R. Metabolic changes in the upper limb during tourniquet ischaemia. Acta Orthop Scand 39:20 1968.
66. Wilgis EFS. Observations on the effects of tourniquet ischemia. J Bone Joint Surg 53A:1343, 1971.
67. Lillie PE, Glynn CJ, Fenwick DG. Site of action of intravenous regional anesthesia. Anesthesiology 61:507, 1984.
68. Colbern EC. Intravenous regional anesthesia: The perfusion block. Anesth Analg 45:69, 1966.
69. Merrifield AJ, Carter SJ. Intravenous regional analgesia: Lignocaine blood levels. Anesthesiology 20:287, 1965.
70. Cotev S, Robin GC. Experimental studies of intravenous regional anaesthesia using radioactive lignocaine. Br J Anaesth, 38:936, 1966.
71. Mazze RI, Dunbar RW. Intravenous regional anesthesia—report of 497 cases with a toxicity study. Acta Anaesth Scand (Suppl) 36:27, 1969.
72. Hargrove RL, Hoyle JR, Boyes M, Beckett AH. Blood levels of local anesthetics following intravenous regional anesthesia. Acta Anesth Scand (Suppl) 36:115–120, 1969.
73. Miles DW, Clark DE, Whitwam JG. Site of action of "intravenous regional anaesthesia." J Neurol Neurosurg 27:574, 1964.
74. Knapp RB, Weinberg M. Distribution of radioactive local anesthetics following intravenous regional anesthesia. Acta Anaesth Scand (Suppl) 36:121, 1969.
75. Raj PP, Garcia CE, Burleson JW, Jenkins MT. The site of action

of intravenous regional anesthesia. Anesth Analg 51:776, 1972.
76. Cotev S, Robin GC. Experimental studies of intravenous regional anaesthesia using radioactive lignocaine. Br J Anaesth 38:936, 1966.
77. Fleming SA, Veiga-Pires JA, McCutcheon RM, Emanuel CI. A demonstration of the site of action of intravenous lignocaine. Can Anaesth Soc J 13:21, 1966.
78. Eksted J, Stalberg E, Thorn-Alquist A. Impulse transmission to muscle fibres during intravenous regional anaesthesia in man. Acta Anesth Scand 15:1, 1971.
79. Harris WH. Choice of anesthetic agents for intravenous regional anesthesia. Acta Anesth Scand (Suppl) 36:47, 1969.
80. Cousins MJ, Mather LE. Clinical pharmacology of local anaesthetics. Anaesth Intens Care 8:257, 1980.
81. Goold JE. Bupivacaine intravenous regional anaesthesia and resuscitation. Anaesthesia 39:612, 1984.
82. McKeown DW, Meiklejohn B, Scott DB. Bupivacaine and prilocaine in intravenous regional anaesthesia. Anaesthesia 39:150, 1984.
83. Hollingworth A, Wallace WA, Dabir R. Comparison of bupivacaine and prilocaine used in Bier's block—a double blind study. Injury 13:331, 1982.
84. Mckeown DW, Duggan J, Wildsmith JAW, et al. Which agent for intravenous regional anaesthesia? Lancet, 24 December:31, 1983.
85. Tryba M, Zens M, Hausmann E. Prolonged analgesia after cuff release following IV regional analgesia with prilocaine. Br J Anaesth 55:631, 1983.
86. Jorfeldt L, Lofstrom B, Pernow B, et al. The effect of local anaesthetics on the central circulation and respiration in man and dog. Acta Anesth Scand 12:153, 1968.
87. Moore DC, Mather LE, Bridenbaugh LD, et al. Bupivacaine (Marcaine): An evaluation of its tissue and systematic toxicity in humans. Acta Anaesth Scand 21:109, 1977.
88. Reynolds F. Bupivacaine intravenous anaesthesia and resuscitation. Anaesthesia 39:105, 1984.
89. Wheeler DM, Bradley EL, Woods WT. The electrophysiologic actions of lidocaine and bupivacaine in the isolated perfused canine heart. Anesthesiology 68:201, 1988.
90. Tucker GT, Boas RA. Pharmacokinetic aspects of intravenous regional anesthesia. Anesthesiology 34:538, 1971.
91. Brown BR. The site of action of intravenous regional anesthesia. Anesth Analg 51:786, 1972.
92. Bromage PR, Robson JG. Concentrations of lignocaine in the blood after intravenous, intramuscular, epidural, and endotracheal administration. Anaesthesia 16:461, 1961.
93. Lehman WL, Jones WW. Intravenous lidocaine for anesthesia in the lower extremity. J Bone Joint Surg 66A:1056, 1984.
94. Brown EM, McGiff JT, Malinowski RW. Intravenous regional anaesthesia (Bier block): Review of 20 years' experience. Can J Anaesth 36:307, 1989.
95. Bowes DN, Dalton MT. Personal communication.

Section VI

•

Gastrointestinal, Obstetric, and Renal Procedures

Chapter 39

•

James W. Davis, MD

Nasogastric Intubation

OUTLINE

I. Introduction

The history of nasogastric and duodenal tubes stretches back to the time of the Roman emperor Claudius, when various devices were used to induce vomiting at the end of a feast. In 1790, John Hunter devised an eel-skin tube covering a probang of whalebone for the delivery of "food and medicines" to the stomach. In the 1800s, these tubes were used for the evacuation of ingested poisons, and in 1867, Kussmaul introduced the use of the nasogastric (NG) tube in the treatment of gastric outlet obstruction from peptic ulcer disease.[1] Although the uses of evacuation, decompression, and delivery of nutrition and drugs are unchanged, the "simple" NG tube has evolved into an array of tubes with different lengths, calibers, pliability, and specialty purposes. This chapter describes the most widely used tubes and their indications, use, and complications.

II. Indications

A. General

Nasogastric tubes are primarily indicated for decompression of the stomach. Gastric dilatation is common after trauma and postoperatively; it occurs with sepsis, small bowel obstruction, or ileus and with upper gastrointestinal hemorrhage. This can lead to respiratory embarrassment and aspiration.[2] Additional indications include evacuation of clot and toxic or poisonous substances, nutritional supplementation, tamponade of bleeding esophageal and gastric varices, and treatment of hypothermia, where the NG tube can be used as a warming conduit.

As the indications for nasogastric intubation have expanded, the number of specialized tubes has increased. Many of these tubes, named for their inventor, have been developed, only to be replaced after a few years with a newer, slightly different (and differently named) successor. A complete listing of these tubes is next to impossible. Table 39–1 lists the most common types of tubes in each category, along with representative examples.

B. *Specific Tubes*

1. Nasogastric (Standard)

The Levin tube (Kaslow Pharmaseal) is a simple argyle tube designed to decompress the stomach and proximal small bowel primarily of gas and some liquid.[3] Because of its single lumen, gastric mucosa can occlude the suction orifice if the tube is placed on constant rather than intermittent suction. The Levin tube has largely been replaced with the salem sump type of tube (Sherwood Medical), with a second lumen.[4] This allows for intake of enough air to prevent the suction seal effect on the gastric wall (see Fig. 39–3D). If the sump becomes occluded (or iatrogenically plugged), this distinction between the salem sump and the Levin tubes is lost. It is commonly believed that the sump tubes are more effective than the single-lumen variety, but there is no scientific evidence to support this view.[4]

2. Nasogastric/Orogastric (Large Bore)

Ewald (Danol) and Lavacuator (Mallinkrodt Anesthesia Products) tubes are used to remove large particles (food, blood clot, poisons) from the stomach rapidly with gavage irrigation. They are used when the standard NG tube is of too small a caliber to function and are the tubes of "stomach pump" infamy.

3. Long Intestinal

Long intestinal tubes are usually placed in patients with partial small bowel obstruction, in an effort to decompress the distal small bowel. Their effectiveness is controversial, with some authors favoring their use to decrease frequency of surgery in partial small bowel obstructions and others noting complications from delayed necessary surgery because of the use of long intestinal tubes.[5–8] The distal balloon is filled with mercury and allowed to pass through the small bowel by peristalsis. The Baker tube is another long intestinal tube; however, the balloon is air or saline filled. This tube will not pass with gravity and peristalsis; it must be placed at laparotomy and advanced by the surgeon through the small intestine to the ileocecal valve.

Table 39–1 • Nasogastric Tube Types

General	Example	Indications
Nasogastric—standard	Levin, salem sump	Decompress gas, liquid (most commonly used)
Nasogastric/orogastric—large	Ewald, Lavacuator	Evacuation; clots, poisons
Long intestinal	Miller-Abbot/Cantor, Baker	Decompression small bowel, especially with partial small bowel obstruction
Nutrition	Keofeed, Panda tube Dobhof, Pedifeeding tube, Moss	Nutritional support, smaller caliber, less aspiration
Tamponade	Sengstaken-Blakemore, Minnesota, Linton	Upper gastrointestinal hemorrhage tamponade varices

4. Nutritional

Nutritional tubes are generally of small caliber and are therefore more comfortable to the patient and questionably decrease the risk of aspiration (see complications). The most common examples are the Keofeed (Corpak), Dobhoff (Biosearch Medical Products), and Panda (O'Brian Pharmaceuticals) (all with fine wire stylet) and the Pedi-feeding tube (Kaslow Pharmaseal). The Moss tube has lumina for gastric suction and simultaneous duodenal feeding[9] (Fig. 39–1).

5. Tamponade

Tamponade tubes are used for control of hemorrhage in patients with esophageal, and in some cases gastric, variceal hemorrhage. The diagnosis of bleeding varices should be confirmed endoscopically before the tube is inserted and the balloon inflated to tamponade the bleeding site. The use of this type of tube has decreased with the advent of endoscopic variceal sclerotherapy. Examples include the Sengstaken-Blakemore (National Catheter), Linton (Danol), and Minnesota (Danol) tubes (see Fig. 39–14).

III. How to Insert Nasogastric Tubes

A. *General*

The placement of an NG tube is usually straightforward, but at times it may be extremely difficult. Inspect the nares to detect obstruction or asymmetry before starting the procedure (Fig. 39–2). The naris that is largest or that the patient can breathe through most easily (unilateral sniff test) should be used. If the patient is a trauma victim, a careful examination for midface fractures is essential. If present these patients should have *orogastric,* not nasogastric, tubes. The tube should be lubricated with a water-soluble agent. It is then gently advanced along the floor of the nasal cavity in a directly posterior (not superior) direction (Fig. 39–3A). Any resistance encountered in the posterior pharynx

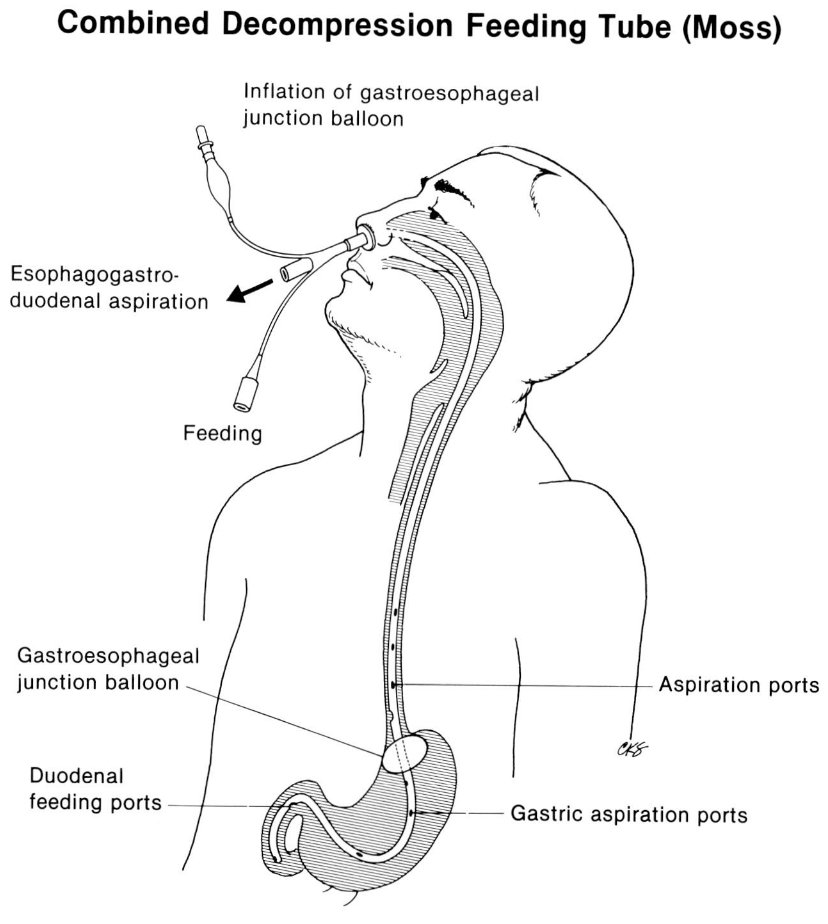

Figure 39–1 • Nasogastric (NG) intubation. The Moss decompression/feeding tube allows for esophagogastroduodenal suction and duodenal feeding (nutrition).

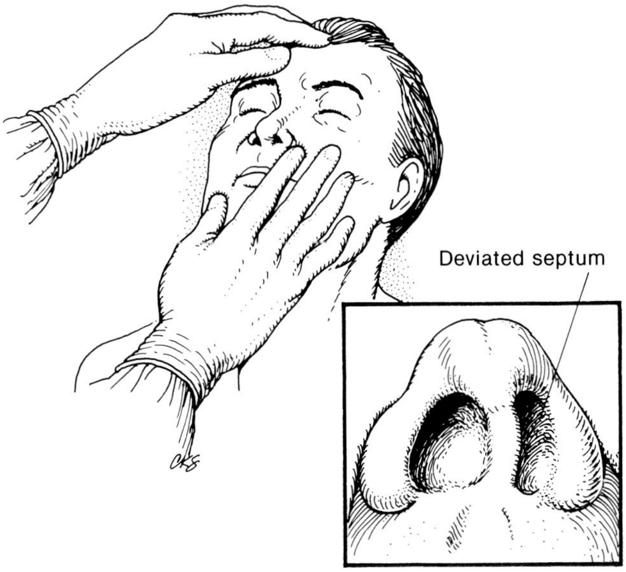

Figure 39–2 • Use the larger naris for tube insertion or check nostril patency with the unilateral sniff test.

should be overcome with firm but gentle pressure. If passage requires more effort than this, the tube may be curling or may be incorrectly located. Patients who are anxious or have an active gag response can be instructed to drink a small volume of water through a straw as the NG tube is being advanced from the pharynx (Fig. 39–3B). Additionally, the use of viscous lidocaine 2% as the lubricant and spraying the posterior pharynx with a topical agent (Cetacaine, tetracaine) may be helpful. In patients undergoing a general anesthetic, vasodilation is common and epistaxis may occur. This risk can be diminished by use of phenylephrine (Afrin) nasal spray. In patients who require gastric decompression during surgery, but not postoperatively, the tube should be placed orally and removed at the end of the procedure.

Advance the tube until it is in the stomach, as evidenced by the return of gastric contents with aspiration, and gurgling can be auscultated over the stomach with injection of air through the tube (Fig. 39–3C). This distance can be approximated before insertion by placing the tube tip at the patient's earlobe and extending the tube to the bridge of the nose and from there to the tip of the xiphoid process.[10] Note this distance on the tube by using a piece of tape or by using the marks on the Salem sump (at 46, 56, 66, and 76 cm from the tip of the tube [Fig. 39-3D]). The tube should be secured with adhesive or twill tape without any pressure placed on the columella of the nose or nostrils (Fig. 39–4). Alternative methods of securing NG tubes include tying a heavy suture around the tube where it exits the naris and taping the suture loosely to the bridge of the nose and to the forehead (Fig. 39–5)[11] or by using the circle tie method. With the circle tie method, the tube is passed in the usual manner and the position is confirmed. A gloved finger is then inserted into the pharynx and is hooked around the tube; a loop of tube is then brought out. An umbilical tape or heavy suture is tied to the loop (usually near the 46-cm mark on the salem sump or Levin tube) and the loop of NG tube is replaced in the posterior pharynx. The free end of the umbilical tape is then tied to the NG tube below the nares (Fig. 39–6A–D).[12]

In patients with endotracheal tubes in place, a number of maneuvers may be necessary to advance the NG tube beyond the cuff of the endotracheal tube (Fig. 39–7A). The simplest of these is to firmly grasp the thyroid cartilage and pull it anteriorly, away from the esophagus (Fig. 39–7B).[13] As the trachea is pulled anteriorly, the NG tube is advanced and can usually be felt to slide by the previous area of resistance. It may be necessary to partially deflate the cuff of the endotracheal tube as well. If these techniques are unsuccessful, a laryngoscope is inserted into the oropharynx to confirm the position of the NG tube in the posterior pharynx and possibly to visualize the esophageal opening. It is

(Text continued on p. 829)

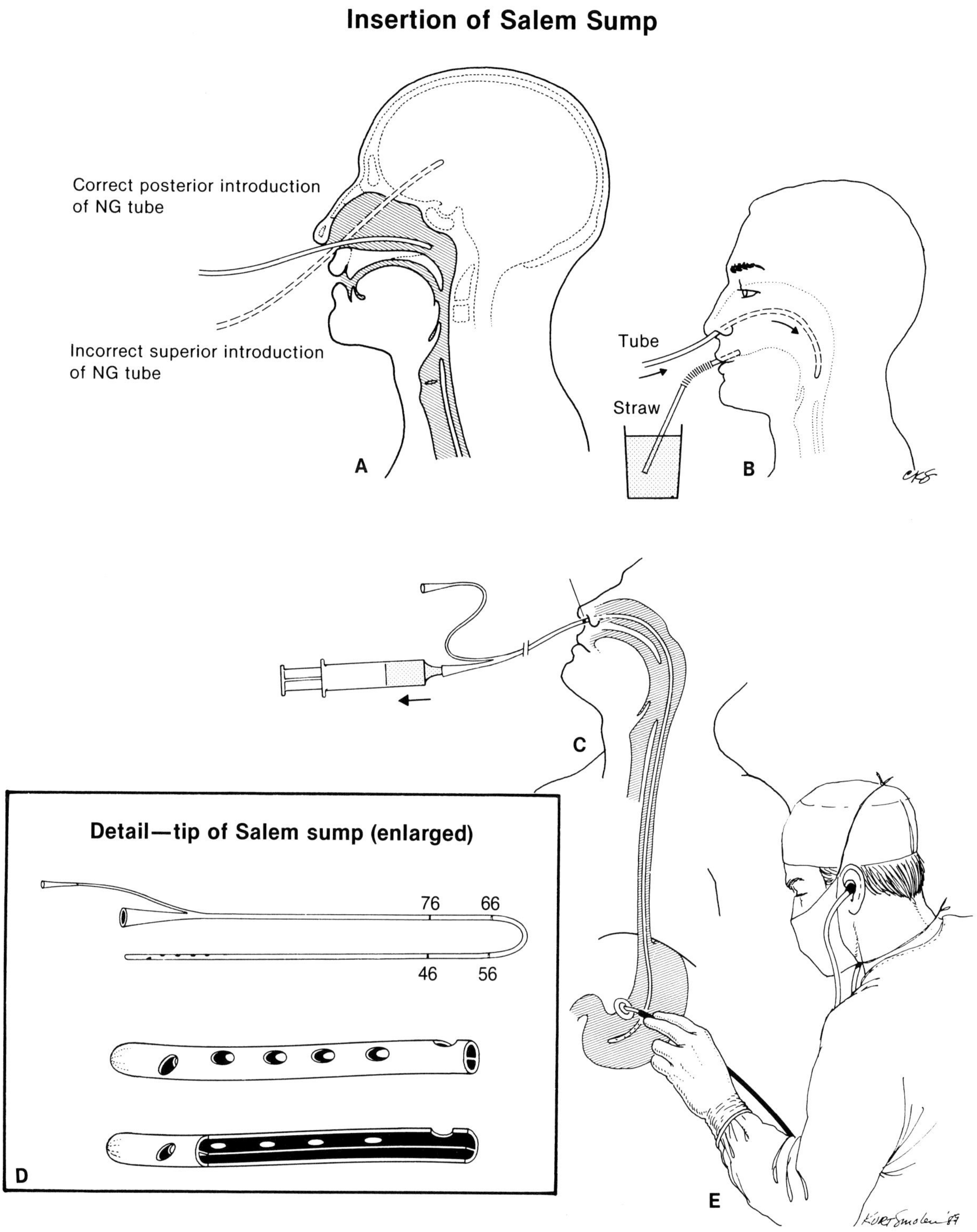

Figure 39–3 • (***A***) Advance the salem sump in a posterior, not superior, direction. (***B***) The patient can drink through a straw to make NG insertion easier. (***C,E***) With the Salem sump in place, aspirate stomach contents and auscultate for gurgling over the epigastrium with injection of air into the tube to confirm position. (***D***) Salem sump with suction and sump ports. The small intraluminal sump port prevents mucosa from being drawn into the suction ports. Black rings mark the distance from the distal tip of the tube.

Simple Tape Fixation of NG Tube

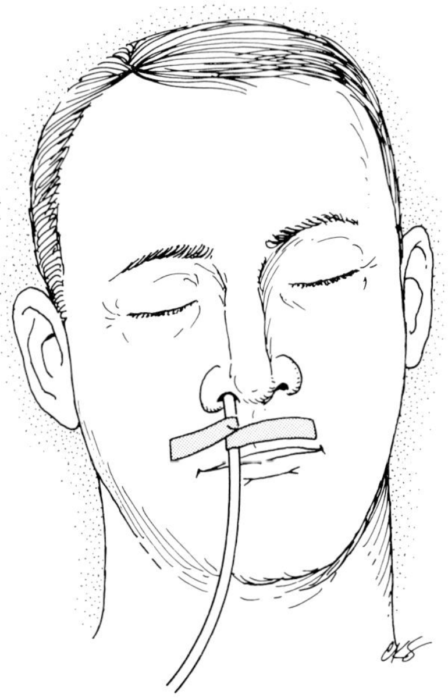

Figure 39-4 • NG tube secured to the upper lip with tape.

Suture and Tape Fixation of NG Tube

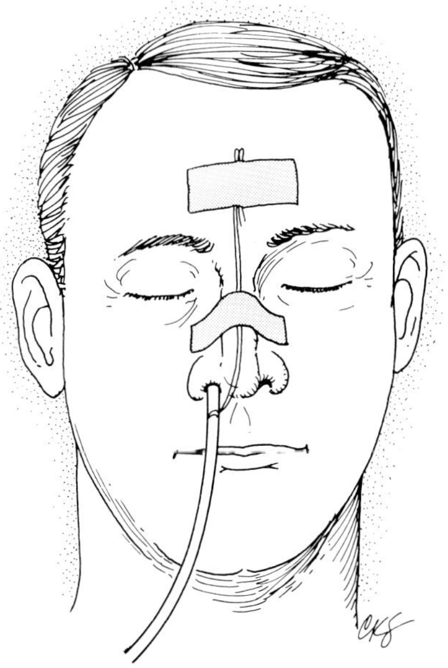

Figure 39-5 • Alternative method of securing an NG tube by tying heavy suture to it and taping the suture to the nose and forehead.

Circle Tie Method

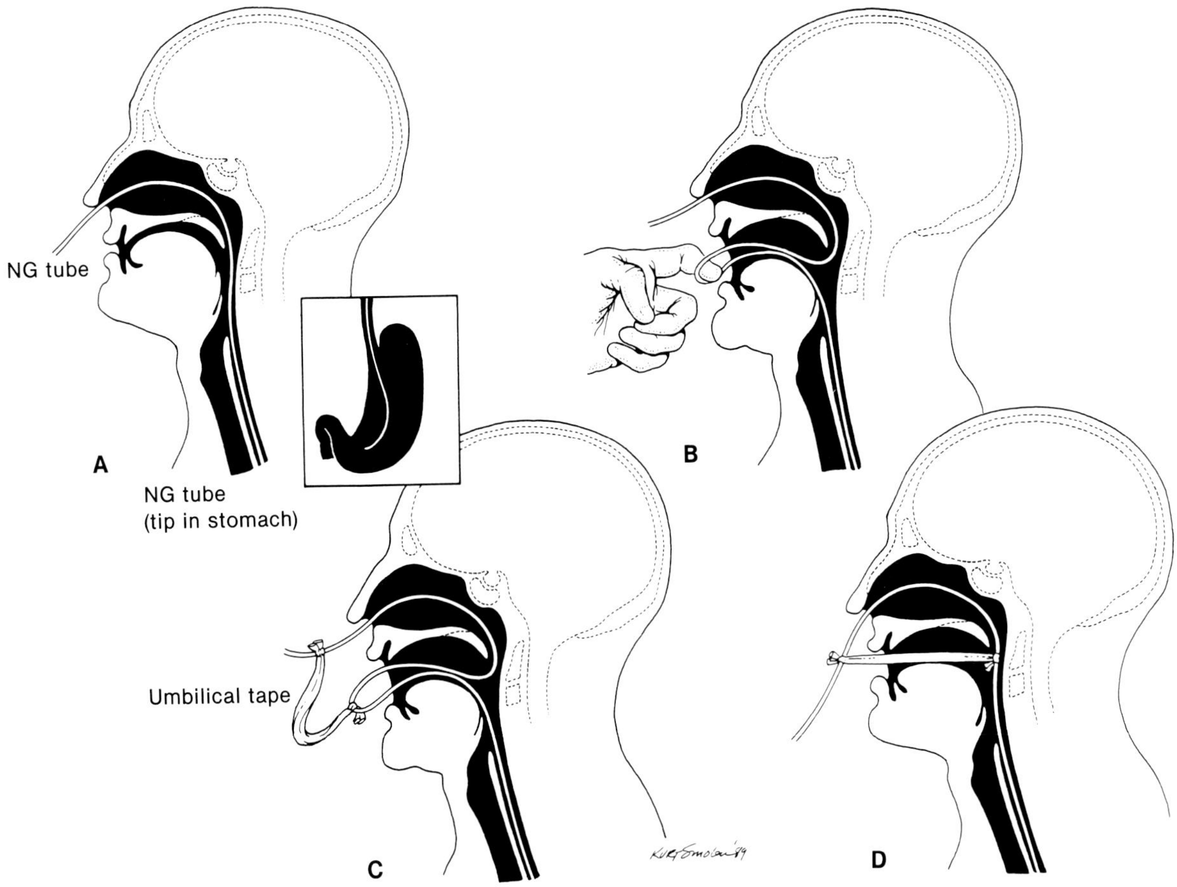

Figure 39-6 • The circle tie method of securing NG tubes. (***A***) The tube is advanced into position. (***B***) A gloved finger is inserted into the mouth and hooked around the tube, pulling a loop out. (***C***) An umbilical tape is tied to the NG tube at the nares and the loop coming from the mouth. (***D***) The tube is repositioned.

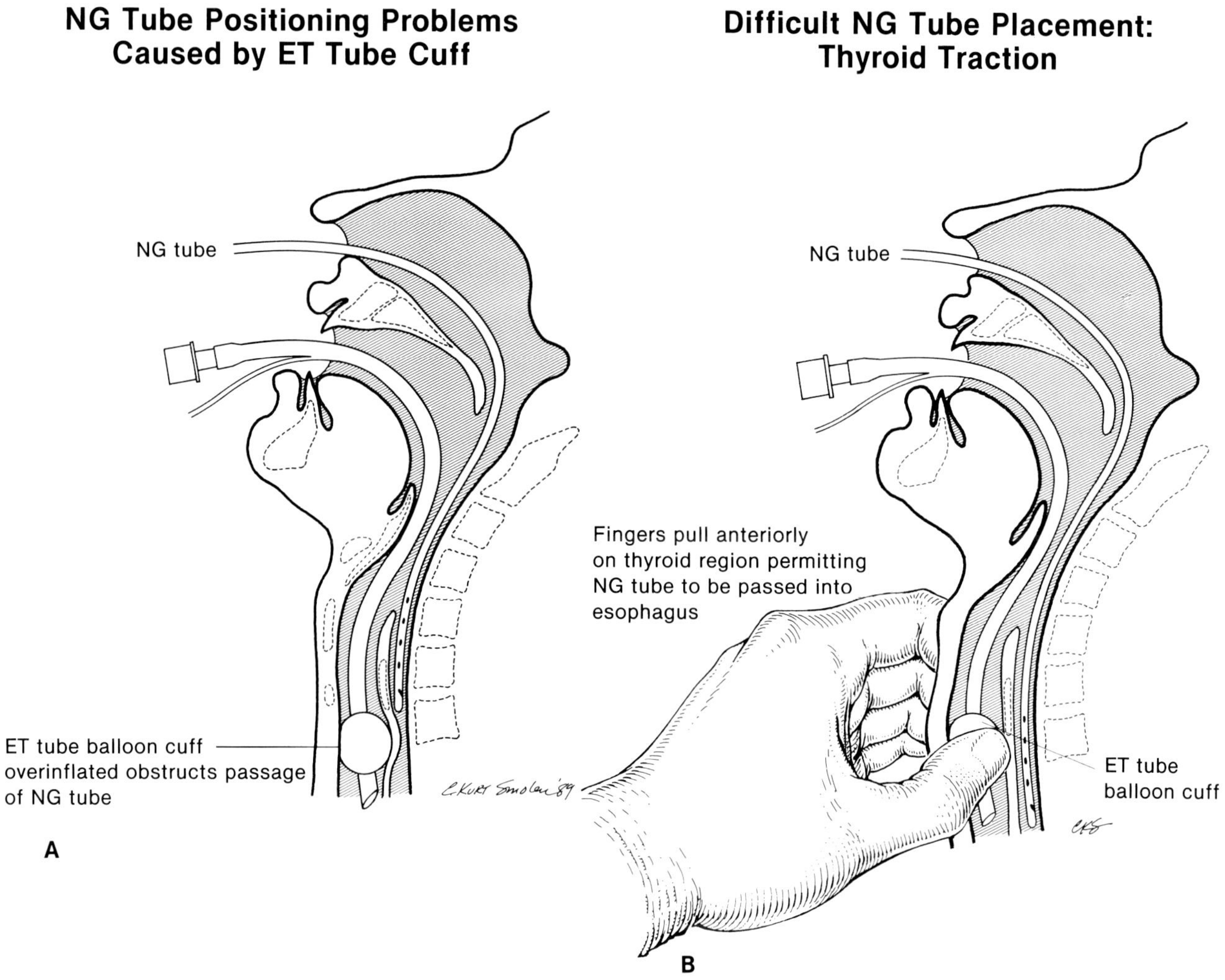

Figure 39–7 • (*A*) In intubated patients, the esophagus may be occluded by an overinflated endotracheal (ET) tube cuff and interfere with NG tube passage. (*B*) The NG tube can be passed by grasping the thyroid cartilage and pulling the trachea anteriorly while advancing the NG tube.

not necessary to view the larynx and cords (Figs. 6–5D and 6–9A). When this is accomplished, the NG tube can be passed into the esophagus under direct vision using McGill forceps (Fig. 39–8). Alternatively, the NG tube can be passed inside a ''split'' endotracheal tube that is then peeled away (Fig. 39–9).[14]

B. *Specialty Tubes*

1. Large Nasogastric/Orogastric

The larger caliber of the large nasogastric/orogastric tube increases patient discomfort (Fig. 39–10). The tube is placed in the same manner as the standard NG tubes. However, adequate lubrication is a must and a phenylephrine nasal spray (Afrin) should be used prior to nasal insertion. In smaller patients and children, it may be necessary to pass this tube via the oral route. A bite block may be necessary in an awake patient for oral insertion.

2. Long Intestinal

The balloon on a long intestinal tube is generally a soft latex one and is not inflated prior to insertion. It is then advanced into the stomach as previously described (Fig. 39–11A–D). Once the tube is in the stomach, the balloon is inflated with 5 mL of mercury (see Fig. 39–11D). The patient is placed in a right lateral decubitus position with the foot of the bed elevated for up to 2 hours to facilitate the passage of the balloon through the pylorus (Fig. 39–11E). After the balloon has passed through the pylorus (confirmed by plain abdominal radiograph), the

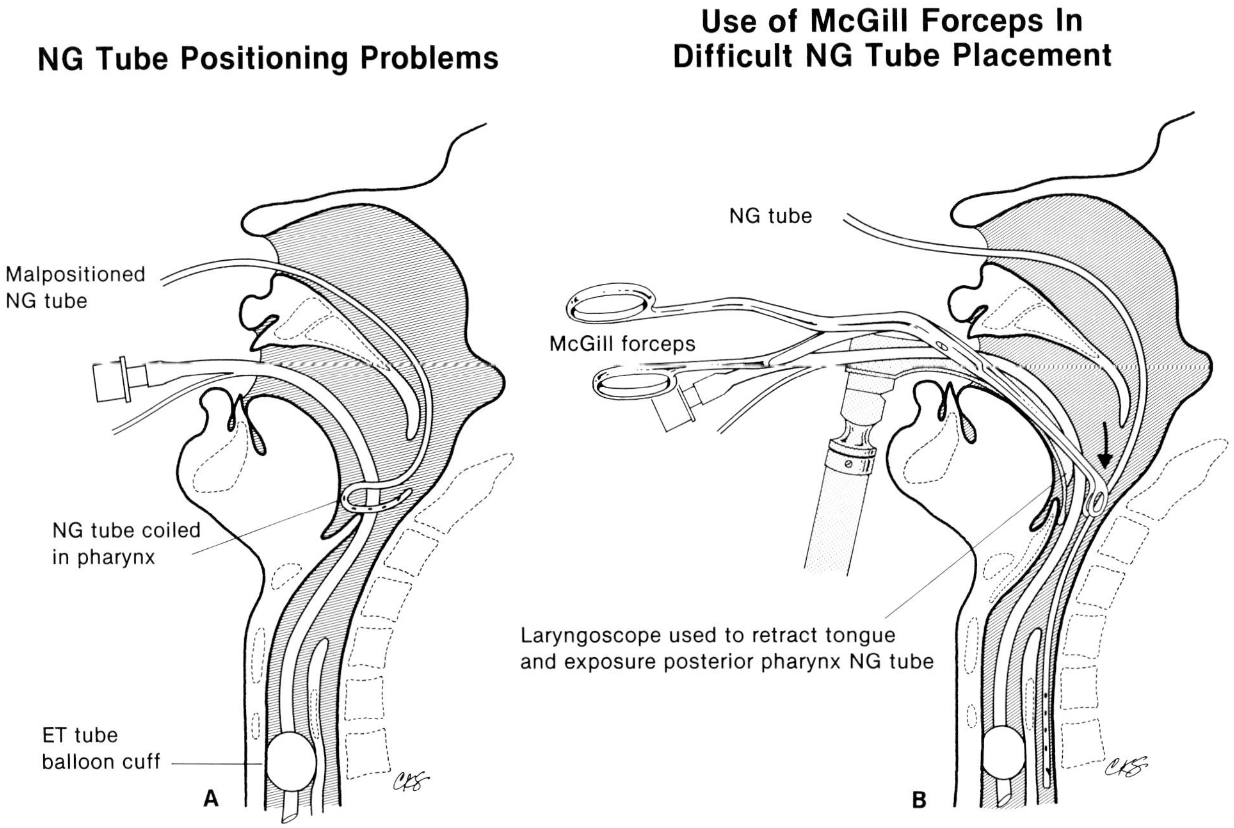

Figure 39–8 • (***A***) The NG tube is coiled in the oropharynx. (***B***) The McGill forceps can be used to advance the NG tube under direct vision.

patient should "swallow" (spontaneously advance) 15 cm of tube every 30–60 minutes (Fig. 39–11F). If faster advancement is desired or if there is difficulty in passing the tube through the pylorus, the procedure can be carried out under fluoroscopy.[15] The tube should be kept well lubricated at the nares until it has reached the correct site in the small intestine (area of obstruction or maximum dilatation on plain film) and then taped or tied in position at this depth of insertion. The tube should be kept on low intermittent suction during the entire time it is being advanced. The lumen of the long intestinal tube should be irrigated with 30–50 mL of saline every 6–8 hours to maintain patency.

3. Nutritional

The Keofeed, Dobhoff, and Panda tubes have an internal wire stylet making them stiffer and, despite their small size, passed with the same facility as the standard NG tube (Fig. 39–12). The pediatric-sized, or pedifeeding, tubes lack this stylet and may be more difficult to pass because of their pliability. The straight end of a long "J" guide wire (for intravascular catheters) can be used as a stylet for these tubes. The pedifeeding tube can also be passed by attaching it to a standard NG tube with half of a dissolvable gelatin capsule at the distal end (Fig. 39–13A). The combined tubes are then passed (Fig. 39–13B) and the NG tube is removed after 20 or 30 minutes (after the retaining gelatin capsule cap has dissolved) and the feeding tube remains in the stomach. An alternative but mechanically similar method involves cementing the fingertip of an exam glove to an esophageal stethoscope and placing the feeding tube in the manufactured "cuff." This assembly is then passed into the stomach. Once in place in the stomach, the esophageal stethoscope is advanced while the feeding tube is held. The stethoscope is then turned 180°, freeing the cuff from the tip of the feeding tube, and the esophageal stethoscope is then carefully removed.[16]

4. Tamponade

The Minnesota tube is a four-lumen tube, with separate gastric and esophageal aspiration ports, and separate in-

(Text continued on p. 835)

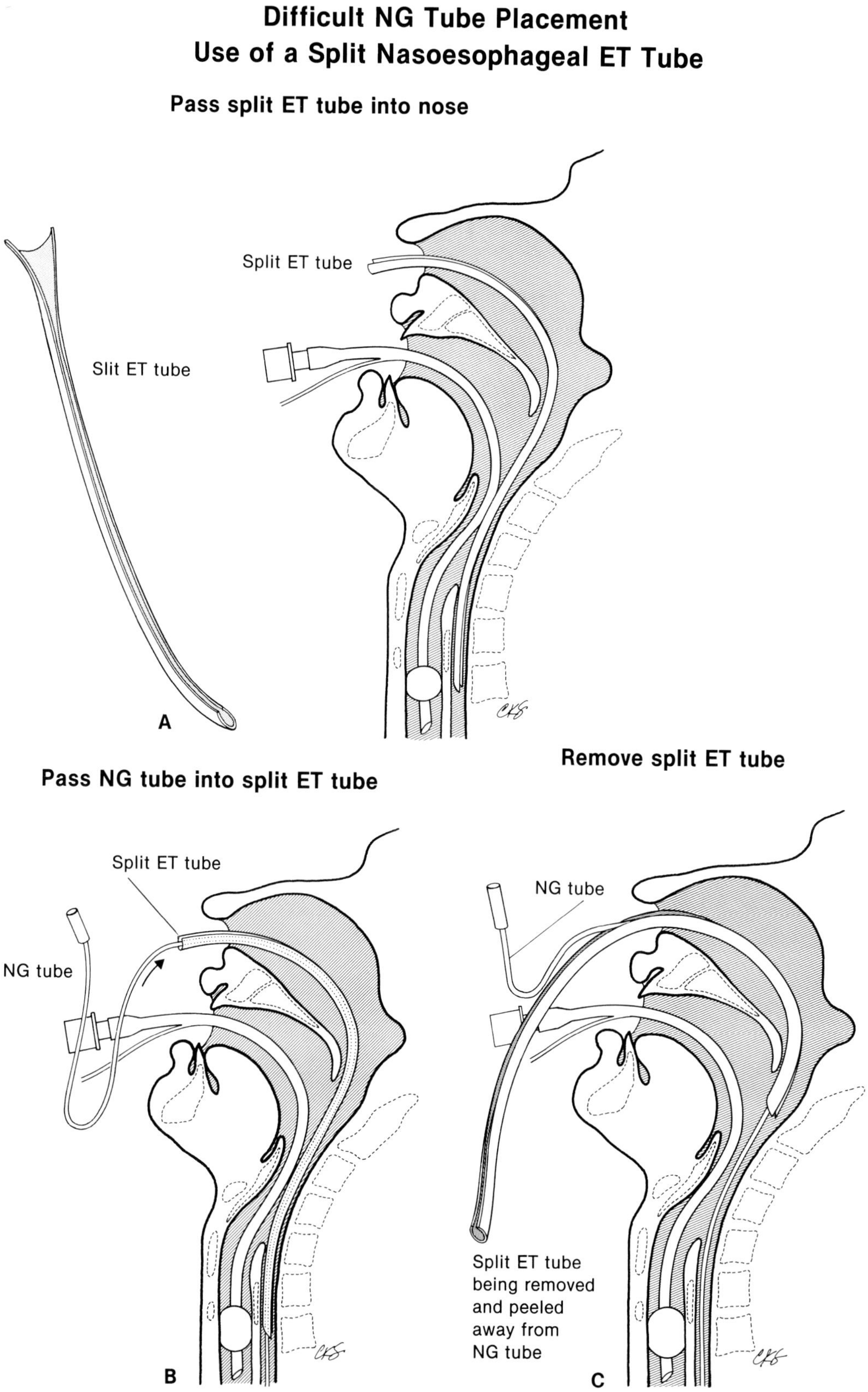

Figure 39–9 • (*A*) An ET tube can be slit longitudinally and passed nasoesophageally. (*B*) A well-lubricated NG tube is then passed through the split ET tube. (*C*) The split ET tube is then peeled away from the NG tube as the ET tube is being removed.

Large Evacuation Tube (Ewald)

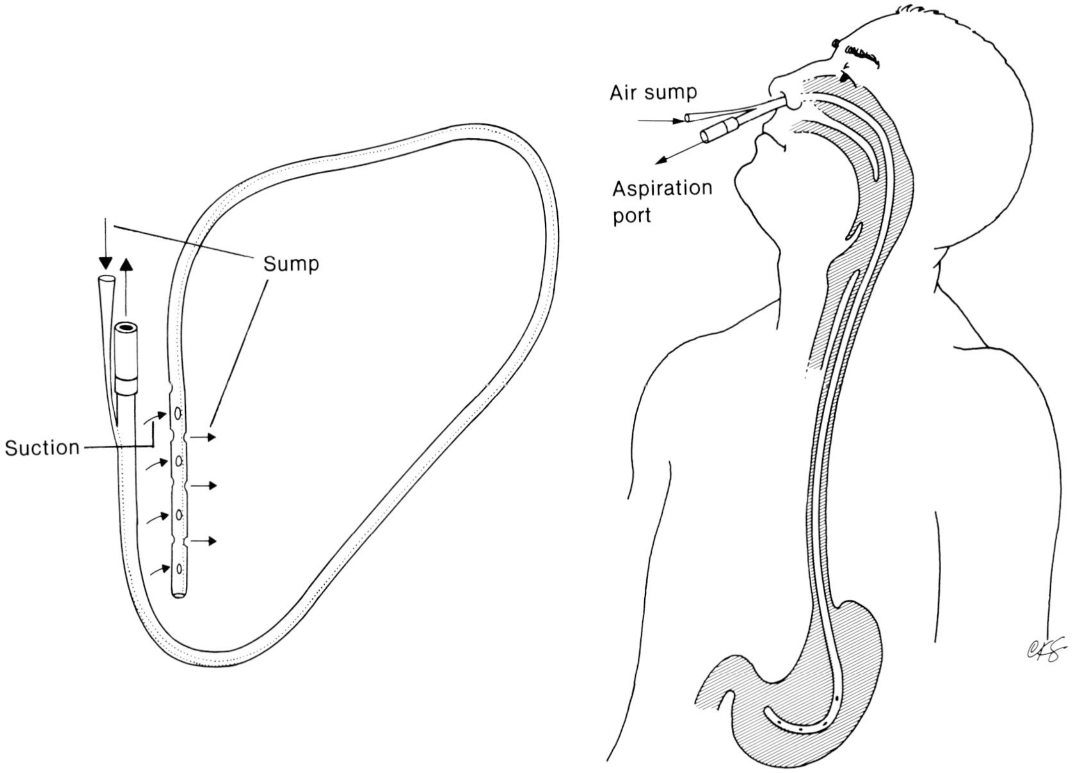

Figure 39–10 • Large evacuation tube (Ewald) with sump and aspiration ports. The sump and suction ports function as in a salem sump tube.

Insertion of Long Intestinal Tube (Miller-Abbot)

Hold tube at distal end to pass into nares

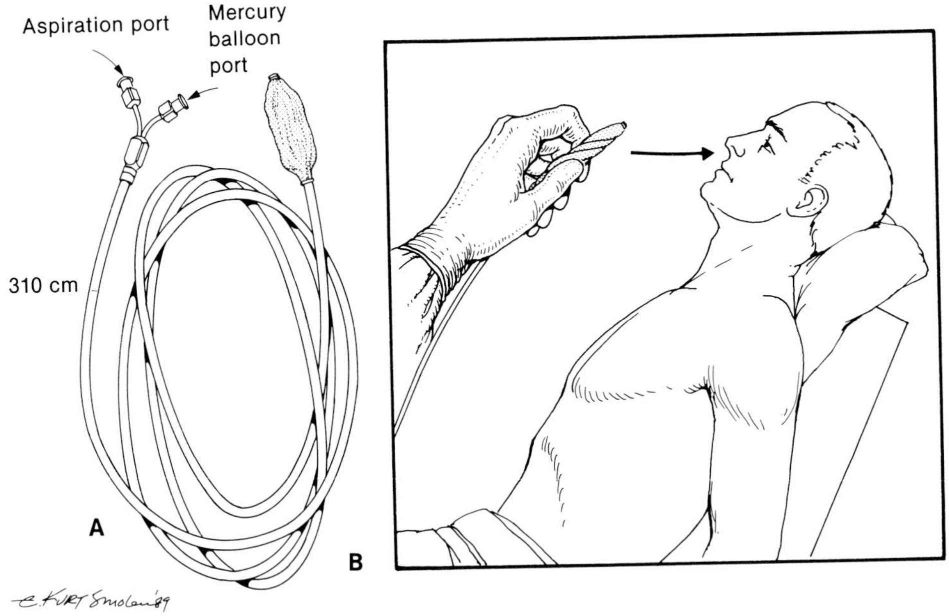

Figure 39–11 • (***A***) Long intestinal tube is shown with aspiration and mercury balloon inflation ports. (***B***) The patient is placed in a semiupright position and the tube held at the distal end.

(continued)

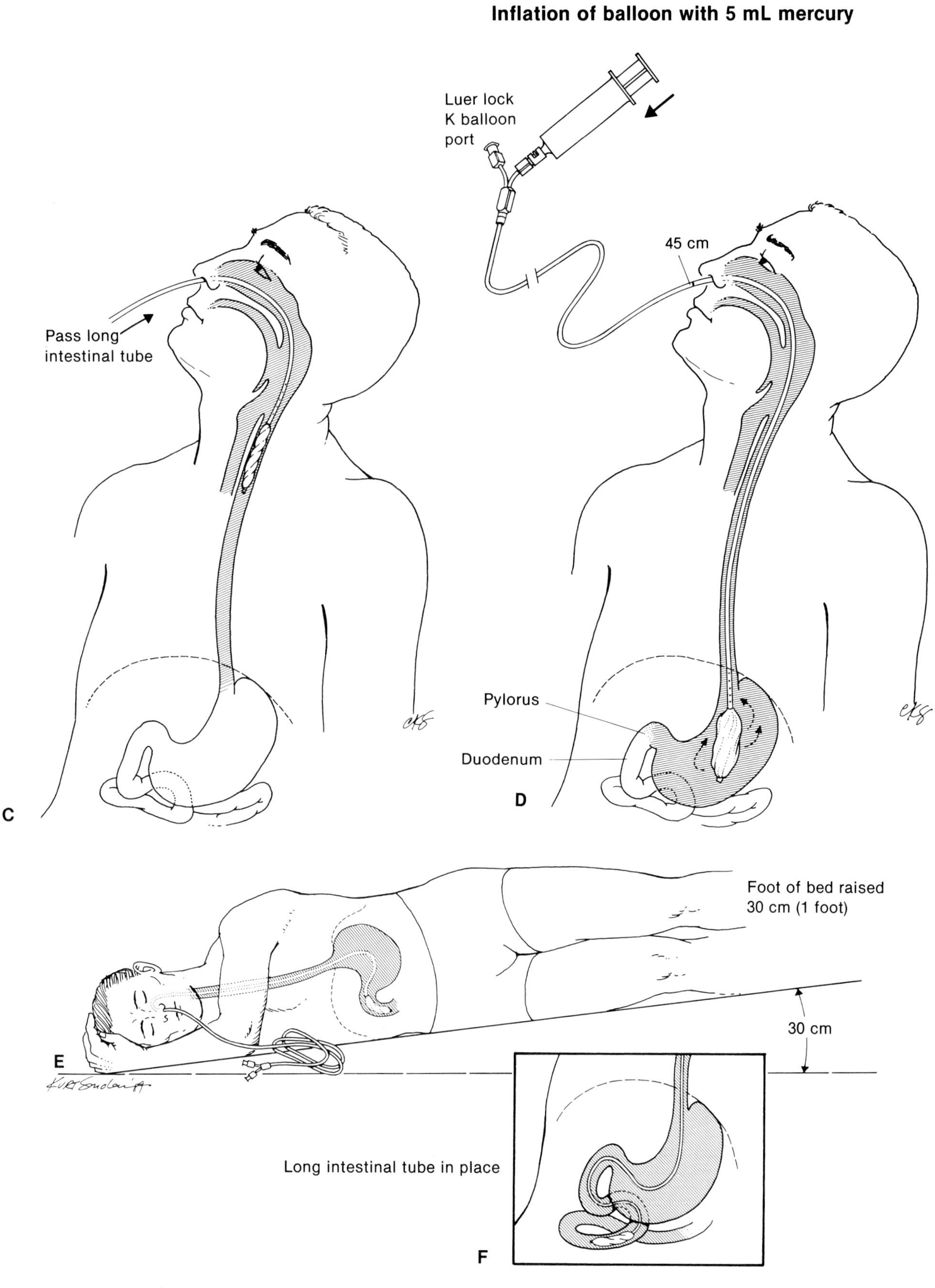

Figure 39–11 *(continued)*
(***C***) The well-lubricated tube is inserted. (***D***) When the 45-cm mark is reached and position in the stomach confirmed, the balloon is inflated with 5 mL of mercury. (***E***) The patient is placed in the right lateral decubitus position to facilitate passage of the tip past the pylorus. (***F***) The tube is advanced 15 cm every 30 to 60 minutes until reaching the desired area as confirmed with fluoroscopy or plain radiograph. The tube is then secured in this position.

Stylet-Type Feeding Tube

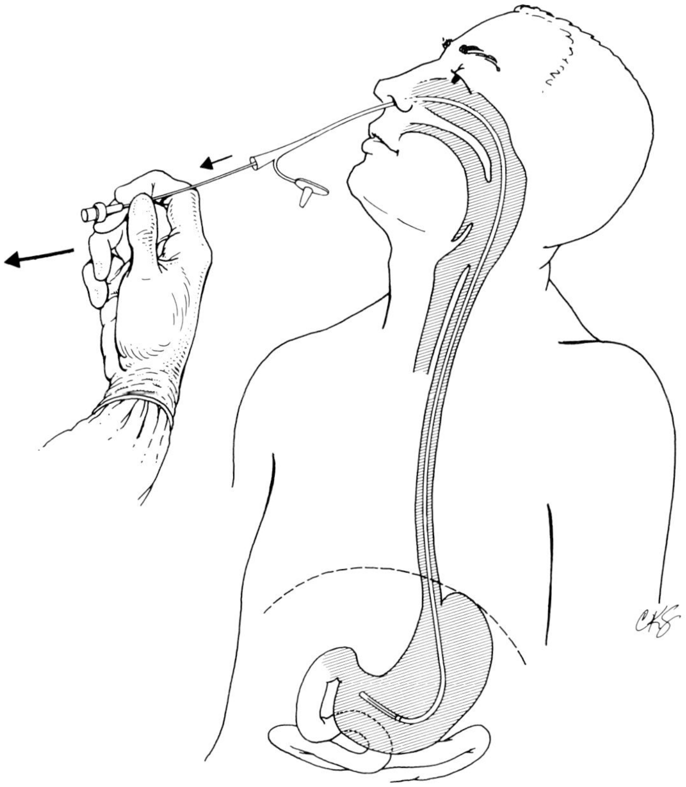

Figure 39–12 • The stylet-type feeding tube is advanced into the stomach or duodenum, its position confirmed radiographically, and the stylet removed.

Insertion of Nonstylet (Pediatric) Feeding Tube

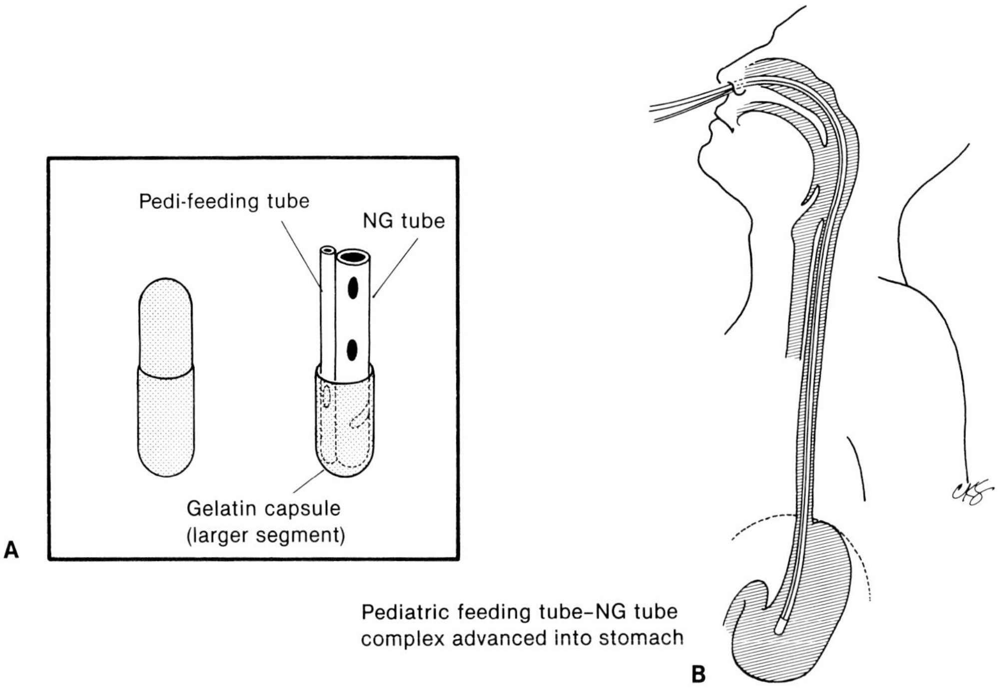

Figure 39–13 • (***A***) The larger segment of a gelatin capsule is used to hold the ends of a regular NG tube and a pediatric feeding tube together. (***B***) The NG/pediatric tube complex is then advanced into the stomach. After 20 to 30 minutes the capsule dissolves and the NG tube is removed, leaving the smaller tube in place for feedings.

flation and pressure monitoring ports for both the gastric and esophageal balloons (Fig. 39–14A). Before the tube is inserted, the balloons should be carefully checked for leaks and the gastric balloon sequentially inflated with 100, 200, 300, 400, and 500 mL of air, with balloon pressures being measured at each inflation. Both balloons are then aspirated completely flat and clamped prior to insertion. The tube and balloons should be thoroughly lubricated to decrease the trauma to tube, balloons, and patient.

The patient should have gavage and emptying of the stomach with a salem sump and the head of the bed elevated 45°. The Minnesota tube is advanced to the 50-cm mark, indicating that the tube tip is in the stomach (Fig. 39–14B). This should be confirmed fluoroscopically before continuing. Aspiration of gastric contents from the gastric port is done at this time to assure tube placement and decrease regurgitation. The esophageal aspiration port is likewise placed to suction. The gastric balloon pressure monitor is then connected to a mercury manometer and the gastric balloon inflated with 100-mL increments of air to a total of 400–500 mL (Fig. 39–14C). At each inflation increment the gastric balloon pressure is checked. If the balloon pressure with the tube in place is more than 15 mmHg greater than the pressure at equal volumes before insertion, it indicates that the gastric balloon is intraesophageal (Fig. 39–14D). Further inflation of the gastric balloon at this point could cause esophageal rupture. The balloon should be deflated, the tube advanced, and the process of inflation restarted. Once the balloon has been placed in the stomach and inflated to 400–500 mL, the gastric balloon inflation and pressure monitoring ports are clamped (or may be ligated with silk suture). The tube is then gently pulled back until resistance (from the balloon at the gastroesophageal junction and diaphragm) is met. The tube is then secured with a nasal guard of sponge rubber as the tube exits the naris. The nasal guard is taped to the Minnesota tube. The stomach and esophageal lumina are aspirated. If blood is continually aspirated from the esophageal lumen, the esophageal balloon is inflated to a pressure of 35–45 mmHg (Fig. 39–14E–F) to control the esophageal variceal hemorrhage. If the bleeding is from a gastric varix, traction will need to be maintained on the tube for tamponade by the gastric balloon. Such traction can cause ulceration of the nares within a few hours; external traction should therefore be employed for only a few hours or the tube must be attached to an external frame device. The gastric aspiration lumen should be placed to intermittent suction (no-sump lumen) of 60–120 mmHg. The esophageal lumen should be on continuous suction at 120–2000 mmHg, to remove swallowed saliva and regurgitated blood.

Because continual balloon pressure of 25–35 mmHg may cause esophageal necrosis, the esophageal balloon should be maintained at the lowest pressure level necessary to stop bleeding and should be completely deflated for 5 minutes every 6 hours. Additionally, the pressure in the esophageal balloon should never exceed 45 mmHg. Once the bleeding has been stopped, with the esophageal balloon inflated to 25 mmHg, the balloon is left inflated at this level (except for the every-6-hour deflations) for at least 12 hours. The balloon is then deflated and the tube is left in place. If there is no recurrent hemorrhage after 4 hours, the tube is removed after complete deflation of all balloons (Fig. 39–14G). During this time the patient should be appropriately volume resuscitated and have any deficits in the coagulation cascade (fresh frozen plasma, platelets) corrected. The use of a tamponade tube for control of variceal hemorrhage is, at best, only a temporizing maneuver until the patient can be definitively treated with endoscopy and sclerotherapy or surgery with portasystemic shunting as needed.

IV. DISCUSSION

A. *Suction/Aspiration of Stomach Contents*

Tubes placed for decompression and evacuation of the stomach and upper gastrointestinal tract should be placed to suction and irrigated with 20–50 mL of saline as needed. Tubes with a sump port should be to continuous, not intermittent, suction, at 30–40 mmHg. The sump port should not be clamped or occluded. The sump port can be tested for patency by listening for the suction sound at its orifice. If the sump lumen is occluded, it should be irrigated with air until it is patent. Tubes without sump lumina should be placed to intermittent suction at 60–120 mmHg.

B. *Removal of NG Tubes*

Nasogastric tubes should remain in place for decompression until there is evidence that the ileus has resolved. The resumption of normal bowel sounds, decreased na-

(Text continued on p. 839)

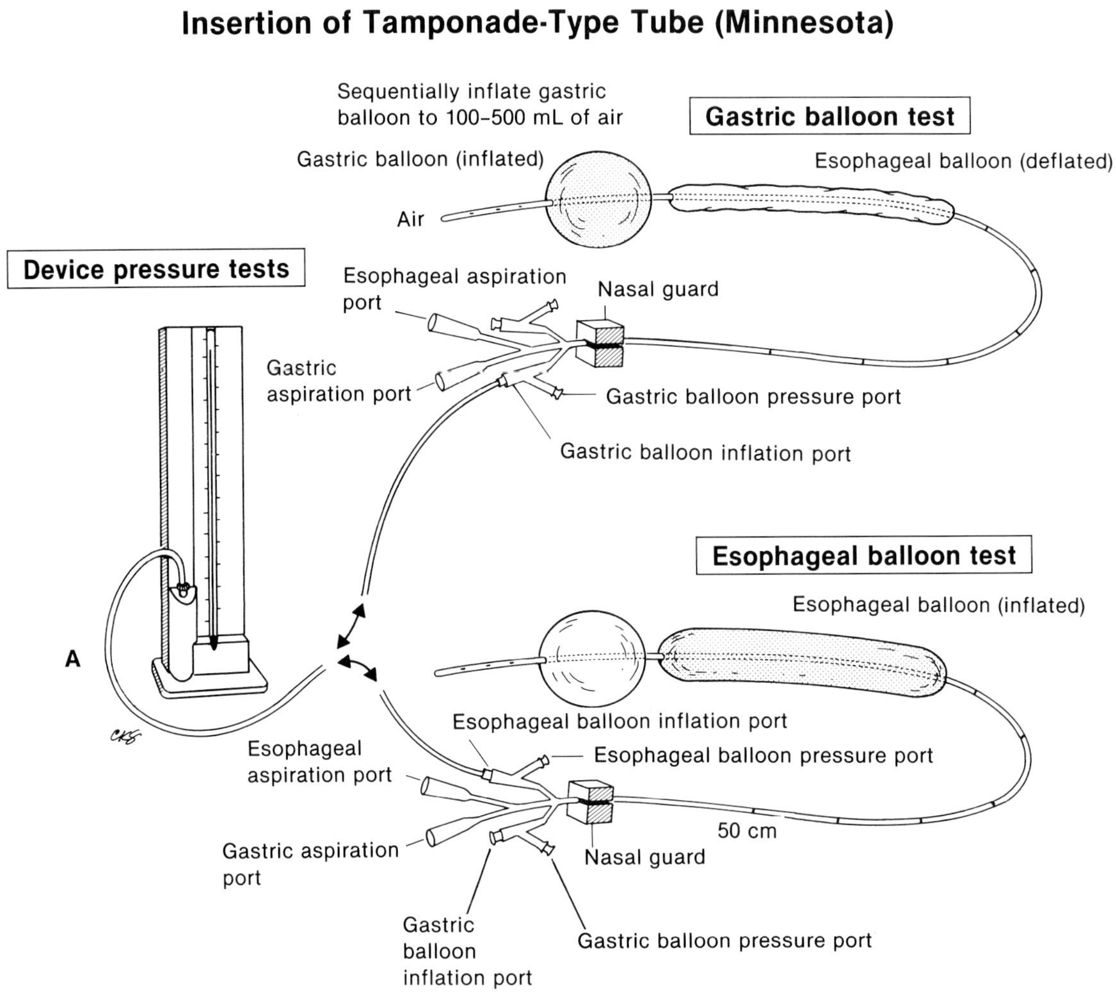

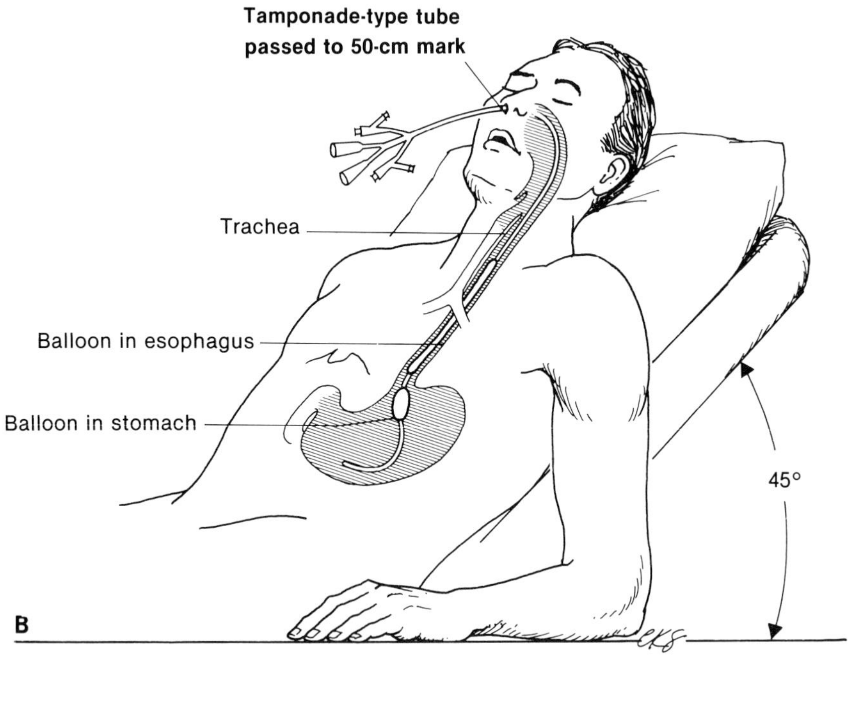

Figure 39–14 • (***A***) The four-lumen Minnesota tube should be tested prior to insertion. The gastric and esophageal balloons should be inflated sequentially to 500 mL of air in 100-mL increments and balloon pressure checked after each increment. (***B***) The tube is then passed to the 50-cm mark (with balloons deflated) and gastric position confirmed with auscultation and radiograph. Both the gastric and esophageal aspiration ports should be placed to suction.

(continued)

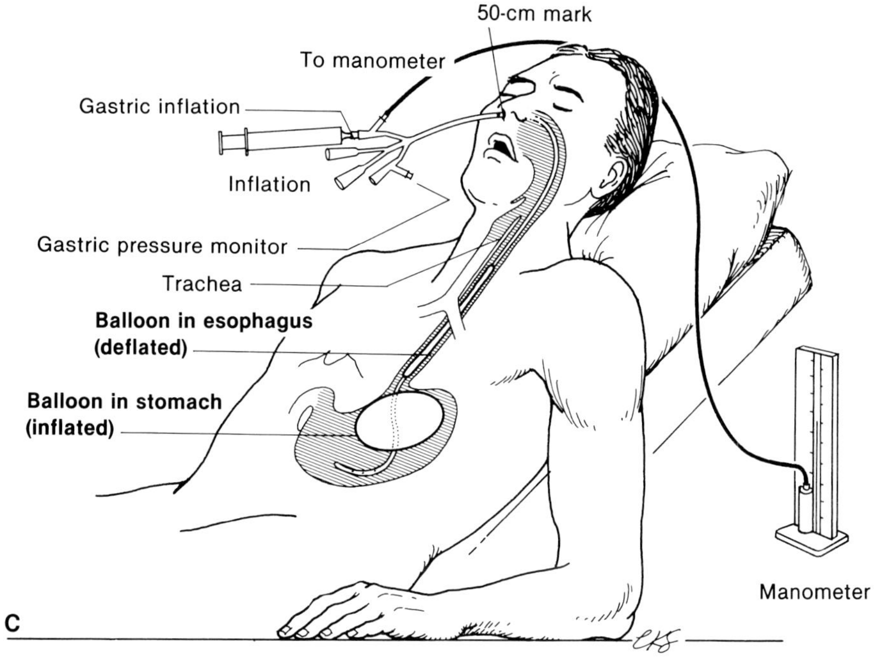

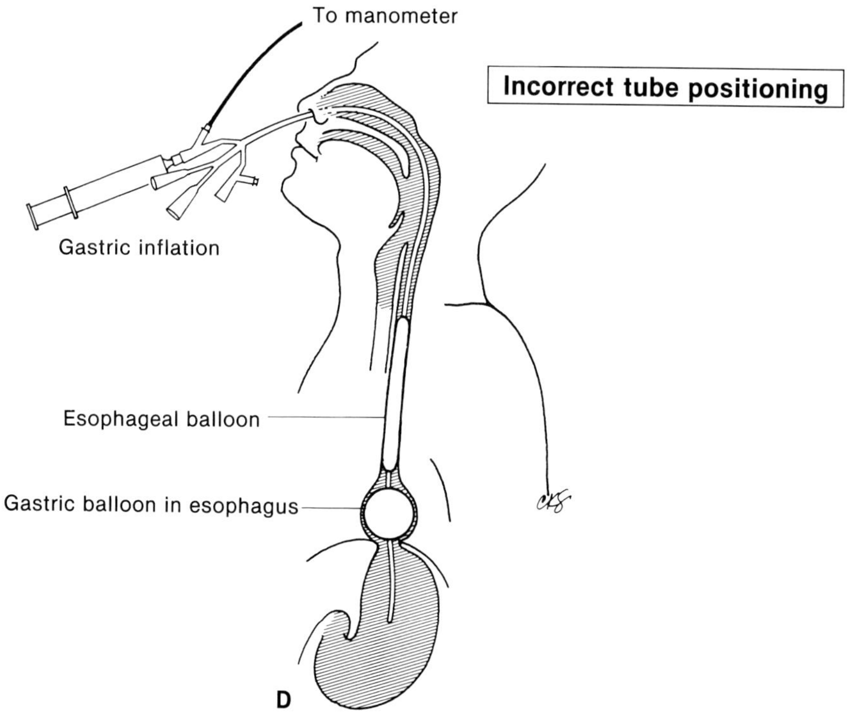

Figure 39–14 *(continued)*
(***C***) The gastric balloon is inflated sequentially to 400–500 mL with continuous balloon pressure monitoring. The tube is gently pulled back until resistance from the balloon is met at the gastroesophageal junction. The tube is then secured in position using the nasal guard and tape. (***D***) If the balloon pressure at any inflation volume is more than 15 mmHg greater than the pressure before tube insertion, it indicates intraesophageal location of the gastric balloon. Orientation of the tube is rotated 180° compared to (***C***)

(continued)

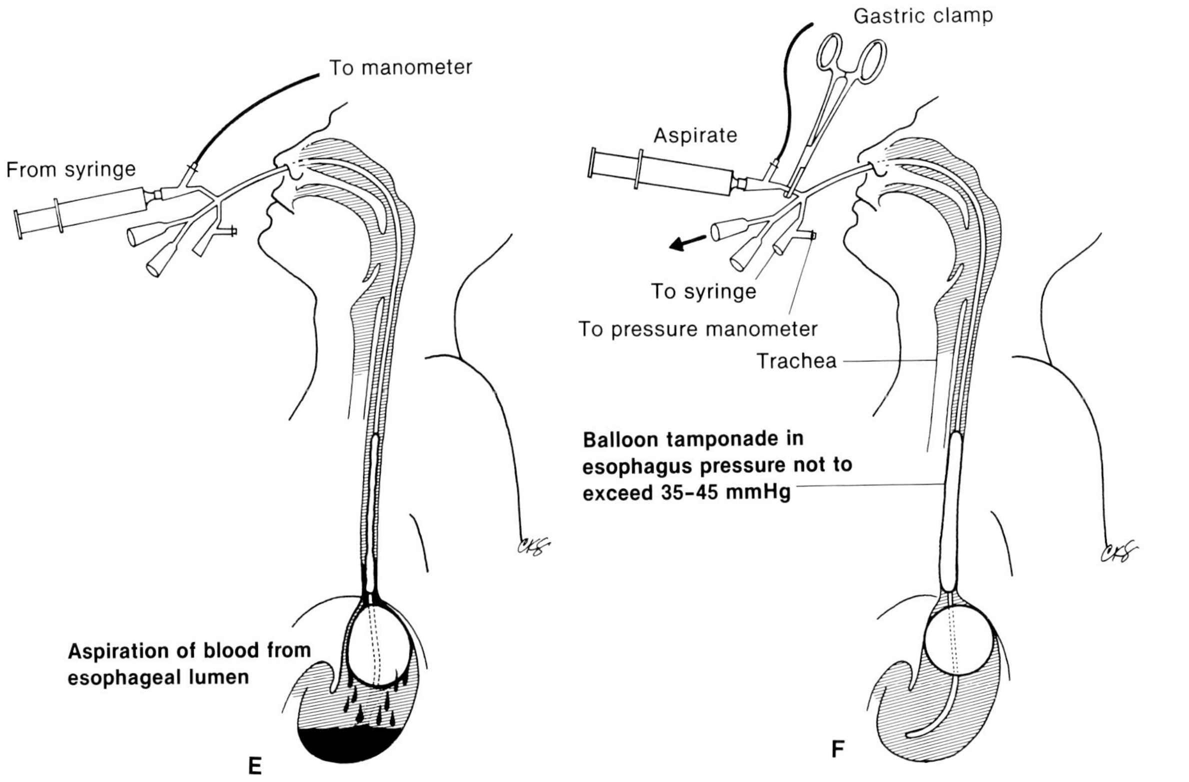

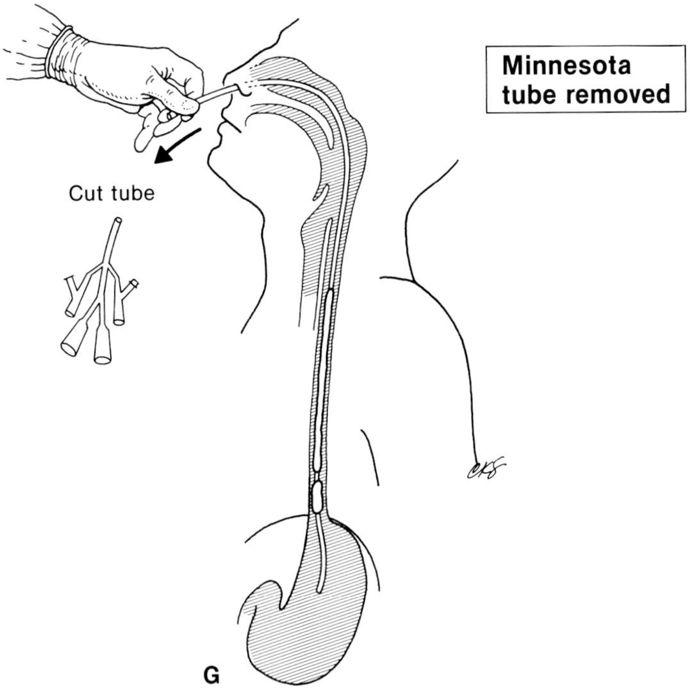

Figure 39–14 *(continued)*
(***E,F***) If blood is aspirated continually from the esophageal lumen, the esophageal balloon is inflated to 35–45 mmHg. (***G***) Deflate all balloons or cut the Minnesota tube prior to removal.

sogastric outputs (less than 400–500 mL/day), and passage of flatus and stool have been used singly and in combination as indications for NG tube removal. In patients where a long intestinal tube was necessary for decompression, a slower, more conservative approach is advocated. Once the decision to remove the tube is reached, the balloon port should be completely aspirated and the tube withdrawn 20–30 cm at a time. If the resistance increases markedly, the operator should pause for several seconds and then resume withdrawing the tube. When the 45-cm mark is reached on the long intestinal tube, the lumen is occluded, the patient is instructed not to breathe, and the tube is rapidly removed. There are no special instructions for removal of feeding or large-bore (Ewald) tubes. Recommendations for the removal of tamponade-type tubes (Minnesota) were previously described.

C. *Fluid and Electrolyte Balance*

Patients with NG tubes require careful monitoring of their fluid balance. Nasogastric and intestinal tube outputs are pathologic fluid losses. As such, they should be replaced on a ''milliliter-for-milliliter'' basis with appropriate intravenous fluids, usually 0.9% or 0.45% normal saline with dextrose and potassium (20–40 mEq/L). Failure to replenish these losses may result in a hypokalemic, hypochloremic metabolic alkalosis.

Intracranial NG Tube

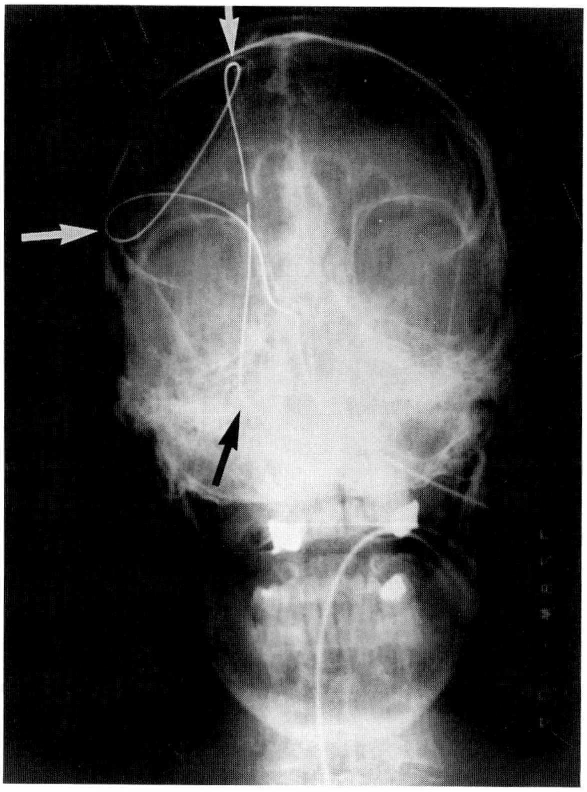

Figure 39–15 • Nasocranial intubation with NG tube (*arrow*). (Courtesy L.A. Shore, MD, Phoenix, AZ.)

V. COMPLICATIONS

Complications from insertion and use of nasogastric and enteric tubes cover a wide range of anatomic locations and severity. This section discusses the most common and most challenging complications.

A. *Head and Neck*

Perhaps the most dreaded complication of attempted NG tube placement is nasocranial intubation (Fig. 39–15).[17–20] This is associated with cribriform plate fractures, allowing the tube to pass cephalad instead of posteroinferiorly (Fig. 39–16). Trauma patients with midface fractures or severe maxillofacial injuries should have these tubes placed via the oral route.

Epistaxis is a very common complication of attempted NG tube insertion. The use of phenylephrine (Afrin) nasal spray to constrict nasal tissues along with careful technique and adequate lubrication will usually prevent its occurrence. Other head and neck complications include gagging and vomiting with airway compromise (aspiration), sinusitis, and tracheal intubation with an NG tube. These are usually readily identified and corrected and do not usually cause major morbidity.[21] Additionally, long-term NG tubes have been associated with laryngeal injuries, including vocal cord paralysis[22] and cricoid chondritis.[23]

The details of securing the NG tube are frequently overlooked, leading to pressure on the nares or the nasal cartilage from the tape or ties. This can lead to pressure necrosis (Fig. 39–17). Corrective cosmetic surgery may be required. This complication can be prevented by securing the NG tube as described previously in this chapter (see Figs. 39–4 and 39–5), with tape to the upper lip (Fig. 39–18), or by a suture placed through the septum (Fig. 39–19).[24]

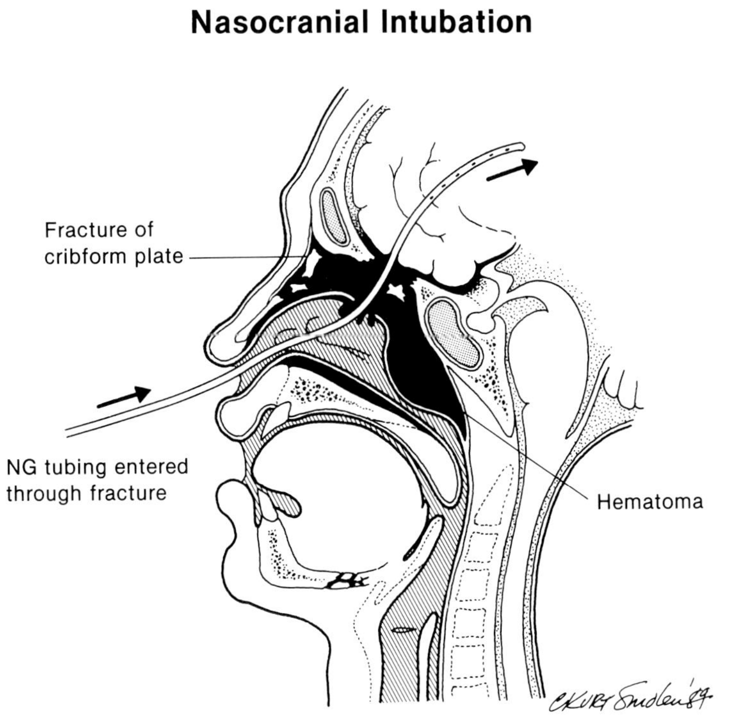

Figure 39–16 • Fracture of the cribriform plate allows nasocranial intubation in trauma patients.

B. *Tracheoesophageal*

Tracheoesophageal fistulas are rare complications of nasogastric intubation and may be associated with concurrent endotracheal intubation. The diagnosis should be suspected when there is evidence of pulmonary aspiration from the esophagus (tube feedings, wheezing, unexplained infiltrates, etc). Barium swallow under fluoroscopy, biplanar cineesophagography, or triple endoscopy provide confirmation of the diagnosis.[25] Initial management should include removal of the NG tube, with placement of a gastrostomy if necessary.[26] Definitive management of the tracheoesophageal fistula is beyond the scope of this text but is well described.[26,27]

Additionally, these tubes can perforate the esophagus (cervical or thoracic), the stomach or intestine, and, with tracheal intubation, the pulmonary parenchyma.[28,29] Perforation of the lung substance should be managed by removal of the tube. Serial chest radiographs should be obtained for diagnosis of delayed pneumothorax or hemothorax.[28,30]

Esophageal perforation in the cervical region requires operative exploration, possible closure, and appropriate drainage.[30] Thoracic esophageal perforation may be diagnosed on routine chest radiograph (Fig. 39–20), but definitive diagnosis requires a contrast study. In patients with small perforations and no local or systemic symptoms, conservative management may be attempted. The presence of pneumothorax or pneumomediastinum, sepsis, shock, or respiratory failure is an indication for operative intervention.[31,32] If the balloon tamponade tubes (Minnesota) are positioned improperly and the balloon inflated, the esophagus can be ruptured. This requires operative repair and possibly esophageal diversion, depending on time delay, contamination, and other factors.[32]

C. *Gastrointestinal*

The presence of an NG tube can cause local irritation, giving rise to ''tube gastritis.''[21] This is usually self-limiting but can go on to ulceration and hemorrhage. The treatment of this consists of standard ''ulcer'' therapy, with H-2 blockers, antacids, or gastric coating agents (sucralfate).

Nasogastric or nasoenteric tubes, if advanced under too much force, can perforate the stomach or small bowel. These injuries are managed with laparotomy, repair of the involved bowel, and irrigation of the perito-

Necrosis of Nasal Septum

Lateral view

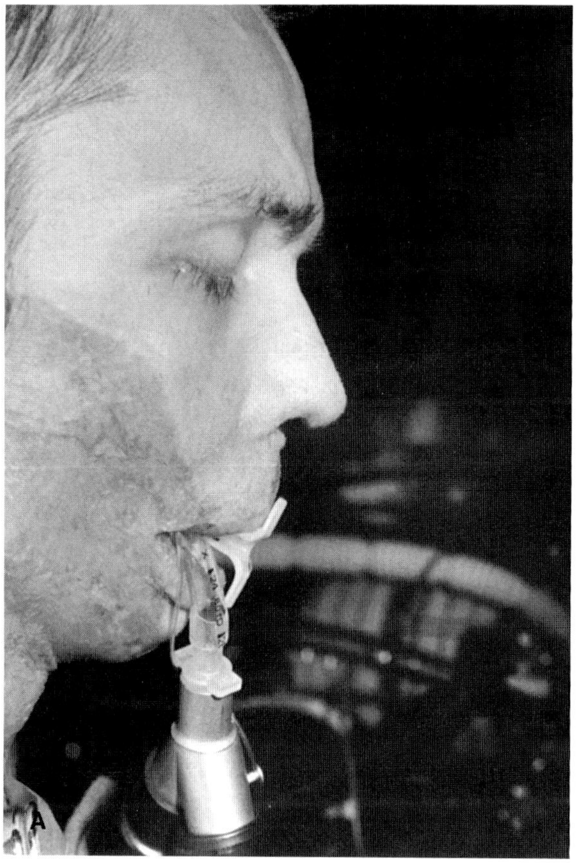

Frontal view

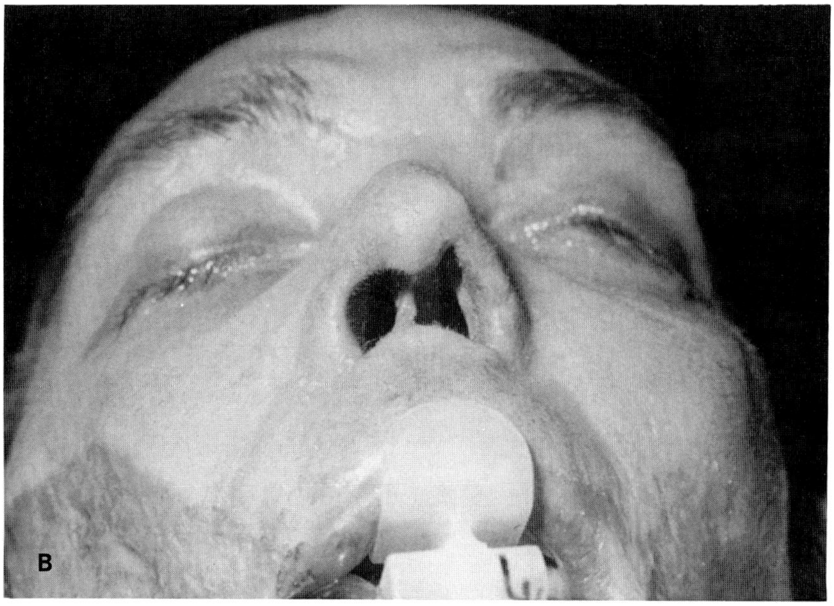

Figure 39–17 • Pressure necrosis of the nasal septum from an incorrectly secured NG tube. (***A***) Lateral view. (***B***) Frontal view. (Courtesy D.H. Frank, MD, University of California–San Diego Medical Center, San Diego, CA.)

NG and ET Tubes Tied Together

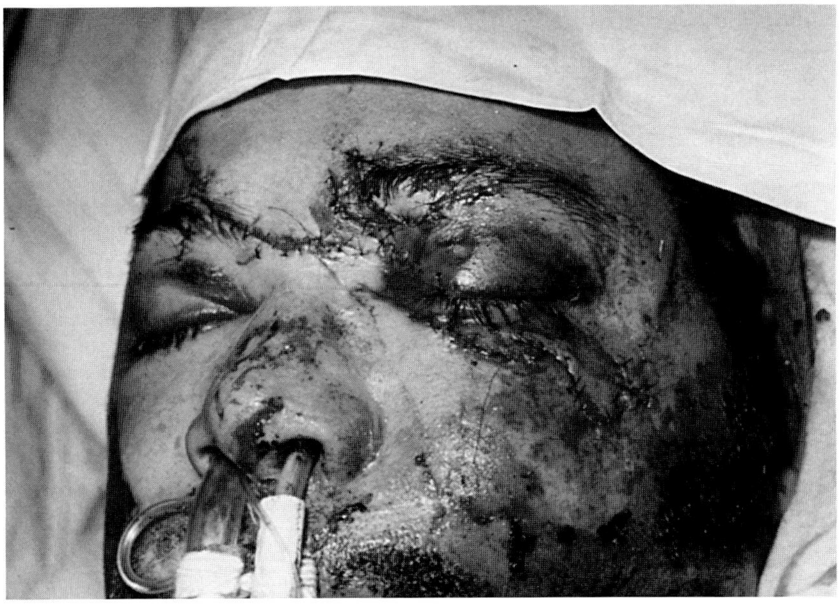

Figure 39–18 • NG and ET tubes are tied together with twill tape and secured to the upper lip. (Courtesy D.H. Frank, MD, University of California–San Diego Medical Center, San Diego, CA.)

neal cavity. Obstructive phenomena can occur with intestinal tubes as well. The tubes can become knotted,[33] the balloon or mercury bag can become overdistended with gas (passive diffusion), or intussusception can occur around the tube. Rupture of the mercury balloon can lead to elemental mercury spilled into the gut. Mercury will generally pass through the GI tract without absorption or toxic effect unless there is a perforation of the intestine as well. Aspiration of mercury after balloon rupture has also been reported.[21]

D. Other

The use of NG tubes has been linked with an increased frequency of aspiration pneumonitis.[34,35] This may be

NG Tube Securement with Suture

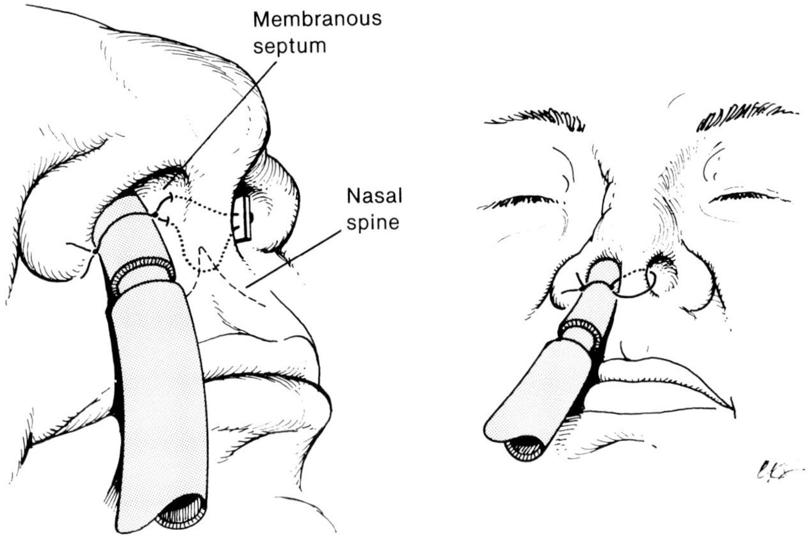

Figure 39–19 • NG tube is secured with a suture placed through the nasal septum.

Perforation of Esophagus by NG Tube

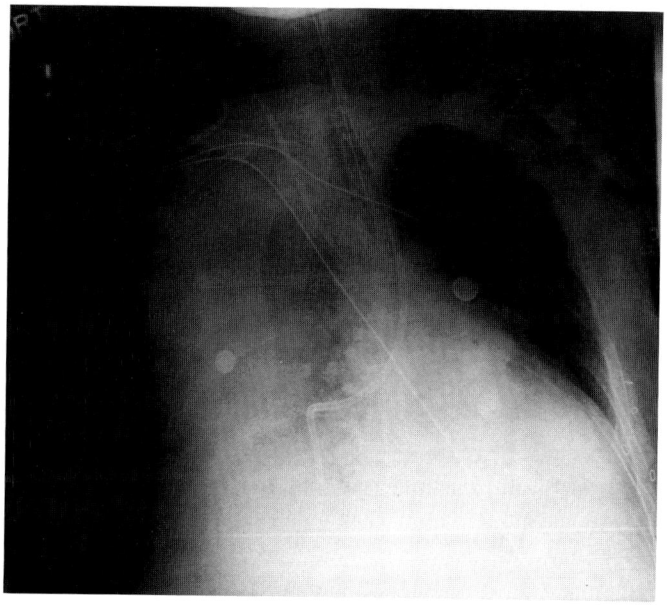

Figure 39-20 • Thoracic esophageal perforation by NG tube is shown. Note right hemithorax filled with nutritional supplement.

Knotted NG and ET Tubes Causing Simultaneous Extubation

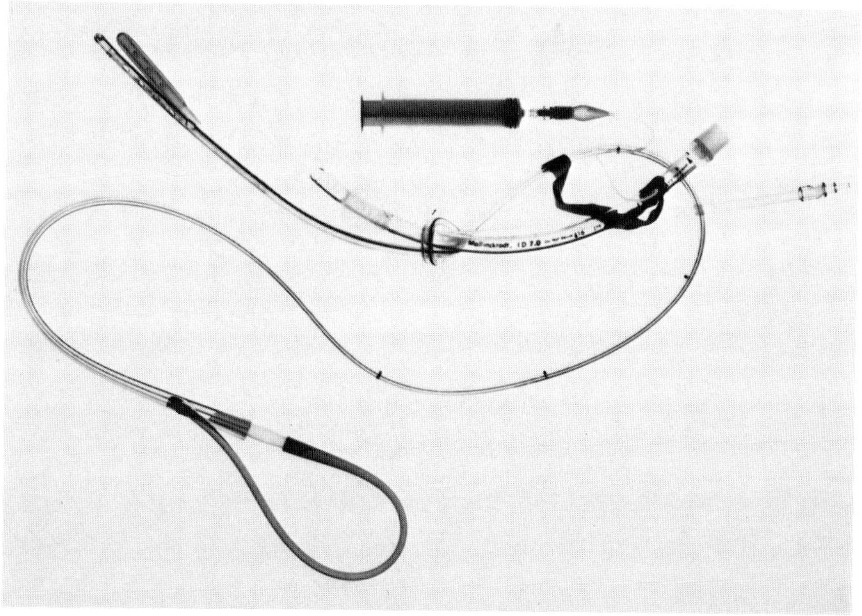

Figure 39-21 • The NG tube became knotted around the ET tube and esophageal stethoscope, leading to extubation with NG removal. (Courtesy J.L. Benumof, MD, University of California, San Diego, Medical Center, San Diego, CA.)

due in part to the tube acting as a wick for regurgitation through the esophageal sphincters.[34,36] In the anesthetized patient, this risk is particularly increased after muscle paralysis and before intubation. However, the use of adequate cricoid pressure has been shown to effectively obliterate the esophageal lumen and prevent regurgitation of gastric contents into the pharynx even in the presence of an NG tube.[37] Additionally, patients with NG tubes in place may be at increased risk for pneumonia because they are less mobile and have a poorer cough effort than those without tubes.[38]

Lastly, NG tubes can become knotted around other tubes in place in the oropharynx, leading to inadvertent removal of these tubes with extubation (Fig. 39–21). If this includes an endotracheal tube, ventilatory compromise can result.[39]

VI. References

1. Paine JR. The history of the invention and development of the stomach and duodenal tubes. Ann Intern Med 8:752–763, 1934.
2. Cogbill TH, Bintz M, Johnson JA, Strutt PJ. Acute gastric dilatation after trauma. J Trauma 27:1113–1117, 1987.
3. Levin AL. A new gastroduodenal catheter. JAMA 76:1007, 1921.
4. Ikard RW, Federspiel CF. A comparison of Levin and sump nasogastric tubes for postoperative gastrointestinal decompression. Am Surg 53:50–53, 1987.
5. Wolfson PJ, Bauer JJ, Gelernt IM, et al. Use of the long tube in the management of patients with small-intestinal obstruction due to adhesions. Arch Surg 120:1001–1006, 1985.
6. Brolin RE. The role of gastrointestinal tube decompression in the treatment of mechanical intestinal obstruction. Am Surg 49:131–137, 1983.
7. Brolin RE. Partial small bowel obstruction. Surgery 95:145–149, 1984.
8. Brolin RE. Long tubes vs. nasogastric tubes in the treatment of intestinal obstruction. Arch Surg 122:118, 1987.
9. Moss G, Friedman RC. Abdominal decompression: Increased efficiency by esophageal aspiration utilizing a new nasogastric tube. Am J Surg 133:225–228, 1977.
10. McConnell EA. 10 problems with nasogastric tubes and how to solve them. Nursing 9:78–81, 1979.
11. Sader AA. New way to stabilize nasogastric tubes. Am J Surg 130:102, 1975.
12. Carr GC, Heimlich HJ. Circle tie to prevent removal of nasogastric tube by patient. Surg Gynecol Obstet 134:317–318, 1972.
13. Mundy DA. Another technique for insertion of nasogastric tubes. Anesthesiology 50:374, 1979.
14. Siegel IB, Kahn RC. Insertion of difficult nasogastric tubes through a nasoesophageally placed endotracheal tube. Crit Care Med 15:876–877, 1987.
15. Sax HC, Hurst JM. Fluoroscopic placement of nasoenteric tubes. Crit Care Med 15:802–803, 1987.
16. Ohn KC, Wu WH. A new method for nasogastric tube insertion. Anesthesiology 51:568, 1979.
17. Bouzarth WF. Intracranial nasogastric tube insertion. J Trauma 18:818–819, 1978.
18. Fremstad JD, Martin SH. Lethal complication from insertion of nasogastric tube after severe basilar skull fracture. J Trauma 18:820–822, 1978.
19. Galloway DC, Grudis J. Inadvertent intracranial placement of nasogastric tube through a basilar skull fracture. South Med J 72:240, 1979.
20. Gregory JA, Turner PT, Reynolds AF. A complication of nasogastric intubation: Intracranial penetration. J Trauma 18:823–824, 1978.
21. Hunter TB, Fon GT, Silverstein ME. Complications of intestinal tubes. Am J Gastroenterol 76:256–261, 1981.
22. Sofferman RA, Hubbell RN. Laryngeal complications of nasogastric tubes. Ann Otol 90:465–468, 1981.
23. Friedman M, Baim H, Stobnicki M, et al. Laryngeal injuries secondary to nasogastric tubes. Ann Otol 90:469–474, 1981.
24. Frank DH. Reconstruction of head and neck burn injury. In Wachtel TL, Frank DH (eds). Burns of the Head and Neck. Philadelphia, WB Saunders, 1984, 153–186.
25. Feliciano DV, Bitondo CG, Mattox KL, et al. Combined tracheoesophageal injuries. Am J Surg 150:710–715, 1985.
26. Grillo HC, Moncure AC, McEnany MT. Repair of inflammatory tracheoesophageal fistula. Ann Thorac Surg 113:112–119, 1976.
27. Geha AS, Seegers JV, Kodner IJ, Lefrack S. Tracheoesophageal fistula caused by cuffed tracheal tube. Arch Surg 113:338–340, 1978.
28. McDanal JT, Wheeler DM, Ebert J. A complication of nasogastric intubation: Pulmonary hemorrhage. Anesthesiology 59:356–358, 1983.
29. McWey RE, Curry NS, Schabel SI, Reines HD. Complications of nasoenteric feeding tubes. Am J Surg 155:253–257, 1988.
30. Holliman PW, McFee AS. Pneumothorax attributable to nasogastric tube. Arch Surg 970, 1981.
31. Tiller HJ, Rhea WG. Iatrogenic perforation of the esophagus by a nasogastric tube. Am J Surg 147:423–425, 1984.
32. Michel L, Grillo HC. Esophageal perforation. Ann Thorac Surg 33:203–209, 1982.
33. Morris HH. Nasogastric intubation: A potentially knotty problem. JAMA 237:1432, 1977.
34. Argov S, Goldstein I, Barzilai A. Is routine use of the nasogastric tube justified in upper abdominal surgery? Am J Surg 139:849–850, 1980.
35. LeFrock JL, Clark TS, Davies B, Klainer AS. Aspiration pneumonia: A ten-year review. Am Surg 45:305–313, 1979.
36. Fanning GL. The efficacy of cricoid pressure in preventing regurgitation of gastric contents. Anesthesiology 32:553–555, 1970.
37. Salem MR, Joseph BS, Heyman HJ, et al. Cricoid compression is effective in obliterating the esophageal lumen in the presence of a nasogastric tube. Anesthesiology 63:443–446, 1985.
38. Bauer JJ, Gelernt IM, Salky BA, Kreel I. Is routine nasogastric decompression really necessary? Ann Surg 201:233–236, 1985.
39. Dorsey M, Benumof JL. Unintentional endotracheal extubation by oralgastric tube extubation. Anesth Rev 15:30–33, 1988.

Chapter 40

•

John A. Weigelt, MD

Parenteral Nutrition

OUTLINE

I. INTRODUCTION

A. *History*

The history of intravenous nutrition has been traced in an excellent article.[1] The astonishing aspect of intravenous parenteral nutrition is its relatively recent arrival. Although intravenous therapy has a 50-year history as an accepted medical practice, central venous nutrition has a history of less than 25 years. Dudrick and Vars demonstrated in 1966 that glucose and protein given intravenously to growing animals could support growth and development. In 1967, Dudrick suggested using a central vein access procedure originally described by Aubaniac in 1952.[2] This allowed hyperosmolar solutions to be injected directly into the central veins where flow was sufficient to dilute the solutions and avoid thrombosis of the veins. In 1968, Dudrick and Wilmore,[1] using only intravenous nutrition, supported growth in a child born with small bowel atresia. This clinical success brought acceptance of hyperalimentation as a useful and practical approach to nutrition when the gastrointestinal tract could not be used.

It is readily apparent that adequate nutrition is necessary to maintain or restore a healthy body. Nutrition provides energy, allows growth, and is necessary for tissue repair. Adult intensive care patients expend energy and have tissue in need of repair, and pediatric patients may also need nutrition for growth. If nutritive support of an injured or sick individual is ignored, progressive catabolism occurs with resulting organ dysfunction (Fig. 40-1). When 30% of the lean body mass is lost, death will occur. This concept is simple, yet adequate nutrition for hospitalized patients is often neglected.[3]

Confusion exists in terms of when, what, and how nutritional support should be provided in an individual patient. This is particularly true when considering parenteral nutrition in terms of its cost and associated risks.[4] This chapter discusses when (nutritional assessment), what (nutrients used), and how (delivery methods) to provide nutrition to critically ill patients. Parenteral and enteral nutrition will be reviewed as well as some unique problems associated with nutritional support.

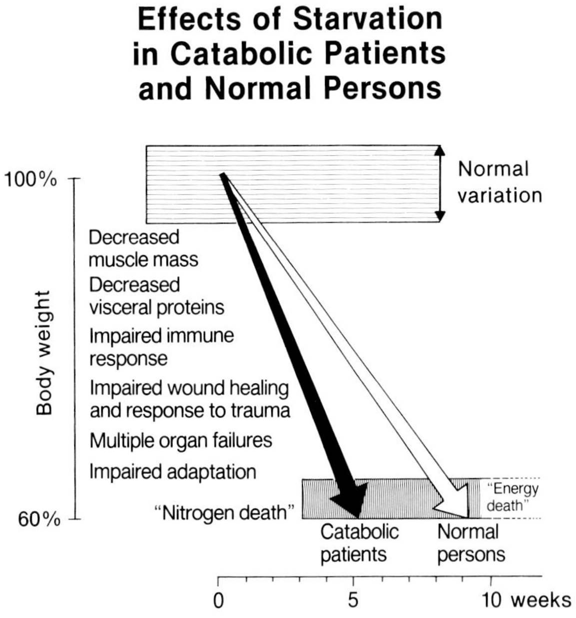

Figure 40-1 • The figure shows results of progressive catabolism in an injured patient. Lean body mass, predominantly protein, is used as an energy source if alternative sources are not provided, producing various organ dysfunctions depending on the degree of lean body mass loss.

II. INDICATIONS

A. *Nutritional Assessment*

Nutritional assessment attempts to use some measurements that correlate with the nutritional status of the patient. Nutritional assessment of hospitalized patients demonstrates that a large number of these patients are undernourished. Furthermore, protein–calorie malnutrition is associated with increased morbidity and mortality.[5] (The term *kwashiorkor* is used to indicate severe protein deficiency; *marasmus* indicates severe protein and calorie deficiency.)

A number of nutritional assessment systems have been devised to identify patients with malnutrition, including percent of ideal body weight, creatinine–height index, serum albumin, serum transferrin, total lymphocyte count, and delayed hypersensitivity to skin antigens.[6] The efficacy of these parameters as compared to clinical assessment for preoperative patients has been questioned.[7,8] Clinical assessment implies a physical examination by an experienced physician. Nutritional assessment systems lose further value when used to evaluate early postoperative, traumatized, or critically ill patients.[9] Intensive care (ICU) patients have medical and surgical conditions that often elevate basal metabolic rate and complicate the patient's handling of exogenous substrates. Most of these patients are catabolic, indicating that they are using their body stores of carbohydrate, fat, and protein to produce energy.

In these patients, adequate nutrition is essential, regardless of preexisting nutritive states. Selection of ICU patients for some form of nutritional support is relatively simple. Patients are candidates if (1) the degree of acute weight loss is greater than 10% of usual body weight, (2) a catabolic state exists, or (3) the length of time without adequate nutrition is estimated at longer than 7 days. Murray and associates evaluated 16 nutrition-related parameters in intensive care patients.[9] A serum albumin concentration of less than 3.2 g/dL clearly identified a group of patients with an increased morbidity as well as, perhaps, an increased mortality. Thus, serum albumin is suggested as a means to select ICU patients for nutritional support. The ease of obtaining serum albumin and its correlation with outcome (level less than 3.2 g/dL) makes it an attractive method to apply. Once the decision to provide nutritional support is made, a determination of the energy and protein requirements must follow.

B. *Metabolic Measurements*

1. Caloric Requirements

Energy is measured in units of calories or, more commonly for metabolic studies, kilocalories. A kilocalorie (kcal) is equal to the heat required to raise the temperature of 1 kg H_2O 1°C. A small calorie (cal) is the amount of heat required to raise the temperature of 1 g H_2O 1°C. Direct and indirect calorimetry can be used to measure energy. Direct calorimetry measures heat production as a temperature change of a medium. It is based on the postulate that all energy expended in the body is released as heat. In a resting person, the metabolic rate is equal to the heat liberated. Indirect calorimetry measures energy expenditure from the amount of oxygen consumed. It is less cumbersome than direct calorimetry and has become the most practical method for measuring energy expenditure in critically ill patients.

Metabolic carts are available that are portable, easy to use, and offer automatic calibration and data management systems (Fig. 40–2). These carts measure heat production indirectly by measuring oxygen consumption and carbon dioxide production once a steady state has been reached. The technique is operator dependent and is inaccurate in ventilated patients on an inspired oxygen of 60% or greater. Care must be taken to insure a stable accurate oxygen concentration in any ventilated patient, since varying or inaccurate inspired oxygen levels will produce erroneous oxygen consumption values.[10] The metabolic cart provides a respiratory quotient (RQ) and a measured energy expenditure (MEE). The respiratory quotient is the production of carbon dioxide divided by the oxygen consumed:

$$RQ = \frac{C0_2 \text{ produced moles}}{0_2 \text{ consumed moles}}$$

where RQ = respiratory quotient, CO_2 = carbon dioxide, and O_2 = oxygen. The RQ is unique for each type of fuel: fat, 0.7; protein, 0.8; and glucose, 1.0. An RQ greater than 1.0 indicates net lipogenesis, since fat forms when more carbon dioxide is produced than oxygen is consumed. The MEE represents the actual energy expenditure at the time of measurement. Despite the improvements in this technology, it is still too cumbersome for routine use and is best used when patients are not responding appropriately in terms of nutrition at calculated levels of energy requirements.

More routine, estimates of caloric or energy requirements are based on basal metabolic measurements. The basal metabolic rate (BMR) is defined as the rate of energy expenditure at complete rest and 12–18 hours after the ingestion of any food. Food ingestion raises energy expenditure approximately 10%. The resting energy expenditure (REE) is measured with the patient supine at complete rest and at least 2 hours after food ingestion. The Harris-Benedict equation is used to estimate the REE from commonly available measurements. The advantages of this calculation are its ease, rapidity, low cost, and lack of technology needed. Its major disadvantage is that it is fairly inaccurate in assessing energy needs under major stress.[11,12]

The energy required by a patient (recommended energy intake [REI]) can be divided into three components: (1) REE, (2) muscle activity, and (3) stress-induced metabolic activity. The REE has already been discussed and muscle activity is usually quite limited in ICU patients and not considered more than an additional 25% of BMR. The stress-induced metabolic activity is a result of the hypermetabolism that accompanies critical illness. A major portion of this increased caloric need results from the increase in resting body temperature associated with hypermetabolism. An increase in body temperature of 1°C causes a 5% to 8% increase in metabolic rate. A decrease in body temperature requires heat production and energy consumption. Other estimated stress factors remain controversial but are nevertheless used to increase the REE (Table 40–1).

Some conditions and their estimated stress factors are starvation (0.9–1.0), peritonitis (1.1–1.3), sepsis (1.3–1.5), multiple organ failure (1.5–1.7), and burns (1.5–2.0).[13,14] A stress factor of 1.0 is used for maintenance nutrition; 1.5–1.75 is satisfactory for repletion nutrition in critically ill patients. Some less obvious stress factors include hypermetabolism, increased heat loss (requiring heat production), pain, and anxiety.

It is important to remember that there is a wide variability in caloric expenditure in critically ill patients.

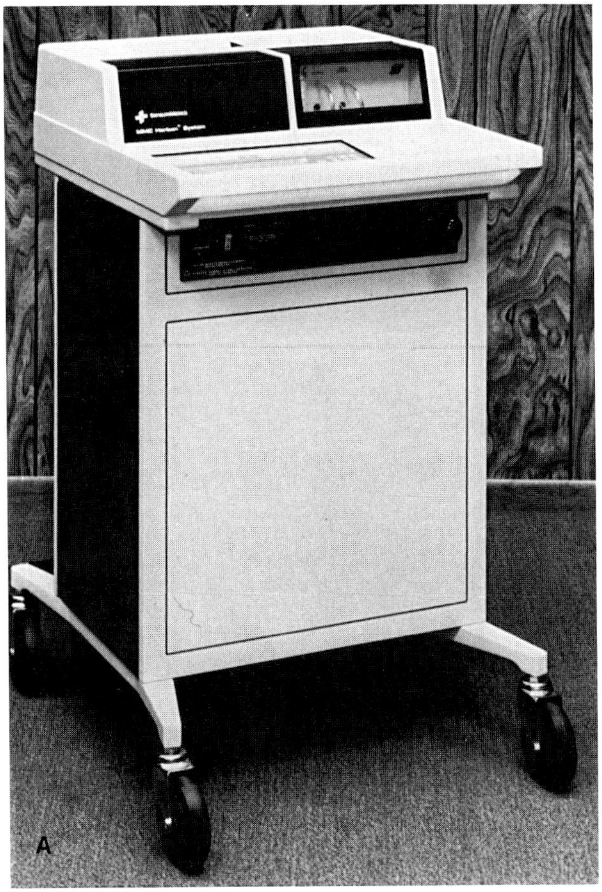

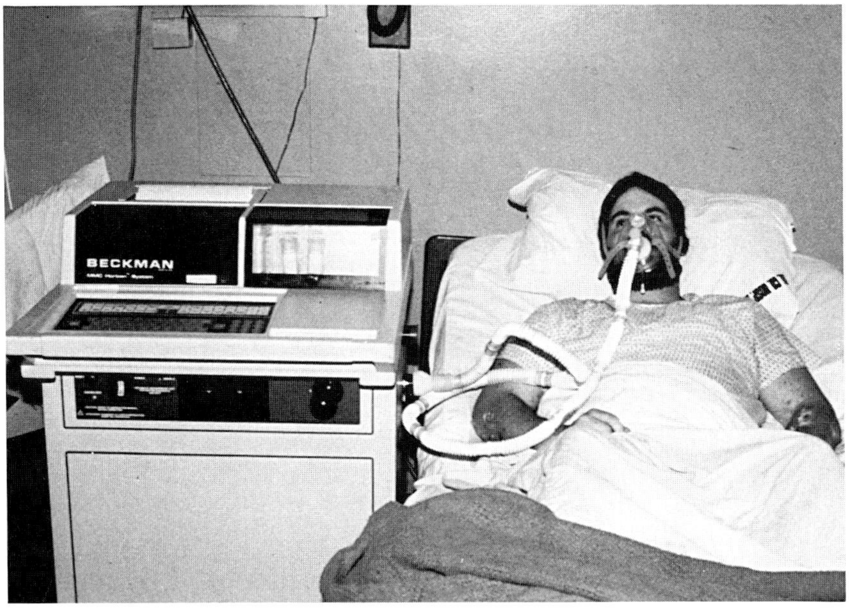

Figure 40–2 • (***A***) Metabolic cart that can be used at the patient's bedside to measure energy expenditure. (***B***) Metabolic cart at the bedside connected to a patient for measurement.

The equations used to calculate the energy requirements give estimates, and each patient must be assessed continually and the attempt made to identify the correct energy requirement. Useful guidelines for various energy states are listed in Table 40–2.

2. Protein Requirements

Protein requirements vary with the degree of illness and catabolism of the patient. Nitrogen excretion is used to identify the catabolic level of the patient. Normal humans excrete up to 5 g of nitrogen every 24 hours.

Table 40–1 • Factors that Increase and Decrease Energy Needs

Factors	Increased Energy	Decreased Energy
REE kcal/day/m2	Young age	Old age
	Male sex	Female sex
Muscle activity	Exercise	Sedation
	Work of breathing	Paralysis
	Ventilator dysnchrony	
	Combative state	
Stress factor	Hypermetabolism	Analgesics
	Pain	Adequate sleep
	Anxiety	Communication
	Excess heat loss	Heat conservation

Nitrogen excretion for mild stress is 5–10 g; moderate stress, 10–15 g; and severe stress, greater than 15 g every 24 hours. Daily protein recommendations range from 1.0 to 2.0 g/kg body weight. Most patients can be managed by administering 1.0–1.5 g/kg body weight every 24 hours. Protein administration is monitored by measuring urinary nitrogen excretion. The urinary urea nitrogen (UUN) in a 24-hour urine collection multiplied by 6.25 yields the protein content.

In starvation, protein sources are conserved, slowing the loss of lean body mass, and fat and ketone bodies from the liver are used for energy production. This process results in approximately 1.0 g protein/kg/day usage with a 150:1 nonprotein calorie–nitrogen ratio. In hypermetabolism, protein is catabolized from the lean body mass and the released amino acids are used as energy sources. This may approach 30% in severe stress states representing 2.5 g protein/kg/day usage with a 100:1 nonprotein calorie–nitrogen ratio. Administration of exogenous amino acids will increase total protein synthesis but may do little to reduce catabolism, especially in advanced stress or sepsis.[15]

III. How to Administer Parenteral Nutrition

A. *Nutritional Components*

1. Carbohydrate

Dextrose is the most commonly used energy source for parenteral nutrition. Each gram of dextrose monohydrate provides 3.4 kcal. Hypertonic glucose solutions are used to increase caloric density. Most adult formulas for parenteral nutrition use a final concentration of 25% to 35%, which is equivalent to a dextrose osmolarity of 1200–1700 mOsm/L.

Fructose is a monosaccharide that may be used as an energy source. It is widely used in Europe mixed with glucose and xylitol. Its advantage is that it does not require insulin for phosphorylation and conversion to glucose. In patients with insulin deficiency it is more efficiently metabolized into glycogen and produces lower serum glucose levels and less glycosuria than dextrose. A 10% solution is available that provides 3.75–4.00 kcal/g. A dose of 0.25 g/kg/hr is suggested, and if the amount or rate is too fast uricemia, lactic acidosis, and hypophosphatemia may occur. Invert sugar is composed of equal parts dextrose and fructose. It has a caloric density of 4 kcal/g. This combination is infrequently used as a calorie source for parenteral nutrition.

Glycerol is a naturally occurring sugar alcohol. It has a caloric density of 4.32 kcal/g and small amounts of glycerin are present in fat emulsions. It is not commonly used as a sole energy source in parenteral nutrition.

Other energy sources include alcohol, sorbitol, and xylitol. At present, none are suggested as replacements for the previously listed carbohydrates.

Table 40–2 • Estimates of Energy Requirements for Different Metabolic States

Metabolic Condition	kcal/kg/day estimate
Normal resting metabolic rate	25 kcal/kg/day
Septic patients	30–40 kcal/kg/day
Multiply injured patients	25–35 kcal/kg/day
Burn patients	25–50 kcal/kg/day

2. PROTEIN

Nitrogen is provided as crystalline amino acids. Solutions of these amino acids contain 40% to 50% essential amino acids and 50% to 60% nonessential amino acids. The concentration of amino acid in the solution ranges from 3% to 11% and the solutions are provided in 500- or 1000-mL volumes. Special amino acid formulas have been suggested for certain disease conditions. A high percentage of essential amino acids is suggested for patients with renal failure. For patients with hepatic disease, a product with a high concentration of branched-chain amino acids (BCAA), including leucine, isoleucine, and valine, is suggested. This product was well tolerated by protein-intolerant patients with no worsening or some improvement in hepatic encephalopathy.[16] A different formula with BCAA is suggested for patients under maximum stress or trauma. This formula achieved nitrogen balance sooner than balanced amino acid solutions.[17] Other data suggest that either a balanced or an enriched BCAA solution improves protein balance in sepsis, but one or the other does not seem to be superior.[18] The benefits of these special formulas remain controversial and are still being evaluated.

In the critically ill hypermetabolic patient, the goal is positive nitrogen balance. This is often difficult if not impossible to achieve. These patients will require 1.5–2.5 g protein/kg/day with a calorie–nitrogen ratio of 100:1 or less.[17]

3. FAT

Lipid metabolism furnishes 9 kcal/g and meets 20% to 50% of the daily caloric requirement in normal adults. Linoleic, linolenic, and arachidonic acids are essential fatty acids, and if not provided in a nutritional regimen will cause a fatty acid deficiency.[19] This condition is characterized by impaired wound healing, thrombocytopenia, hair loss, anemia, and a dry, scaly dermatitis. Thus, it is appropriate to use lipid as a calorie source and an essential nutritional element.

A major obstacle to incorporating fat as a calorie source into nutritional programs was early skepticism about the ability of severely ill patients to use it. However, it is now clear that septic and traumatized patients can use fat as an energy source.[20] Their metabolic response is characterized by hyperglycemia, insulin resistance, and rapid mobilization of all energy sources, including fat. Evidence exists that fat can provide as much as 70% to 80% of the energy requirements in patients with sepsis, although it is not usually used to provide more than 50% of the calories in these patients.[21]

Fat is provided as an emulsion for intravenous use. The particle size measures between 0.1 and 0.5 mm in diameter. The preparation most often used intravenously is Intralipid 10% or 20%. The 10% solution is isotonic, contains 54% linoleic acid, and can be given in a peripheral vein. The 20% solution is hypertonic, contains 50% linoleic acid, and is given by central venous access. Essential fatty acid deficiency can be avoided if at least 6% of the total calories are from linoleic acid. This number of essential fatty acid calories is provided by 122 mL of the 10% solution or 67 mL of the 20% solution per 1000 nonfat calories.

Fat is given intravenously as an intermittent or continuous infusion. When used with a hypertonic glucose solution, 500 mL of the 20% mixture is usually given twice weekly. It is also given as fat-admixture, triple-mix, or all-in-one (AIO) nutrition solutions.[22] This method mixes the fat, carbohydrate, amino acids, electrolytes, trace elements, and vitamins in one container. Mixing all components has the potential for precipitating the fat particles. However, solubility of the AIO solution is excellent at recommended additive concentrations if the solution is stored at 4°C and used within 24 hours.[23]

4. ELECTROLYTES

The goal of electrolyte supplementation is to maintain ionic equilibrium. Guidelines for the overall amount of

Table 40-3 • Electrolyte Additions

Electrolyte	Daily Intake (Adult)
Sodium	130 mEq
Sodium chloride	
Sodium acetate	
Sodium phosphate	
Potassium	60 mEq
Potasium chloride	
Potassium acetate	
Potassium phosphate	
Phosphate	20 m*M*
Sodium phosphate	
Potassium phosphate	
Calcium	5 mEq
Calcium gluconate	
Calcium chloride	
Magnesium	16 mEq
Magnesium sulfate	

electrolytes to be included in parenteral nutrition solutions are listed in Table 40–3. Sodium may have to be increased if excessive gastrointestinal losses are present or reduced if the patient is elderly or has cardiopulmonary disease. Potassium should be decreased in patients with renal insufficiency. An increase in potassium is often needed early in malnourished patients, as intracellular stores are replenished. A number of sources of magnesium loss have been identified and are likely to occur in the critically ill patient.[24] Increased gastrointestinal losses are a major problem and may require increased amounts of magnesium supplementation. Positive phosphorus balance is easily achieved with 15 mEq/day of phosphate.[25] Phosphate additions should be reduced if renal insufficiency is present.

5. Trace Elements

Seven trace elements are important for health: iron, zinc, copper, chromium, selenium, iodine, and cobalt. Chromium, copper, iron, manganese, selenium, and zinc are routinely given as intravenous additives in parenteral nutrition (Table 40–4). Manganese is given, although no deficiencies have been identified with parenteral nutrition. Other trace elements that have been supplemented include fluorine (0.35 mg/day), iodine (0.12 mg/day), and molybdenum (0.075 mg/day).[22] Iron is often included in parenteral nutrition regimens, although some questions remain regarding the ability of acutely ill patients to use it.[26]

Each of the essential trace elements have an identified metabolic function.[27] Chromium is important to glucose metabolism because it mediates the effect of insulin on cell membranes. Copper is required for cytochrome oxidase function. Manganese is a cofactor for pyruvate carboxylase, which is key to oxidative phosphorylation. Selenium is associated with glutathione peroxidase found in erythrocytes. Zinc is a cofactor in a number of enzyme systems, including carboxypeptidase and DNA polymerase. Fluorine may be important for iron absorption. Molybdenum is a cofactor for pyruvate carboxylase involved with oxidative phosphorylation. Iodine is required for thyroglobulin production.

6. Vitamins

Vitamins are essential nutrients that are active in minute quantities. When they are not given in a parenteral nutrition regimen, deficiency states have been identified.

Table 40–4 • Trace Element Additives

Trace Element	Recommended Daily Intake (Adult)
Zinc sulfate	4000 μg
Copper sulfate	1600 μg
Manganese sulfate	400 μg
Selenious acid	40 μg
Chromium chloride	16 μg
Iron dextran	1 mg

Legend–Recommendations for trace element replacement for a patient on parenteral nutrition[75].

Exact requirements are not known, although standard recommendations are available (Table 40–5).

7. Nutrient Mixes

A number of nutrient mixes are possible. The percentage of glucose ranges from 20% to 40%, the percentage of amino acids ranges from 2.5% to 7%, and the percentage of fat ranges from 0 to 5% in the final solution. Some guidelines for using these formulations are helpful. Carbohydrate should provide at least 50% of the nonprotein calories, but should not exceed 7 mg/kg/min. Protein should provide 1.5–2.0 g/kg/day, assuming adequate nonprotein calories are provided. Approximately 20% of calories should come from protein. Fat may supply up to 50% of nonprotein calories as long as the serum triglycerides are less than 250 mg/dL.

Standard parenteral solutions have 25% to 35% glucose and 5% amino acids. These are supplemented with fat emulsions twice weekly. High-nutrient-density

Table 40–5 • Vitamin Supplementation

Vitamin	Recommended Intake
Vitamin A	2500 IU/day
Vitamin D	400 IU/day
Vitamin E (alpha tocopherol)	50 IU/day
Thiamine	5 mg/day
Riboflavin	5 mg/day
Niacin	50 mg/day
Pantothenic acid	15 mg/day
Pyridoxine	5 mg/day
Folic acid	5 mg/day
Vitamin B_{12}	12 μg/day
Vitamin C	500 mg/day
Biotin	60 μg/day
Vitamin K	10 mg/week

parenteral solutions contain 20% glucose and 7% amino acids.[28] The purpose of this formulation is to increase anabolism rather than simply to decrease catabolism. A fat-admixture or triple-mix solution is also used that contains 17.5% dextrose, 5% amino acids, and 5% fat.[29,30] This solution is indicated when (1) hyperglycemia is not controlled with up to 60 units of regular insulin/1000 mL of standard solution, (2) an RQ greater than 1.0 exists, and (3) glucose administration exceeds 7 mg/kg/min. This solution should not be given faster than 2 mL/kg/hr to avoid hypertriglyceridemia. If serum triglycerides are greater than 250 mg/dL, the proportion of fat should be reduced.

8. Other Additives

Insulin should be used to control hyperglycemia. Blood glucose should be kept below 200 mg % to avoid hyperosmolar complications. Insulin is not routinely added to the parenteral nutrition solution unless hyperglycemia is documented or a history of insulin-dependent diabetes mellitus is present. An initial starting point for nondiabetics is 10–20 units/1000 mL. Insulin administration can be guided by monitoring urinary glucose or serum glucose. Regular insulin is given intermittently until a steady state is reached. This total daily dose of insulin can then be added to the total amount of daily parenteral nutrition solution.

Heparin may prevent central vein thrombosis when added to parenteral nutrition solutions. It is added at doses ranging from 1000 to 3000 units/1000 mL of solution. Fabri and associates reported subclavian thrombosis in 32% of patients without heparin and in 8% of patients with heparin in the parenteral nutrition.[31] Other low-dose heparin regimens must be assessed when heparin is used in the parenteral nutrition to avoid dangerous levels of anticoagulation. Heparin-induced thrombocytopenia may also occur when heparin is used in parenteral nutrition solutions.[32]

Appendix A includes a listing of the commonly used parenteral nutrition solutions. Standard and special formulas are included.

B. *How to Order and Manage the Patient on Total Parenteral Nutrition*

Parenteral nutrition is administered through a central venous catheter (CVC). The catheter is dedicated to the nutritive solution and is not used for other infusions except in severe emergencies requiring immediate venous access. Acute temporary central venous access methodology is presented in Chapter 18.

1. Beginning Infusions

An initial rate of 50 mL/hr is suggested to test for glucose intolerance. In patients with no history of glucose intolerance, diabetes mellitus, or metabolic state promoting glucose intolerance (ie, sepsis), higher initial rates are possible, although beginning at more than 2000 mL/day is usually poorly tolerated. Infusion rate is increased every 12–24 hours by 25 mL/hr until the goal rate is reached. Increases should not be made if serum glucose is greater than 200 mg %.

The goal rate is based on the REI or protein requirement. The REI is divided by the caloric concentration of the parenteral solution and the result is divided by 24 to identify the hourly goal rate. If protein requirement is used, the UUN is multiplied by 6.25, determining the daily protein requirement. An hourly rate is calculated by dividing by 24.

An order sheet can be helpful to physicians when writing orders for parenteral nutrition. Such a sheet is easily used by members of a nutritional support team or an individual physician writing orders for a single patient. A sample of an order sheet designed and used by the Nutritional Support Team at Parkland Memorial Hospital (Dallas, TX) is illustrated (Fig. 40–3).

2. Monitoring

Until a steady state is reached on the patient's goal rate of parenteral nutrition, daily laboratory studies are necessary. These include blood glucose, creatinine, sodium, potassium, carbon dioxide, and chloride. Glucose is monitored every 6 hours by urine dipsticks or fingerstick blood glucose. Other blood chemistries needed when beginning parenteral nutrition include calcium, phosphate, magnesium, albumin, prothrombin time, alkaline phosphatase, total bilirubin, and AST (SGOT). These are not daily studies but are obtained to help guide initial electrolyte replacement and follow the efficacy of nutritional support.

Once a steady state has been reached the initial daily studies can be done every 3 days and the other studies are checked once weekly. Triglyceride level is checked once weekly if the patient is receiving fat.

DALLAS COUNTY HOSPITAL DISTRICT
ADULT PARENTERAL NUTRITION
VIA CENTRAL VENOUS CATHETER
NUTRITIONAL SUPPORT TEAM (NST)

Date/Time:

Nursing unit:

INSTRUCTIONS: Complete all parts. Orders must be into the Pharmacy by 1400.

BASE FORMULA - Select one. Non-standard formulas will be reviewed by NST.

☐ **STANDARD**	☐ **FAT ADMIXTURE**	☐ **DILUTE**	☐ **NON-STANDARD FORMULA**
Amino Acids 5%	Amino Acids 5%	Amino Acids 2.5%	Amino Acids ____%
Dextrose 35%	Dextrose 17.5%	Dextrose 20%	Dextrose ____%
	Fat Emulsion 5%		Fat Emulsion ____%
			________ ____%

RATE AND VOLUME - Specify.

____ml/hr x 24 hours = ____ ml of base formula

TOTAL ADDITIVES PER 24 HOURS			Daily Recommendations (Adult)	Max./1000 ml of Fat Admix.
SODIUM	as chloride	____ mEq	130	130
	as acetate	____ mEq		
• **PHOSPHATE**	as sodium	____ mM	20	20
	as potassium	____ mM		
(each mM contributes 1.5 mEq of Na or K)				
POTASSIUM	as chloride	____ mEq	60	100
	as acetate	____ mEq		
• **CALCIUM**	as gluconate	____ mEq	5	10
MAGNESIUM	as sulfate	____ mEq	16	13
ZINC		____ mcg	4000	4000
MANGANESE		____ mcg	400	400
COPPER		____ mcg	1600	1600
CHROMIUM		____ mcg	16	16
SELENIUM		____ mcg	40	40
MULTIVITAMIN - 12		____ ml	10	10
HEPARIN		____ units	heparin 1 unit/ml of base formula	
REGULAR INSULIN		____ units	insulin to control blood glucose < 200 mg/dl	
OTHER ____		____		
____		____		

☐ **SEPARATE IV PIGGYBACK FAT EMULSION 20% 500 ml** (Mon. & Thur. except with Fat Admixture)

Rate = ____ ml/hr (not to exceed 63 ml/hr)

☐ **VITAMIN K 10 mg** added to parenteral nutrition solution (on Monday)

* CALCIUM AND PHOSPHATE **can** be mixed in the recommended amounts in the same bag.

SIGNATURES Physician ________________ MD

Order Sent RN Soln Verified LVN/RN

Special Instructions:

003

57050 (7-86) WHITE – CHART COPY CANARY – PHARMACY COPY

Figure 40–3 • Physician order sheet for parenteral nutrition is shown. Solutions are ordered for a 24-hour period based on caloric requirements. Options for different mixtures appear on the same sheet although standard mixtures are most commonly used.

3. Perioperative Use

Patients receiving total parenteral nutrition often require surgical procedures. Management of the catheter and solution during operative procedures is simple, since it uses the principles already discussed. The catheter should not be used for any other purpose than the infusion of the nutritive solution. If a multilumen catheter is in place, care must be taken to secure the port receiving parenteral nutrition. Asepsis for this line is always important (see Chapter 18).

The parenteral nutrition is infused at a constant rate throughout the operation. This is best achieved by a volumetric pump so constant attention to the flow rate is not necessary. The rate should be the same as the patient has been receiving in the intensive care unit.

Since the patient is receiving hypertonic glucose solution, attention is given to the patient's blood glucose. Measurement of serum glucose every 2 hours is appropriate during the operative procedure. Other laboratory determinations should be done as indicated. If the patient's hyperalimentation is being managed adequately, electrolyte abnormalities should be minimal, since they should already be constantly looked for and corrected.

C. *Permanent Venous Access*

Central venous access for parenteral nutrition is often necessary in a patient with limited central venous sites or with a need for months or years of access because of the disease process. A number of catheter options are available for this type of patient and a brief review of their design, care, and management is appropriate.

1. Indwelling Silastic Catheters

Broviac (18 gauge) or Hickman (16 gauge) catheters are made from Silastic and are implanted via a subcutaneous tunnel. They are transfixed to the subcutaneous tissue via a Dacron cuff placed a short distance from the skin entrance site (Fig. 40–4). The lifespan of these catheters when used for hyperalimentation is 4 to 9 months.[33]

2. Subcutaneous Reservoir Systems

The second type of long-term device is the subcutaneous port system. These systems include an implantable reservoir constructed of stainless steel and Silastic (Figs. 40–5 and 40–6). This reservoir is connected to a silicone catheter that is placed similarly to other central venous catheters. The reservoir is placed in a subcutaneous pocket just inferior to the clavicle. The reservoir is affixed to the underlying pectoral fascia with nonabsorbable sutures and can be palpated. A septum is identifiable that is punctured through the skin by a special atraumatic Huber needle. All the systems guarantee a 2000-plus puncture rate. Since there is no external catheter, patient freedom is increased and infectious complications may be decreased. The incidence of complications associated with indwelling catheters is 3/1000 catheter days and that for subcutaneous ports is 0.3/1000 catheter days.[34,35]

These catheters and reservoirs may be used for continuous or intermittent infusion of parenteral nutrition solutions. Adherence to a care plan for the catheters is essential to avoid catheter clotting and catheter infection. Occlusion of the catheter is often due to clotting of blood in the end of the catheter. This can be avoided by proper flushing of the catheter (Table 40–6).

All catheters require meticulous care of the entrance site. Catheter breaks do occur at the hub and can be repaired easily (Fig. 40–7). The indwelling catheter requires scheduled dressing changes for catheter maintenance, whereas the subcutaneous ports obviate this need (Table 40–7). Dressing change frequency varies from daily to three times a week. Aseptic technique is always used, and a standard protocol is effective in keeping the incidence of infection low.[36]

Figure 40–8A illustrates an improperly dressed CVC. It is obvious that the dressing is not occlusive and the entrance site can be easily contaminated or a leak can develop underneath the dressing (Fig. 40–9). Figure 40–8B illustrates a properly dressed CVP catheter. Note that an occlusive dressing fixes the catheter to the chest wall. This dressing does not need to be massive, nor does it always need to be done with the type of tape illustrated. However, it must be occlusive and secure.

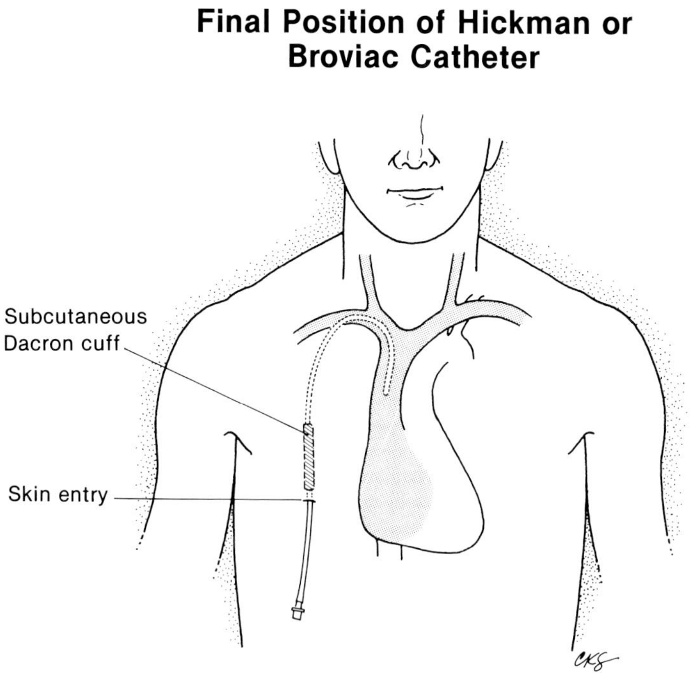

Figure 40–4 • Properly placed Hickman or Broviac catheter permits for long-term venous access. Dacron cuff should lie under the skin 4–5 cm from the entrance site.

Proper Position of Implantable Access System

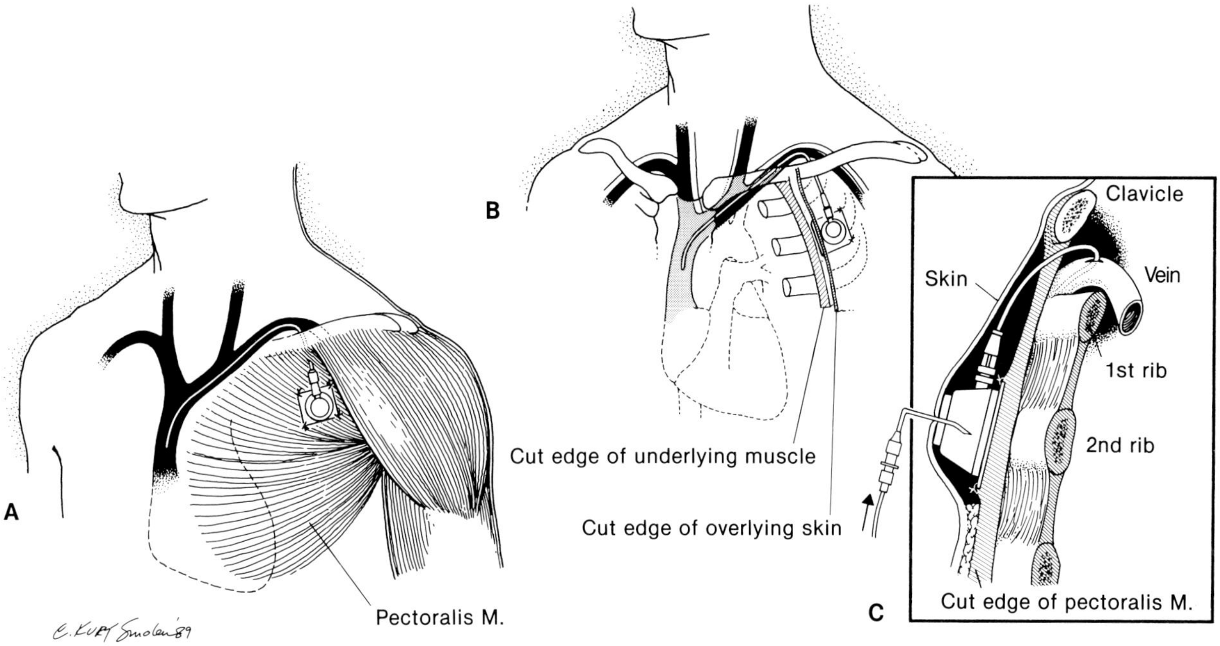

Figure 40–5 • Location of an implantable subcutaneous venous access system is shown. The reservoir lies in a subcutaneous pocket on the chest wall. (***A***) Superficial anatomy. (***B***) Deep anatomy. (***C***) Sagittal view.

Needle Access of Implantable Access System

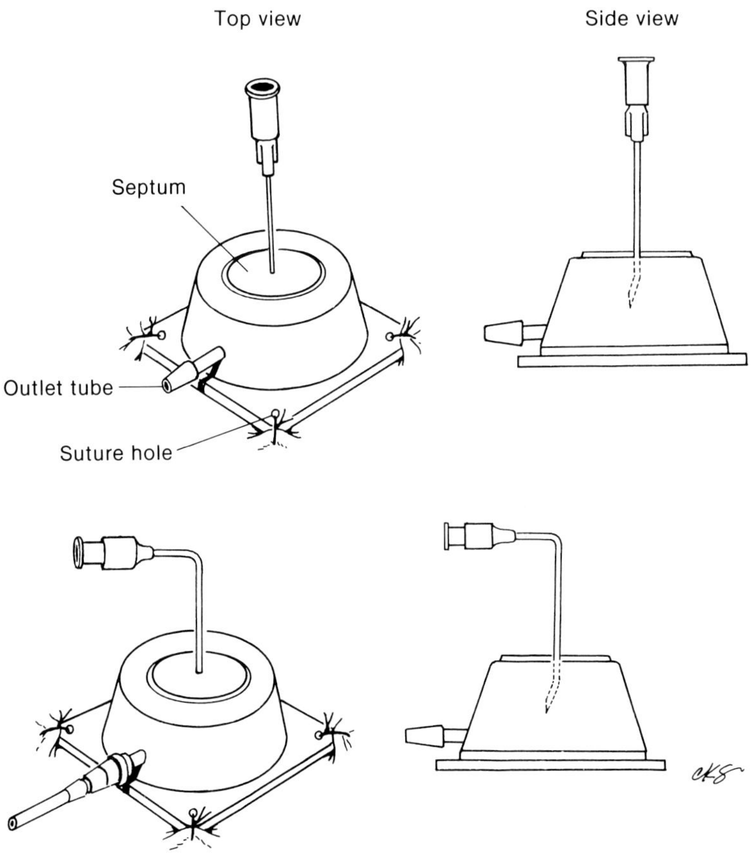

Figure 40–6 • Huber type needles are used with implantable venous access system. The reservoir is penetrated by the Huber needles.

Table 40–6 • Flushing and Heparinizing an Indwelling Hickman or Broviac Catheter

1. Following administration of intravenous nutrition, flush the catheter with 10 mL of normal saline. The catheter should be flushed until there is no grossly visible blood in the tubing.
2. Prepare a 2.5-mL syringe of heparin (100 units/mL).
3. Wash hands and put sterile gloves on.
4. Cleanse the injection plug wth povidone iodine and inject the 2.5 mL of heparin.
5. No needle longer than 1 in should be used for injection into long-term venous access catheters. Longer needles increase the risk of catheter perforation distal to the hub.

D. *Enteral Nutrition*

Enteral feedings should always be considered before parenteral nutrition methods are started. The advantages of enteral feeding include the maintenance of gastrointestinal function, the avoidance of catheter-related sepsis, decreased dependence on hospitalization, and lower cost. A number of trials have demonstrated that enteral nutrition is equivalent to, if not better than, parenteral nutrition.[37–39] Recent evidence suggests that enteral nutrition may support more normal neutrophil function and improve host resistance to infection better than intravenous nutrition.[40]

1. Gastrointestinal Access

Administration is accomplished through a number of different tubes into either the stomach, duodenum, or upper jejunum (Fig. 40–10). These can be placed surgically, placed endoscopically, or passed blindly. The position of all tubes passed blindly should be confirmed radiographically before use. Nasogastric or nasoduodenal tubes have been placed into the lungs or pleural spaces.[41] Successful placement of small bowel feeding tubes (SBFT) is successful in 60% of ICU patients compared to 95% of ward patients,[42] perhaps because of differences in gastrointestinal motility. Metoclopramide is helpful in getting a small-bowel feeding tube to pass through the pylorus into the duodenum in ICU patients.[43] Twenty mg of Metoclopramide is given over 5 minutes and 10 minutes later an SBFT is inserted. The effect on SBFT passage into the duodenum should be immediate. A radiograph is always taken to verify SBFT placement. Tubes that are difficult to place or that are being removed by the patient should be secured with a bridle.

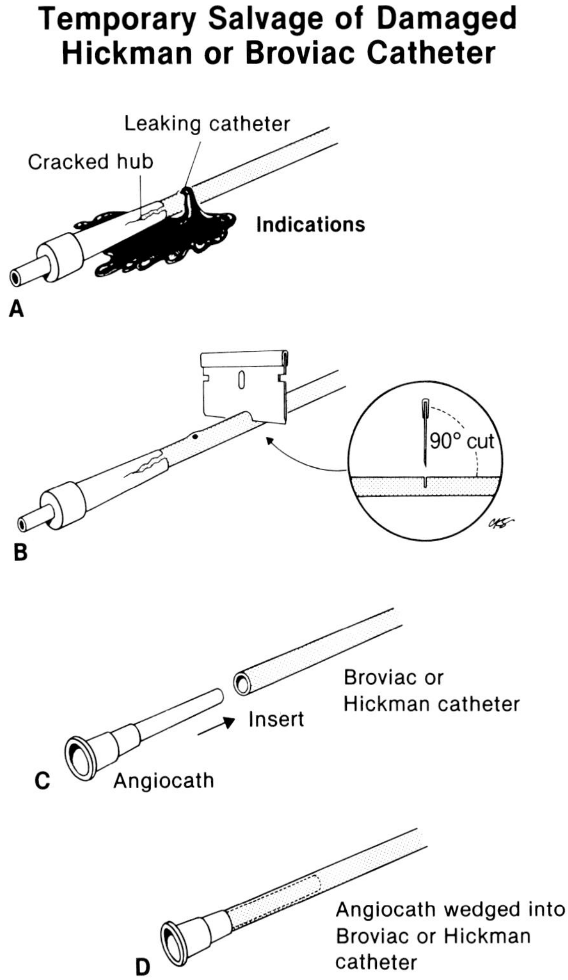

Figure 40–7 • Damage can occur to a catheter from faulty management. (***A***) Damage usually occurs around the hub when clamps and needles are used improperly. The hub can crack or the catheter can actually develop a hole. Whenever a leak is present the catheter sterility is violated and the leak must be repaired as quickly as possible. (***B***) The catheter should be washed with Betadine or some other type of antibacterial solution. It is then cut sharply and squarely proximal to the damaged area. This can be accomplished with a scalpel blade or Weck single-edged razor blade. (***C***) An angiocath is then wedged into the cut end of the catheter. An 18 French angiocath is used for a Broviac catheter; a 14 French angiocath is used for a Hickman. (***D***) The angiocath is inserted into the silicone catheter up to the hub until it is firmly wedged and watertight. This technique should be done under sterile conditions and allows the temporary salvage of a damaged Broviac or Hickman catheter. The catheter should be repaired formally as soon as a repair kit can be obtained.

This is a loop of 8 French plastic tubing (a pediatric feeding tube can be used) passing around the internasal septum (Fig. 40–11). The SBFT is secured to this tube.[43]

Table 40-7 • Dressing Change for Long-Term Catheter Exit Site

1. Remove old dressing from catheter exit site. Inspect skin for signs of inflammation and/or drainage.
2. Open a sterile dressing kit using sterile technique.
3. Wash hands and put sterile gloves on.
4. Scrub a 2-in length of catheter and a 2 × 2-in area around the exit site with acetone swabs, working from the catheter exit site to the periphery.
5. Repeat this process with povidone-iodine.
6. Apply povidine-iodine ointment to the catheter exit site.
7. Cover the catheter exit site with a slit 2 × 2 gauze. Place another one or two 2 × 2's over the exit site and tape occlusively.
8. Coil the remaining catheter on the dressing and tape in place. Allow the infusion plug to remain exposed.
9. If the catheter dressing becomes soiled, wet, or loosened between regularly scheduled dressing changes, it must be changed according to this procedure.
10. A transparent dressing may be indicated in patients who are known to react to any of the components used during the standard technique.

2. FORMULAS

The formulas used for enteral nutrition are usually complete diets with all essential ingredients. Certain special formulations are available.[41] The major differences are in calorie density and osmolarity. Formulas with 1 kcal/mL are commonly isotonic (300 mOsm). High-energy-density formulas have 1.5–2.0 kcal/mL and are hypertonic (690 mOsm). All the formulas are lactose-free. Appendix B includes a listing of many of the available enteral formulas.

Administration should be by an enteral pump to provide a continuous constant rate. Isotonic solutions are started full strength at a base rate of 25–50 mL/hr. The higher rate is considered a base rate; lower rates are only used if the patient does not tolerate the base rate. The rate is increased to the goal rate based on estimated energy needs (REI). Hypertonic solutions are usually diluted to half strength when first given unless the patient is already tolerating an isotonic formula. No more than an 8-hour volume should be hung at one time. Longer hanging times increase bacterial growth and may produce an increase in diarrhea.[44,45]

Diarrhea should be controlled, as the increased water and electrolyte losses can be detrimental. Additionally, the nutritional value of the formula with an increased transit time is diminished. Paregoric, 5–20 mL every 8 hours, can be added to the tube feedings to control the diarrhea.

IV. COMPLICATIONS OF PARENTERAL NUTRITION

A. *Catheter-Related Complications*

Technical complications of central vein access are discussed in Chapter 18. Figure 40-12 summarizes the

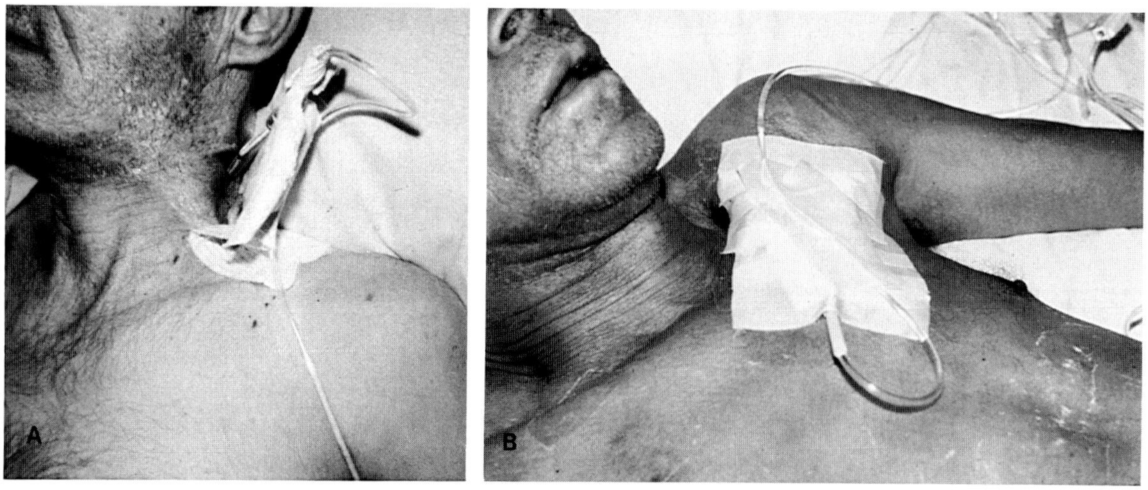

Figure 40-8 • (*A*) Improperly dressed central venous access catheter. (*B*) Properly dressed central venous access catheter.

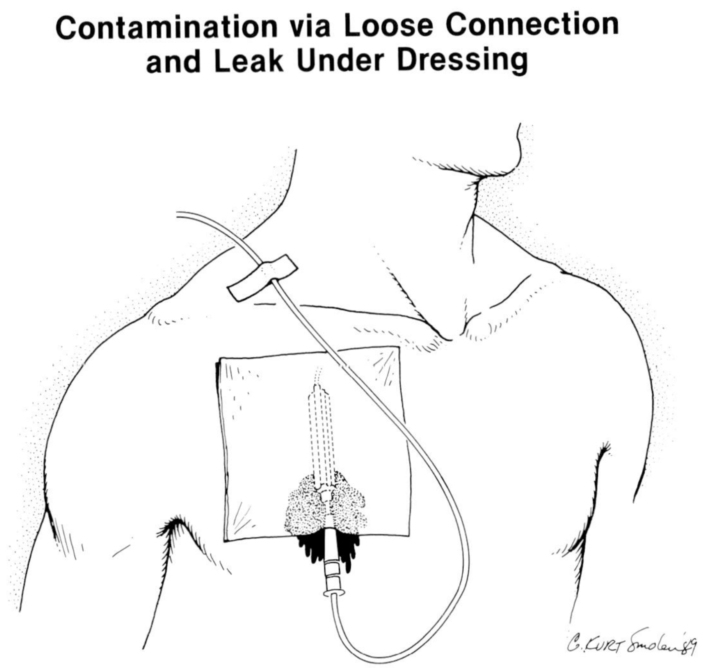

Figure 40–9 • A loose connection under a dressing can cause a leak.

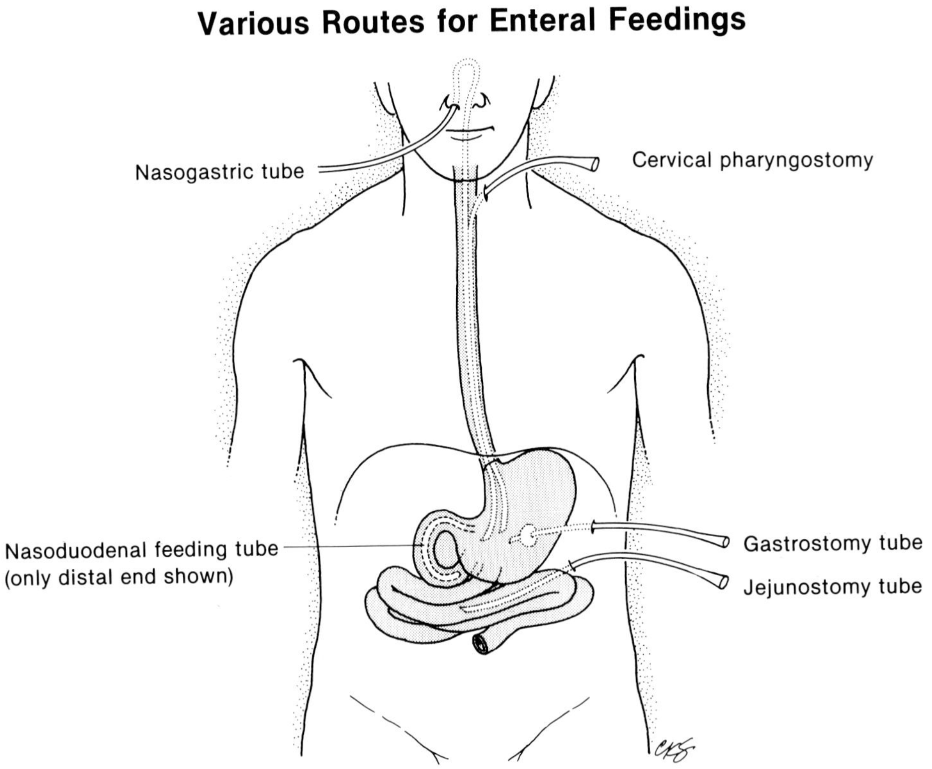

Figure 40–10 • The locations of various enteral feeding tubes are shown. The nasogastric and nasoduodenal tubes are placed without surgical procedures.

Procedure for Placing Nasopharyngeal Bridle for Feeding Tube

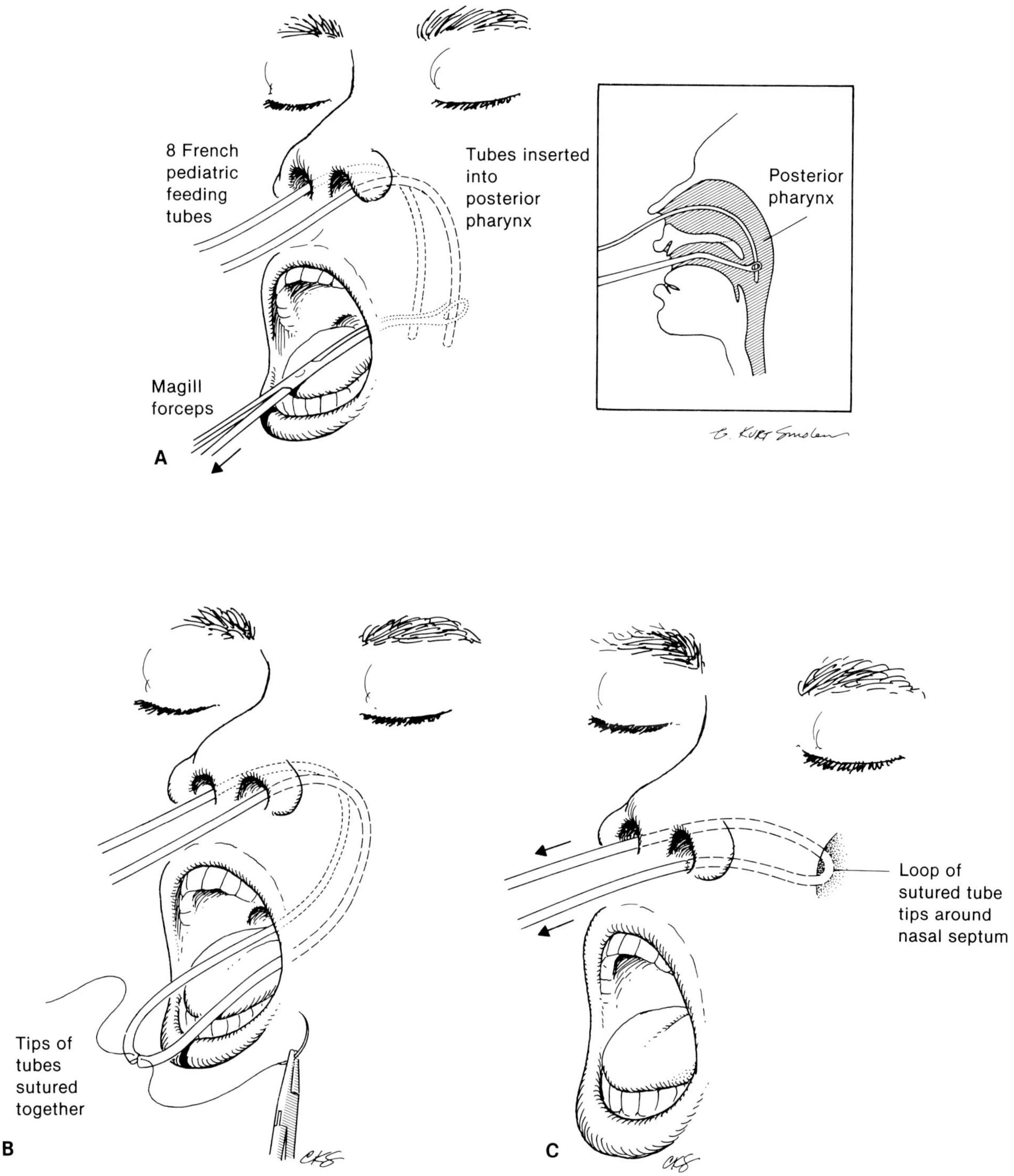

Figure 40–11 • The figure schematically shows the procedure for placing a bridle for a nasoenteric feeding tube. (***A***) Place an 8 French pediatric feeding tube into each nostril and advance these tubes into the posterior pharynx. Grasp each tube with a Magill forceps and pull out of the mouth. A laryngoscope may help locate the tube ends. (***B***) Suture the tips of the tubes together. A 2-0 silk suture on a cutting needle is used. (***C***) Slowly pull the sutured tubes from either nostril until the sutured portion of the two tubes is outside one nostril. At this time, one tube should pass completely around the internasal septum.

(continued)

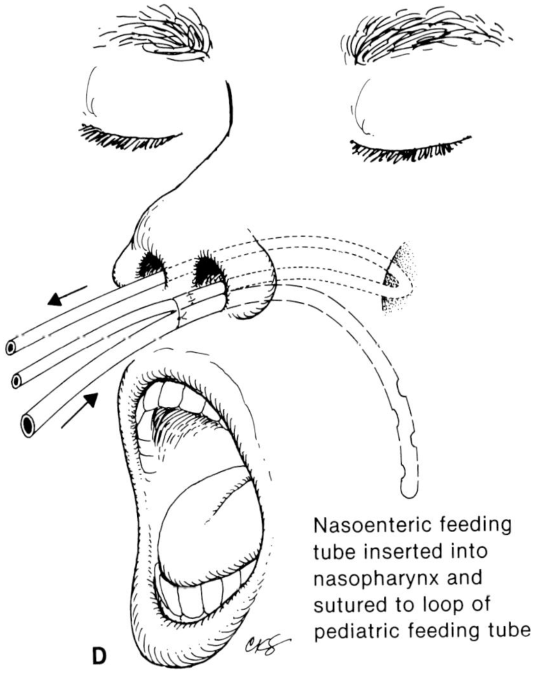

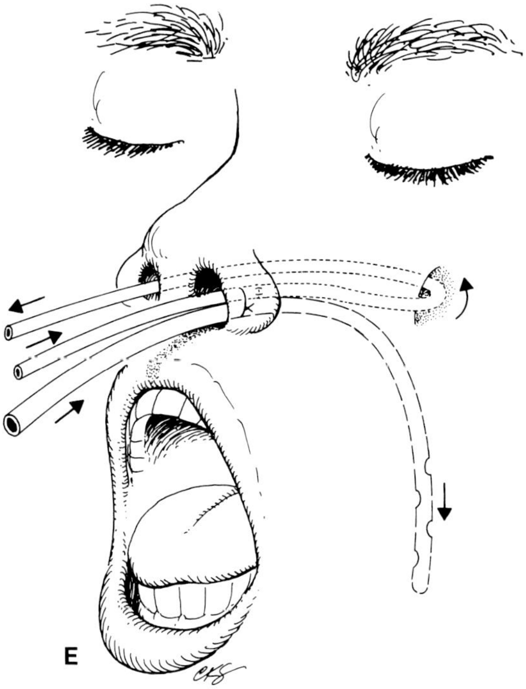

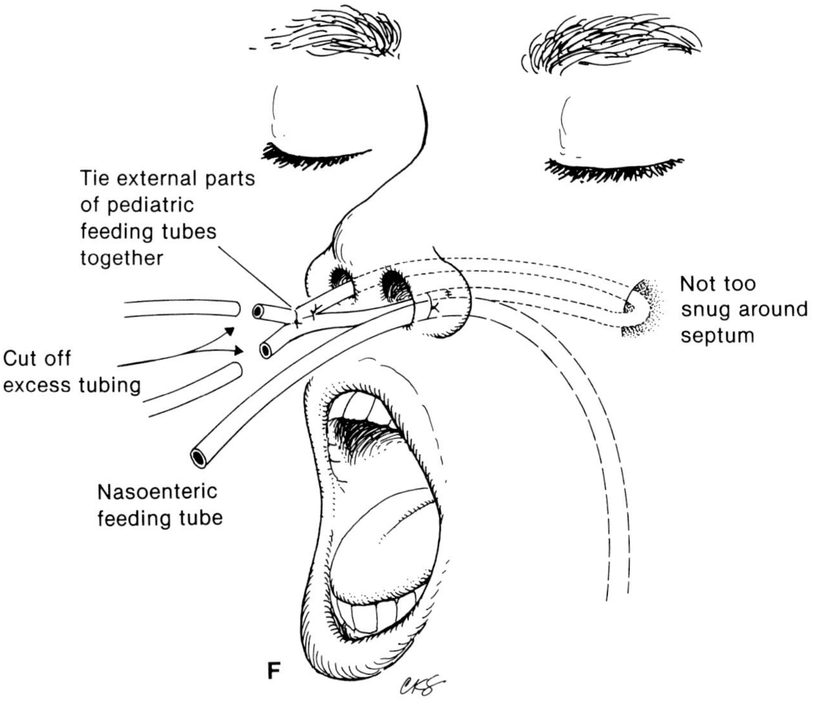

Figure 40–11 *(continued)*
(***D***) Insert a nasoenteric feeding tube without dislodging the bridle tubes. Suture the nasoenteric tube to the bridle just tightly enough to not crimp the feeding tube. (***E***) Pull on the bridle tubing that is not sutured so the suture holding the feeding tube passes into the nostril. (***F***) Suture the two ends of the bridle tubing together. Put a second suture 0.5 cm below the first. Take care not to tighten the bridle too snugly around the septum as this could produce necrosis. Cut the loose ends of the bridle distal to the second suture. (Adapted from Pursell T, Turner WW. Handbook of Intensive Nutritional Support. Dallas, UT South Western Press, 1987.)

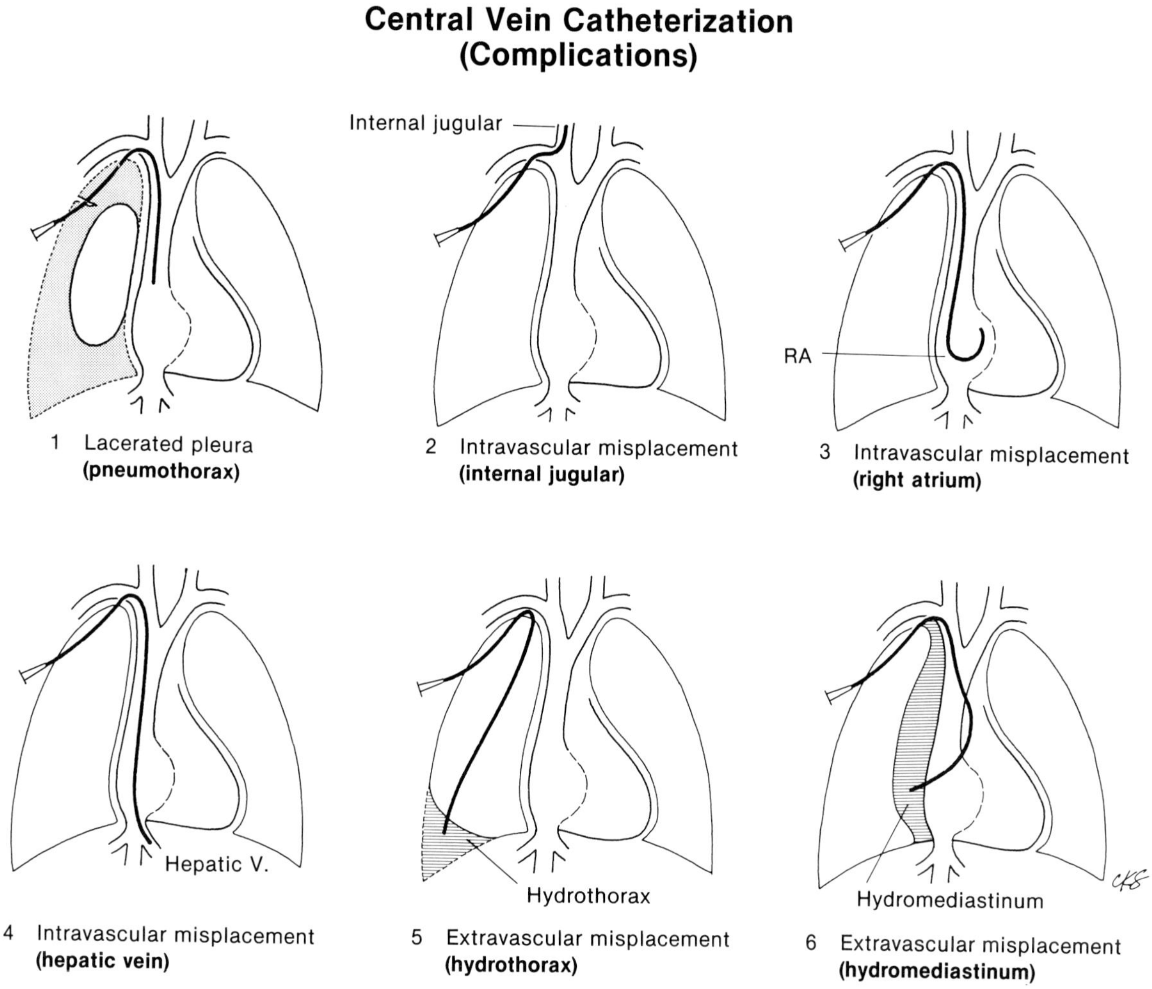

Figure 40–12 • Various complications can occur in central venous catheterization.

important technical central vein catheterization complications as they relate to parenteral nutrition (hyperalimentation). Three complications specifically related to total parenteral nutrition will be reviewed. These are catheter sepsis, catheter occlusion, and central vein thrombosis.

1. CATHETER SEPSIS

Evaluation of the patient who is receiving parenteral nutrition and has signs and symptoms of infection is always difficult. The catheter itself is usually not responsible for the septic episode, but other sites of the infusion system are more likely sources of infection (Fig. 40–13). Indeed, in one prospective series, 25% of 200 catheters were thought to be possible infectious sites.[46] A standard approach to the patient with a parenteral nutrition line and signs of sepsis is helpful. The search is usually triggered by a temperature spike. The patient must be thoroughly evaluated for other sites of infection. This evaluation should include current intravenous solutions, including blood products. The timing of new intravenous solutions and fever spikes should be noted. Intravenous sites, central and peripheral, are inspected. Blood cultures and cultures of abnormal body fluids are obtained. If an obvious source of infection is discovered, treatment is begun. If the patient improves clinically, the catheter can be left in place and treatment can be completed. However, if the patient remains febrile, has a positive blood culture without a recognized site, or has continued deterioration of vital signs, including decreasing mental orientation, then the catheter should be removed. The catheter should be cultured semiquantitatively.[47] If 15 or more bacterial colonies are discovered

Potential Sources of Contamination During Central Parenteral Nutrition

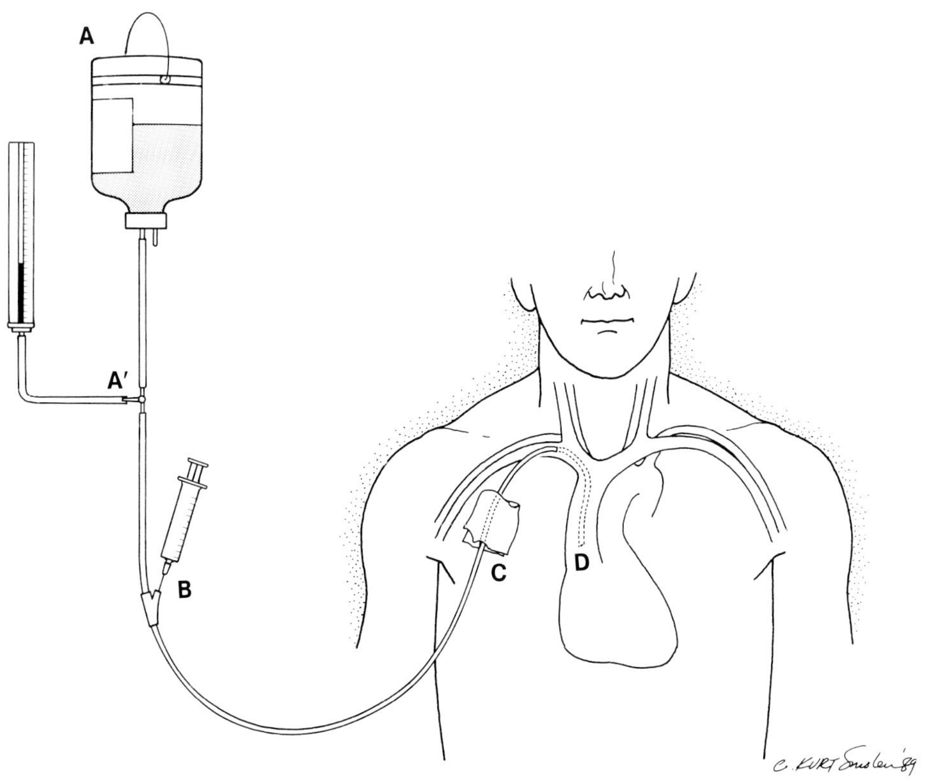

(A,A′) Hyperalimentation solution; connections
(B) Injection sites—use of catheter for other drugs, blood sampling, pressure measurement
(C) Poor dressing techniques

Figure 40–13 • Contamination can occur from several sources in parenteral nutrition. (*A*) Parenteral solution and connections. (*B*) Catheter use for other injections, blood sampling, or pressure measurement. (*C*) Poor dressing techniques. (*D*) Tip of indwelling intravenous catheter.

by this method, then the catheter is infected and antibiotic therapy is appropriate. If fewer than 15 colonies are discovered, then the catheter is contaminated but not considered infected and other infection sites must be sought. Cooper and Hopkins use Gram stains of the catheters to detect infection.[48] Catheters with one organism per 20 oil-immersion fields were more likely to have more than 15 colonies on plate culture. Most catheters had many more than one organism. The sensitivity of the Gram stain was 100% and the specificity was 96.9%.

Since the skin surrounding the catheter entrance site and the subcutaneous tunnel are the potential sources of bacteria causing catheter infection, a different site is usually favored when a catheter is removed. However, if the same site can be used, a guide wire change is a technically safe way to place a new catheter.[49,50] Guide wire exchanges do reduce the risk of technical morbidity, but if catheter infection is documented, insertion of a new, guide wire–placed catheter is discouraged. Prevention of sepsis by weekly guide wire change is also suggested, although in a recent study, a significant reduction in catheter sepsis did not occur.[50]

Host factors must be considered when estimating the risk of catheter infection and applying a protocol to avoid infection (Table 40–8). In patients with a low risk of infection, routine exchanges are not indicated and guide wire changes during febrile evaluations are helpful to decrease technical complications. In immunocompromised hosts with a high risk of infection, routine changes may be indicated. Our policy is to change central venous catheters every 3 days in this type of patient. A prospective study documented fewer infected catheters when a new site was used compared to guide wire

Table 40–8 • Factors to Consider when Central Venous Access Changes are Necessary

Routine changes new site every three days	High Infection Risk
Other infection sites	
Abnormal host immunity	
Fever common	
Multiuse catheter	
Routine guidewire changes 3–5 days	
No other infection site	
Normal host immunity	
Febrile episode	
Single-use catheter	
Elective changes	
No infection sites	
Normal host immunity	
Single-use catheter	
Febrile episode	
No catheter changes	
No infection sites	
Normal host immunity	
Single-use catheter	
No fever	Low Infection Risk
No local inflammatory signs	

The need to change central venous access lines used for total parenteral nutrition depends on the risk of infection from the venous line. Various factors must be used to estimate the infectious risk in each patient. A scale of increasing risk can be identified with a number of these factors.

changes.[51] Routine changes were associated with a 2.4% pneumothorax incidence. Familiarity with the procedure minimizes the technical risk, considering that the increased frequency of line changes diminishes the infection risk. Suggestions for catheter changes in high- and low-risk patients are outlined in Table 40–8.

Signs of sepsis occurring in a patient with a Broviac or Hickman catheter are handled slightly differently.[52] The patient is usually given antibiotics for 36 to 48 hours after initial cultures and evaluation. If no improvement is noted, then a contrast study of the catheter may be performed. A thrombolytic agent is often used if a thrombin sheath is found and other sources of sepsis are sought. If sepsis is controlled, then the antibiotics are continued for at least 14 days. This course of antibiotics is repeated if recurrent sepsis occurs after stopping antibiotics. However, the catheter is removed if sepsis does not abate with initial antibiotic therapy (48–96 hours) or if sepsis recurs after the second course of antibiotics. The indwelling subcutaneous systems are handled similarly.

2. CATHETER OCCLUSION

Occlusion of a parenteral nutrition central venous access line usually results in catheter removal and reinsertion. This problem is especially distressing to physician and patient when the occlusion occurs in one of the more permanent access lines, such as a Broviac or Hickman. Fortunately, the use of thrombolytic agents is very often successful in salvaging these catheters without removal. Streptokinase or urokinase is used to flush the catheters and dissolve the thrombus.[53] Streptokinase (125,000 IU/mL) is used to fill the occluded catheter and allowed to dwell for 2 hours. Aspiration is attempted to remove any clot. Once the catheter is open, it is irrigated with heparinized saline. A quicker alternative is 1 mL of urokinase (5000 IU/mL) placed into the catheter, and 5 minutes later the catheter is aspirated. If results are poor, the sequence can be repeated and the dwell time of the urokinase can be increased to 30 to 60 minutes. The catheter is irrigated with heparin once flow is reestablished.

Sluggish flow in these catheters should not be ignored. Thrombolytic therapy in partially occluded catheters is more successful than in totally occluded catheters. Fibrinolytic therapy was successful in restoring patency in 351 of 352 occluded catheters.[54] In catheters that are unresponsive to thrombolysis, a guide wire aspiration technique is described.[55] Under radiographic guidance, balloon thrombectomy is another possible option.

3. CENTRAL VEIN THROMBOSIS

Thrombosis of the subclavian or internal jugular vein after central vein catheterization occurs 4% to 26%.[56] Three types of thrombosis are described: (1) fibrin sleeve formation, (2) mural thrombosis, and (3) occlusive thrombosis. Fibrin sleeve formation is common (14% to 100%) around central vein catheters. During pull-out venography, this sleeve has been shown to embolize. The clinical importance of this finding remains unknown, although some minor symptoms of pulmonary emboli have been noted following catheter removal.[57]

Even with mural or occlusive thrombosis, most patients remain minimally symptomatic or asymptomatic. Neck pain, arm swelling, fever, and leukocytosis are possible. Diagnosis is often made by sonography or computed tomography. The risk of pulmonary embolus is estimated at 5% and warrants anticoagulation therapy unless this is contraindicated.[58] The incidence of thrombosis with Hickman catheters is 10%, which is not significantly different from that with other catheter types.[59]

B. *Metabolic Complications*

1. Glucose

The most common metabolic abnormalities are associated with glucose and include hyperglycemia, hypoglycemia, hyperosmolar coma, fatty infiltration of the liver, and excessive carbon dioxide production. Glucose intolerance happens in 25% of patients receiving parenteral nutrition.[60] Patients with diabetes, sepsis, shock, elective surgery, or major trauma have a decrease in glucose use and are prone to hyperglycemia. Careful monitoring and adherence to the guidelines for beginning and advancing the infusion rate for these solutions should decrease the incidence of hyperglycemia.

Hyperosmolar coma is now less common than when hyperalimentation was first introduced. Hyperglycemic, hyperosmolar, nonketotic coma is identified by glucose levels greater than 1000 mg/dL, osmolarities greater than 350 mOsm/L, and coma. It results in a mortality rate of 50%. If this syndrome is identified, the parenteral nutrition solution should be stopped immediately, insulin infused as a continuous intravenous drip (10–20 units/hr), and half normal (0.45%) saline infused at 250 mL/hr. Fluid and insulin administration must be adjusted for the severity of the clinical syndrome. Volume repletion is always required and bicarbonate administration is occasionally needed.

Hypoglycemia may occur if the glucose infusion is suddenly discontinued. Guidelines for stopping parenteral nutrition involve tapering the infusions over a few days. This is done to avoid rebound hypoglycemia from excess insulin produced by a stimulated pancreas. Wagman and associates studied 48 patients during a 2-hour tapering of a 25% dextrose and 4.25% amino acid solution.[61] No hypoglycemic symptoms were produced in these patients, although one blood glucose below 60 mg/dL was recorded. Thus, a 2-hour tapering period is suggested as safe. If other sugar sources are available, such as intravenous D5W or enteral nutrition, prolonged tapering is certainly not indicated.

Abnormal liver function secondary to steatosis of the liver may occur in 60% to 90% of patients given glucose-based parenteral nutrition. These abnormalities become evident after 1–3 weeks and correlate most closely with the rate and concentration of glucose infusion. The addition of fat as 25% of the calories avoids the development of hepatic steatosis.[62] Conversely, too much fat has been associated with elevated liver enzymes.[63] A balanced mix of calories with fat providing at least one third is the best way to produce better glucose tolerance and fewer hepatic complications.

Prolonged hyperalimentation may affect gallbladder function secondary to decreased intestinal hormone output. An increased incidence of cholelithiasis is documented in these patients.[64] Stasis of the gallbladder can be prevented by cholecystokinin, and daily injection of this hormone has been suggested as one way to decrease gallbladder stasis and, it is hoped, prevent gallstones in these patients.[65] A more practical approach is to begin enteral nutrition as quickly as possible.

Infusions of calories in excess of demands may be harmful to pulmonary function. When glucose is the primary source of calories, there is an increased level of carbon dioxide production, which can require an increase in minute ventilation. This increase averaged 26% when compared to patients receiving a glucose–lipid mix.[66] This increased demand may become obvious during attempts to wean critically ill patients. Nutritional management of these patients should include increasing fat calories to 40% to 50%.[67]

2. Amino Acids

Abnormalities of protein metabolism were common before crystalline amino acids were introduced. The derangements attributed to protein metabolism included azotemia, hyperchloremic acidosis, and hyperammonemia. These are rare today.

3. Fat

When fat is not used in a nutritional program, essential fatty acid (EFA) deficiency will develop in most patients within 2 to 6 weeks. Linoleate, an 18-carbon chain fat, is the major essential fatty acid in humans. Linoleate is used to synthesize eicosatrienoate and arachidonate. As linoleate is depleted, endogenous fatty acids are used. Unfortunately, endogenous fatty acids (such as Palmitate and stearate) cannot be metabolized to eicosatrienoate and arachidonate (as is linoleate in the diet) but result in a fatty acid unique to essential fatty acid deficiency: 5,8, 11-eicosatrienoate (Fig. 40–14). A triene-tetraene ratio (20:3w9/20:4w6) greater than 0.40 is used to indicate an essential fatty acid deficiency. Low levels of linoleic and arachidonic acid are associated with

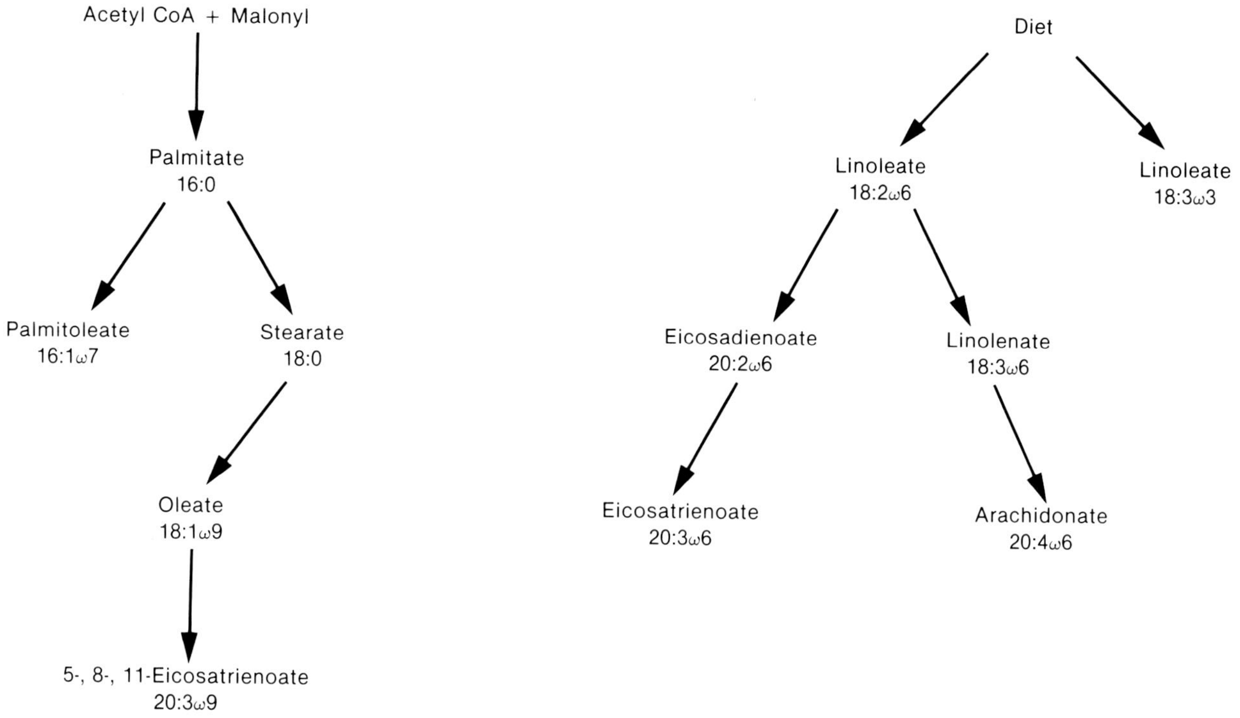

Biosynthetic pathways of the major fatty acids. The endogenous fatty acids are derived from palmitate and stearate. Linoleate is the major essential fatty acid in humans.

Figure 40–14 • Metabolic pathways are shown for the major fatty acids. (*Right*) Dietary linoleate pathway. (*Left*) Endogenous palmitate and stearate pathways.

high levels of 5,8,11-eicosatrienoate producing an increase in the serum triene-tetraene ratio greater than 0.4 (Fig. 40–15).

Routine measurement of fatty acids is not done and EFA deficiency will occur within 2 weeks of fat-free nutrition.[68] This deficiency can be prevented by providing linoleate at 2% to 3% of total calories.

Other possible complications with fat infusions include hyperlipemia, liver enzyme changes, and decreases in respiratory function. These problems are all seen when too much fat is given or when it is given too rapidly. The pulmonary effect is characterized by a reduced P_aO_2, decreased carbon monoxide diffusion capacity, and increased pulmonary artery pressure. The hyperlipidemia associated with fat emulsion administration has been suggested as the cause. However, very recent studies demonstrate that alterations in vascular tone resulting in ventilation–perfusion inequalities secondary to fat-induced increases in prostaglandin production are a more likely explanation.[69]

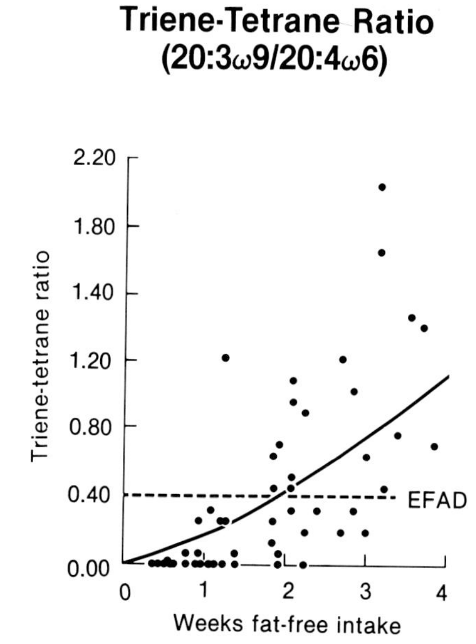

Figure 40–15 • Free fatty acid deficiency states are associated with a triene–tetraene ratio greater than 0.4. EFAD = essential fatty acid deficiency.

Table 40–9 • Biochemical Functions and Manifestations Deficiency of Essential Trace Elements

Element	Sites of Action	Key Biochemical Functions	Deficiency
Cr	"Glucose tolerance factor"	Glucose metabolism (?); mediates insulin effect on membranes	Impaired glucose clearance (many species); impaired growth, reproduction, and lifespan (rats and mice)
Co	Coenzyme B_{12}	Biological methylation (eg, methionine synthesis)	Pernicious anemia (humans) methylmalonic aciduria (humans)
Cu	Metalloenzymes (eg, cytochrome oxidase, lysine oxidase, and tyrosinase)	Mitochondrial function; collagen metabolism; melanin formation	Menkes' syndrome (man); anemia, leukopenia, neutropenia (animals and humans)
Fl	Unknown	(?) Iron absorption	Anemia (mice); impaired growth and re production (rats)
I	Thyroglobulin; thyroxine; triiodothyronine	Cellular oxidation processes	Thyroid diseases (animals and humans)
Mn	Pyruvate carboxylase; activates many intracellular enzymes	Oxidative phosphorylation; fatty acid metabolism, synthesis of proteins, mucopolysaccharides, and cholesterol	Defective growth, bony anomalies, reproductive dysfunction, and central nervous system abnormalities in many species
Mo	Flavoenzymes (eg, xanthine oxidase)	Xanthine; hypoxanthine metabolism	Growth retardation; impaired urate clearance (chicks)
Ni	Ribonucleic acid; serum "nickeloplasmin"	(?) Nucleic acid stabilization; (?) membrane structure and function	Impaired reproduction (rats); deranged liver lipid and phospholipid metabolism (chicks)
Se	Glutathione peroxidase (erythrocytes); "cytochrome" (muscle)	Degradation of intracellular peroxids; oxidation of glutathione	Liver necrosis (rats); "white-muscle disease" (lambs); exudative diathesis (chicks)
Si	Mucopolysaccharides	(?) Connective-tissue structure	Impaired growth and connective-tissue formation
Sn	Fatty tissue	?Redox catalyst	Growth and dentition (rats)
V	Hemovanadin	Oxygen transport; (?) redox catalyst	Impaired growth, reproduction, bone, and lipid metabolism (chickens, rats)
Zn	Metalloenzymes (eg, alcohol dehydrogenase, carboxypeptidase, and DNA polymerase)	Metabolism of lipids, protein, carbohydrates, and nucleic acids	Parakeratosis (swine); acrodermatitis enteropathica (humans); (?) hypogonadism

Ref: Cerda JJ, Baumgartner TG: ASPEN 4:7, 1982.

4. ELECTROLYTES AND TRACE ELEMENTS

Hypophosphatemia may cause lethargy, anorexia, muscle weakness, paresthesias, and coma. Acute hemolytic anemia and platelet dysfunction are also reported. Myocardial depression is also described with severe phosphate depletion.[70] Phosphate is used intracellularly for synthesis of ATP, DNA, and membrane phospholipids. Approximately 1–2 mol of phosphate are incorporated into each gram of nitrogen synthesized. Metabolism of glucose, phosphate, and insulin is closely linked and a phosphate deficiency will increase insulin resistance.[71]

Hypomagnesemia is manifested by weakness, nausea, vomiting, and irritability.[72] Convulsions can occur in severe cases. Signs and symptoms are similar to those of hypocalcemia. The body contains approximately 2000 mEq of magnesium, of which 60% is in bone. Gastrointestinal losses account for most of the losses in deficiency states.

Zinc is an essential trace element required for RNA and DNA synthesis and for a variety of zinc-dependent enzymes. It is the most commonly encountered trace element deficiency during parenteral nutrition.[73] Clinical manifestations of zinc deficiency include impaired wound healing, growth retardation, impaired immunity, diarrhea, and acrodermatitis. (Acrodermatitis is crusting skin lesions, especially around the eyes, nose, mouth, buttocks, and scrotum.[74])

Copper depletion is the second most common trace element deficiency during total parenteral nutrition.[73] Inadequate copper levels are associated with anemia, leukopenia, and neutropenia. Other electrolyte and vitamin deficiencies are listed in Table 40–9.

V. APPENDIX A

Table 40–A1 • Composition of Four Commercial Amino Acid Solutions (8.5% Concentrations)

	Aminosyn (Abbott)	Freamine III (McGaw)	Novamine (Cutter)	Travasol (Travenol)
L-Amino acids (g/100 mL)	8.5	8.5	8.5	
Total nitrogen (g/100 mL)	1.3	1.3	1.35	1.4
Osmolarity (mOsm/L) (calculated)	850	810	785	860
Approximate pH	5.3	6.5	5.6	6.0
Essential amino acids (mg/100 mL)				
L-Leucine	810	770	590	526
L-Isoleucine	620	590	420	406
L-Valine	680	560	550	590
L-Phenylalanine	380	480	590	526
L-Tryptophan	150	130	140	152
L-Methionine	340	450	420	492
L-Threonine	460	340	420	356
L-Lysine	624	620	673	492
Nonessential amino acids (mg/100 mL)				
L-Alanine	1100	600	1200	1760
L-Arginine	850	810	840	880
L-Histidine	260	240	500	372
L-Proline	750	950	500	356
L-Serine	370	500	340	—
L-Tyrosine	44	—	20	34
L-Glutamic acid	—	—	420	—
L-Aspartic acid	—	—	250	—
Glycine (AAA, USP)	1100	1190	590	1760
Cysteine	—	20	40	—
Electrolytes				
Sodium (mEq/500 mL)	—	5	—	—
Potassium (mEq/500 mL)	2.7	—	—	—
Magnesium (mEq/500 mL)	—	—	—	—
Chloride (mEq/500 mL)	17.5	1.5	—	17
Acetate (mEq/500 mL)	45	36	—	26
Phosphate (mM/L)	—	5	—	—

Table 40–A2 • Composition of High-Essential Amino Acid Formulas

Content	Aminosyn RF, 5.2% (Abbott)	Nephramine, 5.4% (McGaw)	Renamin (Travenol)
Essential amino acids (mg/100 mL)			
L-Leucine	726	880	600
L-Isoleucine	462	560	500
L-Phenylalanine	726	880	490
L-Methionine	726	880	500
L-Threonine	330	400	380
L-Valine	528	640	820
L-Lysine	535	640	450
L-Tryptophan	165	200	160
Nonessential amino acids (mg/100 mL)			
L-Arginine	600	—	630
L-Histidine	429	250	420
L-Cysteine	—	20	—
L-Alanine	—	—	560
L-Proline	—	—	350
L-Serine	—	—	300
L-Tyrosine	—	—	40
Glycine (AAA, USP)	—	—	300
Electrolytes (mEq/100 mL)			
Acetate	10.5	4.4	6.0
Chloride	—	—	3.1
Sodium	—	0.6	—
Potassium	0.54	—	—
L-Amino acid content (g/100 mL)	5.2	5.4	6.5
Total nitrogen (g/100 mL)	0.79	0.65	1.0
Approximate pH	5.2	6.5	6.0
Approximate osmolarity (mOsm/L)	475	440	600

Table 40–A3 • Composition of High-BCAA Products

	Hepatamine 8% (McGaw)	Freamine HBC 6.9% (McGaw)
Essential amino acids (mg/100 mL)		
L-Isoleucine	900	760
L-Leucine	1100	1370
L-Valine	840	880
L-Lysine	610	410
L-Methionine	100	250
L-Phenylalanine	100	320
L-Threonine	450	200
L-Tryptophan	66	90
Nonessential amino acids (mg/100 mL)		
L-Alanine	770	400
L-Arginine	600	580
L-Histidine	240	160
L-Proline	800	630
L-Serine	800	330
Glycine (AAA, USP)	900	330
L-Cysteine	20	20
Electrolytes		
Sodium (mEq/L)	10	10
Acetate (mEq/L)	62	57
Chloride (mEq/L)	3	3
Phosphate (mEq/L)	10	—
L-Amino acid content (g/100 mL)	8.0	6.9
Approximate pH	6.5	6.5
Osmolarity (mOsm/L)	785	625

Table 40-A4 • Commercial Fat Emulsion Products

	Intralipid 10% (KABI) (Vitrum)	Liposyn II 10% (Abbott)	Soyocal 10% (Alpha Therapeutic)	Travamulsion 10% (Travenol)	Intralipid 20% (KABI Vitrum)	Liposyn II 20% (Abbott)	Soyocal 20% (Alpha Therapeutic)
Oil	Soybean	Safflower and soybean	Soybean	Soybean	Soybean	Safflower and soybean	Soybean
Fatty acid Content (%)							
Linoleic	54.0	65.8	49.0–60.0	56.0	50.0	65.8	49.0–60.0
Oleic	26.0	17.7	21.0–26.0	23.0	26.0	17.7	21.0–26.0
Palmitic	9.0	8.8	9.0–13.0	11.0	10.0	8.8	9.0–13.0
Linolenic	8.0	4.2	6.0– 9.0	6.0	9.0	4.2	6.0–9.0
Stearic	0	3.4	3.0– 5.0	0.0	0	3.4	3.0–5.0
Calories/mL	1.1	1.1	1.1	1.1	2.0	2.0	2.0
Osmolarity (mOsm/L)	280	320	280	270	330	340	315

VI. Appendix B

Table 40-B1 • Categorization of Enteral Feeding Formulas in Therapeutically Comparable Groups

- Nuritionally complete, lactose-free formulas
  - 1 kcal/mL
    - Standard protein
      - Tube/oral
        - Ensure, Travasorb, Nutri-Aid, Ensure HN
      - Tube only
        - Osmolite, Isocal, Osmolite HN, Compleat Modified
      - Low-fat, oligomeric
        - Travasorb STD, Criticare HN, Standard Vivonex, Vital HN, Travasorb HN, Vivonex HN
      - Fiber-containing
        - Enrich
    - High-protein
      - Sustacal, Isotein HN
  - 1.5 kcal/mL
    - Standard protein
      - Ensure Plus, Sustacal HC, Ensure Plus HN
    - High protein
      - TraumaCal
  - 2 kcal/mL
    - Standard protein
      - Magnacal, Isocal HCN
- Milk-based oral supplements
  - Meritene, Sustagen, Carnation Instant Breakfast
- Specialized formulas
  - Hepatic encephalopathy
    - Hepatic-Aid, Travasorb Hepatic
  - Renal failure
    - Amin-Aid, Travasorb Renal
    - Trauma (44–50% branched-chain amino acids)
    - Traum-Aid HBC, Stresstein
- Modular supplements
  - Protein
    - Propac, Pro-Mix, Casec, Gevral
- Carbohydrate
  - Polycose, Moducal, Sumacal, Cal Plus
- Fat
  - MCT Oil
  - Long-chain triglycerides
    - Microlipid, Lipomul oral

(Adapted from Heimburger DC, Weinsier RL. Guidelines for evaluating and categorizing enteral feeding formulas according to therapeutic equivalence. Parenteral Enteral Nutr 9:61–67, 1985.)

Table 40–B2 • Composition of Nutritionally Complete, Lactose-free Enteral Formulas

Category and Product	kcal/mL	mOsm/kg Water	Non protein kcal/g	Composition/L Protein kcal% Total	Fat kcal% Total	Carbohydrate kcal% Total	Na mg/1000 kcal	K mEq/1000 kcal
Standard protein (1 kcal/mL)								
Ensure	1.06	450	153	14	31.5	54.5	797	38
Travasorb	1	450	144	15	33	58	736	30
Nutri-Aid	1.1	290	142	15	31.5	54	690	30
Ensure HN	1.06	470	124	17	30	53	877	38
Osmolite	1.06	300	153	14	31	55	518	25
Isocal	1.06	300	167	13	37	50	498	32
Osmolite HN	1.06	310	124	17	30	53	877	38
Compleat-modified	1.07	300	131	16	31	53	636	34
Low-fat, Oligomeric								
Standard Vivonex	1	550	286	8	1	91	468	30
Vivonex HN	1	810	127	18	1	81	529	30
Fiber-containing								
Enrich	1.1	480	148	15	30	55	773	36
Standard protein (1.5 kcal/mL)								
Ensure Plus	1.5	600	146	15	32	53	761	40
Sustacal HCs	1.5	650	134	16	34	50	563	25
Ensure Plus HN	1.5	650	125	17	30	53	789	31
High-protein								
Traumacal	1.5	550	89	22	41	38	800	24
Standard protein (2 kcal/mL)								
Magnacal	2	590	154	14	36	50	500	16
Isocal HCN	2	740	145	15	40	45	400	18

Table 40–B3 • Composition of Oral Supplements and Specialized Enteral Formulas

Category and Product	kcal/mL	mOsm/kg Water	Nonprotein kcal/g Nitrogen	Protein kcal% Total	Fat kcal% Total	Carbohydrate kcal% Total	Na mg/1000 kcal	K mEq/1000 kcal
Specialized formulas								
Hepatic encephalopathy (high in BCAA, low in aromatic amino acids)								
Hepatic-Aid	1.6	1158	215	10	20	70	201	<3
Travasorb, hepatic	1.1	690	218	11	12	77	395	26
Renal failure (essential amino acids)								
Amin-Aid	1.9	1095	800	4	21	75	169	<3
Travasorb, renal	1.35	590	362	7	12	81	0	0
Trauma (44–50% BCAA)								
Traum-Aid HBC	1	675	102	22	11	67	529	30
Stresstein	1.2	910	97	23	20	57	660	28

VII. REFERENCES

1. Rhoads JE, Dudrick SJ, Vars HM. History of intravenous nutrition. In Rombeau JL, Caldwell MD (eds). Parenteral Nutrition. Philadelphia, WB Saunders, 1986, 1–8.
2. Aubaniac R. L'injection intraveineuse sous-claviculaire: Avantages et technique. Presse Med 60:1456- , 1952.
3. Steffee WP. Malnutrition in hospitalized patients. JAMA 244:2630–2635, 1980.
4. Sarr MG, Mayo S. Needle catheter jejunostomy: An unappreciated and misunderstood advance in the care of patients after major abdominal operations. Mayo Clin Proc 63:565–572, 1988.
5. McLaren DS. A fresh look at protein-energy malnutrition in the hospitalized patient. Nutrition 4:1–6, 1988.
6. Abbott WC, Echenique MM, Bistrian BR, et al. Nutritional care of the trauma patient. Surg Gynecol Obstet 157:585—595, 1983.
7. Baker JP, Detsky AS, Wesson DE, et al. Nutritional assessment. A comparison of clinical judgment and objective measurements. New Engl J Med 306:969–972, 1982.
8. Muller JM, Keller HW, Brenner U, et al. Indications and effects of preoperative parenteral nutrition. World J Surg 10:53–63, 1986.
9. Murray MJ, Marsh M, Wochos DN, et al. Nutritional assessment of intensive-care unit patients. Mayo Clin Proc 63: 1106–1115, 1988.
10. Feurer ID, Mullen JL. Measurement of energy expenditure. In Rombeau JL, Caldwell MD (eds). Parenteral Nutrition. Philadelphia, WB Saunders, 1986, 225–235.
11. Turner WW, Ireton CS, Hunt JL, et al. Predicting energy expenditures in burned patients. J Trauma 25:11–16, 1985.
12. Saffle JR, Medina E, Raymond J, et al. Use of indirect calorimetry in the nutritional management of burned patients. J Trauma 25:32–39, 1985.
13. Shizgal HM, Martin MF. Caloric requirement of the critically ill septic patient. Crit Care Med 16:312–317, 1988.
14. Brandi LS, Oleggini M, Lachi S, et al. Energy metabolism of surgical patients in the early postoperative period: A reappraisal. Crit Care Med 16:18–22, 1988.
15. Cerra FB, Siegel JH, Coleman B, et al. A failure of exogenous nutritional support. Ann Surg 192:570–580, 1980.
16. Freund H, Dienstag J, Lehrich J, et al. Infusion of branched-chain enriched amino acid solution in patients with hepatic encephalopathy. Ann Surg 196:209–220, 1982.
17. Cerra FB, Blackburn G, Hirsch J, et al. The effect of stress level, amino acid formula, and nitrogen dose on nitrogen retention in traumatic and septic stress. Ann Surg 205:282–287, 1987.
18. Pedersen P, Li S, Hasselgren P, et al. Administration of balanced or BCAA-enriched amino acid solution in septic rats. Ann Surg 208:714–720, 1988.
19. Barr LH, Dunn GD, Brennan MF. Essential fatty acid deficiency during total parenteral nutrition. Ann Surg 193:304–311, 1981.
20. Nordenstrom J, Carpentier YA, Askanazi J, et al. Metabolic utilization of intravenous fat emulsion during total parenteral nutrition. Ann Surg 196:221–231, 1982.
21. MacFie J. Metabolic properties of intravenous fat emulsions during total parenteral nutrition. Nutrition 3:351–352, 1987.
22. Kleinberger G. New aspects of parenteral nutrition with fat emulsions in injured patients. World J Surg 10:20–32, 1986.
23. Tengborn J. Technical aspects on the all-in-one administration technique. Nutrition 3:353–354, 1987.
24. Chernow B, Smith J, Rainey TG, et al. Hypomagnesemia: Implications for the critical care specialist. Crit Care Med 10:193–196, 1982.
25. Sloan GM, White DE, Brennan MF. Calcium and phosphorus metabolism during total parenteral nutrition. Ann Surg 197:1–6, 1983.
26. Hamstra RD, Block MH, Schocket AL. Intravenous iron dextran in clinical medicine. JAMA 243:1726–1731, 1980.
27. Cerda JJ, Baumgartner TG. Trace element requirements during total parenteral nutrition. ASPEN 4:1–7, 1982.
28. Echenique MM, Bistrian BR, Blackburn GL. Theory and techniques of nutritional support in the ICU. Crit Care Med 10:546–549, 1982.
29. Pursell T, Turner WW. Handbook of Intensive Nutritional Support. Dallas, UT Southwestern Press, 1987.
30. Leutenegger AF, Frutiger A. All-in-one: Conventional versus two different all-in-one solutions for total parenteral nutrition of surgical intensive care patients. World J Surg 10:84–94, 1986.
31. Fabri PJ, Mirtallo JM, Ruberg RL, et al. Incidence and prevention of thrombosis of the subclavian vein during total parenteral nutrition. Surg Gynecol Obstet 155:238–240, 1982.
32. Laster J, Cikrit D, Walker N, et al. The heparin-induced thrombocytopenia syndrome: An update. Surgery 102:763–770, 1987.
33. Pessa ME, Howard RJ. Complications of Hickman-Broviac catheters. Surg Gynecol Obstet 161:257–260, 1985.
34. Wachs T, Watkins S, Hickman RO. No more pokes: A review of parenteral access devices. J Nutritional Support Services 7:12–18, 1987.
35. Bothe A, Piccione W, Ambrosino JJ, et al. Implantable central venous access system. Am J Surg 147:565–569, 1984.
36. Forlaw L, Torosian MH. Central venous catheter care. In Rombeau JL, Caldwell MD (eds). Parenteral Nutrition. Philadelphia, WB Saunders, 1986, 316–330.
37. Jacobs DL, Rikkers LF, Forst CF, et al. Effects of enteral vs parenteral nutrition on reticuloendothelial function. J Surg Res 42:661–664, 1987.
38. McArdle AH, Palmason C, Morency I, et al. A rationale for enternal feeding as the preferable route for hyperalimentation. Surgery 90:606–623, 1981.
39. Adams S, Dellinger EP, Wertz MJ, et al. Enteral versus parenteral nutrition support following laparotomy for trauma: A randomized prospective trial. J Trauma 26:882–891, 1986.
40. Meyer J, Yurt RW, Duhaney R, et al. Differential neutrophil activation before and after endotoxin infusion in enterally versus parenterally fed volunteers. Surg Gynecol Obstet 167:501–509, 1988.
41. Hand RW, Kempster M, Levy JH, et al. Inadvertent transbronchial insertion of narrow-bore feeding tubes into the pleural space. JAMA 251:2396–2397, 1984.
42. Levenson R, Turner WW, Dyson A, et al. Do weighted nasoenteric feeding tubes facilitate duodenal intubations? J Parenteral Enteral Nutr 12:135–137, 1988.
43. Levenson RK, Turner WW. Nasoenteral intubation: A guide to techniques. Nutr Clin Pract 1:259–261, 1986.
44. Anliker AW. Bacterial contamination of continuous-infusion enteral feedings. J Nutritional Support Services 8:11–12 & 32, 1988.
45. Crocker KS, Krey SH, Markovic M, et al. Microbial growth in clinically used enteral delivery systems. Am J Infect Control 14:250–256, 1986.
46. Ryan JA, Abel RM, Abbott WM, et al. Catheter complications in total parenteral nutrition: A prospective study of 200 consecutive patients. New Engl J Med 290:757–761, 1974.

47. Maki DG, Weise CE, Sarafin HW. A semiquantitative culture method for identifying intravenous-catheter-related infection. New Engl J Med 296:1305–1309, 1977.
48. Cooper GL, Hopkins CC. Rapid diagnosis of intravascular catheter-associated infection by direct gram staining of catheter segments. New Engl J Med 312:1142–1147, 1985.
49. Sitzmann JV, Townsend TR, Siler MC, et al. Septic and technical complications of central venous catheterization. Ann Surg 202:766–770, 1985.
50. Bozzetti F, Terno G, Bonfanti G, et al. Prevention and treatment of central venous catheter sepsis by exchange via a guide wire. Ann Surg 198:48–51, 1983.
51. Synder RH, Archer FJ, Endy T, et al. Catheter infection: A comparison of two catheter maintenance techniques. Ann Surg 208:651–653, 1988.
52. Schuman ES. Outpatient management of Hickman catheter sepsis. Infect Surg February:103–106, 1987.
53. Faubion WC, Bollish SJ, Wesley JR. Central venous catheter occlusion treated by thrombolytic agents. J Nutritional Support Services 3:24–26. 1983.
54. Hurtubise MR, Bottino JC, Lawson M. Restoring patency of occluded central venous catheters. Arch Surg 115:212–213, 1980.
55. Hawkins IF, Paige RM. Restoring patency of central venous catheters. AJR 140:391--392, 1983.
56. Efsing HO, Lindblad B, Mark J, et al. Thromboembolic complications from central venous catheters: A comparison of three catheter materials. World J Surg 7:419–423, 1983.
57. Brismar B, Hardstedt C, Jacobson S. Diagnosis of thrombosis by catheter phlebography after prolonged central venous catheterization. Ann Surg 194:779–783, 1981.
58. Cohen JP, Persky MS, Reede DL. Internal jugular vein thrombosis. Laryngoscope 95:1478–1482, 1985.
59. Wagman LD, Kirkemo A, Johnston MR. Venous access: A prospective, randomized study of the Hickman catheter. Surgery 95:303–308, 1984.
60. Meguid MM, Akahoshi MP, Jeffers S, et al. Amelioration of metabolic complications of conventional total parenteral nutrition. Arch Surg 119:1294–1298, 1984.
61. Wagman LD, Newsome HH, Miller KB, et al. The effect of acute discontinuation of total parenteral nutrition. Ann Surg 204:524–529, 1986.
62. Buzby GP, Mullen JL, Stein TP, et al. Manipulation of TPN caloric substrate and fatty infiltration of the liver. J Surg Res 31:46–54, 1981.
63. Salvian AJ, Allardyce DB. Impaired bilirubin secretion during total parenteral nutrition. J Surg Res 28:547–550, 1980.
64. Pitt HA, King W, Mann LL, et al. Increased risk of cholelithiasis with prolonged total parenteral nutrition. Am J Surg 145:106–112, 1983.
65. Doty JE, Pitt HA, Porter-Fink V, et al. Cholecystokinin prophylaxis of parenteral nutrition-induced gallbladder disease. Ann Surg 201:76–80, 1985.
66. Askanazi J, Nordenstrom J, Rosenbaum SH, et al. Nutrition for patients with respiratory failure. Anesthesiology 54:373–376, 1981.
67. Askanazi J, Weissman C, Rosenbaum SH, et al: Nutrition and the respiratory system. Crit Care Med 10:163–172, 1982.
68. McCarthy MC, Cottam Gl, Turner WW. Essential fatty acid deficiency in critically ill surgical patients. Am J Surg 142: 747–751, 1981.
69. Skeie B, Askanazi J, Rothkopf MM, et al. Intravenous fat emulsions and lung function: A review. Crit Care Med 16:183–194, 1988.
70. Swaninathan R, Bradley P, Morgan DB, et al. Hypophosphatemia in surgical patients. Surg Gynecol Obstet 148: 448–454, 1979.
71. DeFronzo RA, Lang R. Hypophosphatemia and glucose intolerance: Evidence for tissue insensitivity to insulin. New Engl J Med 303:1259–1263, 1980.
72. Juan D. Clinical review: The clinical importance of hypomagnesemia. Surgery 91:510–517, 1982.
73. McClain CJ. Trace metal abnormalities in adults during hyperalimentation. J Parenteral Enteral Nutr 5:424–429, 1981.
74. Hamit HF, David HE, Stevens JC. Dermatitis due to zinc deficiency associated with prolonged malnutrition and total parenteral nutrition. World J Surg 4:693–700, 1980.
75. Lemoyne M, Jeejeebhoy KN. Total parenteral nutrition in the critically ill patient. Chest 89:568–575, 1986.
76. Heimburger DC, Weinsier RL. Guidelines for evaluating and categorizing enteral feeding formulas according to therapeutic equivalence. J Parenteral Enteral Nutr 9:61–67, 1985.

Chapter 41

•

Robert C. Mackersie, MD

Diagnostic Peritoneal Lavage

OUTLINE

I. INTRODUCTION

The rapid and accurate diagnosis of serious intraabdominal injury is crucial to the successful management of both blunt and penetrating torso trauma. The abdominal examination following trauma is frequently unreliable in determining the presence or absence of injury,[1-4] particularly in patients with a depressed level of consciousness. As a first step in developing a more accurate, objective method for the diagnosis of abdominal injury, abdominal paracentesis was used, but was found to have a high incidence of false-negative results. In 1965, Root and associates[5] introduced the technique of diagnostic peritoneal lavage (DPL), which involved the instillation of crystalloid solution into the peritoneal cavity and examination of the fluid that was returned from the catheter. Since that time, DPL has become a well-established and widely used method for the early diagnostic evaluation of the abdomen. Although used principally for trauma, DPL is occasionally useful in the diagnosis of nontraumatic disease, such as ectopic pregnancy, and acute bacterial peritonitis from a variety of causes[6-8]. Placement of lavage catheters into the peritoneal cavity for continuous lavage may also have therapeutic purposes, such as peritoneal dialysis or lavage following acute hemorrhagic pancreatitis. The indications, catheters, and technical methods used for therapeutic lavage differ somewhat from those used for diagnostic lavage, however, and are beyond the scope of this discussion.

Although DPL is a surgical procedure, it is frequently performed by nonsurgeons, and in settings usually remote from the operating room environment. Patients with indications for DPL are often severely ill with underlying disease or associated injuries. It is important that strict adherence to aseptic technique and to the technical principles described be maintained in order to insure both accurate results and minimal morbidity.

II. INDICATIONS AND CONTRAINDICATIONS

The indications and contraindications for the performance of DPL following traumatic injury are shown in Table 41–1. The vast majority of patients for whom

Table 41–1 • Indications and Contraindications to Diagnostic Peritoneal Lavage Following Trauma

Indications, blunt trauma	
	Hypotension on arrival
	History of hypotension in field
	Abdominal tenderness
	Major associated injuries:
	Multiple rib fractures
	Pelvic fractures
	Axial spine fractures
	Large arterial base deficit (> −3 mEq/L)
	Depressed level of consciousness and major mechanism of injury
Indications, penetrating trauma	
	All stab wounds to anterior abdomen found to penetrate the anterior fascia on local wound exploration.
Relative contraindications	
	Previous abdominal surgery
	Evisceration (requires laparotomy)
	Hypovolemic shock hemodynamically unstable (instability and other sources of hemorrhage excluded) (requires emergent laparotomy)
	Gunshot wounds to the abdomen (requires laparotomy)

DPL is indicated will have sustained acute thoracoabdominal trauma. Mechanisms for these injuries may be either blunt (falls, vehicular accidents, etc) or penetrating (stab and gunshot wounds).

The major purpose of DPL is to detect intraperitoneal blood. Used appropriately, DPL is useful in reducing morbidity and mortality by greatly decreasing the number of missed intraabdominal injuries. In general, any patient suspected of having sustained intraabdominal injury, as judged by a combination of physical findings and associated injuries, should undergo peritoneal lavage. For blunt trauma, hypotension, large arterial base deficit (reflecting tissue hypoperfusion), or abdominal tenderness are indicators of possible intraabdominal injury. Associated injuries, such as pelvic, axial spine, or rib fractures, significantly increase the likelihood that intraabdominal injury is also present; in most cases, associated injuries should prompt the performance of DPL.[9]

Patients with a depressed level of consciousness as a result of head injury, drugs, or alcohol will have a blunted response to the elicitation of pain, and therefore will have an unreliable physical examination. In these patients, DPL should also be strongly considered.

The indications for DPL following penetrating trauma are substantially different. All patients sustaining stab wounds to the torso (from groin to nipple level) are candidates for DPL if local wound exploration demonstrates anterior fascial penetration. Because gunshot wounds to the abdomen are associated with a 95% incidence of serious intraabdominal injury,[10] all of these patients should undergo immediate exploratory laparotomy. Diagnostic peritoneal lavage is contraindicated in these patients because it is both unnecessary and has been reported to have a 25% false-negative rate.[11] Patients who have sustained either stab wounds to the abdomen or blunt abdominal trauma and have clear signs of peritonitis, or who have demonstrated hemodynamic instability attributable to an abdominal injury, also require expeditious laparotomy, not DPL.

Previous abdominal surgery, particularly midline incisions, contraindicates the performance of DPL because of the possibility of catheter penetration into bowel adhesed to the anterior abdominal wall and the possible loculation of intraabdominal hemorrhage by intraabdominal adhesions, producing false-negative lavage results. Occasionally an "open" technique for DPL[12] may be used in patients with a limited or remote site of previous surgery.

Pelvic fractures or a gravid uterus are contraindications to the performance of an infraumbilical lavage and should instead mandate its performance above the umbilicus. In patients with advanced pregnancy, an open technique for DPL is preferable.

III. How to Perform Diagnostic Peritoneal Lavage

Diagnostic peritoneal lavage frequently involves the blind passage of a catheter into the peritoneal cavity. Because of the possibility of injury to adjacent structures, a number of steps must be taken in order to avoid either complications or false-positive results. Gastric and bladder distention should be relieved prior to performing DPL (Fig. 41–1). A Foley catheter will provide bladder decompression in the vast majority of patients, although a few patients with urethral strictures or urethral tears will require suprapubic decompression. A chest radiograph, taken prior to the performance of DPL, will delineate any gastric dilatation. If gastric dilatation is present, a nasogastric tube is indicated, particularly for supraumbilical lavages.

Many patients with pelvic fractures will have significant retroperitoneal hemorrhage. With larger hematomas, blood may dissect into the preperitoneal space between the abdominal muscles and the peritoneum.

Gastric and Bladder Distention Should be Alleviated Prior to Performing DPL

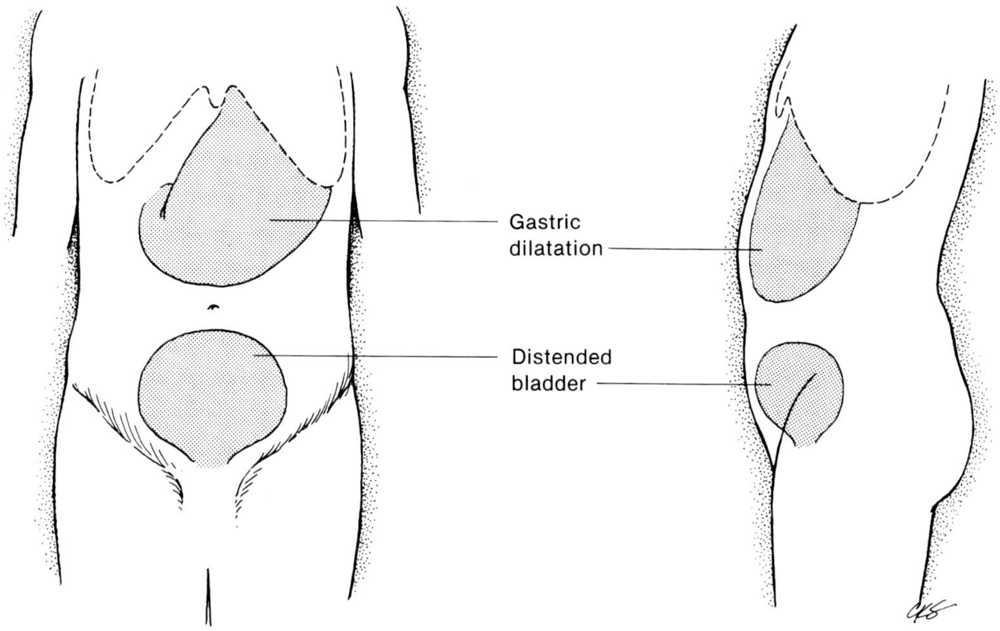

Figure 41–1 • Gastric and bladder distention should be alleviated prior to performing DPL to prevent injury.

Passage of the DPL catheter into the hematoma is common under these circumstances and will result in a high incidence of false-positive lavage results (Fig. 41–2). For this reason, any patient who has sustained a pelvic fracture should have the catheter inserted through a supraumbilical site.[13]

Diagnostic peritoneal lavage may be performed through a variety of abdominal sites, but passage of the lavage catheter through relatively avascular tissue, and placement into the most dependent portion of the abdomen, the pelvis, is generally simplified by the use of one of three incisions (Fig. 41–3). We prefer the standard infraumbilical midline incision, but the paraumbilical incision is also frequently used.[14] Accurate placement of the DPL catheter into the most dependent portion of the abdomen may be more difficult when performed through a supraumbilical site. Because of this, the use of supraumbilical incisions should be reserved for patients with pelvic fracture.

Diagnostic peritoneal lavage is, in effect, a minilaparotomy and should be treated as such with respect to skin preparation and adequate draping. Using strict aseptic technique, with mask, cap, sterile gloves, and preferably sterile gowns, the anterior abdominal wall is prepped with a standard 10% povidone iodine solution (Fig. 41–4A). Wide draping to prevent catheter or instrument contamination is then performed using either multiple sterile towels or eye or thyroid sheets (Fig. 41–4B).

The generous administration of local anesthetic is important for a number of reasons. In addition to patient comfort, the relief of any pain with the procedure is important to avoid sudden motion by the patient who, because of alcohol, drugs, or head injury, may be unable to understand specifically what is happening (Fig. 41–4C). Patients with severe closed head injury also require a local anesthetic because the noxious stimuli caused by the abdominal incision and passage of the catheter to the peritoneum may produce elevations in intracranial pressure. The addition of epinephrine to the lidocaine solution (1:100,000) is essential in preventing local wound hemorrhage from "contaminating" the lavasate, thus producing false-positive results, particularly with penetrating trauma, where the cell count criterion for a positive lavage is substantially less.

Following prepping, draping, and the administration of local anesthetic, a 3- to 5-cm incision is made

(Text continued on p. 878)

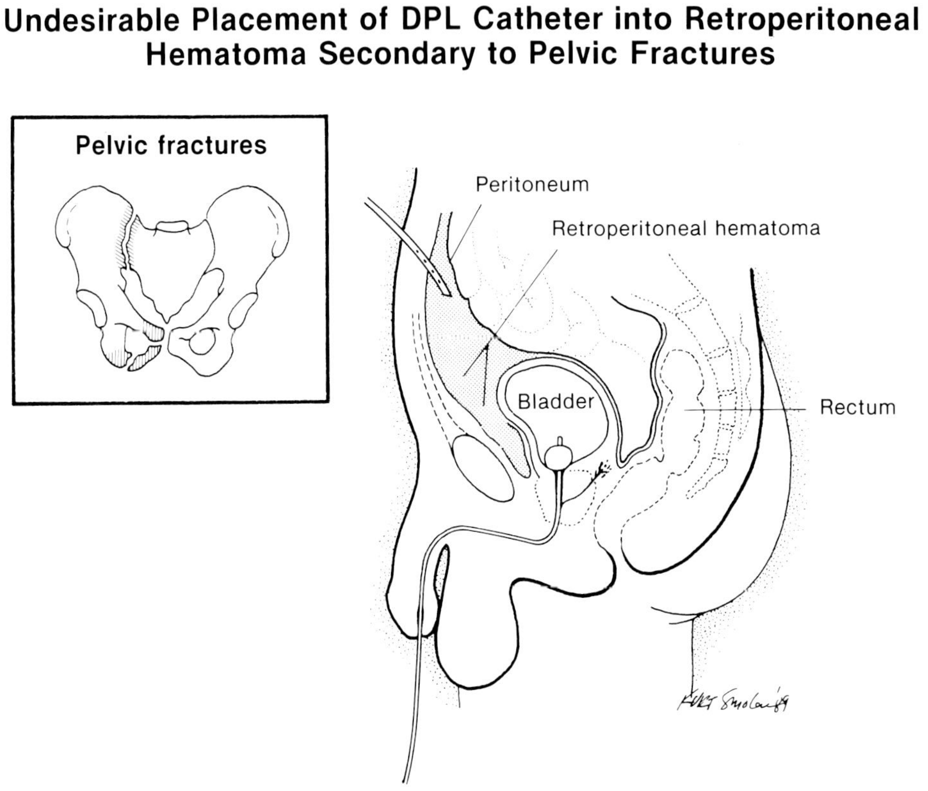

Figure 41–2 • Undesirable placement of DPL catheter into retroperitoneal pelvic fracture hematoma may produce false-positive results.

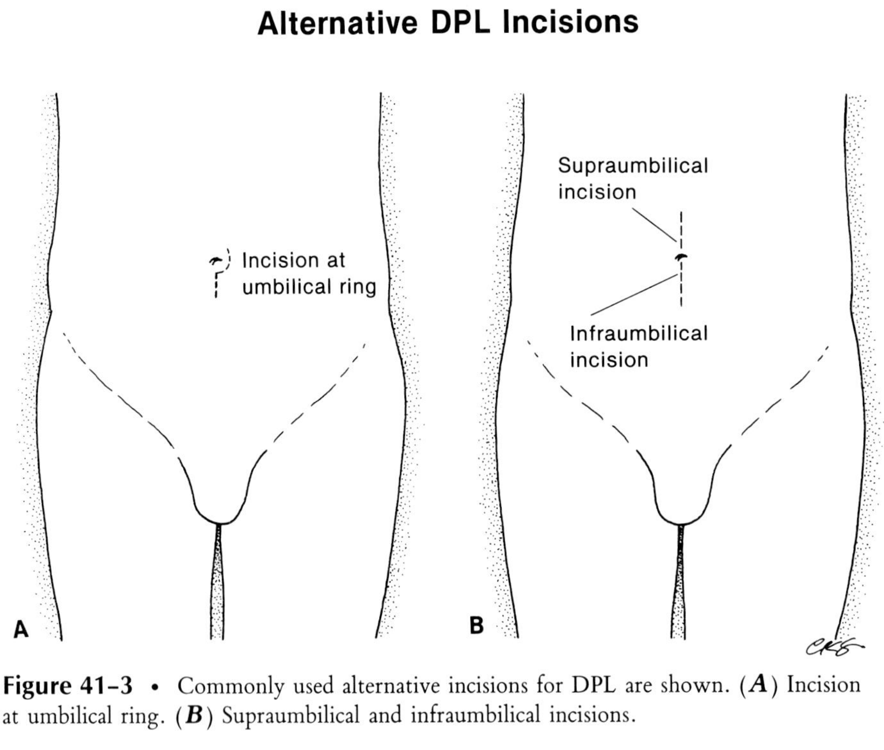

Figure 41–3 • Commonly used alternative incisions for DPL are shown. (***A***) Incision at umbilical ring. (***B***) Supraumbilical and infraumbilical incisions.

Wide abdominal preparation using aseptic technique

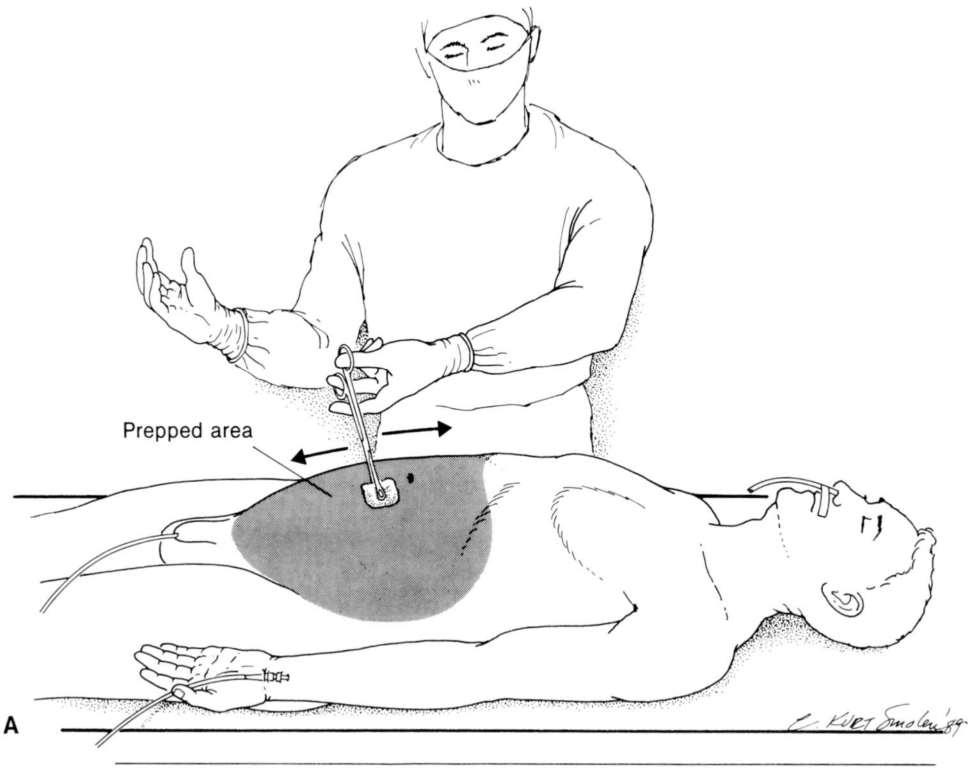

Wide draping to prevent catheter and wound contamination

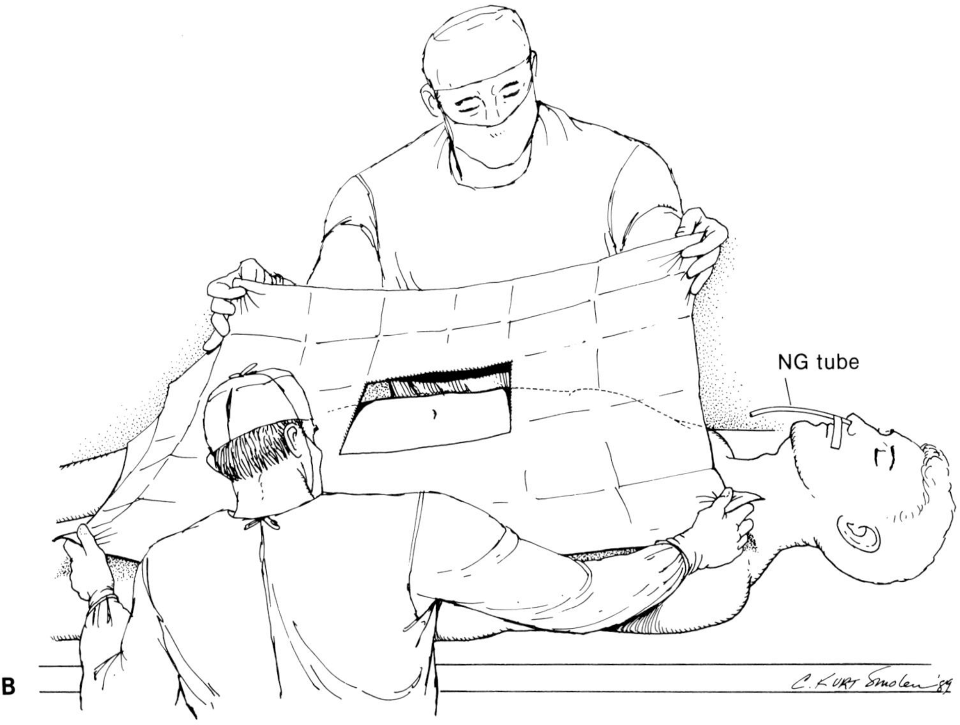

Figure 41–4 • Preparation and draping for DPL should be similar to that for a surgical procedure. (***A***) Wide abdominal preparation is performed using aseptic technique. (***B***) Generous draping is used to prevent catheter and wound contamination.

(continued)

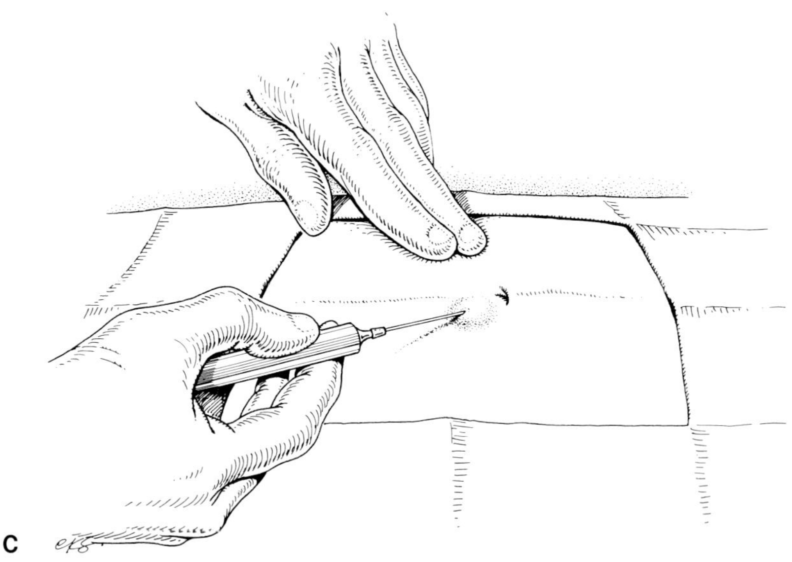

Figure 41–4 *(continued)*
(**C**) Local anesthetic is injected into all layers of the abdominal wall and peritoneum to avoid discomfort and sudden movement.

and carried down sharply to expose the anterior abdominal fascia. Towel clips may be applied to the fat on either side of the incision and removed and repositioned in succession to facilitate exposure as the incision is deepened. Once the fascia is exposed, a small incision slightly larger than the peritoneal lavage catheter is made. The size of this fascial incision is important. Incisions too large will require closure to prevent subsequent hernia formation. Incisions too small will increase resistance to catheter passage, thereby increasing the risk of "plunging" and producing injury to underlying structures. Towel clips placed into the anterior wall fascia are then used to both stabilize the anterior abdominal wall and aid exposure of the small fascial defect (Fig. 41–5).

The most crucial maneuver in the performance of the DPL is the passage of the catheter through the posterior abdominal fascia and the peritoneum. With one assistant holding both towel clips in order to stabilize the anterior abdominal fascia, the catheter is gently inserted vertically into the peritoneum using two hands for precise control. One hand is used to firmly grasp the catheter close to the wound to prevent "plunging"; the second hand is used to determine the direction of passage. In most patients, there will be two small pops felt as the catheter penetrates the posterior abdominal fascia and then the peritoneum (Fig. 41–6A). Once the catheter tip has been passed into the peritoneum, the angle is rotated to approximately 45°, and the catheter is gently directed into the pelvic portion of the peritoneal cavity. There should be very little resistance to catheter passage. Resistance to passage or inappropriate pain experienced by the patient should prompt withdrawal of the catheter and redirection.

After the catheter is gently inserted into peritoneal cavity, a syringe is attached to the catheter and aspirated for blood (Fig. 41–6B). Gross aspiration of blood (more than 10–15 mL) constitutes a grossly positive tap, making the subsequent infusion and return of fluid unnecessary for diagnostic purposes. In the absence of gross blood on aspiration, 1 L of normal saline or Ringer's lactate is infused, either by gravity or under pressure, into the abdominal cavity (Fig. 41–7A). Because the lavasate is returned by a siphon effect only, it is important that a small amount of crystalloid solution be left in the bottom bag and lavage tubing. Lavage fluid return is effected by lowering the level of the infusate bag below the level of the table. The drip chamber should be monitored, particularly in the early moments of lavasate return, to insure a good flow in return (Fig. 41–7B). In the event of poor return of lavasate fluid, the catheter should be gently repositioned within the abdominal cavity.

The technique for DPL catheter placement just described is best termed the semi-open technique. A skin and small fascial incision is made, but the catheter is passed blindly. Two alternative methods for DPL catheter placement have been used.

Exposure and Passage of Catheter Through Small Fascial Incision

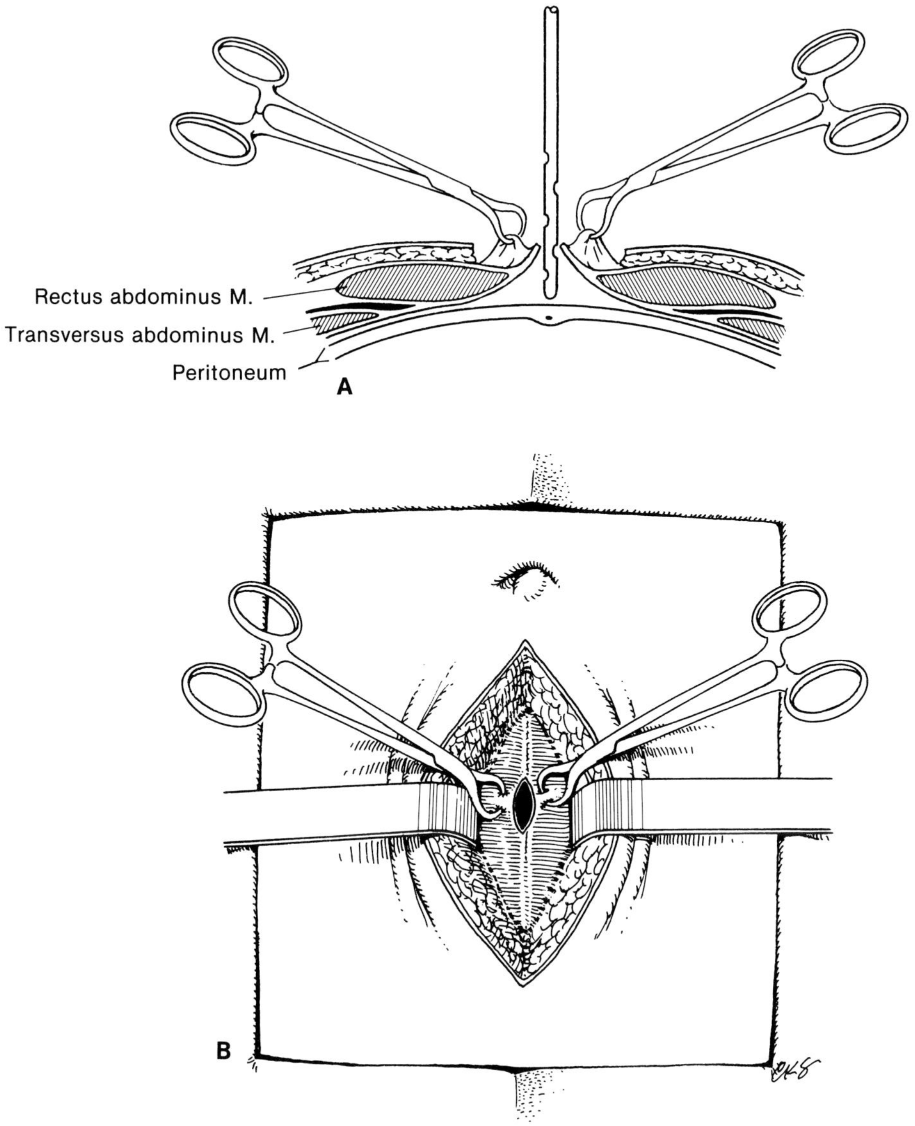

Figure 41–5 • Towel clips facilitate exposure and passage of the DPL catheter through a small fascial incision. (***A***) Cross-sectional view. (***B***) Frontal view.

Closed Method. This technique involves making only a tiny skin incision with blind passage of the lavage catheter over a trochar through fat, fascia, and peritoneum. The use of a guide wire passed through a needle into the peritoneal cavity and subsequent passage of a DPL catheter over the guide wire is a variant of the closed technique found to have a low incidence of complications.[15]

Open Method. The open technique uses a skin incision comparable to that used in the semi-open technique, with a larger incision in the fascia. Through the fascial incision, the peritoneum is identified and opened. The lavage catheter is then passed under direct vision without the use of a trochar.

The disadvantage of the open technique is mainly the average of 55 minutes[16] that it takes to complete the lavage. In obese patients this is a particular problem because of the thickness of the preperitoneal fat layer. The open technique, however, has the advantages of

(Text continued on p. 882)

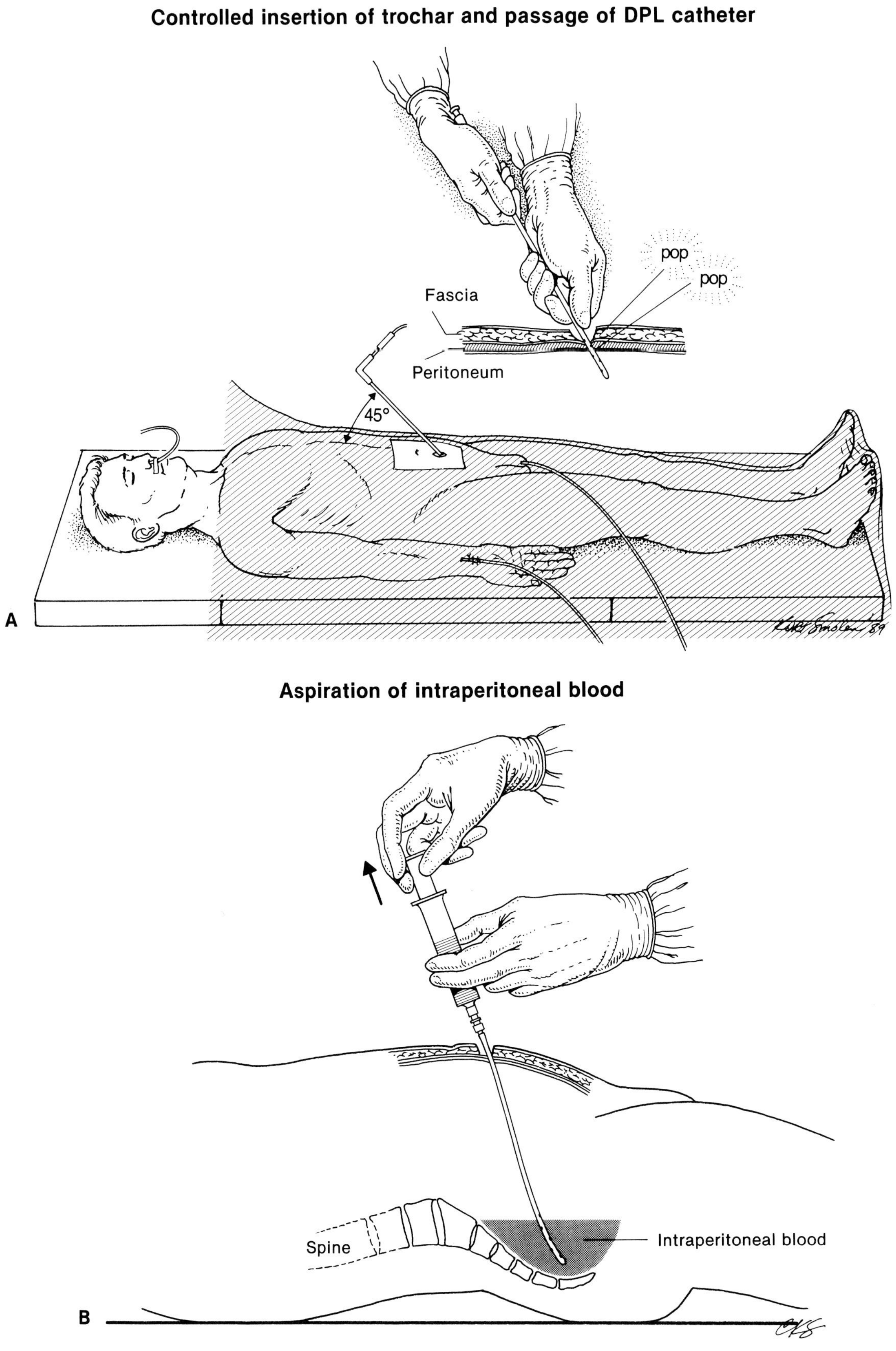

Figure 41-6 • A lavage catheter is passed into the dependent portion of the peritoneal cavity and aspirated for blood. (***A***) Controlled insertion of the trochar is necessary to avoid injuring abdominal organs. The two "pops" are caused by passage of the trochar through the posterior abdominal fascia (first) and the peritoneum (second). (***B***) Intraperitoneal blood is aspirated before infusion of fluid.

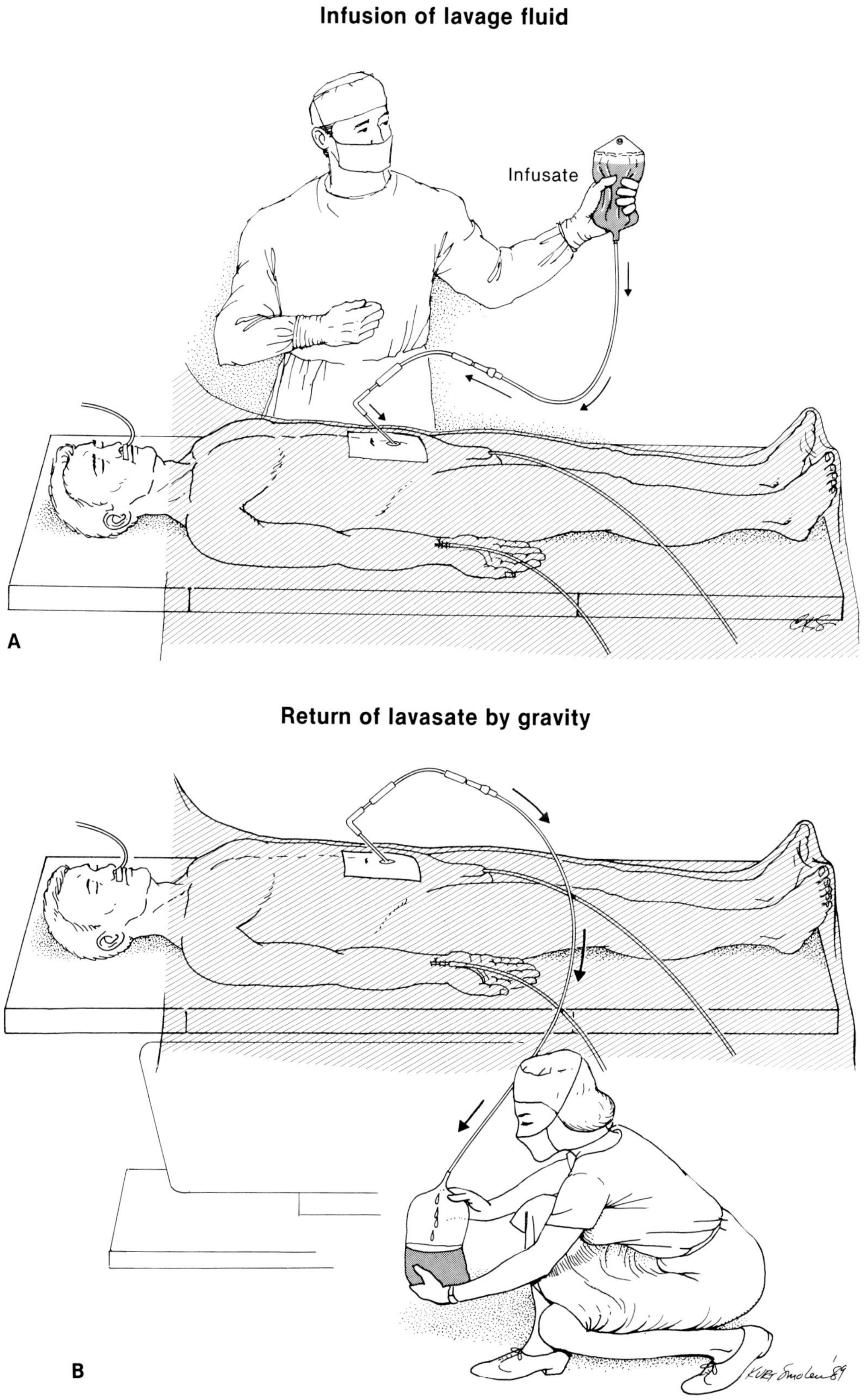

Figure 41–7 • Infusion and return of lavasate. (***A***) Fluid may be infused under pressure to shorten the duration of DPL. (***B***) Return drip rate should be monitored to ensure good return flow of lavasate.

identifying any retroperitoneal hematoma or abdominal wall adhesions and allowing more accurate and safe placement of the DPL catheter. The closed technique involves passage, by force, of the trochar and catheter through the anterior abdominal fascia. This has been associated with a higher incidence of iatrogenic injuries, including lacerations to bowel, mesentery, and iliac vessels.[17] The semi-open procedure combines the advantages of being easier and faster to perform (average time, 10–20 minutes) and avoiding the complications associated with the purely closed method. There does not appear to be any significant difference in terms of diagnostic accuracy between the open and closed methods.[18]

With the open and semi-open methods, wound closure is accomplished using a running 2-0 nylon suture, and may be performed at the same time that infusion is being instilled (Fig. 41–8). Because the fascial incision is less than 3 or 4 mm, it is not necessary that this be closed. Larger fascial incisions such as those used for open lavages should be closed with two or four interrupted fascial sutures of absorbable material. In patients who are in need of additional diagnostic procedures, such as computed tomography (CT) scanning or angiography, the process of infusion and return of lavasate may be performed while in transit or in the radiology department. In patients with significant other injuries, particularly closed head injury requiring CT scan, and in whom a relatively low index of suspicion for hemoperitoneum exists, lavasate infusion and return may be performed with the patient in transit or in the radiology department.

Lavage incision sutures should be replaced with sterile strips at approximately 3 to 5 days or left in place for a total of 10 days to allow adequate wound healing.

IV. Discussion

The interpretation of DPL results has been the subject of much discussion over recent years. Most centers rely on an analytic approach, using red and white blood cell counts in the lavasate. For blunt trauma or the diagnosis of acute peritonitis in an obtunded patient, red blood cell (RBC) counts in excess of 100,000/μL or white blood cell (WBC) counts in excess of 500/μL are considered positive results and indications for exploratory laparotomy.[19,20] These RBC/WBC criteria have been found, in a number of studies, to be associated with a minimal number of missed injuries and an acceptable incidence of negative laparotomies. Although there are reports of the utility of lavasate analysis for amylase, bile, or enzymes,[21,22] such analysis is costly and has not been demonstrated to add enough to the overall diagnostic accuracy of DPL in addition to the use of white and red cell counts to justify its routine use.

False-negative DPL results have been reported to occur with retroperitoneal injuries involving the pancreas, duodenum, retroperitoneal colon, kidney, bladder, or diaphragmatic rupture with hemorrhage into the thoracic cavity.[17,23] DPL is not a foolproof diagnostic method, and diaphragmatic or retroperitoneal or even intraperitoneal injuries suspected on the basis of clinical course or associated injuries may require additional diagnostic studies such as CT, intravenous pyelography (IVP), or cystography. The overall missed injury rate (false negative DPL/total positive DPL) for DPL used following blunt trauma has been reported between 2% and 5%,[18,20,24] and depends on the specific lavage criteria used.

Interpretation of DPL results in penetrating

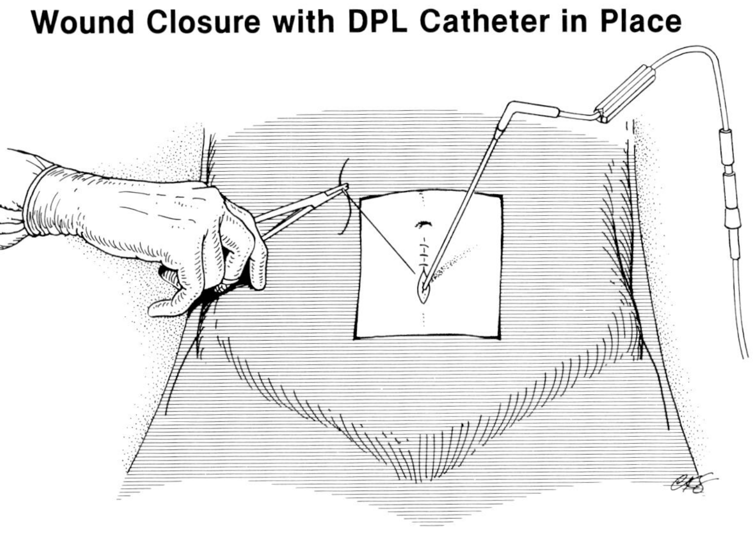

Figure 41–8 • DPL wound may be closed with the catheter in place.

trauma (stab wounds) has been more controversial. Most centers use a lower criterion for red cell count, because the degree of associated hemorrhage with hollow viscous injury may be substantially less than with blunt trauma. The use of 100,000 cells/μL may lead to an unacceptably high incidence of false-negative results. As the criteria for red cell count are lowered, the incidence of missed injury drops, but the incidence of unnecessary laparotomy, as prompted by minimal hemoperitoneum, increases.[20] Oreskovich and Carrico[25] documented a 43% incidence of visceral injury in patients with 1,000 to 50,000 RBCs/μL, and recommend exploratory laparotomy for patients with greater than 1,000 cells/μL. They had no incidence of missed injury and suggested that the unnecessary laparotomy rate should be less than 10%. Using a variety of DPL criteria, most centers report an accuracy rate of 96% to 98%, a missed injury rate of 0% to 5%, and a false-positive rate of 13% to 22% for penetrating injuries.[20,26,27]

The usefulness of DPL for the diagnosis of peritonitis has been reported by several studies.[7,8] Indications for DPL under these circumstances include the suspicion of intraabdominal pathology in an obtunded, debilitated, or elderly patient in whom physical examination and noninvasive imaging studies are inconclusive. Diagnostic accuracy of approximately 97% and a low incidence of false-negative results have been reported. The techniques for the performance of DPL for nontrauma are similar, except perhaps that an open technique is more frequently indicated.

V. Technical Problems of Diagnostic Peritoneal Lavage and Complications

The overall complication rate for diagnostic peritoneal lavage, not including technical problems, varies widely in the literature and is reported to be 1% to 2%.[17,24,28] The incidence of complications varies with the level of expertise of the person performing the lavage, the environment under which it is performed, and the specific type of technique used (open, semi-open, closed). Infectious complications are usually limited to wound infections and can be prevented largely by strict adherence to aseptic technique. Bladder or gastric perforations are entirely preventable with adequate decompression of these organs. Small-bowel and colon perforations and injury to mesenteric or iliac vessels can be largely eliminated by the use of an open or semi-open technique, adequate administration of local anesthetic to prevent any sudden patient movement, and careful controlled passage of the DPL catheter through the peritoneum.

Inadvertent placement of lavage catheters into pelvic fracture hematomas may be avoided by routinely obtaining a pelvic radiograph and by performing lavage in the supraumbilical position for patients with pelvic fractures. Passage of the peritoneal lavage catheter into the space of Retzius (preperitoneal space) in the absence of pelvic fracture hematoma occurs occasionally. Sensitivity to the increased resistance of passing the catheter through the preperitoneal space should reduce the incidence of this problem. In addition, the "froth" test may be applied by vigorously shaking the returned lavasate. The small amount of protein contained in the peritoneal cavity is usually sufficient to produce a frothing appearance. The absence of this should give rise to the suspicion of a misplaced catheter.

Inadequate or incomplete return of lavasate is a common technical problem and is usually related to a large, thin omentum wrapping around the DPL catheter, allowing inflow but preventing lavasate return. Occasionally it is necessary to infuse a second liter of crystalloid solution into the peritoneum. Under these circumstances, the diagnostic cut-off for cell count should be reduced by one half. The average return for lavasate fluid should normally be 650–750 mL/1 liter infused.

False-positive results (caused by hemorrhage produced by the peritoneal catheter) may be reduced by the use of epinephrine in the local anesthetic and careful attention to wound hemostasis following the incision. This is particularly true of DPL performed for penetrating trauma, where the cell count criteria for a positive test is low.

VI. Summary

Diagnostic peritoneal lavage is a rapid, simple, and effective means of determining the presence of intraabdominal hemorrhage or serious intraabdominal infection. It is, however, an invasive surgical procedure capable of producing serious complications. Strict attention to aseptic technique and the details of surgical technique are necessary to maximize diagnostic accuracy and minimize complications.

VII. REFERENCES

1. Powell DC, Bivins BA, Bell RM. Diagnostic peritoneal lavage. Surg Gynecol Obstet 155:257–264, 1982.
2. Perry JF, Strate RG. Diagnostic peritoneal lavage in blunt abdominal trauma: Indications and results. Surgery 71:898–901, 1972.
3. Rodriguez A, DuPriest RW Jr, Shatney CH. Recognition of intra-abdominal injury in blunt trauma victims. Am Surg 48:456–459, 1982.
4. Bivins BA, Sachatello CR, Daugherty ME, et al. Diagnostic peritoneal lavage is superior to clinical evaluation in blunt abdominal trauma. Am Surg 44:637–641, 1978.
5. Root HD, Hauser CW, McKinley CR, et al. Diagnostic peritoneal lavage. Surgery 57:633–637, 1965.
6. Roberts MR, Jackimczyk K, Marx J, Rosen P. Diagnosis of ruptured ectopic pregnancy with peritoneal lavage. Ann Emerg Med 11:556–558, 1982.
7. Lobbato V, Cioroiu M, LaRaja RD, et al. Peritoneal lavage as an aid to diagnosis of peritonitis in debilitated and elderly patients. Am Surg 51:508–510, 1985.
8. Richardson JD, Flint LM, Polk HC. Peritoneal lavage: A useful diagnostic adjunct for peritonitis. Surgery 94:826–829, 1983.
9. Mackersie RC, Tiwary AD, Shackford SR, Hoyt DB. Intraabdominal injury following blunt trauma: Identifying the high risk patient using objective risk factors. Arch Surg 7:809–813, 1989.
10. Moore EE, Moore JB, Van Duzer Moore S, Thompson JS. Mandatory laparotomy for gunshot wounds penetrating the abdomen. Am J Surg 140:847–851, 1980.
11. Thal ER, May RA, Beesinger D. Peritoneal lavage. Its unreliability in gunshot wounds of the lower chest and abdomen. Arch Surg 115:430–433, 1980.
12. DuPriest RW, Khaneja SC, Rodriguez A, Cowley RA. A technique for open diagnostic peritoneal lavage. Surg Gynecol Obstet 147:241–243, 1978.
13. Lazarus HM, Nelson JA. Technique for peritoneal lavage when a pelvic fracture and suspected hematoma are present. Surg Gynecol Obstet 153:403–404, 1981.
14. Felice PR, Morgan AS, Becker DR. A prospective randomized study evaluating periumbilical versus infraumbilial peritoneal lavage: A preliminary report. Am Surg 53:518–520, 1987.
15. Lazarus HM, Nelson JA. A technique for peritoneal lavage without risk or complication. Surg Gynecol Obstet 149: 889–892, 1979.
16. Myers RA, Agarwal NN, Cowley RA. A safe, semi-open procedure for diagnostic peritoneal lavage. Surg Gynecol Obstet 153:739–740, 1981.
17. Soderstrom CA, DuPriest RW, Cowley RA. Pitfalls of peritoneal lavage in blunt abdominal trauma. Surg Gynecol Obstet 151:513–518, 1980.
18. Cochran W, Sobat WS. Open versus closed diagnostic peritoneal lavage. Ann Surg 200:24–28, 1984.
19. Thal ER, Shires GT. Peritoneal lavage in blunt abdominal trauma. Am J Surg 125:64–69, 1973.
20. Alyono D, Morrow CE, Perry JF. Reappraisal of diagnostic peritoneal lavage criteria for operation in penetrating and blunt trauma. Surgery 92:751–757, 1982.
21. Alyono D, Perry JF. Value of quantitative cell count and amylase activity of peritoneal lavage fluid. J Trauma 21:345–348, 1981.
22. McLellan BA, Hanna SS, Montoya DR, et al. Analysis of peritoneal lavage parameters in blunt abdominal trauma. J Trauma 25:393–399, 1985.
23. Brotman S, Shatney CH, Cowley RA. False negative peritoneal lavage. Am Surg 47:309–310, 1981.
24. Engrav LH, Benjamin CI, Strate RG, Perry JF Jr. Diagnostic peritoneal lavage in blunt abdominal trauma. J Trauma 15:854–859, 1975.
25. Oreskovich MR, Carrico CJ. Stab wounds of the anterior abdomen. Analysis of a management plan using local wound exploration and quantitative peritoneal lavage. Ann Surg 198:411–419, 1983.
26. Feliciano DV, Bitondo CG, Steed G, et al. Five hundred open taps or lavages in patients with abdominal stab wounds. Am J Surg 148:772–777, 1984.
27. Griffin JB, Reines HD. Diagnostic criteria for peritoneal lavage in penetrating trauma. Curr Surg 40(5):351–353, 1983.
28. Fischer RP, Beverlin BC, Engrav LH, et al. Diagnostic peritoneal lavage: Fourteen years and 2,586 patients later. Am J Surg 136:701–704, 1978.

Chapter 42

George M. Shumaik, MD

Treatment of Poisoning and Overdose

OUTLINE

I. INTRODUCTION

The poisoning of our world by a myriad of man-made toxins is an issue at the forefront of our current social and political consciousness. The contamination of the earth has lead to a renewed and expanding interest in the field of toxicology. A discussion of the effects of chronic environmental pollution, however, is beyond the scope of this chapter. The goal of this chapter is to provide the reader with the principles of diagnosis and management in acute human poisoning as it presents to the clinician in the emergency department or intensive care setting. This overview will outline the commonly employed procedures for patient decontamination, stressing the importance of standard supportive medical care as the primary therapeutic modality. Classical techniques for the prevention of absorption and elimination of toxins will be described in detail. Antidotal therapy will be reviewed, emphasizing its limited clinical applicability.

Poison, from the Latin *potio* (a draft or drink), is any substance taken into the body by ingestion, inhalation, injection, or absorption that interferes with normal physiologic functions.[1] "All substances are poisons; there is none which is not a poison; it is the right dose that differentiates a poison": a truism of medical toxicology today, taught by Paracelsus during the middle ages.[2] Numerous potential poisons lurk in the average household medicine cabinet, in the garage, and under the kitchen sink.

The number of human poisonings per year in the United States is unknown. The American Association of Poison Control Centers (AAPCC) began its National Data Collection System in 1983. In 1987, 63 poison centers reported nearly 1.2 million human exposure cases.[3] A total population of 137.5 million was served by the participating centers, including portions of 35 states and the District of Columbia. The authors extrapolated that 4.6 million exposures would have been reported if the entire population had been served at a penetrance of the most active reporting center.

Table 42–1 summarizes the medical outcome of the reported exposures. The majority were in children with very low mortality. Overall, there were only 397 deaths reported, the majority occurring in adults. Table 42–2 summarizes the distribution of these deaths by reason for exposure and age. It is important to note that 304 deaths resulted from intentional exposure or overdose. Although these data are incomplete, it is a reasonable conclusion that poisoning and overdose is a "disease" of low mortality when patients receive appropriate medical treatment.

Most of the common therapeutic interventions discussed in this chapter have been and continue to be controversial. Gastric emptying, the use of cathartics, or the administration of activated charcoal have not been "proven" beneficial by standard scientific methods. The reason for this is understandable. Poisoning has a mortality of 1% or less in those patients who survive to access the health care system.[3] A study designed to show a statistically significant decrease in mortality based on a single therapeutic intervention would require thousands of patients. Although these large prospective studies do not exist, the data from trials, the anecdotal literature, and laboratory studies have given rise to the general collective opinion of clinical toxicologists that these "unproven" managements *are* beneficial when ap-

Table 42–1 • Medical Outcome of Human Poison Exposure Cases by Patient Age

Outcome	<6 Yr; no. (%)	6–12 Yr; no. (%)	13–17 Yr; no. (%)	>17 Yr; no. (%)	Unknown; no (%)	Total; no. (%)
No effect	436,805 (59.7)	23,945 (38.3)	13,399 (26.3)	58,051 (18.6)	2,889 (30.3)	535,089 (45.9)
Minor effect	102,168 (14.0)	19,930 (31.9)	21,002 (41.2)	136,080 (43.6)	2,609 (27.4)	281,789 (24.1)
Moderate effect	5,232 (0.7)	1,335 (2.1)	3,027 (5.9)	21,654 (6.9)	339 (3.6)	31,587 (2.7)
Major effect	422 (0.0)	86 (0.0)	335 (0.7)	2,740 (0.9)	48 (0.5)	3,631 (0.3)
Death	22 (0.0)	3 (0.0)	30 (0.1)	341 (0.1)	1 (0.0)	397 (0.0)
Unknown, nontoxic*	160,842 (22.0)	12,982 (20.8)	5,892 (11.6)	41,773 (13.4)	1,343 (14.1)	222,832 (19.1)
Unknown, potentially toxic†	14,991 (2.1)	2,444 (3.9)	6,065 (11.9)	37,859 (12.1)	1,900 (19.9)	63,259 (5.4)
Unrelated effect	9,760 (1.3)	1,617 (2.6)	1,104 (2.2)	13,132 (4.2)	241 (2.5)	25,854 (2.2)
Unknown	1,383 (0.2)	106 (0.2)	125 (0.3)	718 (0.2)	170 (1.8)	2,502 (0.2)
Total	731,625(100.0)	62,448(100.0)	50,979(100.0)	312,348(100.0)	9,540(100.0)	1,166,940(100.0)

Note: Column percentages are provided in this table; data in parentheses are percentages.
*No follow-up provided as exposure was assessed as nontoxic.
†Patient lost to follow-up. Exposure was assessed as potentially toxic.

Litovitz TL, Schmitz BF, Matyunas N, Martin TG. 1987 annual report of the American Association of Poison Control Centers National Data Collectection System. Am J Emerg Med 6:479–515, 1988.

Table 42-2 • Distribution of Reason for Exposure and Age for 397 Human Fatalities

Reason	<6 Yr	6-12 Yr	13-17 Yr	>17 Yr	Total
Accidental					
General	7	2	0	6	15
Environmental	6	0	1	14	21
Misuse	5	0	1	14	20
Occupational	0	0	0	6	6
Unknown	1	0	1	2	4
Total	19	2	3	42	66
Intentional					
Suicide	0	1	15	210	226
Misuse	1	0	0	8	9
Abuse	0	0	10	30	40
Unknown	1	0	2	26	29
Total	2	1	27	274	304
Adverse Reaction	0	0	0	6	6
Unknown	1	0	0	20	21
Total	22	3	30	342	397

plied in individual situations. The majority of these interventions are not typically associated with complications and will continue to be used in the absence of absolute scientific proof.

As individual therapies are debated, one fact remains incontrovertible: *The majority of poisoning victims who present alive to a health care facility will survive if they receive standard supportive medical care.*

II. RESUSCITATIVE CARE

The abrupt presentation of patients in extremis is the nature of emergency medicine. They often arrive without benefit of medical history and require resuscitative intervention in advance of definitive diagnosis. The general contour of priorities in resuscitative care are reviewed below and are applicable to any patient presenting with obtundation, airway compromise, or cardiovascular collapse, including those with toxic etiologies.

A. *Airway*

Immediate attention should be given to securing and maintaining an airway for adequate ventilation and oxygenization. The clinical situation will dictate the type of airway management. Simple maneuvers, such as head positioning and the addition of supplemental oxygen, may suffice (see Chapter 5). If there is doubt about the patency of the airway or if the patient is at risk for aspiration, tracheal intubation should be performed. This can be accomplished via either the nasotracheal or orotracheal route. The techniques for tracheal intubation are discussed in Chapter 6. In addition to clinical assessment, arterial blood gases should be frequently obtained to document adequate gas exchange and to monitor trends.

B. *Vascular Access*

Venous access should be achieved as quickly as possible. Two large-bore (16 or 18 gauge), indwelling catheters at peripheral sites are the norm for the critically ill patient. Central venous lines can be used in the absence of peripheral sites or as a port for the placement of a pulmonary artery catheter. If the fluid requirements of the patient are not known or if there is frank hypotension, isotonic electrolyte solutions should be administered, either 0.9% normal saline or Ringer's lactate solution. Infusion rates will depend on physiologic assessment and hemodynamic monitoring parameters. In general, patients with hypotension should have intravascular volume (preload) assured prior to the administration of pressors.

C. *Monitoring*

Vital signs should be monitored frequently to measure responses to specific therapeutic interventions. Overdoses of certain drugs (narcotics, barbiturates) may cause aberration of temperature regulation, necessitating continuous measurement of core body temperature through a rectal probe thermometer. Blood pressure can be monitored using a traditional arm cuff initially, with consideration given to invasive arterial monitoring if the accuracy of the cuff pressure is questionable or if vasoactive drugs that require continuous monitoring are administered. Cardiac rhythm should be monitored with an external recording device. A Foley catheter should be inserted to measure urine output and to obtain samples for routine and toxicologic analysis. The placement of a pulmonary artery catheter is not typically an early priority in resuscitation.

D. *Laboratory*

Arterial blood gases should be obtained at presentation and again after definitive airway management to document adequate ventilation, oxygenation, and acid-base status. Cooximetry should be ordered if the presence of an abnormal hemoglobin is suspected, such as carboxyhemoglobin (carbon monoxide) or methemoglobin (nitrates, nitrites). Venous blood should be obtained for standard laboratory studies dictated by the clinical situation (complete blood count, electrolytes, blood urea nitrogen, creatinine, liver function tests), as well as for toxicologic analysis (see the section entitled ''Using the Toxicology Laboratory'').

E. *Empiric Therapy*

Obtunded patients should routinely receive (1) glucose 25 g by rapid intravenous injection (unless hypoglycemia can be quickly ruled out by bedside testing of whole blood), (2) thiamine 100 mg intravenously, and (3) naloxone 2 mg intravenously.

A hypoglycemic patient will quickly improve with the administration of glucose, while a hyperglycemic patient is unlikely to have his or her condition worsened by the additional sugar. The administration of thiamine has no morbidity and may prevent the development of Wernicke's encephalopathy in nutritionally depleted alcoholic patients. The narcotic antagonist, naloxone, reverses the effects of essentially all narcotics and is risk free (see section on antidotal therapy).

These initial interventions should take no more than 10 minutes to complete. Although presented as a step-by-step algorithm, adequate professional staffing should allow these procedures to be performed simultaneously. Once these resuscitative and supportive measures have been undertaken, attention can be turned toward diagnosis.

III. Recognizing the Poisoned Patient

A. *History*

Poisoned patients can present because of accidental or intentional exposure. If immediate resuscitation is not required, a detailed history of the exposure is a valuable aid in management. An alert, cooperative patient or unbiased third parties can help direct therapy toward known intoxicants. Important basic information includes type of toxin, amount of toxin, route of exposure, time of exposure, and any subjective complaints of the patient. Past medical history, current medications, and other classical components of a medical history should be included as adjunctive information.

Unfortunately, many patients present to the emergency department with absent or unreliable histories. Patients with altered levels of consciousness may not be able to provide accurate information. Patients poisoned by suicidal intent also cannot be relied on for accurate histories and frequently are overdosed on more than one drug. Ethyl alcohol is frequently combined with other drugs in intentional exposure. If the victim is brought against his or her will by legal authorities, an adversarial relationship may develop with the health care system. In these circumstances, it is important to seek as much third-party information as possible from family, friends, police, and paramedics. For example, an obtunded patient found in a closed garage with the engine of a car running would be highly suspect of carbon monoxide poisoning. The retrieval of empty pill bottles by prehospital personnel could help direct a search for additional toxins.

B. *Physical Signs: Toxidromes*

The physical examination cannot be overlooked in the management of the poisoning victim. In the case of the identified toxin, it can track the onset or confirm the absence of anticipated clinical symptoms. In the case of the unidentified toxin, the presence of physical signs can lead the clinician to suspect specific compounds or categories of intoxicants. Particular attention should be paid to the patient's vital signs, mental status, pupillary reaction, and cardiac rhythm.

Constellations of physical signs and symptoms that suggest poisoning are called toxidromes. Table 42–3 presents ten classical toxidromes and a limited list of possible toxic causes. This represents only one construct and is not comprehensive. It is important to note that many drugs participate in more than one toxidrome (eg, tricyclic antidepressants). Toxidromes can help in defining a management strategy and be a guide for the toxicology laboratory in the search for causes.

Table 42–3 • Toxidromes

Toxidrome	Possible Toxic Agents
Anticholinergic (dry mouth, flushing, mydriasis tachycardia, psychosis)	Atropine, scopolamine, antihistamines, tricyclic antidepressants, Jimson weed
Cholinergic (salivation, lacrimation, bradycardia, bronchoconstriction, muscle fasciculations)	Organophosphate and carbamate insecticides, nicotine
Coma—hypotonic, hypodynamic	Narcotics, barbiturates, benzodiazepines, ethanol, phenothiazines, glutethamide
Coma—hypertonic, hyperdynamic	Tricyclic antidepressants, phencyclidine, amphetamines, cocaine, strychnine
Dysrhythmias	Tricyclic antidepressants, digoxin, propranolol, amphetamines, cocaine, theophylline, phencyclidine
Hyperthermia	Salicylates, phencyclidine, cocaine, amphetamines, neuroleptics
Hypothermia	Ethanol, barbiturates, benzodiazapines, opiates, phenothiazines, tricyclic antidepressants
Psychosis, behavioral aberration	Phencyclidine, amphetamines, cocaine, LSD, anticholinergics, glue sniffing, ethanol, drug withdrawal syndromes
Metabolic acidosis	Salicylates, methanol, ethylene glycol, iron, INH, alcoholic ketoacidosis
Pulmonary edema (noncardiac)	Salicylates, opiates, organophosphates, propoxyphene
Seizures	Tricyclic antidepressants, cocaine, theophylline, amphetamines, alcohol and barbiturate withdrawal

C. *Using the Toxicology Laboratory*

The role of the toxicology laboratory in the management of a poisoned patient is difficult to define. When physicians are faced with the dilemma of a critically ill patient without an obvious cause, a desperate search often ensues for possible causes. Included in a "shotgun" approach to diagnosis is typically an order for a comprehensive laboratory toxicology screen. Implicit in this strategy may be an unfounded faith that the laboratory will search for *all* possible toxins. This misconception may be compounded by the erroneous conclusion that a "negative tox screen" rules out all possible toxic causes. Although it has been shown that the toxicology screen can detect the presence of substances not suspected by history or physical examination,[4] finding a drug does not necessarily define the degree of clinical expression or alter patient management. The exception would be the discovery of a toxin known to have a delay in the onset of its toxicity (acetaminophen, methanol).

Although the technology exists for the detection of literally hundreds of chemicals in bodily fluids, toxicology laboratories must of necessity limit their screens to the most commonly encountered drugs. There are variations in the components of the comprehensive toxicology panel, and it is the responsibility of a managing physician to know which studies are performed locally.

It is also important to know how long it will take for the information to be returned. Not all facilities are equipped for on-site, broad-spectrum screening. If a specimen has to be sent out, there may be a significant delay until the clinician receives the results. This may alter management. For example, if the in-house lab does not perform the study, the ingestion of a large quantity of acetaminophen may require the empiric institution of acetylcysteine therapy prior to laboratory confirmation of a toxic serum level.

Table 42–4 summarizes the comprehensive toxicology panels currently performed at the University of California San Diego Medical Center. To obtain the maximum amount of information from the broad-spectrum screen, samples of whole blood, serum, and urine should be submitted.[5] Gastric fluid obtained by lavage or spontaneous or induced emesis may also be sent for analysis. Many drugs can be identified quantitatively in whole blood and serum. Quantitative data are most useful when the blood level correlates well with clinical toxicity. For example, if a patient with a metabolic acidosis were found to have a whole blood methanol level of greater than 50 mg/dL, hemodialysis would be considered. It is critical that the units of measurement in a quantitative analysis are understood. A theophylline level of 2 mg/dL and 20 μg/mL are equivalent and in the therapeutic range. It is obvious that a serious error in management could be made if a theophylline level of 20 was interpreted as therapeutic when the units of measurement are mg/dL, a level of 10 times greater.

Many of the most commonly encountered drugs (tricyclic antidepressants, narcotics, cocaine, amphetamines) are difficult to detect in blood and are found only qualitatively in the urine. This information may add little to the clinical management of the patient. If a patient overdoses on a cyclic antidepressant prescribed for him or her on a chronic basis, the qualitative presence of the drug in the urine is neither a surprise nor helpful in therapeutic decision-making. In this case, signs of clinical toxicity would be the sole determinant of the management strategy.

Comprehensive toxicology screening is expensive and time consuming. The greatest impact on patient care will come from quantitative analysis for compounds whose clinical toxicity correlates well with measurable levels. Ordering selective studies based on clinical evalu-

Table 42–4 • Toxicology Panels

Alcohol panel, Blood
Quantitative (acetone, ethanol, methanol, isopropanol)

Barbiturate panel, Blood
Quantitative (amobarbital, barbital, butabarbital, butalbital, mephobarbital, pentobarbital, phenobarbital, secobarbital, thiopental)

Drug panel, Blood
Quantitative (alcohol panel, barbiturate panel, acetaminophen, 4-aminoantipyrine, chlordiazepoxide, diazepam, glutethimide, meprobamate, methaqualone, methyprylon, salicylate)

Drug panel, Gastric
Qualitative (alprazolam, 4-aminoantipyrine, amitriptyline, amobarbital, amoxapine, amphetamine, barbital, brompheniramine, butabarbital, butalbital, chlorpheniramine, cocaine, codeine, desipramine, dextromethorphan, diazepam, diphenhydramine, doxepine, ephedrine, flurazepam, glutethimide, H_2-receptor antogonist, hydrocodone, hydromorphone, hydroxyzine, imipramine, ipecac, lidocaine, lorazepam, loxapine, maprotiline, meperidine, methadone, methamphetamine, methaqualone, morphine, N-acetylprocainamide, N-desalkylflurazepam, norpropoxyphene, nortriptyline, oxazepam, oxycodone, pentazocine, pentobarbital, phenazopyridine, phencyclidine, pheniramine, phenmetrazine, phenobarbital, phenothiazines, phenylpropanolamine, phenytoin, primidone, procainamide, propoxyphene, protriptyline, pseudoephedrine, pyrilamine, quinidine, quinine, scopolamine, secobarbital, thiopental, thiothixene, trazodone, trimethobenzamide, trimethoprim, tripelennamine, tripolidine)

Drug panel, Urine
Qualitative (Same agents as gastric drug panel plus benzoylecgonine, ethchlorvynol, salicylate)

University of California–San Diego Medical Center Toxicology Laboratory, David N. Bailey, M.D., Director, 1989; with permission.

ation will increase efficiency and achieve a greater yield of useful information. For example, in a patient who has ingested automobile antifreeze, obtaining a specific ethylene glycol level will yield more useful information than doing a comprehensive toxicology screen.

IV. PREVENTION OF ABSORPTION

Patients can absorb poisons through the skin, conjunctiva, lung, or gastrointestinal tract. The amount of toxin and the duration of exposure relate directly to the severity of the injury. It is intuitive to limit the amount of toxin to which a patient is exposed. For dermal and ophthalmic exposure, it is logical to wash away the offending agent. This should be accomplished as quickly as possible, preferably at the geographic site of exposure. Removal of contaminated clothing and a plain soap-and-water wash is sufficient in most cases of cutaneous exposure. Severe injury can occur with eye exposures, particularly with highly alkaline solutions. The hallmark of initial therapy is irrigation. One to two L of a balanced salt solution would be typically used in the emergency department, but plain tap water is acceptable in the home or work place. For inhalational exposures, removing the victim from the hostile environment is paramount in limiting further absorption.

Table 42–5 summarizes the distribution of human poisonings by route of exposure as reported by the American Association of Poison Control Centers in 1987.[3] Ingestion was the most frequent route of exposure, implicated in three quarters of the reported deaths. Unlike the straightforward initial therapies for cutaneous, ophthalmic, and inhalational exposures, the techniques for gastrointestinal decontamination are controversial. Because the bulk of human poisonings occur via ingestion, these controversies and techniques will be covered in detail.

A. *Gastric Emptying*

For ingested poisons, it is a reasonable premise that toxicity can be limited by removing unabsorbed drug from the stomach. The methods for removing unabsorbed drug from the stomach are the induction of emesis or gastric lavage. Although both have been debated extensively, there is no mandate for either technique.[6–10] Animal models can be criticized as not necessarily being extrapolatable to humans. Experiments involving human subjects have ethically required administration of either nontoxic compounds or subtoxic doses, and therefore do not mimic the clinical circumstances of overdose. Variables such as time of ingestion, phamacokinetic interactions, and polydrug exposures may complicate the management of actual cases. There is no controlled study in the literature that definitively demonstrates an impact of induced emesis or gastric lavage on morbidity or mortality. However, some generalizations about their use can be made.

Neither induced emesis or gastric lavage can completely empty the stomach. It is generally accepted that either technique can evacuate between 30% and 50% of the stomach contents. It is logical that the greatest return of toxin will be achieved with the shortest elapsed

Table 42–5 • Distribution of Route of Exposure for Human Poison Exposure Cases and 397 Fatalaties

Route	All Cases (%)		Fatalities (%)	
Ingestion	944,603	(77.5)	310	(75.2)
Dermal	83,912	(6.9)	4	(0.9)
Ophthalmic	72,180	(5.9)	0	(0.0)
Inhalation	64,190	(5.3)	60	(14.6)
Bites and stings	42,026	(3.4)	2	(0.5)
Parenteral	3,452	(0.3)	22	(5.3)
Other/unknown	7,882	(0.6)	14	(3.4)

Multiple routes of exposure were observed in many poison exposure victims. Percentage is based on the total number of exposure routes (1,218,245 for all patients, 412 for fatal cases) rather than the total number of human exposures (1,166,940) or fatalities (397).

time from ingestion to evacuation. Drugs that delay gastric emptying, however, such as tricyclic antidepressants, may extend the window of efficacy to several hours. Neither technique is recommended in patients who have ingested caustics or low-viscosity hydrocarbons, or who cannot protect their own airway.

Because gastric lavage is limited to the hospital setting, induction of emesis has been a favored maneuver for home care, its primary advantage being the avoidance of delay in therapy. Mechanical stimulation of the pharynx, although safe, has been shown to be a technique of low efficacy.[11] An ideal emetic would be rapid in its onset and free of intrinsic morbidity. Numerous compounds have been used to induce vomiting, including dry mustard powder, table salt, and metallic salts such as copper sulfate and zinc sulfate. They have been abandoned because of variable efficacy and because they can cause significant morbidity. Seemingly innocuous preparations of table salt and water have been associated with death in children.[12] The mainstay for inducing emesis in the home and hospital setting has been syrup of ipecac.

1. Ipecac-Induced Emesis

Ipecac (*Cephaelis ipecacuanha*) was introduced to Europe in 1648 from Brazil, where it had been used by South American natives for the treatment of amebic dysentery. It contains two primary alkaloids, emetine and cephaeline. Cephaeline is primarily responsible for producing the emetic effect by a combination of direct gastric and central nervous system (CNS) stimulation. Emetine is responsible for the antiamebic activity and the majority of the toxicity of the compound.

Ipecac is very effective in inducing emesis, with about 95% of subjects vomiting within 20 minutes of administration. Because there is direct gastric stimulation, vomiting is not significantly inhibited by CNS-active antiemetic drugs.[13] *Patients who are obtunded, at risk for seizures, or who have swallowed caustics or low-viscosity hydrocarbons should not undergo induced emesis.* The absence of a gag reflex is a contraindication to induced vomiting. The presence of the gag reflex is not, however, a guarantee of safety. A patient with a sedative-hypnotic overdose may become rapidly obtunded, and seizures may occur without warning in a cyclic antidepressant ingestion.

Recently, induction of emesis in the hospital setting has been called into question in favor of the early administration of activated charcoal. Although emesis usually occurs within 20 minutes of administration of ipecac, vomiting may continue for up to 2 hours after, particularly if the stomach is redistended by the delivery of a charcoal-fluid slurry. Proponents of the early administration of activated charcoal argue that induced emesis wastes precious time in delivering charcoal to the gastrointestinal tract, where it may *adsorb* drugs before they are *absorbed* by the patient. An attractive theoretical alternative would be to administer charcoal, followed by ipecac to remove charcoal-bound toxin from the stomach. It has been traditional dogma, however, that ipecac and charcoal cannot be administered together because charcoal may adsorb the ipecac. This has been challenged in one small clinical trial.[14]

Dose. Syrup of ipecac is generally not recommended for children under 1 year of age, although it has been used in a population of 9- to 12-month-old infants without complications.[15] From age 1 to 5 years, the recommended dose is 15 mL, followed by 4 ounces of water. From age 5 years to adult, the dose is 30 mL, followed by 8 ounces of water. If there is no response in 20 minutes, an additional 4–8 ounces of fluid may be given. There is no evidence that large volumes of fluid increase efficacy. A second dose of ipecac may be administered in 30 minutes if there is no effect. If the patient fails to vomit, it is not necessary to retrieve the ipecac by gastric lavage.

Adverse Effects. Thousands of doses of syrup of ipecac are delivered in the outpatient and inpatient setting each year without significant morbidity. Early on, there were several reported deaths from the administration of the fluid extract of ipecac, which is 14 times more potent than the syrup of ipecac.[16,17] As a result, the fluid extract of ipecac was removed from the pharmacopeia. The chronic abuse of ipecac for self-purging in patients with eating disorders has been associated with significant toxicity.[18] The emetine alkaloid is notably cardiotoxic when taken either in high doses or over a prolonged period. The majority of other rarely reported complications of ipecac are related to protracted vomiting or complications of emesis including gastric rupture, Mallory-Weiss syndrome, and pneumomediastinum.[19–21]

2. Apomorphine-Induced Emesis

Apomorphine is chemically related to morphine and is a potent inducer of emesis by direct CNS stimulation. It has a diverse and curious history of medical application. It has been used in aversion therapy in the treatment of alcoholism[22] and as an emetic prior to the induction of general anethesia in obstetrics.[23] Given parenterally, it has a rapid onset of action (5 minutes or less). Because of its short latency, it would appear to be an attractive alternative to syrup of ipecac. It has fallen into general disuse, however, because of inconvenience and a reputation for adverse effects.

Apomorphine hydrochloride is available only as a 6.5-mg tablet that must be crushed and dissolved in water immediately before use. This time-consuming and cumbersome process may offset the advantage of its shorter latency. Although there have been attempts at developing a stable solution of apomorphine,[24] there is no such product commercially available. Because it is a parenteral preparation, it has no utility as an emetic in the home setting.

Dose. Apomorphine is given subcutaneously or intravenously at a dose of 0.07-0.1 mg/kg.

Adverse Effects. As an opiate receptor agonist, apomorphine can create CNS depression in both adults[25] and children.[26] A decrease in alertness is clearly undesirable in a patient who is vomiting. There is little documentation, however, that this has caused significant morbidity in clinical practice. Theoretically, CNS depression could be reversed by the delivery of a narcotic antagonist. Although the older narcotic agonist–antagonist drug levallorphan has been used successfully to ameliorate CNS depression,[27] the pure antagonist naloxone failed to reverse these symptoms in a small series of adult patients. [25] A large trial would be necessary to determine the true efficacy and complications of apomorphine-induced emesis in a population of suitable toxic ingestions. With the broad experience with syrup of ipecac as a reasonably rapid and safe emetic, there appears little interest in exploring the apomorphine alternative further.

3. GASTRIC LAVAGE

The alternative to the induction of emesis is gastric lavage. There is no other area of poison management more controversial than the indications for performing gastric lavage. Some clinicians feel that gastric lavage is more efficacious than emesis and recommend its use in patients who are awake as well as those who are obtunded. There is no compelling medical literature to support this position. It can be argued that gastric lavage eliminates the delay in delivery of activated charcoal caused by induced emesis. In an awake patient, gastric lavage requires their full cooperation and is uncomfortable. Unfortunately, "pumping" someone's stomach appears to be a concept accepted by some as not only medically sound, but somehow instructive to the victim of intentional overdose. The punitive approach to therapy has no foundation in either medicine or psychiatry. Gastric lavage is indicated primarily when induced emesis is not, usually because of a risk of aspiration and airway compromise. This typically occurs in the unconscious or obtunded overdose patient.

The key factors in determining the efficacy of lavage are the size of the lavage tube and the amount of lavage fluid. Early comparative studies of lavage vs. emesis[28,29] used small-diameter nasogastric type tubes with poor results. It is now clear that the best return of gastric contents can be achieved with large-bore 34 to 36 French orogastric tubes.[30] This is especially relevant when attempting to retrieve particulate matter such as pill fragments. Figure 42–1 demonstrates the difference in diameter between the routine 16 French nasogastric tube and the large-bore 36 French orogastric tube. Figure 42–2 demonstrates the technique of gastric lavage as it would be applied in a typical obtunded adult overdose patient. The technique is less commonly performed in pediatric patients, essentially reserved only for those situations where induction of emesis is contraindicated because of neurologic impairment and then only with definitive airway protection.

Procedure. As with all seriously ill patients, attention should be directed initially to the issues of resuscitation and stabilization discussed previously. Placement of an orogastric tube can itself be associated with regurgitation of gastric contents and aspiration. A patient who is not a candidate for induced emesis for fear of airway compromise is at the same risk during gastric lavage. The airway should be protected by the placement of a cuffed endotracheal tube. In spontaneously breathing patients, the nasotracheal route is typically used.

In semi-awake or uncooperative patients, passing a large-bore lavage tube through the mouth may be difficult. A bite block (Fig. 42–3) placed between the teeth facilitates passage and prevents the patient from biting the tube. If, however, the patient has his or her teeth tightly clenched, there is no reasonable way to pry them open without risking trauma to the patient or the physician. Under this circumstance, the only alternative is to sedate or paralyze the patient. Further sedation in an already obtunded overdose patient appears illogical. It can be empirically argued that a short-acting benzodiazepine (midazolam) or barbiturate (thiopental) would be

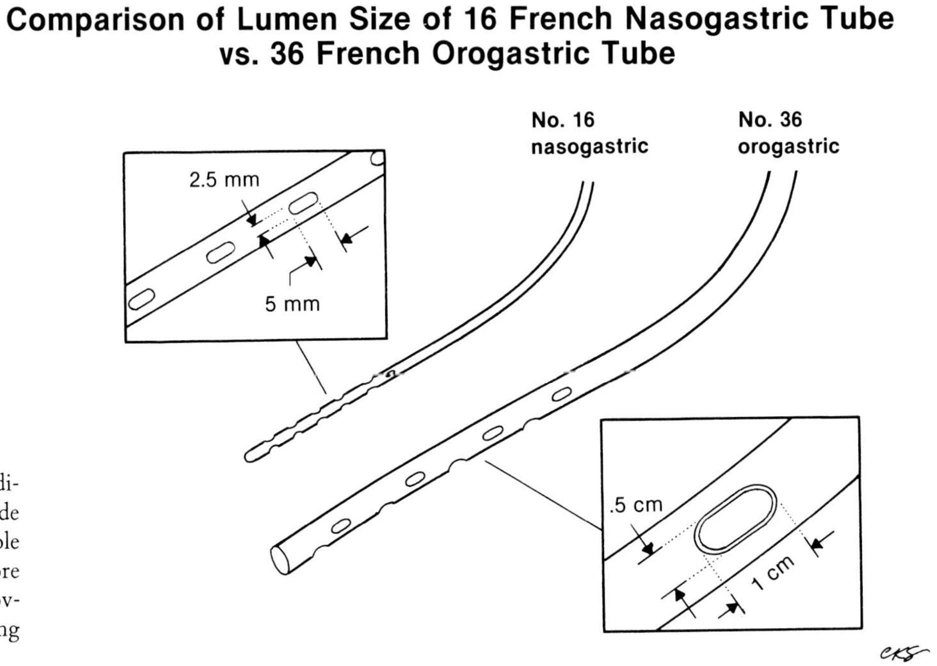

Figure 42–1 • Note the diameter of the lumen and side holes of the two tubes. Whole pills and fragments are more likely to be successfully recovered during gastric lavage using the larger tube.

unlikely to significantly compromise the patient further. A safer approach might be paralysis with a neuromuscular blocking agent such as pancuronium, although this commits the patient to mechanical ventilation. These aggressive interventions must be applied in a considered fashion, balancing their risks against the debated efficacy of gastric lavage in impacting the patient's outcome. The orogastric tube should be lubricated with a small amount of surgical lubricant and advanced gently to avoid injury to the pharynx and esophagus. Correct placement of the tube can be confirmed by the instillation of a bolus of air and auscultating over the left upper quadrant of the abdomen.

The lavage fluid is typically 0.9% NaCl. Plain tap water has been used without creating disturbances in fluid and electrolyte balance.[31] The fluid is directly instilled from a reservoir of 2000–4000 mL in aliquots of 250–500 mL (4mL/kg/cycle). The fluid is returned by gravity drainage, as indicated in Fig. 42–2. This procedure is repeated until the reservoir is depleted with large total volumes being mandatory. A minimum of 2000 mL should be instilled, even if the return is clear, because it may contain dissolved toxin. If obvious toxin, pills, or fragments are being returned, the procedure should continue until clear. Return can be facilitated by placing the patient in the left lateral decubitus position, with the head down. Using warmed lavage fluid (45°C) and external massage over the stomach theoretically may improve efficacy. After the final cycle, the orogastric tube can be used for the delivery of the initial dose of charcoal and then be removed.

Complications. There are few reported complications of gastric lavage when properly performed. Aspiration associated with vomiting during the procedure is the most common hazard.[32] Protection of the airway cannot be overemphasized. Other complications are primarily mechanical problems with the lavage tube, including kinking in the esophagus[33] and esophageal perforation.[34]

B. Activated Charcoal

In 1831, Touery, a French pharmacist, ingested a lethal dose of strychnine mixed with charcoal before the French Academy of Medicine. His survival is the most classically cited early demonstration of the adsorptive properties of charcoal. It has only been in the last 20 years, however, that the administration of activated charcoal has become widely accepted in the management of poisoning. Over the last 5 years, the weight of available evidence suggests that activated charcoal is the most clinically efficacious of the decontamination procedures.[35,36] Many clinicians have stopped the routine use of induced emesis and gastric lavage in favor of the early delivery of activated charcoal.

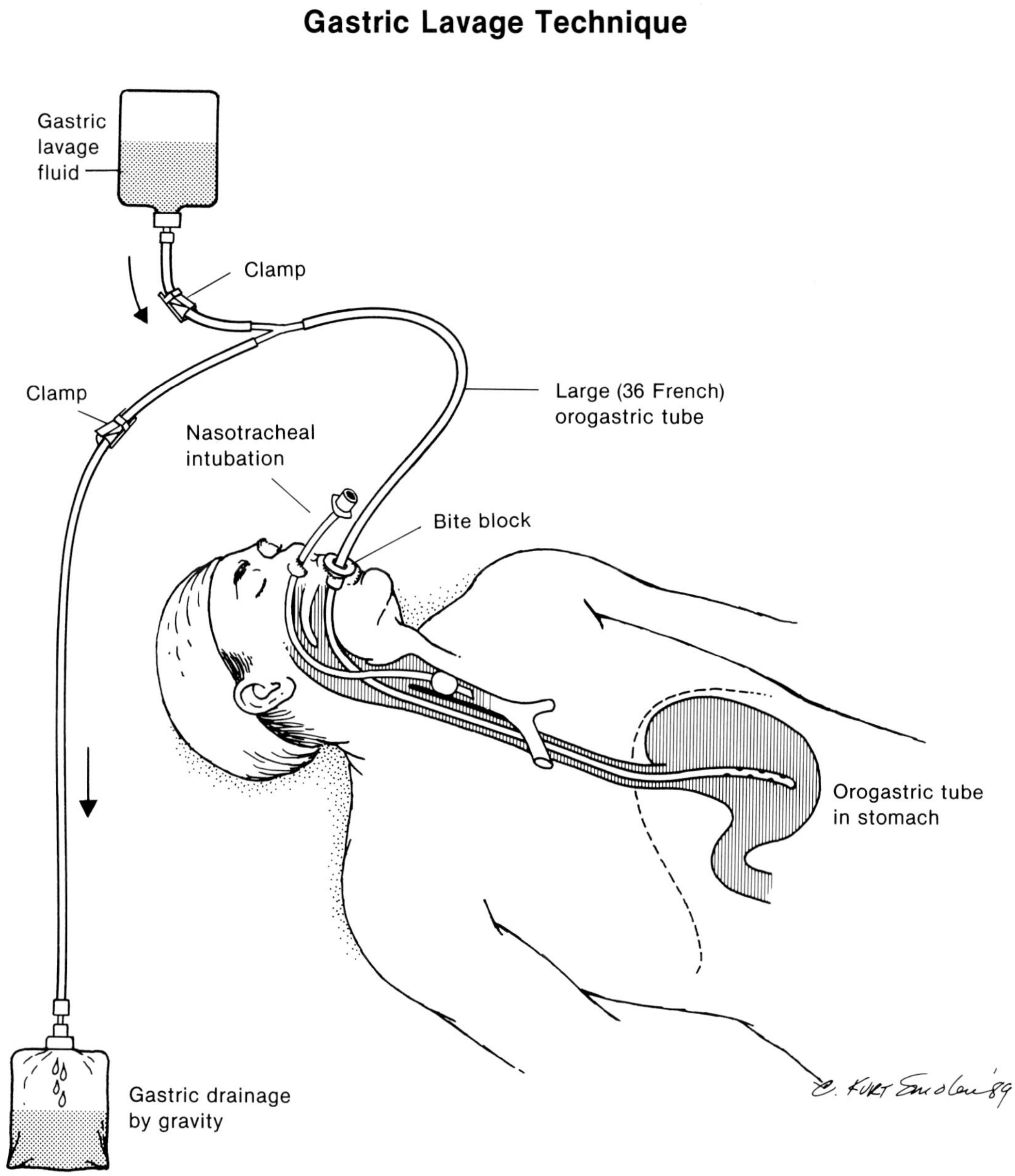

Figure 42–2 • The technique of gastric lavage is ideally performed with airway protection via nasotracheal intubation. Lavage is performed with a large-lumen orogastric tube via gravity instillation and drainage.

Activated charcoal is created by the combustion of various organic materials, including wood pulp, coal, and petroleum bases. The carbon residue is then "activated" by treatment with steam and strong acids. Activation results in a marked increase in surface area by creating a fine powder of porous granules. Early preparations had surface areas of 1000 m^2/g. Newer preparations of "super-activated" charcoal (Super-Char®) have surface areas of 2,500 to 3,500 m^2/g. The pores in the activated charcoal granule have the capacity to bind a vast variety of toxins. There are few categories of toxins that do not adsorb to charcoal. Acids, alkalis, aliphatic hydrocarbons, heavy metals, and highly ionized salts make up the bulk of the poorly adsorbed chemicals.

Because activated charcoal is not itself absorbable through the gut, the rationale for its oral administration in poisoning is to sequester toxin in the gastrointestinal tract by adsorption, allowing for excretion through the feces. This intraluminal binding of ingested toxin is only one of the pharmacokinetic mechanisms of charcoal. Several drugs are secreted into the gastrointestinal tract unchanged or as active metabolites. Some may be se-

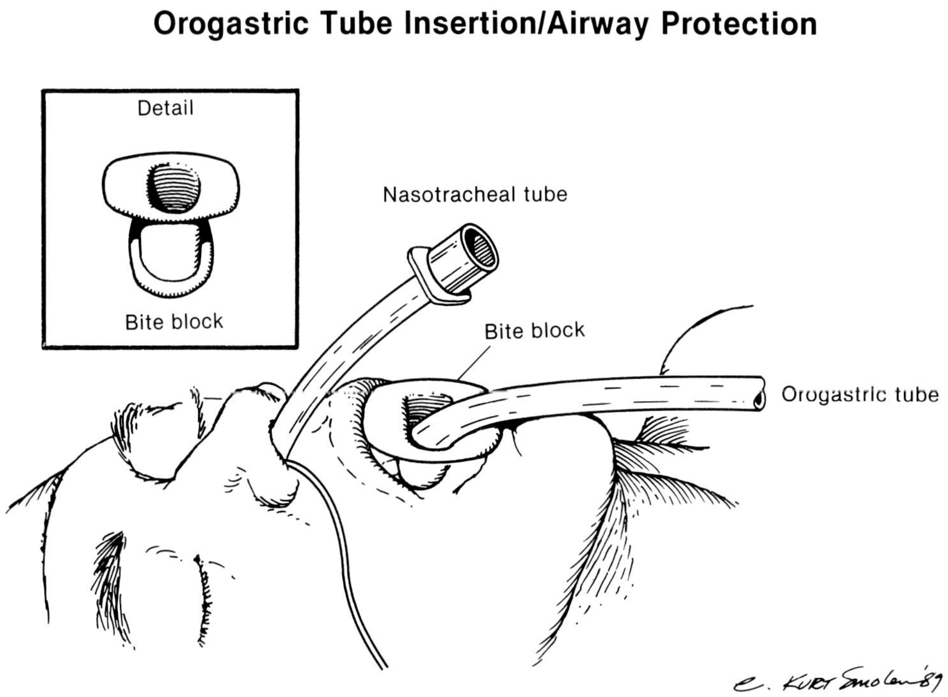

Figure 42–3 • A nasotracheal tube will protect the airway from aspiration. A bite block will facilitate the passage of the orogastric tube.

creted into gastric fluid (phencyclidine) or bile (tricyclic antidepressants) and then reabsorbed. Multiple doses of activated charcoal have decreased the halflife of enterohepatically circulated drugs, such as digoxin, in experimental models.[37] Activated charcoal has also been shown to attract drug from the plasma into the small intestine. The clearance of intravenous phenobarbital and theophylline has been shown experimentally to increase by repetitive dosing with activated charcoal.[38,39] Because neither of these two drugs has significant enterohepatic secretion, it has been proposed that the drug is "dialyzed" across the lumen of the small intestine, bound intraluminally by charcoal, and excreted in the stool. There are many reports in clinical overdose situations of charcoal increasing the clearance of numerous drugs. Although it cannot be unequivocally concluded that charcoal was responsible for favorable patient outcome, the weight of the available evidence argues for its efficacy.

Charcoal is tasteless and most patients can tolerate its slightly gritty consistency. Palatability can be improved if patients cannot see what they are drinking or if the charcoal is mixed with sweet-tasting sorbitol as a cathartic. Cathartics have been intuitively used to deliver the charcoal throughout the gut as quickly as possible to "catch up" with drug beyond the stomach. There is evidence that toxins can *desorb* from charcoal if sustained in the bowel lumen for prolonged periods.[40] Increasing transit time could ameliorate this problem. Cathartics should not be given repetitively, because fluid and electrolyte abnormalities have been documented (see the section entitled "Cathartics").

Dose. The initial dose of activated charcoal is 1 g/kg of body weight delivered as a slurry mixed with enough water or a cathartic to create a drinkable solution (8 to 12 ounces). The slurry can be ingested or delivered down a nasogastric or orogastric tube. Repetitive dosing is at 0.5 g/kg body weight every 4 hours. The initial dose may be lowered to 0.5 g/kg if the charcoal being used is of high surface area (Super-Char®).

Adverse Effects. Complications of activated charcoal therapy are rare. Charcoal has no biologic activity and cannot be absorbed. Reported complications have been essentially limited to aspiration and mechanical obstruction of the bowel. Patients frequently vomit after the delivery of the charcoal slurry, usually because of the prior administration of ipecac. Inhalation of charcoal itself produces no significant effect in experimental animals. Aspiration of gastric contents is associated with airway compromise and significant morbidity in general. The fact that death has been reported with the aspiration of gastric contents containing charcoal[41] is more of an admonition for scrupulous attention to airway management than a condemnation of charcoal. Charcoal can accumulate in the bowel lumen, forming concretions that can be associated with obstruction.[42,43] A typical predisposing factor for this complication is a decrease in gastrointestinal motility as a result of narcotic or anticholinergic drug effect. It is, therefore, important to document the presence of charcoal in the stool, particularly if repetitive doses are given.

C. *Cathartics*

Cathartics are commonly recommended in the management of toxic ingestions. There is an appealing logic to their use that overshadows their lack of proven efficacy. It makes sense to hasten passage of an ingested poison through the gastrointestinal tract, thereby limiting the time the toxin is in contact with the absorptive lining of the gut. Because toxins are not irreversibly bound to charcoal, it is logical to enhance transit time to limit the possibility of desorption. In addition to shortened transit time, the development of charcoal concretions may be prevented by the increased intraluminal fluid caused by an osmotic cathartic. There are several cathartic options available, including oil-based preparations, milk of magnesia, disodium phosphate solution (Fleets®), saline cathartics, and sorbitol. For the most part, cathartics are effective and safe, but they are not completely without hazard.

Oil-based cathartics (mineral oil, castor oil) act as direct irritants. Although there was some enthusiasm for their use in the treatment of lipophilic toxins (glutethimide), there has been no proven efficacy for their use. There is a significant risk of the development of lipoid pneumonia if aspiration should occur. Therefore, oil-based cathartics are not recommended under any circumstance. Milk of magnesia is given in 1- to 2-ounce dosages for the home therapy of constipation, and is rarely used in the medical setting.

Disodium phosphate solution (Fleets®) has been recommended in iron ingestion as a gastric lavage to convert ferrous sulfate to the nonabsorbable ferrous phosphate. It contains 1600 mEq/L of sodium and 4,000 mEq/L of phosphate and has caused hypocalcemia, hypernatremia, and hyperphosphatemia. Its use in iron ingestion has been abandoned in favor of a safer 5% sodium bicarbonate lavage to convert ferrous sulfate to ferrous carbonate.

Saline cathartics have been the mainstay of purgative therapy for many years. Their primary mechanism is osmotic, drawing fluid into the lumen of the gut stimulating peristalsis. The three commonly used saline cathartics are magnesium sulfate, magnesium citrate, and sodium sulfate.

1. SALINE CATHARTIC DOSE

There is great variability in dosing recommendations for the saline cathartics. The sulfates are delivered at a dose of 250 mg/kg or 15–30 g. Magnesium citrate comes prepared as a flavored carbonated beverage dosed at 0.5 mL/kg or 4 to 8 ounces.

2. SALINE CATHARTIC ADVERSE EFFECTS

The magnesium salts contain between 8 and 16 mEq/g of magnesium. Normal magnesium homeostasis is maintained by the kidney with 20% to 30% of an ingested dose being rapidly excreted by the patient with normal renal function. Severe cathartic-induced hypermagnesemia has been reported requiring hemodialysis.[44] Magnesium salt cathartics are not recommended in patients with known kidney disease or who are at risk for developing renal insufficiency (trauma, seizures, myoglobinuria). Osmotic-induced hypernatremia has been reported as well with magnesium citrate.[45] Sodium sulfate contains 14 mEq/g of sodium and should not be used in patients with restricted salt intakes (hypertension, congestive heart failure).

In recent years, the mostly widely used cathartic has become sorbitol. It is a hexahydric alcohol that has been used extensively as an inert ingredient in various pharmaceutical preparations. It is poorly absorbed from the gastrointestinal tract, creating a purgative effect by increasing osmotic pressure in the intestinal lumen. It induces diarrhea three to four times more rapidly than saline cathartics, often within 1 hour of delivery.[46] When mixed with activated charcoal, its sweet taste and syrupy consistency improves palatability. It is available as a 70% solution, the minimal bacteriostatic concentration. There are also commercially available, premixed sorbitol-charcoal preparations.

3. *Sorbitol Dose*

There is wide variability in dosing recommendations for sorbitol, ranging from 2 to 4 mL/kg of the 70% solution, with diarrhea being reported in doses of as little as 0.5 mL/kg. Single doses of 30 grams of charcoal mixed with 150 mL of 70% sorbitol have not caused significant electrolyte disturbances in healthy adult volunteers.[47] There have been reports of severe hypernatremic dehydration with the repetitive use of sorbitol in adults and children.[45,48] It is recommended that sorbitol be used with great care in young children and older adults. In patients receiving multiple-dose charcoal therapy, sorbitol should not be given with every dose of charcoal. Once the patient has passed a charcoal stool, sorbitol should be given, at most, every other cycle. Scrupulous attention must be paid to fluid and electrolyte balance.

D. *Whole Bowel Irrigation*

Whole bowel irrigation is a widely used bowel preparation prior to colonoscopy or colonic surgery. The rapid ingestion or instillation of large volumes of a polyethylene glycol electrolyte solution (eg, Golytely®, Braintree Laboratories, Braintree, MA) causes a brisk mechanical flushing of the bowel. Several studies have demonstrated the efficacy and safety of the technique.[49,50] There is negligible fluid or salt absorption or secretion across the gastrointestinal epithelium. It is not a cathartic in the same sense as a saline cathartic or sorbitol, because there is little intraluminal fluid shift. It has only been recently proposed as an alternative to other gastrointestinal decontamination techniques in the management of selected overdose situations.

Tenenbein has suggested application of whole bowel irrigation in the following circumstances[51]: (1) ingestion of a massive amount of toxic substance; (2) late presentation after ingestion with potentially large amounts of toxin well beyond the pylorus; (3) ingestion of a sustained release preparation, such as theophylline; and (4) overdoses of substances not adsorbed by charcoal, such as iron.

There is documentation of decreased absorption of an ampicillin marker in adults volunteers undergoing whole bowel irrigation.[52] The technique has also been used in theophylline and iron poisoning.[51]

Procedure. The recommended procedure is to pass a nasogastric tube, seat the patient on a commode, and instill the solution at a rate of 2.0 L/h for adults and 0.5 L/h for small children. This obviously requires a completely alert and cooperative patient. End point is reached when there is a clear rectal effluent, usually after 4 to 6 hours. Activated charcoal can be added prior to the procedure, but there are no data on the efficacy of this combined therapy.

Complications. The procedure is apparently well tolerated but requires a cooperative subject and a patient nursing staff. The only significant complication is emesis related to the ingested toxin, the prior use of ipecac, or excessively rapid instillation of the solution. The same caveats about airway management apply here as in the other techniques of gastrointestinal decontamination. Problems with fluids and electrolytes have not been encountered with limited usage in toxic exposures. It is anticipated that whole bowel irrigation in poisoning would have a similar record of safety as it has had as elective bowel purgative. Because the technique is relatively cumbersome and time-consuming to perform, it will likely achieve only limited clinical applicability.

V. Enhancement of Elimination

An ingested toxin residing within the stomach or gut is still outside the body in a physiologic sense. The goal of gastrointestinal decontamination outlined above in the previous section is the prevention of absorption. Once a drug has been absorbed into the bloodstream, it is then available for tissue binding, where its toxic effects can be manifest. Employing techniques to enhance the elimination of absorbed toxin is the next logical step in attempting to limit toxicity.

A. *Pharmacokinetics*

It is beyond the scope of this chapter to engage in a detailed discussion of pharmacokinetics. Defining some of the basic concepts and terminology will be useful, however, in understanding the strategies that follow.

An ingested drug is absorbed, distributed in the blood and tissues, metabolized, and eliminated. The factors affecting absorption are numerous, including the type of drug, the amount ingested, the length of time in contact with the surface of the gut, and the pH of gastric fluid. Once absorbed, the drug has to move through the body. A mathematical description of this process can be developed if the body is divided into a classical two-compartment model. The central compartment consists primarily of the plasma, and the peripheral compartment consists primarily of the tissues.

The plasma concentration of a drug (*Cp*) is equal to *A*/*Vd*, where *A* is the total amount of active drug in the body and *Vd* is the volume of distribution of the drug. The volume of distribution (*Vd*) is fluid that would be necessary if the total amount of drug were distributed at the same concentration as plasma. Drugs such as tricyclic antidepressants and digoxin have large volumes of distribution (more than 1 L/kg) because they are highly tissue or protein bound. Drugs with large *Vds* are generally not effectively cleared by hemodialysis or hemoperfusion. Although plasma concentration (*Cp*) can often be measured in clinical situations, its correlation to clinical toxicity may be problematic because the *Cp* alone may not reflect the entire body burden of drug nor its effect at the tissue level.

If a drug is eliminated in a linear fashion directly proportional to the plasma concentration, it is cleared by *first-order kinetics*. This is typical for drugs that undergo strictly renal elimination. The greater the amount of drug being filtered from the plasma, the greater the amount eliminated from the body. *Zero-order kinetics* is the nonlinear elimination of drug from the plasma and is typical of hepatic metabolism. The elimination is nonlinear because the metabolic pathways are enzyme mediated and therefore saturable. Regardless of the amount of drug present, it can be eliminated only at the rate allowable by the amount of available enzyme. The clearance of ethanol is a classical example of zero-order elimination.

The *halflife (T 1/2)* of a drug is the amount of time required to reduce the peak concentration by half. The meaning of halflife can only be accurately assessed if applied to a specific compartment. The halflife of a drug in the plasma may be very different than in the cerebrospinal fluid. The concept of halflife has its greatest clinical applicability when dealing with drugs with strictly first-order kinetics. In drugs demonstrating zero-order kinetics, the *T 1/2* is not constant, but changes with the amount of drug left in the body. In many situations, the kinetics of drug elimination changes with concentration, limiting the entire concept of halflife as a useful clinical parameter. Salicylates, for example, are eliminated primarily by first-order k inetics in low doses. In higher doses, elimination becomes zero-order with small changes in amount ingested causing large increases in plasma and tissue concentration. Halflives are derived from animal or human models with a single compound under investigation. The clinical situation in the emergency department is often a polydrug ingestion, which may markedly alter the pharmacokinetics of the individual toxins.

B. Repeat-Dose Activated Charcoal

The traditional role of activated charcoal in the management of poisoning has been the adsorption of intraluminal toxin prior to absorption by the gut. Enthusiasm for the use of charcoal has increased further with the discovery that it may also be useful in enhancing the elimination of previously absorbed drugs. Drugs that undergo enterohepatic or enteroenteric circulation (tricyclic antidepressants, glutethimide) are absorbed and then reexcreted into the bowel. Additional doses of charcoal may adsorb further toxin as it reenters the bowel lumen. It has been shown that repeat-dose or "pulse" charcoal shortens the halflife of intravenously administered phenobarbital, theophylline, and salicylate.[38,39,53] The bowel mucosa may act as a "dialysis" membrane in this situation, with drug being drawn across from an area of higher concentration in the plasma to an area of lower concentration in the gut, where it becomes adsorbed by the charcoal (see the section entitled "Activated Charcoal").

Dose. The dose of repeat charcoal is one half the initial dose every 2 to 4 hours, typically 15–40 g. It can be delivered with a cathartic to enhance gastrointestinal transit time. Because cathartics have been associated with fluid and electrolyte abnormalities, caution should be used. If the patient has already developed a charcoal diarrhea, cathartics should be eliminated or used only in every other cycle.

Adverse Effects. Complications of activated charcoal therapy are rare. Adverse effects are essentially limited to aspiration and mechanical obstruction of the bowel. See the section on activated charcoal above.

C. Urine Alkalinization and Acidification

Drugs can be classified as either weak acids or weak bases, depending on their ability to donate or accept a hydrogen ion when placed in solution. When dissolved in solution, a drug establishes an equilibrium in ionized and nonionized forms. The amount of ionized or polar form depends on the dissociation constant *Ka* of the drug and the pH of the solution. The pKa of a drug is the pH at which one half of the compound is ionized and the other half is nonionized. Weak acids are classified as having a pKa of 3.0–7.5, while weak bases have a pKas of 7.5–10.5. A weak acid will increase its ionization when placed in an alkaline environment. A weak base will increase its ionization when placed in an acidic environment.

Drugs cross cellular membranes most efficiently in their nonionized form. In the body, pH varies from one physiologic compartment to another. If the pH could be manipulated so that a drug was in a highly ionized state in a particular compartment, the drug could be trapped in that space. Alkalinization or acidification of the urine theoretically uses this concept of ion-trapping to enhance elimination of drugs. Figure 42–4 illustrates the principle of alkalinization to trap a weak acid such as salicylate (pKa 3.5) in the urine. Nonionized drug moves from the tissue to the plasma to the urine, where it becomes highly ionized and excreted.

Although this technique is appealing theoretically, its application is limited due to the risk of complications and the small number of drugs that have appropriate chemistry. Drugs must have small volumes of distribution, high urinary clearance, limited metabolism, and a pKa that allows for reasonable alterations of urine pH to enhance excretion.

1. Alkaline Diuresis

Alkaline diuresis can be achieved by the administration of 1–2 mEq/kg of sodium bicarbonate in 15 mL/kg of 5% dextrose in 0.45% saline over 3 to 4 hours to create a urinary pH of 7.5–8.0.

Complications. Great caution should be used because complications of pulmonary edema, cerebral edema, and electrolyte disturbances can occur with the haphazard delivery of large quantities of this hypertonic solution. Hypokalemia is a common side effect of salicylate overdose that can be exacerbated by the delivery of alkali. If the patient has a significant preexisting metabolic acidosis, alkalinization of the urine may not be achievable without the delivery of unacceptable amounts of sodium bicarbonate. Patients with renal insufficiency should not undergo alkaline diuresis. Urine volumes need to be adequate (2–4 mL/kg/h). There is little evidence that forced diuresis with large volumes of fluid enhances excretion of drug and may contribute to volume overload. Although alkaline diuresis is commonly considered in the management of salicylate (pKa 3.5) and phenobarbital (pKa 7.2) overdose, most patients do well with conservative management. Hemodialysis is an effective and safer method of treatment in patients with severe intoxication.

2. Acid Diuresis

Urine acidification has extremely limited applicability and is uncommonly performed. Acidification can be achieved by the delivery of ammonium chloride, 75 mg/kg/24 h divided into four to six oral doses or a 2% intravenous solution. An alternative is the administration of 0.2 mEq/kg/h of a 0.1-M hydrochloric acid solution through a central venous line. Urinary pH should reach 5.5–6.0 as an end point.

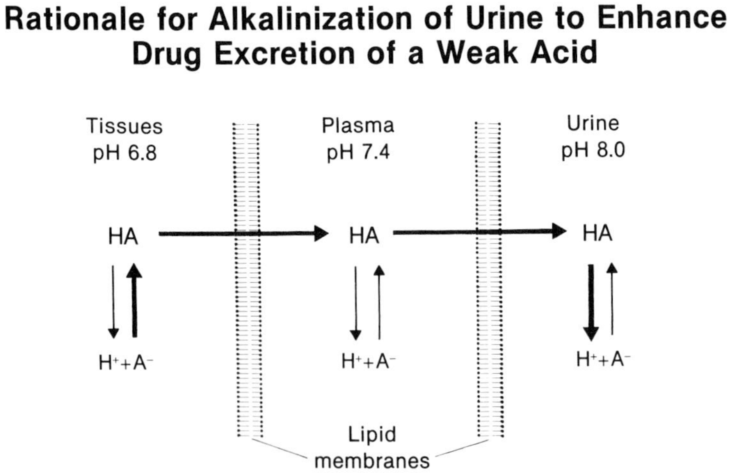

Figure 42–4 • Only nonionized drug will freely cross the lipid membrane. Alkalinization of the urine will cause a weak acid such as salicylate to become "trapped" in the urine, enhancing excretion.

Complications. Phencyclidine (PCP) and amphetamine are both drugs of abuse commonly seen in overdose. As weak bases, they are both theoretically candidates for acid diuresis. However, both are hepatically metabolized, PCP has a large volume of distribution, and neither is excreted significantly in the urine. Both drugs create a hyperadrenergic, hyperdynamic state, often with profound muscle rigidity that may result in rhabdomyolysis. Myoglobin precipitates in an acidic environment, which may contribute to the development of acute tubular necrosis.

D. *Extracorporeal Methods*

Cleansing the blood of absorbed toxins through hemodialysis or hemoperfusion is a theoretically useful intervention for a large number of exposures. Table 42–6 is an abbreviated list of poisons whose elimination may be enhanced by extracorporeal means. In clinical practice, however, relatively few patients benefit from this therapy, and the indications for hemodialysis and hemoperfusion are controversial. The fact that a drug or toxin can be eliminated more rapidly by these techniques does not mandate their use. Hemodialysis and hemoperfusion are relatively complicated techniques, with a potential for significant morbidity in their own right. They should be employed only in selected circumstances.

Table 42–6 • Drugs Eliminated by Extracorporeal Means

Hemodialysis	Hemoperfusion
Amphetamines	Amanitin
Barbiturates	Barbiturates
Bromides	Carbamazapine
Chloral hydrate	Ethchlorvynol
Ethanol	Glutethimide
Ethylene glycol	Meprobamate
Isopropanol	Methaqualone
Lithium	Paraquat
Methanol	Propoxyphene
Salicylates	Theophylline
Theophylline	
Thiocyanate	

The fact that a drug may have its elimination enhanced by an extracorporeal technique does not necessarily demand its employment in clinical situations (see text).

1. HEMODIALYSIS

The first question to answer in considering hemodialysis is whether clearance of drug or toxin will be enhanced over what can be achieved by normal physiologic processes or other, less complicated techniques. Clearance depends in large degree on the physical characteristics of the toxin. In general, toxins must have small volumes of distribution, be of low molecular weight, and have low protein binding and high water solubility. In addition, plasma levels must correlate well with clinical toxicity so that following blood levels will be useful in confirming the effectiveness of the procedure.

Patient selection is based primarily on clinical criteria. Severely intoxicated individuals with marked aberration of vital signs not responding to supportive measures are the prime candidates for hemodialysis. Others include patients with hepatic or renal insufficiency and patients with prolonged coma. Individuals with underlying hepatic or renal disease may not be able to eliminate toxins by normal metabolic or excretory mechanisms. Patients in prolonged coma may develop complications of the intensive care unit, such as nosocomial pneumonia. The documentation of a potentially lethal drug level may argue for hemodialysis, regardless of the immediate clinical state of the patient.

Absolute indications for hemodialysis do exist. For example, severe intoxication with methanol and ethylene glycol are mandates for hemodialysis. Both chemicals are metabolized into toxic compounds. Methanol is metabolized into formate, which causes metabolic acidosis and retinopathy. Ethylene glycol is metabolized into oxalate, which also causes metabolic acidosis and is nephrotoxic. Because the first step in the metabolism of both chemicals is mediated by alcohol dehydrogenase, administering ethanol may block immediate toxicity by ''occupying'' the enzyme. In severe intoxication, this is only a temporizing maneuver, because efficient alternate pathways for elimination do not exist.

Complications of hemodialysis include hypotension, electrolyte imbalances, osmolar shifts, and mechanical problems such as bleeding at the vascular access sites. These will be minimized in the hands of a nephrologist and trained technicians who perform the procedure routinely.

2. HEMOPERFUSION

The principle of hemoperfusion is to pass anticoagulated blood through an adsorbent column that binds toxin. In the mid 1960s, Yatzidis demonstrated that barbiturate, salicylate, and glutethimide could be adsorbed from plasma by perfusion through a charcoal column.[54] Enthusiasm for the technique was initially high, because charcoal columns could theoretically be efficacious for elimination of any of the literally hundreds of compounds capable of being adsorbed by charcoal. It was also attractive because the limiting factors in hemodialysis, such as molecular weight, water solubility, and protein binding, were not a problem. The development of non–charcoal-containing polystyrene Amberlite resin columns were shown to bind highly lipid soluble drugs such a glutethimide and methaqualone more efficiently than the charcoal columns.[55,56] Although hemoperfusion may clear the plasma, if the drug has a large volume of distribution (glutethimide), rebound is likely once tissue stores equilibrate with the plasma, necessitating retreatment. The fact that a resin or charcoal column may effectively adsorb a given compound does not mean that hemoperfusion will have an impact on clinical outcome. Although tricyclic antidepressants are effectively bound to charcoal, so little of the drug is distributed to the plasma that clearance is not appreciably increased. It has been suggested, however, that in severe toxicity, even a small shift in drug level may prevent a life-threatening dysrhythmia. Hemoperfusion has been proposed in exposures with compounds with delayed toxicity, such as the mushroom *Amanita phalloides* or the herbacide paraquat. There are no data showing definitive efficacy in these ingestions.

Over time, clinical use of the hemoadsorbtive techniques has not been extensive. The American Association of Poison Control Centers Annual Report of 1987[3] documented only 124 cases of charcoal hemoperfusion and 35 cases of resin hemoperfusion in a population of 1.2 million poison exposures.

Procedure. Figure 42–5 illustrates a classical hemoperfusion circuit. Blood is withdrawn from an arteriovenous or venous–venous shunt using a blood pump at a rate of flow of approximately 300 mL/min. An

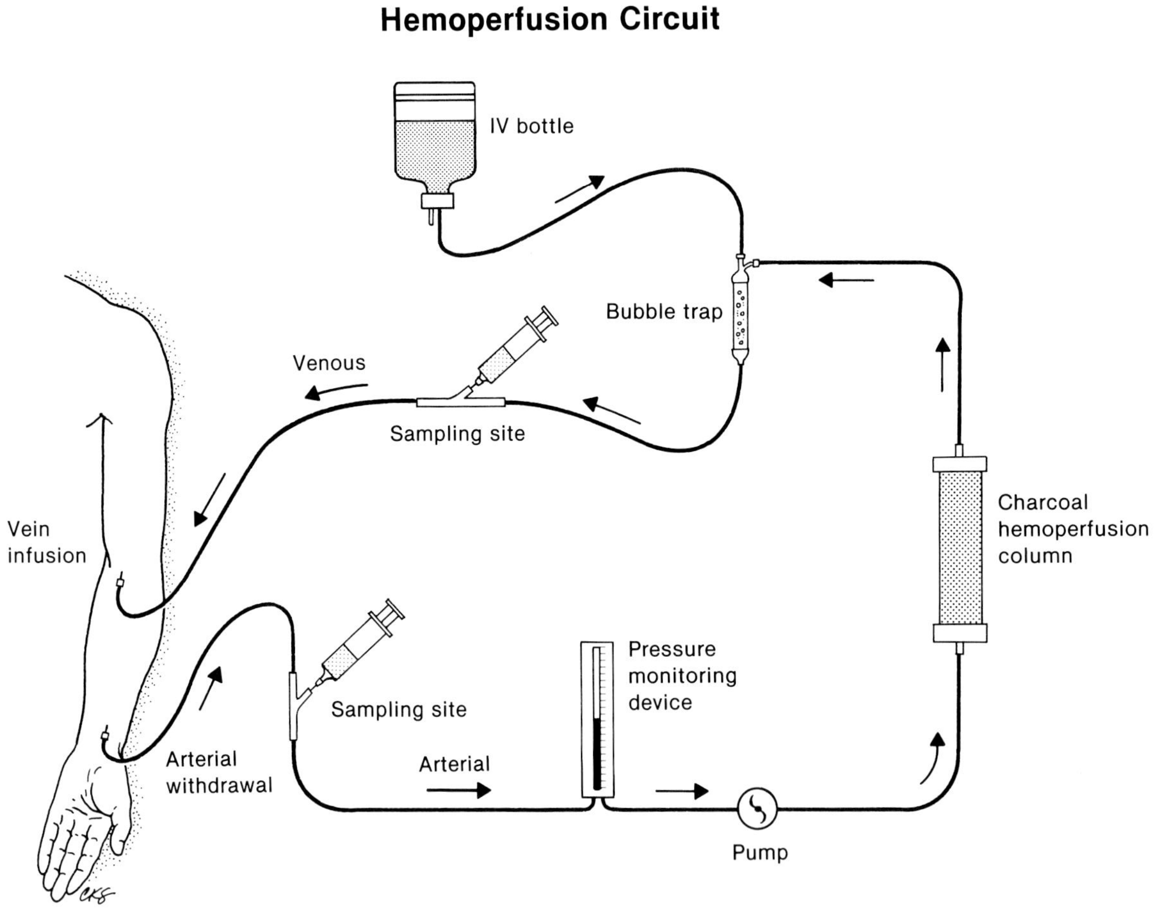

Figure 42–5 • The figure shows a hemoperfusion circuit. See text for details of application.

in-line pressure monitoring device detects increases in perfusion pressure, implying clotting in the device. A bubble trap is placed to prevent the possibility of air embolism. Priming volume is dependent on the device used, but is typically 100 mL. The patient requires heparinization for the procedure. The length of time the patient is hemoperfused ranges from 1 to 30 hours,[57,58] but is usually 3 to 4 hours, depending on the type of drug and clinical response. Repeat hemoperfusion may be necessary if the patient deteriorates because of reequilibration of drug from tissue depots.

Although conceptually simple, the circuit requires constant monitoring in an intensive care setting. One practical consideration to explain the limited use of this technique is the unfamiliarity of the devices among intensivists and intensive care nurses. In contrast, hemodialysis is commonly performed for renal insufficiency, making the transitional application to poisoning an easier one. Even in the situation where hemoperfusion has been shown to be more efficacious in clearance of drug (theophylline, phenobarbital), hemodialysis may be chosen because of greater clinical familiarity with the technique.

Complications. The principal complication of the columns is that they absorb platelets and, to a lesser degree, leukocytes.[59] As much as a 30% reduction in platelets can be seen and, coupled with the obligatory heparinization, bleeding may become a problem. Particulate embolization was a problem of the early charcoal columns. Coating the charcoal columns with a polymer limited this problem and reduced the amount of platelet and leukocyte loss.[60] Hemolysis has been reported with the use of a polymer-coated charcoal column.[61]

VI. ANTIDOTAL THERAPY

For Snow White, the delivery of a kiss was sufficient to reverse the coma induced by the poisoned apple. Unfortunately, the notion that every poison has an antidote is limited to the storybook world. The brief list of toxins for which specific antidotal therapy is available is presented in Table 42–7. An antidote in this context is a specific agent that uniquely reverses or limits the effect of a single type of toxin. Activated charcoal may be antidotal in the broad sense, but is usually categorized as a decontaminant. The distinction is largely a semantic one.

Table 42–7 • Antidotal Therapies

Toxin	Antidote
Acetaminophen	N-acetylcysteine
Anticholinergics	Physostigmine
Carbamate insecticides	Atropine
Cyanide	Lilly® CN antidote kit
Digoxin	Fab fragments
Ethylene glycol	Ethanol
Heavy metals	Penicillamine, dimercaprol
Iron	Deferoxamine
Isoniazid	Pyridoxine
Methanol	Ethanol
Narcotics, opiates	Naloxone
Nitrates, nitrites	Methylene blue
Organophosphate insecticides	Atropine, pralidoxime

The "universal antidote" of tea and burnt toast has no efficacy and should not be recommended even for home use. Analeptics (picrotoxin, nikethamide) stimulate respirations in CNS-depressed patients. In overdose, they may precipitate seizure activity and are not recommended. Patients with hypoventilation or at risk for aspiration should have mechanical airway management. Several of the commonly administered antidotes are discussed in greater detail below.

A. *Naloxone*

Naloxone is a pure opiate antagonist derived from thebaine. It is useful in reversing the effect of essentially all opiate-receptor agonists by competitive inhibition. It is the most commonly administered antidote[3] and is part of the routine resuscitative management of all patients with CNS depression of unknown cause.

Dose. Naloxone comes in single- and multidose vials in concentrations of 0.4 mg/mL or 1 mg/mL. In children the dose is 0.03–0.1 mg/kg intravenously. In adults, starting dose is usually 2 mg intravenously followed by further 2- to 10-mg boluses, depending on effect. Some opiate overdoses (propoxyphene, fentanyl derivatives) may require multiple boluses or continuous infusion for reversal. In patients without intravenous access, the drug may be given intramuscularly, subcutaneously, or via an endotracheal tube. There is no maximum dose. The total amount administered is dictated by clinical response.

Adverse Effects. There are anecdotal reports of hypertension, dysrhythmias, and pulmonary edema occurring after the administration of naloxone.[62,63] These usually occurred postoperatively or in patients with abstinence syndrome. Literally thousands of doses are administered yearly by paramedics and in emergency rooms without reported complications. A predictable effect of the drug is precipitation of withdrawal in some narcotic addicts. Although uncomfortable to experience, narcotic abstinence syndrome is generally not associated with severe medical complications.

B. *N-acetylcysteine*

In overdose, acetaminophen is hepatotoxic, with intermediate metabolites rapidly exhausting intrinsic glutathione stores. N-acetylcysteine (NAC) is a glutathione substitute, providing sulfhydryl groups, which are avid for these toxic metabolites.[64] N-acetylcysteine (Mucomyst®) has been commercially available as a mucolytic agent since the 1950s. Only the oral preparation is available in the United States. In Europe, an intravenous preparation is available, which is under investigation in the United States. N-acetylcysteine is relatively unpalatable because of its offensive sulfur odor. The precipitation of vomiting may limit its administration. Palatability can be improved by mixing with a soft drink or fruit juice. Controversy exists about the use of charcoal in acetaminophen overdose. Charcoal may potentially adsorb the NAC, and generally they should not be given together.

Dose. Potential hepatotoxicity can be predicted by determining a serum level and applying the Rumack/Matthew nomogram (Fig. 42-6) as adapted by Smilkstein.[64] (*Note*: The terms "probable" and "high" risk defined groups within the study, and only the solid line in the nomogram should be used for clinical decision-making.) Ideally, NAC should be administered no later than 16 hours from the time of ingestion. If there is delay in obtaining a serum level, the loading dose should be administered in a large ingestion. The loading dose of NAC is 140 mg/kg diluted with a soft drink or juice, followed by 70 mg/kg every 4 hours for 17 additional doses.[64] Any dose that is vomited within 1 hour of administration should be repeated.

Adverse Effects. Allergic reactions have been seen with the intravenous preparation. Oral administration of NAC is not associated with significant adverse reactions.

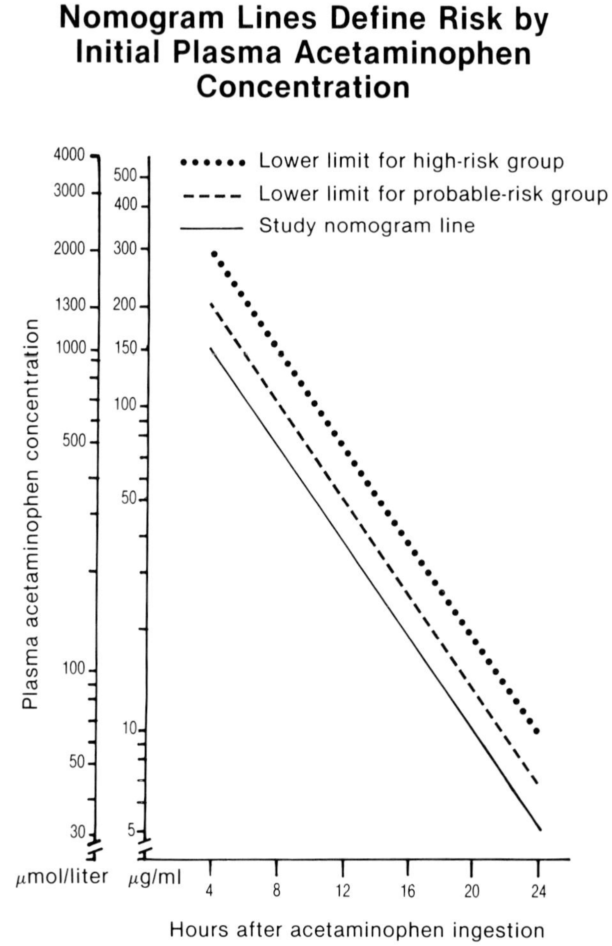

Figure 42-6 • Nomogram lines are used to define risk according to initial plasma acetaminophen concentration. Only the solid line should be used in clinical decision making. The terms "probable-risk" and "high-risk" are only used to define study classifications and have no direct clinical applicability. (From Smilkstein MJ, Knapp GL, Kulig KW, Rumack BH. Efficacy of oral N-acetylcysteine in the treatment of acetaminophen overdose: Analysis of the national multicenter study (1976 to 1985). (N Engl J Med 319:1557–1562, 1988; with permission.)

C. *Atropine and Pralidoxime*

Organophosphate and carbamate insecticides have largely replaced the chlorinated hydrocarbons (DDT) because they do not accumulate in the environment. They do, however, possess significant toxicity in acute exposure.

Acetylcholine is the synaptic neurotransmitter at postganglionic parasympathetic terminals, preganglionic sympathetic and parasympathetic nerve endings, and at the motor end plates of skeletal muscle. After release and binding to the postsynaptic effector site, acetylcholine is enzymatically degraded by the action of acetylcholine. Organophosphate and carbamate insecticides bind to acetylcholinesterase, rendering the enzyme inactive. The accumulation of acetylcholine causes excessive postsynaptic stimulation. Classical muscarinic symptoms usually occur first, including abdominal cramps, vomiting, diarrhea, bronchorrhea, increased salivation, and lacrimation. Miosis is a classical sign but may not always be present. Nicotinic effects typically occur later and include muscle twitching and fasiculations. Central nervous system effects are more common with organophosphates. Death is usually caused by respiratory failure.

Organophosphate toxicity can be reversed by the delivery of atropine and pralidoxime. Atropine binds competitively at postsynaptic sites, blocking the effects of the excess acetylcholine. The administration of atropine will quickly reverse muscarinic symptoms, but does not deal with the underlying biochemical lesion. Pralidoxime (2-PAM) cleaves the bond between the organophosphate and the enzyme, restoring the cholinesterase activity. Pralidoxime should be administered early in the course of therapy, because the bond between toxin and enzyme matures with time.

Carbamate toxicity is treated with atropine alone, because the bond between carbamate and cholinesterase is not reversible by the administration of pralidoxime.

Dose. Atropine is administered in relatively high doses. In adults, 2–4 mg is delivered intravenously every 5 to 10 minutes, titrated to the disappearance of cholinergic symptoms or the development of anticholinergic effects. The dose in children is 0.015–0.05 mg/kg.[65]

Pralidoxime in adults is administered in a dose of 1–2 g intravenously over 15 to 20 minutes. In face of severe or recurrent symptoms, it can be delivered as an infusion of 500 mg/h. The initial pediatric dose is 25–50 mg/kg IV.

Adverse Effects. Excessive administration of atropine will cause anticholinergic symptoms, including tachycardia, dry mouth, mydriasis, urinary retention, and decreased gastrointestinal motility. Serious side-effects have not been reported with the use of pralidoxime.

D. *Physostigmine*

Anticholinergic effects can be seen with a large number of drugs including antihistamines, antipsychotics, cyclic antidepressants, over-the-counter cold remedies, and synthetic belladonna alkaloids. All create their atropine-like effect by the competitive inhibition of acetylcholine at cholinergic receptor sites. Peripheral effects of parasympathetic blockade include dry mouth, sinus tachycardia, mydriasis, urinary retention, decreased gastrointestinal motility, and hyperpyrexia. Central nervous system effects include disorientation, hallucinations, anxiety, delirium and, rarely, coma and death.

A logical strategy in treating these symptoms would be to increase the amount of acetylcholine present in the synapse to actively compete for binding sites. Blocking the action of the enzyme acetlycholinesterase would achieve this end. There are several noninsecticide carbamate drugs that are acetylcholinesterase inhibitors, including neostigmine, pyridostigmine, and edrophonium. Edrophonium and pyridostigmine are useful in the diagnosis and management of myesthenia gravis. These compounds can be used to reverse peripheral anticholinergic effects but do not cross into the CNS. Physostigmine, however, does cross and can be used to treat both peripheral and central anticholinergic symptoms. Physostigmine has significant side effects. Because most anticholinergic symptoms in overdose tend not to be severe and can be managed supportively, the risks of physostigmine delivery usually outweigh the potential benefit. As a result, *physostigmine is not considered a first-line drug* and should be used only when severe symptoms are present.

Dose. In adults, the initial dose is 0.5–1 mg given intravenously at a rate not to exceed 1 mg/min. The dose in children is 0.02 mg/kg. Because of a short half-life, the initial dose may need to be repeated every 30 to 60 minutes.[66]

Adverse Effects. The use of physostigmine is associated with significant side effects, including the precipitation of seizures, bradycardia, heart block, asystole, and potential cholinergic excess.[67–69]

E. *Ethanol*

Methanol (wood alcohol) is a ubiquitous chemical with myriad industrial uses. It can be found in a number of cleaning solutions and as a common ingredient in most automobile windshield washing fluid. Historically, it is well known as an adulterant in "moonshine" whiskey, with the infamous toxic corollary of "O sweet blindness." Methanol itself is not toxic. It is oxidized by alcohol dehydrogenase to formic acid, which causes metabolic acidosis and retinal toxicity. There may be a significant delay in the onset of toxic symptoms from the time of ingestion, because metabolism is rate limited by the amount of available enzyme (zero-order kinetics).

Ethylene glycol is most commonly found as the primary ingredient in automobile antifreeze. Its sweet taste and easy availability make it a popular agent for intentional ingestion.[3] Like methanol, ethylene glycol is not toxic in its own right. It is oxidized by alcohol dehydrogenase into a number of toxic intermediate compounds that share a common end product, oxalic acid. The oxalate contributes to the creation of a metabolic acidosis and, with the other intermediates, causes nephrotoxicity. As with methanol, the onset of clinical toxicity may lag significantly behind the time of ingestion.

The treatment strategy in ingestions of methanol and ethylene glycol is to limit the creation of the toxic metabolites from the parent compound. Ethyl alcohol has a greater affinity for alcohol dehydrogenase than either methanol or ethylene glycol. Administration of ethanol in sufficient amounts to fully saturate available enzyme allows for the renal elimination of the unchanged toxic compounds. This works well for relatively small ingestions. In large exposures, however, the maintenance of ethanol intoxication for extended periods of time becomes unpalatable for the patient and expensive for the health care system. Fortunately, serum levels correlate well with toxicity, and hemodialysis effectively removes both compounds. In general, a serum level of 50 mg/dL or greater of either methanol or ethylene glycol would mediate for dialysis.

Dose. Alcohol dehydrogenase should be completely saturated at an ethanol level of 100 mg/dL. This can be achieved by the administration of a loading dose followed by a maintenance dose. Oral administration is easier but may be limited because of vomiting, patient compliance, or variable absorption. Intravenous therapy is generally preferred. Using absolute alcohol (95%), a loading dose of 1 mL/kg in 5% dextrose in water over 10 to 15 minutes should achieve a blood ethanol level of 100 mg/dL.[70] This level can be maintained by continuous infusion of 0.1 mL/kg/h. Other dosing regimens using lower concentrations of ethanol are available by contacting a regional poison center. Because hemodialysis effectively removes ethanol as well as the target chemicals, maintenance therapy must be adjusted in patients undergoing dialysis.

Adverse Effects. There are no unique complications for ethanol intoxication when used for this therapeutic indication.

F. *Cyanide Antidote Kit*

Cyanide can be found in various formulations in a broad range of industrial products, such as metal polishes, electroplating solutions, and synthetics. Combustion of various polymers can result in the liberation of cyanide. Amygdalin occurs naturally in the pits of peaches, apricots, plums, and other members of the plant family Rosaceae. Laetrile is the amygdalin-containing drug that relies on the liberation of hydrocyanic acid by cellular enzymes to purportedly kill cancer cells. Oral ingestion can cause toxicity by the liberation of hydrogen cyanide by gastric juice. Hydrogen cyanide gas is used in some states for judicial executions, and cyanide salts are well known as the poisons ingested in the Jonestown, Guyana, incident and the Tylenol® tampering cases in Chicago.

Cyanide can cause death in a matter of minutes by creating cellular hypoxia. It binds avidly to iron in the ferric (trivalent) state. It combines with cytochrome oxidase, inhibiting the final step of oxidative phosphorylation, blocking aerobic metabolism and, in effect, causing the suffocation of the victim. Ingestion of the cyanide salts or inhalation of hydrogen cyanide gas creates this precipitous course. Cyanide liberated by enzymatic degradation may cause a more insidious toxicity.

The aim of therapy is to prevent the cyanide ion from binding to cytochrome oxidase or to reverse the bond if it has occurred. In the United States, the only commercially available antidote kit is manufactured by Eli Lilly and Company (Indianapolis, IN). The kit contains amyl nitrate perles, sodium nitrite, and sodium thiosulfate.

Nitrates and nitrites cause the oxydation of ferrous hemoglobin to ferric hemoglobin (methemoglobin). The ferric ion in the methemoglobin provides an alternate binding site for the cyanide ion. The inhalation of amyl nitrate produces a relatively low level of methemoglobin. It is included in the kit primarily to allow therapy to begin rapidly. The sodium nitrite is more effective in inducing methemoglobinemia. The goal is to induce a 25% to 30% methemoglobinemia. In the presence of the enzyme rhodinase and a sulfur donor (thiosulfate), thiocyanate is created, which is relatively nontoxic and excreted by the kidneys. Although this is a naturally occurring reaction, the body cannot store thiosulfate, and the amount available would be quickly depleted in a large exposure. Thisosulfate is essentially nontoxic.

In Europe, dicobalt edetate is available as a direct chelator of cyanide, as is hydroxycobalamin (vitamin

B12a). These are thought by many experts to be a safer alternative to the induction of methemoglobinemia. Hydroxycobalamin is currently under investigation in the United States.

Dose. Amyl nitrate is inhaled directly for 30 seconds of each minute. If intravenous access is available, amyl nitrate inhalation can be bypassed in favor of the administration of the sodium nitrite. For adults, the dose of sodium nitrite is 300 mg or 10 mL of the 3% solution delivered no faster than 5 mL/min. For children, the dose is 10 mg/kg or 0.2 mL/kg, not to exceed 10 mL. Sodium thiosulfate is administered in adults at a dose of 12.5 grams or 50 mL of the 25% solution. In children the dose is 375 mg/kg or 1.5 mL/kg.

Adverse Effects. Fatal methemoglobinemia has been induced by the excessive administration of sodium nitrite in children.[71] Rapid administration of sodium nitrite may cause hypotension.

G. *Fab Antibody Fragments*

The use of exogenous antibodies in the treatment or prevention of infectious disease is not new. Diphtheria, tetanus, rabies, and infectious hepatitis are classical examples. Using antibodies to treat drug intoxication is conceptually the same. Antibodies to digoxin were successfully produced in 1967 and were successfully used in the treatment of experimentally induced digoxin toxicity in animals in 1971.[72] The mechanism of action is binding of drug in extracellular fluid, preventing or reversing tissue binding. The delivery of whole antibodies is associated with a predictable incidence of immediate and delayed hypersensitivity. A complete gamma-globulin molecule can be split into two antigen-binding Fab fragments and one Fc fragment by enzymatic digestion. The Fc portion contains antigenic determinants and complement binding sites. The Fc fragments can be removed, leaving the less antigenic Fab fragments, which can act in the same manner as the intact immunoglobulin. Digoxin-specific Fab fragments are commercially available (Digibind®, Burroughs-Wellcome, Research Triangle Park, NC). There is excellent documentation for the reversal of life-threatening digitalis toxicity without evidence of immediate or delayed hypersensitivity.[72,73]

The diagnosis of digitalis toxicity can be difficult. Digitalis glycosides inhibit the action of Na-K ATPase, paralyzing the Na-K pump. Toxic cardiac effects are common, including varying degrees of heart block, as well as atrial and ventricular tachyarrhythmias. The cardiac effects may be potentiated by the presence of hypokalemia. In cases of massive overdose, however, refractory hyperkalemia may be present.[74] Although hypokalemia is more commonly seen, empiric potassium should be administered cautiously.

In general, there is good correlation between serum drug level and toxicity. Severe pulmonary, coronary, or valvular heart disease, as well as old age, may predispose a given patient to toxicity at a lower serum level. Digoxin levels must be interpreted in a complete clinical context. As a guideline, a therapeutic level is in the range of 1–2 ng/mL. Toxic effects are typically seen at two to three times the therapeutic levels. Patients with mild digitalis toxicity usually do well with supportive management, correction of hypokalemia, and by holding further glycoside until the level falls. Patients with severe toxicity or with massive overdose are candidates for Fab fragments. Dosing regimens are complicated and are based on amount ingested or serum levels. The package insert contains detailed dosing information. A regional poison center should be contacted for advice in any severe intoxication.

H. *Hyperbaric Oxygen*

Carbon monoxide (CO) is a byproduct of incomplete combustion with an affinity for hemoglobin approximately 200 times that of oxygen. There is a widely held misconception that the toxicity of CO is only related to the formation of carboxyhemoglobin (COHb) and the blockage of oxygen transport. There is ample scientific evidence that CO is toxic well beyond what can be explained by simple hypoxemia alone. The definitive study was conducted by Goldbaum et al[75]; they transfused blood from fatally injured dogs with COHb levels of 80% into partially exsanguinated normal animals, resulting in COHb levels of greater than 50%. The transfused animals tolerated a 50% carboxyhemoglobinemia without symptoms. The mechanism of cellular toxicity of CO is unknown, but is postulated to be related to lipid peroxidation or cytochrome binding.

Late neurologic sequelae have been associated with CO poisoning in untreated patients as well as those who received 100% oxygen therapy.[76] These sequelae are myriad and are often subtle in nature. Changes in personality or cognition may require formal psychometric testing for documentation. Recent clinical experience indicates that treatment of CO poisoning with hyberbaric oxygen (HBO) may be useful in limiting these late sequelae.[76] COHb levels of greater than 25% to 30% are associated with an increased risk of cardiovascular compromise, but COHb levels do not correlate with the development of neurologic sequelae.

The guidelines for the use of HBO in the treatment of CO poisoning are in flux, and the reader is encouraged to consult a regional poison center or HBO treatment facility for contemporary guidance. In general, consideration for HBO should be given to patients with high initial levels (greater than 25%), those with loss of consciousness, and those with overt or subtle neurologic deficits.

VII. SUMMARY

This chapter has attempted to review the general approach to the management of acutely poisoned patients as they would present to an emergency department. Typical decontamination procedures have been described in detail, with a review of the current controversies surrounding their use. In general, poisoning and overdose is a "disease" of low mortality, with the majority of patients doing well with standard supportive care. There is a vast array of potential toxins in the environment. It is impossible for any text to be contemporary in the management of every poison. The American Association of Poison Control Centers provides a network of up-to-date information with around-the-clock accessibility. A regional poison center should be contacted whenever there is uncertainty about the proper management of a toxic exposure.

VIII. REFERENCES

1. Thomas Tl (ed). Taber's Cyclopedic Medical Dictionary. Philadelphia, FA Davis, 1985, pp 1332–1333.
2. Von Howeheim TB. Paracelsus, Von der Besucht. Dillingen, 1567.
3. Litovitz TL, Schmitz BF, Matyunas N, Martin TG. 1987 annual report of the American Association of Poison Control Centers National Data Collection System. Am J Emerg Med 6:479–515, 1988.
4. Bailey DN, Manoguerra AS. Survey of drug abuse patterns and toxicology analysis in an emergency-room population. J Anal Toxicol 4:199–203, 1980.
5. Bailey DN. The role of the laboratory in treatment of the poisoned patient: Laboratory perspective. J Anal Toxicol 7:136–141, 1983.
6. Amitai Y, Mitchell AA, McGuigan MA, Lovejoy FH. Ipecac-induced emesis and reduction of plasma concentrations of drugs following accidental overdose in children. Pediatrics 80: 364–367, 1987.
7. Tandberg D, Diven BG, McLeod JW. Ipecac-induced emesis vs. gastric lavage: A controlled study in normal adults. Am J Emerg Med 4:205–209, 1986.
8. Auerbach PS, Osterloh J, Braun O, et al. Efficacy of gastric emptying: Gastric lavage vs. emesis induced with ipecac. Ann Emerg Med 15:692–698, 1986.
9. Comstock EG, Faulkner TP, Boisaubin EV, et al. Studies on the efficacy of gastric lavage as practiced in a large metropolitan hospital. Clin Toxicol 18:581–597, 1981.
10. Tennenbein M. Inefficacy of gastric emptying procedures. J Emerg Med 3:133–136, 1985.
11. Dabbous IA, Bergman AB, Robertson WO. The ineffectiveness of mechanically induced vomiting. J Pediatr 66:952–954, 1965.
12. Barer J, Hill LL, Hill RM. Fatal poisoning from salt used as an emetic. Am J Dis Child 125:889–890, 1973.
13. Manoguerra AS, Krenzelok EP. Rapid emesis from high-dose ipecac syrup in adults and children intoxicated with antiemetics or other drugs. Am J Hosp Pharm 35:1360–1362, 1978.
14. Freedman GE, Pasternak S, Krenzelok EP. A clinical trial using syrup of ipecac and activated charcoal concurrently. Ann Emerg Med 16:164–166, 1987.
15. Gaudreault P, McCormick MA, Lacouture PG, Lovejoy FH. Poisoning exposures and use of ipecac in children less than 1 year old. Ann Emerg Med 15:808–810, 1986.
16. Smith RP, Smith DM. Acute ipecac poisoning. N Engl J Med 265:523–525, 1961.
17. Miser JS, Robertson WO. Ipecac poisoning. West J Med 128:440–443, 1978.
18. Adler AG, Walinsky P, Krall RA, Cho SY. Death resulting from ipecac syrup poisoning. JAMA 243:1927–1928, 1980.
19. Knight KM, Doucet HJ. Gastric rupture and death caused by ipecac syrup. South Med J 80:786–787, 1987.
20. Tandberg D, Liechty EJ, Fishbein D. Mallory-Weiss syndrome: An unusual complication of ipecac-induced emesis. Ann Emerg Med 10:521-523, 1981.
21. Wolowodiuk OJ, McMicken DB, O'Brien P. Pneumomediastinum and retropneumoperitoneum: An unusual complication of syrup-of-ipecac-induced emesis. Ann Emerg Med 13:1148–1151, 1984.
22. Parr D. Cardiovascular collapse during apomorphine treatment. Br Med J 2:860–862, 1956.
23. White RT. Apomorphine as an emetic prior to obstetric anesthesia: The prevention of inhaled vomitus. Obstet Gynecol 14:111–115, 1959.
24. Decker WJ, Corby DG, Combs HF. A stable parenteral solution of apomorphine. Clin Toxicol 18:763–772, 1981.
25. Schofferman JA. A clinical comparison of syrup of ipecac and apomorphine use in adults. JACEP 5:22–25, 1976.
26. MacLean WC. A comparison of ipecac syrup and apomorphine in the immediate treatment of ingestion of poisons. J Pediatr 82:121–124, 1973.
27. Berry FA, Lambdin MA. Apomorphine and levallorphan tartrate in acute poisonings. Am J Dis Child 105:160–163, 1963.
28. Abdallah AH, Tye A. A comparison of the efficacy of emetic drugs and stomach lavage. Am J Dis Child 113:571–575, 1967.
29. Boxer L, Anderson FP, Rowe DS. Comparison of ipecac-induced emesis with gastric lavage in the treatment of acute salicylate Ingestion. J Pediatr 74:800–803, 1969.
30. Fane LR, Combs HF, Decker WJ. Physical parameters in gastric lavage. Clin Toxicol 4:389–395, 1971.
31. Rudolph JP. Automated gastric lavage and a comparison of 0.9% normal saline solution and tap water irrigant. Ann Emerg Med 14:1156–1159, 1985.
32. Matthew H, Mackintosh TF, Tompsett SL. Gastric aspiration and lavage in acute poisoning. Br Med J 1:1333–1337, 1966.

33. Calvanese JC. Complications of gastric lavage, including a case report of mid-esophagus kinking and lodgement of a #36 Fr Ewald tube (abstract). Vet Hum Toxicol 25:286, 1983.
34. Reid DHS. Treatment of the poisoned child. Arch Dis Child 45:428–433, 1970.
35. Kulig K, Bar-Or D, Cantrill SV, et al. Management of acutely poisoned patients without gastric emptying. Ann Emerg Med 14:562–567, 1985.
36. Tenenbein M, Cohen S, Star DS. Efficacy of ipecac-induced emesis, orogastric lavage, and activated charcoal for acute drug overdose. Ann Emerg Med 16:838–841, 1987.
37. Lalonde RS, Deshpande R, Hamilton PP, et al. Acceleration of digoxin clearance by activated charcoal. Clin Pharmacol Ther 37:367–371, 1985.
38. Berg MJ, Berlinger WG, Goldberg MJ, et al. Acceleration of the body clearance of phenobarbital by oral activated charcoal. N Engl J Med 307:642–644, 1982.
39. Kulig KW, Bar-Or D, Rumack BH. Intravenous theophylline poisoning and multiple-dose charcoal in an animal model. Ann Emerg Med 16:842–846, 1987.
40. Filiponne G, Fish SS, Lacouture PG, et al. Desorption of aspirin from activated charcoal (abstract). AAPCC/AACT ABMT/CAPCC Annual Scientific Meeting, September 1986.
41. Harsch HH. Aspiration of activated charcoal (letter). N Engl J Med 314:318, 1986.
42. Watson WA, Cremer KF, Chapman JA. Gastrointestinal obstruction associated with multiple-dose activated charcoal. J Emerg Med 4:401–407, 1986.
43. Ray MJ, Padin DR, Condie JD, Halls JM. Charcoal bezoar, small-bowel obstruction secondary to amitryptyline overdose therapy. Dig Dis Sci 33:106–107, 1988.
44. Jones J, Heiselman D, Dougherty J, Eddy A. Cathartic-induced magnesium toxicity during overdose management. Ann Emerg Med 15:1214–1218, 1986.
45. Caldwell JW, Nava AJ, DeHaas DD. Hypernatremia associated with cathartics in overdose management. West J Med 147:593–596, 1987.
46. Krenzelok EP, Keller R, Stewart RD. Gastrointestinal transit times of cathartics combined with charcoal. Ann Emerg Med 14:1152–1155, 1985.
47. Minocha A, Herold DA, Bruns DE, Spyker DA. Effect of activated charcoal in 70% sorbitol in healthy individuals. Clin Toxicol 22:529–536, 1984.
48. Farley TA. Severe hypernatremic dehydration after use of an activated charcoal-sorbitol suspension. J Pediatr 109:719–722, 1986.
49. Ambrose NS, Johnson MJ, Burdon DW, Keighley MRB. A physiological appraisal of polyethylene glycol and a balanced electrolyte solution as bowel preparation. Br J Surg 70:428–430, 1983.
50. Ernstoff JF, Howard DA, Marshall JB, et al. A randomized blinded clinical trial of a rapid colonic lavage solution (Golytley) compared with standard preparation for colonoscopy and barium enema. Gastroenterology 84:1512–1516, 1983.
51. Tenenbein M, Cohen S, Sitar D. Whole bowel irrigation as a decontamination procedure after acute drug overdose. Arch Intern Med 147:905-907, 1987.
52. Tenenbein M. Whole bowel irrigation as a gastrointestinal decontamination procedure after acute poisoning. Med Toxicol 3:77–84, 1988.
53. Barone JA, Raia J, Yih CH. Evaluation of the effects of multiple-dose activated charcoal on the absorption of orally administered salicylate in a simulated toxic ingestion model. Ann Emerg Med 17:71-74, 1988.
54. Yatzidis H, Voudiclari S, Oveopoulus D, et al. Treatment of severe barbiturate poisoning. Lancet ii:216–217, 1965.
55. Rosenbaum JL, Kramer MS, Raja R. Resin hemoperfusion for acute drug intoxication. Arch Intern Med 136:263–266, 1976.
56. Rosenbaum JL, Kramer MS, Raja R, Boreyko C. Resin hemoperfusion: A new treatment for acute drug intoxication. N Engl J Med 284:874–877, 1971.
57. Vale JA, Rees AJ, Widdop B, Goulding R. Use of charcoal hemoperfusion in the management of severely poisoned patients. Br Med J 1:5–9, 1975.
58. DeBroe ME, Bismuth C, DeGroot G, et al. Haemoperfusion: A useful therapy for a severely poisoned patient? Human Toxicol 5:11–14, 1986.
59. Russo ME. Management of theophylline intoxication with charcoal-column hemoperfusion. N Engl J Med 300:24–26, 1979.
60. Chang TMS. Coated charcoal haemoperfusion. Life Supp Syst 2:99–106, 1984.
61. Gallagher EJ, Howland M, Greenblatt H. Hemolysis following treatment of theophylline overdose with coated charcoal hemoperfusion. J Emerg Med 5:19–22, 1987.
62. Michaelis L, Hickey P, Clark T. Ventricular irritability associated with the use of naloxone hydrochloride. Ann Thorac Surg 18:608–614, 1974.
63. Tanaka G. Hypertensive reaction to naloxone. JAMA 228: 25–26, 1974.
64. Smilkstein MJ, Knapp GL, Kulig KW, Rumack BH. Efficacy of oral N-acetylcysteine in the treatment of acetaminophen overdose: Analysis of the national multicenter study (1976 to 1985). N Engl J Med 319:1557–1562, 1988.
65. Milby T. Prevention and management of organophoshate poisoning. JAMA 216:2131–2133, 1971.
66. Ellenhorn MJ, Barceloux DG. Selection, Medical Toxicology: Diagnosis and Treatment of Human Poisoning. New York, Elsevier Science, 1988, p 83.
67. Levy R. Arrhythmias following physostigmine administration in jimson weed poisoning. JACEP 6:107–108, 1977.
68. Pentel P, Peterson CD. Asystole complicating physostigmine treatment of tricyclic antidepressant overdose. Ann Emerg Med 9:588–590, 1980.
69. Newton RW. Physostigmine salicylate in the treatment of tricyclic antidepressant overdose. JAMA 231:941–943, 1975.
70. McCoy HG, Cipolli RJ, Ehlers SM. Severe methanol poisoning: Application of a pharmacokinetic model for ethanol therapy and hemodialysis. Am J Med 67:804–807, 1979.
71. Berlin C. The treatment of cyanide poisoning in children. Pediatrics 46:793–796, 1970.
72. Wenger TL, Butler VP, Haber E, Smith TW. Treatment of 63 severely digitalis-toxic patients with digoxin-specific antibody fragments. J Am Coll Cardiol 5:118A–123A, 1985.
73. Smith TW, Butler UP, Haber E, et al. Treatment of life-threatening digitalis intoxication with digoxin-specific Fab antibody fragments: Experience in 26 cases. N Engl J Med 307:1357–1362, 1982.
74. Bismuth C, Gaultier M, Conso F, Efthymiou ML. Hyperkalemia in acute digitalis poisoning: Prognostic significance and therapeutic implications. Clin Toxicol 6:153–162, 1973.
75. Goldbaum LR, Ramirez RG, Absalon KB. What is the mechanism of carbon monoxide toxicity? Aviat Space Environ Med 46:1289–1291, 1975.
76. Myers RA, Snyder SK, Emhoff TA. Subacute sequelae of carbon monoxide poisoning. Ann Emerg Med 14:1163–1167, 1985.

Chapter 43

•

Laurence S. Reisner, MD
D. Jill Ellis, MD

Fetal Monitoring

OUTLINE

I. INTRODUCTION

The assessment of fetal heart rate and uterine activity during labor has been recognized as an important and useful evaluation by obstetricians for nearly a century. Until the advent of the electronic age in the 1960s, these functions were carried out by intermittently auscultating the fetal heart rate with a fetoscope and palpating the uterine contractions. This was fraught with difficulties, particularly during contractions. The patient would often move and the fetal heart rate would be lost until after the contraction. The intensity and duration of contractions were an estimate; moreover, it was virtually impossible to relate fetal heart rate changes to uterine contractions. Modern electronics first brought us the high quality microphone and then the Doppler device, both of which were capable of picking up the fetal heart rate in utero, but suffered from some of the same limitations as auscultation and palpation. In the mid-1960s

Hon and Quilligan applied space-age electronic knowledge to a device capable of being directly attached to the fetus in utero that captured the fetal electrocardiogram (ECG), averaged the interval between R waves, and displayed the fetal heart rate on a meter and on a paper strip chart in a continuous fashion. An auditory signal was also provided. These outputs were also coupled with a standard physiologic pressure transducer that was connected to a saline-filled catheter placed directly into the uterine cavity. The result was the ability to continuously monitor uterine contractions and fetal heart rate in a beat-to-beat, second-to-second fashion and to relate the fetal heart rate directly to uterine activity. Caldeyro-Barcia had already identified two classic fetal heart rate deceleration patterns, and the advent of the modern fetal monitor provided the research tool to enhance and enlarge upon this knowledge and to provide the clinician with the ability to accurately follow the events of labor.[1] Further refinements of fetal monitors have evolved over the last two decades, and now external devices with nearly the sensitivity and reliability of the internal fetal heart rate monitor are available.

But why is this of interest to the anesthesiologist? Obstetric anesthesia is now routinely used in labor and delivery suites. The analgesic techniques administered during labor may affect the fetal heart rate and uterine contractions both directly (by placental transfer of drugs or alterations in uterine artery tone) and indirectly (by changes in blood pressure induced by the anesthetic technique itself or by supine positioning). Preexisting conditions may alter our approach to providing analgesia for labor or anesthesia for delivery. Although not always considered optimum, there are periods of time in some labor suites when the anesthesiologist is the only physician immediately available. It therefore behooves the anesthesiologist providing services in a labor and delivery suite to become familiar with fetal monitoring and its interpretation. Familiarity with the interpretation of the fetal heart rate tracing may also help the anesthesiologist anticipate obstetric emergencies and thus prepare for them. Finally, it is recommended that the fetal monitor be applied to pregnant patients undergoing nonobstetric surgical procedures, although the information gained is often of limited usefulness.

This chapter deals only minimally with the technical aspects of applying the fetal monitoring devices, because this is universally performed by the obstetric care provider, and will concentrate on the interpretation of the tracings and their importance to anesthesiologists.

II. How to do Fetal Monitoring

A. *Application of the Fetal Monitor*

1. The Internal Monitors

The internal monitors, although invasive, provide the most reliable information. The fetal heart rate is monitored by attaching a silver/silver chloride electrode to the fetal presenting part and a ground plate to the mother's leg. The fetal electrode (Fig. 43–1) is currently a spiral that is rotated clockwise through a tubular plastic insertion device that is held firmly against the presenting part, usually the vertex. Because the fetal electrode is a spiral, the rotation essentially screws the electrode into the skin (Fig. 43–2). The tube is then removed and the two wires attached to the maternal leg plate, which is connected to the fetal monitor (Fig. 43–3). The fetal ECG is detected by the monitor. Some versions will display the ECG waveform on a screen. The uterine pressure monitor is a piece of plastic tubing inserted manually through an introducer that is passed into the cervix and past the fetal presenting part (Fig. 43–4). It must lie within the amniotic cavity to work effectively. It is filled with sterile physiologic saline and attached to a pressure transducer. The transducer is calibrated at the height of the uterus. This yields a direct intrauterine pressure reading in millimeters of mercury (Fig. 43–5).

2. The External Monitors

Current, state-of-the-art electronics allows for accurate continuous detection of the fetal heart rate externally. Highly sensitive Doppler ultrasound transducers attach to the maternal abdomen with an elastic strap (Fig. 43–6). The sensor head is moved about the abdomen until the maximum audible signal is attained, and then it is secured. These sensors do not sense the fetal ECG, but rather actual fetal heart activity. Beat-to-beat variability is not as reliably interpreted as with the internal monitor, because an artificial variability of about 5 beats/minute is inherent in the function of this device. Uterine activity is monitored by a tocodynamometer, an external pressure transducer (Figs. 43–7 and 43–8). This senses overall abdominal wall activity, and the height of the waveform can be adjusted by the observer. It therefore can yield reasonable information as to the frequency and duration of contractions, but cannot yield accurate information about amplitude.

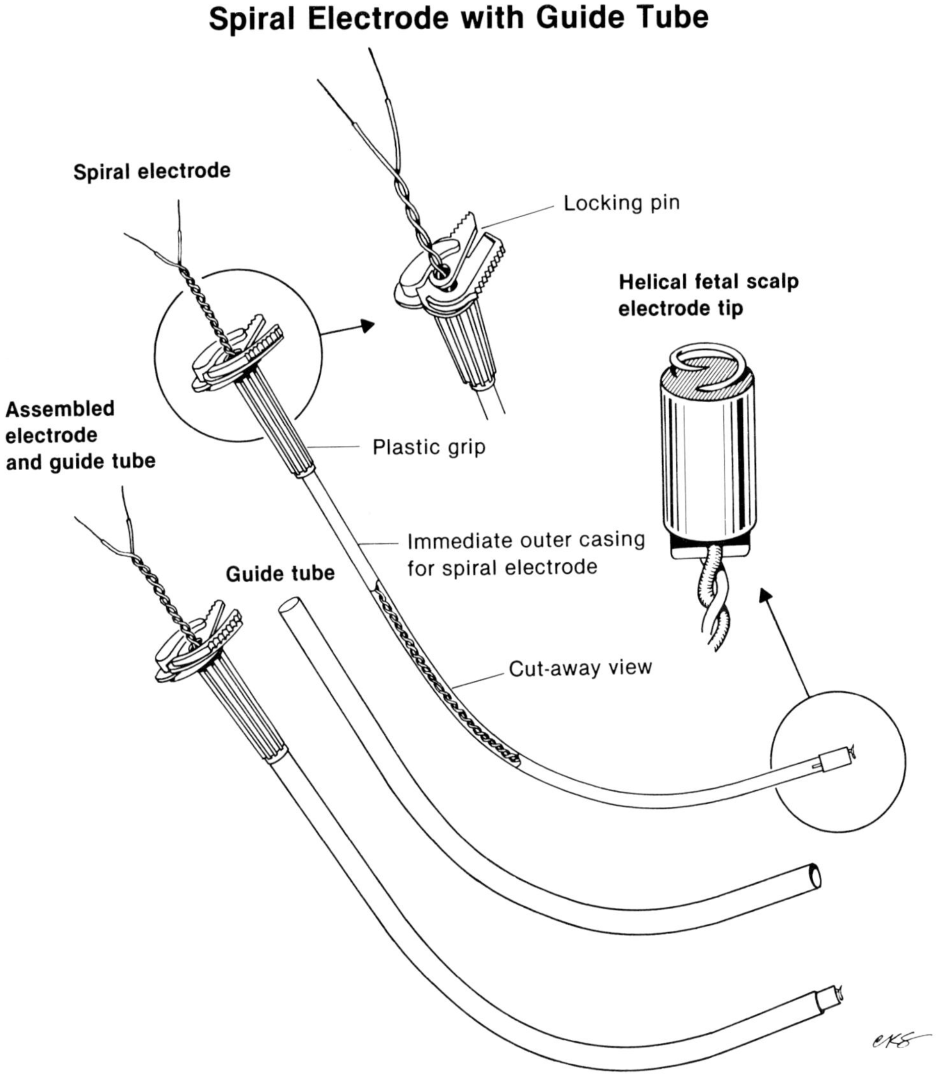

Figure 43–1 • Spiral fetal scalp electrode with applicator is shown. The spiral electrode resembles a small corkscrew. It is attached by a twisted pair of wires to the main input cable. The assembly is inserted into the vagina through a plastic guide tube which is removed after insertion.

External monitoring is useful for routine and oxytocin-induced labors with intact membranes, and situations where an internal electrode might be desired but cannot be applied, eg, the second of twins. If the fetus is at high risk, if doubt as to the fetal status exists, or when the external tracing is difficult to interpret, then internal monitoring is preferred.

B. *Interpreting the Fetal Monitor Tracing*[2,3]

The strip chart recorder used by the fetal monitor is reminiscent of the type commonly used in the operating room for cases where invasive monitoring is used (Fig. 43–9). It is divided into two sections. The upper section is the continuous output of fetal heart rate, and the paper is graduated vertically with the fetal heart rate in beats per minute (Fig. 43–10). The range is from 30 to 240, with a center of 140, the mean for term fetal heart rates. An additional scale appears at regular intervals on some monitors to display the amount of beat-to-beat variability. The pen is deflected to mark this scale on command or at scheduled intervals. The lower half of the paper displays uterine contractions. The vertical scale is calibrated from 0 to 100 mmHg. This scale is valid

(Text continued on p. 916)

Technique for Application of Spiral Electrode

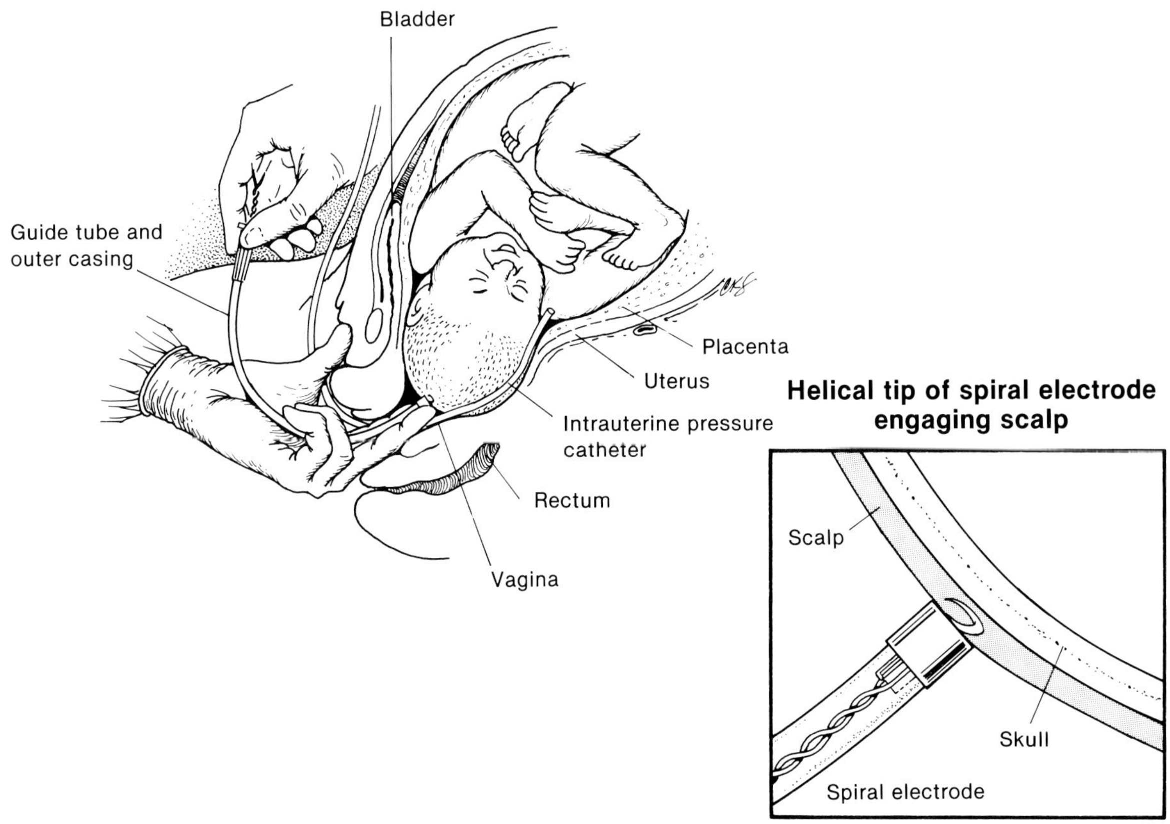

Figure 43–2 • The spiral electrode is gently guided to the infant's head and screwed into place with a clockwise motion. The locking mechanism on the outer casing is released; it and the guide tube are then removed and the wires on the external end connected to the maternal leg plate apparatus.

Fetal Scalp Electrode Properly Attached for ECG (Heart Rate) Monitoring

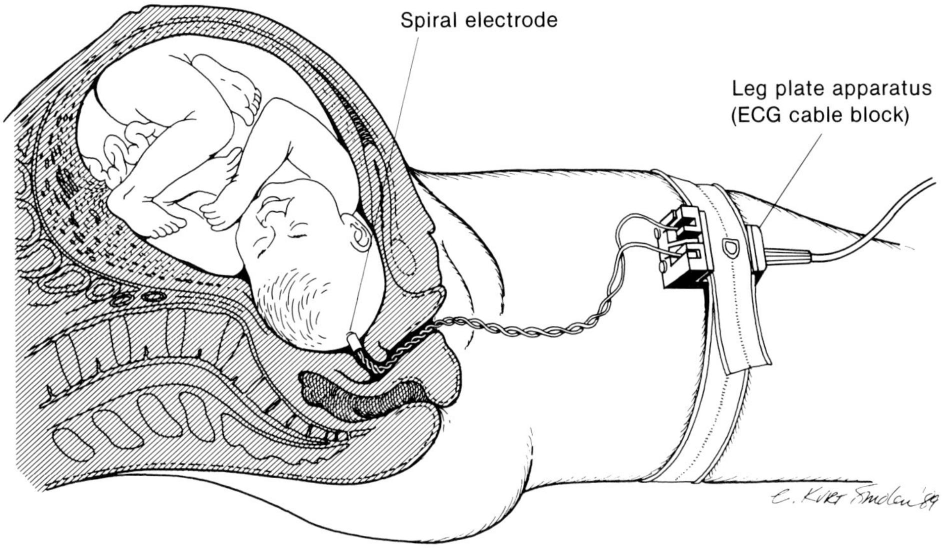

Figure 43–3 • The fetal heart rate electrode is properly attached and ready for ECG recording. Note the leg plate apparatus strapped to the mother's thigh. The underside is a metal plate to which conductive gel is applied before attachment. This serves as an electrical ground.

Technique of Uterine Pressure Catheter Insertion

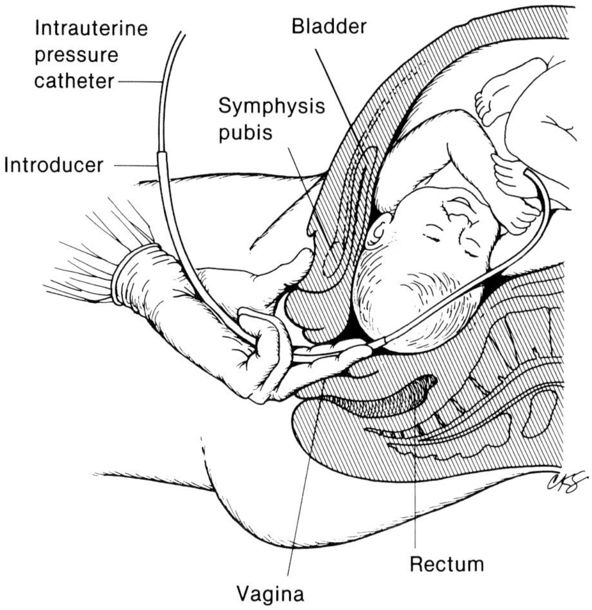

Figure 43-4 • Uterine pressure catheter is inserted. The catheter and guide are inserted into the vagina manually as shown and then the catheter is advanced until a mark on the catheter lines up with the external end of the applicator. The applicator is then removed. The external end of the catheter is attached to a standard fluid-filled strain gauge apparatus and the catheter and transducer filled with sterile saline.

Fetal Heart Rate Monitor with Scalp Electrode and Uterine Pressure Catheter Attached

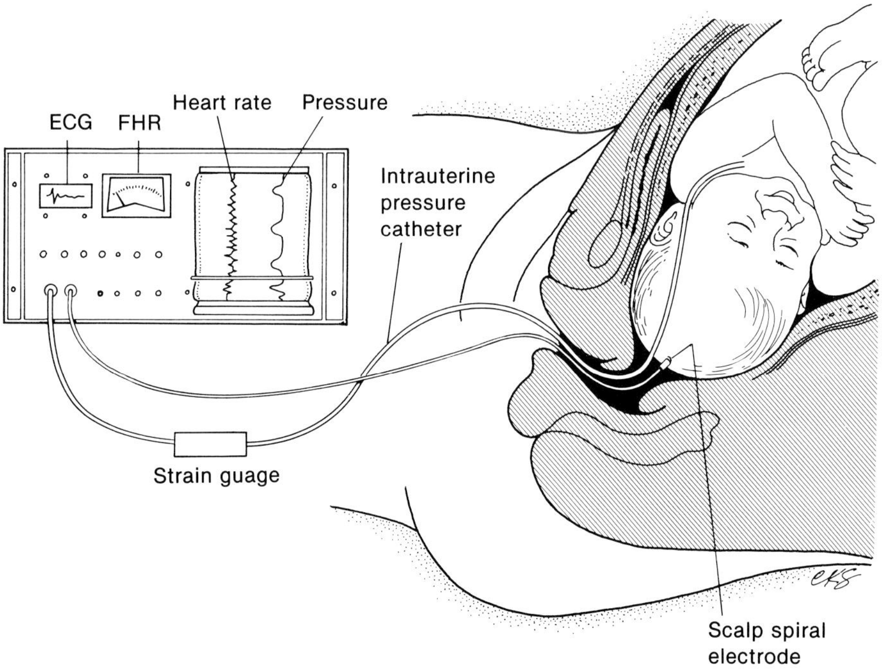

Figure 43-5 • The fetal heart rate electrode and the intrauterine pressure catheter are attached to the fetal heart rate monitor and recording. Note that this monitor has a screen for viewing fetal ECG and that the fetal heart rate is displayed on a sweep needle meter. More modern machines use a digital readout for the fetal heart rate and some do not display the ECG complex.

External Fetal Heart Rate Transducer

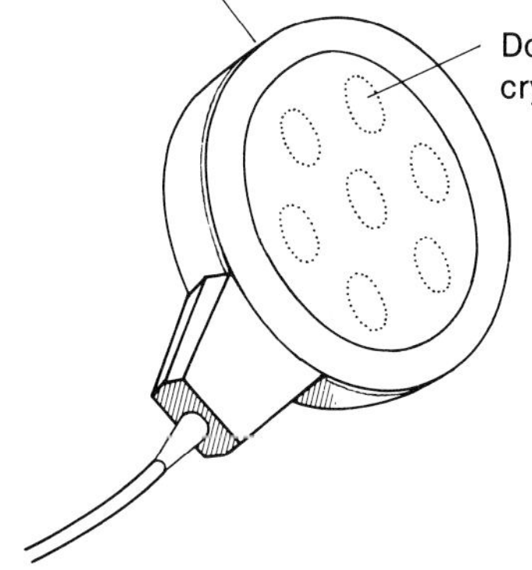

Figure 43-6 • The external fetal heart rate transducer allows monitoring of the fetal heart rate transabdominally by employing a Doppler ultrasound transducer system. This is less invasive but not as reliable as the scalp electrode in some situations.

only when an internal monitor is used. The external monitor writes out on this section, but the amplitude cannot be calibrated. The horizontal scale of the paper is calibrated in major divisions of 1 minute and minor divisions of 20 seconds.

1. Definition of Normal Fetal Heart Rate

The mean heart rate of a term fetus is approximately 140 beats per minute (bpm). This will vary from 120 to 160 bpm; this is considered the normal range. A fetal heart rate between 100 and 120 is considered a moderate bradycardia, and below 100 a severe bradycardia. Bradycardia is often the first recognized response of the fetus to acute hypoxia. Fetal heart rates between 160 and 180 are called a moderate tachycardia, and above 180 a severe tachycardia.

There is a constant variation in the fetal heart rate in a normal fetus. This is due to a frequent readjustment of both sympathetic and vagal tone in response to environmental conditions. This gives an irregular appearance to the heart rate tracing (a jagged or zigzag appearance), and this variation is known as beat-to-beat variability. The range of this variability is from 3 to 10 bpm. A lack of variability or a decrease in its degree may indicate fetal distress.[4]

2. Definition of Normal Uterine Activity

Although there is considerable variation, a normal labor pattern consists of regular uterine contractions occurring at 3- to 5-minute intervals. The contraction should last from 45 seconds to 1 minute. The baseline pressure reading between contractions should be between 0 and 15 mmHg, and the amplitude should not exceed 70 mmHg (Fig. 43-11). Contractions in excess of this are said to be hypertonic. An elevation of the baseline pressure to greater than 15 mmHg is considered abnormal. A sustained hypertonic contraction significantly reduces uteroplacental blood flow and requires immediate administration of a uterine relaxant.

External Uterine Activity Transducer (Tocodynamometer)

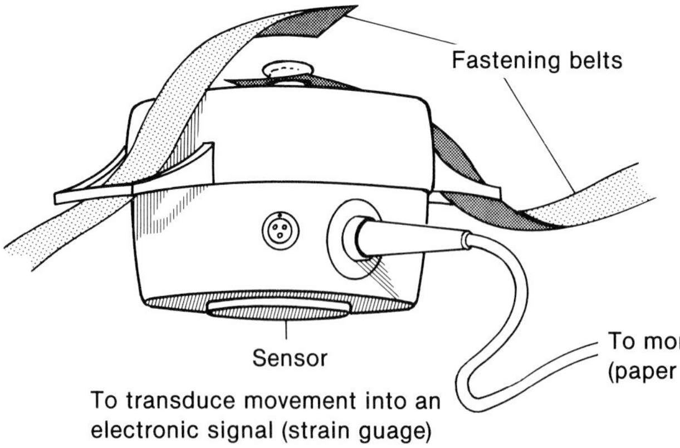

Figure 43-7 • The external uterine activity transducer (tocodynamometer) attaches to the maternal abdomen with a circumferential elastic strap. The abdomen expands with uterine contractions as the uterus lifts towards the anterior abdominal wall. This increase in girth presses the sensing plunger inward. This motion is changed into an electrical signal and a waveform is generated. The size of this waveform is user adjustable and does not directly relate to the intensity of uterine contractions.

External Monitoring of Uterine Contractions and Fetal Heart Rate

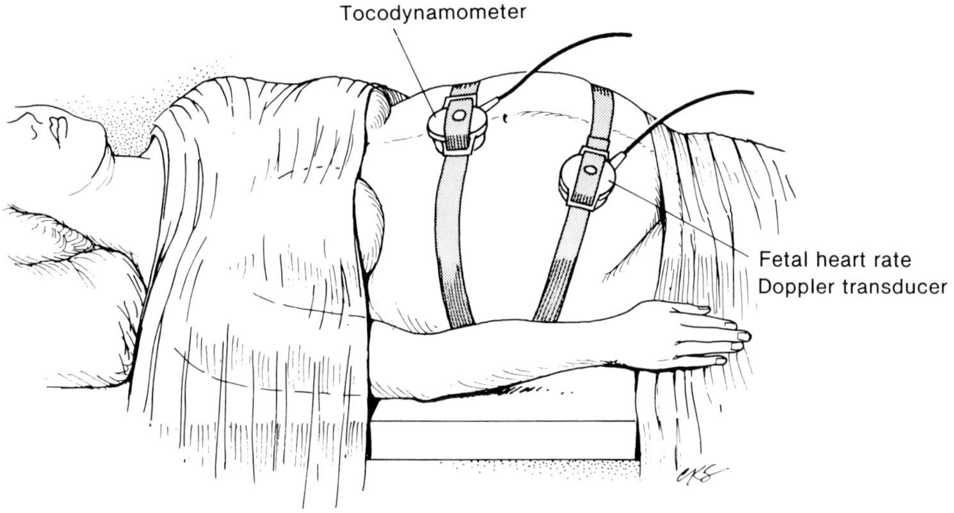

Figure 43-8 • The external detectors of fetal heart rate and uterine contractions are properly attached and situated. Their locations may have to be moved as labor progresses and the position of the fetus changes.

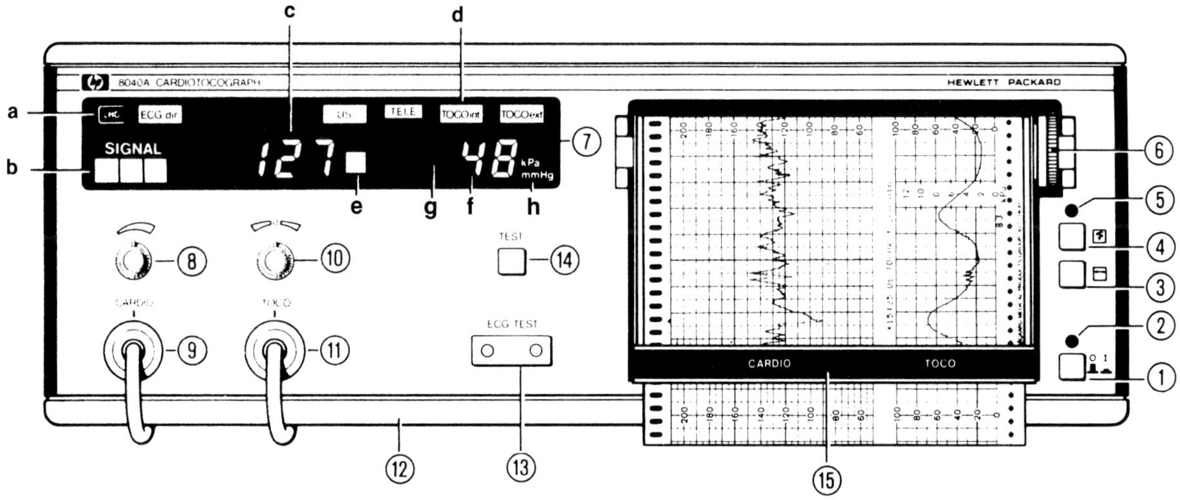

Figure 43-9 • The figure shows the modern fetal heart rate monitor (Hewlett-Packard 8040A). (*1*) Instrument power ON/OFF button. (*2*) Instrument ON lamp: lit when the instrument is switched on. (*3*) Mark button: can be pressed up to 10 times/mark sequence. Each time it is pressed, a line is drawn across both channels. (*4*) Recorder ON/OFF button. (*5*) Recorder ON lamp: lit when the recorder is switched on. (*6*) Thumbwheel: permits manual paper advance. (7) Display. Contains the following functions: (*a*) When on, this indicates that the fetal heart rate logic is disabled, in order to record fetal arrhythmias. Operative only in the direct ECG mode. (*b*) Signal quality indicator: relates to fetal heart rate signal quality. (*c*) Fetal heart rate numeric display. (*d*) Selected monitoring method will light up when the transducer is plugged in. TELE lights when instrument is being used with rear-panel input telementry. (*e*) Acceptance lamp: flashes when measurements of fetal heart rate are made. (*f*) Uterine activity numeric display. (*g*) Flashing +: indicates recorder upper limit is exceeded on TOCO channel. Flashing −: indicates recorder lower limit is exceeded on TOCO channel. (*h*) Indicates intrauterine pressure measurement units (kPa or mmHg). (*8*) Adjusts loudspeaker volume. (*9*) CARDIO Socket (blue) accepts any fetal heart rate transducer plug (blue). (CARDIO input is *not* electrically isolated for ultrasound). (*10*) Sets TOCO (labor) channel baseline on recorder and numeric display. (*11*) TOCO Socket (brown) accepts any uterine activity transducer plug (brown). (TOCO input is *not* electrically isolated for external TOCO method.) (*12*) Instructions, Test, and Error Messages/Additional Information cards. (*13*) ECG test pins: tests direct ECG mode and cable. (*14*) Test button. (*15*) Paper magazine Recorder operates with magazine locked vertically or at 20° or 45°. Magazine is removed by swinging to horizontal position and pulling. (Diagram courtesy of Hewlett-Packard Corporation, Palo Alto, CA; with permission. Legend information also provided by Hewlett-Packard.)

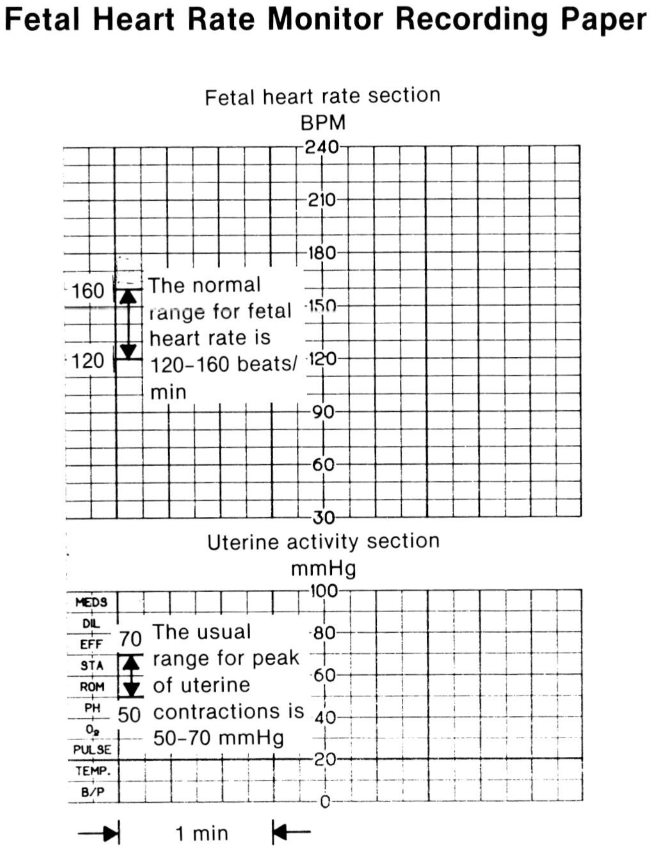

Figure 43–10 • Fetal heart rate monitor recording paper is divided into two sections, the uppermost for recording fetal heart rate in beats-per-minute (bpm) and the lower portion for recording uterine activity. This is in millimeters of mercury when the patient has an intrauterine pressure catheter in situ; there is no scale for the external pressure transducer. Note the normal range for fetal heart rate of 120–160 bpm, the normal peak height for uterine contractions of 50–70 mmHg, and the normal duration of contractions of up to one minute.

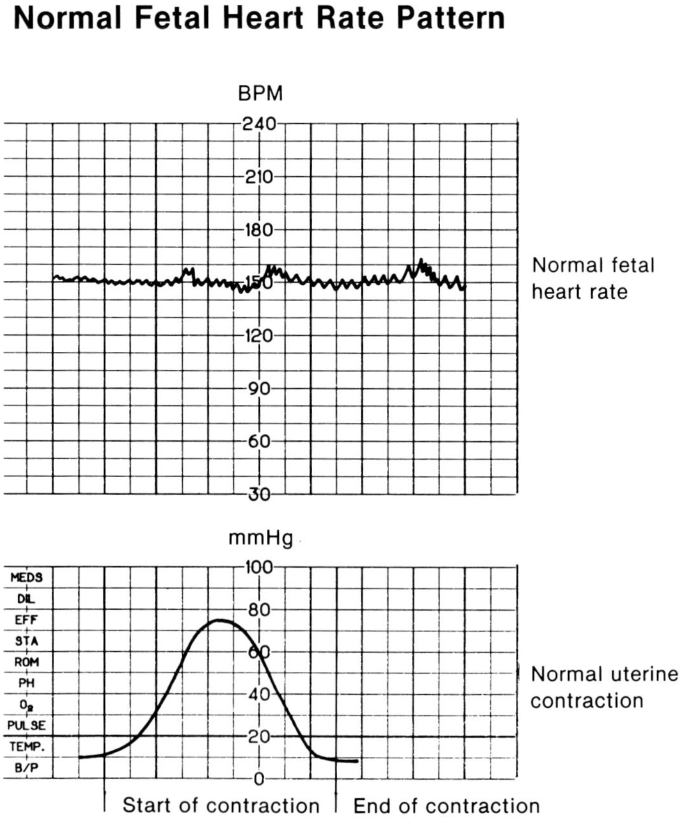

Figure 43–11 • Note the normal fetal heart rate of 150 bpm. The line has a wavy character which is not artifact. This is normal beat-to-beat heart rate variability. This is a sign of a healthy fetus. The uterine contraction shown is of 1 minute's duration, with a normal baseline tone of 10 mmHg and a peak intensity of 75 mmHg.

3. Periodic Heart Rate Patterns

There are four periodic heart rate patterns that should be recognized and distinguished from each other. Although in many cases this distinction is fairly obvious, at times the changes may be fairly subtle.

a. *Early Uniform Decelerations*

Early uniform decelerations (EUD) begin with the onset of a uterine contraction and end with the contraction (Fig. 43–12). The degree of deceleration may be as much as 30–40 bpm. They appear as a mirror image of the uterine contraction. They may be caused by pressure of the fetal head against the cervix or the bony portions of the birth canal. This would lead to increased pressure on the dura and a vagal response. Parer alternatively and currently suggests that the vagal response is initiated by mild fetal hypoxia not associated with clinically apparent compromise.[5] The EUD pattern is often seen during the second stage of labor. Although usually of no consequence to the infant, if it is sustained and severe, the fetus may become acidotic because fetal cardiac output is rate dependent. Because this is a vagally mediated reflex, it can be attenuated or eliminated by the administration of maternal atropine. This pattern corresponds to the type I dip of Caldeyro-Barcia and is also known as a head compression (HC) pattern.

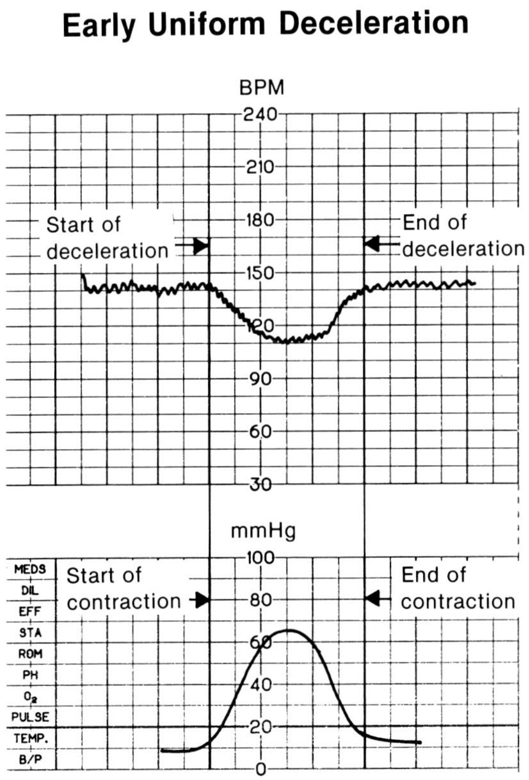

Figure 43–12 • Early uniform deceleration begins and ends with the uterine contraction. The nadir is above 100 bpm. Heart rate variability is not lost. The deceleration appears to be a mirror-image of the uterine contraction. This type of deceleration is thought to be caused by head compression and does not signify fetal distress.

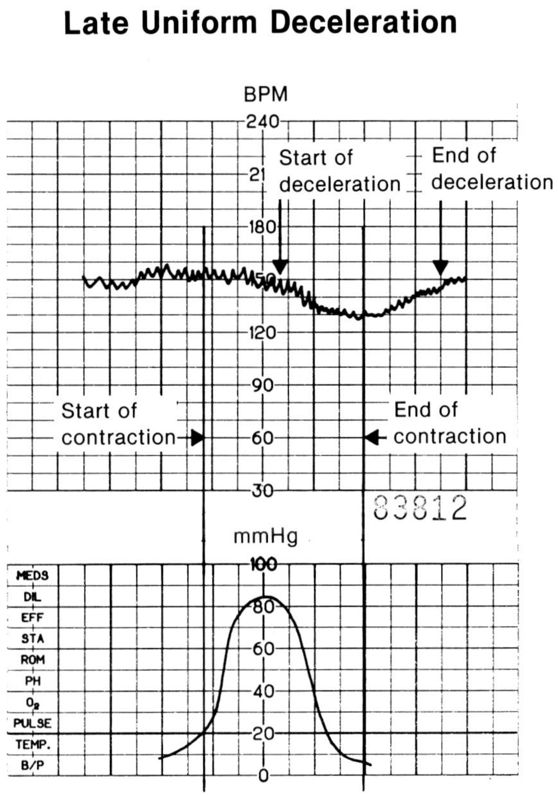

Figure 43–13 • Late uniform deceleration begins during the peak intensity of the contraction and persists for 20–30 seconds after the contraction is over. Variability is decreased but not lost in this example. This type of pattern is associated with uteroplacental insufficiency and may indicate fetal distress in labor. Hypotension from epidural anesthesia may cause this pattern. Administration of oxygen and left uterine displacement are indicated. Head-down position and vasopressors may be necessary if hypotension is the cause.

b. *Late Uniform Decelerations*

Late uniform decelerations (LUD) are frequently less severe in the degree of heart rate decline than other patterns but are of greater concern in terms of fetal welfare. They typically begin after the onset of a uterine contraction, usually near its peak, and are sustained after the contraction is over (Fig. 43–13). They are caused by decreases in uteroplacental perfusion. When the uterus contracts and reaches pressures of 60–70 mmHg, this exceeds the usual mean uterine artery pressure and flow temporarily ceases. A normal fetus can tolerate this short decrease, but an abnormal fetal–placental unit has limited reserve and thus becomes hypoxic and acidotic and indicates its distress with this type of pattern.[6] However, this pattern is not always associated with significant acidosis. This pattern corresponds to the type II dip of Caldeyro Barcia and is also known as a uteroplacental insufficiency pattern (UPI).

Parer has distinguished two types of late uniform decelerations, a reflex type and a nonreflex type. The former is associated with a previously normal fetus that is exposed to an acute intrapartum event decreasing uteroplacental blood flow or fetal oxygenation.[6] This pattern is distinguished by the presence of normal heart rate variability, which indicates normal fetal cerebral and myocardial oxygenation. The nonreflex pattern includes a significant decrease or loss of fetal heart rate variability, and this probably represents a chronic condition with a fetal cerebral and cardiovascular system that has limited or no reserve, ie, inadequate oxygenation.

c. *Variable Decelerations*

Variable decelerations have no distinctive relationship to uterine contractions. They may occur before, during, or after a contraction. They are typically abrupt in the fall of fetal heart rate and often abrupt in return to baseline. Occasionally, there is some overshoot of return to resting heart rate and then a decline to previous values (Fig. 43–14). This pattern is believed to be due to umbilical cord compression and vagal reflect pathways. It is often seen during the second stage of labor, and in this circumstance may be caused by increased fetal dural pressure from head compression from pushing. This pattern may reflect a state of fetal distress, particularly if the degree of heart rate decline is severe and persistent. Goodlin's rule of 60 defines severe variable decelerations as those that result in a heart rate below 60 bpm, those that are 60 beats below baseline, or those that exceed 60 seconds in duration.[7] This pattern is also known as the cord compression pattern (CC). As with any deceleration, if it is sustained, fetal acidosis may develop.

d. *Accelerations with Contractions*

Accelerations with contractions are indicative of a healthy fetus that is reacting to its environment with greater sympathetic than vagal activity (Fig. 43–15).

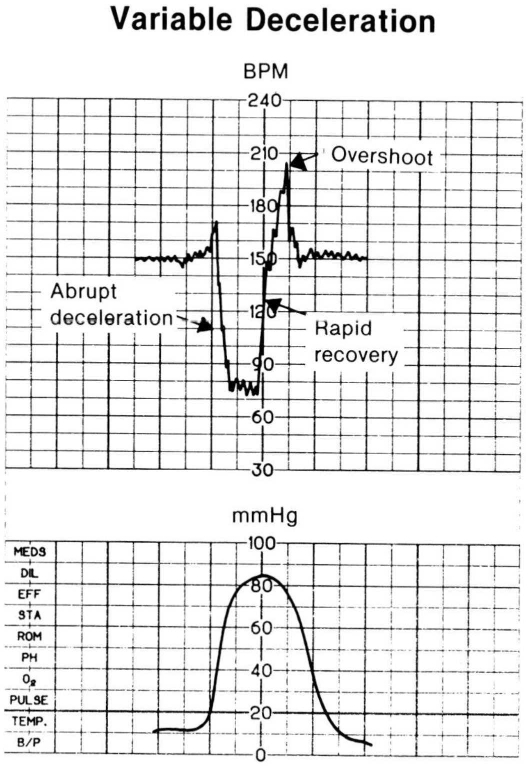

Figure 43–14 • Variable deceleration is characterized by its sudden descent and equally rapid recovery. Beat-to-beat variability is maintained. It does not always appear at the same place in reference to uterine contractions. There is occasionally some overshoot as recovery occurs. This pattern is associated with transient umbilical cord compression and, as long as rapid recovery occurs, is not associated with fetal acidosis. If the nadir is below 100 bpm for prolonged periods of time the fetus may become acidotic.

C. *Prenatal Predictive Use of the Fetal Heart Rate Monitor*

1. The Nonstress Test

The nonstress test (NST) (Table 43–1) is employed when a patient has a condition such as diabetes or hypertension that is known to adversely affect the fetal environment. This is one of a few tests that can be used to evaluate the well-being of the fetoplacental unit and assist in the decision of when to deliver the patient, as well as raise an alert to a potentially high-risk labor. The test is performed by applying the external fetal monitor and observing the fetal heart rate and the presence and frequency of fetal movement and uterine activity. The tracing is marked when the mother notes a fetal movement. A normal fetus is expected to increase its heart rate by at least 15 bpm with these movements. A non-

Fetal Heart Rate Accelerations with Contractions

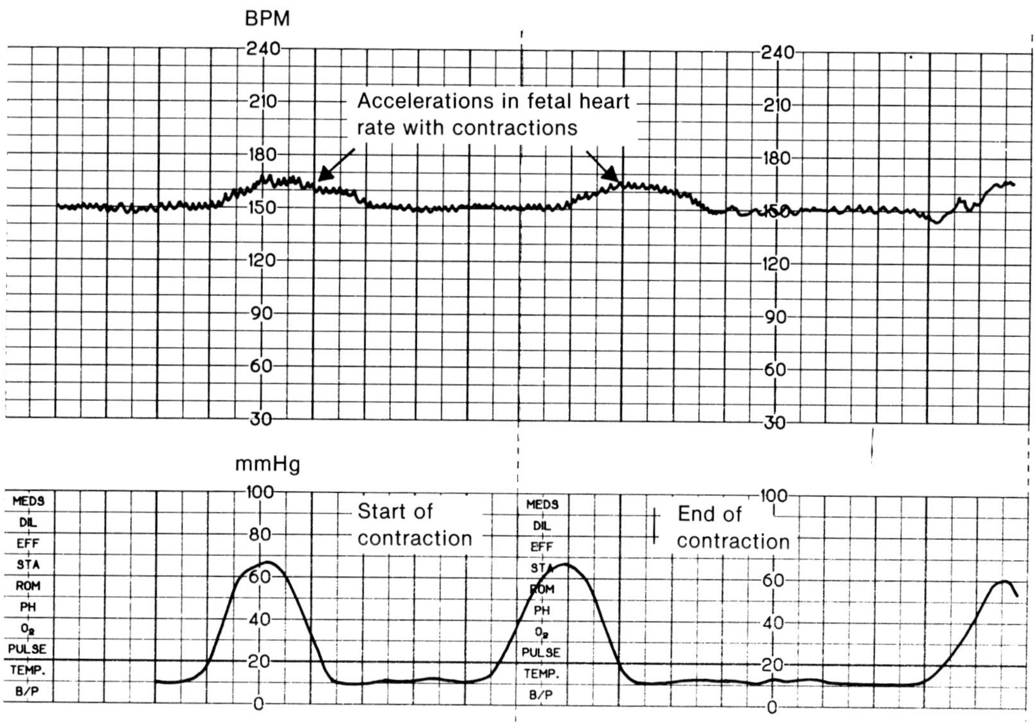

Figure 43–15 • Fetal heart rate accelerations with contractions are shown. Note the mild accelerations in fetal heart rate with uterine contractions and the presence of good variability. This tracing reflects a very healthy fetus.

stress test is considered *reactive* if at least two fetal movements occur in a 20-minute period with the normal acceleration in heart rate mentioned above. The baseline heart rate should be in the normal range, and the long-term variability should be about 10 bpm. A *nonreactive* test is one in which there are no fetal movements felt or no accelerations in heart rate occur with fetal movement. This fetus generally has no long-term heart rate variability. An *uncertain* test is one in which there are fewer than two movements per 20 minutes or the heart rate increase is less than 15 bpm with movement, or long-term variability is below 10 bpm and/or the baseline heart rate is abnormal.

A reactive test is associated with good fetal outcome and neonatal survival of greater than 1 week in greater than 99% of cases. It reliably indicates a healthy fetus and normal placental function. A nonreactive test is associated with poorer fetal outcome in approximately 20% of cases. The affected infants typically experience late decelerations during labor, low Apgar scores, or perinatal death. Therefore, a reactive test is reassuring, but a nonreactive test requires further evaluation, ie, the contraction stress test (CST), also previously known as the oxytocin challenge test (OCT).[6]

Table 43–1 • The Nonstress Test

Reactive
1. At least 2 fetal movements in 20 min
2. Normal acceleration in FHR with fetal movements
3. Baseline fetal heart rate of 120–160 beats/min
4. Long-term variability of approximately 10 beats/min

Nonreactive
1. No fetal movements
2. No acceleration in FHR
3. No long-term variability

Uncertain
1. Fewer than 2 fetal movements in 20 min
2. Increase of FHR of less than 15 beats/min
3. Long-term variability of less than 10 beats/min

FHR, fetal heart rate

2. The Contraction Stress Test

The contraction stress test (Table 43–2) was initially the only assessment of its kind. However, careful observation of patients being prepared for this study led to the development of the nonstress test, which requires very little intervention. The CST is now reserved for those situations in which the NST has yielded an uncertain or nonreactive result. The external fetal heart rate and uterine monitors are applied and the patient is observed for

Table 43–2 • The Contraction Stress Test

Negative	
	Three contractions in a 10-min period with:
	1. No late uniform decelerations
	2. Normal baseline FHR
Positive	
	Persistent late uniform decelerations with contractions
Suspicious	
	1. Late uniform decelerations, but not with every contraction
	2. Variable decelerations
	3. Abnormal baseline FHR
Unsatisfactory	
	1. Excessive fetal movement
	2. Cannot achieve 3 contractions in a 10-min period

FHR, fetal heart rate

a 10-minute period. If three spontaneous contractions should occur during this period, then the test is considered completed and the heart rate strip is analyzed. If there are not three contractions, then uterine activity is stimulated by either manual nipple stipulation to cause the endogenous release of oxytocin or the administration of a low-dose oxytocin intravenous infusion. A *negative* test is one in which there were three contractions with no late uniform fetal heart rate decelerations and during which a normal baseline heart rate was maintained. Accelerations with the contractions are considered normal. A *positive* CST demonstrates persistent late decelerations with the uterine contractions. Fetal heart rate variability may be decreased or absent. A *suspicious* test is one in which there are late decelerations but not with every contraction, or one with variable decelerations. The test is also deemed suspicious if there is an abnormal baseline heart rate, ie, >160 or <120 bpm. The test is *unsatisfactory* if there is excessive fetal movement or if three contractions during a 10-minute period cannot be achieved.

A negative CST is associated with fetal survival of greater than 1 week in greater than 99% of cases. A positive CST is associated with a poor neonatal result in about 50% of cases. Suspicious and unsatisfactory tests obviously should be repeated at a later time if possible.[6]

The importance of these tests is that they can predict which fetuses should fare well during labor; they will also identify those patients who require more intense observation and monitoring. This information should assist the anesthesiologist in preparing an analgesic or anesthetic plan, and also identify those patients who are more likely to have an operative delivery.

III. Discussion

A. *Etiology and Management of Abnormal Heart Rate Patterns*

Each of the abnormal patterns may have several etiologies. An understanding of the patient's clinical condition and the events occurring in labor will lead to a more rapid diagnosis and possible correction of the problem.

1. Fetal Heart Rate Variability

Fetal heart rate variability is affected by several factors. Although a decrease in variability in association with decelerations identifies a fetus that is quite likely hypoxic and acidotic, a decrease in variability alone may reflect a fetal resting state or be the effect of a drug (Fig. 43–16). The fetal resting state usually lasts about 20 minutes. Because virtually any drug that causes central nervous system depression in the mother will cross the placenta, it is commonly believed that these agents may decrease fetal heart rate variability. Drugs often associated with this phenomenon are magnesium sulfate, meperidine and other narcotic analgesics, barbiturates, benzodiazepines, phenothiazines, atropine, and local anesthetics. Local anesthetics used in appropriate doses for analgesia during labor should not have this effect unless injected intravascularly. The larger doses used for vaginal delivery or cesarean section may decrease variability, because the blood levels from absorption are higher. Heart rate variability may be artificially increased by the administration of ephedrine or catecholamines to the mother.

2. Fetal Tachycardia

Fetal tachycardia may be caused by hypoxia, but is probably short in duration and usually not observed. Maternal fever and maternal–fetal sepsis may result in fetal tachycardia (Fig. 43–17). Drugs such as atropine, catecholamines, and ephedrine induce an increase in fetal heart rate as they cross the placenta. Glycopyrrolate does not cross the placenta readily and does not produce this change. A fetus with congestive heart failure or severe anemia may also exhibit tachycardia. Fetal tachyarrhythmia, such as paroxysmal atrial tachycardia, may also be

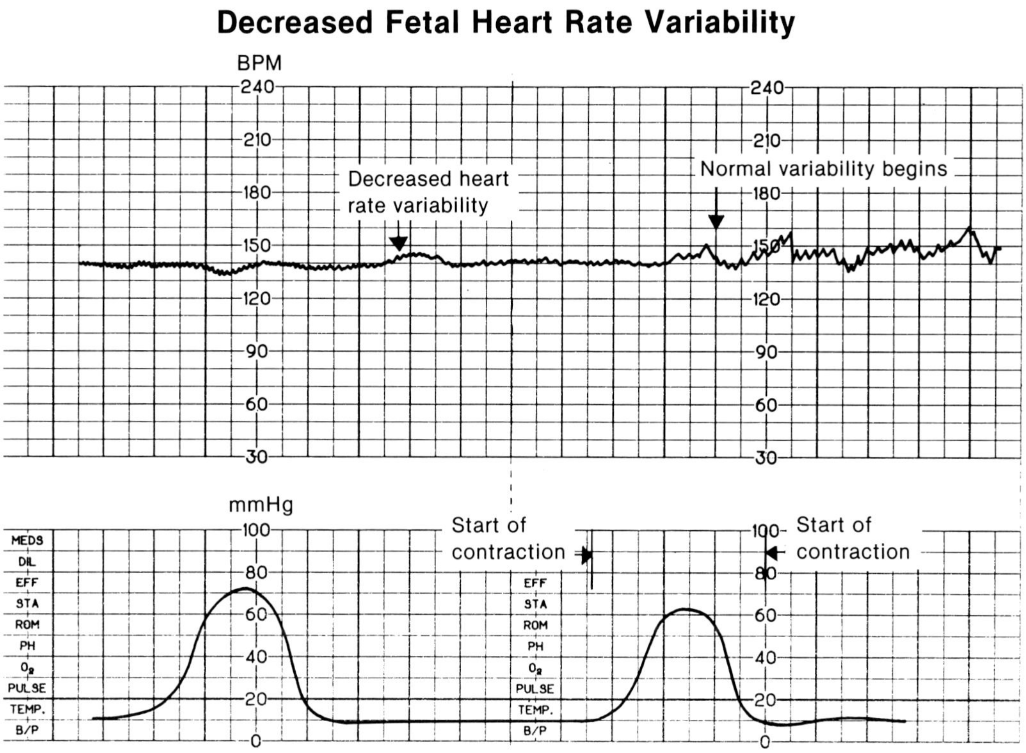

Figure 43–16 • This tracing demonstrates decreased fetal heart rate variability. Observe the flattening out of the fetal heart rate variability for the first 4 1/2 minutes of this tracing. This may occur spontaneously for up to 20-minute periods as the result of sedative drug administration or as a sign of fetal distress. Because the tracing shows a return to normal variability, this was probably a fetal "resting" period. Continued lack of variability requires further fetal assessment.

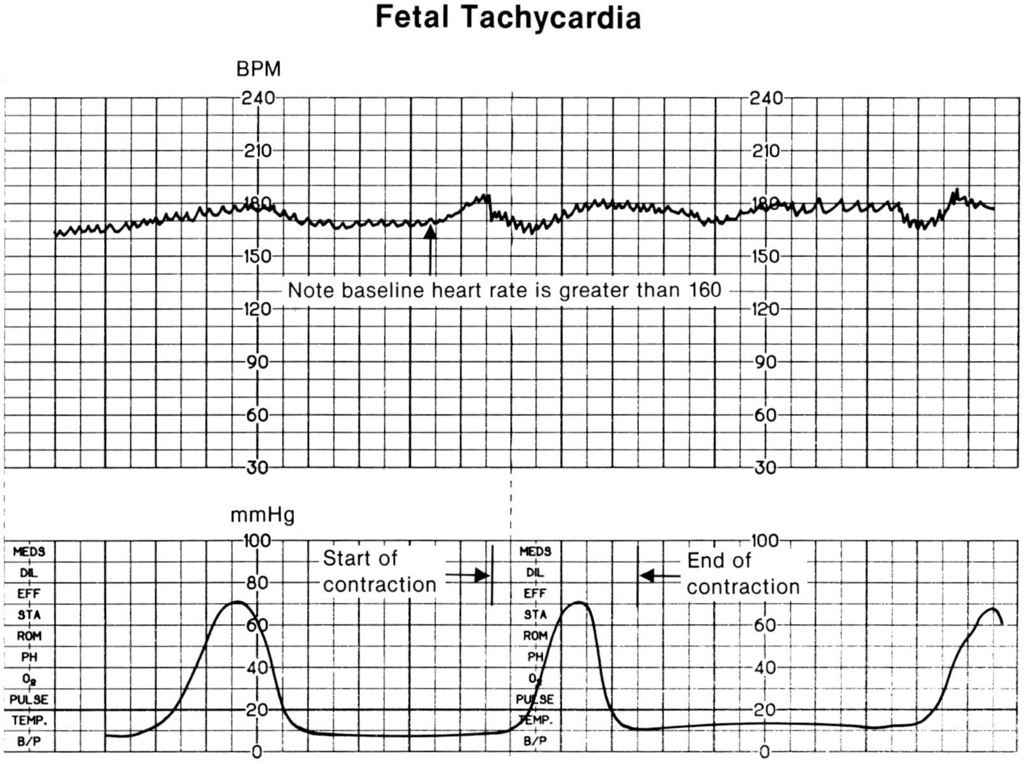

Figure 43–17 • This tracing demonstrates a fetal tachycardia of 170–180 bpm. Variability is normal. This may be due to maternal fever, fetal distress, maternal atropine or ephedrine administration, or merely a normal variation.

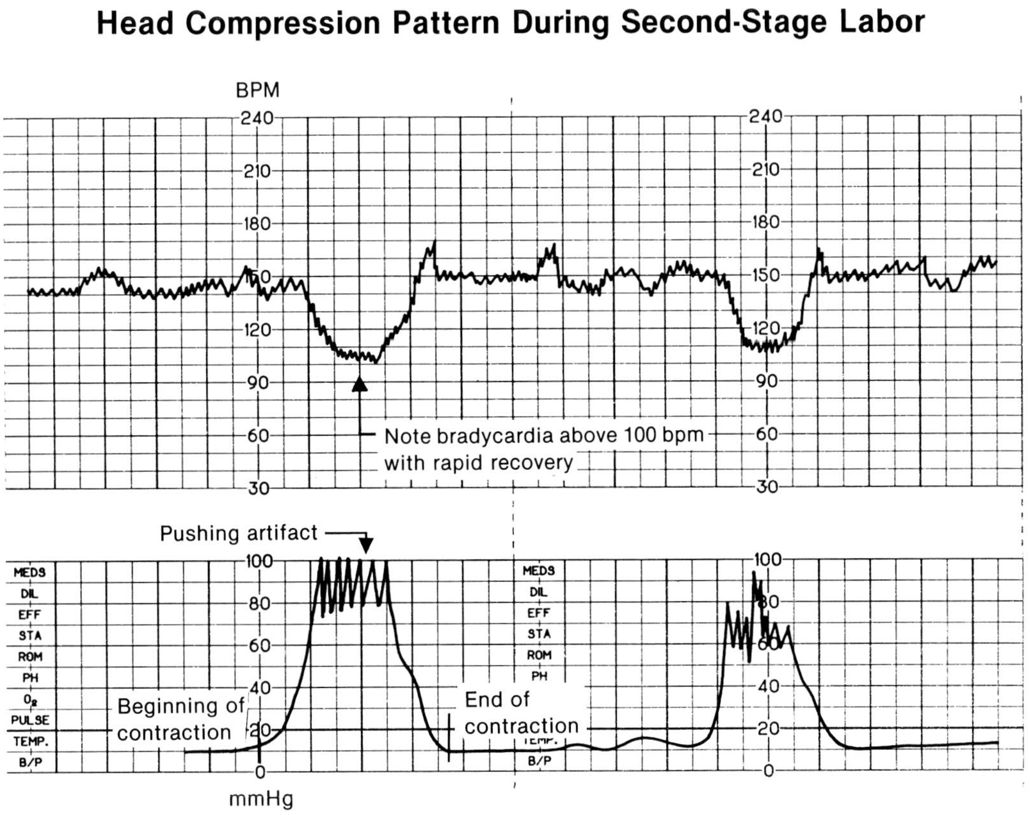

Figure 43–18 • Head compression pattern during second-stage labor is shown. Note the exaggerated uterine activity associated with maternal pushing. The fetal bradycardia recovers rapidly and maintains good variability. This is not a sign of distress at this time. The pattern is the result of head compression during expulsive efforts. If this persists for a prolonged period of time, fetal acidosis may ensue secondary to decreased fetal cardiac output.

detected. Management is directed at the underlying cause whenever possible.

3. Fetal Bradycardia

Fetal bradycardia, that is, a decrease in fetal heart rate that is sustained and not part of a periodic deceleration, may or may not represent fetal acidosis. A sustained bradycardia that is not less than 100 bpm and associated with good variability may be a vagal response to continuous head compression (Fig. 43–18). Fetal scalp blood sampling to determine the pH would be appropriate if the pattern persisted. A prolonged bradycardia may be precipitated by maternal hypoxia, decreased uteroplacental blood flow (eg, from hypotension, vasoconstriction, or sustained uterine contraction), decreased umbilical blood flow from cord compression, or loss of functional placental area (eg, a placental abruption) (Fig. 43–19). Another cause is the use of paracervical block, which may cause uterine artery constriction as well as elevated local anesthetic levels in the fetus.

Treatment should be instituted immediately on recognition of bradycardia and is oriented at optimizing the fetal environment (Table 43–3). Steps to be taken are (1) administration of maternal oxygen, (2) position change (usually onto the left side), (3) maintenance of maternal blood pressure over a systolic of 100 mmHg or within 20% of baseline values, (4) maternal hydration, and (5) avoidance or elimination of excessive uterine activity by stopping or decreasing oxytocin infusion, if present, or the administration of a tocolytic agent such as terbutaline. If these measures and any treatable underlying cause do not resolve the problem, scalp sampling or expeditious delivery of the infant may be necessary. Finally, intrinsic bradyarrhythmia due to a cardiac conduction defect may exist. These may occasionally respond to maternal drugs but usually are not a problem until after delivery, when treatment may be administered directly to the infant.

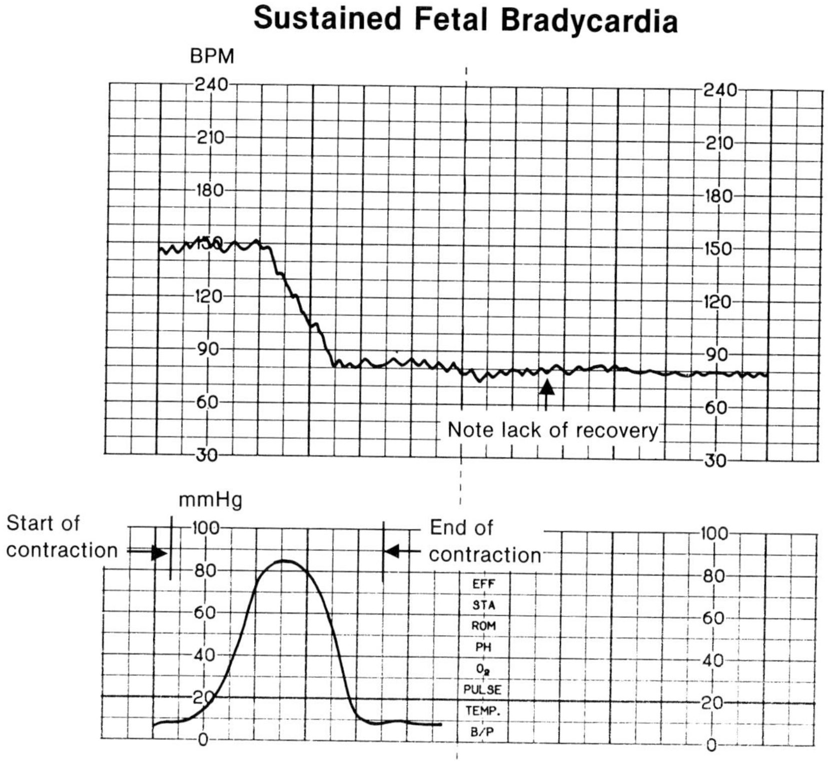

Figure 43–19 • This tracing shows sustained fetal bradycardia. This bradycardia is sustained and not recovering after a contraction. This is often an indicator of severe fetal compromise or persistent umbilical cord compression and generally results in rapid diagnostic and therapeutic maneuvers including immediate delivery by the most expeditious route.

4. EARLY UNIFORM DECELERATIONS

Early uniform decelerations are usually of no clinical significance and usually require no intervention. If they are severe during the second stage of labor, decreased pushing efforts by bearing down on alternate contractions, maternal oxygen, and left lateral positioning may prove helpful to the fetus.

5. LATE UNIFORM DECELERATIONS

Late uniform decelerations may be caused by chronic uteroplacental insufficiency or by acute decreases in uteroplacental perfusion (Fig. 43–20). Chronic insufficiency is frequently associated with hypertension, preeclampsia, diabetes, and postmaturity. Acute causes include excessive oxytocin stimulation, hypotension from regional anesthesia, and aortocaval compression from supine positioning. Initial treatment is the same as that outlined above for bradycardia. If there is a treatable inciting cause identified, it should be corrected, eg, by discontinuing oxytocin infusion (Fig. 43–21). Scalp sampling blood pH is often employed if the pattern persists and delivery effected if the fetus becomes hypoxic and acidotic.

Table 43-3 • Treatment of Fetal Bradycardia

1. Administer maternal oxygen.
2. Change maternal position.
3. Maintain adequate maternal blood pressure.
4. Ensure adequate maternal intravascular volume with intravenous fluids.
5. Eliminate excessive uterine activity, if present:
   a. Stop oxytocin infusion.
   b. Administer a tocolytic agent.

B. *Anesthetic Implications of Fetal Heart Rate Patterns*

1. THE LABORING PATIENT

It has been estimated that approximately 25% of parturients with no risk factors will develop abnormal fetal heart rate tracings during labor. Should these patterns be considered a contraindication to the use of epidural analgesia? Generally, no. The underlying cause for the aberrant pattern should be identified and corrected if possible. Maternal oxygen administration and proper positioning should be effected. Early uniform decelerations and moderate variable decelerations rarely repre-

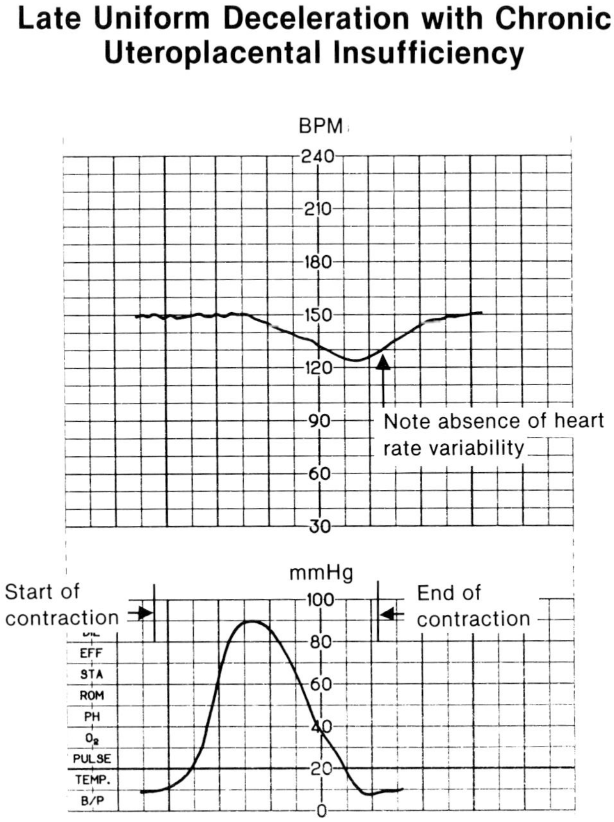

Figure 43-20 • Late uniform deceleration with chronic uteroplacental insufficiency is shown. The marked lack of fetal heart rate variability associated with this late uniform deceleration suggests that the fetal reserve is exhausted and that the sympathetic and parasympathetic nervous systems are at their maximum compensatory state. This is indicative of a chronic uteroplacental insufficiency. This pattern may not recover with the usual therapeutic maneuvers and immediate delivery may become necessary.

sent a problem for the fetus, and any appropriately administered form of analgesia is in order. Late uniform decelerations, although more disconcerting, are not a contraindication to epidural analgesia, particularly if labor is to continue. Careful attention must be paid to avoid hypotension, because a fetus with late uniform decelerations has demonstrated that it has no reserve. Aortocaval compression must be prevented. The judicious use of epidural analgesia may reduce maternal catecholamine secretion in response to painful contractions. It has been demonstrated that uteroplacental blood flow is reduced significantly in the presence of a painful stimulus and the subsequent release of catecholamines, especially norepinephrine. Proper use of epidural analgesia has been demonstrated to improve intravillous blood flow as much as 70% in humans with pregnancy-induced hypertension, as long as hypotension is avoided. Therefore, skillful application of epidural analgesia in a segmental fashion should not compromise and may actually improve the situation for the fetus.

Epidural analgesia may lead to the occurrence of late uniform decelerations if the maternal systolic blood pressure is allowed to decrease more than 25% from baseline or to less than 100 mmHg. Uterine blood flow is pressure dependent because the uteroplacental vasculature is maximally dilated at term due to high levels of estrogen. A mean arterial pressure of approximately 70 mmHg is considered the lowest at which normal uterine blood flow may be maintained. Therefore, a significant reduction in uterine blood flow will lead to acute fetal hypoxia and late uniform decelerations. Beat-to-beat variability is usually not abolished, and these decelerations should resolve with appropriate therapy to restore maternal blood pressure and uteroplacental perfusion. The maneuvers are to place the mother in the left lateral position with a head-down tilt, administer intravenous fluids, administer oxygen, and frequently assess the blood pressure. If a suitable response does not occur quickly, the use of a vasopressor is indicated. The vasopressor of choice is ephedrine or the pharmacologically similar mephentermine. These drugs do not cause uterine artery constriction and have been demonstrated to return both maternal blood pressure and uterine blood flow to near normal. Drugs with primarily direct alpha-adrenergic agonist activity, such as phenylephrine and methoxamine, are not advised because they cause uterine artery constriction. Thus, although these drugs can increase maternal blood pressure toward normal, they also cause uterine blood flow to remain at its decreased level or to be depressed even further. Although ephedrine does cause the release of endogenous catecholamines and although there are alpha-receptors on the uterine vessels, there appear to be few uterine nerve endings capable of releasing norepinephrine in the vicinity. Hypotension from nonanesthetic causes will also reduce uterine blood flow, eg, arrhythmias, dehydration, vasodilator drugs, or hemorrhage.

Although arterial pressure is a critical factor in maintaining uteroplacental perfusion, the entire equation can be expressed as:

$$UBF = \frac{UAP - UVP}{UVR}$$

Late Uniform Decelerations Associated with Oxytocin Administration

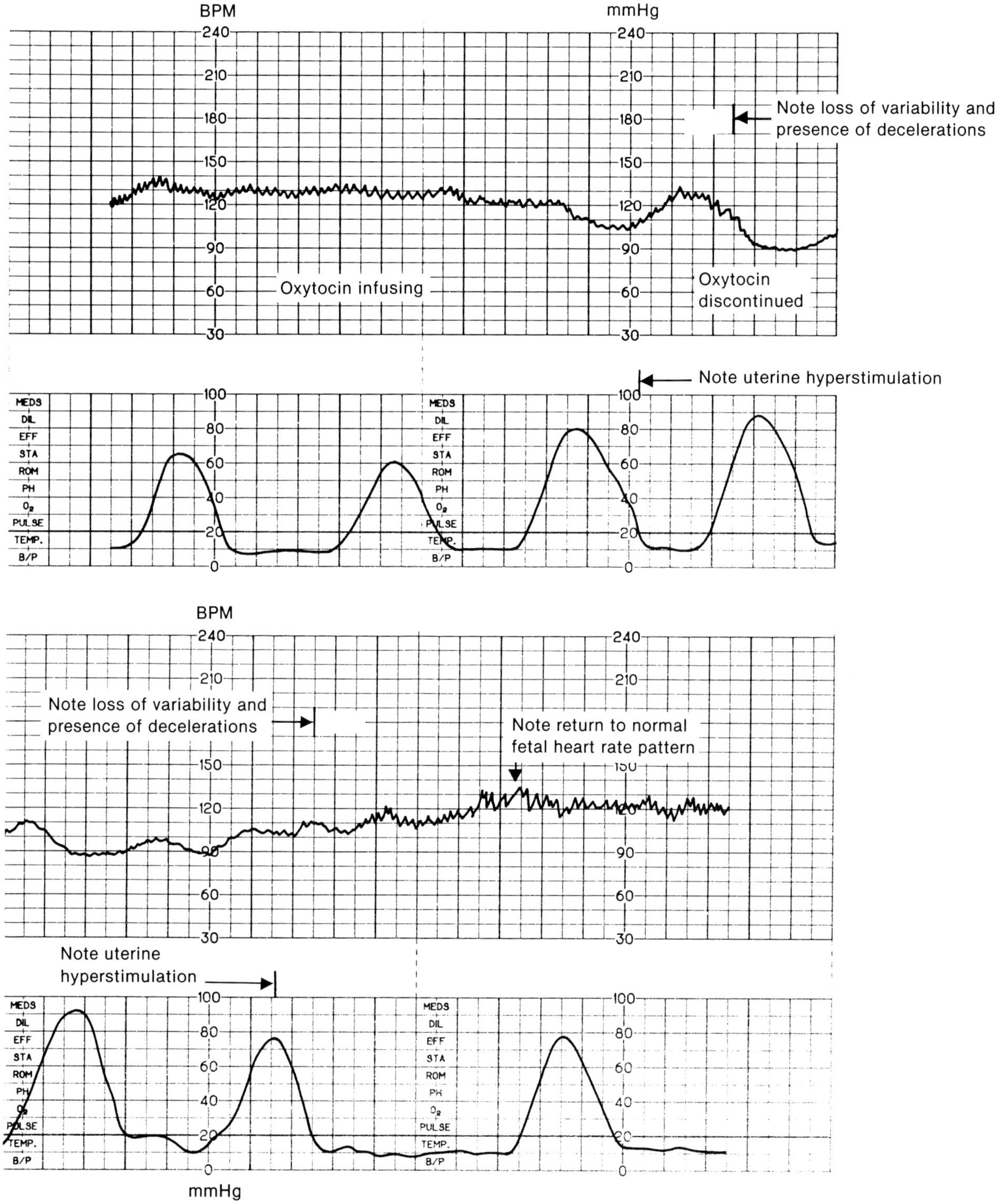

Figure 43–21 • Late uniform decelerations are associated here with oxytocin administration. The period of uterine hyperstimulation does not allow uteroplacental blood flow to return to normal and thus the fetus becomes compromised. Discontinuing the oxytocin as well as oxygen administration and left uterine displacement should result in prompt recovery. If hypertonus persists, a tocolytic may be indicated.

Using the Fetal Heart Rate Monitor to Record Maternal Heart Rate During an Epidural Test Dose

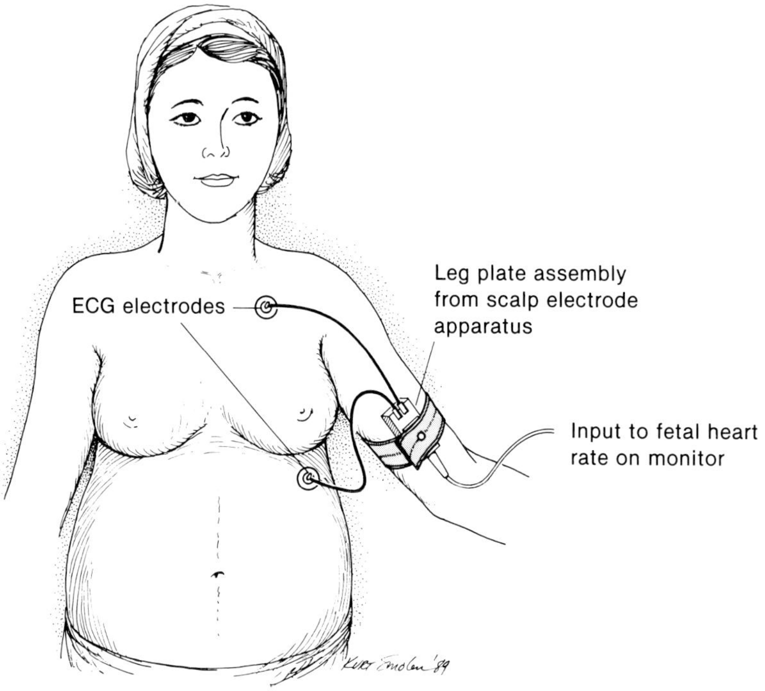

Figure 43–22 • The fetal heart rate monitor is used to record maternal heart rate during an epidural test dose. The upper electrode is placed at the left sternal border and the lower one just beneath the left breast in the left anterior axillary line. This should yield a good ECG complex and heart rate indication. This should only be done with a dual trace monitor designed for monitoring twins or with an additional monitor. The fetus should not be disconnected to observe maternal heart rate.

where

UBF = uterine blood flow
UAP = mean uterine arterial pressure
UVP = uterine venous pressure
UVR = uterine vascular resistance

Uterine vascular resistance is determined by two components, arteriolar constriction and vascular compression by the myometrium. Although the effect of various anesthetics on uteroplacental flow has been extensively studied in animals, it is now possible to accurately assess this in humans as well by use of the xenon clearance technique. It is apparent from the formula that uterine blood flow may be reduced by decreasing arterial pressure, increasing uterine venous pressure, constricting the uterine arteries, or by increasing myometrial tone. Uterine vascular resistance will be increased by elevating myometrial tone. This will occur in response to overstimulation with oxytocin, abruptio placenta, and perhaps with an increase in endogenous catecholamines. Therefore, increased uterine tone from oxytocin administration in concert with hypotension from epidural anesthesia is a combination destined to produce late decelerations and has been observed. Hypertension, both chronic and pregnancy induced, increases uterine artery resistance. Human uterine arteries have also been shown to constrict in the presence of high levels of local anesthetic drugs. These levels would only be reached by direct application, eg, paracervical block, or from unintentional intravascular injection of a very large epidural dose of drug. Arteriolar constriction may also occur as the result of sympathetic stimulation in response to hypercarbia or hypoxia.

Supine positioning should be strictly avoided, because aortocaval compression can lead not only to the supine hypotensive syndrome but to decrease uterine artery pressure without systemic hypotension from compression of the aorta or the common iliac artery. Obstruction of the inferior vena cava not only reduces maternal cardiac return, but results in an elevation in uterine venous tone that adversely affects the equation for uteroplacental blood flow. It should be remembered that once the patient is comfortable, she may be more likely to remain in the supine position and therefore must be encouraged to assume the left lateral position.

2. Vaginal Delivery

If the patient is to undergo a vaginal delivery, the choice of anesthesia should encompass the information presented above. If the delivery becomes emergent and an epidural anesthetic suitable for delivery is not present, saddle block (low spinal anesthesia) is a prompt and efficient way to provide conditions for an instrumented delivery in the face of a sustained bradycardia or another worrisome pattern with little risk of hypotension. If regional anesthesia is not an option and an immediate forceps-assisted delivery is required, low-dose ketamine (0.2–0.5 mg/kg) will provide analgesic conditions suitable for delivery and produce amnesia for the event. General endotracheal anesthesia for vaginal delivery is rarely dictated by a fetal heart rate tracing unless it suggests cord compression of severe degree for a second twin requiring breech extraction, or shoulder dystocia in a patient without another form of anesthesia.

3. CESAREAN SECTION

When cesarean section is planned for failure to progress in labor or for cephalopelvic disproportion with a normal heart rate tracing, there are no particular anesthetic implications. However, some of these patients will undergo cesarean section with a diagnosis of fetal distress because of significant recurrent variable decelerations or late decelerations. It is essential that the tracing be evaluated in the context of when the decelerations began and whether they are still present when the patient is prepared for the operative delivery. They may have been the result of oxytocin stimulation with a marginally compromised fetus, one that recovers a normal pattern when the oxytocin is discontinued. There also may have been uterine hypertonus as a result of oxytocin use with resultant decelerations in a normal fetus, which will again recover after discontinuation of oxytocin (see Fig. 43–21). The use of regional anesthesia with measures to avoid hypotension and aortocaval compression is appropriate under these circumstances. Patients with variable decelerations that are severe and persistent are occasionally rushed to the operating room; by the time the monitor is reattached, the pattern has resolved. Patients with variable, severe, persistant decelerations are also candidates for carefully conducted regional anesthesia.

Patients who present with tracings or fetal scalp sample pH indicating severe fetal distress will receive general anesthesia under many, albeit not all, circumstances. This is usually when there is no prior epidural catheter in place or when the heart rate is so persistently slow that the time to initiate regional block and the possibility of hypotension are believed to be inappropriate.

4. NONOBSTETRIC SURGERY

Although not always feasible, the external fetal monitor and external contraction monitor can be useful for nonobstetric surgical procedures during pregnancy.[8] Although some cases of fetal bradycardia during surgery have alerted anesthesiologists to the presence of maternal hypoxia or hypotension, current monitoring practices that include a pulse oximeter should make this unlikely. Variability is decreased and can be abolished by hypoxia and by sedative drugs, as well as periods of fetal sleep. Slowing of the fetal heart rate in the operative setting suggests hypoxia and acidosis, but may also be related to the administration of drugs or anesthetic agents, which tend to slow the heart rate. Thus, interpretation of slight changes in fetal heart rate can be difficult. Because the fetus has little ability to adjust its stroke volume, cardiac output is rate dependent. If the heart rate falls to 80 bpm, cardiac output is significantly reduced; at a rate of 60 bpm, the fetus is in jeopardy. The presence of periodic or sustained fetal heart rate changes may indicate aortocaval compression or decreasing uterine blood flow from other causes, eg, induced hypotension for neurosurgical procedures[9] or decreased flow from the pump-oxygenator during cardiac procedures.[10] Hypothermia and alpha-agonists can slow the fetal heart rate as well.[11,12] This usually recovers satisfactorily with rewarming of the patient.

Uterine activity may be monitored with an external tocodynamometer. If preterm labor develops in the perioperative period, tocolysis may be necessary to preserve the pregnancy. Some authors have suggested using the potent volatile anesthetics because they relax the uterus. This may prove effective intraoperatively as long as an excessive decrease in blood pressure does not occur, but other drugs, such as ritodrine, will be required postoperatively.

Placement of the external fetal heart rate transducer and the tocodynamometer can be problematic for an intraabdominal procedure. Intermittent determination of fetal heart rate by a sterile Doppler probe may be substituted, although this is a limited evaluation. The most important tracings are those obtained preoperatively, during the induction of anesthesia, and the immediate postoperative period. This establishes a baseline with which to compare intraoperative events, and allows for postoperative assessment of uterine activity.

Hyperventilation is commonly used during neuroanesthesia because the decrease in carbon dioxide reduces cerebral blood flow. The potential adverse effects on the fetus of decreased placental oxygen transfer due to leftward shift of the oxyhemoglobin dissociation curve and umbilical vessel vasoconstriction in the presence of alkalosis should not be a problem for a healthy fetus whose mother receives moderate hyperventilation, ie, to a CO_2 of approximately 25 mmHg. Fetal heart rate monitoring should alert the anesthetist to compromises in fetal oxygenation, and adjustments should be made accordingly. Similarly, the fetal heart rate tracing should indicate if induced hypotensive techniques have reduced uteroplacental blood flow below the critical point.

C. *Maternal Heart Rate Monitoring*

A unique use of the fetal monitoring equipment is to monitor maternal heart rate and heart rate variability during the administration of an epidural test dose containing epinephrine or isoproterenol. The catecholamine marker is supposed to increase maternal heart rate if the test dose is injected intravascularly. Chestnut has described a technique wherein an ECG lead is placed at the upper left sternal border and in the left anterior axillary line just beneath the breast (Fig. 43-22).[13] The wires are inserted into the fetal heart rate monitor cable block and the block is secured to the patient's arm. The fetal heart rate monitor is set on direct ECG mode (Model 8040A, Hewlett-Packard Corporation, Palo Alto, CA). The maternal heart rate and its variability are recorded on the standard strip chart recorder. If there is a tachycardia, it will be recorded and thus can easily be quantified. This same group has employed this technique in laboring as well as elective cesarean section patients, and has discovered that laboring patients have cyclic accelerations in heart rate with uterine contractions.[16] This would suggest that the catecholamine-containing epidural test dose is less reliable in the laboring patient.

IV. COMPLICATIONS

Maternal complications from application of the internal monitor are the result of either injury or infection. The spiral scalp electrode can be misplaced onto the uterine cervix or vaginal wall and cause bleeding. Such an application would also record the maternal heart rate rather than the fetal heart rate and could obviously lead to misinterpretation of the clinical situation. The internal uterine catheter or its introducer could perforate the lower uterine segment or dissect between the muscle layers, causing bleeding or hematoma formation. Fortunately, these are rare occurrences. Infection may occur as a result of a foreign body remaining in the uterine cavity for a long period of time, leading to chorioamnionitis in labor or endometritis in the postpartum period.[14] Infection might also be introduced by injection of contaminated saline through the intrauterine catheter.

The external monitors have no direct complications associated with their use. The only significant complication would be misinterpretation of the data displayed.

The fetus also faces risk of injury from the scalp electrode placement in the form of cephalohematoma. Infection may occur at the site of the electrode placement. Chorioamnionitis also presents a significant threat to the fetus, thereby reinforcing the concept that the more invasive procedures should be reserved for those situations where the information to be gained will significantly alter the therapeutic or management plan.[15]

A major problem with fetal monitors is the size of the console, which is usually mounted on a cart. Patients who have infants at risk are disconnected from the monitor for transport to a delivery room or cesarean section suite, and the instrument may not be reconnected. The fetus then remains unmonitored save for intermittent auscultation until delivery. This may be a critically significant period of time. It is in everyone's best interest to leave the monitor attached and functioning for as long as possible.

V. REFERENCES

1. Hon EH, Quilligan EJ. The classification of fetal heart rate. II: A revised working classification. Conn Med 31:779–784, 1967.
2. Paul RH, Petrie RH. Fetal Intensive Care: Current Concepts. Los Angeles, USC Press, 1973.
3. Parer JT. Handbook of Fetal Heart Rate Monitoring. Philadelphia, WB Saunders, 1983.
4. Paul RH, Suidan AK, Yeh SY, et al. Clinical fetal monitoring. VII: The evaluation and significance of intrapartum baseline variability. Am J Obstet Gynecol 123:206–210, 1975.
5. Parer JT. Fetal heart rate. In Resnik R, Creasy R (eds). Maternal-Fetal Medicine. Philadelphia, WB Saunders, 1989, pp 314–343.
6. Kubli FW, Hon EH, Khazin AF, Takemura H. Observations

on heart rate and pH in the human fetus during labor. Am J Obstet Gynecol 104: 1190, 1969.
7. Goodlin RC. Inappropriate fetal bradycardia. Obstet Gynecol 48:117, 1976.
8. Katz JD, Hook R, Barash PG. Fetal heart rate monitoring in pregnant patients undergoing surgery. Am J Obstet Gynecol 125:267–269, 1976.
9. Rigg D, McDonogh A. Use of sodium nitroprusside for deliberate hypotension during pregnancy. Br J Anaesth 53:985–987, 1981.
10. Levy DL, Warriner RA, Burgess GE. Fetal response to cardiopulmonary bypass. Obstet Gynecol 56:112–114, 1980.
11. Hess OW, Davis CD. Electronic evaluation of the fetal and maternal heart rate during hypothermia in a pregnant woman. Am J Obstet Gynecol 89:801–807, 1964.
12. Chestnut DH, Weiner CP. Monitoring maternal heart rate during epidural injection of a test dose containing epinephrine. Anesthesiology 64:839–840, 1986.
13. Chestnut DH, Owen CL, Brown CK, et al. Does labor affect the variability of maternal heart rate during induction of epidural anesthesia. Anesthesiology 68:622–625, 1988.
14. Emmons SL, Krohn M, Jackson M, Eschenbach DA. Development of wound infections among women undergoing cesarean section. Obstet Gynecol 72:559–564, 1988.
15. McCusker J, Harris DR, Hosmer DW Jr. Association of electronic fetal monitoring during labor with cesarean section rate and with neonatal morbidity and mortality. Am J Public Health 78:1170–1174, 1988.

Chapter 44

Alan M. Demby, MD
Joseph D. Schmidt, MD

Bladder Catheterization

OUTLINE

I. Introduction

In general, indwelling urinary catheters are placed for two reasons. First, urine output is one of the more physiologic and sensitive indicators of intravascular volume status and can usually be measured with minimal risk or morbidity. In the acutely ill or anesthetized patient, continuous monitoring of the urinary output can be accomplished with an indwelling bladder catheter. Consequently, preoperative placement of such catheters is a routine procedure for many operations. Second, patients under general or spinal anesthesia cannot empty their bladder. If drainage is not instituted, the bladder may become overdistended during surgery, resulting in transient or permanent damage to the detrusor muscle. In addition, the high pressures created by an overdistended bladder can cause hydroureteronephrosis and a decrease in renal function. In some instances, urinary extravasation may occur via a forniceal tear of the calyx. Less likely, rupture of the bladder (intraperitoneal) may occur.

Catheterization is also common in the intensive care unit setting for both of the above reasons, and is especially useful for hemodynamically unstable patients.

A. *Anatomy and Physiology*

Normal bladder function depends on an intact and coordinated nerve supply.[1] The micturition center is located in the brainstem (pons) and is under inhibitory influence from the cerebral cortex. The lower urinary tract, including bladder, prostate, urethra, and pelvic floor musculature, is innervated by the sympathetic, parasympathetic, and somatic nerves.

The bladder is a muscular bag that both stores urine and infrequently eliminates urine under voluntary control. The bladder detrusor is composed of interlacing bundles of smooth muscle cells without discrete layers. The major motor innervation of the detrusor emanates from the pelvic nerves (splanchnics), which are part of the parasympathetic system arising from the sacral spinal cord levels S-2 to S-4. The sympathetic nerves arising from the spinal cord levels T-10 to L-2 give sensory innervation (pain and temperature) to the bladder.

The pudendal nerve is a somatic motor and sensory nerve that supplies the external sphincter and pelvic floor musculature. It arises from the sacral cord levels S-2 to S-4.

Thus, both the detrusor motor nucleus and the pudendal nerve nucleus are located in the sacral spinal cord. Under normal circumstances, these nuclei, under influence from the micturition center, work in a coordinated manner during micturition. However, even in the absence of innervation from above, the bladder may empty via the spinal reflex arc, "the micturition reflex."

Urine is expelled via the urethra. In the adult man, this is a conduit approximately 25 cm long, composed of mucosa and submucosa, the anterior part of which is surrounded by spongy tissue (corpus spongiosum) (Fig. 44–1). The male posterior urethra is composed of membranous and prostatic segments. The former portion, lying in the urogenital diaphragm, is surrounded by skeletal muscle, which is partially under voluntary control. The prostatic urethra extends from the bladder neck to just distal to the verumontanum, and is completely surrounded by smooth muscle and the glandular substance of the prostate.

The female urethra measures only 3–4 cm in length and has no corpus spongiosum. It is surrounded by a network of longitudinally aligned smooth muscle fibers (Fig. 44–2).

II. INDICATIONS

Regional (spinal and epidural) or general anesthesia that is adequate for major abdominal operations effectively paralyzes the detrusor muscle and the micturition reflex. Under these conditions, continence is usually maintained by the normally high compliance of the bladder wall and the mechanical resistance of the urethral tube. However, as the bladder reaches capacity, the intravesical pressure will rise and exceed that of the urethra, usually resulting in overflow incontinence. Damage to the detrusor may precede overflow decompression, as mentioned earlier.

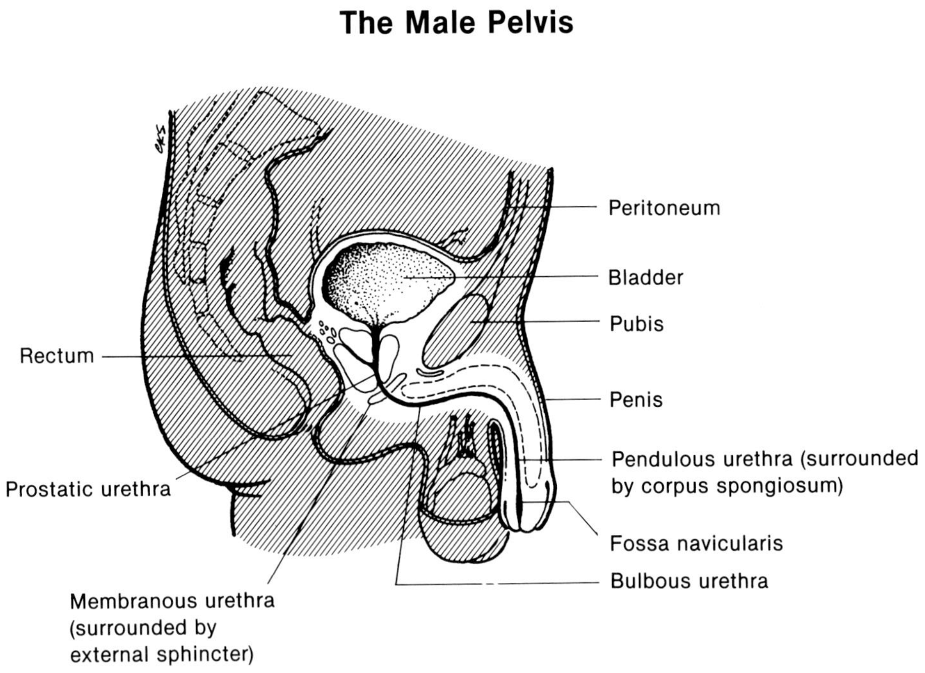

Figure 44–1 • The male pelvis is shown. The male urethra has four parts (prostatic, membranous, bulbous, and pendulous) and is 25 cm long.

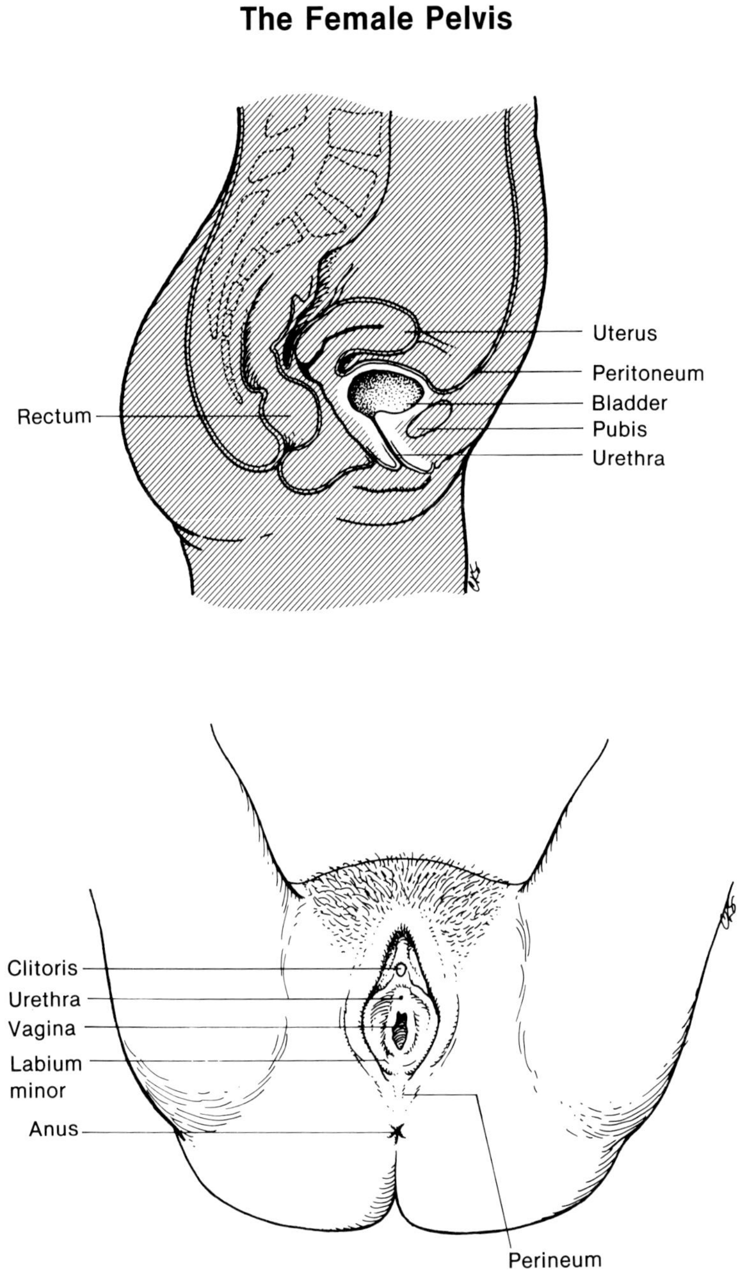

Figure 44–2 • The female pelvis is shown. The female urethra is only 3–4 cm long.

The bladder capacity in the awake individual is approximately 350–550 mL, but under anesthesia this may reach as high as 1500 mL. To avoid overdistention and possible detrusor damage, a catheter should be placed prior to starting any procedure where the detrusor will be paralyzed for more than several hours.

Other indications for indwelling or continuous bladder drainage are:

1. Monitoring urine output for volume status
   a. Perioperatively
   b. For hemodynamically unstable patients
2. Urinary retention secondary to
   a. The effects of anesthesia
   b. Bladder outlet obstruction, including prostatism, urethral stricture, or trauma (urethral disruption)
   c. Spinal cord injury including trauma and disc disease
   d. Neurologic disorders including head trauma, cerebrovascular accidents, brain tumor, and multiple sclerosis
3. Bladder trauma secondary to
   a. Pelvic fracture with bladder rupture
   b. Drainage after surgical procedures on the lower urinary tract

4. Urinary diversion to avoid contamination of lower abdominal, upper thigh, or buttock wounds
5. Incontinence of any type in which conservative measures have failed

III. How to Catheterize the Bladder

A. *Types of Indwelling Catheter*

The most commonly used catheter is (Fig. 44–3) the Foley type. This is a tube composed usually of rubber, plastic, or silicone with an inflatable balloon near the tip, which serves to keep the catheter in the bladder. The balloon is inflated via a separate port located near the end of the catheter. Other types of indwelling catheters include a coudé (from the French for "elbow"), which has a 45° bend near its tip. The coudé catheter is helpful in negotiating the posterior urethra of a patient who has an enlarged prostate or hypertrophied bladder neck. Council-tip catheters are similar to Foley catheters, with the exception of a preformed hole in the tip that allows it to be passed over a filiform or guide wire. Emmett catheters are especially useful for patients with hemorrhage from the prostate. These catheters have an extended tip proximal to the balloon with more side holes, affording better drainage.

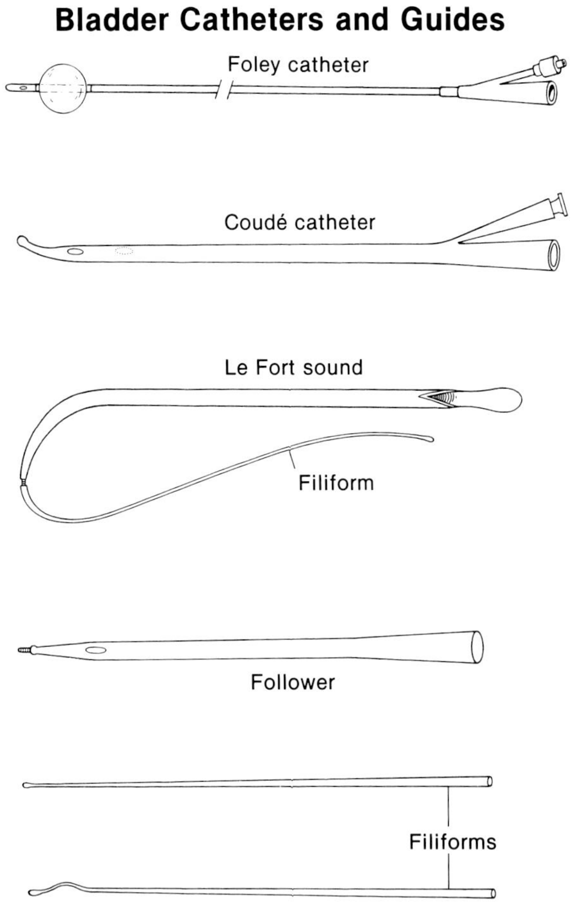

Figure 44–3 • Various bladder catheters and guides are illustrated.

For noncontinuous monitoring of urinary output, there is a large number of straight catheters available; the most commonly used is the Robinson type (a.k.a. "red rubber Robinson"). The advantage to this catheter is that it is soft and thin walled, and therefore has a larger lumen than other similarly sized catheters. Tiemann catheters are made of a hard, clear plastic material. They are usually employed for women who are on a self-catheterization program. Men with stricture disease can also use this catheter for self-dilation.

For patients who will have a catheter for more than 2 weeks, a pure silicone catheter should be chosen, because this causes the least amount of inflammatory reaction in the urethra. The disadvantage of pure silicone catheters is that they are soft, and therefore their walls must be thicker and the lumen of the catheter is then smaller for any given French size. They are also slightly more difficult to pass. Silastic or silicone-coated plastic catheters are somewhat stiffer, and therefore their walls are thinner and their lumina are larger for any given French size. They are thus easier to pass, but are more reactive in causing urethral inflammation. Plastic or rubber catheters are even more irritating and should only be used for short-term drainage or for intermittent catheterization.

B. *Routine Placement of a Foley Catheter*

Although placement of a Foley catheter is routine, simple, and often performed by nursing personnel, it should be considered a procedure and treated as such. Therefore, as with any procedure, it is important to first insure that all necessary equipment is readily available, sterile, and open.

Bladder catheterization kits are available containing a sterile field, rubber gloves, Betadine solution, cotton swabs, forceps, lubricating jelly, a 16 French Foley catheter, and a syringe with 10 mL of saline. It is suggested that additional lubricating jelly be available when performing this procedure. A separate Mayo stand to place the kit on when opened is also helpful and strongly recommended.

The following is a step-by-step description of the suggested method for placing a Foley catheter using a bladder catheterization kit (Fig. 44–4).

1. Open the kit on a Mayo stand. Sterile gloves should be the first item on the top of the kit and should be worn at this time.
2. Remove the sterile field and place it over the penis with the dull side (absorbent side) face up. All the sterile drapes provided should be used. The larger the sterile field, the easier it is to work without contamination.
3. Open the lubricant and empty the packet onto the sterile field or another convenient sterile part of the kit. Also at this time, open the Betadine solution and pour it over the cotton swabs.
4. Retract the foreskin, if present, with the left hand (to be

Catheterization of the Male Bladder

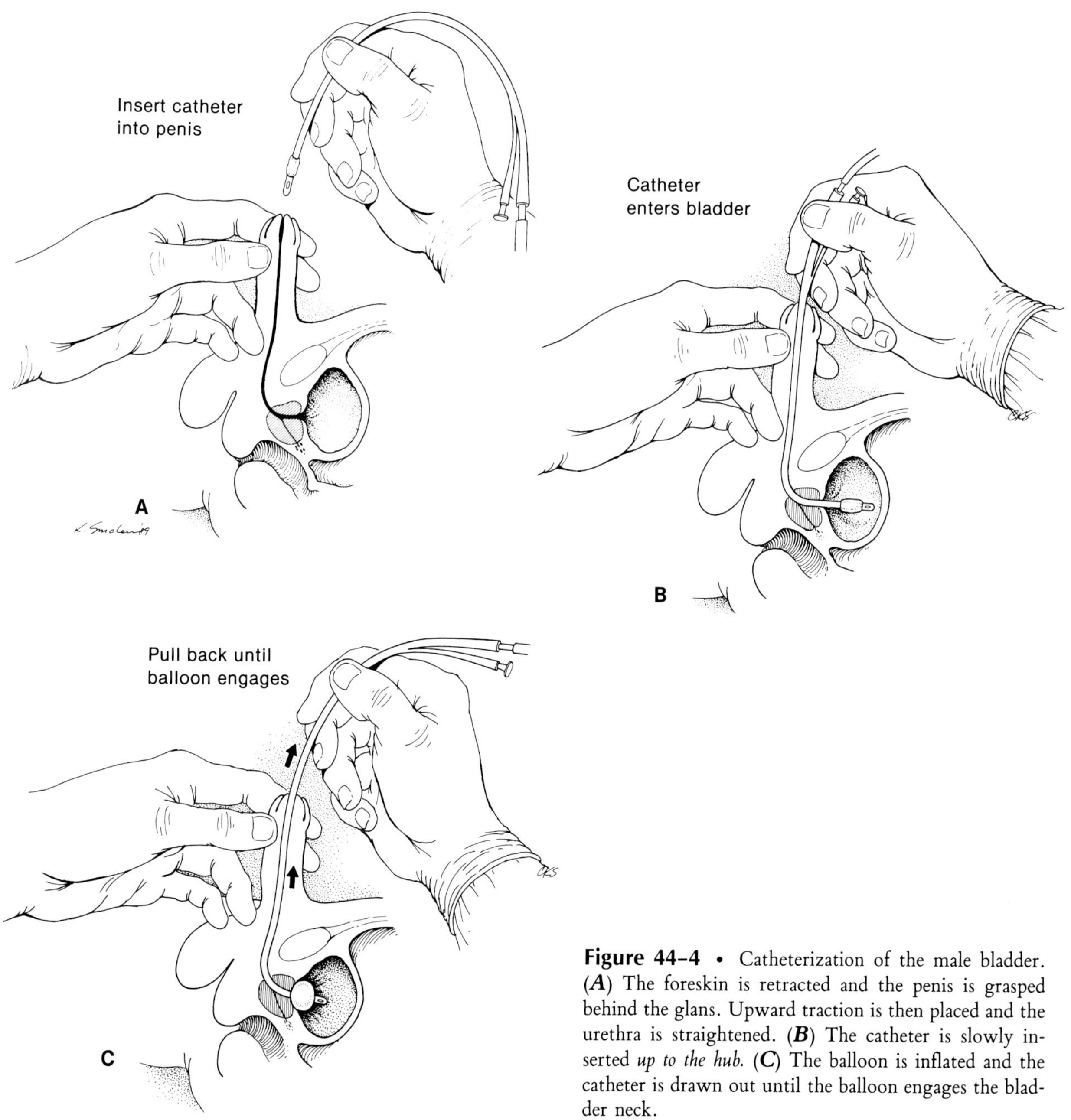

Figure 44–4 • Catheterization of the male bladder. (***A***) The foreskin is retracted and the penis is grasped behind the glans. Upward traction is then placed and the urethra is straightened. (***B***) The catheter is slowly inserted *up to the hub.* (***C***) The balloon is inflated and the catheter is drawn out until the balloon engages the bladder neck.

known as the "nonsterile hand"). Grasp the penis behind the glans with the left hand and telescope the penis straight up to extend the urethra. The contents of the kit should now only be touched using the right (clean) hand.

5. Use the forceps to grasp the Betadine-soaked cotton swabs. Using a circular motion, apply the Betadine to the meatus and the glans of the penis. Make sure to dispose of the used cotton swabs in an area outside of your sterile field.
6. Lubricate the catheter with the jelly provided. Some kits have injectable lubricant in a catheter-tip syringe, which can be *gently* instilled into the penile urethra for less traumatic catheterization.
7. With the urethra extended (Fig. 44–4A), slowly pass the catheter into the meatus up to the hub (Fig. 44–4B). *Note:* Urine may be obtained from the prostatic urethra; therefore to insure correct placement into the bladder, the catheter should be advanced up to its hub. Inflation of the balloon in the prostatic urethra may cause pain and bleeding, and results in inadequate bladder drainage.
8. Inflate the balloon with 7–8 mL of saline. Pull the catheter back until the balloon engages the bladder neck (Fig. 44–4C).
9. If no urine is obtained at this time, gently compress the bladder suprapubically (Credé maneuver), since the catheter may be obstructed with lubricating jelly. If the catheter is correctly placed into the bladder lumen, irrigation with saline via a catheter tip syringe should show easy in-and-out flow.

Important points:

1. Adequate lubrication is essential. Inadequate lubrication results in difficulty or inability to pass the catheter and painful catheterizations.
2. The external sphincter is under voluntary control. Many patients will contract this muscle during catheterization, making negotiation of the membranous urethra difficult. Gentle, steady pressure usually overcomes this obstacle. In addition, instructing the patient to relax by taking a deep breath is helpful.

C. *Potential Problems*

Difficulty in catheterizing the male urethra usually arises because of three specific problems: (1) narrowing or stricture in any part of the urethra, eg, meatal stenosis or bulbar urethral stricture disease; (2) enlargement of the prostate, especially median lobe or bladder neck hypertrophy; and (3) false passage of the urethra (usually iatrogenic).

1. Urethral Stricture and Meatal Stenosis

The caliber of the normal adult male urethra is approximately 24–28 French in diameter. The urethral meatus is usually the most narrow portion of the urethra. On occasion, the meatus may be less than 16 French, making passage of a catheter difficult. This situation can be remedied by meatal dilation with successively larger metal sounds (Van Buren; similar to the Le Fort sound shown in Fig. 44–3). However, sometimes the meatus is so tight (less than 12 French) that a meatotomy is required. This procedure is easily performed at the bedside. The equipment necessary includes local anesthesia, a small hemostat, and fine scissors. *Please note:* Urologic consultation should be obtained prior to performing this procedure.

a. Ventral Meatotomy

1. The patient should be prepped in a manner similar to that previously described for insertion of a Foley catheter.
2. Lidocaine, 1% or 2% is used to anesthetize the area to be incised. This should be directly ventral from the most inferior aspect of the meatus.
3. A hemostat is used to crush the area to be incised after adequate anesthesia is obtained. This should be no more than a few millimeters in length, just enough to enable passage of a catheter. The hemostat should be left in place for several minutes prior to incision to insure adequate hemostasis (Fig. 44–5).
4. The hemostat is removed and the crushed area is incised with the fine scissors. Bleeding should be minimal.
5. The catheter is passed as previously described.
6. Local wound care includes topical antibiotic ointment.

2. Urethral Stricture Disease

Strictures of the urethra can be the result of trauma, infectious or inflammatory lesions, or neoplasia. The most common cause of stricture disease today is iatrogenic (ie, previous urethral manipulation or instrumention including catheterizations). The most common site for stricture is the bulbous urethra. On occasion, difficulty in passing a catheter may be the only manifestation of a urethral stricture. Often, however, a history of voiding symptoms can be elicited. These may include hesitancy, weak stream, splaying of the stream, or incomplete emptying.

During attempted catheterization, the catheter will "hang up" in the area of the stricture, usually the

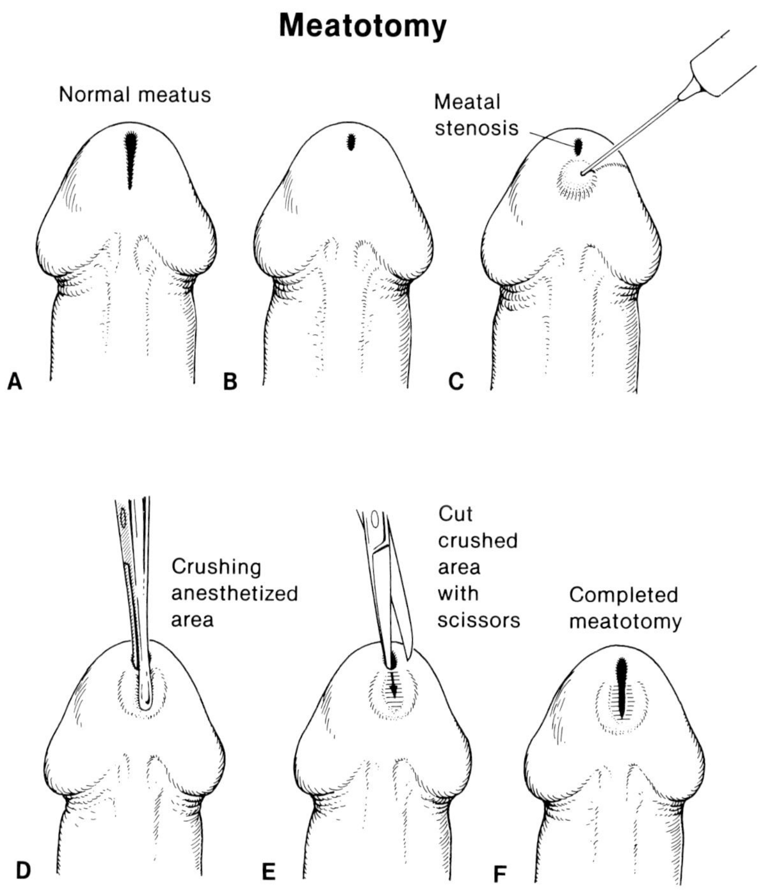

Figure 44–5 • If the meatus is too small to accept a catheter, a ventral meatotomy may be needed. See text for description.

bulbous urethra just beyond or at the penoscrotal junction. In this case, filiforms and followers will be required. Because this is not a routine part of bladder catheterization, it is suggested that urologic consultation be obtained at this time.

Filiforms are guides that are usually 3–5 French in diameter and have no lumen. They may have a straight, coudé, or spiral-tip, as in Fig. 44–3. The end of the filiform can be attached onto various types of "followers" (see Fig. 44–3). Followers are straight, stiffer catheters with a lumen, and range in size from 8 to 32 French.

Le Fort sounds are similar to Van Buren sounds, with the exception of their having "male" threads on their proximal tip that can be attached to the "female" filiforms (see Fig. 44–3). They have no lumen and are used strictly for dilating purposes, ranging in size from approximately 12 to 32 French.

a. *Filiform and Follower Technique*

1. The patient is prepped and draped as for placement of a Foley catheter. Adequate lubricating jelly should be available. It is often helpful to use 2% xylocaine jelly that comes with a catheter tip and can be gently injected directly into the urethra. It is important that this be done *gently* in patients with stricture disease, because high-pressure injection can cause urethral disruption and intravasation of the lubricant.
2. A single filiform is passed to the area of the stricture. If the stricture can be negotiated, the filiform is then passed into the bladder up to its hub. The 12 or 14 French follower is then attached to the filiform. The follower is then passed beyond the stricture into the bladder behind the filiform (the soft filiform coils in the bladder), thus dilating the strictured area. Drainage of the bladder at this time can be accomplished because the followers have a lumen (Fig. 44–6).
3. The 12 or 14 French follower is then pulled back until the end of the filiform is just outside the meatus. This follower is removed and successively larger followers are placed onto the filiform and passed beyond the stricture. In this manner, the urethra can be dilated up to 24 or 26 French.
4. If the dilation was easily performed, the filiform can be removed and a 16 or 18 French catheter passed into the bladder. If this is not the case, the filiform should not be

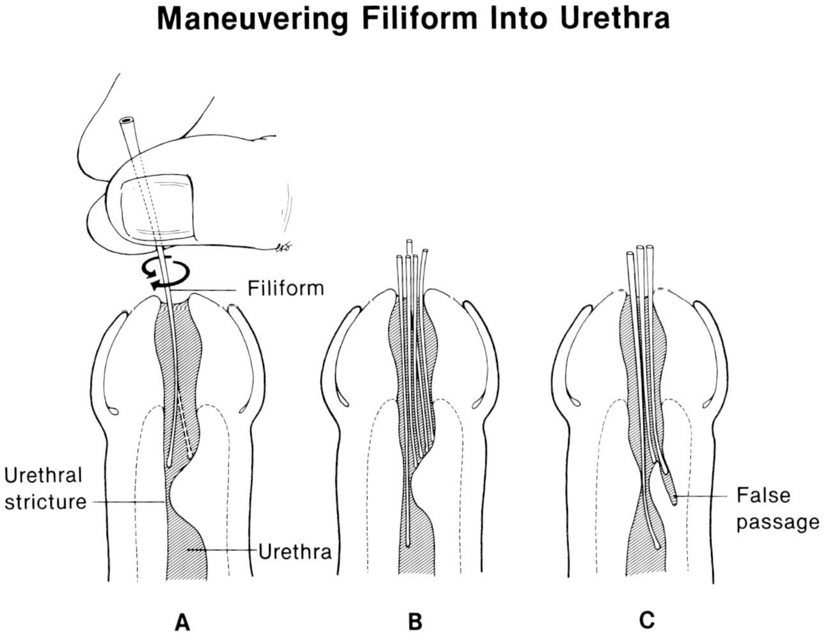

Figure 44–6 • The filiform is maneuvered into the urethra. (***A***) In the case when the caliber of the urethral lumen is decreased, such as with a stricture or a false passage, filiforms and followers are required. (***B***) Often multiple filiforms are needed to "fill in" the incorrect channels, allowing a single filiform to follow the correct path. (***C***) After a filiform is successfully passed, the others are removed, and successively larger followers are then used to delete the narrowed area(s).

removed and instead a catheter should be passed over the filiform.

5. A metal catheter guide (mandarin) with a preloaded Council-tip catheter can be attached to the filiform and passed into the bladder (Figs. 44–7 and 44–8). Once inside the bladder, the catheter can then be slipped over the filiform. The metal guide and the attached filiform are then withdrawn through the preformed hole in the tip of the Council catheter. *Metal catheter guides can perforate the urethra, prostate, bladder, or rectum! They should be used* **only** *by trained personnel.*
6. If the first filiform cannot negotiate the stricture, it should be left in place at the site of obstruction. Subsequent filiforms can then be placed into the urethra, filling the incorrect channels until one filiform finds the correct channel (see Fig. 44–6). After the correct channel is found and the filiform is passed up to its hub, the other filiforms are removed. The urethra may then be dilated using the followers in a manner already described.

3. False Passages

False passages are usually created by traumatic instrumentation. Commonly, this is associated with an attempted catheter passage in a patient with urethral stricture disease. The false passage occurs just proximal to the scarred urethra. False passages may also occur in the posterior part of the prostatic urethra during attempted

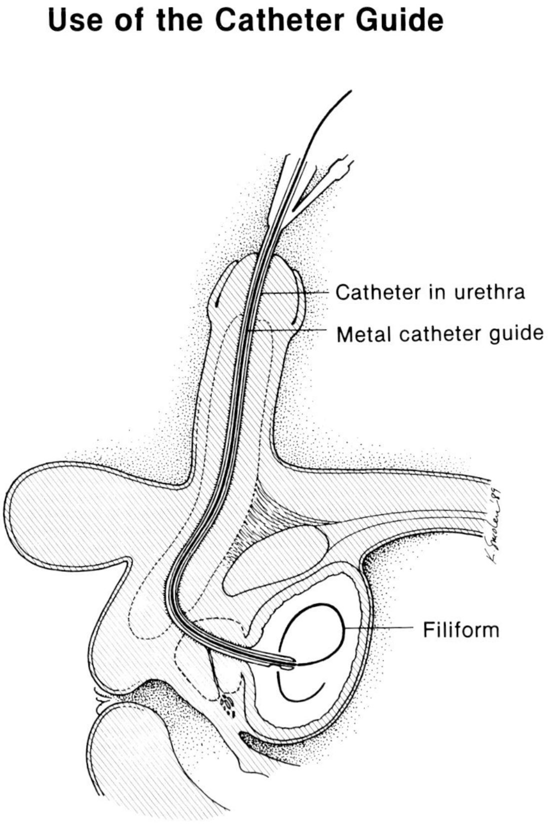

Figure 44–7 • The catheter guide is used. If a catheter does not pass easily into the bladder after stricture dilation, or if there is an abnormality of the bladder neck, a metal catheter guide (Mandarin) may be used.

Catheter Guide with Filiform

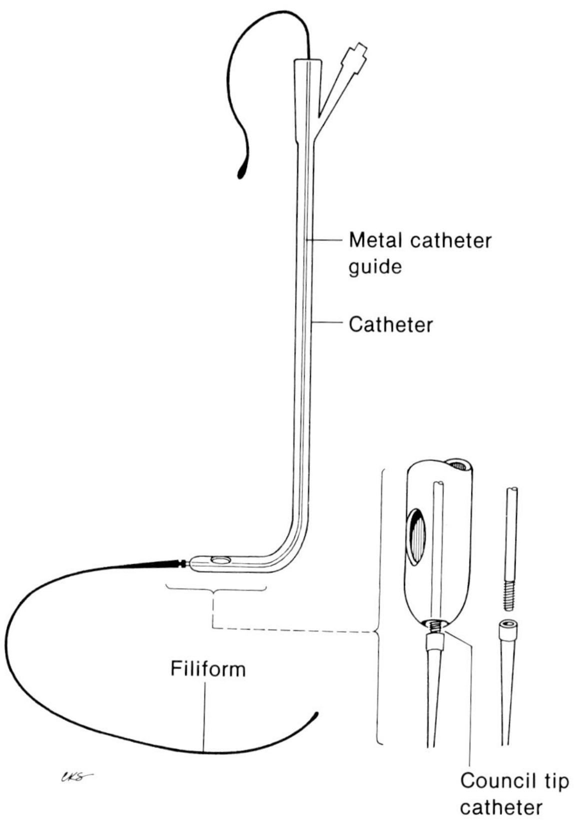

Figure 44–8 • Catheter guide is shown with filiform.

catheterization, especially in patients with enlarged prostates. False passages should be managed in the same fashion as previously described for urethral stricture disease.

4. Prostatic Enlargement

Enlargement of the benign or malignant prostate, especially the median lobe, can make catheterization difficult. This is usually overcome with adequate lubrication and a stiffer coudé catheter. A 20 or 22 French coudé catheter is best suited for this situation. Gentle injection of 2% xylocaine jelly, as previously described, is also quite helpful. However, if this is unsuccessful, then elevation of the prostatic urethra with an index finger in the rectum is helpful. This directs the tip of the catheter up and over the median lobe or hypertrophied bladder neck. As depicted in Fig. 44–9, an assistant is required for this technique. The assistant grasps the penis behind the glans and telescopes the urethra upward. The operator then inserts the catheter with one hand while elevating the prostatic urethra with the index finger of the other hand.

With the index finger in the rectum, the tip of the catheter can usually be felt in the prostatic urethra. At this point, the catheter is withdrawn several centimeters. The index finger elevates the prostatic urethra anteriorly, after which the catheter should pass easily.

D. *Suprapubic Cystostomy*

If the bladder cannot be drained via the urethra for any reason, then punch suprapubic cystostomy is indicated. This again is not a routine procedure, and urologic consultation should be obtained.

Relative contraindications to punch suprapubic cystostomy include previous lower abdominal or pelvic surgery, because this distorts normal anatomy and may cause the peritoneum or peritoneal contents to extend over the anterior wall of the bladder. Small contracted or

Use of Catheter with Rectal Maneuver

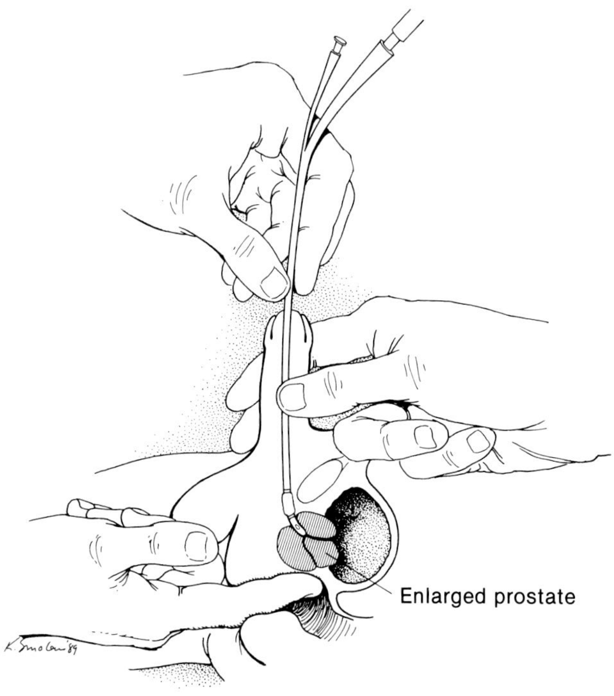

Figure 44–9 • The catheter with the rectal maneuver. Elevation of the prostate with the index finger can sometimes help negotiate an enlarged median lobe. As above, this maneuver requires assistance.

nondilated bladders are also a relative contraindication. Under these conditions, open cystostomy or endoscopic placement of a catheter is recommended.

The most common type of punch suprapubic tube is a 12 or 14 French Malecot-type catheter. A hollow trochar can be passed through the tip of the catheter. The end of the trochar can be screwed down into the end of the catheter. This creates tension on the wings of the Malecot, effectively straightening them. When the trochar is unscrewed and released, the wings of the Malecot expand and maintain the catheter in the bladder lumen.

Punch suprapubic tubes are temporary devices only. The wings of the Malecot are not strong; thus the catheter can be easily dislodged from the bladder. Long-term suprapubic drainage should be performed with a large-bore (24–26 French) catheter. The technique of placement of this type of catheter is beyond the scope of this chapter. Punch suprapubic cystostomy tubes are of small diameter and thus may become easily obstructed with debris. They are therefore also inadequate for patients with significant hematuria or blood clots.

1. Technique for Punch Suprapubic Cystostomy

Prior to performing a punch cystostomy, the bladder should be full and percussible above the pubis. If this is not the case, hydrating the patient and waiting until the bladder is distended is appropriate.

a. The patient's lower abdomen should be prepped and draped in the usual manner for any lower abdominal or pelvic procedure.
b. Lidocaine, 1% or 2%, is used to anesthetize the anterior abdominal wall in the midline, approximately two fingerbreadths above the symphysis pubis.
c. Preload the catheter onto the trochar.
d. A #11 blade is used to make a small vertical midline incision down through the skin and subcutaneous tissue, *not* entering the anterior rectus fascia (Fig. 44–10A).
e. The catheter and trochar are then placed into the incision and advanced at approximately a 30° angle aimed toward the hollow of the sacrum (Fig. 44–10B). The trochar is used to penetrate the anterior rectus fascia and the bladder wall. There should be no intervening bowel or peritoneum in the course of the trochar.
f. Aspiration with a 12-mL syringe is recommended during passage of the trochar to assure proper placement into the bladder lumen. After urine is aspirated, the trochar and catheter should be advanced another 2 cm, because urine may be aspirated when only the tip of the trochar is in the bladder lumen. The entire tip of the Malecot needs to be in the bladder lumen prior to releasing the wings.
g. The trochar may be disengaged and removed, thus expanding the wings of the catheter.
h. The catheter is secured to the skin with heavy silk.

It is important that the catheter *not* be pulled back snug to the anterior abdominal wall. If significant traction is placed on the wings of the Malecot, the catheter may be dislodged as the bladder empties and collapses.

Excessive length of catheter within the bladder may also be detrimental. The catheter may lodge in the bladder neck and not drain adequately. In addition, a large amount of catheter in the bladder lumen or on the trigone causes significant urgency and suprapubic discomfort.

A properly placed suprapubic catheter irrigates easily. If this is not the case, the catheter should be repositioned or the procedure repeated. Occasionally, a cystogram is needed to assess adequate placement.

Bleeding is rarely a problem. If significant hemorrhage does occur, then the catheter should be repositioned or the procedure repeated. As previously stated, these small-caliber catheters are inadequate for patients with gross hematuria because they become obstructed easily. Irrigation of the bladder with normal saline may be employed. If significant hemorrhage continues despite the above maneuvers, open cystostomy with control of hemorrhage and bladder drainage should be undertaken.

IV. Discussion

Figure 44–11 shows an algorithm for problem catheterizations.

If passing a 16 French Foley catheter is unsuccessful for any reason, the first step is to check your technique. Adequate lubrication is a must. Most kits are now supplied with KY jelly or 2% lidocaine jelly for injection directly into the urethra. Very often, one small packet of KY jelly is inadequate for lubrication. If a kit is not available with injectable lubricant, then a Toomey syringe can be filled with sterile lubricant and gently injected into the urethra.

It is also important to insure that the urethra is telescoped and extended upward. This straightens and

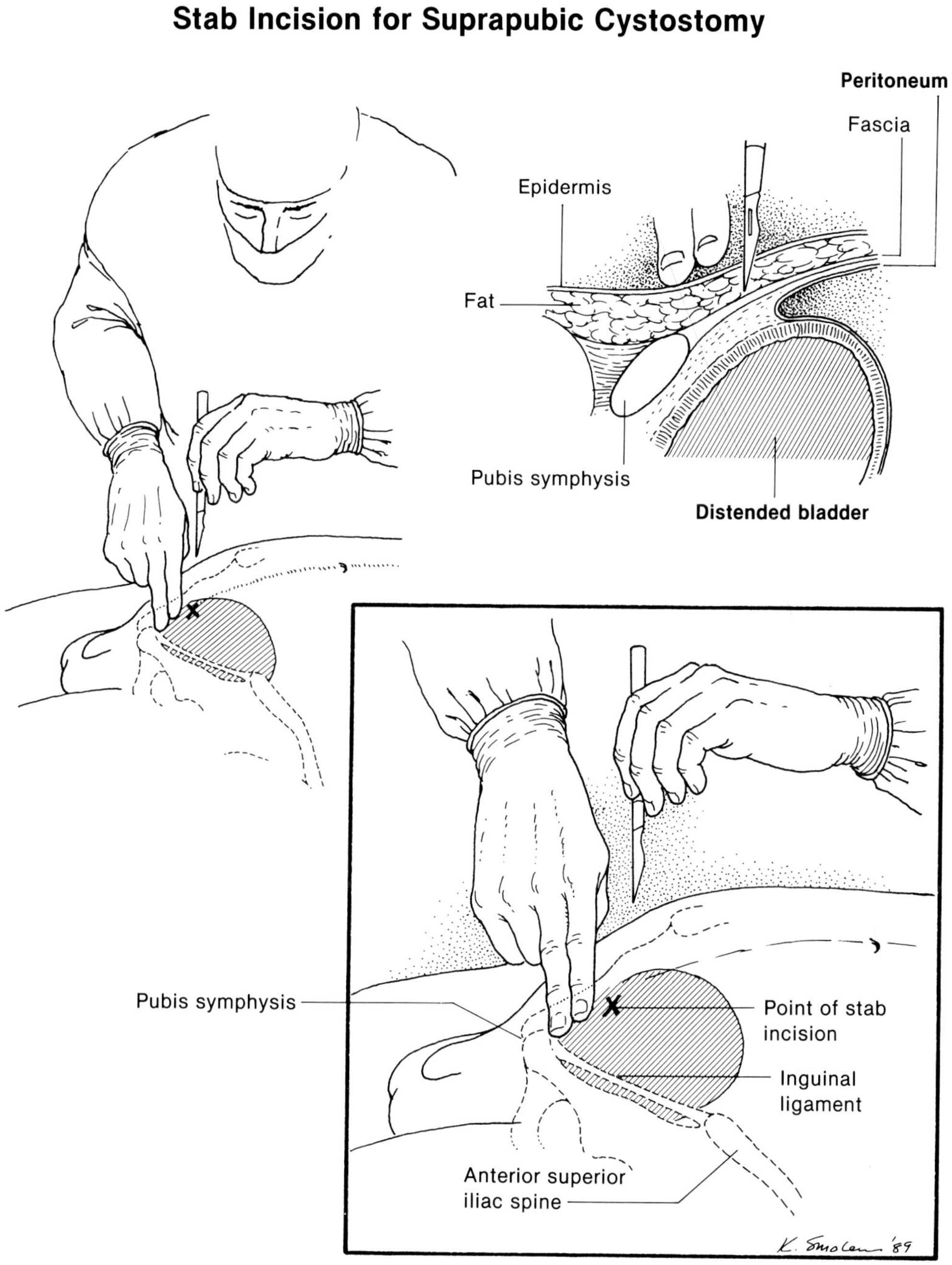

Figure 44–10 • A stab incision is made for suprapubic cystostomy. (*A*) A midline vertical stab incision through the skin (not fascia) is made approximately 2 fingerbreadths above the pubis.

(continued)

elongates the urethra, facilitating the passage of a catheter.

There is often resistance at the membranous urethra (external sphincter). Gentle continuous pressure on the membranous urethra is usually successful in negotiating this segment. Reassurance to the patient with instructions to relax is also helpful.

If the above maneuvers are still unsuccessful, then the next step depends on where the catheter is hung up. This is easily checked by palpation. The bulbous urethra is palpated at the penoscrotal junction or through the median "raphe" of the scrotum. The membranous and prostatic urethra can be palpated through the rectum.

If the hang-up is at the prostate and palpation re-

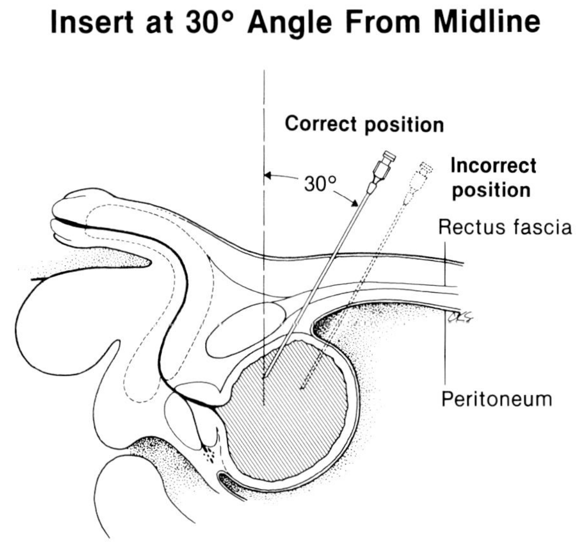

Figure 44–10 *(continued)*
(***B***) The catheter and trochar are advanced at approximately a 30° angle from the vertical, toward the balloon of the sacrum. Aspiration of urine with a 12-mL syringe assures proper placement.

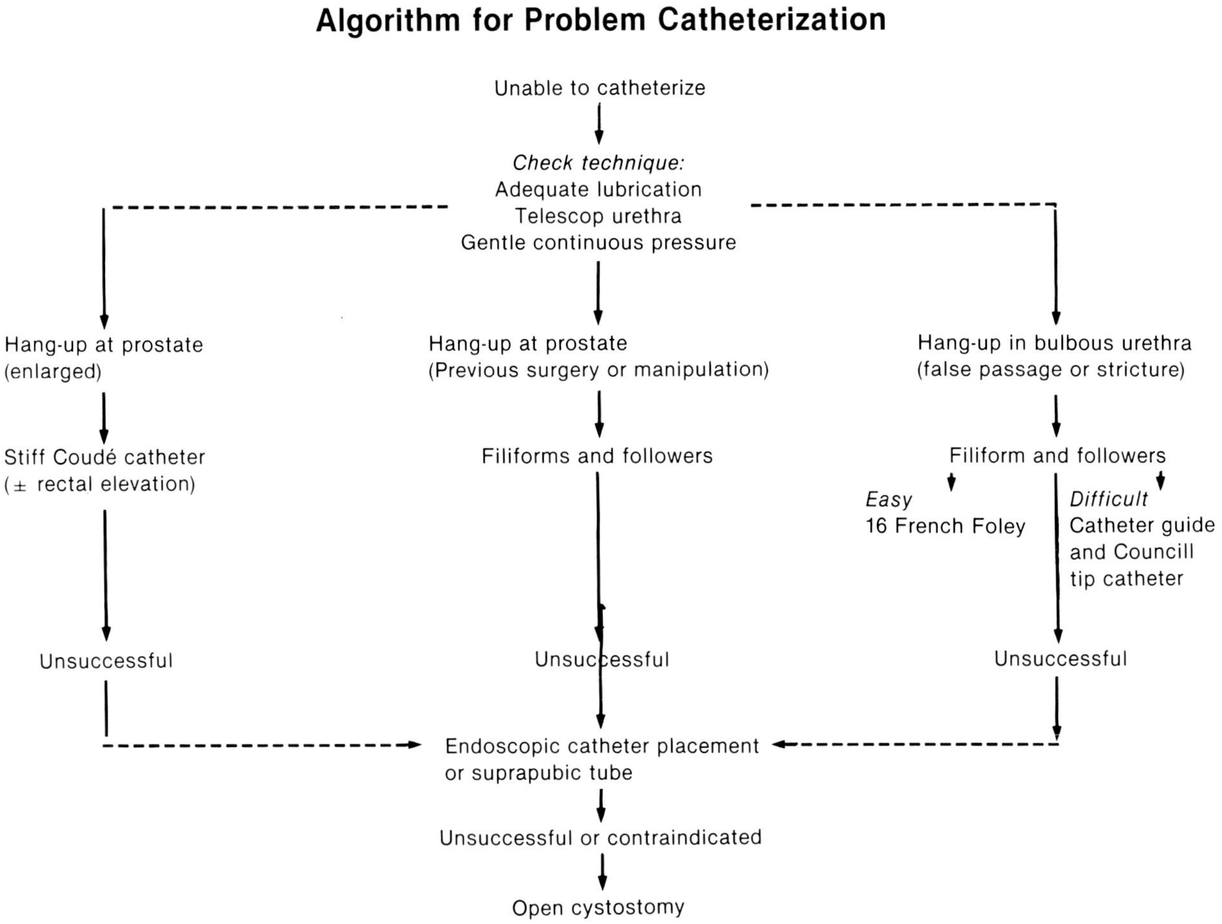

Figure 44–11 • Management algorithm is given for problem catheterization.

veals an enlarged prostate, a stiffer catheter with a coudé tip is recommended. Stiffer catheters will negotiate an enlarged prostate much easier than smaller diameter, softer catheters. A 20 French size is recommended. The coudé tip enables the catheter to better negotiate an enlarged median lobe. With adequate lubrication and correct technique, a 20 French coudé can be passed the majority of times in patients with enlarged prostates.

If, however, the patient has had previous surgery on the prostate or instrumentation of the urethra, one must suspect that there is a stricture. This may be manifested by a bladder neck contraction or a stricture in the membranous bulbous or penile urethra. Under these conditions, filiforms and followers are recommended.

If the catheter hangs up in the bulbous urethra, the tip of the catheter can be palpated at or near the penoscrotal junction. This most commonly represents a urethral stricture. Often, a history of previous urethritis or urethral catheterizations or instrumentations can be elicited. Filiforms and followers are then recommended for placement of a catheter, as described in the text.

During dilation, often there is slight resistance to the first follower, after which a "pop" is felt and subsequent followers pass easily. This would be considered an "easy" dilatation. After such a dilatation, a 16 French Foley catheter should be placed after removing the filiform.

If, however, during dilation, successive followers have been difficult to pass and the stricture is rather tight, the filiform should not be removed ("difficult" dilation). If urethral access is lost in this case, it may be impossible to regain. Rather, a catheter guide and Council-tip catheter should be employed under these circumstances.

If all the above maneuvers are unsuccessful in gaining access to the bladder via the urethra, endoscopic catheter placement or placement of a punch suprapubic tube should then be considered.

Certainly in emergency situations placement of a suprapubic tube is much easier and quicker than endoscopic placement of a catheter. The equipment is more readily available, and placement of a punch suprapubic tube in the hands of a trained physician usually takes only minutes. The cause of obstruction in the area of the urethra can then be evaluated and treated electively.

If, however, more time is available (eg, elective placement of a Foley catheter for 24-hour collection of urine), one can consider endoscopic catheter placement. Flexible endoscopes with a light source are portable and can be brought to the patient's bedside. Flexible endoscopy can be easily performed under local anesthesia. In this way, a filiform or guide wire can be passed under direct vision. A Council-tip catheter can then be passed over a catheter guide and into the bladder after urethral dilation, if necessary.

Endoscopic catheter placement should only be considered when adequate time and equipment are available. This should not be considered an urgent or emergent procedure, especially after previous manipulation. Multiple attempts at placement of a filiform or catheter often produces false passages and bleeding, which obscures the view during endoscopy. This makes the procedure less likely to be successful.

Finally, if placement of a suprapubic tube or endoscopic catheter placement is unsuccessful or contraindicated, open cystostomy should be pursued (see text for contraindications for punch cystostomy). Relative contraindications to bedside endoscopic catheter placement include severe penile trauma (urethral laceration or disruption), excessive bleeding per urethra, or history of known severe stricture disease.

Open cystostomy is an operative procedure and usually requires regional or general anesthesia. It is best done under the sterile conditions of an operating room, where the appropriate equipment is readily available. It is most easily performed through a lower abdominal midline incision. The linear alba is incised and the rectus muscles are separated. An incision is then made in the transversalis fascia, and the space of Retzius is entered. The bladder is then directly visualized and grasped with Allis forceps. A large-bore, Malecot-type catheter can then be placed directly into the bladder. This should be secured to the bladder and brought out through a separate stab incision. As with placement of a percutaneous suprapubic tube, it is much easier to perform when the bladder is distended and is more easily recognized.

This procedure is most often used in patients with small capacity bladders, patients who have undergone previous abdominal or pelvic surgery, or patients with pelvic trauma and severe hematuria in which punch suprapubic cystostomy is contraindicated.

V. REFERENCE

1. Mundy AR, Stephenson, TP, Wein, AJ (eds). Urodynamics: Principles, Practice and Application. New York, Churchill Livingstone, 1984.

Index

Page numbers followed by *f* indicate figures; those followed by *t* indicate tabular material.

C

O

P

ISBN 0-397-50950-2